WORMINGTON

DICTIONARY
OF
VISUAL SCIENCE

A modern comprehensive dictionary covering the terminology of the visual sciences, including the fields of ocular anatomy, ocular physiology, ocular pathology, ocular embryology, neuro-ophthalmology, ocular histology, ocular genetics, comparative anatomy of the eye, ocular prosthetics, physiological optics, psychological optics, ophthalmic optics, geometrical optics, ocular refraction, orthoptics, vision therapy, dispensing, aniseikonia, perimetry, contact lenses, low vision aids, occupational vision, and motorists' vision, and also including the phases of remedial reading, illumination, and physical optics that relate closely to vision.

Third Edition

DICTIONARY
OF
VISUAL SCIENCE

DAVID CLINE, B.S., O.D

HENRY W HOFSTETTER, O.D., PH.D.

JOHN R. GRIFFIN, O.D., M.S.ED.

CHILTON BOOK COMPANY
RADNOR, PENNSYLVANIA

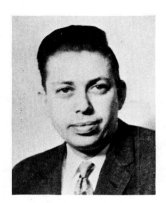

DR. MAX SCHAPERO
1921–1972

This volume is dedicated to the late Professor Max Schapero of the Southern California College of Optometry. The *Dictionary of Visual Science* became a reality only because of his years of dedicated research into the field of terminology.

His many accomplishments in research and teaching, as well as in the writing of numerous articles and the book *Amblyopia*, published just prior to his death, would have been remarkable for a strong, healthy person. Max Schapero, however, in his short lifespan was never without pain, suffering from arthritis and an intestinal ailment from childhood. Only his family and a few close associates knew of his poor health and even they never heard a complaint from him.

The need for a modern, meaningful, and concise dictionary of the terminology of the visual sciences became apparent to him and his friend, David Cline, when they were preparing a glossary to be appended to a visual training manual. The manual was abandoned and, after years of research, together with his two associate editors and over sixty collaborators and contributors, Max Schapero witnessed publication of the first and second editions of the *Dictionary of Visual Science*, accomplishments for which he always will be honored and remembered.

Preface

Our knowledge of the eye, its structure and function, and the diseases and problems that afflict it, has greatly expanded in the twelve years since publication of the second edition of the *Dictionary of Visual Science*. Thus, approximately three thousand new terms had to be added to this edition; and the definition of each term which was retained from preceding editions had to be closely scrutinized, updated, and, often, expanded. We have in the first instance tried to do justice to the emergence or rapid growth of such fields as contact lens technology, vision therapy, aids to low vision, detection of ocular disease, and diagnostic ocular pharmacology; and, in the second, to include relevant new developments in such specialties as ocular genetics, syndromes with ocular manifestations, intraocular implant lenses, physical and geometrical optics, and visual-perceptual-motor dysfunctions.

Countless new terms could be included in a dictionary such as this, but a realistic limit had to be imposed. As in previous editions, terms considered remote from the field of visual science and found in other readily available dictionaries are not included. Some entries from the first and second editions have been omitted, such as statistical terms which have broad-based applications and are more appropriately presented in other reference books.

Emphasis throughout is placed on succinct definition, rather than on encyclopedic elaboration. The sequence of definitions for terms with several meanings represents the editors' view of greater and lesser currency.

The editors are indebted to many for their aid and cooperation: to the contributors for their authoritative assistance in highly specialized areas; and to the Southern California College of Optometry, formerly the Los Angeles College of Optometry, which bore some of the financial cost of the original edition and has continued, through grants-in-aid, clerical assistance, library facilities and working and storage space, to support this ongoing project.

For help in the preparation of previous editions, grateful appreciation is extended to Mrs. Grace Weiner and Mrs. Winifred Hirsch for technical assistance; to the American Optometric Foundation, the

American Academy of Optometry, and the Southern California Chapter of the AAO for grants-in-aid used to defray manuscript preparation expenses.

For their work on this new edition, special thanks are extended to the SCCO librarian, Patricia Carlson, M.S.L.S., and to the library staff; to Kenneth G. Steuck, M.A., Director, Audio-Visual Services; to students James Eddleman, Jeffrey Jacob, and Donald Guido for aid in manuscript preparation; and to Kathryn Conover and the staff at Chilton for help in editing.

Contributors to the Third Edition

AFANADOR, ARTHUR J., O.D., PH.D.
Assistant Professor, School of Optometry, Indiana University. Special field: electrodiagnostic methods

ALLEN, MERRILL JAMES, M.SC., PH.D.
Professor, School of Optometry, Indiana University. Special field: strabismus; amblyopia; vision and highway safety

BACKMAN, HOWARD A., L.SC.O., O.D.
Optometric consultant, Department of Ophthalmology, McGill University, Montreal Children's Hospital and Montreal General Hospital. Special field: pediatric neuro-optometry; contact lenses; aviation vision

BAILEY, JAMES E., B.S., M.OPT., PH.D.
Assistant Professor, Southern California College of Optometry. Special field: physiological optics; color vision

BALDWIN, WILLIAM R., O.D., PH.D.
Dean, College of Optometry, University of Houston. Special field: ocular pathology; visual optics

BARTLETT, ROBERT E., M.D.
Clinical Professor of Ophthalmology, University of California at Los Angeles. Special field: ophthalmology

BARTLEY, S. HOWARD, B.S., M.A., PH.D.
Distinguished Research Professor, Memphis State University. Special field: neurophysiology of the visual pathway; visual perception; fatigue

BORISH, IRVIN M., O.D., D.O.S., L.L.D.
Professor, School of Optometry, Indiana University. Special field: contact lenses; binocular functions

BRAFF, SOLON M., A.B., O.D.
Private practice, El Monte, California. Special field: corneal and scleral contact lenses

BRAZELTON, FRANK A., B.V.S., O.D., M.S.ED.
Professor, Southern California College of Optometry. Special field: low vision; visual fields

BRISBANE, WILLIAM N., B.A., O.D.
Professor, Southern California College of Optometry. Special field: optometry; tonometry

BROOKS, CLIFFORD W., JR., B.A., O.D.
Assistant Professor, Indiana University. Special field: optometric technology

BRUNGARDT, TOM F., A.B., M.S., O.D.
Assistant Professor, Southern California College of Optometry. Special field: contact lenses

CHASE, WALTER WILLIAM, B.SC., M.OPT., M.SC.
Professor, Southern California College of Optometry. Special field: physiological optics; ocular motility; electrophysiology

CLINE, DAVID, B.S., O.D.
Co-Editor, *Dictionary of Visual Science*. Special field: physiological optics; ophthalmic optics; pediatric optometry

COHEN, MICHAEL M., B.A., B.S., O.D.
Associate Professor, Pennsylvania College of Optometry. Special field: optometry

DINSDALE, HOWARD A., A.B., M.D.
Private practice, Lincoln, Nebraska. Special field: ophthalmology

EARLE, ROBERT W., B.A., M.S., PH.D.
Professor, Southern California College of Optometry, and Senior Lecturer, University of California, Irvine, California College of Medicine. Special field: pharmacology

ESKRIDGE, JESS BOYD, O.D., M.SC., PH.D.
Professor, School of Optometry, University of Alabama in Birmingham. Special field: ocular motility; binocular vision; aniseikonia

FISHER, EDWARD J., M.A., O.D., D.SC.
Professor, School of Optometry, University of Waterloo, Waterloo, Ontario, Canada. Special field: ophthalmic optics; contact lenses; education

FLORA, MARK ROBERT, O.D.
Resident in Optometric Primary Care, Southern College of Optometry. Special field: ocular diseases

FRIEDMAN, MELVIN A., B.S., O.D.
Resident in Optometric Primary Care, Southern College of Optometry. Special field: ocular diseases

FRY, GLENN A., A.B., M.A., PH.D., D.O.S.
Regents Professor, College of Optometry, The Ohio State University. Special field: physiological optics; color vision; illumination

GAFFNEY, WILLIAM L., M.D.
Assistant Professor, Southern California College of Optometry, and Clinical Associate in Ophthalmology, Jules Stein Institute. Special field: ophthalmology

GELLMAN, MARTIN, O.D., M.S.
Associate Professor, Southern California College of Optometry. Special field: contact lenses

GILIO, ERNEST JOSEPH, B.S., M.S., O.D.
Private practice, Bernardsville, New Jersey. Special field: ultrasonic research

GOLDBERG, JOE B., O.D.
Private practice, Virginia Beach, Virginia. Special field: contact lenses

GREENE, HENRY A., B.S., O.D.
Consultant, Industrial Home for the Blind, Brooklyn, New York. Special field: low vision

GREENSPAN, STEVEN B., B.S., M.S., O.D., PH.D.
Assistant Professor, Illinois College of Optometry. Special field: psychology of perception; child development; learning disabilities

JAMES R. GREGG, O.D.
Professor, Southern California College of Optometry. Special field: optometric history

GRIFFIN, IVAN VINCENT, B.S., M.S.
Meteorologist, Cassville, Missouri. Special field: meteorology

GRIFFIN, JOHN R., B.S., M.OPT., O.D., M.S.ED.
Associate Professor, Southern California College of Optometry, and Co-editor, *Dictionary of Visual Science*. Special field: binocular vision; visual fields; learning disabilities

GUTH, SYLVESTER K., B.S., E.E., D.O.S.
Manager, Radiant Energy Effects Laboratory, General Electric Company. Special field: psychophysical and psychological effects of light and lighting; illuminating engineering

HARWOOD, LORANCE W., O.D., M.OPT.
Private practice, Mill Valley, California. Special field: ophthalmic instruments; contact lenses

HEARD, HOWARD M., JR.
Optician, Southern California College of Optometry. Special field: opticianry

HILL, RICHARD M., O.D., PH.D.
Professor, College of Optometry, The Ohio State University. Special field: contact lenses; corneal physiology

HOFFMAN, LOUIS G., B.A., O.D., M.S.
Assistant Professor, Southern California College of Optometry. Special field: binocular vision and perception

HOFSTETTER, HENRY W, B.S., M.S., O.D., PH.D.
Rudy Professor, School of Optometry, Indiana University, and Co-Editor, *Dictionary of Visual Science*. Special field: physiological optics; optometry; environmental optics

HOPPING, RICHARD L., B.S., O.D., D.O.S.
President, Southern California College of Optometry. Special field: administration in optometric education

JAANUS, SIRET DESIRÉE, B.S., M.A., PH.D.
Associate Professor, Southern California College of Optometry. Special field: ocular pharmacology; autonomic control of visual function; actions of corticosteroid hormones

JUNGSCHAFFER, OTTO H., M.D.
Private practice, North Hollywood, California. Special field: ophthalmology; diseases and surgery of the retina

KAVNER, RICHARD S., B.S., O.D.
Private practice, New York City. Special field: binocular vision and perception

KIRSCHEN, DAVID GARY, O.D., PH.D.
Assistant Professor, Southern California College of Optometry. Special field: binocular vision; orthoptics

KNOLL, HENRY A., B.S., M.S., PH.D.
Senior Scientist, Bausch and Lomb, Inc., Rochester, New York. Special field: geometrical optics; physiological optics; contact lenses

LEBENSOHN, JAMES ELZAR, M.D., PH.D.
Associate Professor of Ophthalmology, Emeritus, Northwestern University. Special field: ophthalmology

LONG, WILLIAM F., M.S., PH.D., O.D.
Assistant Professor, School of Optometry, University of Waterloo, Ontario, Canada. Special field: optics

MICHAELS, DAVID D., M.S., O.D., M.D.
Associate Clinical Professor of Ophthalmology, University of California, Los Angeles. Special field: ophthalmology

MOHINDRA, INDRA, O.D., M.S.
Private practice, South Brookline, Massachusetts. Special field: binocular vision; pediatric optometry

MORGAN, MEREDITH W., M.A., O.D., PH.D.
Dean Emeritus, School of Optometry, University of California, Berkeley. Special field: ophthalmic optics; binocular vision

RENIER, GARY L., B.S., O.D.
Private practice, Fargo, North Dakota. Special field: geriatric optometry; aphakia

RICHMAN, JACK E., B.S., O.D.
Associate Professor, Ferris State College of Optometry. Special field: binocular vision and perception

RIMOIN, DAVID L., M.D., PH.D.
Professor of Pediatrics and Medicine and Chief, Division of Medical Genetics, University of California, Los Angeles, Harbor Medical Center. Special field: medical genetics

ROBERTS, BERTRAM L., B.S., O.D., M.A., M.P.A.
Assistant Professor, Southern California College of Optometry. Special field: visual fields

ROSENBLOOM, ALFRED A., B.A., M.A., O.D., D.O.S.
President, Illinois College of Optometry. Special field: low vision, learning disabilities

SALADIN, J. JAMES, O.D., PH.D.
Associate Professor, Ferris State College of Optometry. Special field: binocular vision; accommodation

SARVER, MORTON D., O.D., M.S.
Professor of Optometry, School of Optometry, University of California, Berkeley. Special field: contact lenses

SCHMIDT, INGEBORG, M.D.
Professor Emeritus, School of Optometry, Indiana University. Special field: physiological optics; color vision; aerospace medicine

SHANDELING, PHILIP D., B.S., M.D.
Chairman, Department of Ophthalmology, Mount Sinai Hospital, Los Angeles. Special field: ophthalmology

SHARP, JAMES F., M.D.
Assistant Clinical Professor of Ophthalmology, University of California, Los Angeles. Special field: ophthalmology

STARK, LAWRENCE, A.B., M.D.
Professor, School of Optometry, University of California, Berkeley. Special field: neurology; bioengineering

STELLA, S. VICTOR, B.S., O.D.
Private practice, Huntington Beach, California. Special field: contact lenses

VODNOY, BERNARD E., O.D.
Private practice, South Bend, Indiana. Special field: binocular vision; contact lenses; optical instrumentation

WALD, GEORGE, B.S., D.SC., PH.D., M.D.(hon.)
Professor, Harvard University. Special field: retinal physiology; color vision

WALTON, HOWARD N., M.S., O.D., D.O.S.
Associate Professor, Southern California College of Optometry. Special field: learning disabilities

WEI, TED CHAU-PO, M.D., PH.D.
Chief of Glaucoma Service, Department of Ophthalmology, University of California, Irvine. Special field: ophthalmology

WEINER, GRACE C., B.A.
Former Librarian, Southern California College of Optometry, and The University of Alabama in Birmingham. Special field: visual science

WELSH, ROBERT C., M.D.
Private practice, Miami, Florida. Special field: ophthalmology; aphakia; special lens design

WILD, BRADFORD W., M.S., O.D., PH.D.
Professor, School of Optometry, University of Alabama in Birmingham. Special field: geometrical optics; physiological optics

WILEY, NORMAN C., O.D.
Associate Professor, Southern California College of Optometry. Special field: physical optics

Contributors to the
First and Second Editions

ABEL, CHARLES A., B.S., O.D.

ADAMS, ANTHONY J., B.APP. SC., L.O.SC., PH.D.

ALLEN, MERRILL JAMES, M.SC., PH.D.

ALPERN, MATHEW, O.D., B.M.E., M.S., PH.D.

BABER, WILMA R., B.S.ED., B.S.OPT., O.D.

BAGLIEN, JAMES W., B.S., O.D.

BALDWIN, WILLIAM R., O.D., PH.D.

BANNON, ROBERT E., B.S., D.O.S.

BARTLETT, ROBERT E., M.D.

BARTLEY, S. HOWARD, B.S., M.A., PH.D.

BECHTOLD, EDWIN W., B.S., M.A.

BENNETT, IRVING, O.D.

BLOOM, HARRY W., B.S., B.S.OPT., O.D.

BORISH, IRVIN M., O.D., D.O.S., L.L.D.

BRAFF, SOLON M., A.B., O.D.

BRECHER, GERHARD A., M.D., PH.D.

CARTER, DARRELL B., A.B., O.D., M.S., PH.D.

CARTER, JOHN H., O.D., M.S., PH.D.

CHASE, WALTER WILLIAM, B.SC., M.OPT., M.S.

CLINE, DAVID, B.S., O.D.

D'ARCY, DANIEL L., B.S., D.O.S.

ESKRIDGE, JESS B., O.D., M.SC., PH.D.

FINKELSTEIN, ISIDORE SIGMUND, B.S., PH.D.

FISHER, EDWARD J., O.D., M.A., D.SC.

FLOM, MERTON CLYDE, B.S., M.OPT., PH.D.

FREEMAN, EUGENE, A.B., O.D., PH.D., D.O.S.

FRY, GLENN A., A.B., M.A., PH.D., D.O.S.

GRAHAM, ROBERT, A.B., B.SC.

GREEN, RALPH H., O.D., D.O.S., D.SC.

GUTH, SYLVESTER K., B.S., E.E., D.O.S.

HAYNES, PHILLIP ROBERT, O.D.

HEATH, GORDON G., B.V.S., O.D., M.S., PH.D.

HESTER, MARGARET, B.S., O.D.

HILL, RICHARD M., O.D., PH.D.

HIRSCH, MONROE J., O.D., PH.D.

HOFSTETTER, HENRY W., B.S., M.S., O.D., PH.D.

HUTCHINSON, ERNEST A., O.D.

JAMPOLSKY, ARTHUR, A.B., M.D.

JANKIEWICZ, HARRY A., D.O.S., PH.D.

JUNGSCHAFFER, OTTO H., M.D.

KEMENY, STUART S., O.D.

KNOLL, HENRY A., B.S., M.S., PH.D.

KNOX, GEORGE W., B.A., B.S., M.A., O.D., PH.D.

KORB, DONALD R., B.S., O.D.

KRAMER, PAUL W., B.S., M.OPT.,
M.D.
KRATZ, J. DONALD, A.B., O.D.
LAUER, ALVHH R., B.M., A.B., M.A.,
M.S., PH.D.
LEVENE, JOHN R., D. PHIL., M.SC.
LEVY, O. ROBERT, B.S.
LYLE, WILLIAM M., O.D., M.S., PH.D.
MANAS, LEO, CH.E., M.A., O.D.,
D.O.S.
MANDELL, ROBERT B., O.D., M.S.,
PH.D.
MARG, ELWIN, A.B., PH.D.
MARGACH, CHARLES B., B.S., M.S.,
O.D.
MESSIER, J. ARMAND, B.A.
MICHAELS, DAVID D., M.S., O.D.,
M.D.
MORGAN, MEREDITH W., M.A., O.D.,
PH.D.
NADELL, MELVIN CHARLES, B.A.,
M.A., O.D., PH.D.
NELSON, IRVING K., O.D.
NICHOLAS, JOHN P., M.D.
NUGENT, MAURICE WILFRED, M.D.
NYE, ARTHUR W., B.S., M.E., PH.D.
PASCAL, JOSEPH I., B.S., O.D., M.A.,
M.D.
PHEIFFER, CHESTER H., A.B., M.S.,
O.D., PH.D.
PIERCE, JOHN R., B.S., O.D., M.S.,
PH.D.
PITTS, DONALD GRAVES, O.D., M.S.,
PH.D.

RAFALKO, J. STANLEY, A.B., M.S.,
PH.D.
RICHARDS, OSCAR W., PH.D.
ROSENBLOOM, ALFRED A., B.A., M.A.,
O.D., D.O.S.
ROTH, NILES, O.D., PH.D.
SCHAPERO, MAX, B.S., O.D.
SCHMIDT, INGEBORG, M.D.
SCHUBERT, DELWYN G., B.S., M.S.,
PH.D.
SCOWN, LESLIE W., O.D., D.O.S.
SHANEDLING, PHILIP D., B.S., M.D.
SHLAIFER, ARTHUR, B.S., M.S., O.D.,
PH.D.
SIMMERMAN, HAROLD, O.D.
SINN, FREDERICK WM., O.D.
SLOAN, LOUISE L., PH.D.
SMITH, WILLIAM, O.D., D.O.S.
STEWART, CHARLES REESE, B.S.,
M.S., PH.D.
STIMSON, RUSSELL L.
TENNANT, E.R., O.D., D.O.S.
TOWER, PAUL, M.D.
WALTON, HOWARD N., M.S., O.D.,
D.O.S.
WESTHEIMER, GERALD, A.S.T.C.,
F.S.T.C., B.S., PH.D.
WEYMOUTH, FRANK WALTER, A.B.,
A.M., PH.D.
WILD, BRADFORD W., M.S., O.D.,
PH.D.
WOOLF, DANIEL, A.B., B.S., PH.D.

Notes on Use of the Dictionary

In order to facilitate the use of this dictionary, terms of more than one word are listed alphabetically by nouns, rather than by the modifying adjectives. For example, *asymmetric convergence, fusional convergence,* and *proximal convergence* are all found as subentries under *convergence.* Similarly, eponymic terms are cross-filed to the nouns and are listed thus: "*Hall's test.* See under *test,*" "*Hamilton slide.* See under *slide.*" When the entry includes many terms, the instruction is to *See under the nouns.* Thus, "*Donders' experiment; law; line; method.* See under the nouns" indicates that the specific definitions will be found as subentries under *experiment, law, line,* and *method,* respectively. Nouns with extensive subentries are set off by a large, centered head and diamond ornament (◆), with the diamond repeated at the end of the noun entry, to help the dictionary user locate major entries quickly and easily.

When two adjectives modify a noun and the significant adjective is second, the term may occur in one of two ways: if it is a subentry, the first adjective is inverted, as for example, *deep punctate keratitis* is listed under *keratitis* as *punctate k., deep;* if the term occurs as a sub-subentry, it is alphabetized by adjective under the subentry, as for example, *partial color blindness* occurs under *blindness,* then under *color b.,* where it is alphabetized in normal reading order as *partial c.b.* When three adjectives modify a noun, the least significant adjective is listed in parentheses, as for example, *anterior principal focal length* is listed as a sub-subentry under *length,* then under *focal l.,* as *principal (anterior) f.l.*

For certain phrases, it may be necessary to look under more than one listing. For example, a term may be variously designated a syndrome or a disease; a test or a method; a reaction or a reflex; etc. Grammatical identifications and etymology are not included unless particularly important in denoting the true connotation of a word, or for clarification.

Key to Pronunciation

A phonetic respelling, enclosed in parentheses, follows those entries whose pronunciation is not readily apparent. If more than one pronunciation is in common usage, all are given. None is given for very simple English words or for most adjectives. The basic rule to indicate vowel sound is: a vowel, without a diacritical mark, is short if followed by a consonant within the same syllable, and an unmarked vowel ending a syllable is long. The letter *h* is added to a short vowel which comes at the end of a syllable to indicate the short sound. For example, in "**exophoria** (eks″o-fo′re-ah)" the first *e* is short, the second *e* long, the *a* is short, and both *o*'s are long.

No attempt has been made to indicate fine gradations of sound by diacritical marks. However, certain diacritical marks are used. The macron (¯) is used to indicate a long vowel when the vowel is followed by a consonant in the same syllable; for example, "**acetone** (as′e-tōn)." The breve (˘) is used to indicate the short sound of a vowel in cases where confusion might otherwise arise; for example, the initial *a* in the word "**acopia** (ă-ko′pe-ah)." The *h* is also used after *a* in certain syllables ending with a consonant to indicate a broad *a* sound; for example, "**far-sighted** (fahr-sīt′ed)."

A syllable followed by a hyphen is unstressed and the primary (′) and the secondary (″) accents are indicated in polysyllabic words as follows, "**platycoria** (plat″ih-ko′re-ah)."

DICTIONARY
OF
VISUAL SCIENCE

A

A; Å. Symbol for *angstrom unit.*

A. Angle of anomaly.

a. Abbreviation for *accommodation.*

α. The Greek letter *alpha* used as a symbol for (1) *angle alpha;* (2) *alpha movement;* (3) *absorptance.*

AACO. See *American Association of Certified Orthoptists.*

AAO. See *American Academy of Ophthalmology; American Academy of Optometry; American Association of Ophthalmology.*

A case. See *case, type A.*

Abadie's sign (ah″bah-dēz′). See under *sign.*

abathic (ah-băth′ik). See *distance, abathic.*

abaxial (ab-ak′se-al). Situated out of, or directed away from, the axis.

abaxile (ab-ak′zīl). Abaxial.

Abbe's (ab′ēz) **condenser; condition; constant; eyepiece; number; prism; refractometer; theory.** See under the nouns.

abducens (ab-du′senz). 1. External rectus muscle. 2. Sixth cranial nerve.

    a. oculi. External rectus muscle.

abducent (ab-du′sent). Abducting.

abduct (ab-dukt′). To turn away from the midline, as in abduction.

abduction (ab-duk′shun). 1. The rotation, temporally, of an eye away from the midline. 2. A commonly used, but incorrect, definition: The diverging of the eyes away from each other, especially as determined by clinical tests with prisms, measured in terms of one or more of the criteria establishing the divergence limits of binocular vision, such as blurring, diplopia, or recovery from diplopia. Clinically, the base-in prism limits of clear and single binocular vision.

abductor (ab-duk′tōr). A muscle which rotates the eye away from the medial plane (templeward). The lateral rectus muscle is primarily an abductor, the inferior and the superior oblique muscles secondarily so.

    a. oculi. External rectus muscle.

ABERRATION

aberration (ab″er-a′shun). Failure of the rays from a point source to form a perfect or single point image after traversing an optical system. Optical aberration may manifest itself in the formation of multiple images or in the formation of a single imperfectly defined image. In Seidel's formula, it is the deviations from the path of light prescribed by Gauss's theory.

    chromatic a. Aberration produced by unequal refraction of different wavelengths or colors. The typical manifestation of chromatic aberration in a simple optical system is a colored fringe on the border of an image. Syn., *color aberration; Newtonian aberration.* **axial c.a.** Longitudinal chromatic aberration. **lateral c.a.** Chromatic aberration, manifested as a change in size of the image of a point formed by a lens or an optical system, due to differences of incident wavelengths. (See Fig. 1.) **longitudinal c.a.** Chromatic aberration, manifested as a displacement of the image formed by a lens or an optical system along the axis, due to differences of incident wavelengths. Syn., *axial chromatic aberration.*

    color a. Chromatic aberration.

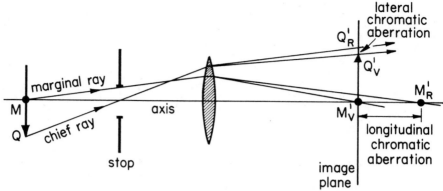

Fig. 1 Lateral and longitudinal chromatic aberration of a single lens. (From Jenkins and White, *Fundamentals of Optics*, 3d ed. New York: McGraw-Hill, 1957; copyright © 1957; used with permission of McGraw-Hill Book Co.)

curvature a. 1. Aberration attributable to curvature characteristics of the refracting surfaces in an optical system. 2. Aberration manifesting itself in curvature of the image field. See *curvature of the field.*

dioptric a. Aberration peculiar to, or characteristic of, dioptric systems. Sometimes synonymous with *spherical aberration.*

distantial a. Blurredness or loss of definition attributable to factors related to distance of viewing, one factor being atmospheric haze.

lateral a. The amount of aberration expressed as the lateral deviation of a ray from a point of reference on the axis, ordinarily from an assumed or empirical focal point.

least circle of a. The circle representing the smallest cross section of a bundle of rays manifesting aberration, especially spherical aberration. Cf. *circle of least confusion.*

longitudinal a. 1. A displacement of the image, or of a series of images, formed by a fixed lens or optical system along its axis. Ex.: *longitudinal spherical aberration; longitudinal chromatic aberration.* 2. Aberration expressed in terms of the distance between the axial crossing point of an aberrant ray and a point of reference on the axis, the point of reference ordinarily being a focal point.

marginal a. Aberration encountered in the use of the peripheral areas of a lens, frequently mentioned in reference to ophthalmic lenses.

meridional a. 1. Aberration produced in the plane of a single meridian of a lens. 2. Differences in type or amount of aberration in two different meridians of a lens.

monochromatic a. 1. A defect of image formation in a lens or an optical system for a constant index of refraction, i.e., a single wavelength of incident light. Ex.: *spherical aberration; oblique astigmatism; coma; curvature of the field; distortion.* 2. Aberration exclusive of chromatic aberration; aberration present when monochromatic light is used.

negative a. See *spherical aberration.*

Newtonian a. Chromatic aberration.

peripheral a. 1. Aberration encountered in image formation on the peripheral retina. 2. Marginal aberration.

positive a. See *spherical aberration.*

spherical a. A monochromatic aberration occurring in simple refraction at a spherical surface, characterized by peripheral and paraxial rays focusing at different points along the axis. In the Gauss theory, the focus of the system is identified with the paraxial rays, the peripheral rays being regarded as aberrant when they fail to intersect at the focal point of the paraxial rays. **against the rule s.a.** Negative spherical aberration. **lateral s.a.** Variation in size of an image of a point, formed by a lens or an optical system, due to spherical aberration. **longitudinal s.a.** The difference measured along the axis between the distance from a lens or an optical system to the focus of peripheral rays and the distance to the focus of paraxial rays from an object point on the axis; commonly called *spherical aberration*. **negative s.a.** Spherical aberration in which the paraxial rays show greater refraction than the peripheral rays. Syn., *against the rule spherical aberration*. **positive s.a.** Spherical aberration in which the peripheral rays show greater refraction than the paraxial rays. Syn., *with the rule spherical aberration*. **with the rule s.a.** Positive spherical aberration.

◆

aberrometer (ab″er-om′eh-ter). An instrument for measuring aberration.

aberroscope (ab-er′o-skōp). An instrument for observing aberration. Especially, an instrument for observing aberrations in one's own eye.

Tscherning's a. An instrument constructed by Tscherning for measuring aberrations, consisting of a plano-convex lens mounted on a handle which has on its plano side a micrometer grid in the form of little squares.

abient (ab′e-ent). Tending to remove the organism from the source of stimulation.

abiotrophy (ab″ih-ot′ro-fe). A postnatal degeneration of an anatomical structure which was normal at the time of birth, as occurs in retinitis pigmentosa.

ablatio falciformis congenita (ab-la′she-o fal″se-fōr′mis kon-jen′ih-tah). A condition of the retina characterized by folds or ridges which project into the vitreous. They arise from the disk, involving the inner layer of the optic cup, and usually are found in the lower temporal quadrant of the retina. Syn., *congenital retinal septum*.

ablatio retinae (ab-la′she-o ret′ih-ne). Detachment of the retina.

ablepharia (ab″ble-fa′re-ah). Ablephary.

ablepharon (ă-blef′ah-ron). Ablephary.

ablepharous (ă-blef′ah-rus). Without eyelids.

ablephary (ă-blef′ah-re). Congenital absence, complete or partial, of the eyelids. Syn., *ablepharia; ablepharon*.

partial a. Eyelids of reduced size. Syn., *microblepharon*.

ablepsia (ă-blep′se-ah). Lack or loss of vision; blindness. Syn., *ablepsy*.

ablepsy (ă-blep′se). Ablepsia.

Abney's (ab′nēz) **colorimeter; effect; formula; law; phenomenon; photometer; sensitometer.** See under the nouns.

ABO. See *American Board of Opticianry*.

abrasio corneae (ab-ra′ze-o kōr′ne-e). A scraping away of part of the surface of the cornea. It usually implies a superficial injury to the cornea by a physical agent, as differentiated from lacerations of the cornea extending deeper than Bowman's membrane.

abridgment of response. See under *response*.

abscess. A localized, circumscribed collection of pus.

orbital a. Suppuration in the orbit.

ring a. A yellow ring of purulent infiltration at the periphery of the cornea surrounding necrotic tissue and surrounded by about 1 mm of clear cornea. Syn., *peripheral annular infiltration*.

vitreous a. Accumulation of pus in the noncellular vitreous. True abscess should involve solid tissue.

abscissa (ab-sis′ah). The horizontal or the x axis of reference in a graph of rectilinear co-ordinates. See also *ordinate*.

abscissio bulbi (ab-sis′e-o bul′bi). Enucleation of the eyeball.

abscission, corneal (ab-sish′un). Surgical removal of the prominence of the cornea in staphyloma.

absolute impression; judgment. See under the nouns.

absorbance (ab-sorb′ans). The logarithm of the reciprocal of spectral internal transmittance.

absorbancy (ab-sōrb′an-se). The logarithm of the reciprocal of transmittancy.

absorptance (ab-sōrp′tans). The ratio of absorbed radiant flux to incident radiant flux. Syn., *absorption factor*.

spectral a. The ratio of the amount of light of a given wavelength absorbed by a medium to that incident upon it.

absorptiometer (ab-sōrp″te-om′eh-ter). An instrument for determining the light or gas-absorbing properties of a substance. Syn., *absorption meter*.

absorption (ab-sōrp′shun). The process in which radiant energy is converted into other forms, usually heat, by passage through, or reflection from, a medium. The absorbing of light by a blackbody or any light-absorbing substance. Absorbed light is that which is neither transmitted nor reflected in an optical system, but may be re-emitted as light of another wavelength, as in fluorescence or luminescence.

a. band. See under *band.*

a. factor. See under *factor.*

general a. The reduction of intensity, in approximately the same amount, of all wavelengths of light entering a given medium.

neutral a. The absorption of radiant energy uniformly throughout the spectrum.

resonance a. Resonance radiation.

selective a. Absorption in selected or specific segments of the spectrum.

absorptivity (ab″sōrp-tiv′ih-te). 1. The absorption per unit thickness of an absorbing medium. Syn., *coefficient of absorption.* 2. The transmissivity of an absorbing medium subtracted from unity.

abtorsion (ab-tōr′shun). Extorsion.

abversion (ab-vur′zhun). Templeward rotation of the eye. A term used categorically to identify the rotation of the eye templeward irrespective of the mechanism or its association with other functions.

AC/A ratio. See under *ratio.*

acalculia (a-kal-ku′le-ah). Inability, or loss of ability, to perform simple mathematical functions.

acanthosis nigricans (ak″an-tho′sis nig′re-kanz, ni′gre-kanz). A rare condition presenting numerous superficial, pigmented, papillomatous growths on many portions of the body and occasionally on the conjunctiva. A marked conjunctivitis occurs, characterized by a diffuse papillary hypertrophy; the palpebral conjunctiva, especially, may be heavily pigmented. Syn., *keratosis nigricans.*

acanthrocytosis (ah-kan″thro-si-to′sis). A rare, simple recessive hereditary disease characterized by malformation of the erythrocytes, faulty absorption of fat in the intestines, neuromuscular degeneration, and atypical retinitis pigmentosa.

acatamathesia (a-kat″ah-mah-the′ze-ah). 1. The inability to comprehend conversation. 2. Mental deterioration of the senses, as in psychic blindness.

acc. Abbreviation for *accommodation* or *accommodative.*

◆

ACCOMMODATION

accommodation (ă-kom″o-da′shun). Specifically, the dioptric adjustment of the eye (to attain maximal sharpness of retinal imagery for an object of regard) referring to the ability, to the mechanism, or to the process. The effecting of refractive changes by changes in shape of the crystalline lens. Loosely, ocular adjustments for vision at various distances.

absolute a. 1. Accommodation specified with reference to, or measured from, the zero level of accommodation. 2. The accommodation of either eye separately; hence, the accommodation elicited independently of the inhibitory or facilitative influence of convergence or binocular vision.

amplitude of a. See under *amplitude.*

apparent a. A semblance of accommodation by virtue of ability to accomplish usable, clear vision through a considerable range of distances, the clear vision being a matter of depth of focus rather than dioptric change. Applied especially to apparent accommodation in aphakia.

astigmatic a. Unequal accommodation in different meridians of the eye, ordinarily exclusive of differences in optical effectivity dependent on choice of a reference plane. Typically applied to differential changes in curvature of the surfaces of the crystalline lens in different meridians. Syn., *meridional accommodation.* **innervational a.a.** Accommodation resulting in an astigmatic surface of the crystalline lens caused by meridional or sectional differences in innervation to the accommodative musculature.

a. of attention. *Psychology:* The adjustment or readjustment of the individual which is essential for the maximal clearness of an impression.

available a. 1. Amplitude of accommodation. 2. Reserve accommodation.

binocular a. 1. Accommodation in the two eyes regarded as a single unitary response. Clinically, the accommodative response when both eyes receive the dioptric stimulus. 2. Rarely, the convergence response of the eyes to a binocular fixation object.

breadth of a. Range of accommodation.

center of a. See under *center.*

consensual a. Simultaneous accommodation in the two eyes occurring in accordance with Hering's law of equal innervation to the two eyes. Accommodation in one eye occurring as a correlated response with the accommodation of the other eye, especially when only one eye receives the dioptric stimulus.

convergence a. Accommodation changes induced by, or associated with, changes in convergence.

deficiency of a. Absence of, or reduced, ability to accommodate. Cf. *insufficiency of accommodation.*

distal a. Distant accommodation.

distant a. Active accommodation for distant fixation, distinguished from the concept of relaxation of accommodation for distant fixation, with the implication or assumption of an effector mechanism for accomplishing this. Syn., *negative accommodation.*

excessive a. 1. Accommodation in excess of the amount required for sharpest imagery of the stimulus object. 2. The tendency to maintain or sustain accommodation in the absence of a dioptric stimulus.

far point of a. The conjugate focus of the retina (fovea) when the accommodation is relaxed or at its minimum. In emmetropia, the far point is said to be at infinity; in myopia, it is at some finite distance in front of the eye; in hyperopia, it is at some finite (virtual) distance behind the eye. Syn., *punctum remotum of accommodation.*

focus a. 1. Accommodation in response to the desire for clear imagery. 2. Negative relative accommodation. 3. Retinal accommodation. 4. Accommodation changes necessary for clear imagery after convergence for a finite point has taken place, with the assumption that convergence reflexly stimulates accommodation.

ill-sustained a. Weakened or fluctuating accommodation resulting from prolonged use or due to extreme dioptric demand.

inertia of a. Slow or difficult accommodative response to dioptric change in stimulus; especially, sluggish accommodative response to changes in fixation distance.

inhibition of a. See under *inhibition.*

insufficiency of a. 1. Insufficient amplitude of accommodation to afford clear imagery of a stimulus object at a specified distance, usually the normal or desired reading distance.

2. One of several theoretical clinical types of cases identified by a syndrome of refractive findings. Definitions vary. 3. Less accommodative ability than expected for the patient's age.

lag of a. 1. The extent to which the accommodative response is less than the dioptric stimulus to accommodation. The failure to accommodate the full amount demanded for the sharpest imagery of the stimulus object. The phenomenon is quite general and often referred to as the *lazy lag of accommodation.* 2. In binocular fixation, the failure to accommodate for the full amount of the dioptric stimulus when the convergence response is normal. Hence, called the *lag of accommodation behind convergence.* 3. The additional lag sometimes induced by dissociating the two eyes. *Rare.* 4. *Optometric Extension Program:* By special definition, an index, expressed in diopter units, obtained by application of a formula using numerical values of several clinical findings. These formulas vary. Most commonly, "that amount of accommodation free of association with convergence as determined by the net of the unfused and fused cross-cylinder findings."

latent a. 1. That accommodation not manifested, elicited, or demonstrated by tests of the amplitude of accommodation. Accommodation in excess of the apparent near point of accommodation. The term also applies to the accommodation in play when all subjective attempts have been put forth to relax accommodation. 2. Neuromuscular accommodative action not eliciting a dioptric change in the crystalline lens, theoretically occurring beyond the limits of functional flexibility of the crystalline lens.

lazy lag of a. See *lag of accommodation.*

lenticular a. Accommodation attributable to dioptric changes in the crystalline lens of the eye, to be distinguished from other theoretical mechanisms of accommodation, such as corneal, axial, etc.

line of a. See under *line.*

manifest a. That accommodation measurable by conventional clinical tests or by demonstrable changes in the dioptric mechanism; distinguished from *latent accommodation.*

meridional a. Astigmatic accommodation.

monocular a. 1. Accommodation measured in one eye without regard to that occurring in the other eye. 2. Accommodation elicited when the stimulus is presented to one eye only. 3. Accommodation elicited when convergence factors are eliminated by clinical dissociation techniques.

a. muscle. Ciliary muscle.

near point of a. The point representing the maximum dioptric stimulus to which the eye can accommodate. Hence, usually the nearest point anteriorly on which the eye can focus. In absolute hyperopia, it may be a virtual point represented schematically as posterior to the eye. **absolute n.p. of a.** The conjugate focus of the retina (fovea) under maximum accommodation; clinically, the nearest point of clear vision. **relative n.p. of a.** The conjugate focus of the retina (fovea) under maximum accommodation attainable with a given amount of convergence; conventionally, measured by the maximum amount of minus lenses (or minimum plus) permitting clear vision at a fixed convergence distance, usually 33 or 40 cm.

negative a. 1. Negative relative accommodation. 2. Relaxation of accommodation below apparent zero level obtained by conventional clinical techniques, or below that level of accommodation manifested in the absence of any positive visual stimulus. 3. That reduction in accommodation accomplished by denervation, shock, or tonus-reducing experimental techniques. 4. Distant accommodation.

optical a. Physical accommodation.

painful a. of Donders. Accommodative spasms associated with hysteria, or as a hysterical manifestation.

paralysis of a. See under *paralysis.*

physical a. Accommodation changes as manifested in the lenticular body. Syn., *optical accommodation.*

physiological a. Accommodation referred to as a myologic function concerned with the innervation of the ciliary muscle and its contraction without regard to concomitant lenticular changes.

positive a. 1. Accommodative response normally associated with a positive dioptric stimulus. 2. Normal accommodation, distinguished only from the phenomenon of negative accommodation.

posture of a. The state of accommodation under specified stimulus or test conditions. Quantitative specifications may be in terms of diopters of accommodation, lag of accommodation, or the given clinical test finding itself.

power of a. Amplitude of accommodation.

proximal a. Accommodation induced by the apparent nearness, or awareness of nearness, of the fixation object, independent of the actual dioptric stimulus. Syn., *psychic accommodation.*

psychic a. Proximal accommodation.

range of a. The linear distance from the nearest point of accommodation or clear vision to the farthest point of accommodation or clear vision. Syn., *breadth of accommodation.* **absolute r. of a.** An expression employed by Donders to represent the maximum monocular amplitude of accommodation. **binocular r. of a.** The range or amplitude of accommodation that can be elicited with binocular fixation of the test object. **relative r. of a.** The dioptric range of change in accommodation that can be elicited with convergence held constant; clinically, measured binocularly with minus or plus lenses to the limit of clear vision, with convergence held at a specified point, usually 33 or 40 cm.

reflex a. 1. Accommodation changes occurring in direct response to reduced quality, or to blurredness, of the perceived image. 2. Accommodation induced reflexly by convergence or any other physiologically associated function.

region of a. Donders' term for *range of accommodation.*

relative a. Changes in accommodation that can be elicited with convergence held constant. **negative r.a.** Relaxation or reduction of accommodation below that normally demanded for a given binocular fixation distance, with convergence fixed; clinically, measured subjectively by the maximum amount of plus lens power permitting clear, single, binocular vision at a given distance, usually 33 or 40 cm, or objectively by dynamic retinoscopic techniques. **positive r.a.** Increase of accommodation in excess of that normally demanded for a given binocular fixation distance, with convergence fixed; clinically, measured subjectively by the maximum amount of minus lens power permitting clear, single binocular vision at a given distance, usually 33 or 40 cm.

reserve a. The amplitude of accommodation minus the amount of accommodation needed for clear imagery at a given fixation distance. **negative r.a.** Negative relative accommodation. **negative fusional r.a.** Accommodation changes induced by changes in fusional divergence. **negative relative r.a.** Negative relative accommodation. **positive r.a.** Positive relative accommodation. **positive fusional r.a.** Accommodation changes induced by changes in positive fusional convergence. **positive relative r.a.** Positive relative accommodation.

resting state of a. The state of accommodation under the influence of normal muscle tonus, in the absence of any stimulus to accommodation and convergence.

retinal a. Accommodation reflexly induced by an out-of-focus retinal image.

sectional a. Astigmatic accommodation.

spasm of a. See under *spasm.*

static a. Zero level of accommodation.

a. time. See under *time.*

tonic a. 1. Accommodation attributable to the normal tonus of the ciliary muscle. 2. A rare condition in which the posture of accommodation is prolonged so that change in focus from one distance to another is delayed; occasionally reported in diabetes, alcoholism, Graves's disease, syphilis, measles, and after trauma.

unequal a. Unequal simultaneous accommodation in the two eyes, or unequal accommodation in two meridians of the same eye.

vergence a. Accommodation induced by binocular disparity of the retinal images.

voluntary a. Accommodation induced by voluntary effort. **negative v.a.** Accommodation reduced or relaxed through voluntary control. **positive v.a.** Voluntary accommodation.

zero level of a. Clinically, the state of accommodation in the absence of any accommodative effort or stimulus to accommodation; relaxed accommodation, identified as that obtained in the subjective or objective determination of the distance correction of refractive error. Experimentally, the state of accommodation with third cranial nerve denervation or cycloplegia. Syn., *static accommodation.*

◆

accommodative (a-kom′o-da″tiv). Pertaining to accommodation.

a. convergence. See under *convergence.*

a. reflex. See under *reflex.*

a. rock. An accommodative exercise consisting of a series of accommodative responses to alternate monocular increases and decreases in dioptric stimulus to accommodation. Clinically performed by having the right and the left eye alternately view a target through lenses which present different dioptric stimuli to each of the two eyes. **inhibitory phase of a. r.** The phase of accommodative rock corresponding to decrease of dioptric stimulus. **stimulatory phase of a. r.** The phase of accommodative rock corresponding to increase of dioptric stimulus.

accommodometer (ă-kom″o-dom′eh-ter). An instrument to measure ability or facility to accommodate.

accuracy. Correctness; conformity to truth or to a model or standard; without mistake or error; exactness.

acetazolamide (ah-set″ah-zōl-am′ĭd). A generic name for 2-acetylamino-1, 3, 4-thiadiazole-5-sulfonamide, a carbonic anhydrase inhibitor, supplied under the trade name *Diamox.* It is a diuretic used to control fluid retention in certain systemic conditions and also to reduce intraocular pressure in the treatment of glaucoma.

acetone (as′e-tōn). A liquid ketone, CH_3COCH_3, also called dimethyl ketone and propanone, used as a solvent for many organic compounds and, frequently, for glazing or repairing plastic spectacle frames.

acetylcholine (as″e-til-ko′lin). A chemical substance with excitatory properties, formed by cholinergic nerve fibers at synaptic and neuro-effector junctions during the transmission of nerve impulses. Fibers producing acetylcholine include all autonomic preganglionics, most parasympathetic postganglionics, motor fibers to skeletal muscle, and probably the neurons of the central nervous system. Acetylcholine is synthesized and liberated by action of the enzyme choline acetylase and normally exists only momentarily after formation, being rapidly hydrolyzed by the enzyme cholinesterase which is present in high concentration in surrounding tissues.

achievement, visual. 1. *Optometric Extension Program:* The ability to get meaning out of the external world through vision. 2. Improvement in performance of a visual task or tasks.

achloroblepsia (a"klo-ro-blep'se-ah, ak"lor-). Green blindness.

achloropsia (ak"klo-rop'se-ah, ak"-lor-). Green blindness.

achroma (a-kro'mah). 1. Lack of color. 2. Lack of normal pigmentation, as in albinism.

    congenital a. Albinism.

achromasia (ak"ro-ma'se-ah). 1. Absence of pigment, as in albinism or vitiligo. 2. Total color blindness.

    atypical a. Achromasia that is acquired and not inherited.

    typical a. Achromasia that is inherited as a simple recessive, not sex-linked.

achromasy (a-kro'mah-se). Achromatism.

    atypical a. Photanopia.

achromat (ak'ro-mat). An achromatic lens.

achromate (ak'ro-māt). One who is totally color blind, perceiving colors as black, white, and grays.

achromatic (ak"ro-mat'ik). 1. Pertaining to a lens or an optical system corrected for, or free from, chromatic aberration. 2. Pertaining to a totally color-blind individual. 3. Colorless.

achromaticity (a-kro"mah-tis'ih-te). The state, quality, or degree of being achromatic.

achromatism (a-kro'mah-tizm). 1. The condition of a lens or an optical system corrected for, or free from, chromatic aberration. 2. The condition of being totally color blind. 3. The condition of being colorless.

    actinic a. The condition of a lens or an optical system corrected for chromatic aberration of actinic wavelengths for photographic purposes.

    optical a. The condition of a lens or an optical system corrected for, or free from, chromatic aberration of the visible wavelengths.

achromatize (a-kro'mah-tīz). To render achromatic.

achromatope (a-kro'mah-tōp). One having achromatopsia.

achromatopsia (a-kro"mah-top'se-ah). Total color blindness.

    cone a. Cone monochromatism.

    incomplete typical a. Photanopia.

    rod a. Rod monochromatism.

achromatosis (a-kro"mah-to'sis). A deficiency of pigmentation in the tissues, as in the iris.

achromatous (a-kro'mah-tus). Colorless.

achromia (a-kro'me-ah). Achroma.

achromic (a-kro'mik). Colorless.

achromoderma (a-kro"mo-der'mah). Albinism.

achromodermia (a-kro"mo-der'me-ah). Albinism.

achromous (a-kro'mus). Colorless.

achroous (ak'ro-us). Achromatic.

achropsia (a-krop'se-ah). Color blindness.

acid, ascorbic. A water-soluble vitamin found in citrus fruits, tomatoes, salad greens, apples and new potatoes necessary in the maturation and maintenance of teeth, bone, and vascular walls. A severe deficiency in the diet is a cause of scurvy with the symptoms of spongy gums, extreme weakness, swollen joints, and petechial hemorrhages of the skin and mucous membranes and of ocular structures. Syn., *vitamin C.*

acid, nicotinic. Niacin.

acinesia (as"ih-ne'ze-ah). Akinesia.

aclastic (a-klas'tik). Nonrefracting.

acne (ak'ne). An affection of the skin, especially of the face, the back, and the chest, due to chronic inflammation of the sebaceous glands and the hair follicles, forming either papules, pustules, or nodules.

    ciliary a. Inflammation or infection of the glands of the margins of the eyelids.

    a. mentagra. An inflammatory disease of the hair follicles characterized by papules or pustules that are perforated by the hairs and surrounded by infiltrated skin. It may affect the eyebrows or the margins of the eyelids. Syn., *sycosis vulgaris.*

    a. rosacea. A chronic inflammatory disease affecting the skin of the nose, the cheeks, the forehead, and, occasionally, the cornea and the conjunctiva. It is characterized by a red coloration of the skin due to dilatation of the capillaries and the presence of acnelike pustules; it is common in alcoholics.

a. tarsi. An inflammatory affection of the Meibomian glands.

acopia (ă-ko'pe-ah). The inability to copy written material.

acorea (ak"o-re'ah). Absence of the pupil.

Acosta syndrome (ah-kos'tah). See under *syndrome*.

Acoustic Localizer. A visual training instrument designed by Bangerter to teach spatial localization with the assistance of auditory clues, in the preliminary treatment of amblyopia ex anopsia. It consists essentially of a plate containing a series of holes which may be individually illuminated. A hand-held electrically connected stylus is used to locate and touch the illuminated hole and is guided by a humming sound which increases as the target is approached and ceases when the target is contacted.

acritochromacy (ă-krit"o-kro'mah-se). Total color blindness.

acrocephalosyndactyly (ak"ro-sef"ah-lo-sin-dak'til-e). Congenital malformation of the skull, tower-shaped anteriorly and shortened anteroposteriorly, in association with complete or partial webbing of the fingers and toes. Eye symptoms include strabismus, reduced visual acuity, exophthalmos, and ophthalmoplegia. Syn., *acrosphenosyndactylia; Apert's syndrome.*

acrodermatitis chronica atrophica (ak"ro-der"mah-ti'tis kron'ih-kah a-tro'fih-kah). A rare disease characterized by a thinning of the skin causing the venous network to stand out prominently; associated with scar formation in the conjunctiva.

acroisa (ă-croy'sah). Blindness.

acropachy (ak'ro-pak"e). Clubbing of the fingers and pretibial myxedema accompanied by exophthalmos in thyroid disease.

acrosphenosyndactylia (ak"ro-sfe"-no-sin"dak-til'e-ah). Acrocephalosyndactyly.

acrylic (ah-kril'ik). The generic name for the family of transparent thermoplastic resins made by polymerizing esters of acrylic or methacrylic acid.

actinic (ak-tin'ik). Pertaining to wavelengths of radiant energy which produce chemical changes, especially those beyond the violet end of the spectrum.

actinism (ak'tin-izm). The property of radiant energy (especially ultraviolet) which produces chemical changes.

actinograph (ak-tin'o-graf). An instrument for measuring the actinic or chemical influence of solar rays.

actinology (ak"tin-ol'o-je). That branch of science which investigates the chemical action of light.

actinometer (ak"tin-om'eh-ter). An instrument for measuring the intensity of the sun's heat rays.

actinometry (ak"tin-om'eh-tre). The measurement of the intensity of solar radiation.

actinophthalmic (ak-tin"of-thal'mik). Having eyes with a highly reflective tapetum lucidum, as in cats.

activity, optical. The property of certain substances to rotate the plane of polarization. Substances which rotate the plane (looking against the oncoming light) to the right are called dextrorotatory, and those which rotate to the left are called levorotatory. Syn., *optical rotation.*

◆

ACUITY

acuity (ă-ku'ih-te). Clearness, distinctness, sharpness, or acuteness.

visual a. Acuteness or clearness of vision (especially of form vision) which is dependent on the sharpness of the retinal focus, the sensitivity of the nervous elements, and the interpretative faculty of the brain. Involved are the minimum visible (light sense), the minimum separable (resolving power), and psychological interpretations. Visual acuity varies with the region of the retina stimulated, the state of light adaptation of the eye, general illumination, background contrast, the size and the color of the object, the effect of the refraction of the eye on the size and the character of the retinal image, and the time of the exposure. Clinically, it is usually measured with a Snellen chart in terms of the Snellen fraction, and, occasionally, with the Landolt broken ring chart. Both methods are calibrated on a standard resolution threshold of 1 minute of arc. **absolute v.a.** Visual acuity as measured in an ametropic eye when accommodation is completely relaxed and the refractive error is corrected by a spectacle lens situated at the anterior focal point of the eye. It is expressed as the angle subtended at the anterior focal point of the corrected eye by the detail of the letter recognized. (Gullstrand) **angular v.a.** Visual acuity measured in a manner such that the identification of the target is free from influence of neighboring contours and is thus considered to be solely dependent on the subtense of the visual angle. Clinically, it is usually determined with single, isolated targets. Cf. *cortical visual acuity.* Syn., *letter visual acuity.* **apparent v.a.** Relative visual acuity. **binocular v.a.** 1. Visual acuity as measured with both eyes viewing the test target simultaneously. 2. Stereoscopic visual acuity. **contour v.a.** Vernier visual acuity. **cortical v.a.** Visual acuity measured in a manner such that the identification of targets may be influenced by the contours of neighboring targets. Clinically, it is usually determined by the simultaneous presentation of grouped targets, such as a line of letters on a Snellen chart. Cf. *angular visual acuity.* Syn., *line visual acuity; morphoscopic visual acuity; separation visual acuity.* **darkness v.a.** Visual acuity of the dark-adapted eye. **decimal v.a.** Visual acuity expressed as a decimal derived by reducing the Snellen fraction, e.g., 20/40=0.5. **displacement threshold v.a.** Vernier visual acuity. **dynamic v.a.** Visual acuity as determined for test targets in motion. Syn., *kinetic visual acuity.* **grating v.a.** Visual acuity based on the ability to resolve fine parallel lines in a test object. **kinetic v.a.** Dynamic visual acuity. **letter v.a.** Visual acuity measured by the presentation of single isolated letter or equivalent targets free from influence of neighboring contours. Cf. *line visual acuity.* Syn., *angular visual acuity.* **line v.a.** Visual acuity measured by the simultaneous presentation of one or more lines of targets such that identification may be influenced by the proximity of contours of neighboring targets. Cf. *letter visual acuity.* Syn., *cortical visual acuity; morphoscopic visual acuity; separation visual acuity.* **minimal v.a.** Visual acuity based on the ability to distinguish form under the condition of threshold illumination. **minimum separable v.a.** Resolution visual acuity. **morphoscopic v.a.** Cortical visual acuity. **naked v.a.** Unaided visual acuity. **natural v.a.** 1. Unaided visual acuity. 2. The visual acuity of an eye not corrected by a spectacle lens,

expressed as the angle subtended at the anterior principal point of the eye by the detail of the letter recognized with the object at the punctum remotum in myopia, at infinity in emmetropia, and with accommodation active in hypermetropia. (Gullstrand) Syn., *true visual acuity.* **peripheral v.a.** Visual acuity of the extrafoveal or the peripheral regions of the retina. **primary v.a.** Visual acuity based solely on the resolving power of the eye, exclusive of psychological factors. Cf. *secondary visual acuity.* **relative v.a.** Visual acuity as measured in an ametropic eye when accommodation is completely relaxed and the refractive error is corrected by a spectacle lens which is not situated at the anterior focal point of the eye. It is expressed as the angle subtended at the anterior principal point of the correcting lens by the detail of the letter recognized. (Gullstrand) Syn., *apparent visual acuity.* **resolution v.a.** Visual acuity based on the ability to distinguish two parallel lines or two points as two, and not as a single line or one point. **secondary v.a.** Visual acuity based on the minimum cognoscible, including the influence of the higher brain centers and, especially, such psychological factors as experience and judgment. Cf. *primary visual acuity.* **separation v.a.** Visual acuity measured in a manner such that the identification of test targets is influenced by the contours of neighboring targets, being related to the distance between the targets. **Snellen v.a.** Visual acuity as measured with Snellen test letters. **stereoscopic v.a.** The smallest difference in distance of two objects, perceivable by stereopsis cues, ordinarily specified as *angle of stereopsis.* **true v.a.** Natural visual acuity. **unaided v.a.** Visual acuity as measured without a spectacle lens or any other corrective device before the eye. Syn., *naked visual acuity.* **vernier v.a.** Visual acuity based on the ability to detect the alignment or the nonalignment of two lines, as in the reading of a vernier scale. Syn., *displacement threshold visual acuity.*

◆

acutance (ah-ku'tans). The sharpness of the optical or photographic image gradient for an object intensity step function, as by a knife edge, expressed quantitatively as the mean of the squares of the ratios of intensity or density differences to corresponding differences in distances across the edge function.

acutometer (ak"u-tom'eh-ter). An instrument for measuring visual acuity.

acyanoblepsia (a-si"ah-no-blep'se-ah, ă-si"-). Acyanopsia.

acyanopsia (a-si"ah-nop'se-ah, ă-si"-). The inability to distinguish blue tints. Syn., *acyanoblepsia*.

adacrya (a-dak're-ah, ă-dak'-). Deficiency or absence of tears.

Adair-Dighton syndrome (ă-dār'di'-ton). Van der Hoeve's syndrome.

Adams' (ad'amz) **diagram; theory.** See under the nouns.

◆

ADAPTATION

adaptation. 1. Any adjustment of an organism to the conditions of its environment. 2. The change in sensitivity to continuous or repeated sensory stimulation.

   alpha a. A term devised by Schouten to designate the neuro-electrical reaction of the retina to a light stimulus which results in almost instantaneous light adaptation, or reduced light sensitivity,.of the entire retina (although it is more marked at the site of stimulation). Cf.*beta adaptation.*

   amplitude of a. See under *amplitude.*

   beta a. A term devised by Schouten to designate the local photochemical reaction of the retina to a light stimulus which results in very rapid light adaptation, or reduced light sensitivity, only in the stimulated area of the retina. Cf. *alpha adaptation.*

   chromatic a. An altered sensitivity to color which produces apparent changes in hue or saturation. It may be induced, for example, by varying levels of illumination or by prolonged exposure to a specific color. **general c.a.** Adaptation in viewing objects through a colored filter so that these objects seem of normal or true color, i.e., as if the colored filter were not placed before the eye. **special c.a.** The apparent loss of saturation, hence of hue, in a color stimulus which is fixated steadily.

   dark a. The adjustment occurring under reduced illumination in which the sensitivity to light is greatly increased or the light threshold is greatly reduced. The process is slower than light adaptation. Syn., *scotopic adaptation.*

   lateral a. The effect of a specific, sharply defined retinal stimulus on adjoining areas of the retina, a factor in simultaneous color contrast.

   light a. The adjustment occurring under increased illumination in which the sensitivity to light is reduced or the light threshold is increased. Syn., *photopic adaptation.* **direct l.a.** The decrease in sensitivity to light of a region of the retina previously stimulated by light. **indirect l.a.** The decrease in sensitivity to light of one, usually more central, region of the retina when another region, usually more peripheral, has been just previously or simultaneously stimulated by light. The term was introduced by Schouten and Ornstein, who found that this effect varied with the angular separation of the two retinal regions and with retinal illuminances. It is closely related to direct light adaptation in that light striking a peripheral region of the retina may simultaneously strike the central region as a consequence of light scattering within the eye.

   local a. Adaptation produced by a stimulus that has been confined to a specific, more or less sharply defined, region of the retina, involved in after-images and successive color contrast.

   photopic a. Light adaptation.

   pupil a. Adjustment of pupil size to the intensity of light, the quality of light, and/or the level of accommodation and convergence.

   retinal a. A process in which the light threshold of the retina is shifted in relation to the level of illumination to which the eye is exposed.

   scotopic a. Dark adaptation.

   visual a. Any alleviatory, escape, or avoidance adjustment or response of the visual apparatus to an anomaly, defect, or condition, e.g., horror fusionalis, amblyopia, or suppression in strabismus.

◆

adaption (ah-dap'shun). Adaptation.

adaptometer (ad"ap-tom'eh-ter). An instrument for measuring the temporal course or degree of retinal adaptation in terms of change of light threshold. Most adaptometers are designed to investigate dark adaptation.

   Crookes a. An adaptometer used in a dark room with or without a fixation point, consisting essentially of a transilluminated white field subtending 7° at a viewing distance of 2 feet, with luminance controlled in steps by neutral density filters, and with a rotatable, four-position arrow on the test field to be identified at each luminance level and the elapsed time recorded.

Della Casa a. An adaptometer designed primarily as a quick and easily operated screening instrument in a somewhat darkened room and consisting essentially of an interiorly illuminated cylinder 40 cm long with a 13.0 X 2.5 cm viewing aperture at one end, with a cloth cover for the subject's head, and a low contrast, variable position, Landolt ring on a slightly luminous disk at the inner surface of the opposite end. The elapsed times, following preadaptation, for successive detection of the disk, the ring, and the gap in the ring are compared to norms for classification into normal and deficient dark adaptation.

Feldman's a. A dark adaptometer consisting primarily of a luminous slot to be identified after a bright preadaptation field is turned off, the time indicating the quality of dark adaptation.

Goldmann-Weekers a. An instrument consisting essentially of an interiorly and variably illuminated sphere with an open sector which confronts the subject's face as he looks into the sphere, a fixation light and test objects of variable reflectance and pattern at the surface opposite the subject's face, a constant speed rotating drum with a perforating marker for recording response times, and various incidental controls and attachments. It is variously used for measuring, during dark adaptation following preadaptation, the absolute threshold of a selected part or whole of the retina, the brightness contrast threshold, or the visual acuity by various techniques.

Hecht-Shlaer a. An adaptometer with controlled variability of the duration and intensity of the preadapting field and of the brightness, retinal location, size, time of exposure, and color of the threshold test light.

Nagel's a. An instrument consisting essentially of a box 80.0 cm long divided into three compartments in sequence, with a circular opal glass 10.0 cm in diameter on the front end face to serve as the test object in a darkroom in combination with a red fixation light. A

second opal glass and an adjacent variable square shutter aperture separate the front and middle compartments, and a blue glass plate with immediately adjacent changeable plates of different proportions of perforation separate the middle from the rear compartment in which are housed three incandescent light sources. The range of intensity of the resultant white test object luminance is from 1 to 80,000,000.

add. Abbreviation for *addition.*

Addison's disease (ad'ih-sunz). See under *disease.*

addition. The difference in spherical power between the distance and the near corrections in a bifocal or trifocal lens; usually referred to as the "add."

adducens (ă-du'senz). The branch of the third cranial nerve which supplies the internal rectus muscles.

  a. oculi. Internal rectus muscle.

adducent (ă-du'sent). Performing adduction.

adduct (ă-dukt'). To turn toward the midline, as in adduction.

adduction (ă-duk'shun). 1. The rotation of an eye toward the midline (nasally). 2. A commonly used, but incorrect, definition: The converging of the eyes toward each other, especially as determined by clinical tests with prisms, measured in terms of one or more of the criteria establishing the convergence limits of binocular vision such as blurring, diplopia, or recovery from diplopia. Clinically, the base-out prism limits of clear and single binocular vision.

  true a. *Optometric Extension Program:* The base-out–prism-to-blur finding during binocular fixation of a test object at a distance of 6 m.

adductor (ă-duk'tor). A muscle which rotates the eye toward the medial plane (nasally). The medial rectus muscle is primarily an adductor, the superior and the inferior rectus muscles secondarily so.

adenologaditis (ad'e-no-log"ah-di'tis, -lo"gah-di'tis). 1. Inflammation of the conjunctiva and the glands of the eyes. 2. Ophthalmia neonatorum.

adenoma (ad"e-no'mah). A benign tumor originating from, or having the appearance of, glandular epithelium; of endocrine or exocrine origin.

adenophthalmia (ad"e-nof-thal'me-ah). Inflammation of the Meibomian glands.

adiactinic (ad″ih-ak-tin′ik, a″di-). Impervious to the actinic or chemical rays of light.

adiaphanous (ad″ih-af′ah-nus). Opaque.

Adie's pupil (a′dēz). Tonic pupil.

Adie's syndrome (a′dēz). See under *syndrome.*

adisparopia (ah-dis″pahr-o′pe-ah). A term coined by Rabkin to identify an adaptation phenomenon variously called "Umstimmung" (Trendelenburg), "tuning" (Walls), chromatic fatigue, color asthenopia, and chromatic adaptation, manifested by an increase in the range of anomaloscope matches by anomalous trichromats with continuing adjustment attempts, as compared to the matches made immediately following pre-exposure to a neutral white surface.

aditus orbitae (ad′ih-tus or′bih-te). The orbital opening.

adjustment, absolute. The mechanical provision for adjusting the two oculars of a binocular instrument separately.

Adler's test (ad′lerz). See under *test.*

adnexa bulbi (ad-nek′sah bul′bi). Adnexa oculi.

adnexa oculi (ad-nek′sah ok′u-li). The appendages of the eye, as the lacrimal apparatus, the eyelids, and the extraocular muscles.

ADO. See *Association of Dispensing Opticians.*

adorbital (ad-ōr′bih-tal). Located in, or near, the orbit. *Rare.*

adrenalin (ad-ren′al-in). Epinephrine.

adtorsion (ad-tōr′shun). Intorsion.

advancement. A corrective surgical procedure for strabismus in which an extraocular muscle is severed from its scleral insertion and reattached to a more anterior position on the sclera within the same plane of action of that muscle. This has the effect of enhancing the mechanical action of the muscle and, theoretically, alters the arc of contact. It is seldom used as an isolated procedure, but more often is combined with a resection of the same muscle, although resection alone, utilizing natural insertion, is employed more commonly.

  capsular a. The surgical attachment of a part of Tenon's capsule to an ocular muscle for the purpose of advancing the insertion of the muscle.

adventitious (ad″ven-tish′us). Nonhereditary, acquired, accidental, or abnormally located.

adversion (ad-vur′shun). The nasal rotation of the eye. A term used categorically to identify the rotation of the eye nasalward, irrespective of the mechanism or its association with other functions.

aegilops (e′jih-lops). Egilops.

aeluropsis (e″loo-rop′sis, el′u-). A nasal inclination of the eyelids or the palpebral fissure.

aesthesiometer (es-the″ze-om′eh-ter). Esthesiometer.

AFB. See *American Foundation for the Blind.*

afferent (af′er-ent). Carrying toward a main structure, as a sensory neuron, or a lymphatic vessel approaching a lymph node.

afixation (a-fik-sa′shun). Absence of fixation, as seen in strabismus when the deviating eye fails to make any fixation movement upon occlusion of the normally fixating eye.

afocal (a-fo′kal). Pertaining to a lens or a lens system with zero focal power, or one in which rays entering parallel emerge parallel.

aftercataract (af′ter-kat′ah-rakt). Remains of the lens capsule following extracapsular cataract extraction which lie in the pupillary area and interfere with vision.

afterdischarge. 1. The persistence of effect or discharge of impulses in a nerve fiber or trunk after stimulation has ceased. As observed in optic nerve studies, the phenomenon is differentiated from the off-effect. 2. A discharge of impulses from a neural center after the removal of the stimulus.

aftereffect. In general, the experience that may follow the removal of the external stimulus. More specifically, it is a synonym for *afterimage* or *after-sensation.*

  figural a. The effect of a previously viewed figure or pattern on the perception of a different, subsequently observed, figure or pattern; especially any one of several classic distortion and illusion effects produced by previewing specially designed geometric patterns. Certain varieties of this phenomenon are also called *visual satiety effects.*

afterimage. A persisting sensation or image perceived after the correlated physical stimulus has been removed. Visually, the afterimage may be the continued perception of the essential form, motion, brilliance, or color qual-

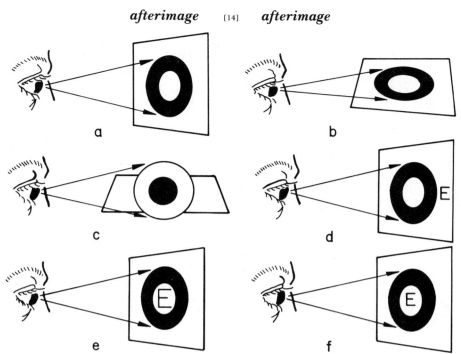

Fig. 2 Afterimages advocated by Cüppers for eccentric fixation therapy. (a) Negative afterimage; (b) afterimage with psychological characteristics of a real object; (c) positive afterimage which violates the psychological characteristics of a real object; (d) nasal eccentric fixation of the right eye; (e) central fixation; (f) central fixation using small letter as fixation target. (From J. R. Griffin, *Binocular Anomalies.* Chicago: Professional Press, 1976)

ities of the removed stimulus, or the perception of qualities of form, motion, color, or brilliance having an apparent relationship to the original stimulus though notably dissimilar. Ordinarily, the primary image is not regarded as an afterimage even though it persists a short period following the discontinuation of the stimulus. (See Fig. 2.)

complementary a. An afterimage in which the color is complementary to the color of the original stimulus.

Hering's a. First positive afterimage.

Hess's a. Third positive afterimage.

homochromatic a. An afterimage in which the hue is the same as that of the original stimulus.

induced a. An afterimage of an original stimulus which has been modified by secondary light stimuli.

motion a. An illusion of movement of an observed stationary object in the opposite direction from a just previously observed moving object.

negative a. 1. An afterimage in which the areas corresponding to the light areas of the original stimulus appear dark, dark areas light, and colors complementary. 2. An afterimage that appears less bright than its surround, regardless of hue.

original a. Any of the afterimages resulting from a single light stimulus, no secondary variations in light stimulus being presented.

positive a. 1. An afterimage in which the areas corresponding to the light areas of the original stimulus appear light, dark areas dark, and colors remain similar. 2. An afterimage that appears brighter than its surround, regardless of hue. **first p.a.** The first afterimage following the primary image of a brief, single, light stimulus of moderate intensity. It is a bright image of less intensity than the original stimulus and of the same hue. Syn., *Hering's afterimage.* **fourth p.a.** An afterimage which, after a long dark interval, may follow the third positive afterimage if the original light stimulus was of high intensity. **second p.a.** An afterimage which, after a dark interval, follows the first positive afterimage. It is less bright than the first, and its hue varies with the intensity of the stimulating light. It is generally considered to be a function of the scotopic mechanism since it is absent in the light-adapted eye. It is seen best with a green light stimulus, worst with red, and rarely with foveal stimulation. Syn., *Purkinje afterimage; Bidwell's ghost; following image of von Kries; pursuant image of von Kries; satellite of Hamaker.* **third p.a.** An afterimage which, after a long dark interval, follows the second positive afterimage. It is less bright than the second and of the same hue as the first. Syn., *Hess's afterimage.*

   Purkinje a. Second positive afterimage.

   pursuant a. Second positive afterimage.

   satellite a. Second positive afterimage.

afternystagmus (af"ter-nis-tag'mus). A vestibular nystagmus manifest after the abrupt cessation of a rotation of the head, due to the tendency of the labyrinthine fluid to persist in its movement. Syn., *secondary nystagmus.*

   optokinetic a. Nystagmus appearing with the eyes closed after a previously elicited optokinetic nystagmus.

aftervision (af'ter-vizh"un). Vision persisting after the exciting visual stimulus has been terminated. Syn., *persistent vision.*

Agamodistomum ophthalmobium (ag"ah-mo-dis'to-mum of"thal-mo'be-um). A trematode parasite occasionally found in the crystalline lens of the human eye.

age. 1. The time elapsed from the beginning or birth of an object or a being to any given time. 2. The latter part of life. 3. A measure of development of an individual in terms of the chronological age of an average individual of corresponding development.

   achievement a. Proficiency in study expressed in terms of what an average child of that chronological age can perform, as determined by tests.

   anatomical a. Age estimated by body developments.

   Binet a. Mental age approximated by Binet tests.

   chronological a. The time elapsed from birth to the present in a living individual, measured in years.

   mental a. The degree of mental development measured in terms of the chronological age of the average individual of corresponding mental ability; usually determined by the score of an intelligence test.

   physiological a. Age estimated by functional development.

   reading a. Proficiency in reading expressed in terms of what an average child of a given chronological age can achieve, as determined by tests.

aglaucopsia (a"glaw-kop'se-ah, ă"-glaw-). Green blindness.

aglaukopsia (a"glaw-kop'se-ah, ă"-glaw-). Green blindness.

aglia (ag'le-ah). A spot or speck on the sclera or the cornea.

agnea (ag-ne'ah). A condition in which objects or persons are not recognized.

agnosia (ag-no'se-ah). Total or partial loss of the perceptive faculty or of the ability to recognize or orientate objects or persons due to a disturbance in the cerebral associational areas, the sensory pathway and the receptor areas being intact. It is classified according to the sense affected, e.g., visual agnosia, auditory agnosia.

   color a. Total or partial inability to recognize or appreciate colors, though the sensory pathway and the receptors are normal, due to a disturbance existing in the integrative cerebral centers. Syn., *amnesic color blindness.*

   corporeal a. The inability of an individual to recognize the existence or the identity of parts of his own body or to appreciate defects of its functions.

   music a. Note blindness.

   spatial a. The inability to orientate oneself in space, usually accompanied by object visual agnosia. **visual s.a.** Spatial agnosia due primarily to an inability to appreciate visual clues. Syn., *space blindness.*

   visual a. The inability to understand or interpret what is seen due to a disturbance in the cerebral associational areas, the retina, the sensory pathways, and the striate area being intact. Syn., *cerebral blindness; cortical psychic blindness; psychic blindness.* **object v.a.** The inability to recognize, by sight, objects previously known, although the objects are seen clearly. Syn., *object blindness.*

agonist (ag′o-nist). Any muscle yielding the desired movement; the opposite of *antagonist;* a prime mover or protagonist. Superior rectus and inferior oblique muscles are agonists when they both elevate the eye.

agraphia (a-graf′e-ah, ă-graf′-). 1. That type of aphasia characterized by an inability to express meaning in written language. 2. A pathological lack or loss of the ability to write, usually resulting from a brain lesion.

   absolute a. Agraphia characterized by the complete inability to write. Syn., *agraphia atactica.*

   acoustic a. Agraphia characterized by the inability to write material which is dictated verbally.

   amnemonic a. Agraphia in which one is able to write letters or words but cannot write complete or meaningful sentences.

   a. atactica. Absolute agraphia.

   cerebral a. Mental agraphia.

   jargon a. Agraphia in which one can write only senseless combinations of letters.

   literal a. Absolute agraphia.

   mental a. Agraphia characterized by an inability to express thoughts in words. The individual can write, but cannot express his ideas in written form. Syn., *cerebral agraphia.*

   motor a. Agraphia in which the inability to write is consequent on muscular in-coordination.

   optic a. Visual agraphia.

   verbal a. Agraphia in which one is able to write letters but not words.

   visual a. Agraphia in which one can write from dictation but not from copy. Syn., *optic agraphia.*

Ahrens′ (ah′renz) **polarizer; prism.** See under *prism.*

aim. The process of placing the axis of reference of an object in line with a point of fixation or intent.

AION. Anterior ischemic optic neuropathy.

airlight. The luminance added to a black surface by the light scattered by air between the surface and the observer.

Airy′s (ār′ēz) **condition; disk.** See under the nouns.

akinesia (ak″ih-ne′se-ah). Lack of movement due to loss or impairment of motor function.

   a. iridis. Immobility or rigidity of the iris.

akinesis (ak″ih-ne′sis). Akinesia.

aknephascopia (ak″nef-ah-sko′pe-ah). Reduced visual acuity in low levels of illumination, such as in twilight or in inadequate artificial illumination. Syn., *twilight blindness; twilight vision.*

akyanoblepsia (a-ki″ah-no-blep′se-ah). Acyanopsia.

Alabaster′s projectionometer (al′ah-bas″terz). See under *projectionometer.*

alacrima (a-lak′ri-mah). Lack of secretion from the lacrimal gland.

Aland disease. Forsius-Eriksson syndrome. See under *syndrome.*

albedo (al-be′do). 1. The whiteness of a surface. 2. The diffuse reflecting power of a surface.

   a. retinae. Edema of the retina.

Albers-Schönberg disease (al′berz-shun′berg). See under *disease.*

Albini′s E test (al-be′nēz). See under *test.*

albinism (al′bin-izm). Congenital deficiency or absence of pigment in skin, hair, choroid, retina, and iris.

Albright′s (awl′brīts) **disease; syndrome.** See under the nouns.

Albright-McCune-Sternberg syndrome. Albright′s syndrome.

albuginea oculi (al″bu-jin′e-ah ok′u-li). The scleral coat of the eye.

albugineous (al″bu-jin′e-us). 1. Whitish. 2. Pertaining to or resembling the sclera.

albuginitis (al″bu-jin-i′tis). Inflammation of a tunica albuginea, as in the scleral coat of the eye.

albugo (al-bu′go). A white corneal opacity.

Alcaine (al′kān). Trade name for *proparacaine hydrochloride.*

alexia (a-lek′se-ah). The inability to recognize or comprehend written or printed words. Syn., *optic aphasia; visual aphasia; word aphasia; word blindness.*

   cortical a. Alexia in which word blindness results from lesions of the left angular gyrus.

   motor a. Alexia in which written words can be comprehended but cannot be read aloud.

   subcortical a. Alexia in which word blindness results from an interruption in the connection between a visual center and the angular gyrus.

Algemene Professionele Opticiensbond van België. See

L'Association Professionnelle des Opticiens de Belgique.

allachesthesia, visual (al″ă-kes-the′ze-ah). Visual allesthesia.

Allard's law. See under *law.*

allel (ă-lēl′). Allelomorph.

allele (ă-lēl′)). Allelomorph.

allelomorph (ă-le′lo-mōrf, ă-lel′o-). One of two or more genes which occupy the same locus in a pair of chromosomes and affect the same parts of the body in regard to inheritance of a trait or traits. Syn., *allele.*

Allen (al′en) **chart; gonioprism; implant; contact prism; theory.** See under the nouns.

Allen-Braley fundus lens. See under *lens.*

Allen-Gulden plunger retractor. See under *retractor.*

Allen-O'Brien contact lens. Allen's contact prism.

Allen-Thorpe gonioprism. See under *gonioprism.*

allesthesia, visual (al″es-the′ze-ah). A rare disorder in which images are transposed from one half of the visual field to the other, occasionally from the lower to the upper quadrant, or vice versa. Syn., *visual allachesthesia.*

alley. A passageway between two structures or an analogous representation.

    Blumenfeld a. The loci of two series of luminous points observed binocularly in a dark room and adjusted to form two rows seen from one end as being parallel or as pairs of lights separated by equal distances, the two criteria producing two different sets of loci, those for the former called the *parallel* or *Hillebrand alley* and those for the latter called the *distance alley.*

    distance a. The Blumenfeld alley resulting from the criterion of equal separation of paired alley points.

    Hillebrand a. The loci of two series of luminous points observed binocularly in a dark room and adjusted to form two rows seen from one end as being parallel. Syn. *parallel alley.* Cf. *Blumenfeld alleys.*

    Hillebrand-Blumenfeld a. Blumenfeld alleys.

    parallel a. Hillebrand alley.

allochroism (al″o-kro′izm). Variation or change in color.

allochromasia (al″o-kro-ma′ze-ah). 1. Change in color of skin or hair. 2. Color blindness. *Obs.*

allochromy (al″o-kro′me). The property of exhibiting, emitting, or reflecting a hue at variance with that ordinarily expected, as may occur in fluorescent or impure substances.

alloesthesia, visual (al″o-es-the′ze-ah). Visual allesthesia.

allokeratoplasty (al″o-ker′ah-to-plas″te). The grafting to the cornea of foreign material.

allometropia (al″o-me-tro′pe-ah). The refraction of the eye along any secondary line of regard. It is equal in magnitude and opposite in sign to the lens or combination of lenses required to bring any extrafoveal region of the retina into conjugate focus with an infinitely distant object.

allophthalmia (al″of-thal′me-ah). Heterophthalmia.

allopsychosis (al″o-si-ko′sis). A psychosis characterized by hallucinations and illusions and caused by disorganization of the external perceptive powers without disorder of the motor powers.

allotransplant, corneal (al″o-trans′plant). The replacement of opaque corneal tissue by a transplant prosthesis, usually acrylic. See also *autotransplant; heterotransplant; homotransplant.*

allowance. In general, the deduction from the gross finding obtained at the end of a given test in order to obtain the net finding. Ex.: 1. *Retinoscopy:* The value of the lens which must be deducted from the total lens power before the eye of the subject at the conclusion of the test in order to change the conjugate focus of the subject's eye lens system from the peephole of the retinoscope to infinity. 2. *Fused and unfused cross cylinder test:* The value to be deducted from the total lens power before the subject's eye at the conclusion of the cross cylinder test in order to determine the net near point finding. 3. *Ophthalmometry:* The deduction which must be made from the keratometric astigmatism in order to determine the total astigmatism of the eye.

all-*trans* retinene₁. An isomer of retinene₁.

Aloe (al′o) **distance unit; reading unit.** See under *unit.*

Alpascope. A trade name for an instrument designed to measure photophobic sensitivity or the need for absorptive spectacle lenses by the intensity level at which a pair of closely aligned, parallel filament images of increasing brightness are seen to merge into one.

alpha [α] (al'fah). The Greek letter used as the symbol for (1) *angle alpha;* (2) *alpha movement;* (3) *absorptance.*

alpha-chymotrypsin (al"fah-ki"mo-trip'sin). See *chymotrypsin, alpha.*

Alport's syndrome (al'pōrtz). See under *syndrome.*

Alström-Hallgren syndrome. See under *syndrome.*

alternation, figural. Retinal rivalry.

Alternator (awl'ter-na"ter). A device which controls the light-dark cycle of intermittent illumination, used in conjunction with Cüppers' afterimage method in the treatment of amblyopia and eccentric fixation. Syn., *Alternoscope.*

alternocular (al'ter-nok"u-lar). Denoting the use of each eye separately instead of binocularly; e.g., one eye for distant vision, the other for near.

Alternoscope (awl-tern'o-skōp). Alternator.

Alvarez lens (al-var'ez). See under *lens.*

alychne (ă-lik'ne). The locus of points on a color mixture diagram which have zero luminosity coefficients; hence the line $y = O$ in the CIE chromaticity diagram.

alypin (al'ip-in). A local anesthetic similar to, but less toxic than, cocaine; not mydriatic when used in the eye.

am. Abbreviation for *ametropia.*

AMA. See *American Medical Association.*

amacratic (am"ak-rat'ik). Amasthenic.

Amalric's syndrome (ah-mal'riks). See under *syndrome.*

amasthenic (am"as-then'ik). Serving to bring a bundle of rays to a point; distinguished from *collimating* (making parallel). Cameras are classified as amasthenic optical systems, whereas microscopes are of the collimating type. Syn., *amacratic.*

Amauroscope (am-aw'ro-skōp). An instrument for aiding the totally blind consisting of photoelectric cells and other electronic equipment fitted into a container approximately the size and shape of a skin diver's mask and fitted over the eyes. Impulses excited by light are conducted by wires to a number of sites around the eyes and behind the ears where the wires are fastened to the surface of the skin. It has been reported that the electrical impulses are capable of stimulating visual receptors of the brain so that dark shadows against a light field can be perceived. (A. del Campo)

◆

AMAUROSIS

amaurosis (am"aw-ro'sis). 1. Partial or total blindness from any cause. 2. Blindness occurring without apparent change in the eye itself, as from cortical lesions.

albuminuric a. Amaurosis due to renal disease.

Burns's a. Temporary amaurosis due to sexual excess.

central a. Amaurosis due to disease of the central nervous system.

cerebral a. Amaurosis due to brain disease.

congenital a. Amaurosis which exists from birth.

diabetic a. Amaurosis associated with diabetes.

epileptiform a. A sudden amaurosis characterized by dilation of the retinal veins; considered by some to be epileptic in nature.

a. fugax. 1. Sudden temporary amaurosis. 2. The blackout or temporary loss of vision resulting from sudden acceleration, as in aviation.

hysteric a. Amaurosis associated with hysteria.

intoxication a. Amaurosis caused by a systemic poison, such as alcohol or tobacco.

Leber's congenital a. A recessive hereditary disease characterized by partial or complete blindness occurring at birth or shortly thereafter. The fundus may appear normal in the first months of life, but diffuse pigmentation typically appears and may develop into the bone corpuscle type, the retinal vessels become attenuated, and the optic nerve becomes atrophic. Photophobia is the rule, and other ocular anomalies may be keratoglobus-like keratoconus, cataract, and night blindness (when some residual vision remains).

a. partialis fugax. A partial amaurosis, sudden and transitory, associated with headache, vertigo, and nausea.

reflex a. Amaurosis caused by reflex action of a remote irritation.

saburral a. Amaurosis occurring in an attack of acute gastritis.

sympathetic a. Amaurosis of

one eye due to transmission of disease from the other eye.

tapeto-retinal a. A rare amaurosis occurring at or shortly after birth in which an atypical form of diffuse pigmentation of the retina appears, retinal vessels are attenuated, optic atrophy is common, zonular cataract and keratoglobus may develop, and when some vision remains photophobia is present.

tobacco a. A toxic amaurosis due to excessive use of tobacco.

toxic a. Amaurosis caused by the toxic effects of the products of metabolic change occurring in uremia or diabetes or by the intake of various endogenous poisons such as ethyl and methyl alcohol, tobacco, quinine, and lead.

traumatic a. Amaurosis due to trauma.

uremic a. Amaurosis due to the products of metabolic change in uremia.

◆

amaurotic (am"aw-rot'ik). 1. Pertaining to blindness. 2. One suffering from amaurosis.

a. cat's eye. Blindness of one eye due to various intraocular conditions such as retinoblastoma, vitreous deposits, exudative choroiditis, etc., in which a bright reflection is observed at the pupil as it would appear from the tapetum lucidum of a cat.

a. family idiocy. A familial lipoid degeneration of ganglionic cells in the central nervous system occurring in three forms: 1. Early infantile, characterized ophthalmoscopically by a cherry red spot at the fovea surrounded by a white edematous macular area, atrophic changes of the disk, and normal surrounding retina. It occurs mainly in Jewish children, beginning at about the fourth month of life; accompanying symptoms are blindness, flaccid muscles, and convulsions. See also *Tay-Sachs disease.* Syn., *Kuf syndrome.* 2. Late infantile, occurs usually in non-Jewish children at about 2 years of age where pigmentary changes in the macula may occur instead of the cherry red spot. Syn., *Bielschowsky-Jansky disease.* 3. Juvenile, begins between 5 and 12 years of age and is characterized by "salt and pepper" pigmentation of the macula, pallor of the disk, reduced vision, and retarded mental development. See also *Batten-Mayou disease.*

a. pupillary paralysis. See under *paralysis, pupillary.*

Ambermatic. A trade name for a photochromic sunglass lens that is amber in misty or overcast weather, brown in warm and sunny weather, and dark silver-gray in bright and cold weather.

ambient (am'be-ent). Pertaining to surroundings, e.g., *ambient light.*

ambiocular (am"be-ok'u-lar). 1. With both eyes. Etymologically, "with both eyes together," and, hence, synonymous with *oculi uniter;* however, the clinical connotation has been "with either eye," that is, synonymous with *oculus uterque.* 2. Pertaining to the absence of ocular dominance.

ambiocularity (am"be-ok"u-lar'ih-te). 1. The faculty of ambiocular vision. 2. In strabismus, the use of either eye at will. 3. In strabismus, a phenomenon reported by Brock in which both eyes are used simultaneously but in which various portions of the image of each eye are utilized to form a single, composite percept without normal sensory fusion.

amblyope (am'ble-ōp). One who has amblyopia.

◆

AMBLYOPIA

amblyopia (am"ble-o'pe-ah). Low or reduced visual acuity not correctable by refractive means and not attributable to ophthalmoscopically apparent structural or pathological anomalies or proven afferent pathway disorders. Generally, it is detected by the measurement of visual acuity after the correction of any refractive error which may be present. Clinically, amblyopia is said to exist if vision is 20/30 (i.e., 6/9) or worse, or if the vision of one eye is significantly less than that of the other.

alcohol a., ethyl. 1. Amblyopia associated with the prolonged intake of ethyl alcohol and attributed to concurrent nutritional deficiencies. See also *nutritional amblyopia.* 2. A toxic amblyopia resulting from the ingestion of impure ethyl alcohol.

alcohol a., methyl. Reduced vision due to the toxic effects of methyl alcohol. The onset is usually sudden and severe after ingestion of the alcohol.

alternating a. The alternating inhibition or suppression of vision which occurs in alternating strabismus. The deviating eye exhibits the suppression.

ametropic a. Refractive amblyopia.

aniseikonic a. Amblyopia attributable to unequal size of the ocular images.

anisometropic a. Refractive amblyopia attributed to previously uncorrected anisometropia, typically in the eye with the greater error of refraction. See also *isoametropic amblyopia*.

a. of arrest. A type of amblyopia ex anopsia in which the reduced vision results from failure in normal development of visual acuity with maturation. Cf. *amblyopia of extinction*.

astigmatic a. Reduced vision resulting from previously uncorrected astigmatism, especially astigmatism of high degree, and characteristically accentuated in the meridian of greatest refractive error.

central a. Reduced vision confined to the macular area.

color a. Partial or complete color blindness.

congenital a. Reduced vision existing since birth with or without any accompanying congenital anomaly. Attributed by various authorities to arrested development of the macular area, to absence of the fovea, or to a fault in the conducting visual pathways.

deficiency a. Nutritional amblyopia.

dental a. Amblyopia resulting from the toxic effects of a dental infection.

disuse a. Amblyopia ex anopsia.

a. ex anopsia. Amblyopia attributable to nonuse or prolonged suppression. It is usually associated with strabismus or anisometropia, and vision may be partially or totally recoverable. Some prefer to reserve *amblyopia ex anopsia* as being due to lack of stimulation by light or form, such as may occur with total occlusion, severe ptosis or very dense cataract. Syn., *disuse amblyopia; obligatory amblyopia; suppression amblyopia*.

a. of extinction. A type of amblyopia ex anopsia in which vision is reduced from that previously attained, and, hence, is recoverable. Cf. *amblyopia of arrest*.

facultative a. Suppression or inhibition of vision in one eye in response to the use of the other eye.

functional a. Amblyopia attributable to functional disorders, the retinal receptors and visual pathways being anatomically intact and free from pathology, as, for example, amblyopia ex anopsia or hysterical amblyopia.

hysterical a. A psychic loss of vision due to a neurosis or a psychosis; often characterized by tubular visual fields.

isoametropic a. Refractive amblyopia occurring bilaterally and in association with relatively high but approximately equal, previously uncorrected, errors of refraction. See also *anisometropic amblyopia*.

Jamaican a. Amblyopia not unlike tobacco amblyopia, occurring among West Indians, accompanied by bizarre and atypical visual field defects; obscure etiology, possibly of dietary or toxic origin. Syn., *West Indian amblyopia*.

light deprivation a. Functional amblyopia attributed to non-use of the visual pathway due to gross insufficiency in light stimulation of the eye during the first few years of life, as may result from congenital cataract, congenital ptosis, traumatic cataract, or corneal opacification. Syn., *stimulus deprivation amblyopia*.

malarial a. Loss of vision resulting from the toxic effects of malaria.

nicotine a. Tobacco amblyopia.

nocturnal a. Night blindness.

nutritional a. Amblyopia due to dietary insufficiencies or malnutrition, especially to lack of the B vitamins. The loss of vision is gradual and the visual fields typically show a bilateral, roughly symmetrical, central, paracentral, or centrocecal scotoma, larger for red than white. Prognosis is good if treatment is instituted early. Syn., *deficiency amblyopia*.

obligatory a. Amblyopia ex anopsia.

occlusion a. Amblyopia ex anopsia which develops in an eye that has been constantly occluded for a period of time.

organic a. Amblyopia attributable to anatomical or pathological anomalies in the visual pathway.

postmarital a. Temporary loss of vision due to sexual excess. Syn., *Burns's amaurosis*.

a. potatorum. Amblyopia associated with excessive intake of ethyl alcohol.

quinine a. Loss of vision from the toxic effects of quinine.

receptor a. Amblyopia attributed to an anomaly in position, density, or composition of the foveal receptors, as, for example, tilting of the foveal receptors, or to a disturbance in their photopigment molecules.

reflex a. Partial or total blindness due to irritation or other disturbances in distal parts of the body, principally in peripheral sensory nerves, and especially in the trigeminal, as in dental amblyopia. Priestly Smith advanced the hypothesis that the irritation causes stimulation to the sympathetic nerve which leads to a contraction of the choroidal blood vessels and thus to an interference with chorioretinal functions.

refractive a. Amblyopia associated with, or attributed to, previously uncorrected high but equal refractive errors (*isoametropic amblyopia*) or significantly unequal refractive errors (*anisometropic amblyopia*).

relative a. Amblyopia ex anopsia coexisting with an organic loss of central vision.

simulated a. A pretense at blindness of varying degree; visual malingering.

stimulus deprivation a. Light deprivation amblyopia.

strabismic a. Amblyopia, usually unilateral, in association with strabismus and generally considered to be a sequel to the onset of strabismus.

suppression a. Amblyopia ex anopsia.

tobacco a. Amblyopia associated with, or attributed to, the prolonged or excessive use of tobacco and considered by some to be due to toxic substances in the tobacco and by others to be due to concurrent nutritional deficiencies. Typically, it occurs in males between the ages of forty and sixty and is characterized by bilateral juxtacecal or centrocecal scotomata which may be more advanced in one eye than the other. Prognosis is good if the use of tobacco is discontinued, the amblyopia is not of long standing, and the patient is in good health.

toxic a. Amblyopia due to exogenous poisons, such as alcohol, or to endogenous poisons, such as focal infections. The visual fields may show either a central or a peripheral loss, depending on the poisonous agent.

traumatic a. Amblyopia as a result of injury.

tropical a. Amblyopia of dietary origin occurring in warm countries in association with bilateral optic atrophy, sensorineural deafness, panmyelopathy, and peripheral neuropathy.

a. of uncorrected ametropia. Refractive amblyopia.

uremic a. Amblyopia resulting from toxic effects of uremia.

◆

amblyopiatrics (am″ble-o″pe-at′riks). The therapeutics, or treatment, of amblyopia.

amblyopic pupillary paresis (am″-ble-op′ik). See under *paresis*.

amblyoscope (am′ble-o-skōp). A reflecting mirror haploscopic device consisting essentially of two angled tubes, held in front of the eyes like opera glasses, which can be turned on a swivel to any degree of convergence or divergence. Originally designed by Claude Worth.

major a. A large, table-supported amblyoscope. Usually greater freedom for adjustments is incorporated in its design than in a simple amblyoscope.

Stanworth a. A major amblyoscope incorporating half-silvered mirrors so that the haploscopically viewed targets may be perceived to be among objects in real space.

Wheatstone a. An amblyoscope using mirrors to change the convergence stimulus. Syn., *Wheatstone stereoscope*.

Worth a. See *amblyoscope*.

Worth-Black a. A modified Worth amblyoscope providing vertical as well as horizontal adjustments.

amebiasis (am″e-bi′ah-sis). Infection with *Endamoeba histolytica*, sometimes producing conjunctivitis.

amentia, nevoid (a-men′she-ah). Sturge-Weber disease.

American Academy of Ophthalmology. An association of ophthalmologists that separated from the American Academy of Ophthalmology and Otolaryngology in 1978 and which publishes the journal *Ophthalmology*, formerly *Transactions of the American Academy of Ophthalmology*. Its membership is limited to board certified ophthalmologists.

American Academy of Optometry. A professional and scientific organization originated in 1922 for the purpose of encouraging the development of optometric science and practice by providing opportunities for the presentation, discussion, and publication of clinical and research papers. The Academy also provides funds for optometric research and graduate fellowships. Membership is confined to practitioners, scientists, and teachers who meet high professional standards.

American Association of Certified Orthoptists. An association founded in 1940 of Orthoptists certified by the American Orthoptics Council.

American Association of Ophthalmology. An association founded in 1956 primarily for public education and promotional purposes. Formerly the National Medical Foundation for Eye Care.

American Board of Opticianry. An association of opticians organized in 1947 to establish standards of education and training and to accredit training programs in opticianry, and to examine and certify individuals for membership.

American Foundation for the Blind. An organization founded in 1921 for the advancement of care for the blind and partially sighted through research, literature, films, lectures, and consultations, and by making available subnormal vision aids.

American Medical Association. An organization formed in 1847 whose membership consists of those who hold medical degrees. Its principal function is to represent the interests of the medical profession, and since 1883 it has published the *Journal of the American Medical Association.* The association's section on ophthalmology, established in 1883, offers an opportunity for the presentation of scientific programs in conjunction with American Medical Association conventions.

American National Standards Institute, Inc. An organization founded in 1918 as a clearing house for nationally coordinated standards.

American Ophthalmological Society. An organization formed in 1869 as the first specialty medical society in America. It has high requirements for membership, including excellent professional performance and adherence to the highest ethical standards.

American Optometric Association. A national organization of optometrists incorporated under the laws of the state of Ohio. Its prime purpose is to unite optometrists into a nationally representative group for the betterment of the optometric profession. It is supported by voluntary membership of individual optometrists, but membership must be accompanied by membership in local and state associations. It publishes the monthly *Journal of the American Optometric Association.*

American Optometric Foundation. An organization incorporated in the state of New York and sponsored by optometrists for the advancement of visual care through research, literature, education, and other related activities. This is accomplished largely through grants-in-aid to individuals and institutions.

American Optometric Student Association. An association founded in 1970 and affiliated with the American Optometry Association. It consists of students enrolled in accredited schools and colleges of optometry for intercommunications purposes and to represent students' interests in matters of professional concern.

American Orthoptic Council. A commission of twelve ophthalmologists and four orthoptists which regulates the training, certification, and practices of orthoptists.

American Osteopathic Association. An association of osteopathic physicians founded in 1897 to represent the professional, political, and educational interests of its members.

American Public Health Association. An organization of persons in the various professions and vocations related to health and health maintenance and of employees in public health related agencies, founded in 1872 to promote the development of activities and programs leading to the improved health of the public.

American Research Council of Optometry. An organization formed in Ord, Nebraska, by George A. Parkins and others and concerned with problems in reading as related to vision.

American School Health Association. An association founded in 1927 of school physicians, nurses, administrators, employees, consultants, and others interested in the improvement of health facilities and programs in schools.

Ames room. See under *room.*

ametrometer (am″e-trom′eh-ter). An instrument used in the refraction of the eye and consisting essentially of a complete set of trial lenses mounted in several rotating disks.

ametrope (am'e-trōp). One who has ametropia.

◆

AMETROPIA

ametropia (am"e-tro'pe-ah). The refractive condition in which, with accommodation relaxed, parallel rays do not focus on the retina; a condition representing the manifestation of a refractive error, specifically *myopia*, *hypermetropia*, or *astigmatism;* hence, a deviation from *emmetropia*.

axial a. 1. Myopia or hyperopia due primarily to a deviation from the average, or some other standard value, of the anteroposterior diameter of the globe. 2. In geometric optics, ametropia due to an axial length other than that of the schematic eye (Gullstrand value, 24.38 mm).

combination a. Ametropia resulting from chance combinations of normal elements of the refracting system of the eye, considered nonpathological in origin. Cf. *component ametropia*. Syn., *correlation ametropia*.

component a. A refractive error attributable to the abnormal development or acquired deviance of some of the optical components of the eye, and therefore considered of pathological origin. Cf. *combination ametropia*.

correlation a. Combination ametropia.

curvature a. 1. Myopia or hyperopia due primarily to a deviation from the average, or some other standard value, of the radius of curvature of one or more of the refracting surfaces of the cornea or the crystalline lens. 2. In geometric optics, ametropia due to differences in the radius of one or more of the refracting surfaces from the values of the schematic eye. 3. Clinically, the anterior surface of the cornea is considered to be the most frequent cause of curvature ametropia of significant amounts; hence, the term frequently implies ametropia due to the deviation of the anterior radius of the cornea from a standard value (Gullstrand value, 7.7 mm).

index a. 1. Myopia or hyperopia due primarily to a deviation from the average, or some other standard value, of the index of refraction of any of the refracting media of the eye. 2. Clinically, since the changes in index are rare or of small degree except in the crystalline lens, the term usually refers to ametropia consequent upon changes in the index of refraction of this body.

position a. Myopia or hyperopia due primarily to a deviation from the average, or some other standard value, of the crystalline lens position, i.e., distance from cornea and from fovea. In the schematic eye, if other things are equal, placing the lens farther back (large anterior chamber) will create hyperopia, while the reverse will cause myopia.

refractive a. 1. Myopia or hyperopia due primarily to a deviation from the average, or some other standard value, of the refractive power of the eye (cornea-aqueous-crystalline system). 2. In geometric optics, ametropia due to a total refracting power greater or less than that of the schematic eye (Gullstrand value, 58.64 D).

simple a. Ametropia due only to refractive anomalies in an otherwise healthy eye.

◆

ametropic (am"e-trop'ik). 1. Relating to ametropia. 2. Having ametropia.

Amici prism (ah-me'che). See under *prism*.

Amici-Bertrand lens (ah-me'che-bār'trahn). See under *lens*.

Amidei's syndrome (am'ah-dēz). See under *syndrome*.

amimia (ă-mim'e-ah). A sensory aphasia characterized by the loss of ability to communicate by gestures or signs.

Ammann's test (am'anz). Dark filter test.

von Ammon's posterior protrusion (fon am'onz). See *protrusion, von Ammon's posterior*.

amnesia (am-ne'ze-ah). Partial or total loss of memory.

color a. The inability to retain memory of color perceptions or to name colors properly.

visual a. The partial or total loss of ability to recall or identify past visual experiences, as the failure to recognize written or printed words or objects previously seen.

amotio retinae (ă-mo'she-o ret'ih-ne). Detachment of the retina.

amphiblestritis (am"fih-bles-tri'tis). Inflammation of the retina.

amphiblestrodes (am"fih-bles-tro'dēz). Retina. *Obs.*

amphiblestroid apoplexia (am"fih-bles'troid ap"o-plek'se-ah). Hemorrhage of the retina.

amphicrania (am"fih-kra'ne-ah). Headache occurring in both sides of the head.

amphodiplopia (am"fo-di-plo'pe-ah). Double vision in both eyes.

amphoterodiplopia (am-foh"te-ro-di-plo'pe-ah). Amphodiplopia.

amplification 1. Optically synonymous with *magnification*. 2. The increase of light intensity or image luminosity by means of an optical amplifier.

amplifier. 1. Optically synonymous with *magnifier*. 2. An instrument that provides an image of greater luminous intensity than that of the object viewed.

◆

AMPLITUDE

amplitude. The range or the extent of a surface, a space, or a capacity.

a. of accommodation. The difference expressed in diopters between the farthest point and the nearest point of accommodation with respect to the spectacle plane, the entrance pupil, or some other reference point of the eye. **absolute a. of a.** The amplitude of accommodation, but distinguished from amplitude of relative accommodation. **binocular a. of a.** The amplitude of accommodation measured with binocular fixation of the test stimulus. **minus lens a. of a.** The amplitude of accommodation measured by increasing the minus lens (or decreasing the plus lens) to the limit of clear vision while the distance of the test object is held constant. **monocular a. of a.** The amplitude of accommodation measured with the test stimulus presented to one eye, the other being absent, occluded, or fusionally dissociated from the first. **negative a. of a.** Negative relative amplitude of accommodation. **positive a. of a.** Positive relative amplitude of accommodation. **push-up a. of a.** The amplitude of accommodation as measured by a push-up test, i.e., moving the test object toward the eye or eyes to the nearest point of clear vision. **relative a. of a.** The total dioptric range of accommodation which can be elicited with convergence fixed. **negative a. of a.** The decrease in accommodation that can be elicited, as by means of convex lenses, with the convergence fixed, usually at a normal reading distance. **positive relative a. of**

a. The increase in accommodation that can be elicited, as by means of convex lenses, with the convergence fixed, usually at a normal reading distance. **reserve a. of a.** The amplitude of accommodation minus the accommodation needed for clear vision at a given fixation distance, usually an assumed reading distance. **usable a. of a.** 1. That portion of the total amplitude of accommodation available for prolonged use without discomfort, usually considered to be from one half to two thirds of the total amplitude. 2. The accommodation changes possible during binocular fixation of an object at a given fixed distance. Syn., *relative accommodation.*

a. of adaptation. The difference between the light sense threshold of a light-adapted eye and the light sense threshold of the same eye when dark-adapted.

a. of convergence. Clinically, the angle of maximum convergence; the angular deviation of the lines of sight from parallelism in converging to the maximum; occasionally synonymous with *absolute amplitude of convergence.* Syn., *amplitude of triangulation.* **absolute a. of c.** The amplitude of convergence measured from the maximum limit of divergence to the maximum limit of convergence. Clinically, it is the range in angular units from the prism base-in to break findings, accommodation relaxed, to the near point of convergence, maximum accommodation in force. **fusional a. of c.** The amplitude of convergence measured from the limit of negative fusional convergence to the limit of positive fusional convergence, with accommodation held constant. **negative a. of c.** Amplitude of negative relative convergence. **positive a. of c.** Amplitude of positive relative convergence. **push-up a. of c.** The amplitude of convergence measured by moving a test object in the median plane of the two eyes to the nearest point of single binocular vision. **relative a. of c.** The total relative convergence which can be elicited; conventionally measured from the prism base-in limit to the prism base-out limit of clear, single, binocular vision at a fixed level of accommodation. **relative, negative a. of c.** That part of the amplitude of relative convergence measured from the normal convergence demand for a given fixation distance to the prism base-in limit. **relative, positive a. of c.** That part of the amplitude of relative convergence measured from the normal convergence demand for a given fixation distance to the prism base-out limit. **reserve a. of c.** 1. Relative amplitude of convergence. 2. The total convergence ability of the eyes, minus the convergence in use.

cyclofusional a. The angle between the limits of excyclofusional and encyclofusional rotation of the eyes.

fusional a. The angle between the maximum convergence and the maximum divergence of the eyes that can be elicited in response to change in convergence stimulus while the accommodation stimulus, but not necessarily the accommodation, remains constant.

size a. In the measurement of aniseikonia, the range of magnifying power through which the patient sees no difference in the appearance of the eikonic test elements. One half of the size amplitude is known as the "sensitivity."

a. of stereopsis. An expression designating the interval between the upper or maximum limit and the lower or minimal limit of retinal disparity producing stereopsis. Cf. *range of stereopsis.*

a. of triangulation. Amplitude of convergence.

wave a. The maximum displacement of any particle in a wave from its equilibrium position. The energy or intensity is proportional to the square of the amplitude.

◆

ampulla, lacrimal (am-pul'ah). A dilatation of the canaliculus at the junction of its vertical and horizontal portions about 2 mm from the lacrimal punctum.

Amsler (amz'ler) **charts; grids.** See under *chart.*

Amsler's degrees of keratoconus. Four grades of keratoconus: 1. Showing an angle of 1° to 3° between the two horizontal radial lines of the photokeratoscope. 2. Showing an angle of 4° to 8°. 3. Easily detected with slit lamp and ophthalmometer. 4. Easily detected by external profile inspection.

Amsler-Huber test (amz'ler hu'ber). See under *test.*

amydriasis (am"ih-dri'ah-sis). Contraction of the pupil.

amygdala (a-mig'dah-lah). A nucleus in the temporal lobe of the brain connecting to the fornix and midbrain, stimulation of which is reported to cause accommodation and pupillary dilation.

amyloidosis (am"ih-loi-do'sis). A disease of unknown etiology characterized by the abnormal deposition of amyloid, a translucent homogenous glycoprotein, in various organs and tissues of the body. In the eye, it may occur as a primary affection, may follow trachoma or other chronic infections, or may occur rarely as part of a systemic involvement. It may affect the bulbar or palpebral conjunctiva, tarsus, cornea, sclera, vitreous humor, optic nerve, or the levator palpebrae muscle, and it leads to tumor formation.

anacamptic (an"ah-kamp'tik). Pertaining to reflection of light or sound.

anacamptics (an"ah-kamp'tiks). The study of reflection of light or sound.

anaclasis (an-ak'lah-sis). Refraction or reflection of light or sound.

anaclastic (an"ah-klas'tik). Pertaining to reflection or refraction of light or sound.

anagenesis (an"ah-jen'e-sis). 1. Regeneration, reparation, or reproduction of tissue. 2. A photochemical regeneration of previously bleached or exhausted color elements, such as rhodopsin of the retina.

anaglyph (an'ah-glif). Two related photographs or drawings, superimposed and laterally displaced, each outlined in a color complementary to that of the other (usually in red and blue-green), to be viewed through filters of the same colors, one to each eye. If the corresponding parts of the drawings have been properly displaced, or the photographs are of a single scene taken from two directions, when properly fused the anaglyph will give rise to the percept of relief or stereopsis.

anaglyphoscope (an"ah-glif'o-skōp). Anaglyptoscope.

anaglyptoscope (an"ah-glip'to-skōp). An instrument used to demonstrate the effect of shadows in the interpretation of perspective by redirecting the light upon an object in relief to an opposite direction, resulting in an apparent reversal of perspective.

anagnosasthenia (an"ag-nōs"as-the'ne-ah). 1. The inability to read although the printed words are distinguishable. 2. Distress at any attempt to read.

Analyser, Automatic Central Field.
Trade name for an electronic automatic visual field testing instrument designed specifically to check the central field by presenting a random program of 128 stimuli, 112 of which are within the 30° area. It utilizes a hemispheric bowl of 33 cm, a stimulus size of 1 mm diameter, and has a monochromatic light source providing a constant wavelength of 583 nanometers.

Analyser, Friedmann Visual Field.
An instrument designed to explore the central visual field, utilizing a single xenon flash tube in an integrating bowl hemisphere, in front of which is a flat, perforated, opaque diaphragm which can produce single or multiple stimuli of variable intensity and of brief duration.

analysis, Fourier's. Resolution of a complex periodic wave form into a series of single components according to Fourier's theory.

analysis, graphic. 1. An analysis of image formation by ray tracing. 2. An analysis of the accommodation and convergence interrelationships by plotting clinical findings on a coordinate graph.

analysis, visual. The analysis of functional visual problems in terms of cause and correction.

analyzer (an'ah-li"zer). 1. A polarizing filter with which it is possible to determine the direction of polarization of a beam of light. 2. One of the two filters in a plane polariscope, the other being the polarizer.

Analyzer, Humphrey Lens. Trade name for an automatic and instantaneous computerized lensmeter which displays the spherical, cylindrical, and prismatic components of an ophthalmic lens digitally in standard prescription form.

Analyzer, Humphrey Vision. A haploscopic projection instrument for deriving the subjective refraction and various supplementary motility, binocular coordination, and image quality measurements of the eyes by utilizing continuously variable (Alvarez) lenses, a mirror which directs light with adjustable vergence, a system for measuring astigmatism which involves subjective judgments of line targets in two pairs of fixed meridians, and the automatic computation of the indicated spherocylinder prescription.

Analyzer, Lovibond Color Vision.
The trade name for an instrument patterned after the Lovibond tintometer utilizing a mixture of three primary colors provided by transillumination of glass filters which can be adjusted to match a reference standard to detect and measure color blindness.

anamorphic (an-ah-mōr'fik). Of different optical magnification in mutually perpendicular meridians.

anamorphoser (an"ah-mor-fo'ser). A device (the simplest form of which is the Brewster prism unit) by which meridional magnification without effective power for distance vision can be obtained. Two identical prisms are placed base to apex and hinged at the base of one and the apex of the other so that the angle between the prisms may be changed. The degree of meridional magnification which occurs in the base-apex meridian varies with the angle between the prisms.

anamorphosis (an"ah-mōr'fo-sis, an"-ah-mōr-fo'sis). A method by which a distorted image is corrected when viewed through a curved mirror or through a pyramidal glass.

   catoptric a. The correction of a distorted image by means of a curved mirror.

   dioptric a. The correction of a distorted image by means of a pyramidal glass.

anaphalantiasis (an"af-ah-lan-ti'ah-sis). Lack of eyebrows or eyelashes. *Obs.*

anaphoria (an"ah-fo're-ah). A tendency of both eyes to turn upward above the horizontal plane in the absence of a stimulus eliciting fixation attention.

anastigmatic (an"as-tig-mat'ik, an-as"-). Without astigmatism; corrected for astigmatism.

anatropia (an"ah-tro'pe-ah). A persistent, abnormal upward turning of the visual axes above the horizontal plane.

anchylops (ang'ki-lops). An abscess at the inner canthus of the eye.

ancoramic (an"ko-ram'ic). Pertaining to viewing distances less than 30 cm from the eye, a classification by Weston. Cf. *mesoramic; teloramic.*

Andersen-Weymouth hypothesis (an'der-sen-wa'muth). See *hypothesis, Weymouth-Andersen.*

Andogsky's syndrome (an-dog'skēz). See under *syndrome.*

anemia (ă-ne'me-ah). A diminution of the

normal blood volume, or a deficiency of the number of red cells, hemoglobin, or both.

glaucomatous a. A localized anemia in the limbal area, characterized by a dead white appearance; seen in cases of chronic glaucoma.

retinal a. Anemia characterized in the retina by a generalized pallor and, occasionally, superficial hemorrhages and slight engorgement of the veins.

sickle-cell a. Sickle-cell disease.

anerythroblepsia (an"e-rith"ro-blep'-se-ah). Protanopia.

anerythropsia (an"e-rith-rop'se-ah). The inability to perceive the color red; red blindness or protanopia.

anesthesia, optic (an"es-the'ze-ah). Temporary loss of vision.

anesthesia, retinal (an"es-the'ze-ah). Temporary amaurosis, usually due to hysteria.

aneurysm (an'u-rizm). A saclike dilatation of the walls of a blood vessel, usually an artery. It is filled with fluid or clotted blood, usually forming a pulsating tumor.

Leber's miliary a's. Telangiectases of the retinal vessels occurring in *Leber's retinal degeneration.*

Angelucci's syndrome (an"jeh-lu'chez). See under *syndrome.*

angioblastomatosis (an"je-o-blas"to-mah-to'sis). Von Hippel-Lindau disease.

angiogliomatosis (an"je-o-gli"o-mah-to'sis). Von Hippel-Lindau disease.

angiogram, fluorescein (an'je-o-gram"). The record of rapid serial photography of the retinal vasculature following the intravenous injection of fluorescein.

angiography, fluorescence. A specialized technique for observing the retinal vasculature in which rapid serial photography records the retinal circulation following the intravenous injection of fluorescein. Syn., *fluorescein angiography; ocular angiography.*

angiography, ocular. Fluorescence angiography.

angioid streaks (an'je-oid). See under *streak.*

angiokeratoma corporis diffusum (an"je-o-ker"ah-to'mah kor-por'is dih-fu'sum). Fabry's disease.

angioma (an"je-o'mah). A tumor composed of lymphatic or blood vessels.

angioma pigmentosum atrophicum (an"je-o'mah pig-men-to'sum ă-tro'fik-um). Xeroderma pigmentosum.

angiomatosis (an"je-o-mah-to'sis). A diseased state of the blood vessels marked by the formation of multiple angiomas.

encephalocutaneous a. Sturge-Weber disease.

encephalofacial a. Phacomatoses.

encephalo-oculo-facial a. Sturge-Weber disease.

encephalotrigeminal a. Sturge-Weber disease.

hereditary hemorrhagic a. Rendu-Osler disease.

meningocutaneous a. Sturge-Weber disease.

a. retinae Von Hippel's disease.

retinocerebral a. Von Hippel-Lindau disease.

angiomegaly (an"je-o-meg'ah-le). Enlarged blood vessels occurring mainly in the eyelids.

angiopathia retinae traumatica of Purtscher (an"je-o-path'e-ah ret'ih-ne traw-mat'ih-kah). Purtscher's disease.

angiopathia retinalis juvenalis (an"je-o-path'e-ah ret"ih-nal'is ju"ven-nal'is). Eales's disease.

angiopathica traumatica of Purtscher (an"je-o-path'ih-kah traw-mat'ih-kah). Purtscher's disease.

angioreticuloma (an"je-o-reh-tik"u-lo'mah). A hemangioma of the retina or the brain. See also *von Hippel-Lindau disease.*

angioscotoma (an"je-o-sko-to'mah). A scotoma due to the blocking of incident light by the larger retinal vessels; characteristically, it is ribbon-shaped and extends from the normal blind spot.

angioscotometry (an"je-o-sko-tom'eh-tre). The plotting of angioscotomata by the use of sufficiently small test objects and accurate fixation.

angiospasm, retinal (an'je-o-spazm"). A spasmodic segmental contraction of a blood vessel of the retina.

◆

ANGLE

angle. 1. The figure formed by the meeting of two lines at a point, or the space bounded by two such lines. 2. The degrees of turning necessary to bring one line or plane parallel to, or coincident with, another. 3. The direction from which an object is viewed.

a. of aberration. The angle between a refracted ray and the extension of the incident ray. Syn., *angle of deviation.*

acceptance a. Field of view.

a. of adaptation. Angle of anomaly.

advancing a. A wetting angle measured on a dry optical surface. Cf. *receding angle.*

a. alpha. 1. The angle formed at the first nodal point by the intersection of the optic axis and the visual axis. 2. The angle between the visual axis and the line normal to the cornea at its geometric center. (Donders) 3. The angle between the visual axis and the major axis of the corneal ellipse. (Landolt) **negative a.a.** The angle formed by the intersection of the visual axis and the optic axis in such a way that the visual axis lies temporal to the optic axis in the plane of the cornea. **positive a.a.** The angle formed by the intersection of the visual axis and the optic axis in such a way that the visual axis lies nasal to the optic axis in the plane of the cornea.

a. of altitude. Angle of elevation.

a. of anomaly. The angle between the line of visual direction of the fovea and the line of visual direction of a retinal area in the same eye which has a common visual direction with the fovea of the other eye. Usually it is represented by the difference between the objective and the subjective angles of strabismus in anomalous retinal correspondence. Abbreviation, *A.* Syn., *angle of adaptation.*

a. of the anterior chamber. The angle at the periphery of the anterior chamber, formed by the uveal meshwork, the ciliary body, and the root of the iris.

aperture a. The angle subtended in an optical system by the radius of the entrance pupil or the exit pupil at the anterior focal point or the posterior focal point, respectively.

apical a. The dihedral angle formed by the meeting of the two plane faces of a prism at its edge. Syn., *angle beta; prism angle; refracting angle.*

a. of azimuth. In a system for specifying the direction of regard in terms of elevation and azimuth, the angle of rotation (μ) of the line of sight right or left from its zero value in the primary position about an axis perpendicular to the primary plane of regard.

a. beta. 1. The angle between the fixation line and that normal to the cornea which goes through the geometric center of the cornea. (Helmholtz) 2. Refracting angle of a prism.

biorbital a. The angle of about 45° formed by the intersection of the orbital axes of the paired bony orbits.

Brewster's a. Angle of polarization.

collimation a. The angle subtended by a projected or signal light source at a point on an irradiated surface.

contact a. Wetting angle.

a. of convergence. The laterally or horizontally oriented angle between the lines of sight of the two eyes. The angle is positive when the lines of sight intersect in front of the centers of rotation, negative when behind. Directional axes other than the lines of sight may be employed as a basis for specifying angle of convergence.

critical a. That angle of incidence which results in the refracted ray traveling along the surface between the two media. Any angle greater than the critical angle results in total reflection. Syn., *limiting angle.*

a. of declination. The total angular difference between (1) the meridians of orientation of the corresponding retinal images in the two eyes which produce a stereoscopic vertical appearance of the fixation object or (2) the meridians of orientation of the same images which produce a given inclination of the perceived (fused) images. Cf. *angle of inclination.*

a. of deviation. 1. In strabismus, the angle by which the visual axis, or foveal line of sight, of the deviating eye fails to intersect the object of fixation, usually subtended at the center of rotation of the deviating eye. 2. The angle through which a ray of light has been deviated by reflection or refraction. **chromatic a. of d.** The angle through which a ray of specific wavelength has been deflected in passing through a refracting surface or prism. **minimum a. of d.** The angle between the incident ray and the emergent ray of an optical prism, when the path of light traversing the prism is that producing the least deviation. This condition exists when the path of light traverses the prism symmetrically, when the (reduced) angles of incidence and emergence are equal, and when the ray which traverses the prism is perpendicular to a bisector of the refracting angle of the prism. **objective a. of d.** The angle of deviation of the visual axes as determined by objective testing procedures, e.g., cover test and making allowance for any eccentric fixation. **primary a. of d.** In strabismus, the angle of deviation when the normally fixating eye is fixating. **secondary a. of d.** In strabismus, the angle of deviation when the normally deviating eye is made to fixate. **true a. of d.** In strabismus, the angle of deviation when it includes consideration of angle kappa.

a. of direction. The angle between the optical axis of an optical system and the chief ray to some object of interest, as measured at the appropriate principal point of the system. In the case of the eye, the point of reference may also be (1) one of the nodal points, (2) the center of the entrance pupil, or (3) the center of rotation.

a. of discrimination. Minimum separable angle.

a. of displacement. The angle between the line of sight when the eye is in the primary position and the line of sight when the eye is in any secondary position.

a. of distinctness. The smallest visual angle at which the form of objects can be distinguished; visual acuity expressed in terms of the angle subtended.

a. of divergence. The angle between the lines of sight when they diverge from parallelism, especially laterally, although it may refer to vertical divergence. Directional axes other than the lines of sight may also be employed as a basis for specifying angle of divergence.

a. of eccentric fixation. The angle between the center of the fovea and the extrafoveal retinal area used for fixation subtended at the center of rotation of the eye.

a. of eccentricity. In a system for specifying the direction of regard in terms of eccentricity and meridional direction, an angle of rotation of the line of sight in a meridian plane containing the lines of sight in both the zero and the eccentric direction. This is the system used in the perimeter in which meridional direction pertains to the position of the arc of the perimeter and eccentricity to the position of the line of sight on the arc.

a. of elevation. In a system for specifying the direction of regard in terms of elevation and azimuth, the angle of rotation (λ) of the line of sight up or down from its zero value in the primary position about an axis lying in the primary plane of regard. Syn., *angle of altitude.*

a. of emergence. The angle formed between the emergent ray and the normal at the point of emergence.

a. epsilon. The angle between the macular axis and the papillary axis, as subtended at the second nodal point. This is equivalent to the angle between the point of fixation and the nasal edge of the blind spot, as subtended at the primary nodal point.

a. eta. The relative binocular parallactic angle or the angle of stereopsis.

external a. The angle formed by the eyelids at the outer canthus.

a. of field of view. The angle subtended by the entrance port at the center of the entrance pupil.

a. of filtration. The peripheral portion of the anterior chamber between the root of the iris, the front surface of the ciliary body, and the sclera; the part of the anterior chamber related to the trabecular spaces and the canal of Schlemm.

focal point a. The angle subtended by an object at the primary focal point of the eye.

a. of Fuchs. A recess or space between the superficial and the deep layers of the anterior surface of the iris along the line of the collarette in the ciliary portion of the iris.

fusion a. In strabismus, the angle through which haploscopic targets must be moved from parallelism for fusion to occur, or the angular displacement of the fixation target by a measuring prism for fusion to occur.

a. gamma. The angle between the fixation axis and the optic axis of the eye.

great a. of the eye. The angle formed by the lid margins at the inner canthus of the eye.

half-field a. One half the angle of field of view.

half-shade a. The angle between the planes of polarization in the field of a polarimeter.

image a. The angle of displacement when a prism is placed between the eye and an object.

a. of incidence. The angle formed between the incident ray and the normal at the point of incidence.

a. of inclination. The angle represented by the fore or aft tilt (or reorientation) of a line of reference which intersects the visual plane at the point of fixation. It is measured from the stereoscopic vertical or from the perpendicular to the visual plane. The angle of inclination bears a simple geometric relationship to the angle of declination. The apparent inclination of the vertical meridian may be created by an oblique meridional aniseikonia or by rotating the vertical meridian of targets in a stereoscope in opposite directions about the axes of fixation.

iridocorneal a. The angle between the iris and the cornea at the periphery of the anterior chamber of the eye. Syn., *angle of the iris; angulus iridis.*

a. of the iris. Iridocorneal angle.

a. kappa. The angle between the visual axis and the pupillary axis of the eye, measured at the nodal point. **negative a. k.** The angle between the visual axis and the pupillary axis when the visual axis is temporal to the pupillary axis. A negative angle kappa is anomalous; if present, the eyes may appear to converge. **positive a. k.** The angle between the visual axis and the pupillary axis when the visual axis is nasal to the pupillary axis; if abnormally large, the eyes may appear to diverge.

a. lambda. The angle subtended at the center of the entrance pupil of the eye by the intersection of the pupillary axis and the line of sight. It is this angle which is measured in routine clinical tests, although it is commonly designated *angle kappa.*

a. of latitude. In a system for specifying the direction of regard in terms of longitude and latitude, the angle of rotation (ϕ) of the line of sight about an axis lying in the primary plane of regard at the center of rotation of the eye.

limiting a. Critical angle.

a. of longitude. In a system for specifying the direction of regard in terms of longitude and latitude, the angle of rotation (θ) of the line of sight about an axis perpendicular to the primary plane of regard at the center of rotation of the eye.

a. of meridional direction. In a system for specifying the direction of regard in terms of eccentricity and meridional direction, the specified angle (κ), clockwise from the subject's point of view, between the plane of regard and the meridian plane in which the angle of eccentricity is measured.

meter a. A unit of convergence; the angular amount of convergence required for binocular fixation of a point on the median line 1 m from the centers of rotation of each eye. The magnitude of the angle varies with interpupillary distance and may be converted into prism diopters by multiplying the number of meter angles by the interpupillary distance in centimeters.

minimum a. of resolution. The minimum separable angle as determined by the identification of form targets and represented by the reciprocal of the Snellen fraction, e.g., 20/40 = 2 minutes of arc.

minimum separable a. The smallest angle subtended at the nodal point, the center of the entrance pupil, or other point of reference of the eye by two points or lines in order that they may be discriminated as separate; a measure of the threshold of form sense. Syn., *angle of discrimination; limiting visual angle; minimum visual angle.*

minimum visible a. The angle subtended at the anterior nodal point, the center of the entrance pupil, or other point of reference of the eye by rays from the extremities of the smallest areal extension of light which can be perceived. It varies with the region of the retina stimulated, the nature of the surround, the state of adaptation, and the duration and the intensity of the stimulus.

nasal a. The angle formed by the lid margins at the inner canthus of the eye.

nasomalar a. The angle of about 145° made by the intersection of lines, extending from the lateral orbital margins through the medial orbital margins.

ocular a. Palpebral angle.

ommatidial a. The angular extent of the visual field encompassed by each ommatidium of a compound eye.

optic a. The angle formed by two lines from the anterior nodal point of the eye to the extremities of the object of regard. Cf. *visual angle.*

orbital a. An angle of about 45° where the orbital axes meet. Syn., *biorbital angle.*

palpebral a. The angle formed by the eyelids at the external or internal canthus. Syn., *ocular angle.*

pantoscopic a. The angle between the plane of a spectacle lens and the frontal plane of the face when the superior margin of the lens is farther away from the frontal plane than the inferior margin. Cf. *retroscopic angle.*

parallactic a. The magnitude of parallax expressed as an angle with reference to the entrance pupils of the two eyes in binocular parallax, or with reference to the entrance pupil of one eye in two separate positions in monocular parallax. **binocular p.a.** The angular difference in direction of a viewed object with respect to the entrance pupils of the two eyes, represented by the angle between the lines connecting the entrance pupils of the two eyes with the object. **monocular p.a.** The angular change in direction of a viewed object with respect to the entrance pupil of the eye when the eye is moved from one location to another, represented by the angle between the lines connecting the center of the entrance pupil of the eye, in the two positions, with the object. **relative binocular p.a.** The angular change of the relative difference in direction of two objects with respect to the centers of the entrance pupils of each of the two eyes considered as viewing the object separately. It is derived by subtracting the binocular parallactic angle for the one object from that of the other. Syn., *angle eta.* **relative monocular p.a.** The angular change of the relative difference in direction of two objects with respect to the center of the entrance pupil of the eye, viewed with the eye first in one position and then in another. It is derived by subtracting the monocular parallactic angle for the one object from that of the other.

a. of parallax. Parallactic angle.

physiological a. The angle formed by the corneal and the visual axes. Syn., *angle alpha.*

a. of polarization. The angle of incidence at which the reflected light is all plane polarized. This occurs when the reflected light is at right angles to the refracted light. Syn., *Brewster's angle.* See also *Brewster's law.*

principal a. The angle between the two refracting surfaces of a prism. Syn., *angle beta; prism angle; refracting angle.*

principal point a. The angle subtended by an object at the primary principal point of the eye.

prism a. The dihedral angle between the sides of a prism. Syn., *angle beta; principal angle; refracting angle.*

a. of projection. The extreme angle between rays emerging from an optical system.

a. of false projection. The angle between the line drawn from the true position of an object through the center of the entrance pupil and the line drawn from the perceived position of the object. It is most apparent in past pointing exhibited by a recent paralytic strabismic; also, it may be apparent in patients with anomalous fixation.

receding a. A wetting angle measured on a wetted surface. Cf. *advancing angle.*

re-entering a. An angle with its apex toward the interior of the figure in which it occurs. Hence, in perimetry, a wedge-shaped sector defect with its acute angle within the seeing field and with the side opposite this angle extending to the limit of the field.

reflecting a. of prism. The angle through which a reflecting prism will turn a ray of light.

a. of reflection. The angle between the incidence normal and the reflected ray.

refracting a. The dihedral angle between the faces of a prism. Syn., *angle beta; principal angle; prism angle.*

a. of refraction. The angle, formed at the point of emergence, between the emergent ray and the normal.

retroscopic a. The angle between the plane of a spectacle lens and the frontal plane of the face when the superior margin of the lens is closer to the frontal plane than the inferior margin. Cf. *pantoscopic angle.*

a. of rotation. The angle through which the plane of polarization is rotated by an optically active substance. See also *optical activity*.

Russell a's. In the *Rousseau construction*, the angle values on the polar coordinate system which correspond to equal sine intervals on the rectilinear coordinate system. For a luminous flux distribution curve of a lamp with symmetrical flux distribution, the simple arithmetical average of the intensities measured on a series of Russell angles covering the 0° to 180° range gives the mean spherical candlepower.

scattering a. The angle between the initial and final paths of a scattered ray.

slope a. The angle between a ray of light and the optical axis of a lens or a lens system.

a. of stereopsis. The difference between the angles subtended, at the centers of the entrance pupils of the two eyes, by two points in space at different distances from the eyes. The binocular relative parallactic angle considered as a stereopsis cue during binocular fixation. Syn., *angle eta*.

a. of strabismus. The objective angle of strabismus, or the subjective angle of strabismus if no anomalous retinal correspondence is present. **objective a. of s.** The angle by which the line of sight or other axis of reference of the deviating eye in strabismus fails to intersect the object of fixation, subtended at the center of rotation of the deviating eye. Usually it is measured by an objective technique such as the corneal reflex method, or by the alternate occlusion test combined with measuring prisms. If measured with an amblyoscope or under infinity testing conditions, it may be considered the angle between the line of sight of the deviating eye and the line of sight of the fixating eye. **residual a. of s.** The angle of deviation remaining after corrective surgery for strabismus. **subjective a. of s.** The angle of separation between the image of the point of fixation as seen by the fixating eye and the image of the point of fixation as seen by the deviating eye, subtended at the center of rotation of the deviating eye; the angle through which dissimilar targets in an amblyoscope must be moved from parallelism for superimposition to occur; the angle through which light to the nonfixating eye is deviated by measuring prisms for superimposition

to occur. As related to the eye, it may be considered to be the angle of separation between the point on the retina of the nonfixating eye stimulated by the image of the point of fixation and the retinal site in the same eye which gives rise to a common visual direction with the fovea of the fixating eye, subtended at the center of rotation.

temporal a. The angle formed by the lids at the outer canthus.

a. of torsion. The dihedral angle between the horizontal meridian of the eye and the plane of regard where they intersect at the line of sight, or line of fixation, depending on how the plane of regard is defined, or for what purpose. **negative a. of t.** The angle of torsion when the horizontal meridian of the eye is displaced counterclockwise with reference to the subject's view. **positive a. of t.** The angle of torsion when the horizontal meridian of the eye is displaced clockwise with reference to the subject's view.

a. of triangulation. Angle of convergence.

a. V of Helmholtz. The angle between the apparent (subjective) vertical meridians of the two eyes.

visual a. The angle subtended by the extremities of an object at the entrance pupil or other point of reference of the eye. Cf. *optic angle*. **limiting v.a.** Minimum separable angle. **minimum v. a.** Minimum separable angle.

wetting a. The fluid-containing angle between the tangent to the surface of a drop of fluid and the tangent to the optical surface on which it rests, as measured at the intersection of the two surfaces. See also *advancing angle; receding angle*. Syn., *contact angle*.

◆

angling. Bending the endpiece of a spectacle frame or mounting to alter the angle between the temple and the plane of the lenses.

anglometer (an'glo-me"ter). An instrument using corneal reflection for measuring the primary and the secondary deviations of strabismus.

angstrom, Angstrom (ang'strum), **Ångström** (ōng'strum) **law; unit.** See under the nouns.

angular gyrus (ang'gu-lar ji'rus). See under *gyrus*.

angulus (ang'gu-lus). Latin for *angle*.

a. iridis. Iridocorneal angle.

a. oculi. Palpebral angle.

anianthinopsy (an″e-an′thi-nop″se). The inability to recognize violet tints.

aniridia (an″ir-id′e-ah, an″i-rid′-). Complete or partial absence of the iris, usually hereditary. Syn., *irideremia.*

aniseikometer (an″is-i-kom′eh-ter). An instrument for the measurement of aniseikonia; usually referred to as an *eikonometer.*

◆

ANISEIKONIA

aniseikonia (an″ih-si-ko′ne-ah). A relative difference in size and/or shape of the ocular images. It may be measured by viewing haploscopically a pair of objects and determining the relative difference in the visual angles which causes the objects to appear equal in size, or equal in distance from the point of binocular fixation.

anatomical a. Aniseikonia due to an anatomical cause, such as unequal distribution of the retinal elements.

anomalous a. Aniseikonia which is clinically significant and which is correctable by clinical means (iseikonic lenses). It is usually referred to simply as aniseikonia, the prefix ''anomalous'' being used to differentiate it from physiological aniseikonia which is due to retinal disparity caused by lateral separation of the eyes.

asymmetrical a. Aniseikonia characterized by a progressive increase or decrease in size across the visual field, as may be produced by a flat prism in front of one eye.

axial a. Aniseikonia due to unequal axial lengths of the two eyes.

crossed-meridional a. Aniseikonia in which the required meridional correction is axis 90° in one eye and axis 180° in the other eye.

induced a. 1. Aniseikonia induced by refractive or size lenses. 2. The stereoscopic effect induced by magnification in the vertical meridian of one eye which corresponds to that which would be produced by magnification in the horizontal meridian of the other eye.

luminance a. Irradiation stereoscopy.

meridional a. Aniseikonia in which there is a symmetrical meridional difference between the size of the ocular images of the two eyes, so that the ocular image in the one meridian is larger or smaller than the corresponding meridian of the other eye.

natural a. Physiological aniseikonia.

optical a. Aniseikonia due to optical (dioptric) factors. **acquired o.a.** Aniseikonia due to the refractive (corrective) lenses worn; their power, position in front of the eyes, curvatures, thicknesses, etc., create the difference in image size. **inherent o.a.** Aniseikonia dependent on the dioptric characteristics of the eyes.

over-all a. Aniseikonia in which the image of one eye is symmetrically larger or smaller than that of the other eye, in all meridians.

over-all-meridional a. A combination of over-all and meridional aniseikonia.

physiological a. The normal relative difference in retinal image size due to image disparities introduced by the lateral separation of the eyes, asymmetrical convergence, or asymmetry of the field of vision. Syn., *natural aniseikonia.*

symmetrical a. Aniseikonia in which the difference in image size is symmetrical, as distinguished from asymmetrical aniseikonia.

◆

anisoastigmatism (an-i″so-ah-stig′-mah-tizm). Compound astigmatic anisometropia.

aniso-accommodation (an-i″so-ah-kom″o-da′shun). Unequal simultaneous accommodation in the two eyes.

anisochromatic (an-i″so-kro-mat′ik). 1. Lacking in uniformity of color; not of the same color throughout. 2. Pertaining to two pigments used for testing color blindness which are distinguished by both the normal and the color-blind eye.

anisochromatopsia (an-i″so-kro″mah-top′se-ah). Deficient color perception affecting only one eye or of an unequal character or severity in the two eyes.

anisochromia (an-i″so-kro′me-ah). Heterochromia iridis.

anisocoria (an-i″so-ko′re-ah). Pupils of unequal diameter; may be physiological, as in antimetropia, or pathological, as in Adie's syndrome or in unilateral Argyll Robertson's pupil.

dynamic a. Unequal pupils during reflex activity; typically pathological.

latent a. of Levatin. Levatin's term for Gunn's pupillary phenomenon as evidenced by the swinging flashlight test.

static a. Unequal pupils during a state of rest; may be physiological or pathological.

anisocycloplegia (an-i″so-si″klo-ple′je-ah). A term used by Beach for a phenomenon of unequal response to cycloplegics by the two eyes.

anisodominance (an″i-so-dom′in-ans). A classification of eye dominance based on the observation that two similar equidistant objects are not seen as equidistant, those seeing the right object nearer being said to be right-eyed and those seeing the left object nearer being said to be left-eyed.

anisohypermetropia (an-i″so-hi″per-me-tro′pe-ah). Compound hypermetropic anisometropia.

anisometrope (an-i″so-met′rōp). One who has anisometropia.

◆

ANISOMETROPIA

anisometropia (an-i″so-me-tro′pe-ah). A condition of unequal refractive state for the two eyes, one eye requiring a different lens correction from the other.

compound astigmatic a. Anisometropia in which both eyes are astigmatic, the degree of astigmatism in one exceeding that of the other. Syn., *anisoastigmatism.*

compound hypermetropic a. Anisometropia in which both eyes are hypermetropic, the degree of hypermetropia of one exceeding that of the other. Syn., *anisohypermetropia.*

compound myopic a. Anisometropia in which both eyes are myopic, the degree of myopia of one exceeding that of the other. Syn., *anisomyopia.*

mixed a. Anisometropia in which one eye is myopic, the other hyperopic, the degree of difference between them being clinically significant. Syn., *antimetropia.*

relative a. Anisometropia in which the total refractive states of each of the two eyes are nearly equal but the components (such as corneal power, axial length, or crystalline lens power) exhibit marked differences.

simple astigmatic a. The presence of astigmatism in one eye but not in the other.

simple hypermetropic a. The presence of hypermetropia in one eye with emmetropia in the other.

simple myopic a. The presence of myopia in one eye with emmetropia in the other.

vertical a. Anisometropia in which there is unequal refraction for the two eyes only in the vertical meridians.

◆

anisometropic (an-i″so-me-trop′ik). Relating to or having anisometropia.

anisomyopia (an-i″so-mi-o′pe-ah). Compound myopic anisometropia.

aniso-oxyopia (an-i″so-ok″se-o′pe-ah). Inequality of acuity of the two eyes fully corrected for ametropia. Cf. *iso-oxyopia.*

anisophoria (an″i-so-fo′re-ah). Heterophoria in which the degree of the phoria varies with the direction of gaze.

essential a. Anisophoria due to paresis or spasm of one or more of the extraocular muscles.

optical a. Anisophoria induced by spectacle correction of anisometropia and caused by the varying prismatic effect as the eyes deviate from the optical axes of the spectacle lenses.

anisopia (an″i-so′pe-ah). Difference of vision of the two eyes.

anisosthenic (an″i-sos-then′ik). Unequal strength of paired muscles.

anisotropic (an″i-so-trop′ik). Doubly refracting; polarizing; birefringent; pertaining to an optical medium in which the index of refraction is not the same for all directions within that medium (not to be confused with inhomogeneous as applied to optical media, for this refers to a difference in index at different points within the medium). An incident ray will be divided within a uniaxial anisotropic medium into two refracted rays, an ordinary ray obeying the usual law of refraction and an extraordinary ray following a different law. A biaxial anisotropic medium produces two extraordinary rays whose wavefronts are more complex than that of the extraordinary ray of the uniaxial medium.

ankyloblepharon (ang″kil-o-blef′ar-on). Partial or total adhesion of the eyelids to each other along their margins. Syn., *blepharocleisis.*

a. adnatum. Congenital ankyloblepharon.

external a. Adhesion of the eyelid margins to each other in the region of the external canthus.

a. filiforme. Ankyloblepharon in which the upper and the lower eyelids are united by filamentous bands.

internal a. Adhesion of the eyelid margins to each other in the region of the internal canthus.

anneal (ă-nēl'). A regulated process of heating materials (glass and metals) and the subsequent slow, controlled cooling to eliminate strains.

annexa oculi (ă-nek'sah ok'u-li). Adnexa oculi.

annulus ciliaris (an'u-lus sil"e-ar'is). The superficial portion of the ciliary body between the iris and the choroid. Syn., *ciliary ring*.

annulus conjunctivae (an'u-lus kon-junk'tih-ve). The dense, raised, limbal conjunctiva where the bulbar conjunctiva approaches the corneoscleral junction. Syn., *conjunctival ring*.

annulus iridis major (an'u-lus i'rid-is ma'jor). A circle composed of anastomosing arteries derived from two long posterior ciliary and seven anterior ciliary arteries, located in the ciliary body about the root of the iris. Syn., *greater arterial circle of the iris; circulus arteriosus iridis major*.

annulus iridis minor (an'u-lus i'rid-is mi'nor). A vascular circle containing both arteries and veins located at the junction of ciliary and pupillary portions of the iris. Branches from the major circle anastomose to form most of the circle. Syn., *lesser arterial circle of the iris; minor vascular circle; circulus arteriosus iridis minor*.

annulus tendineus communis (an'-u-lus ten-din'e-us kom-u'nis). Annulus of Zinn.

annulus tendinosus (an'u-lus ten"dih-no'sus). 1. A rarely used term for the peripheral rim of Descemet's membrane near the limbus. 2. The annular ligament, a term also rarely used for the scleral spur.

annulus of Zinn (an'u-lus). The common tendon of the rectus group of muscles that, as a fibrous cone, surrounds the optic foramen and a portion of the superior orbital fissure, to the anterior margin of which it is attached at the spina recti lateralis. Syn., *annulus tendineus communis; ligament of Zinn; tendon of Zinn*.

anodynes, ophthalmic (an'o-dīnz). Ocular analgesics.

anomalopia (ă-nom"ah-lo'pe-ah). Anomalous color vision.

anomaloscope (ă-nom'ah-lo-skōp"). An instrument to test the color sense. It usually consists of a viewing tube with a circular bipartite field, one half of which is illuminated with yellow, the other with a mixture of green and red. The yellow half is not variable except for brightness, while the other may be varied continuously from red to green. The color sense is tested by mixing the colors of the variable color field until it subjectively matches the yellow field. A certain combination in the variable field is considered normal, and specific variations indicate the type or the degree of anomalous color vision present.

anomalous (ă-nom'ah-lus). Deviating from the usual; existing in an abnormal location, form, or structure; functioning in an abnormal manner.

anomalous (ă-nom'ah-lus). **retinal correspondence; deuteranopia; dichromatism; projection; trichromatism.** See under the nouns.

anomaly (ă-nom'ah-le). A deviation from the usual or norm.

Axenfeld's a. Axenfeld's syndrome.

Peter's a. A congenital developmental anomaly of the anterior segment of the eyeball characterized by a central corneal stromal opacity usually associated with a defect in the posterior stroma and Descemet's membrane and anterior synechiae which extend from the iris to the periphery of the corneal opacity. Glaucoma is frequently associated and less frequently congenital cataract and sometimes microphthalmus.

Rieger's a. Rieger's disease.

anomia (ă-no'me-ah). Loss of ability to recognize names or to name objects. Syn., *nominal aphasia; dysnomia*.

anomoscope, Brock's (ă-nom'o-skōp). An instrument for differentiating anomalous and normal binocular projection.

anoopsia (an"o-op'se-ah). Hypertropia.

anophoria (an"o-fo're-ah). Anaphoria.

anophthalmia (an"of-thal'me-ah). Absence of an eye or eyes in the newborn, due to failure of development of the optic cup or to disappearance of the eyes after partial development. Most clinical cases actually represent extreme microphthalmia and rudimentary extrinsic muscles usually are present. Syn., *anophthalmos; anophthalmus.*

consecutive a. Anophthalmia resulting from atrophy or degeneration of the optic vesicle subsequent to its initial formation.

a. cyclopica. A condition in which the eye and the orbital contents are imperfectly developed.

primary a. Anophthalmia resulting from suppression of the optic primordium during the differentiation of the optic plate and after the formation of the rudiment of the forebrain. It tends to be bilateral and usually occurs without other deformities.

secondary a. Anophthalmia secondary to complete suppression or grossly abnormal development of the entire anterior portion of the neural tube. It is usually accompanied by numerous other abnormalities and therefore usually occurs in a nonviable monster.

unilateral a. Monophthalmia.

anophthalmos (an"of-thal'mos). Anophthalmia.

anophthalmus (an"of-thal'mus). Anophthalmia.

anopia (an-o'pe-ah). 1. Absence of the eye. 2. A rudimentary condition of the eye.

anopsia (an-op'se-ah). A defect or loss of vision from failure to use the visual capacity; differentiated from *anoopsia.*

quadrantic a. Lost or reduced vision in a quarter sector of the visual field of one eye. Syn., *quadrantanopsia.*

anopsis (an-op'sis). Blindness.

anorthopia (an"or-tho'pe-ah). 1. A perceptual anomaly in which objects appear distorted, straight lines do not appear straight, etc. 2. Strabismus. *Rare.*

anorthoscope (an-or'tho-skōp). An apparatus for producing a specific illusion, consisting of a distorted picture on a rotating disk which is seen as not distorted when viewed through a second slotted disk rotating at a different speed.

anosognosia (an-o"sog-no'se-ah, an-o"so-). Inability to recognize loss of function, disease, or defect in a part of one's own body.

visual a. The inability to recognize the partial or total loss of one's own

visual acuity, or the partial loss of one's own visual field.

anotropia (an"o-tro'pe-ah). Anatropia.

ANSI. See *American National Standards Institute, Inc.*

antagonism. The mutually opposing action between two forces, as in the paired extrinsic muscles of the eye.

antagonist. A muscle having opposite primary action to that of another; an opposing muscle. Ex.: The right medial rectus is the antagonist of the right lateral rectus.

contralateral a. A rarely used term indicating a muscle in the fellow eye which acts as an antagonist to the yoke muscle of the other eye. Ex.: The right superior rectus muscle is the contralateral antagonist of the left superior oblique.

anterior. In man, ventral; nearer to the front; the opposite of *posterior.*

anthelion. A rarely observed concentration of diffuse colorless light in cirrus clouds opposite the sun and at the same elevation but never higher than 46°.

antimetropia (an"tih-met-ro'pe-ah). Mixed anisometropia.

antimydriatic (an"tih-mid"re-at'ik). An agent or a drug which prevents dilatation of the pupil or reduces dilation.

antinode (an'tih-nōd). That point of a wave motion at which the particles undergo maximum displacement. It is midway between two adjacent nodes.

antirheoscope (an"tih-re'o-skōp). An apparatus for producing a specific illusion, consisting of a board perpendicular to the line of sight covered with a pattern (usually horizontal stripes) and an endless belt of the same pattern which is seen moving vertically through a window in the board. When the real motion ceases, there is an illusion of movement in the opposite direction (the *waterfall illusion*).

antixerophthalmic (an"tih-ze"rof-thal'mik). Preventive of xerophthalmia, as vitamin A.

Anton's (an'tonz) **symptom; syndrome.** See under the nouns.

antophthalmic (ant"of-thal'mik). Relieving ophthalmia.

antorbital (ant-ōr'bih-tal). Anterior to, or in front of, the orbit.

antrophose (an'tro-fōz). A subjective sensation of light or color originating in the visual centers of the brain.

AOA. See *American Optometric Associa-*

tion; Australian Optometrical Association; American Osteopathic Association.

AOE. See *Optometric Editors Association.*

AOF. See *American Optometric Foundation.*

AOP. See *Association of Optical Practitioners.*

AOS. See *American Ophthalmological Society.*

AOSA. See *American Optometric Student Association.*

apanastema (a″pan-as′te-mah). A wart-like protuberance on the conjunctiva.

Apert's syndrome (a′pertz). Acrocephalosyndactyly.

apertometer (ap″er-tom′eh-ter). An instrument which measures the numerical aperture of an objective.

apertor oculi (ap′er-tōr ok′u-li). Levator palpebrae superioris muscle.

aperture (ap′er-tūr). An opening or hole which admits light.

angular a. The extreme angle between incident rays traversing an optical system.

clear a. The aperture at the entrance of an optical system.

effective a. That part of the aperture of a lens actually used by the bundle of rays contributing to the formation of an image.

numerical a. An expression designating the light-gathering power of microscope objectives; the product of the index of refraction of the object space and the sine of the half-angle of the incident cone.

objective a. Clear aperture.

palpebral a. The opening formed by the margins of the eyelids.

relative a. The ratio of the diameter of the entrance pupil to the primary focal length of an optical system; the reciprocal of the f-number. Syn., *aperture ratio.*

aperture-stop. The stop of an optical system which, by virtue of its size and position with respect to the radiating object, is effective in limiting the bundle of light rays traversing the system.

apex. 1. The vertex of an angle, a cone, or a pyramid. 2. The extreme point of any anatomical structure resembling an angle, a cone, or a pyramid; or the extreme point of any anatomical structure being in any respect a spheroid, a conoid, an ellipsoid, or a combination thereof.

corneal a. The point of the cornea which is most anterior when the eye is in a straightforward or primary position.

a. of prism. 1. The end of a prism at which the two faces intersect. 2. The direction along the base-apex line of a prism opposite the base, or the same direction along the base-apex line as the apparent displacement of the image.

APHA. See *American Public Health Association.*

aphacia (ă-fa′se-ah, -she-ah). Aphakia.

aphakia (ă-fa′ke-ah). 1. Absence of the crystalline lens of the eye; due most frequently to surgical removal, occasionally to a perforating wound or ulcer, rarely to a congenital anomaly. 2. Absence of the lens from the pupillary area, as in dislocation or luxation of the lens.

primary a. Congenital absence of the crystalline lens due to failure of development, usually in association with other congenital ocular abnormalities.

secondary a. Congenital absence of the crystalline lens, partial or complete, due to degeneration or extrusion of a previously formed lens. In the case of degeneration, the lens substance may be absorbed, leaving remnants of the capsule and fibrous tissue to form a membranous cataract (*pseudoaphakia*) or it may be invaded by vascularized mesodermal tissue (*pseudophakia*).

aphakic (ă-fa′kik). One who has aphakia. Pertaining to or having aphakia.

aphasia (ă-fa′ze-ah). The inability, because of a disturbance in the cerebral mechanism, (1) to express oneself in speech or in writing, (2) to comprehend either the spoken or the written word, or (3) to do any combination of these.

motor a. The inability to express oneself in speech or in writing.

nominal a. Anomia.

optic a. Alexia.

semantic a. The inability to appreciate or to give an account of the general significance of what is heard or read, although the meaning of individual words or sentences is understood.

sensory a. The inability to comprehend written or spoken words, or gestures, or any combination of these.

visual a. Alexia.

Wernicke's a. Sensory aphasia in which the comprehension of written and spoken words is lost, although articulation is retained.

word a. Alexia.

aphose (ă-fōz', a'fōz, af'ōz). A subjective shadow or dark spot in the visual field.

aphytria retinae (ă-fit're-ah ret'ih-ne). A condition in which there is a loss of retinal pigment. *Rare.*

aplanasia (ap"lah-na'ze-ah). Absence of spherical aberration and coma in an optical system. Syn., *aplanatism.*

aplanatic (ap"lah-nat'ik). Pertaining to an optical system free from spherical aberration and coma.

aplanatism (ă-plan'ah-tizm). Aplanasia.

aplasia, retinal (ă-pla'se-ah). See *dysplasia, retinal.*

APOB. See *Association Professionnelle des Opticiens de Belgique.*

apochromatic (ap"o-kro-mat'ik). A lens design or condition in which maximum correction has been attained for the spherical aberration of a maximum number of wavelengths.

apodization (ap'o-dih-za"shun). The process of reducing the intensity of, or eliminating the peripheral portions of, a diffraction pattern as may be accomplished by suitably shaped apertures or apertures with nonuniform absorption.

Apollonio lens (ap"ŏ-lo'ne-o). See under *lens.*

aponeurosis (ap"o-nu-ro'sis, a-pon"u-). A tendinous expansion consisting of a fibrous or membranous sheath which serves as a fascia to enclose or bind a group of muscles, or as a means of attachment for muscles at their origin or insertion.

lid a. Septum orbitale.

a. orbito-ocularis. Tenon's capsule.

apoplexy, corneal (ap'o-plek"se). Migration of blood into the cornea.

apoplexy, retinal. Copious hemorrhage into the retina.

apostilb (ă-post'ilb). A unit of luminance equal to $1/10$ millilambert. See also *footlambert.*

apparatus (ap"ah-ra'tus, -rat'us). 1. A system or group of organs, or parts of organs, which collectively perform a common function. 2. A collection of instruments, devices, or implements used for a given work, as an experiment or an operation.

accessory sense a. Those parts of a sense organ, other than the afferent nerve and the receptor cells, which are essential for the functioning of the organ. In the eye, this would include all structures other than the optic nerve and the rods and cones of the retina.

accommodative a. The structures of the eye which are related to accommodation; the ciliary apparatus and the crystalline lens.

ciliary a. The ciliary muscle and processes; the structures other than the crystalline lens which are related to accommodation; the ciliary body.

lacrimal a. The tear-forming and tear-conducting system, composed of lacrimal and accessory lacrimal glands, eyelid margins, conjunctival sac, lacrimal lake, lacrimal puncta, canaliculi or lacrimal ducts, common canaliculus or sinus of Maier, lacrimal sac, nasolacrimal duct, and Hasner's valve at the inferior meatus of the nose.

muscular a. The intraocular and the extraocular musculature of the eye considered collectively. See under *muscle* for the specific muscles involved.

nervous a. The sensory and the motor nerves of the eye and the orbit considered collectively. See under *nerve* for the specific nerves involved.

refractive a. Cornea, aqueous humor, crystalline lens, and vitreous humor considered collectively; the surfaces and the media traversed by light entering the eye and involved in the production of the retinal image.

visual a. The two eyes, their extrinsic muscles and other contents of the orbits, the nerves, the pathways, and the visual cortex, considered collectively. Syn., *visuum.*

apparent. 1. As perceived, or pertaining to the visual percept or mental impression of a visible attribute of a viewed object or pattern. 2. In several optical usages: Pertaining to physically measureable dimensions or attributes of a viewed object or pattern or of its optical image, not necessarily identical to the correspondingly perceived or sensed characteristics.

apparent candlepower; contrast; footcandle; height; luminance; magnification; magnitude; movement; position; pupil; size; strabismus. See under the nouns.

apparition (ap"ah-rish'un). 1. A supernatural visual manifestation. 2. A visual hallucination.

appearance. 1. The distinctive characteristics or features of an object or an individual as noted by visual observation. 2. The originating of an experience, particularly visual. 3. An incorrect visual or other impression.

appendages of the eye (ă-pen'dih-jez). The accessory structures or adnexa of the eye, including the lacrimal apparatus, the conjunctiva, the cilia, the supercilia, the eyelids, and sometimes the extraocular muscles.

apperception (ap"er-sep'shun). The action of past experience upon received sensory stimuli, resulting in individual differences of interpretation of the same sensory stimuli.

applanatio corneae (ap"lah-na'she-o kōr'ne-e). A flattened cornea due to degenerative changes.

applanation (ap"lah-na'shun). An abnormal flattening of a convex surface, especially of the cornea or the crystalline lens.

apraxia (a-prak'se-ah, ă-prak'-). The inability to accomplish an intended or purposeful movement, the nature of which is understood, in the absence of motor paralysis, sensory loss, or ataxia.

constructional a. Apraxia in which there is an inability to arrange objects into a desired pattern or formation.

ocular motor a. Apraxia in which there is an inability to perform intended or purposeful ocular movements.

optical a. Apraxia in which there is an inability to copy or spontaneously draw diagrams or drawings in their proper spatial orientation.

visual a. Optical apraxia.

aprosopia (ap"ro-so'pe-ah). Congenital absence of the eyelids in the newborn, usually occurring with other facial defects.

aqua oculi (ah'kwah, a'kwah ok'u-li). Aqueous humor.

aqueduct of Sylvius. A canal in the midbrain connecting the third and the fourth ventricles and containing cerebrospinal fluid. Syn., *cerebral aqueduct.*

aqueous (a'kwe-us, ak'we-) **chamber; flare; humor.** See under the nouns.

aquocapsulitis (a"kwo-kap"su-li'tis). Serous iritis.

arachnitis, chiasmal (ar"ak-ni'tis). Chiasmal arachnoiditis.

arachnodactyly (ă-rak"no-dak'til-e). 1. A hereditary, familial condition characterized by extreme length and thinness of bones. Syn., *dolichostenomelia; dystrophia mesodermalis congenita hypoplastica.* 2. Marfan's syndrome.

arachnoid (ă-rak'noid). The central, weblike member of the three meninges covering the brain, the spinal cord, and the optic nerve. It is separated from the pia mater by the subarachnoid space, but follows it into all of its folds, and is separated from the dura mater by the subdural space. From the optic nerve it becomes continuous with the sclera.

arachnoiditis, chiasmal (ă-rak"noidi'tis). A localized inflammation at the base of the brain affecting the chiasma, the optic nerve, and the meninges surrounding them, and leading to a rapid loss of visual acuity and to primary optic nerve atrophy. Syn., *chiasmal arachnitis.*

Arago's spot (ar'ah-gōz). See under *spot.*

ARC. Abbreviation for *anomalous retinal correspondence.*

arc. A portion of a curved line, as that of a circle or an ellipse.

blue a's. An entoptic phenomenon elicited by a spot of light stimulating the temporal parafoveal area. The subjective sensation is of two bands of blue light arching from above and below the light toward the blind spot.

a. centune. The angle subtended by 1 cm of arc whose radius is 1 m. Designated by the symbol ∇. Syn., *centrad.*

a. of contact. That portion of an extrinsic muscle in actual contact with the surface of the eyeball, continually changing as the eye rotates.

epithelial a. The fluorescein pattern of an epithelial imprint resulting from, for example, the removing of a small diameter, steeply fitted contact lens.

a. of uncertainty. The angular range of uncertainty of a person in perceiving the gravitational or true vertical when he is tilted.

visual reflex a. The complete anatomical pathway from the retinal receptors, including a centripetal pathway to the lower visual centers and to the cortex, the cortex itself, and a centrifugal pathway to the intrinsic and the extrinsic muscles of the eye and to the skeletal muscles of the body. See also *visual reflex.*

arcade. An anatomical structure composed of a series of arches, usually of blood vessels.

arterial a's., marginal. A group of anastomosing arteries at the margins of both the upper and the lower eyelids which supplies the lids and the conjunctiva. Syn., *tarsal arches.*

arterial a's., peripheral. A group of anastomosing arteries in the upper border of the tarsus of the upper eyelid (sometimes present in the lower eyelid), supplying the eyelid and the conjunctiva.

temporal a., superior. The supraorbital arch.

arch. An anatomical structure having a curved or bowlike shape.

orbital a. Supraorbital arch.

Salus' a. An arch in a retinal venule, above or below a sclerosed arteriole, due to deflection from its normal course by the arteriole. Syn., *Salus' sign.*

supraorbital a. The portion of the frontal bone forming the superior margin of the orbit. Syn., *superior temporal arcade; orbital arch; supraorbital margin.*

tarsal a's. Marginal arterial arcades.

Archambault's loop (ahr″shahm-bōz′). Meyer's loop.

ARCO. See *American Research Council of Optometry.*

arcus (ahr′kus). An arch or an archlike structure.

a. arteriosus palpebrae. Marginal arterial arcades. *Rare.*

a. corneae. A white ring opacity in the periphery of the cornea due to a lipoid infiltration of the corneal stroma. See also *arcus juvenilis* and *arcus senilis.*

a. juvenilis. A white ring opacity in the periphery of the cornea, occurring in early or middle life, due to a lipoid infiltration of the corneal stroma; distinguished from arcus senilis, which occurs in later life. Syn., *anterior embryotoxon; arcus pre-senilis.*

a. lipoides. Any ring opacity in the periphery of the cornea due to a lipoid infiltration of the stroma, such as *arcus juvenilis* or *arcus senilis.*

a. marginale. A thickening of the periorbita at the orbital margin to which the orbital septum is attached.

a. marginalis. Arcus senilis.

a. pinguiculus. Arcus senilis.

a. pre-senilis. Arcus juvenilis.

a. senilis. A grayish-white ring opacity in the periphery of the cornea, occurring in the aged, due to a lipoid infiltration of the corneal stroma. It is separated from the limbus by a zone of clear cornea (lucid interval of Vogt). Syn., *arcus marginalis; arcus pinguiculus; gerontoxon.*

a. senilis lentis. A white ring opacity near the equator of the crystalline lens which sometimes occurs in the aged.

a. superciliaris. The superciliary ridge or arch on the frontal bone above the orbit. Syn., *supraorbital ridge.*

a. tarseus. Marginal arterial arcade.

Arden (ahr′den) **grating; index.** See under the nouns.

◆

AREA

area. 1. A limited space or extent of surface; a region. 2. A portion of the brain or the retina regarded as having a particular function.

anomalous associated a. In a strabismic with anomalous retinal correspondence, the peripheral retinal area in the one eye which corresponds in visual direction with the fovea of the other eye.

a. of attraction to fusion. The area in a graphical representation of retinal disparity within which adequate or inadequate fusional movements of the eyes can be elicited in response to a given pair of disparate retinal stimuli; considered by some to bear a relationship to Panum's area and to stereopsis.

a. B17. Brodmann's area 17.

a. B18. Brodmann's area 18.

a. B19. Brodmann's area 19.

Brodmann's a's. Specific histological areas of the cerebral cortex located by Brodmann and numbered from 1 to over 44. Neurologists have found functional significance for each of these areas. Others, such as Vogt and von Economo, also numbered cortical areas, but they do not correspond to Brodmann's **B.a. 3, 1, 2.** The somesthetic or general sensory receptive area located in the parietal cortex, just posterior to the fissure of Rolando, and extending from the longitudinal sulcus to the Sylvian fissure. **B.a. 6, alpha.** The region of the cerebral cortex used for voluntary mass movements of skeletal muscles, located between areas 4 and 8 in the posterior part of the frontal lobe. Also called the *precentral motor cortex* or *area 6*. **B.a. 6 alpha beta.** The region of the cerebral cortex that controls the rotation of the head, the trunk, and the eyes to the opposite side, located in the posterior part of the frontal lobe, superior to the frontal eye fields in the superior frontal gyrus. Syn., *frontal adversive field*. **B.a. 8, alpha beta delta.** The region of the cerebral cortex that controls voluntary conjugate movements of the eyes and affects the eyelids, the pupils, and the lacrimal glands; the frontal eye fields located in the posterior portion of both middle frontal convolutions in the premotor cortex. Also called *area 8, alpha beta*. **B.a. 8, gamma.** The region of the cerebral cortex that affects the opening and the closing of the eyelids and inhibits mastication activity initiated by the motor cortex in the precentral gyrus, located in the posterior portion of the inferior gyrus, inferior to the frontal eye fields. **B.a. 17.** The area striata on either side of the calcarine fissure, in the occipital lobe of each cerebral cortex. **B.a. 18.** The parastriate area; the visual association area closely surrounding the area striata and located in the cuneus and the lingual gyrus of each occipital lobe. **B.a. 19.** The peristriate area; the visual association area immediately surrounding the parastriate area in each occipital lobe.

a. caeca. Blind spot of Marriotte.

calcarine a. Brodmann's area 17 in the occipital lobe in and about the calcarine fissure. Syn., *area striata*.

a. centralis. 1. The portion of the retina with the greatest number of visual cells per unit area and with a more restricted hookup with ganglion cells. It is located just temporal to the optic disk, is about 6 mm in diameter, and, according to Polyak, includes the fovea centralis and the parafoveal and the perifoveal regions. 2. The portion of the retina called the *macula lutea*, which contains a yellow pigment and has a diameter of about 5 mm; the retina minus the periphery and the optic disk. 3. According to Chievitz, the region of the

retina characterized by the fibers of Henle in the external molecular layer and by a rich number of ganglion cells. This roughly agrees with Polyak. (Until some compromises are made, a general disagreement exists as to size and restrictions of its included parts.)

a. of comfort. Percival's term for the middle third of the range of relative convergence. For example, if, for a fixation distance of 40 cm, the base-out limit of relative convergence is 15 prism diopters and the base-in limit is 15 prism diopters, the total range is 30 prism diopters. The area of comfort then extends from 5 prism diopters base-out to 5 prism diopters base-in. If the convergence stimulus or demand falls within this range, comfort in convergence performance can be anticipated.

cone-pure a. Rod-free area.

a. of confusion. An area of the visual field specified with reference to one eye, occurring especially in strabismus, in which objects are inaccurately or improperly localized.

a. of critical definition. 1. The central portion of the visual field in which objects appear clearly defined. 2. That portion of any optical image in which detail is clearly defined.

dangerous a. The ciliary region of the eye, so called because the most serious results may follow injury to this area.

a. eight alpha beta delta. See *Brodmann's area 8, alpha beta delta*.

a. eight gamma. See *Brodmann's area 8, gamma*.

eye a. The frontal eye fields in the frontal lobes; the midportion of area 8 for voluntary conjugate movements of the eyes.

fusion a. Panum's area.

light a. 1. The entire illuminated area of the retinal image, whether of liminal or subliminal value. 2. The portion of the pupil illuminated by the retinoscopic reflex.

macular a. That portion of the retina containing a yellow pigment and including the rod-free area. Roughly, the portion of the retina that is used for central vision and that appears free of visible vessels when viewed with an ophthalmoscope. It is the part that contains Henle's oblique fibers.

a. of Martegiani. The slightly dilated, posterior segment of the hyaloid canal in the vitreous humor at the optic disk.

mirror a. The reflecting surface of the crystalline lens and the cornea when viewed with the slit lamp.

opticomotor a. Portions of the cerebral cortex which affect the movements of the eyeballs. The voluntary opticomotor area is the frontal eye field located in each frontal cortex in the back of the middle frontal convolution. Also called *Brodmann's area 8, alpha beta delta.* The involuntary opticomotor area is the occipital eye field located in each occipital cortex, possibly in the peristriate or the parastriate area.

Panum's a. An area in the retina of one eye, any point of which, when stimulated simultaneously with a single specific point in the retina of the other eye, will give rise to a single fused percept. Syn., *fusion area; corresponding retinal area.*

parastriate a. Brodmann's area 18, a visual association area in each occipital lobe.

peristriate a. Brodmann's area 19, a visual association area surrounding area 18 in each occipital lobe.

psycho-optic a. Brodmann's areas 18 and 19 in each occipital lobe. Syn., *visual association areas.*

retinal a's., corresponding. 1. A pair of areas, one in each retina, which, when stimulated, gives rise to a percept of common visual direction. 2. Panum's areas.

rod-free a. The central portion of the fovea centralis, about 0.25 mm to 0.5 mm in diameter, containing only cone cells. Syn., *cone-pure area.*

a. of sensitivity. That portion of the retinal image in which the intensity of illumination attains liminal or supraliminal value.

a. six alpha. Brodmann's area 6, alpha.

a. six alpha beta. Brodmann's area 6, alpha beta.

a. striata. Brodmann's area 17 in each occipital lobe, identified by the presence of the line of Gennari. Syn., *calcarine area; visual area; visual projection area; visuosensory area.*

suppression a. An area in the binocular field of vision in which the ocular image from one eye is not perceived in consciousness. This can be plotted in stereocampimetry and des-

ignated as a scotoma of one eye for a certain size target, when binocular vision is stimulated. The scotoma must be shown to be absent when the field of either eye is plotted separately.

a. three, one, two. Brodmann's area 3, 1, 2.

visual a. 1. Striate area. 2. Loosely, all parts of the occipital lobe and the angular gyrus related to visual function.

visual association a's. The parastriate and the peristriate areas, respectively numbered Brodmann's areas 18 and 19, in the occipital lobes that assist in interpreting the impulses received by area 17, the visual area. Syn., *psycho-optic areas; visuopsychic areas.*

visual projection a. Striate area.

visuopsychic a's. Visual association areas.

visuosensory a. Striate area.

Vogt's a. 8. A strip of cortex anterior to the precentral gyrus in the frontal lobe, containing in its central portion the frontal eye fields for voluntary conjugate eye movements. It also has suppressor action.

◆

areola (ă-re′o-lah). 1. The part of the iris surrounding the pupil of the eye. 2. Any interstice or minute space in a tissue.

argamblyopia (ahr-gam″ble-o′pe-ah, ahr″gam-). Amblyopia ex anopsia.

argema (ahr′je-mah). A white ulcer of the cornea.

Argyll Robertson's (ahr′gĭl rob′ert-sonz) **pupil; reflex; sign.** See under the nouns.

argyrosis oculi (ahr″jir-o′sis ok′u-li). Dusky gray or bluish pigmentation of the conjunctival and the corneal tissues, caused by granular deposition of silver from the prolonged use of preparations containing silver compounds.

Arlt's (ahrltz) **line; sign; sinus; theory; trachoma; triangle.** See under the nouns.

arm, guard. That part or extension of a spectacle frame or mounting that connects the guard to the bridge or the front. Syn., *pad arm.*

arm, lens. A portion of a rimless or semirimless mounting, extending along the back upper edge of the lens from the endpiece to the strap.

arm, pad. Guard arm.

Armorlite (arm'or-līt). A trade name for hard resin lenses, made by casting pure, thermoset allyl diglycol carbonate.

Arneson Korector (ahrn'eh-sun). See under *Korector*.

Arnold's (ahr'nuldz) **fold; foramen; notch.** See under the nouns.

Arnold-Chiari syndrome (arn'ōld-ke-ar'e). See under *syndrome*.

Arnold-Pick syndrome (ahr'nuld-pik). See under *syndrome*.

Arroyo's sign (ar-roi'yōz). See under *sign*.

Arruga's implant (ă-ru'gaz). See under *implant*.

arteriography, orbital. A radiological technique for studying the orbital vasculature following the intravenous injection of a radiopaque dye.

arteriolosclerosis (ahr-te″re-o″lo-skle-ro'sis). Thickening and loss of elasticity and contractility of the walls of arterioles, as manifested in the branches of the central retinal artery by increased tortuosity, a copper wire reflex, and A-V crossing defects.

arteriosclerosis (ahr-te″re-o-skle-ro'sis). Thickening and loss of elasticity and contractility of the wall of an artery. A fibrous overgrowth, mainly of the inner coat of an artery, and degenerative change of the middle coat, usually associated with old age.

arteritis, brachycephalic (ar″teh-ri'tis). Pulseless disease.

arteritis, giant cell. Temporal arteritis.

arteritis, temporal (ar″teh-ri'tis). A self-limiting disease of undetermined etiology occurring after the age of 55, in which there is widespread inflammation of the arteries, particularly the temporal arteries. Symptoms include malaise, fever, weight loss, severe headache, tinnitus, deafness, arthralgia, myalgia, and neuralgia. Vision may be mildly or severely impaired as a result of occlusion of the central retinal artery or one of its branches, and other ocular symptoms include ischemic papilledema or retrobulbar neuritis, ophthalmoplegia, pain behind the eye, and retinal hemorrhage. Syn., *giant cell arteritis*.

◆

ARTERY

artery (ahr'ter-e). A tubular vessel which conveys blood from the heart to the various parts of the body. Typically, its wall is composed of an outer fibrous and elastic coat (tunica adventitia), a middle muscular coat (tunica media), and an inner coat (tunica intima) of fibrous and elastic tissue lined with endothelium.

angular a. The terminal branch of the external maxillary artery located between the nose and the eye or the cheek, supplying eyelids, lacrimal sac, orbicularis oculi, and neighboring skin.

annular a. Annular vessel.

basilar a. A vessel formed by the union of paired vertebral arteries located on the ventral surface of the pons. Its terminal branches, the posterior cerebral arteries, enter the arterial circle of Willis.

calcarine a. A branch of the posterior cerebral artery found within the calcarine fissure. It supplies the optic radiations and the visual cortex together with the middle cerebral artery with which it forms an important anastomosis to allow for sparing of the macula from circulatory disturbances to the visual cortex.

carotid a., internal. An important branch of the common carotid artery that travels through the cavernous sinus. After giving rise to the ophthalmic artery, it terminates in the anterior and the middle cerebral arteries.

central a. of optic nerve. A branch of the central retinal artery originating in the optic nerve and giving rise to an anterior branch which accompanies the central retinal artery and a posterior branch which is recurrent.

central retinal a. A direct or indirect branch of the ophthalmic artery which courses below the optic nerve, entering the center of the nerve and supplying it. In the vicinity of the optic disk it divides into superior and inferior branches, the nasal and the temporal branches of which course in the nerve fiber layer to supply capillaries feeding the bipolar and the ganglion cell layers of the retina. Except for a tiny anastomosis with the circle of Zinn or Haller, it is an end artery. **collateral c.r.a.'s** Branches of the central retinal artery which originate within the optic nerve.

cerebral a., anterior. The terminal branch of the internal carotid artery distributed to cerebral hemispheres and basal ganglia. The left and the right arteries are connected by an anterior communicating artery to help form a portion of the arterial circle of Willis.

cerebral a., middle. A terminal branch of the internal carotid artery which supplies the lateral portion of the cortex, the optic chiasm, the optic tract, and the optic radiations. The macular portion of the visual cortex is supplied by it and the calcarine artery, central vision often being spared due to this double blood supply.

cerebral a's., posterior. Terminal branches of the basilar artery which, by the posterior communicating artery, connect with the internal carotid arteries, forming part of the circle of Willis. They supply parts of the forebrain and the midbrain, and the calcarine branch supplies the posterior portion of the visual pathway.

chiasmal a., central. A median branch of the anterior communicating artery that, together with the pre-chiasmal plexus from the anterior cerebral arteries, supplies the anterior optic chiasm.

chiasmal a., inferior. A medial branch of the internal carotid artery which supplies the inferior, lateral portion of the optic chiasm. Syn., *lateral chiasmal artery.*

chiasmal a., lateral. Inferior chiasmal artery.

chiasmal a., superior. A branch of the anterior cerebral artery which supplies the superior, anterior portion of the optic chiasm.

choroidal a., anterior. A branch of the internal carotid artery supplying the basal ganglia, the choroid plexus of the lateral ventricle, the lateral geniculate body, the chiasm, the optic tract, and the optic radiations.

choroidal a., posterior. A branch of the posterior cerebral artery to the choroid plexus of the third ventricle.

choroidal a., recurrent. Any of over a dozen branches of the major arterial circle of the iris, the anterior ciliary arteries, and the long posterior ciliary arteries, which supply the choriocapillaris from the ora serrata to the equator of the eye.

ciliary a's., anterior. Seven branches of the muscular arteries of the rectus muscles. They help form the major arterial circle of the iris, give off anterior conjunctival and episcleral arteries, and enter the eyeball at the anterior scleral apertures.

ciliary a., common. The embryological branch of the internal ophthalmic artery of an 18 mm embryo.

ciliary a., nasal. An artery in an 18 mm embryo which anastomoses with the common ciliary and helps form the nasal of the two long posterior ciliary arteries in the developed eye.

ciliary a's., posterior. Branches of the ophthalmic artery which yield the long and the short posterior ciliary arteries. **long p.c.a's.** Typically, two branches of the posterior ciliary artery or the ophthalmic artery which pierce the posterior sclera and course in the perichoroidal space. They supply the ciliary body and help form the major arterial circle of the iris. **short p.c.a's.** Approximately 12 branches of the two posterior ciliary arteries or of the ophthalmic artery which pierce the posterior sclera to supply the choriocapillaris, the optic disk, the circle of Zinn (Haller), the cilioretinal artery, and the episcleral artery.

ciliary a., temporal. An artery in an 18 mm embryo which becomes the temporal of the two long posterior ciliary arteries in the developed eye.

cilioretinal a. A branch of the circle of Zinn or Haller around the optic nerve, posterior to the optic disk. It leaves the temporal side of the disk and supplies the bipolar and the ganglion cells between the macula and the disk. With this artery, cessation of circulation in the central retinal capillaries does not affect central vision. Roughly one fifth, or less, of human eyes possess one.

communicating a., anterior. An anterior unpaired artery of the circle of Willis that connects the anterior cerebral arteries and gives rise to the central chiasmal artery.

communicating a., posterior. A part of the circle of Willis that connects the internal carotid artery with the posterior cerebral artery of the same side.

conjunctival a's., anterior. Branches of the anterior ciliary artery or episcleral branch which supply the bulbar conjunctiva in the limbal area and do not move with the conjunctiva. They are involved in ciliary injection.

conjunctival a's., posterior.
Ascending branches of the peripheral or marginal arcades formed by the palpebral artery. At the fornix they become the posterior conjunctival arteries of the bulbar conjunctiva.

copper wire a. A retinal artery exhibiting an increased brightness of the reflex, such that it resembles copper wire; a sign of sclerosis. Cf. *silver wire artery.*

episcleral a's. Branches of the anterior ciliary and the short posterior ciliary arteries which supply the outer layer of the sclera.

ethmoidal a., anterior. A branch of the ophthalmic artery that leaves the orbit through the anterior ethmoidal foramen to supply the ethmoidal air cells, the nasal cavity, the skin of the nose, and the frontal sinus.

ethmoidal a., posterior. A branch of the ophthalmic artery that leaves the orbit by the posterior ethmoidal foramen to supply the ethmoidal air cells, the dura mater, and the upper nasal cavity.

frontal a. The terminal branch of the ophthalmic artery which supplies the skin, the muscles, and the pericranium of the forehead.

Heubner's a. The recurrent branch of the anterior cerebral artery which supplies the anterior limb of the internal capsule. When obstructed, the frontopontine tract degenerates and, rarely, the contralateral eyebrow cannot be lowered (frontal muscle) and the eyelids cannot be completely closed for a few days. Contralateral paralyses occur in the face below the eye, in the tongue, and in the arm.

hyaloid a. The fetal branch of the ophthalmic artery which divides in the vitreous humor and supplies the crystalline lens. It buds off retinal arteries, then degenerates down to this point, becoming the central retinal artery. **persistent h.a.** Portions of the hyaloid artery which fail to fully degenerate and which remain in the vitreous, posterior to the crystalline lens or anterior to the optic disk.

hypophysial a., anterior superior. A branch of the internal carotid artery that supplies the inferior, posterior portion of the optic chiasm.

infraorbital a. A branch of the internal maxillary artery which enters the orbit through the inferior orbital fissure and leaves via the infraorbital canal. It supplies the inferior extrinsic muscles, the orbicularis oculi, the lacrimal sac, the maxillary sinus, and the upper teeth.

lacrimal a. A branch of the ophthalmic artery which supplies the lacrimal gland, the superior and the lateral rectus muscles, the eyelids, and the conjunctiva, and gives origin to the lateral palpebral arteries.

lenticulo-optic a. A branch of the middle cerebral artery which supplies the internal capsule, especially its posterior limb; when involved in cerebral hemorrhage, the resulting symptoms are the same as those from hemorrhage of the lenticulo-striate arteries.

lenticulo-striate a's. Branches of the middle cerebral artery which supply the internal capsule, especially its posterior limb, commonly involved in cerebral hemorrhage. If extensive, and the optic radiations become affected, the hemorrhage leads to contralateral homonymous hemianopsia, generally with partial recovery. Other symptoms are a transient deviation of the eyes to the ipsilateral side, contralateral weakness of the frontal and the orbicularis oculi muscles, and contralateral paralysis of the lower face, the tongue, the arm, and the leg.

macular a's. Branches of the temporal arteries of the central retinal system, or of a cilioretinal artery when present, which supply the macula lutea.

meningeal a., anterior. A recurrent branch of the ophthalmic artery that leaves the orbit through the superior orbital fissure to enter the middle cranial fossa.

meningeal a., middle. A branch of the internal maxillary artery which supplies the dura mater, V and VII cranial nerves, and, by orbital branches through the superior orbital fissure, anastomoses with the lacrimal or other branches of the ophthalmic artery.

meningeal a., recurrent. A branch of the lacrimal artery which leaves the orbit through the superior orbital fissure to anastomose with the middle meningeal artery. Rarely, it supplies the orbital branches that ordinarily come from the ophthalmic artery.

muscular a. 1. An artery to a skeletal muscle. 2. Muscular branches of the ophthalmic, the lacrimal, and the infraorbital arteries, and others which supply the extrinsic eye muscles.

nasal a. A terminal branch of the ophthalmic artery which supplies the side of the nose and anastomoses with the angular artery. Syn., *dorsalis nasi.*

nasofrontal a. That portion of the ophthalmic artery which gives rise to the two ethmoidal arteries and a few muscular branches and terminates by dividing into the frontal and the nasal arteries. *Obs.*

oculonuclear a. A small artery between the posterior cerebral and superior cerebellar arteries which helps supply the midbrain and pons in the region of the III, IV, and VI motor nuclei.

ophthalmic a. A branch of the internal carotid artery which enters the orbit through the optic canal. Typically, its branches are: central retinal, posterior ciliaries, lacrimal, recurrents, muscular, supraorbital, posterior and anterior ethmoidals, and medial palpebrals. It terminates by forming the nasal and the frontal arteries and supplies all the tunics of the eyeball, most of the structures in the orbit, the lacrimal sac, the paranasal sinuses, the dura mater, and the nose. **internal o.a.** An artery of a 16 mm embryo which gives origin to the hyaloid, the common ciliary, and the nasal ciliary arteries. **primitive dorsal o.a.** A branch of the primitive internal carotid artery, appearing in the embryo at the 9 mm stage, which, through its branches, is the principal blood supply to the developing eye. **primitive ventral o.a.** A branch of the primitive internal carotid artery, appearing in the embryo at about the 12 mm stage, which supplies the ventral and medial portions of the plexus around the optic cup.

optic a., deep. A branch of the middle cerebral artery to the optic and the auditory radiations.

opticociliary a. An infrequent branch of the central retinal artery (or one of its branches in the region of the optic disk) that dips into the choroid. Syn., *retinociliary artery.*

palpebral a's., lateral. Superior and inferior branches of the lacrimal artery which anastomose with the medial palpebral arteries to supply the eyelids and the conjunctiva.

palpebral a's., medial. Superior and inferior branches of the ophthalmic artery which, with the lateral palpebral arteries, form the marginal and the peripheral (arterial) arcades and supply the eyelids, the conjunctiva, and the lacrimal sac.

prechiasmal a. A branch of the ophthalmic artery that supplies the region of the junction of the optic nerve with the optic chiasm.

recurrent a. An artery which turns back and runs in the opposite direction from its origin. The ophthalmic and the lacrimal arteries and the vessels that form the major arterial circle have such recurrents.

recurrent choroidal a. See *choroidal artery, recurrent.*

recurrent meningeal a. See *meningeal artery, recurrent.*

retinal a., central. A direct or indirect branch of the ophthalmic artery which courses below the optic nerve, entering the center of the nerve and supplying it. In the vicinity of the optic disk it divides into superior and inferior branches, the nasal and the temporal branches of which course in the nerve fiber layer to supply capillaries feeding the bipolar and the ganglion cell layers of the retina. Except for a tiny anastomosis with the circle of Zinn or Haller, it is an end artery.

retinociliary a. Opticociliary artery.

silver wire a. A retinal artery in which the whole thickness appears as a bright white reflex like a silver wire, a late sign of sclerosis. Cf. *copper wire artery.*

stapedial a. An artery arising from the primitive internal carotid artery which supplies the orbital tissues of the embryonic eye through its supraorbital division. In the 20 mm embryo this division forms an anastomosis with the ophthalmic artery which eventually takes over its function.

striate a., lateral. A branch of the middle cerebral artery, superficial to the lentiform nucleus in the forebrain. It is a common site of cerebral hemorrhage.

striate a., medial. A branch of the middle cerebral artery which supplies the caudate and the lentiform nuclei of the forebrain.

supraorbital a. A branch of the

ophthalmic artery to the levator muscle of the upper eyelid and the frontal bone, which, after leaving the orbit by the supraorbital notch (foramen), supplies the upper eyelid and the scalp.

   Zinn's central a. Central retinal artery.

◆

artiphakia (ar"tih-fa'ke-ah). The condition of an eye into which an artificial lens has been placed, following removal of the crystalline lens, in an attempt to duplicate a normal refractive state.

artiphakic (ar"tih-fa'kik). 1. One who has artiphakia. 2. Pertaining to or having artiphakia.

Arundel glass (ar'un-del). See under *glass.*

ARVO. See *Association for Research in Vision and Ophthalmology.*

as. Abbreviation for *astigmatism.*

Ascher's (ash'erz) **outlets; glass rod phenomenon; syndrome.** See under the nouns.

Aschner's(ash'nerz) **phenomenon; reflex; sign.** See under the nouns.

ASCO. See *Association of Schools and Colleges of Optometry.*

asemasia (as"e-ma'ze-ah). Asemia.

asemia (ă-se'me-ah). Aphasia in which there is an inability to employ or understand writing, speech, or gestures as a means of communication. Syn., *asemasia; asymbolia; asymb_oly.*

ASHA. See *American School Health Association.*

Asher's test (ash'erz). See under *test.*

Asher-Law stereoscope (ash'er-law'). See under *stereoscope.*

aspergillosis (as-per"jil-o'sis, as"per-). An infectious disease caused by the *Aspergillus* fungus. In the eye, it is characterized by the development of a necrotic corneal ulcer, surrounded by a yellow line of demarcation, which results in an iridocyclitis and accompanying hypopyon. Orbital involvement is rare and is probably secondary to infection of the accessory nasal sinuses.

aspheric (a-sfer'ik). Not spherical.

aspherize (a'sfer-ize). A hand-polishing process by which various zones of one or both lens surfaces are given different curvatures to reduce spherical aberration.

assimilation. According to the Hering theory of color vision, the reformation

of the three primary substances in the retina by green, blue, and black; the reverse of *dissimilation.*

   color a. The perceptual process by which a gray appears to be tinted by the color bordering it, as when a gray bordered by yellow appears to be a yellowish-gray, or the perceptual process by which the perceived saturation of a chromatic color is influenced positively by an achromatic border, as when a red appears to be a darker red when surrounded by black and a lighter red when surrounded by white.

association, corrective. A procedure advocated by the Optometric Extension Program to determine acceptable lens corrections for distance and near vision. The basic distance correction (No. 7) is determined by standard methods. The basic near correction is determined by the dynamic cross cylinder (14a or 14b) after a deduction (lag) depending on the phoria (15a or 15b) and the amplitude of accommodation (19). This basic near correction is called the *near net.* If either, or both, of the basic distance and the near net corrections indicates the use of convex lenses, comparisons of the ductions (break and recovery) of tests 10, 11, 16b, and 17b determine whether this convex lens power should be prescribed in full or reduced. The reduction may be from the basic distance correction only or from both distance and near. The amount of the reduction cannot be greater than 0.75 D for each and is decided by a comparison of the blur points (16a, 17a, 20, and 21). The amount of reduction should modify these blur points so that their amounts will be closer to the published norms ("expecteds"), but should not reverse their relative values as compared to those obtained through the basic corrections. At no time should the final distance correction be more convex than the final near correction, although they may be equal.

Association for Research in Vision and Ophthalmology. An association founded in 1928 of persons interested in research in visual science and ophthalmology. Formerly Association for Research in Ophthalmology.

Association of Contact Lens Manufacturers, Ltd. A British association of manufacturers of contact lenses and associated products and accessories, inaugurated in 1959 and registered in

1962 to serve their various promotional needs.

Association of Contact Lens Practitioners. An organization formed in 1949 to encourage high standards of practice in the specialty of contact lenses. Membership is open to anyone holding recognized ophthalmic optical qualifications or engaged in the development of contact lenses. See also *British Contact Lens Association.*

Association of Dispensing Opticians. A British organization of employees and principals exclusively engaged in optical dispensing (no sight testing). The association serves the interests of its members, including the qualifying examinations of candidates.

Association of Ophthalmic Opticians (Ireland) An association of ophthalmic opticians in Eire.

Association of Optical Practitioners. An association of mainly British ophthalmic and dispensing opticians and optical students founded in 1946 to replace two older organizations, the Institute of Ophthalmic Opticians and the Joint Council of Qualified Opticians, especially to serve and protect the interest of members in their relations with various governmental and public agencies.

Association of Optometric Editors. See *Optometric Editors Association.*

Association of Optometric Educators. An association of members of the faculties of schools and colleges of optometry founded in 1970 to enhance their professional, academic, and economic status.

Association of Schools and Colleges of Optometry. An organization, founded in 1941, of the institutions teaching optometry in the United States and Canada, for the purpose of advancing the profession of optometry through development of its educational system.

L'Association Professionnelle des Opticiens de Belgique. An association of Belgian optician-optometrists founded in 1923. Syn., *De Algemene Professionele Opticiensbond van België.*

ast. Abbreviation for *astigmatism.*

astaxanthin (as″tah-zan′thin). A derivative of β carotene present in the integument of lower animals and Euglena which makes phototactic responses possible.

asteroid hyalitis (as′ter-oid hi″ah-li′tis). Snowball-like bodies of calcium soaps occurring in a structurally intact vitreous body as an uncommon senile change. The condition is more frequent in males and is usually unilateral. These bodies do not signify inflammation, as "itis" would imply. It is often confused with the similar picture of synchysis scintillans, signifying degenerative changes which show numerous freely floating crystals of cholesterol in a fluid vitreous. Syn., *Benson's disease.*

asth. Abbreviation for *asthenopia.*

asthenocoria (as-then″o-ko′re-ah, as′-the-no-). A condition in which the light reflex of the pupil is sluggish.

asthenope (as′then-ōp). One having asthenopia.

◆

ASTHENOPIA

asthenopia (as″the-no′pe-ah). A term generally used to designate any subjective symptoms or distress arising from use of the eyes; eyestrain.

accommodative a. Asthenopia arising from the use of accommodation, as in uncorrected hypermetropia or low accommodative amplitude.

accommodative-convergence a. Asthenopia attributed to a high or low accommodative-convergence to accommodation ratio.

aniseikonic a. Asthenopia attributed to uncorrected aniseikonia.

anisometropic a. Asthenopia attributed to anisometropia.

aphakic a. Asthenopia attributed to aphakia, especially monocular aphakia.

astigmatic a. Asthenopia attributed to astigmatism.

a. cephalalgica. Asthenopia associated with headache.

color a. See *adisparopia.*

cyclophoric a. Asthenopia attributed to cyclophoria.

a. dolens. Asthenopia associated with ocular pain.

a. dolorosa. Painful spasm of accommodation as may occur after the instillation of eserine.

heterophoric a. Asthenopia attributed to heterophoria.

hyperphoric a. Asthenopia attributed to hyperphoria.

hysterical a. Asthenopia associated with psychosis or neurosis.

integrative a. Asthenopia due to

fusion difficulties, as in aniseikonia or anisometropia.

a. irritans. Asthenopia associated with ocular inflammation and irritation.

motor a. Asthenopia attributed to excessive lateral phoria, cyclophoria, hyperphoria, or deficiency of fusional reserve. Syn., *muscular asthenopia.*

muscular a. Motor asthenopia.

nervous a. 1. Hysterical asthenopia. 2. Asthenopia due to actual organic nervous disease.

neurasthenic a. 1. Asthenopia due to neurasthenia following a debilitating disease. 2. Hysterical asthenopia.

photogenous a. Asthenopia resulting from improper illumination.

presbyopic a. Asthenopia attributed to the low amplitude of accommodation in uncorrected presbyopia. See also *accommodative asthenopia.*

reflection a. Asthenopia attributed to reflections from the surfaces of ophthalmic lenses.

reflex a. Asthenopia in which the exciting cause is remote from the eyes, as in sinusitis.

retinal a. Asthenopia attributed to actual fatigue or exhaustion of the nervous elements of the eyes.

tarsal a. Asthenopia attributed to pressure of the eyelids on the cornea.

◆

asthenopic (as"the-nop'ik). Relating to, or suffering from, asthenopia.

astigmagraph (ă-stig'mah-graf). An instrument for showing or recording the astigmatism of an eye.

astigmatic (as"tig-mat'ik). Affected with, or pertaining to, astigmatism.

astigmatic amblyopia; chart; dial; interval. See under the nouns.

◆

ASTIGMATISM

astigmatism (ă-stig'mah-tizm). A condition of refraction in which rays emanating from a single luminous point are not focused at a single point by an optical system, but instead are focused as two line images at different distances from the system, generally at right angles to each other. In the eye, astigmatism is a refractive anomaly due to unequal refraction of the incident light by the dioptric system, in different meridians. It is generally caused by a toroidal anterior surface of the cornea or, of less degree, by other ocular refracting surfaces or by the obliquity of incidence of the light entering the cornea or the crystalline lens.

accommodative a. Astigmatism induced by the act of the ciliary muscle in accommodation which causes either unequal curvatures of the surfaces of the crystalline lens or a tilt of the crystalline lens; changes in amount of astigmatism associated with changes in accommodation, exclusive of apparent changes in astigmatism due to meridional differences in optical effectivity.

acquired a. Astigmatism which appears after birth as a result of disease or injury, or of normal physiological changes.

against the rule a. Astigmatism in which the meridian of greatest refractive power of the eye is in, or within 30° of, the horizontal. Syn., *indirect astigmatism; inverse astigmatism; perverse astigmatism.*

asymmetrical a. Astigmatism in which the two weakest or the two strongest meridians of both eyes do not total 180° upon addition of their meridional locations. The meridians of greatest, or weakest, power in the two eyes are not located as mirror images of each other with respect to the midline.

bi-oblique a. Astigmatism in which the two principal meridians are not at right angles to each other.

complex a. Astigmatism present in both the cornea and the crystalline lens.

compound a. Astigmatism in which the two principal meridians of an eye are both either hypermetropic or myopic. **c. hypermetropic a.** Astigmatism in which the two principal meridians of an eye are both hypermetropic. **c. myopic a.** Astigmatism in which the two principal meridians of an eye are both myopic.

congenital a. Astigmatism present at birth.

conical a. A condition which may appear as retinoscopy is performed in the presence of a posterior staphyloma of the sclera characterized by a scissors movement of the reflex with the blades in the direction of the staphyloma. Astigmatism said by Batten to be due to an asymmetric distortion of the cornea by a nearby scleral staphyloma optically identifiable by retinoscopic scissors movement with nonparallel blades.

corneal a. Astigmatism due to toroidal curvature of the cornea.

curvature a. Astigmatism due to unequal curvature in the two principal meridians of any surface of refraction.

direct a. With the rule astigmatism.

a. due to obliquity of the visual axis. Astigmatism induced by lack of coincidence of the optical axis of the eye and the foveal chief ray. Incident light therefore strikes the refracting surface obliquely and radial astigmatism results.

dynamic a. Astigmatism which becomes manifest during accommodation. See also *accommodative astigmatism*.

facultative a. Astigmatism attributed to the differential flattening of the cornea by the pull of the extrinsic ocular muscles.

heterologous a. Against the rule astigmatism with the corresponding cylinder axes in the two eyes symmetrical with each other.

heteronymous a. Astigmatism with the meridian of greatest power nearer the horizontal in one eye and with the meridian of greatest power nearer the vertical in the other eye.

homologous a. With the rule astigmatism with the corresponding cylinder axes in the two eyes symmetrical with each other.

homonymous a. Astigmatism in which the meridians of greatest power in the two eyes are within 30° of being parallel.

hypermetropic a. Astigmatism in which one principal meridian is hypermetropic and the other emmetropic, or in which both principal meridians are hypermetropic.

imbedded a. *Optometric Extension Program:* Astigmatism characterized by consistent and repeatable measurability and said to be "structured" or "fixed."

incidence a. Astigmatism caused by incident rays not being normal to a refracting surface. Cf. *radial astigmatism*.

index a. Lenticular astigmatism due to variation in the index of refraction in different areas of the crystalline lens.

indirect a. Against the rule astigmatism.

inverse a. Against the rule astigmatism.

irregular a. 1. Astigmatism in which the two principal meridians of the eye are not at right angles to each other. 2. Variations in refraction in a single meridian of the eye. **abnormal i.a.** Irregular astigmatism due to abnormalities of the cornea caused by injury or disease. **normal i.a.** Irregular astigmatism due to irregularities in the refracting power of the different sectors of the crystalline lens.

latent a. Astigmatism which is hidden or masked by the use of accommodation.

lenticular a. Astigmatism of the crystalline lens due to variations of curvature or to inequalities of refractive index. **dynamic l.a.** Dynamic astigmatism. **static l.a.** Lenticular astigmatism present when accommodation is not active.

manifest a. Astigmatism which can be measured in refraction.

marginal a. Radial astigmatism.

mixed a. Astigmatism in which one principal meridian is hypermetropic and the other myopic.

myopic a. Astigmatism in which one principal meridian is myopic and the other emmetropic, or in which both principal meridians are myopic.

near a. Accommodative astigmatism.

neutral a. An astigmatic refractive error having a mean spherical equivalent value of zero, such as that which would be produced artificially by placing a crossed cylinder lens before an emmetropic eye.

night a. The radial astigmatism manifested with the increased obliquity of incidence when paramacular instead of foveal imagery is used in very low, scotopic, illumination.

nonembedded a. *Optometric Extension Program:* Astigmatism which is characterized by lack of consistency and repeatability in its measurement and which varies in axis and power in different or repeated tests and which is said to be in process of becoming "imbedded."

nonneutral a. An astigmatic refractive error having a mean spherical equivalent value other than zero.

normal a. Physiological astigmatism.

oblique a. 1. Astigmatism in which the two principal meridians of an eye are oblique with respect to the horzontal or the vertical; nominally, between 30° to 60°, and 120° to 150°, on the spectacle axis scale. 2. Radial astigmatism.

pathological a. Astigmatism induced by a disease process, such as corneal disease, lenticular sclerosis, etc.

perverse a. Against the rule astigmatism.

physiological a. 1. Astigmatism of approximately 0.50 D found in the normal eye when the cornea is spherical, or when the corneal astigmatism is neutralized, as with a contact lens. 2. The small amount of corneal astigmatism, usually up to 1.50 D, found frequently, as contrasted to pathological astigmatism, usually of greater magnitude.

postoperative a. Astigmatism created by an operation involving the cornea.

radial a. A monochromatic aberration of spherical surfaces, refracting or reflecting, as a result of small bundles of incident rays being oblique with reference to the optic axis, two line images of a point source being formed. Syn., *marginal astigmatism; oblique astigmatism.*

regular a. Astigmatism produced by normal refraction at a simple toroidal surface.

residual a. 1. The difference between corneal and total astigmatism. Also called *physiological astigmatism.* 2. The ocular astigmatism manifested with a spherical contact lens in place.

retinal a. Schlaer's retinal astigmatism.

Schlaer's retinal a. Apparent astigmatism demonstrated by the fact that resolution is better in certain meridians than in others even after optical astigmatism has been corrected. Described by Schlaer, although first described by Hering, and attributed to elliptical distribution of retinal receptors.

simple a. Astigmatism in which one principal meridian of the eye is emmetropic and the other either myopic or hypermetropic. **s. hypermetropic a.** Astigmatism in which one principal meridian is hypermetropic and the other emmetropic. **s. myopic a.** Astigmatism in which one principal meridian is myopic and the other emmetropic.

symmetrical a. Astigmatism in which the two weakest or the two strongest meridians of both eyes total 180° upon addition of their meridional locations. The principal meridians of the two eyes are as mirror images of each other with respect to the midline. **heterologous s.a.** Against the rule astigmatism in which the total of the degrees representing the two weakest or the two strongest meridians for both eyes equals 180°. **homologous s.a.** With the rule astigmatism in which the total of the degrees representing the two weakest or the two strongest meridians for both eyes equals 180°.

vitreal a. Irregular astigmatism attributed to variations in optical density in the vitreous humor.

with the rule a. Astigmatism in which the meridian of greatest refractive power is in, or within 30° of, the vertical. Syn., *direct astigmatism.*

◆

astigmatizer (ă-stig'mah-ti"zer). Any device which brings a point of light into focus as lines; an astigmatic lens or lens combination.

astigmatometer (ă-stig"mah-tom'eh-ter, as"tig-). Astigmometer.

astigmatoscope (as"tig-mat'o-skōp). Astigmoscope.

astigmatoscopy (ă-stig"mah-tos'ko-pe). Astigmoscopy.

astigmia (as-tig'me-ah). Astigmatism.

astigmic (as-tig'mik). Astigmatic.

astigmism (as'tig-mizm). Astigmatism.

astigmometer (as"tig-mom'eh-ter). An instrument for measuring astigmatism. Syn., *astigmatometer.*

Lebensohn a. A test chart for determining the axis of astigmatism, consisting essentially of a rotatable white disk containing a centered black cross, with two short black lines set at 30° angles in arrowhead formation at the end of one line of the cross. The axis is located when the barbs of the arrowhead are equally blurred.

astigmometry (as"tig-mom'eh-tre). The measuring of astigmatism with the astigmometer.

astigmope (as'tig-mōp). One having astigmatism.

astigmoscope (ă-stig'mo-skōp). An instrument for observing and measuring the astigmatism of an eye. Syn., *astigmatoscope.*

astigmoscopy (as"tig-mos'ko-pe). The measuring of astigmatism with the a-stigmoscope. Syn., *astigmatoscopy.*

astrocyte (as'tro-sīt). A neuroglial cell of a macroglia type with many processes and perivascular feet, found in the central nervous system, the retina, and the optic nerve. Syn., *Cajal's cell; spider cell.*

astrocytoma (as"tro-si-to'mah). A tumor of the retina or of the central nervous system which is derived from astrocytic glial tissue. It does not recur or metastasize after removal. Syn., *glioma.*

astroglia (as-trog'le-ah). A type of neuroglia composed of astrocytes. Syn., *macroglia.*

asyllabia (as"ih-la'be-ah). A form of aphasia in which one cannot form syllables or words, although single letters are recognized.

asymbolia (as"im-bo'le-ah). Asemia.

asymboly (ă-sim'bo-le). Asemia.

asymmetropia (a"sih-met-ro'pe-ah). Anisometropia.

asymmetry (a-sim'eh-tre, ă-sim'-). 1. Lack of similarity in corresponding parts or organs on opposite sides of the body. 2. Lack of equal movement of two co-ordinated parts, as in asymmetrical convergence. 3. Lack of symmetry in the parts of an object or a geometric figure.

   chromatic a. Difference in color in the irides of the two eyes.

   monocular a. The perceiving of a line, bisected by a point which is monocularly fixated, as not being divided into two equal parts. The nature and the amount of the Hering-Hillebrand deviation result from the relationship between the asymmetries of the individual eyes. **Kundt's m.a.** The more common form of monocular asymmetry in which the segment in the temporal field is underestimated, resulting in subjectively locating the midpoint too far nasalward; hence, the temporal segment is longer than the nasal. Syn., *partition of Kundt.* **Münsterberg's m.a.** A less common form of monocular asymmetry, supposedly reported by Münsterberg, in which the segment in the temporal field is overestimated, resulting in subjectively locating the midpoint too far temporalward; hence, the nasal segment is longer than the temporal. Syn., *partition of Münsterberg.*

   visual a. 1. A condition in which one eye converges more than the other, as occurs when the point of fixation is not in the median plane. 2. A condition in which one eye differs from its fellow in visual acuity, refractive error, or size or shape of the ocular image.

asynergia (as"ih-ner'je-ah). Asynergy.

asynergy (ă-sin'er-je). Faulty co-ordination of skeletal muscles in their proper timing, or failure of a muscle to aid another when it would be normal for it to do so.

ataxia (ă-tak'se-ah). An inability to co-ordinate muscular movements.

   Friedreich's spinal a. Friedreich's disease.

   Marie's cerebellar a. Marie's disease.

   Sanger-Brown a. A hereditary degeneration of the cells of the posterior column, Clark's column, and the spinocerebellar tracts, characterized by spasticity and lack of motor co-ordination of the arms and legs, optic atrophy, and usually ptosis and external and internal ophthalmoplegia. The onset is usually between the ages of 16 and 40 and the disease is slowly progressive, resulting in mental deterioration and helplessness.

   a. telangiectatica. Louis-Bar syndrome.

atheroma of the eyelid (ath"er-o'-mah). Steatoma of the eyelid.

atherosclerosis (ath"er-o-skle-ro'sis). A lipoid deposition in the intima of arteries usually occurring as a senile change. Later it affects the deeper layers, producing plaques which obscure the vessel lumen. The ophthalmoscopic picture, according to Friedenwald, is of a narrowed arterial tree, arteries less tortuous than normal, and branches bifurcating at angles more acute than normal. Others state that the arteries become more tortuous.

athetosis, pupillary (ath"e-to'sis). Hippus.

atopognosia (ă-top"og-no'se-ah). Loss of ability to localize a sensation accurately.

atopognosis (ă-top"og-no'sis). Atopognosia.

atresia iritis (ă-tre'ze-ah i-ri'tis). Closure or imperforation of the pupil.

atretoblepharia (ă-tre″to-bleh-fa′-re-ah). Symblepharon.

atretopsia (ă″tre-top′se-ah). Imperforation of the pupil due to a persistent pupillary membrane.

atrophia bulborum hereditaria (ah-tro′fe-ah bul-bor′um her″ed-ih-ter′e-ah). Norrie's disease.

atrophoderma pigmentosum (at″ro-fo-der′mah pig-men-to′sum). Xeroderma pigmentosum.

♦

ATROPHY

atrophy (at′ro-fe). An acquired wasting or decrease in size of a portion of the body, an organ, or a tissue due not to direct injury but rather to faulty nutrition or loss of nerve supply. It may occur physiologically or pathologically; and starvation, senile, disuse, pressure, endocrine, excessive overwork, and, possibly, toxic types exist.

central areolar choroidal a. Atrophy of the choroid with the first ophthalmic appearance between the ages of 20 and 40 being of an exudative-edematous type resembling a macular degeneration which progresses to a pathognomonic, sharply defined circular or oval area in which the choriocapillaris and pigment epithelium disappear and the choroidal vessels are exposed as white strands. When fully developed, usually after age 50, the lesion is 2 to 4 times the size of the optic disk.

essential progressive iris a. A progressive atrophy of the iris without accompanying inflammatory signs or an evident etiologic factor. It is typically unilateral, affects young adults, more commonly females, and is characterized initially by distortion and displacement of the pupil followed by multiple holes in the iris which may coalesce. Secondary glaucoma, which usually does not respond to treatment, gradually develops in the later stages, and the condition may terminate in enucleation.

gyrate a. of choroid and retina. A slowly progressive hereditary atrophy of the choroid and the retina producing irregularly shaped white areas which coalesce into bizarre forms as a result of pigment upset. Centripetal involvement is typical, with the macular area the last to be affected. The symptoms are night blindness (commencing in childhood) and disturbances of vision; etiology is unknown. Syn., *Fuchs disease.*

optic a. Degeneration of the optic nerve fibers, characterized by pallor of the optic nerve head which may appear grayish, yellowish, or white. Visual loss usually accompanies this condition. **ascending o.a.** Consecutive optic atrophy. **cavernous o.a.** Optic atrophy usually associated with glaucoma and characterized by the disappearance of optic nerve fibers and mucoid degeneration of the neuroglia, resulting in a riddling of the optic nerve with spaces filled with clear, mucoid material. Syn., *lacunar optic atrophy.* **choroiditic o.a.** Chorioretinitic optic atrophy. **chorioretinitic o.a.** Optic atrophy characterized by a waxy yellow color of the disk, which follows diffuse chorioretinal disease or degenerative processes, the prototype being optic atrophy as found in retinitis pigmentosa. **consecutive o.a.** 1. Optic atrophy associated with inflammatory or degenerative lesions of the retina and the choroid which have affected the ganglion cell layer of the retina. Syn., *ascending optic atrophy.* 2. Optic atrophy which is secondary to papilledema. **descending o.a.** Optic atrophy which results from a lesion in the intraorbital, intracanalicular, or intracranial portions of the nerve and progresses toward the retina to involve the optic nerve head. **Fuchs′ o.a.** Optic atrophy associated with circumpapillary atrophy, presumably due to choroidal stretching and atrophy subsequent to high myopia. **glaucomatous o.a.** Optic atrophy secondary to glaucoma and characterized by a cupping or excavation of the nerve head which extends to the border of the disk. The retinal vessels are displaced toward the nasal border of the disk and bend sharply over the margins of the disk as they dip down into the excavation. The disk is pale and may be surrounded by an atrophic halo. **inflammatory o.a.** Optic atrophy due to local inflammation of the nerve head, intraocular inflammation, inflammation of the tissues surrounding the nerve fibers, systemic diseases, or diseases of the central nervous system. Syn., *secondary optic atrophy.* **lacunar o.a.** Cavernous optic atrophy. **Leber's o.a.** Optic atrophy, both bilateral and hereditary, of fairly rapid onset, usually in young adult males. As a rule, it involves the entire disk, but occasionally only the papillomacular bundle. It is an atrophy of the primary type, although there may be a papillitis at the onset of the disease. **noninflammatory o.a.** Optic atrophy due to causes other than inflammation, such as physical severance of the conduction path, pressure, or essential atrophy. Syn., *primary optic atrophy.* **postneuritic o.a.** Optic atrophy secondary to inflammation of the nerve head. **primary o.a.** Optic atrophy characterized by a sharply defined pale gray or white disk without excessive glial proliferation and, usually, with unobscured lamina cribrosa; typically seen in lesions affecting the conduction path posterior to the nerve head. Syn., *simple optic atrophy.* **retinitic o.a.** Chorioretinitic optic atrophy. **secondary o.a.** Optic atrophy characterized by a gray disk with obscured margins and glial proliferation filling the physiological cup; typically seen in lesions involving the nerve head directly. **simple o.a.** Primary optic atrophy. **temporal o.a.** Optic atrophy of the temporal portion of the optic disk. It results from involvement of the papillomacular bundle and occurs characteristically in multiple sclerosis. **vascular o.a.** Optic atrophy associated with extreme attenuation of the retinal vessels. It occurs characteristically from arteriosclerosis or embolus or thrombosis of the central retinal artery.

peripheral chorioretinal a. Paving-stone degeneration of the retina.

pigmented paravenous retinochoroidal a. A rare condition of unknown etiology wherein pigment aggregates around retinal vessels, especially around the venules, with chorioretinal atrophy underlying the pigmentation radiating out from the optic disk. Syn., *paravenous retinal degeneration; melanosis of the retina; congenital pigmentation of the retina; retinochoroiditis radiata.*

progressive choroidal a. Choroideremia.

progressive tapetochoroidal a. Choroideremia.

senile circumpapillary choroidal a. A patchy sclerosis particularly evident around the optic disk due to degeneration of arterioles in the choriocapillaris, with thickening of their walls and narrowing of their lumens, and to endothelial cells filled with fatty droplets in the perivascular spaces. Syn., *senile peripapillary halo.*

senile marginal a. Peripheral corneal ectasia.

traumatic macular a. Traumatic macular degeneration of Haab.

◆

atropine (at'ro-pēn, -pin). A poisonous alkaloid derivative of belladonna. Its action is mydriatic, cycloplegic, antispasmodic, sedative, and narcotic. Atropine sulfate, used as a cycloplegic for therapeutic action and for refracting, paralyzes the pupillary sphincter and the ciliary muscle by preventing the action of acetylcholine at the parasympathetic nerve endings. Its action may persist for over 2 weeks after full cycloplegia.

atropinism (at'ro-pin-izm). Atropism.

atropinize (at'ro-pin-īz). 1. To bring under the influence of atropine. 2. To install atropine into the conjunctival sac.

atropism (at'ro-pizm). A condition produced by the use of atropine.

attensity (ă-ten'sih-te). Sensory clearness as distinguished from cognitive clearness; employed by Titchener.

attention. The focusing of conscious activity; conscious adjustment of the senses to facilitate optimal response.

fluctuation of a. The periodic variation of the degree of maximum clearness of the contents of consciousness, regardless of the change in content.

inertia of a. A lag or slowness of the normal shift of attention.

a. reflex. See under *reflex.*

a. span. See under *span.*

visual a. 1. Attention mediated by the visual sense. 2. The conscious or purposeful fixation of the eyes to an object of regard.

attenuation (ah-ten″u-a′shun). 1. In physical optics, the reduction in light flux due to light traveling through an absorbing or scattering medium. 2. Clinically, a procedure used in the treatment of binocular anomalies whereby the dominant eye is occluded with an attenuating lens so as to favor the non-dominant eye. A procedure also referred to as *penalization.*

attolens oculi (at'ol-enz ok'u-li). Superior rectus muscle.

Aubert's (o-bārz') **phenomenon; theory.** See under the nouns.

Aubert-Förster (o-bār'fers'ter) **law; phenomenon.** See under *law*.

Aubineau-Lenoble syndrome. See under *syndrome*.

aura, visual (aw'rah). Visual sensations which precede an attack of epilepsy or migraine. These include flashes of light (photopsia), scintillating scotoma, fortification spectrum (teichopsia), or hallucinations.

Australian Optometrical Association. An association of optometrists organized in 1918 by federations of existing Australian state optometric associations and presently the principal representative body of optometrists in Australia.

Autocluder. Trade name for a battery-driven spectacle frame attachment which automatically shifts an occluder alternately from one eye to the other at adjustable frequencies, usually at about one Hertz.

autocollimation (aw"to-kol-ih-ma'-shun). A procedure for collimating a telescope, or similar optical instrument having an objective and crosshairs, in which the instrument is directed toward a plane mirror and the reflected image of a luminous object or point source in the focal or crosshair plane is seen focused in the same plane by virtue of both the anteriorly exiting and entering pencils being of parallel rays.

Autocross, Matsuura. A phoroptor attachment for performing a crossed cylinder test for astigmatism, consisting essentially of a biprism doubling system and two crossed cylinder lenses, enabling the doubled image of the test object to be seen simultaneously through the two positions of the crossed cylinder lenses instead of sequentially.

Auto-disc, Nutt. An attachment used with the Projectoscope in the treatment of eccentric fixation, housing three graticules which are sequentially projected onto the fundus, the first being a green filter with a lighter green three-degree central area, the second being clear with a centrally located three-degree black spot, and the third, a green filter with a small central clear aperture. When connected to the control unit with the second graticule utilized, an intense light of preset duration illuminates the retina not shielded by the black spot. When the third graticule is in place, the control unit will automatically produce flashing light with preset light and dark phases.

autofundoscope (aw"to-fun'do-skōp). An instrument designed for the self-examination of the macular and the perimacular regions of the eye.

autokeratoplasty (aw-to-ker'ah-to-plas"te). Keratoplasty in which the transplanted tissue is obtained from the other eye of the patient or is rotated in the same eye. Cf. *homokeratoplasty.* Syn., *autogenous keratoplasty.*

autokinesis, visual (aw"to-kih-ne'sis). The apparent motion of a small, single, stationary spot of light when continuously observed in an otherwise dark field. Syn., *autokinetic visual illusion.*

autolenticule (aw"to-len'tih-kūl). The lamellar disk, consisting of epithelium, Bowman's membrane, and some corneal stroma, cut from the patient's cornea in keratomileusis, reshaped on a cutting lathe, and replaced in its original bed of the cornea.

autoluminescence (aw"to-lu"mih-nes'-ens). Luminescence produced by energy within the luminescent substance itself.

auto-ophthalmoscope (aw"to-of-thal'-mo-skōp). An instrument for examining one's own fundus.

auto-ophthalmoscopy (aw"to-of"-thal-mos'ko-pe). The examination of one's own fundus by means of an auto-ophthalmoscope or by means of entoptic imagery.

autoperimetry (aw"to-per-im'eh-tre). The examination of one's own field of vision.

autophthalmoscope (aw"tof-thal'mo-skōp). Auto-ophthalmoscope.

autophacoscopy (aw"to-fa-kos'ko-pe). The viewing of the image of the interior of one's own eye. The apparatus consists of a lens to which adheres a drop of colorless viscous fluid on the outer surface. The lens is held before the eye in the same position as a spectacle lens, and the reflections from the interior of the eye are visible through the drop of fluid. The term is a misnomer, because only the movement of muscae volitantes is seen.

autophakoscopy (aw"to-fa-kos'ko-pe). Autophacoscopy.

Autoplot tangent screen. See under *screen.*

autopsia (aw-top'se-ah). The apparent perception of an external object when no such object is present; a visual hallucination.

autorefraction (aw"to-re-frak'shun). A procedure of refraction in which the patient or subject controls or adjusts the lenses, knobs, or dials on the refractor.

autoretinoscopy (aw"to-ret"ih-nos'ko-pe). Velonoskiascopy.

autoscope (aw"to-skōp). An instrument for visually examining one's own organs, such as the eye or larynx.

autoscopy (aw-tos'ko-pe). 1. Examination of one's own organs by means of an autoscope. 2. Examination of one's own eyes. 3. A vivid sense of one's own organs; a visualization of one's own organs.

autoskiascopy (aw"to-ski-as'ko-pe). Skiascopy of one's own eye by means of a mirror and the other eye.

autotransplant, corneal (aw"to-trans'plant). Transplantation of corneal tissue in which the tissue is obtained from the other eye of the patient or is rotated in the same eye. See also *allotransplant; heterotransplant; homotransplant.*

auxesis, visual (awk-ze'sis). 1. An increase in any specific visual sensibility while under the influence of the original stimulus. 2. Recovery from effects of what is conventionally spoken of as visual fatigue; the opposite of *visual minuthesis.*

auxiometer (awk"se-om'eh-ter). Auxometer.

auxometer (awks-om'eh-ter). An instrument for measuring the magnifying power of lenses.

auxoptician (oks-op-tish'an). One who uses his eyes to aid the blind by reading aloud, guiding, or helping generally by providing auxiliary vision.

A-V nicking. See under *nicking.*

Avellis syndrome (av-el'ēz). See under *syndrome.*

aversion to fusion. Horror fusionis.

Aves's deviograph. See under *deviograph.*

avulsion (ă-vul'shun). The forcible separation, or tearing away, of a part or an organ.

    a. of the bulb. The forcible expulsion of the eyeball with tearing of the conjunctiva, the muscles, and the optic nerve.

    a. of the optic nerve. Traumatic separation of the optic nerve from its attachment to the eyeball.

    a. of the retina. The tearing of the retina away from the ora serrata boundary.

ax. Abbreviation for *axis* (of cylinder).

axanthopsia (ak"zan-thop'se-ah). An inability to distinguish yellow; yellow blindness.

Axenfeld's (ak'sen-feltz) **anomaly; accessory ganglion; follicular conjunctivitis; intrascleral nerve loop; syndrome.** See under the nouns.

Axenfeld-Schurenberg syndrome (ak'sen-felt-shēr'en-burg). See under *syndrome.*

axicon (aks'ih-kon). A type of optic having the structural characteristic of being a figure of revolution and the property that a point source on its axis of revolution is imaged to a range of points along its axis.

axiometer (ak"se-om'eh-ter). A device for determining the axis of a cylindrical lens. It is a boxlike instrument emitting a luminous streak reflected on the lens and rotated until it is parallel with its reflected image.

◆

AXIS

axis. 1. An imaginary straight line passing through a body or a system with respect to which this body or system is symmetrical. 2. An imaginary straight line passing through a body or an object about which this body or object rotates. 3. A line of reference corresponding to a unique diametric dimension of a body or a system.

    anteroposterior a. Sagittal axis.

    azimuthal a. The axis about which azimuthal movements of the eye are made. It corresponds to the Z axis of Fick.

    a. of collineation. 1. The intersection of all corresponding incident and refracted paraxial rays lying in a meridian plane of a single spherical refracting surface or of an infinitely thin lens. 2. A line perpendicular to the optic axis at the optical center of a thin lens, or at the vertex of a single refracting surface, and used to represent the lens or the surface itself in ray diagramming.

    corneal a. A variously defined axis to represent the anteroposterior orientation of the cornea as a discrete anatomical structure. Depending on the assumed or actual structural characteristics of the cornea, it has been variously named the axis of symmetry or the major axis of the corneal ellipsoid. The definitions sometimes stipulate that the axis must pass through the corneal apex or the center of curvature of the optical zone of the cornea.

cylindrical a. 1. Mathematically, the axis of radial symmetry of a cylinder. 2. The meridian of least refractive power or of longest radius of curvature on the toric surface of an astigmatic lens.

Fick, axes of. Primary axes of Fick.

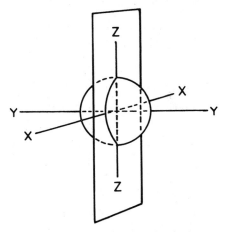

Fig. 3 The primary axes of Fick.

fixation a. The line connecting the point of fixation to the center of rotation of the eyeball. Syn., *fixation line.*

frontal a. The line connecting the centers of rotation of the eyeballs. Syn., *x axis; base line.*

a. of gaze. Visual axis.

geometrical a. The line passing through the anterior and the posterior poles of the eye. If the refractive surfaces are symmetrically located within the eye, then the geometrical axis coincides with the optic axis, which passes through the centers of curvature of the refracting surfaces. **external g.a.** In a schematic topographical representation of the eye, the line joining the most anterior surface of the cornea to the most posterior surface of the episclera. **internal g.a.** In a schematic topographical representation of the eye, the line joining the most anterior surface of the cornea to the most posterior point on the anterior surface of the retina.

Helmholtz axes. In the representation of ocular rotations, a fixed horizontal axis connecting the centers of rotation of the two eyes around which elevation is represented and a variably oriented secondary axis in the vertical plane around which azimuth is represented.

horizontal a. Transverse axis.

lateral a. Transverse axis.

a. of lens. 1. The straight line normal to both surfaces of the lens. Syn., *optical axis; principal axis.* 2. The cylindrical axis of a spectacle lens. 3. The line joining the anterior and the posterior poles of the crystalline lens.

Listing, axes of. Axes which lie in a plane (Listing's plane) passing through the center of rotation of the eye and perpendicular to the line of sight when the eye is in its primary position. Movements of the eyes are referred to these axes in the analysis of torsional movements.

macular a. The line joining the fovea to the second nodal point of the eye.

major a. The horizontal line at the maximum width of a spectacle lens; it may or may not fall on the datum line, depending on the lens shape.

a. marker. See under *marker.*

mechanical a. Datum line.

minor a. The perpendicular to the major axis at its midpoint.

oblique a. 1. An axis which is neither vertical nor horizontal. 2. In ophthalmic lenses, the axis of the cylindrical correction if it is not at 0° or 90° on the spectacle reference scale. 3. In ophthalmometry, the axis of the astigmatism if it lies between 30° and 60°, or between 120° and 150°, on the spectacle reference scale.

optic a. 1. In the eye, the line passing through the centers of curvature of all the optical elements (corneal and lens surfaces), or the best approximation of this line. 2. In doubly refracting crystals, such as calcite and quartz, the direction in which the ordinary and the extraordinary rays behave alike in all respects.

optic a. of Gullstrand. Pupillary axis.

optical a. 1. The straight line normal to both faces of a lens along whose path a ray will pass without being deflected. 2. The straight line joining the centers of curvature of all the refracting surfaces of a centered lens system.

orbital a. The line from the middle of the orbital opening to the center of the optic foramen. In an adult, the orbital axes make an angle of approximately 45° with each other.

papillary a. The line joining the temporal edge of the optic disk and the second nodal point.

primary a. The straight line normal to the surfaces of a lens or a centered lens system which passes through the nodal points.

primary axes of Fick. A system of three mutually perpendicular coordinate axes which intersect at a point specified as the center of rotation of the eye and to which all positions of direction of the eye may be referred. These axes of reference were designated *x*, *y*, and *z* by Fick, and were defined with respect to the frontal plane of the head. (See Fig. 3.)

principal a. 1. A straight line which is normal to both surfaces of a lens. Syn., *optical axis*. 2. A straight line through the center of curvature of a spherical reflecting or refracting surface and through the center of the surface.

pupillary a. The line perpendicular to the cornea and passing through the center of the entrance pupil of the eye. It is the line by means of which the direction of a person's gaze is objectively determined. Syn., *optic axis of Gullstrand; pupillary line.*

rectilinear axes. Axes which are mutually perpendicular to each other.

a. of refraction. The normal to a refracting surface at the point of incidence of a ray of light.

sagittal a. The line connecting the anterior and the posterior poles of the eye. Loosely, the visual axis or the y axis for true torsion or wheel rotation. Syn., *anteroposterior axis.*

secondary a. Any line not coincident with the primary axis which passes through the optical center of an infinitely thin lens or through the nodal points of a thick lens or of a lens system. Any ray not coincident with the primary axis which passes without deviation through an infinitely thin lens will be along a secondary axis. In the case of thick lenses, the path of such a ray will be a pair of parallel lines interconnected by the line connecting the two nodal points.

a. of symmetry of the cornea. The line about which the cornea may be assumed to be symmetrical. The definition may variously be applied to the whole corneal structure or just to the optical zone. See also *corneal axis.*

transverse a. A line passing through the center of rotation of the eyeball, perpendicular to the anteroposterior axis and serving as the x axis for elevation or depression. Syn., *horizontal axis; lateral axis.*

vertical a. 1. A superior-inferior line through the center of rotation of the eyeball which serves as the z axis for abduction and adduction. 2. A line of reference for the whole body, extending from the head to the feet in the midsagittal plane.

visual a. 1. The line joining the point of fixation and the anterior nodal point. 2. The line connecting the fovea to the point of fixation and passing through the nodal points of the eye. Since it connects both nodal points, it is a broken, not a single, straight line. In practice, the two nodal points are regarded as coincident, in which case it is a straight line. Syn., *line of gaze; line of regard; line of vision; visual line.* **binocular v.a.** An arbitrary reference line connecting a binocularly fixated point and a reference point between the two eyes, ordinarily midway between the two eyes. **false v.a.** Any axis which, by reason of the method of determination, seems to be the visual axis but which is in fact not the true visual axis. It is occasionally incurred in subjective determinations in which an anomalously localized visual image of a foveally fixated object is used as a reference point instead of the real fixated point, or when an extrafoveal point is used for fixation.

working a. Datum line.

x axis. A line passing through the centers of rotation of the eyes; one of the primary axes of Fick. Syn., *frontal axis.*

y axis. A line passing through the anterior and the posterior poles and the center of rotation of the eye, perpendicular to the x and the z axes; one of the primary axes of Fick. Syn., *anteroposterior axis; sagittal axis.*

z axis. A vertical line passing through the center of rotation of the eye, perpendicular to the x and the y axes; one of the primary axes of Fick. Syn., *vertical axis.*

◆

axometer (ak-som'eh-ter). 1. An instrument for determining the axis and the optical center of a lens. It is used especially to adjust a pair of spectacles to a patient so that the optical centers are properly placed with respect to the lines of sight of the eyes. 2. An instrument used in the subjective determination of the axis of astigmatism of the eye.

Ferree-Rand a. A visual testing instrument consisting essentially of three small, bright, transilluminated apertures in a row which, in astigmatism, are seen in streaked, meridional distortion and which may be made to coalesce by orientation of the instrument parallel or perpendicular to the axis of astigmatism.

axonometer (ak″so-nom'eh-ter). 1. An instrument for the determination of the axis of a cylindrical lens. 2. An instrument for locating the axis of astigmatism of the eye.

azimuth (az'ih-muth). The horizontal co-ordinate in a system of spherical co-ordinates, measured in a horizontal plane as an angular rotation about a fixed vertical axis.

B

B. Abbreviation for base (of prism).

B₁, B₂, etc., case type. See under *case type, B₁, B₂, etc.*

Babinet's (bah"be-nehz') **compensator; principle; rule.** See under the nouns.

Babinski-Froehlich syndrome (bahbin'skē-fra'lik). Froehlich's syndrome.

Babinski-Nageotte syndrome (bahbin'skē-nazh-yot'). See under *syndrome.*

Bach's (bahks) **test; theory.** See under the nouns.

Bachmaier's method; technique. See under *method.*

background. Neutral surroundings and interstices of a figure; the framework in which a figure is suspended. It may be simple, amorphous, homogeneous, and localized behind the figure, and is characteristically less structured, less penetrating, less independent, and less meaningful than the figure.

backstroke. A specific series of afferent nerve impulses which originate in the sense organ and are of value in correcting for errors in the motor adjustments of the body.

Badal's optometer (bah-dalz'). See under *optometer.*

Baer's nystagmus (bārz). See under *nystagmus.*

Bagolini's (bah'go-le"nēz) **striated glass; test.** See under the nouns.

Bailey's test (ba'lēz). See under *test.*

Bailey-Lovie Distance Acuity Chart (ba'le-luv'e). See under *chart.*

Baillarger's (bi"yar-zhāz') **band; line; sign.** See under the nouns.

Bailliart's (bah'yartz) **test; tonometer.** See under the nouns.

balance, binocular. 1. The condition characterized by the two eyes being simultaneously in focus or equally out of focus. 2. The condition represented in the various ocular muscle functions providing for normal binocular fusion without stress, fatigue, discomfort, etc. E.g., orthophoria is said to indicate binocular balance. See also *muscle balance.*

balance, muscle. 1. Orthophoria, particularly when regarded as an indication of extraocular muscle function. 2. The status of extraocular muscle function as represented in phoria measurements.

Baldwin's (bawl'dwinz) **figure; illusion.** See under the nouns.

Balgrip (bal'grip). A trade name for a rimless spectacle mounting in which the lenses are held in place by tension instead of screws. Brackets, soldered to an arm, fit into notches cut on the nasal and the temporal sides of the lens.

Balint's syndrome (bah-lintz'). See under *syndrome.*

Ball effect (bahl). See under *effect.*

ball, Landolt's. A device designed by Landolt to demonstrate movements of the eyeball, consisting of a simple rubber ball on which are depicted cornea, anterior and posterior poles, horizontal and vertical meridians, etc.

ball, Marsden. A soft rubber ball about 15 cm in diameter with small letters, numbers, and figures imprinted on it, suspended from the ceiling by a string and used for oculomotor fixation and pursuit training.

Ballet's sign (bal-āz'). See under *sign.*

ballottement, ocular (bah"lot-mawn', bah-lot'ment). The falling of opaque particles in a fluid vitreous body, on movements of the eyeball.

Balopticon (bal-op'tih-kon). A trade name for an apparatus which projects enlarged images of opaque objects onto a screen. See also *epidiascope; opaque projector.*

balsam, Canada (bawl'sam). A transparent substance used to cement glass, as in a cement bifocal. It is obtained from the sap of the North American balsam fir and is soluble in xylol. Its index varies, 1.54 being a typical value.

Bancroft's filiariasis (ban-croftz'). See under *filiariasis.*

band. A flat strip, or a section of a surface having the appearance of a flat strip, separated from the adjacent areas by some differing characteristic, as color, texture, etc.

absorption b's. Regions of the spectrum absorbed by liquids or solids in contrast with gases which have absorption lines. The bands are generally continuous in character, fading off gradually at the ends. Salts of certain rare earth metals give narrow bands with fairly sharp limits.

astigmatic b. The band of light seen in the retinoscopic reflex of an astigmatic eye, especially on neutralization of only one of the principal meridians.

Baillarger's outer b. Baillarger's outer line.

Charpentier's b's. A series of alternating light and dark bands which are pulsations of sensation produced by the observation of a moving slit-shaped light stimulus in a dark visual field, e.g., a radial slit in a rotating disk, the center of which is constantly fixated. The magnitude of the effect depends on the intensity of the stimulus, the state of adaptation of the eye, and the region of the retina stimulated.

fusion b. of Langrange. A line horizontally traced, at eye level, on the three sides of a rectangular or square room to measure the horizontal field of binocular fixation, ruled into 5° intervals. With a red glass in front of one eye, the subject fixates a white light source target which is moved along the line until it no longer appears to be of such color as to indicate fusion of the red and white targets.

b. of Gennari. Line of Gennari.

Haidinger's b's. Haidinger's fringes.

interference b. Black bands crossing the various orders of spectra produced when a diffraction grating is held in contact with a plane reflecting surface, due to the interference of the direct and reflected orders of the spectra.

Mach's b. Mach's ring.

neutral b. A band in the spectrum which, to a dichromat, is without hue, appearing as white or gray, and varies in location with the type of dichromat.

b. opacity. See *opacity, Haab's band.*

Talbot b's. Interference bands appearing in a prismatic spectrum when a thin glass plate is mounted in a spectroscope between the collimator and prism, or prism and telescope, so that half of the beam which is nearer the vertex of the prism passes through the glass.

trabecular b. A narrow band seen with the slit lamp or with the gonioscope which represents the meshwork of the angle of the anterior chamber. Syn., *trabecular zone.*

b. of Vicq d'Azyr. Line of Gennari.

bandage, Borsch's. A bandage that covers both the diseased and the healthy eye.

bandpass (band'pas). Pertaining to a multilayer, interference optical filter designed to transmit only within a selected band or narrow range of wavelengths. Also spelled band-pass.

Bangerter's occluders (bang'er-terz). See under *occluder.*

Bannon-Raubitschek chart (ban'un-row'bih-shek). Paraboline chart.

bar. 1. A piece of material, usually rigid, which is proportionately greater in length than in breadth and thickness. 2. A strip, band, or broad line.

Galton b. An instrument for determining the accuracy of judgment of lengths, consisting of a horizontal bar to be bisected by an adjustable vertical line.

Koenig b's. A target used for visual acuity measurements, consisting of two parallel black bars of the same size and shape on a white background. The length of each bar is three times its width and the space between the bars is equal to the width of one bar. The smallest angular subtense (from the eye) for which the bars can be perceived as separate is a measure of the acuity.

prism b. A series of prisms of ascending powers arranged in a convenient barlike mount for rapid successive positioning in front of an eye.

pulley b. Falciform fold.

terminal b. A very thin opening or gap found at the posterior end of the intercellular borders between endothelial cells of the corneal mesothelium which is formed by a densification of neighboring cytoplasm in the terminal web.

bar reader. An appliance which provides for the placement of an opaque septum or bar between a printed page and the reader's eyes so as to occlude different areas of the page for each of the two eyes. Used for diagnosis and training of simultaneous binocular vision. Cf. *Javal's grid.*

bar reading. See *test, bar reading.*

Bar Trainer, Engelmann. A pair of slender vertical bars mounted on a horizontal piece with a central, downward-extending handle, the whole resembling a tuning fork in shape, to be held at given distances in front of the eyes with the plane of the two bars approximately in the median plane of the head. Alternate binocular fixation of test characters on the two bars provides tests and training for physiological diplopia, accommodation, and convergence.

bar-screen. A grid used in conjunction with a stereoscopic camera in order to produce a parallax stereogram so constructed that portions of the image blocked from one view are permitted to reach the film from the other view.

Bárány's (bah′rah-nēz) **chair; nystagmus.** See under the nouns.

Bard's sign (bardz). See under *sign.*

Bardet-Biedl syndrome (bar-da′-be′-del). Laurence-Moon-Biedl syndrome.

baring of the blind spot. See under *spot.*

Barkan (bar′kan) **Focal Illuminator; goniotomy lens; line; membrane.** See under the nouns.

Barlow's (bar′lōz) **disease; lens; method.** See under the nouns.

Barnet's theory (bar-netz′). See under *theory.*

Baron lens (bar′on). See under *lens.*

Barraga visual efficiency scale (bah-rah′gah). See under *scale.*

Barré's sign (bah-rāz′). See under *sign.*

barrel. A usually cylindrical attachment to the eyewire of a metal spectacle frame through which a screw is inserted to fasten it to the hinge, or to another threaded barrel, for the purpose of holding together the ends of the eyewire.

Barré-Liéou syndrome (bar′a-le-a′-oo). See under *syndrome.*

Barrett subnormal vision monocular (bar′et). See under *monocular.*

Bartels' (bar-telz′) **nystagmus; spectacles.** See under the nouns.

Bartenwerfer syndrome (bahr-ten-ver′fer). See under *syndrome.*

Bartholin-Patau syndrome (bar′to-lin-pah′to). Trisomy 13 syndrome. See under *syndrome.*

Bartley phenomenon. See *effect, Brücke-Bartley.*

base. 1. The lowest part of anything, considered as its support; a foundation. 2. The point or line from which actions or operations are performed or calculated. 3. The portion of an organ by which it is attached to a more central structure.

b. curve. See under *curve.*

b. line. The line joining the centers of rotation of the two eyes.

parallactic b. The separation between the optical centers of the two objective lenses in a stereoscopic camera, or the separation between the centers of the entrance pupils of the two eyes. Syn., *stereoscopic base.*

b. of prism. 1. The edge of a prism at which the faces are separated a maximum distance. 2. The direction along the base-apex line of a prism opposite the apex, or the direction along the base-apex line opposite to the apparent displacement of the image.

stereoscopic b. Parallactic base.

vitreous b., Salzmann's. The portion of the peripheral anterior vitreous humor, about 1.5 mm wide, which is attached to the ciliary epithelium in the area of the ora serrata.

Basedow's disease (bas′e-dōz). Exophthalmic goiter.

Basedow's triad (bas′e-dōz). See under *triad.*

basic. Cridland's term, prefixed to the phorias, to denote deviations measured at infinity under the condition of emmetropia. Cf. *basic deviation.*

basket, fiber, Schultze's. See under *fiber.*

Bassen-Kornzweig syndrome (bas'-en-korn'zwīg). See under *syndrome.*

batch. The mixture of raw materials from which glass is made.

Bates chart (bāts). See under *chart.*

bathomorphic (bath″o-mōr'fik). Having an eye of greater than average axial length; used in reference to a myopic eye.

Batten's myotonic dystrophy (bat'-enz). Myotonic dystrophy. See under *dystrophy.*

Batten-Mayou disease (bat'en-ma'o). See under *disease.*

batwing. Pertaining to a distribution of light intensity from a luminaire for which the maximum occurs in the direction of about 35° from straight down with relatively less at 0° and little or none beyond 60°. The resultant graphical representation of the intensity resembles a pair of batwings.

Baumgardt-Segal experiment (bowm'gart-se'gul). See under *experiment.*

Baumgarten's glands (bowm'gar-tenz). See under *gland.*

Baumgartner reflectometer (bowm'-gart-ner). See under *reflectometer.*

Bayshore contact lens (ba'shōr). BT contact lens.

Bazzana syndrome. Angiospastic ophthalmo-auricular syndrome. See under *syndrome.*

BCD. Borderline between comfort and discomfort.

BCLA. See *British Contact Lens Association.*

Beach test chart. See under *chart.*

beading (bēd'ing). A fragmented appearance of the blood stream in the retinal arteries and veins subsequent to retinal artery occlusion.

Beal's (bēlz) **conjunctivitis; syndrome.** Acute follicular conjunctivitis of Beal. See under *conjunctivitis, follicular.*

beam of light. A family of light rays emanating from all points of a given area or source and proceeding to points within another given area, such as the total bundle of rays traversing an optical system from object plane to image plane, or from a projected source to a screen.

beamsplitter (bēm'split-er). A semi-transparent mirror or surface which separates an incident beam of light into two beams of lesser intensity but with the same cross-section dimensions as the incident beam, one reflected and one transmitted, and proceeding in different directions.

beamspread. The amount that a laser beam departs from a perfectly parallel pencil of rays, usually specified in degrees or milliradians.

bear tracks. Unilateral pigmentations on the retina in groups of 4 or 5, like the tracks of a bear, which typically are localized in one sector and not sharply outlined. They are congenital, harmless, and sometimes falsely called nevoid pigmentation.

Bechterew's (bek-ter'yefs) **compensation; disease; nystagmus; reflex.** See under the nouns.

Bechterew-Mendel sign (bek-ter'yef-men'del). See under *sign.*

Becker's (bek'erz) **chart; microscope; phenomenon; sign; system; test.** See under the nouns.

bedewing, corneal (be-du'ing). An edematous condition of the epithelium of the cornea characterized by irregular reflections from a multitude of droplets when viewed with the slit lamp.

Beebe loupe. See under *loupe.*

Beer's law (bārz). See under *law.*

Begbie's disease (beg'bēz). See under *disease.*

Behçet's (beh-shets') **disease; symptom; syndrome.** See under the nouns.

Behr's (bārz) **disease; loupe; phenomenon; sign; syndrome; theory.** See under the nouns.

belladonna (bel″ah-don'ah). The plant *Atropa belladonna*, from the leaves and roots of which may be obtained the poisonous alkaloid precursors of various medically useful narcotics, chief among which is atropine.

Bell's occluder; palsy; paralysis; phenomenon; sign. See under the nouns.

belonoskiascopy (bel″o-no-ski-as'ko-pe). Determination of the refractive error by the elimination of perceived shadow movement when a slender bar or a needle is moved across the front of the eye while a distant point of light is fixated.

bench, optical. An elongated support usually consisting of a horizontal bar or pair of bars which rest on pedestals and on which sliding or clamped supports can be mounted for holding the components and auxiliary apparatus of an optical system or assembly such as lenses, mirrors, prisms, screens, light sources, and other objects. Frequently, the bars are graduated for measuring distances between components.

bend, Kohlrausch's. The transition point in the two segment curve of dark adaptation, representing a shift from cone adaptation to rod adaptation as the eye becomes increasingly dark adapted.

Bender's test (ben'derz). See under *test.*

Benedikt's syndrome (ben'e-dikts). See under *syndrome.*

Benham's (ben'amz) **disk; top.** See under *top.*

benign (be-nīn'). Applied to tumors; nonfatal unless in a vital organ; nonmalignant, innocent, tending to be localized or encapsulated.

benoxinate (ben-ok'sih-nāt). A topical corneal anesthetic having similar time of onset and duration of action as *proparacaine* or *tetracaine.* Generally available in a 0.4% solution and used for applanation tonometry under the trade name *Fluress* when combined with 0.25% sodium fluorescein.

Benson's disease (ben'sunz). Asteroid hyalosis.

Benton right-left discrimination test (ben'tun). See under *test.*

benzalkonium chloride (ben"zal-ko'ne-um). A detergent acting on the walls of bacteria used for the preservation of eye drops and for sterilization of instruments. With prior instillation it is known to enhance corneal penetration of certain ophthalmic drugs.

benzene ring schema. Any one of several mnemonics, invented by Pascal, and resembling the conventional benzene ring of chemistry, used to represent such functions as the interrelationships of the cardinal optical points, extraocular muscle actions, etc.

Béraud's valve (ba-rōz'). Valve of Krause.

Berens (ber'ens) **chart; test.** See under *chart.*

Berens-Tolman Ocular Hypertension Indicator (ber'ens-tōl'man). See under *indicator.*

Berger's (ber'gerz) **loupe; sign; postlenticular space.** See under the nouns.

Bergmeister's papilla (berg'mi-stirz). See under *papilla.*

Berlin's (ber'linz) **disease; edema; opacity.** See under the nouns.

Bernard's syndrome (ber-narz'). See under *syndrome.*

Bernard-Horner syndrome (ber-nar'hōr'ner). Horner's syndrome.

Bernell Tranaglyphs. Trade name of a variety of training and test targets similar to anaglyphs, consisting of various red and green details on transparencies to be viewed in combination with a red filter in front of one eye and a green filter in front of the other.

Berry's circles (ber'ēz). See under *circle.*

Berson device (bur'sun). See under *device.*

Bertrand lens. Amici-Bertrand lens. See under *lens.*

besiclometer (bes-e-klom'eh-ter). An instrument for measuring the forehead to determine the proper width of spectacle frames.

Besnier-Boeck disease (bes-ne-a'-bek). Sarcoidosis.

Besnier-Boeck-Schaumann disease (bes-ne-a'-bek-shaw'man). Sarcoidosis.

Best's disease. See under *disease.*

beta (β) (ba'tah). The Greek letter used as the symbol for (1) *angle beta;* (2) *beta movement.*

Beta Sigma Kappa. An international optometric honorary fraternity, founded in 1925 to provide membership, titles, awards, and honors for achievements in optometry.

Better Vision Institute. A nonprofit corporation supported by and representing subscribing ophthalmic manufacturers, distributors, ophthalmologists, optometrists, and dispensing opticians. Its main function is to provide speakers and educational literature, displays, movies, etc., concerning matters of eye care which are of direct interest to the public.

Betts's reading readiness charts. See under *chart.*

Betz's cells (betsz). See under *cell.*

bevel. 1. The V-shaped edge of a lens to be inserted in a frame. 2. To shape the edge of a lens to a V-shape. 3. The most peripheral curve on the posterior surface of a contact lens, usually narrow in width and of a radius considerably longer than that of the base curve. 4. A taper at the edge of a contact lens on the anterior surface to contour the edge and reduce its thickness. 5. To cut a taper or curve at the edge of a contact lens.

CN b. A taper at the periphery of the anterior surface of a contact lens to reduce edge thickness.

safety b. A slight flattening or rounding out of the otherwise sharp corners at the edge of a rimless spectacle lens.

bezel (bez'el). The grooved rim or flange of the spectacle frame or eye wire in which a lens is set.

Bezold spreading effect (ba'zold). See under *effect, spreading.*

Bezold-Brücke phenomenon (ba'-zold-bre'keh). See under *phenomenon.*

BFP. Binocular fixation pattern.

BI. Abbreviation for *base-in (prism).*

BIO. See *Bundesinnung der Optiker.*

Bianchi's valve (be-ang'kēz). Plica lacrimalis.

biastigmatism (bi"ah-stig'mah-tizm). A condition of the eye in which corneal and lenticular astigmatism coexist.

bicentric (bi-sen'trik). Pertaining to or having two optical centers.

Bickel-Bing-Harboe syndrome (bik'el-bing-har'bo). See under *syndrome.*

biconcave (bi-kon'kāv). As applied to lenses, having two concave surfaces on opposite faces.

biconvex (bi-kon'veks). As applied to lenses, having two convex surfaces on opposite faces.

bicylinder (bi-sil'in-der). See *lens, bicylindrical.*

Bidwell's experiment (bid'welz). See under *experiment.*

Bidwell's ghost (bid'welz). Second positive afterimage.

Biedl's (be'dlz) **disease; syndrome.** See under the nouns.

Bielschowsky's (be-el-show'skēz) **heterophorometer; phenomenon; sign; test.** See under the nouns.

Bielschowsky-Jansky disease (be-el-show'ske-yan'ske). See under *disease.*

Bielschowsky-Lutz-Cogan syndrome (be-el-show'ske-luts-ko'gan). Anterior internuclear ophthalmoplegia. See under *ophthalmoplegia.*

Biemond's syndrome (be'munz). Laurence-Moon-Biedl syndrome.

Bier contact lens (bēr). See under *lens, contact.*

Bietti's (be-et'ēz) **corneal dystrophy; lens.** See under the nouns.

bifixation (bi"fik-sa'shun). The fixation of a single object by both eyes simultaneously so that the image on each retina is on the fovea.

bifocal (bi-fo'kal). 1. Pertaining to a lens system having two focal lengths. 2. A bifocal lens.

bifocals, rising front. See *rising front spectacles.*

bilateral (bi-lat'er-al). Affecting or pertaining to both sides or halves of the body with reference to the midsagittal plane.

Billet's split lens (bil'ets). See under *lens.*

Binkhorst (bink'hōrst) **formula; implant; lens.** See under the nouns.

Binkhorst-Weinstein-Troutman lens (bink'hōrst-wīn'stīn-trawt'man). See under *lens.*

binocular (bin-ok'u-lar, bi-nok'u-). 1. Pertaining to both eyes. 2. The use of both eyes simultaneously in such a manner that each retinal image contributes to the final percept.

binocular balance; contrast; flicker; fusion; imbalance; instability; color mixture; parallax; rivalry; summation; vision. See under the nouns.

binoculars (bin-ok'u-larz, bi-nok'-). A double telescope, one for each eye; field glasses.

prism b. Binoculars equipped with Porro prisms to lengthen the light path in short telescope tubes.

binoculus (bin-ok'u-lus). 1. Cyclopean eye. 2. A figure eight bandage covering both eyes. Syn., *oculus duplex.*

binophthalmoscope (bin"of-thal'mo-skōp). Binocular ophthalmoscope.

binoscope (bin'o-skōp). A visual training instrument employed especially in correcting strabismus, in which both foveae may be simultaneously stimulated by one object.

biocular (bi-ok'u-lar). 1. Pertaining to two eyes, but not implying a paired function of two eyes as does *binocular.* 2. Bioptic.

bioluminescence (bi"o-lu"mih-nes'ens). The emission of light by living organisms such as the firefly, certain mollusks, beetles, fish, bacteria, fungi, and protozoa.

Biometer, van der Heijde (bi-om'eh-ter). A circular slide rule based upon the van der Heijde formula to determine the power of an intraocular implant to replace the crystalline lens after cataract surgery.

biometry (bi-om'eh-tre). The branch of statistics which applies to biological data.

biometry, ocular. Measurement of the eye or its structures.

biomicroscope (bi"o-mi'kro-skōp). An instrument containing a magnifying lens system for examining living tissues of the body, as used with a slit lamp.

Bionite. Trade name for a hydrophilic material of which contact lenses are made.

biophotogenesis (bi"o-fo"to-jen'e-sis). The production of bioluminescence.

biophotometer (bi"o-fo-tom'eh-ter). An instrument for measuring the rate and degree of dark adaptation.

bioptic (bi-op'tik). 1. Pertaining to a single optical system or aperture which permits simultaneous viewing by both eyes. 2. Pertaining to a combination of optical systems or lenses in a singly mounted unit to provide two foci or two viewing areas, such as in a *Bioptic telescopic lens.*

Bioptic lens (bi-op'tik). See under *lens.*

Bioptor (bi-op'tor). A trade name for a Brewster type stereoscope for vision skills testing and training.

biphakia (bi-fa'ke-ah). A rare congenital anomaly in which two crystalline lenses are present in an eye.

biorbital (bi-ōr'bih-tal). Pertaining to or affecting both orbits.

biprism, Fresnel's (bi'prizm). An optical device for obtaining two virtual, coherent sources of light which are very close together, consisting of a piece of optical glass, about two inches square, optically flat on one side and ground and polished on the other side to form two prisms of very small refracting angle, set base to base. It is used to form interference fringes from monochromatic light coming from a narrow slit.

birefractive (bi"re-frak'tiv). Birefringent.

birefringence (bi"re-frin'jens). The property of nonisotropic media, such as crystals, whereby a single incident beam of light traverses the medium as two beams, each plane-polarized, the planes being at right angles to each other. One beam, the ordinary, obeys Snell's law; the other, the extraordinary, does not. Along the optical axis the two beams travel at the same speed;

in other directions the extraordinary beam travels at different speeds. Syn., *double refraction.*

  allogyric b. A difference of velocity of right and left circularly polarized light.

  circular b. Birefringence in which the right circularly polarized light travels at a different velocity than that of the left circularly polarized light.

  electro-optical b. Kerr electro-optic effect.

  Faraday b. The difference of index of refraction of a medium in a magnetic field for right and left circularly polarized light.

  stress b. Birefringence induced by stress in the medium.

birefringent (bi"re-frin'jent). Having the property of birefringence. Syn., *birefractive.*

Birren's constant hue triangle (bēr'enz). See under *triangle.*

Bishop Harman (bish'up har'man) **magnifier; diaphragm test.** See under the nouns.

bispherical (bi-sfēr'ih-kal). As applied to lenses, spherical on both sides.

Bitot's spots (be'tōz). See under *spot.*

Bjerrum's screen (byer'oomz). Tangent screen.

Bjerrum's (byer'oomz) **scotoma; scotometer; sign; test types.** See under the nouns.

black. 1. An achromatic color of minimum lightness or maximum darkness representing one limit of the series of grays. The complement or opposite of white. 2. A visual sensation, arising from some portion of a luminous field which is of extremely low luminosity. Though typically a response to zero or minimal stimulation, black appears always to depend upon contrast.

Black bifocal contact lens. See under *lens, contact, bifocal.*

blackbody. A thermal source of radiant energy, or temperature radiator, whose radiant flux in all parts of the spectrum is the maximum obtainable from any such source at the same temperature. Such a radiator is called a blackbody because it will absorb all the radiant energy that falls on it. All other temperature radiators may be classed as nonblackbodies. They radiate less in some or all wavelength intervals than a blackbody of the same size and the same temperature. Syn., *complete radiator; ideal radiator; Planckian radiator; standard radiator; total radiator.*

black-eye. Ecchymosis of the eyelid.

blackness. 1. A positive perceptual attribute of any surface or part thereof which has lower reflectance than its surroundings. Blackness is "induced" by the brighter surround. When the reflectance of a spot and surround differ sufficiently, the spot is accepted as "black." The color of any "dark" object has a content of blackness which leaves it if the object is spotlighted in a lightless surround. This converts the surface color to a film color having a brightness aspect but no lightness-darkness aspect. Conversely, a patch of colored light projected on a screen is invaded by blackness and converted to an object color if the patch is surrounded by an annulus of white light much brighter than the patch. 2. The degree of approach to that extreme or limit of the series of grays known as *black.* 3. Suggesting *black,* e.g., the shade of a color.

blackout. Loss of central vision due to positive gravitational acceleration; attributed to restriction of blood supply to the eye. It occurs at 4.7 ± 0.8 g to unprotected subjects seated upright. Cf. *grayout; redout.*

Blackowski's experiment (blah-kof'skēz). See under *experiment.*

blank. 1. A piece of glass pressed, while hot, into its approximate finished shape and thickness so that it can be fabricated later into a lens, prism, or mirror. 2. A plastic disk, cut from a rod or flat sheet, from which a contact lens is fabricated.

 dropped b. A glass blank shaped by heating it and allowing it to settle into a curved former.

 fused b. A blank for the preparation of a fused multifocal lens at the stage when the contact surfaces have been ground and polished and fused together.

 semifinished b. A blank, one side of which has been completely finished, that is, ground and polished to desired curvature specifications.

blanking, perceptual. The phenomenon of obliteration of the perception of tachistoscopically presented information by a subsequently presented brief flash of light.

blastomycosis (blas"to-mi-ko'sis). A fungus disease caused by yeast-like organisms that attack skin, eyelids, or lungs. Rarely, the uvea may be affected. Actually, the organism is a related *Monilia* yeast and not a true *Blastomyces.*

Blaxter's test (blax'ters). Bulbar pressure test.

blaze. In a diffraction grating, the shape of the groove, or the angle of the flatter side of the groove, so designed as to concentrate most or almost all of the reflected or transmitted radiant energy into a single spectral order, as, for example, in the *echelette diffraction grating.*

Blegvad-Haxthausen syndrome. See under *syndrome.*

blend, color. A color perceived as a composite of two adjacent colors in the color circle, e.g., purple is red-blue, or aquamarine is blue-green. Cf. *color fusion.*

blending. 1. A gradual or imperceptible change from one color to another. 2. The process of fusion, that is, the undifferentiated product of intermittent or multiple stimulation. 3. The removal of the sharp junction formed between curves of unlike radii on the surface of a contact lens, usually by polishing with a tool having an intermediate radius.

blennophthalmia (blen"of-thal'me-ah). Catarrhal conjunctivitis.

blennorrhagia ocularis (blen"o-ra'je-ah ok'u-lar"is). 1. A particularly profuse blennorrhea. 2. Gonococcal conjunctivitis.

blennorrhea (blen"o-re'ah). A general term including any inflammatory process of the external eye which gives a mucoid discharge. More exactly, a discharge of mucus; popularly, purulent discharges from a variety of etiological factors, bacterial, allergic, and physical.

 inclusion b. A specific type of conjunctivitis, occurring chiefly in the newborn, caused by a virus which produces a follicular response of a hyperemic conjunctiva with intracellular inclusion bodies. Characteristically, it gives preauricular adenopathy and is supposedly transmitted via the genital system. In the adult it is usually called *swimming pool conjunctivitis.* Syn., *paratrachoma.*

 b. neonatorum. Any blennorrhea of the newborn; usually meant to describe ophthalmia neonatorum or gonorrheal neonatorum; often confused with *inclusion blennorrhea*.

blephar- (blef′ar-). A combining form denoting the eyelid.

blephara (blef′ah-rah). The eyelids.

blepharadenitis (blef″ar-ad″e-ni′tis). Inflammation of the glands of the eyelids. Although usually referring to involvement of the Meibomian gland, it may also apply to the marginal glands of Moll or Zeis.

blepharal (blef′ah-ral). Pertaining or relating to the eyelids.

blepharectomy (blef″ah-rek′to-me). Excision of all or part of an eyelid.

blepharedema (blef″ar-e-de′mah). An abnormal collection of excess watery fluid in the tissue spaces of the eyelid which produces a swelling and, often, a baggy appearance.

blepharelosis (blef″ah-rel-o′sis). Entropion.

blepharemphysema (blef′ar-em″fise″mah). An abnormal collection of air in the tissues of the eyelid which produces a crackling sensation of the eyelids when palpated, usually caused by a communication between the sinuses and the orbital tissues through a defect in the bone wall.

blepharis (blef′ah-ris). An eyelash. *Obs.*

blepharism (blef′ah-rizm). Rapid involuntary winking due to spasm of the orbicularis oculi muscle.

blepharitis (blef′ah-ri′tis). Any inflammation of the eyelid without reference to any particular part of the eyelid, but commonly meaning the margin. Syn., *blepharophlegmasia; palpebritis.*

  b. acarica. Inflammation of the eyelid margin caused by an acarid or a mite. Syn., *demodectic blepharitis.*

  b. angularis. Inflammation of the margins of the eyelids involving especially the canthi laterally, less so medially; it is caused by the diplobacillus of Morax-Axenfeld. A slight maceration sometimes extends over the skin of the lateral canthus.

  b. ciliaris. 1. Blepharitis marginalis. 2. Inflammation of the root of a cilium on the eyelid margin, producing a small abscess called a sty or a hordeolum.

  demodectic b. Blepharitis acarica.

  furunculous b. An acute and severe staphylococcal infection of an eyelid in which cellulitis and purulent inflammation involve the glands associated with the follicles.

  b. gangraenosa. A circumscribed, deep-seated, suppurative inflammation of the subcutaneous tissue of the eyelid discharging pus from several points.

  hypertrophic b. A condition in which the eyelid margins are hypertrophied, rounded, and thickened as a sequela to inflammation, and droop because of their own weight. Syn., *tylosis.*

  b. marginalis. A common chronic inflammation of the eyelid margin, usually bilateral and accompanied by crusts or scales, characteristically caused by a staphylococcus infection, although it may be due to various organisms or allergies. Syn., *blepharitis ciliaris; blepharitis simplex; psorophthalmia.*

  mycotic b. Inflammation of the eyelid resulting from a fungus infection. Syn., *tinea tarsi.*

  b. oleosa. A form of blepharitis squamosa in which a yellow, waxy crust forms about the bases of the cilia.

  b. pediculosa. Inflammation of the eyelids due to infestation with pediculi or lice on the shafts of the cilia.

  rosacea b. Inflammation and scaling of the eyelid margins, with frequent chalazia, occasionally accompanying acne rosacea of the skin of the face.

  b. sicca. Blepharitis squamosa.

  b. simplex. Blepharitis marginalis.

  b. squamosa. A scaling or crusting of the eyelid margins commonly caused by a bacterial infection, usually staphylococcus or diplobacillus, but may be seborrheic. Removal of the scales does not leave, characteristically, an ulcerated base. Syn., *blepharitis sicca.*

  sudoriparous b. An acute or subacute infection of the glands of Moll associated with generalized infection of the ciliary border characterized by minute, red, inflammatory papules along the ciliary border which develop rapidly and usually disappear without suppuration or ulceration.

  sycotic b. Inflammation of the eyelid margins accompanied by an infection of the hair follicles of the eyelashes. The condition is usually recurrent and may result in permanent loss of the eyelashes.

ulcerative b. Inflammation of the eyelid margins producing numerous small ulcers which may be covered by crusts, generally caused by a staphylococcus infection.

vaccinial b. An accidental infection of the eyelids with the vaccinia virus, occurring only on the eyelid margins as a widespread ulceration which tends to spread over the palpebral conjunctiva.

vasomotor b. A common affection in which the eyelid margins are red and slightly swollen, giving the appearance of red-rimmed eyes, due to engorgement of the blood vessels.

blepharo- (blef′ah-ro). A combining form denoting the *eyelid.*

blepharo-adenitis (blef″ah-ro-ad″e-ni′tis). Blepharadenitis.

blepharo-adenoma (blef″ah-ro-ad″e-no′mah). Adenoma of the eyelid.

blepharo-atheroma (blef′ah-ro-ath″er-o′mah). An encysted tumor in the eyelid, such as a sebaceous cyst.

blepharoblennorrhea (blef″ah-ro-blen′o-re-ah). Conjunctivitis with a profuse purulent discharge.

blepharochalasis (blef′ah-ro-kal′ah-sis). Atrophy of the skin of the upper eyelids, usually bilateral and equal, following chronic or recurrent edematous swellings of the upper eyelids; characterized in its later stages by loose folds of wrinkled and venuled skin overhanging the upper eyelid margin. Syn., *ptosis atrophica.*

blepharochromidrosis (blef′ah-ro-kro″mid-ro′sis). A condition in which colored sweat, usually bluish, is excreted from the eyelids.

blepharocleisis (blef′ah-ro-kli′sis). Ankyloblepharon.

blepharoclonus (blef′ah-ro-klo′nus). A spasm of the muscles that close the eye.

blepharocoloboma (blef″ah-ro-kol′o-bo′mah). A notch- or cleft-shaped coloboma of the eyelid.

blepharoconjunctivitis (blef′ah-ro-kon-junk″tih-vi′tis). Inflammation of both the conjunctiva and the eyelids.

b. rosacea. Inflammation of the eyelids and the conjunctiva occurring in most cases of ocular rosacea, characterized by a desquamation of the eyelid margins and either a diffuse hyperemia of the conjunctiva or a nodular conjunctivitis.

blepharodenitis (blef′ah-ro-de-ni′tis). Blepharadenitis.

blepharodermachalasis (blef′ah-ro-der″mah-kal′ah-sis). Blepharochalasis.

blepharodermatitis (blef″ah-ro-der″mah-ti′tis). Inflammation of the skin of the eyelids.

blepharodiastasis (blef″ah-ro-di-as′-tah-sis). 1. A condition in which the eyelids cannot be completely closed. 2. Excessive separation of the eyelids.

blepharodyschroia (blef″ah-ro-dis-kroy′ah). Discoloration of the eyelid, as from a nevus.

blepharoedema (blef″ah-ro-e-de′mah). Blepharedema.

blepharolithiasis (blef′ah-ro-li-thi′ah-sis). A condition in which chalky concretions are formed in or on the eyelid.

blepharomelasma (blef″ah-ro-me-las′mah). A condition of excessive secretion of the sebaceous glands of the eyelids, resulting in a dark, oily appearance.

blepharomelena (blef′ah-ro-meh-le′-nah). The secretion of blue or black sweat, a rarity characterized by the appearance of blue-black spots on the eyelids, preferentially the lower, although all four eyelids may be affected, and only rarely does the condition spread to the nose and face.

blepharon (blef′ah-ron). The eyelid.

blepharoncus (blef-ah-rong′kus). A tumor of the eyelid.

blepharopachynsis (blef″ah-ro-pah-kin′sis). A pathological thickening of an eyelid.

blepharophimosis (blef′ah-ro-fi-mo′-sis). A condition in which the palpebral aperture is abnormally small.

blepharophlegmasia (blef″ah-ro-fleg-ma′zhe-ah). Blepharitis.

blepharophryplasty (blef′ah-rof′re-plas″te). Plastic surgery of the eyelid and/or eyebrow.

blepharophyma (blef″ah-ro-fi′mah). A tumor of the eyelid.

blepharoplasty (blef″ah-ro-plas′te). Plastic surgery of the eyelid.

blepharoplegia (blef′ah-ro-ple′je-ah). Paralysis of an eyelid.

blepharoptosis (blef″ah-ro-to′sis). Drooping of an upper eyelid. Syn., *ptosis.*

blepharopyorrhea (blef′ah-ro-pi″o-re′ah). A purulent discharge from the eyelid; purulent ophthalmia.

blepharorrhaphy (blef′ah-ror′ah-fe). 1. The suturing of a lacerated eyelid. 2. Tarsorrhaphy.

blepharorrhoea (blef″ah-roh-re′ah). Blepharopyorrhea.

blepharosis (blef″ar-o′sis). A degenerative condition of the eyelids, to be distinguished from blepharitis.

blepharospasm (blef′ah-ro-spazm″). Excessive winking; tonic or clonic spasm of the orbicularis oculi muscle.

clonic b. Blepharospasm in which there is a twitching or vibratory movement within the eyelid.

essential b. Tonic blepharospasm occurring in the hysterical or the elderly.

symptomatic b. Tonic blepharospasm occurring in conjunction with ocular pathology (particularly that of the anterior portion of the eye), albinism, chorea, or tetanus.

tonic b. Blepharospasm in which there is a convulsive closure of the eyelids.

blepharosphincterectomy (blef″-ah-ro-sfing″ter-ek′to-me). Surgical removal of fibers of the orbicularis oculi muscle, together with the overlying skin, to lessen the pressure of the upper eyelid on the cornea.

blepharostat (blef′ah-ro-stat″). An instrument for holding the eyelids apart. Cf. *eye speculum.*

blepharostenosis (blef′ah-ro-ste-no′-sis). A pathological narrowing of the palpebral aperture.

blepharosymphysis (blef′ah-ro-sim′-fih-sis). Blepharosynechia.

blepharosynechia (blef′ah-ro-si-nek′-e-ah). An adhesion of the eyelids. Syn., *blepharosymphysis.*

blepharotomy (blef″ah-rot′o-me). Surgical incision of the eyelid.

blepsopathia (blep″so-path′e-ah). Eyestrain. *Obs.*

blepsopathy (blep-sop′ath-e). Eyestrain. *Obs.*

Blessig's (bles′igz) **cysts; groove.** See under the nouns.

blind. Wholly or partially unable to see; *amaurotic.*

◆

BLINDNESS

blindness. The inability to see; absence or severe reduction of vision. Syn., *amaurosis.*

absolute b. Total blindness; complete amaurosis.

apperceptive b. A kind of blindness presumed to be of cortical or functional origin in which patterns in, or attributes of, the observed field of view cannot be grasped or perceived as structural or otherwise organized entities.

blue b. A form of partial color blindness or dichromatism characterized by the inability to distinguish the color blue; *tritanopia.*

blue-yellow b. A rare type of dichromatic vision about which detailed information is lacking, but in which the relative luminosity of blue stimuli is believed to be much less than normal, leading to confusion of blues with dark shades of other colors. Also, a neutral point occurs in the yellow region of the spectrum, leading to the confusion of yellow with other desaturated colors. See also *tritanopia* and *tetartanopsia.*

Bright's b. Partial or total loss of vision associated with uremia.

cerebral b. Visual agnosia.

color b. A misleading, but commonly used, term which includes all forms of defective color vision, however mild or severe. Usually a sex-linked hereditary defect, color blindness occurs in about 8% of all males and 0.4% of all females. See also *achromatism; deuteranomaly; deuteranopia; dichromatism; protanomaly; protanopia; anomalous trichromatism; tritanomaly; tritanopia.* **amnesic c.b.** Color agnosia. **partial c.b.** Any form of defective color vision except total color blindness, thus including the various types of dichromatism and anomalous trichromatism. **total c.b.** A rare form of defective vision, either congenital or acquired, characterized by total inability to discriminate any of the ordinarily differentiated hues. Presumably all hues are seen as varying shades of gray, black, or white. The condition is usually believed to be due to total absence, or inactivation, of the cones in the retina, since the photopic relative spectral sensitivity of affected individuals appears identical to that of the normal scotopic relative spectral sensitivity, no Purkinje shift is observable, and dark adaptation ordinarily shows no transitional change from cone to rod vision. The condition is typically accompanied by lowered visual acuity, nystagmus, and photophobia. Syn., *achromatism; achromatopsia; monochromatism; achromatic vision.*

concussion b. Functional blindness caused by the shock of an explosion, as from a bomb or a shell.

congenital b. Absence of vision from the time of birth.

cortical b. Total loss of vision in all or part of the visual field due to a lesion in the striate area, characterized by the patient's subjective unawareness of his disability and the absence of cortical functions of vision, with the subcortical functions intact. Syn., *mind blindness.*

cortical psychic b. Visual agnosia.

Craik's b. A temporary loss of vision produced by external pressure on the eyeball.

day b. Reduced vision in daylight or in comparable illumination associated with normal, or relatively better, vision in dim light, variously synonymous with *nyctalopia* and *hemeralopia.*

desert b. Partial or complete loss of vision, usually temporary, caused by excessive exposure to brilliant sunlight reflected from the desert sands.

eclipse b. Partial or complete loss of central vision due to a foveal lesion caused by direct fixation of the sun, as in viewing a partial eclipse.

economic b. Industrial blindness.

educational b. A degree of blindness, specifically referring to school children, necessitating special teaching facilities and methods. That loss of vision defined by statutory, or other, provisions which is necessary for admittance to sight-saving or to similar special educational classes. Syn., *pedagogical blindness.*

electric light b. Dimness of vision due to prolonged exposure to intense electric illumination.

flash b. Visual loss during and following exposure to a light flash of extremely high intensity.

flight b. Amaurosis fugax.

functional b. Loss of vision not due to an organic cause; considered to be of psychogenic origin with the visual mechanism intact.

green b. A form of dichromatic vision in which the relative spectral luminosity does not differ noticeably from normal, but in which the only hues seen are blue and yellow (as reported by unilateral deuteranopes) and all colors can be matched by a mixture of blue and yellow stimuli. A neutral point occurs at about 497 mμ. Light of shorter wavelengths appears blue, of longer wavelengths, yellow, with saturation increasing to the ends of the spectrum. A sex-linked hereditary defect, it occurs in about 1% of all males and 0.01% of all females. Syn., *achloropsia; aglaucopsia; deuteranopia.*

hysterical b. Functional blindness associated with, or characterized by, hysteria.

industrial b. Loss of vision considered necessary to render a worker unable to compete or perform normally in industry. The degree of loss is usually defined by statute, industrial commissions, or insurance provisions, to be 20/200 or less, though various criteria apply. Cf. *educational, occupational,* and *vocational blindness;* also *visual efficiency.*

lactation b. Reduced vision of a mother during the time her child is a suckling.

legal b. Such degree or type of blindness as is defined in, or recognized by, the statutes to constitute blindness.

letter b. A type of aphasia in which individual letters are seen but have no meaning.

methyl-alcohol b. Loss of vision resulting from the consumption of methyl alcohol.

mind b. Cortical blindness.

moon b. Reduced vision, superstitiously said to be caused by exposure to the moon's rays during sleep.

negative b. Total loss of vision in all or part of the visual field which is not recognized subjectively by the affected individual. See also *cortical blindness.*

night b. Abnormal or complete loss of vision in dim light, characteristically associated with loss of rod function, variously synonymous with *nyctalopia* and *hemeralopia.*

note b. Alexia in which musical notes cannot be read.

object b. Object visual agnosia.

occupational b. Blindness resulting from occupational disease or as a result of injury from occupational hazards.

organic b. Absence of vision due to an organic cause; differentiated from *psychic* or *functional blindness.*

pedagogical b. Educational blindness.

psychic b. 1. Partial or total loss of vision due to a mental aberration. 2. Visual agnosia.

quinine b. Loss of vision, usually temporary, associated with excessive doses of quinine.

red b. A form of partial color blindness or dichromatism characterized by the inability to distinguish the color red; protanopia. Syn., *aneryth-ropsia*.

red-green b. 1. A general term for the most common types of defective color vision; it includes *protanopia* and *deuteranopia* as well as *protanomaly* and *deuteranomaly*, since these are not differentially diagnosed by means of pseudo-isochromatic charts or the various yarn tests or their modifications. 2. According to the Hering theory of color vision, a form of partial color blindness in which red and green cannot be distinguished because of total or partial absence of the red-green photochemical substance in the retina.

river b. Blindness resulting from onchocerciasis, so called because the black fly, *simulium damnosum*, which may deposit tiny infectious parasitic worms into the skin when sucking blood from a human, thrives in fast-moving foamy river water; endemic in the savanna zones of West Africa and occurring also in Yemen and in parts of Central and South America.

simulated b. Feigned inability to see; a type of malingering.

snow b. Partial or complete loss of vision, usually temporary, caused by excessive exposure to brilliant sunlight reflected from snow. Syn., *nivialis ophthalmia*.

soul b. Visual agnosia.

space b. Visual spatial agnosia.

sun b. Partial or total loss of vision, either temporary or permanent, due to overexposure to the rays of the sun.

total b. Complete inability to see; lack of the light sense.

twilight b. Abnormally reduced vision in low levels of illumination, as in twilight. Syn., *aknephascopia*.

violet b. Partial color blindness characterized by reduced sensitivity to violet or the confusion of violet with other hues; considered by some to be

the same as *blue blindness* or *tritanopia*. Syn., *anianthinopsy*.

vocational b. Such degree or type of blindness as to prevent the continued pursuit of the vocation for which one is trained or otherwise qualified.

water b. Partial or complete loss of vision, usually temporary, caused by excessive exposure to brilliant sunlight reflected from water.

word b. A type of aphasia in which there is an inability to recognize or comprehend written or printed words. Syn., *alexia*.

yellow b. A rare type of dichromatic vision which occurs only as *blue-yellow blindness (tritanopia, tetar-tanopia)*. A neutral point occurring in the yellow region of the spectrum in this form of dichromatism leads to confusion of yellows with light tints of other hues.

◆

blink. 1. A momentary closure of the upper and lower eyelids. 2. To close the eyelids momentarily.

blinking. 1. The brief closing of the eyelids; winking. Blinking usually applies binocularly; winking, monocularly. 2. Flashing (of a light) on and off.

Bloch's law (bloks). See under *law*.

Bloch-Sulzberger syndrome (blok-sulz'ber-ger). See under *syndrome*.

block. A tool, or part of a jig, usually a solid piece of iron, to which a lens (or lenses) is cemented or clamped during the grinding and polishing operations. Syn., *body*.

block, pupillary. A closure of the pupil which prevents the flow of aqueous humor from the posterior to the anterior chamber, as may occur in iridocyclitis from annular synechiae, in spherophakia from bulging forward of the small lens into the pupil, or in surgical aphakia from iridic adhesions to residual lens or capsule substance or to the vitreous.

blocking. The fastening or cementing of blanks or partially fabricated lenses to metal tools for grinding or polishing. The cementing agent is usually pitch.

blondel (blon-del'). A unit of luminance equal to $1/10$ millilambert; an apostilb.

Blondel-Ray law (blon-del'ra). See under *law*.

bloom. 1. An antireflection film. 2. A tarnish of a lens surface as a result of chemical action from exposure to the atmosphere.

blooming. The process of depositing a very thin film of a transparent substance on the surface of glass to create interference of light rays striking the surface, in order to prevent or reduce reflection. By varying the thickness of the film the reflection of specific wavelengths may be eliminated. Lenses so treated are referred to as *coated.*

blue. 1. The hue attribute of visual sensations typically evoked by stimulation of the normal human eye with radiation of wavelengths approximately 476 mμ. 2. Any hue predominantly similar to that of the typical blue. 3. One of the psychologically unique colors. 4. The complement of yellow.

blue arc; spike. See under the nouns.

blue sclerotic (blu′ skle-rot′ik). See under *sclerotic.*

blue-sighted. Displaying an abnormally high color sensitivity to blue. Congenital or acquired, the condition may occur alone or in combination with other defects of color vision (perhaps as a consequence of these other defects).

Blumenfeld alleys (bloo′men-feld). See under *alley.*

blur. 1. Diffuseness at the borders in any pattern involving lines, points, and areas, the transition across a given border being gradual instead of abrupt, resulting in a vague or indistinct appearance. 2. A form of degradation of an image formed by an optical system in which points, lines, and borders are less sharply or distinctly defined than in the original. It may result from lack of sharp focus, aberrations, diffusion by the scattering surfaces or media near the plane of the image, or by spread of the image in the retina or in a photographic film.

    spectacle b. Reduction in visual acuity experienced with spectacle lenses after the wearing of contact lenses and due to transient alterations in corneal curvature or index of refraction.

blur-image. An image of less than optimal quality for which the optically reproduced counterparts of sharp object borders are diffuse or gradientlike, variously due to out-of-focus conditions, refractive errors, vibrations, light scattering, diffraction, and optical aberrations.

blur-point. See under *point.*

BOA. See *British Optical Association.*

Board, Posture, Brock's. See under *Posture Board.*

bobbing, ocular. A motor anomaly characterized by a periodic downward movement of the eyes of a comatose person with pontine disease.

Boberg-Ans (bo′berg-ans). **implant; sensibilitometer; test.** See under the nouns.

Bochdalek's valve (bok′dal-eks). See under *valve.*

Bochenek's (bo-hen′eks) **anterior accessory optic bundle; anterior accessory fasciculus; anterior accessory optic tract.** See *tract, optic, anterior accessory, of Bochenek.*

Bodal's test (bo′dalz). See under *test.*

Boder-Sedgwick syndrome (bo′der-sedj′wik). See under *syndrome.*

body. 1. A mass of matter distinct from other masses. 2. The physical structure of a man or an animal. 3. The largest and primarily central part of a structure. 4. A block used in lens grinding.

    amyloid b's. Microscopic, round, hyaline bodies occurring as a degenerative change in the prostate, meninges, lungs, and occasionally in the nerve fiber layer of the retina and the optic nerve head. Syn., *corpora amylacea.*

    asteroid b's. Small, discrete, disk-shaped or spherical bodies in the vitreous humor in asteroid hyalitis. Syn., *nivea; scintillatis albescens.*

    bigeminal b. The tectum of the midbrain in lower vertebrates receiving optic and spinotectal fibers and acting as a visual input and output center. In amphibia and in higher animals having hearing, it is replaced with a quadrigeminal body with superior and inferior colliculi.

    ciliary b. The part of the uvea or vascular tunic, anterior to the ora serrata between the iris and the choroid, with the sclera outside and the vitreous and the posterior chamber inside. A longitudinal section is approximately the shape of a triangle, the outer side of which is formed by the ciliary muscle; the anterior portion of the inner side (pars plicata) includes the ciliary processes (corona ciliaris), and the posterior portion (pars plana or orbiculus ciliaris) is smooth.

    colloid b's. Drusen.

    cytoid b's. Sharply defined, shiny, white spots in the retina, due to localized degeneration of the nerve fibers. Syn., *Cajal's nodes.*

Elschnig b's. Rounded or oval, transparent globules, each formed by a swollen and vacuolated epithelial cell, in the remains of the capsule of the crystalline lens following extracapsular cataract extraction. They usually occur in grapelike clusters. Syn., *globular cells of Elschnig; Elschnig pearls.*

geniculate b's., external. Ovoid protuberances lateral to the pulvinar of each thalamus in the diencephalon of the forebrain. They are one of the lower or primary visual centers, consisting of alternating white and gray areas. The white areas are formed by the medullated fibers of the optic tract, the gray areas are the nuclei in which these terminate and from which arises a new relay of visual fibers which form the optic radiations. The geniculate bodies also contain fibers which pass through without synapsing and go to the surface of the pulvinar and thence to the superior colliculus.

geniculate b's., internal. Bilateral protuberances below the pulvinar of the thalamus and medial to the lateral geniculate bodies in the diencephalon of the forebrain which function as a relay station for the auditory pathway to the temporal lobes.

geniculate b's., lateral. External geniculate bodies.

geniculate b's., medial. Internal geniculate bodies.

Hassall-Henle b's. Rounded wartlike elevations of the posterior surface of Descemet's membrane at the periphery of the cornea which tend to increase in old age. Syn., *Hassall-Henle warts.*

Henle's b's. Hassall-Henle bodies.

hyaline b's. Drusen.

hyaloid b. Vitreous body.

pineal b. An unpaired protuberance from the roof of the diencephalon of the forebrain which suggests a rudimentary midsagittal eye. It is often listed with the endocrine system, but it forms no known hormone. Syn., *epiphysis cerebri.*

quadrigeminal b. Corpora quadrigemina.

vitreous b. A noncellular, transparent, colorless gel filling the posterior $^4/_5$ of the eyeball between the retina and the crystalline lens. It is sphere-shaped with an anterior concave depression, the patellar fossa. The hyaloid canal, which in the fetus carries the hyaloid artery, traverses it centrally from the optic disk to the patellar fossa. It is adherent at the optic disk, more firmly to the ciliary epithelium adjacent to the ora serrata, less firmly to the capsule of the crystalline lens. Syn., *hyaloid body.*

Boeck's sarcoid (beks). Sarcoidosis.

Boettcher chart (bet'sher). See under *chart.*

van Bogaert's disease. Subacute sclerosing panencephalitis.

Bogorad syndrome. Crocodile tears syndrome. See under *syndrome.*

bolometer (bo-lom'eh-ter). A very sensitive thermometer for the detection and measurement of radiant energy, especially infrared.

bone. An element or an individual member of the skeleton or the material of which it is composed.

ethmoid b. An unpaired cranial bone which helps form the medial walls of the orbits and contains the ethmoidal air cells which drain into the nose.

frontal b. An unpaired cranial bone which forms the region of the forehead and the greater part of the roofs of the orbits and contains the frontal sinuses, which drain into the nose.

lacrimal b's. Paired facial bones in the medial walls of the orbits which help form the fossa for the lacrimal sac and the nasolacrimal canals.

malar b. Zygomatic bone.

maxillary b's. Paired facial bones which unite to form the upper jaw and help form the floor and medial wall of the orbits and the walls of the nasolacrimal duct. Each contains one of the two large maxillary sinuses.

nasal b's. Paired facial bones, located between the orbits, that form the upper part of the bridge of the nose.

palatine b's. Paired facial bones that help form the hard palate, lateral walls of the nose, and the floor of each orbit.

Soemmering's b. The marginal process of the zygomatic bone.

sphenoid b. An unpaired cranial bone with a body containing the sphenoid sinus and forming the posterior part of the medial walls of the orbits. It has paired great wings found in the lateral walls and paired small wings in the upper orbital walls.

zygomatic b's. Paired facial bones that help form the lateral and lower orbital walls. Syn., *malar bones.*

Bonnet's (bo-nāz') **capsule; syndrome.** See under the nouns.

Bonnet-Cochet law (bo-na'-ko-sha'). See under *law.*

Bonnevie-Ullrich (bon've-ul'rik) **status; syndrome.** See under *status.*

Bonvue (bon'vu). A trade name for a corrected curve series of lenses; also for a flat-top bifocal.

boopia (bo-o'pe-ah). A dazed, dull expression of the eyes in hysterical individuals; an oxlike eye.

border. 1. The outer part, the margin, or the edge of an area or a surface. 2. The boundary between a figure and its background or between two figures in the perceptual field. Borders may interfere with and inhibit each other according to the organization of the perceptual field.

    b. contrast. See under *contrast.*

    posterior zonular b. A ridge, approximately 1.5 mm anterior to the ora serrata on the pars plana of the ciliary body, that gives rise to thick and strong fibers of the suspensory ligaments of the crystalline lens.

    b. tissue of Elschnig. See under *tissue.*

borderline between comfort and discomfort. In psychophysical tests of lighting design, the luminance of one or more eccentrically located light sources in the field of view which are judged to separate the intensity levels deemed comfortable from those deemed uncomfortable. Abbreviation *BCD.*

Bordier-Fränkel sign (bōr-dya'-freng'kel). See under *sign.*

Borish near point test chart. See under *chart.*

BOSA. See *British Optical Students Association.*

Boston's sign (bos'tonz). See under *sign.*

Boström's (bost'remz) **charts; plates; test.** See under the nouns.

Boström-Kugelberg (bos'trem-kōō'-gel-berg) **charts; plates; test.** See under the nouns.

bothrion (both're-on). A deep ulcer of the cornea. *Obs.*

Bouguer's law (boo-garz'). See under *law.*

boundary, purple. The straight line drawn between the ends of the spectrum locus on a chromaticity diagram.

bouquet of central cones of Rochon-Duvigneaud. The group of longest and thinnest cone cells, located in the center of the rod-free area of the fovea, which provide maximal visual acuity.

Bourdon's (boor'donz) **figure; illusion.** See under the nouns.

Bourneville's disease (boor'ne-vēz). See under *disease.*

Bouwers' optical system (bōō'werz). See under *system, optical.*

bow. The sidepiece or temple of a spectacle frame.

Bowen's disease (bo'enz). See under *disease.*

Bowman's (bo'manz) **lamina; layer; membrane; muscle; shadow; tubes.** See under the nouns.

box. A container with four sides, a bottom, and a top, or any similar structure.

    Brock's scotoma b. A small optical instrument for detecting a central scotoma; when the box is properly strapped to the patient's head, and directly in front of the nonamblyopic eye, a 2° transilluminated red disk with a central black fixation dot is superimposed on a small bright spot of white light seen by the other, amblyopic, eye in a dark room. Disappearance of the spot of light indicates a central scotoma. Syn., *projection box.*

    Chauvel's b. A pseudoscope designed to make it difficult to determine with which eye one is observing, thus to detect malingering.

    Fles's b. A pseudoscope used to detect malingering, consisting of a box in which targets located inside the front corners are seen by reflection from two plane mirrors in the rear of the box, set at an obtuse angle with each other. (See Fig. 4.)

    Kühne's optical b. A schematic eye filled with water, having a cornea, an iris, and a crystalline lens of glass.

    Maréchal's b. A pseudoscope used to detect malingering, consisting of a box in which targets on the inside front are seen by reflection from a plane mirror in the rear of the box.

    Maxwell's color b. An instrument for the physical mixing of color, consisting essentially of an L-shaped box containing a mirror, prisms, a lens, three adjustable slits, and a viewing aperture. The three slits allow three

box [76] **Brewster's fringes**

different wavelengths to impinge upon the prisms, so that they are seen superimposed when viewed through the aperture and lens. A mixture of any three colors may be obtained by varying the position of the slits, and the intensity of each color can be varied by adjusting the width of the slits. White light is reflected by the mirror to an area adjacent to the color mixture for comparison.

Prato's b. A pseudoscope used to detect malingering, consisting of a box containing two viewing tubes which cross each other in an *x* pattern.

projection b. Brock's scotoma box.

smoke b. An airtight box with a glass side into which smoke is pumped. It is used to demonstrate the paths of light through lenses, prisms, apertures, and other optical elements.

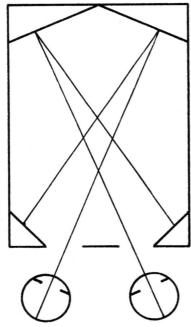

Fig. 4 Fles's box.

Bozzi's foramen (bot'tsēz). Macula lutea. *Obs.*

brachium, superior (bra'ke-um). A bundle of nerve fibers connecting the optic tract to the superior colliculus for photostatic function and to the pretectal nuclei for pupillary reflex activity to light.

brachium tecti (bra'ke-um tek'ti). A bundle of nerve fibers from the ventral nucleus of the lateral geniculate body that synapses in the superior colliculus and may have a photostatic function.

brachydactylia (brak"e-dak-til'e-ah). Extremely short fingers and toes. In one syndrome, it may be inherited along with an abnormally small, spherical crystalline lens. Syn., *brachydactyly.*

brachydactyly (brak"e-dak-til'e). Brachydactylia.

brachymetropia (brak"e-met-ro'pe-ah). Myopia.

brachymetropic (brak"e-me-trop'ik). Myopic.

Bradley's method (brad'lēz). See under *method.*

bradyesthesia (brad"e-es-the'ze-ah). Abnormally slow perception.

bradylexia (brad"e-lek'se-ah). Abnormally slow reading.

bradypsychia (brad"e-si'ke-ah). Abnormally slow mental reaction.

Braid's strabismus (brādz). See under *strabismus.*

Braille (bra'il). A system of printing for blind persons, devised by Louis Braille, in which points raised above the surface of paper are used as symbols to designate the letter of the alphabet. Reading is accomplished through the sense of touch as the fingertips are moved over the points.

Brailsford syndrome (brālz'fōrd). Morquio's disease. See under *disease.*

Brain's syndrome (brānz). See under *syndrome.*

Braley dystrophy (bra'le). See under *dystrophy.*

Branchaud wand (bran'shōd). See under *wand.*

breadth of fusion. See under *fusion.*

break, alpha. Cone-rod break.

break, cone-rod. The point of intersection of the rod and cone dark adaptation curves. Syn., *alpha break.*

Brevet de Technicien Supérieur Opticien-Lunetier. In France, the ministry of education certificate of eligibility to practice ophthalmic optics. Abbreviation *BTSOL.*

brevissimus oculi (breh-vis'ih-mus ok'u-li). Inferior oblique muscle.

Brewster's angle (bru'sterz). Angle of polarization.

Brewster's (bru'sterz) **fringes; law; prisms; stereoscope.** See under the nouns.

bridge. That part of a spectacle front which connects the two eyewires, the lens arms, or the nasal straps. Its name stems from the early type of saddle bridge which rested on the bridge of the nose.

blanked b. A metal spectacle or eyeglass bridge stamped from flat stock.

braced b. 1. The bridge of a plastic spectacle front which has a metal implant for reinforcement. 2. The bridge of a metal spectacle front having an added reinforcing member.

form-fit b. A type of bridge used in plastic spectacle frames and shaped to fit the contour of the bridge of the nose.

high bar b. A type of bridge construction in which the bridge fastens near the top of the eyewires.

inset b. A saddle bridge having its apex behind the plane of the eyewires of the frame.

keyhole b. A type of bridge construction used in plastic spectacle frames, the outline as seen from the front resembling a keyhole. It differs from the saddle type in that only the sides touch the nose.

on-line b. A saddle bridge having its apex in the plane of the eyewires of the frame.

outset b. A saddle bridge having its apex in front of the plane of the eyewires of the frame.

pad b. A bridge of a spectacle frame to which pads are attached to act as the resting surface on the nose.

reversible b. An x-shaped bridge formed of two arches joined at their apices, used in reversible spectacle frames.

saddle b. A type of bridge construction used in metal and plastic spectacle frames without nose pads. It is a simple curved piece that conforms to and rests on the bridge of the nose.
modified s.b. A saddle bridge on a plastic spectacle frame to which nose pads are attached to carry some of the weight.

wire b. A metal spectacle or eyeglass bridge stamped or drawn from wire stock.

Bright's blindness (brīts). See under *blindness.*

Bright's retinitis (brīts). Renal retinopathy.

bright. Said of light sensation or psycho-logical light; having relatively high brightness; the opposite of *dim.* See also *light.*

brightness. The subjective attribute of any light sensation giving rise to the percept of luminous intensity, including the whole scale of qualities of being *bright, light, brilliant, dim* or *dark.* More popularly, brightness implies the higher intensities, dimness the lower. Cf. *luminance.*

b. contrast. See under *contrast.*

minimum field b. The brightness of an area or field which has been reduced in size so that it matches the brightness of a fixed comparison standard.

normal b. The brightness or luminance of a retinal image provided by an optical system when it is the same as that obtained without the optical system. This condition is met when the exit pupil of the optical system is not smaller than the entrance pupil of the eye.

photometric b. Luminance.
b. ratio. See under *ratio.*
specific b. The brightness value characteristic of a given hue.

brill (bril). A suggested unit of photometric brightness or luminance applying to the dark-adapted eye and for a 10° field. Luminance in brills = 10 $\log_{10}$ [(1000 × luminance) + 1], luminance being in footlamberts.

brilliance (bril'yans). 1. Brightness, especially as a subjective attribute of a light source; hence, differentiated from luminance. 2. The attribute of being *brilliant.*

brilliant (bril'yant). 1. Characterized by relatively high brightness. 2. Shining, glistening, lustrous, or sparkling.

brillmeter (bril'me-ter). An instrument to measure the luminance of a surface in brills.

Brinker-Katz method (brink'er-katz). See under *method.*

British Contact Lens Association. An association of persons connected with any professional or technological aspect of contact lens practice. It was founded in 1977 as an amalgamation of the Contact Lens Society, the Association of Contact Lens Practitioners, and the Association of Dispensing Opticians Contact Lens Study Group.

British Optical Association. An organization founded in London in 1895 to advance the science and profession of ophthalmic opticians. Eligibility for membership includes passing the association's qualifying examination or the equivalent.

British Optical Students Association. An association founded in 1962 and consisting of ophthalmic and dispensing optics students in the United Kingdom.

Broca's (bro'kahz) **orbital index; plane; pupillometer.** See under the nouns.

Broca-Sulzer (bro'kah-sul'zer) **curve; effect; phenomenon.** See under the nouns.

Brock's (broks) **projection box; scotoma box; method; Posture Board; rings; test.** See under the nouns.

brocken bow. Brocken specter.

brocken specter. The perceived projection of one's figure on a cloud or fog bank, especially when encircled by spectral colors, which may be observed from a high elevation with the sun behind the observer. Syn., *brocken bow.* Cf. *glory.*

Brock-Givner test (brok-giv'nur). See under *test.*

Brooke's cystic adenoid epithelioma (brookz). See under *epithelioma.*

brow. 1. The superciliary ridge and the eyebrow. 2. The forehead.

brown. 1. The hue attribute of visual sensations typically aroused by stimulation with radiation of wavelength approximately 593 mμ of relatively low luminance. 2. Any color which manifests a hue predominantly similar to that of brown, such as a mixture of red and dark yellow, or dark orange.

Brown's tendon sheath syndrome. See under *syndrome.*

Bruch's (brooks) **glands; layer; membrane.** See under the nouns.

Brücke's (bre'kez) **disk; lens; loupe; muscle; theory.** See under the nouns.

Brücke-Bartley effect (bre'keh-bart'le). See under *effect.*

Brungardt magnifier (brun'gart). See under *magnifier.*

Brunswik ratio (bruns'wik). See under *ratio.*

brushes, Haidinger's. A transient, entoptic phenomenon observed when polarized light, particularly blue light

from a large homogeneous surface, is viewed. It consists of a pair of yellow, brushlike shapes which appear to radiate from the point of fixation; believed to be due to double refraction by the radially oriented fibers of Henle around the fovea.

Brushfield's spots (brush'feldz). See under *spot.*

BSK. See *Beta Sigma Kappa.*

BTSOL. See *Brevet de Technicien Supérieur Opticien-Lunatier.*

Bundesinnung der Optiker. The representative ophthalmic optical organization of Austria, through which the member retail firms negotiate with the national and other social security insurance agencies and conduct promotional and educational programs.

Bückler's corneal dystrophy (bek'-lerz). See under *dystrophy, corneal.*

buckling, scleral. A surgical procedure for the repair of detachment of the retina in which the deep sclera and choroid are indented in the region of the tear to impress them toward the retina, as by infolding a flap of superficial sclera, or by imbedding a silicone rod in the sclera.

Buerger's disease (ber'gerz). See under *disease.*

Buffon's theory (bu-fonz'). See under *theory.*

bufilcon A. The nonproprietary name of a hydrophilic material of which contact lenses are made.

bulb. A rounded mass or structure, especially one at the end of a part.

    end b. The end of a rod cell of the retina, located in the outer molecular layer, which synapses with bipolar and horizontal cells. Syn., *end knob; rod spherule.*

    b's. of Krause. End bulbs or corpuscles which act as cold receptors, formed by concentric layers spherically surrounding a sensory fiber, located in dermis, external genitalia, limbus corneae, and conjunctiva.

bulbus oculi (bul'bus ok'u-li). The eyeball.

bulbus quadratus (bul'bus kwod-rat'us). Phthisis bulbi, in which the rectus muscles mold the shrunken eyeball into a mass of four segments.

Buller's shield (bul'erz). See under *shield.*

Bumke's (boom'kez) **pupil; symptom.** See under the nouns.

bundle. A band, cluster, or group of relatively parallel lines or fibers, as of nerves or muscles; a fasciculus; a tract.

Druault's marginal b. In the 48 mm embryo, a bundle of fibrils in the vitreous body, peripheral to the equator of the crystalline lens and somewhat parallel to the optic cup. It disappears when the iris and the zonule of Zinn develop. Syn., *faisceau isthmique.*

fiber b. A bundle of very fine flexible cylindrical glass or plastic fibers used to conduct light or optical images by internal reflection. **coherent f.b.** A fiber bundle capable of transmitting images throughout its entire length. **incoherent f.b.** A fiber bundle that transmits light only, not optical images.

medial longitudinal b. One of a pair of medullated nerve fiber bundles on each side of the brain stem, extending from the midbrain to the cervical spinal cord, consisting of ascending and descending fibers contributed primarily by the superior vestibular nucleus of Bechterew, lateral vestibular nucleus of Deiter, third, fourth, and sixth cranial nerve nuclei, nucleus of Darkschewitsch, and interstitial nucleus of Cajal. It is involved in integrating the eye muscle nuclei with each other, with the facial nuclei, the vestibular nuclei (for maintaining equilibrium), and the head-turning nuclei. Syn., *medial longitudinal fasciculus; posterior longitudinal bundle.*

optic b., anterior accessory, of Bochenek. Anterior accessory optic tract of Bochenek.

papillomacular b. A well-defined, oval-shaped bundle of ganglionic axons in the nerve fiber layer of the retina, extending from the region of the macula lutea to the optic disk, entering it from the temporal side. All other temporal fibers course around this bundle as they approach the disk.

posterior longitudinal b. Medial longitudinal bundle.

b. of rays. See under *ray.*

Spitzka's b. Nerve fibers from the cerebral cortex which pass through the cerebral peduncles to supply the contralateral oculomotor nuclei.

Bunsen's photometer (bun'sens). See under *photometer.*

Bunsen-Roscoe law (bun'sen-ros'ko). See under *law.*

buphthalmia (būf-thal'me-ah). Hydrophthalmos.

buphthalmos (būf-thal'mos). Hydrophthalmos.

buphthalmus (būf-thal'mus). Hydrophthalmos.

Burch interferometer (berch). See under *interferometer.*

Bürger-Grütz disease (bēr'ger-grētz). Essential familial hyperlipemia.

Burnett syndrome. See under *syndrome.*

Burnham-Clark-Munsell color memory test. See under *test.*

Burns syndrome. See under *syndrome.*

Burton lamp. See under *lamp.*

Busacca's (bus-ah'kaz) **nodules; phenomenon.** See under the nouns.

BUT. Abbreviation for *breakup time.*

butt. The anterior, thickened portion of a spectacle temple.

button. 1. In a multifocal lens, that component of a selected index of refraction which is fused to the main blank of another index and then partly ground away, the remainder forming the segment or segments for near seeing. In flat-top bifocal or trifocal constructions the button is made of two or more glasses of different refractive index which are fused together before being fused to the main blank. 2. A small disk of plastic from which a contact lens is fabricated.

butyn (bu'tin). A chemical compound which acts as a surface anesthetic when instilled in the eye.

BVI. See *Better Vision Institute.*

C

C. Symbol for *coefficient of facility of aqueous outflow*.

c. Abbreviation for *cylinder*.

C case. See *case, type C*.

CAB. Cellulose acetate butyrate.

cae- (se). For words beginning thus, see also *ce-*.

caecanometer (se"kan-om'eh-ter). An instrument for plotting the blind spot of Mariotte. Its essential feature is the movement, over the indirect field of vision, of a metal ball by a concealed, manually controlled magnet.

Caffey's disease (kaf'ēz). Infantile cortical hyperostosis. See under *hyperostosis*.

Caffey-Silverman syndrome (kaf'e-sil-vur'man). Infantile cortical hyperostosis. See under *hyperostosis*.

Cajal's (ka-halz') **cell; nodes; interstitial nucleus.** See under the nouns.

calcar avis (kal'kar a'vis). A ridge in the posterior horn of the lateral ventricle of the brain formed by the anterior indentation of the calcarine fissure.

calcinosis oculi (kal"sih-no'sis ok'u-li). Deposits of calcium salts in tissues of the eye.

calcite (kal'sīt). Calcium carbonate ($CaCO_3$), a doubly refracting crystal found in a variety of forms, transparent to visible and ultraviolet radiation and used to produce polarized light.

calculator, Maddox torsion. A mechanical analog incorporating the system of axes of rotation of the eye and demonstrating the apparent torsion produced when conventional methods of specification of torsion are employed. It consists of a disk at whose center a rod protrudes perpendicular to the surface. A plumb line, attached to the rod, indicates the true vertical and its position is compared to the vertical meridian of the eye as it is diagrammed on the disk.

caligo (kah-li'go). Obscure vision.

    c. corneae. Obscure vision due to corneal opacity.

    c. lentis. Obscure vision due to cataract.

    c. pupillae. Obscure vision due to an occluded pupil.

calisthenics, ocular. The exercising of the extraocular or intraocular muscle function for the purpose of developing strength, coordination, speed, or amplitude of action.

calorescence (kal"o-res'ens). Tyndall's term for the transference of heat radiations into visible radiations.

calyculus ophthalmicus (kah-lik'-u-lus of-thal'mih-kus). Optic cup.

camera. A chamber closed except for a relatively small aperture, through which light from external objects enters to form an image on an inner surface, usually one of light sensitive material. The aperture usually contains a lens, an adjustable diaphragm, and a shutter to time the exposure.

    c. aquosa. The aqueous chamber of the eye.

    fundus c. A camera with optics and an illumination system which permit photography of the ocular fundus.

    c. lucida. An instrument, invented by Wollaston, consisting essentially of a prism or a mirror through which an object may be viewed so as to

[80]

appear on a plane surface seen in direct view and on which the outline of the object may be traced. The direct view of the plane surface may be accomplished with the other eye, or with the same eye if the mirror or prism aperture is semitransparent, perforated, or divided so as to permit visual superimposition of the direct and indirect views.

c. obscura. A relatively dark chamber, on the interior surface of which is (invertedly) imaged a relatively luminous external scene by means of a stenopaic aperture or pinhole (sometimes provided with a lens); hence, a type of pinhole camera.

c. oculi. A chamber of the eye. **anterior c.o.** The anterior chamber of the eye. **minor c.o.** The posterior chamber of the eye. **posterior c.o.** The posterior chamber of the eye.

pinhole c. A camera having a pinhole aperture instead of a lens. See also *Abney's formula.*

Camp bifocal contact lens. See under *lens, contact, bifocal.*

campanula (kam-pan'u-lah). A ligamentous condensation of vitreous, of variable size and shape, attached to the crystalline lens of teleosts, considered by some to be involved in accommodation.

campimeter (kam-pim'eh-ter). Any one of several types of instruments for measurement of the field of vision, especially of the central or paracentral region. Ex.: *perimeter; tangent screen; stereocampimeter.*

campimetry (kam-pim'eh-tre). Investigation of the integrity of the field of vision with a campimeter.

black light c. Campimetry performed under ultraviolet light and with luminescent targets.

flicker fusion c. Determination of the integrity of the visual field by plotting of the critical fusion frequency (cff) throughout its extent.

kinetic c. Exploration of the visual field with a moving test object of fixed luminance.

projection c. Campimetry performed with optically projected luminous targets.

static c. Exploration of the visual field in which test objects of various sizes, located at fixed positions, are gradually increased in luminance to the threshold of visibility.

Campos' ligament (kam'pos). See under *ligament.*

◆
CANAL

canal. A tubular channel or passageway; a duct.

central c. Hyaloid canal.

ciliary c. The spaces of Fontana in the pectinate ligament.

Cloquet's c. Hyaloid canal.

corneal c's. Channels that appear to connect lacunae which harbor the corneal corpuscles of the stroma.

ethmoidal c., anterior. A bony channel connecting the medial wall-roof junction of the orbit with the anterior cranial fossa of the cranial cavity and transmitting the nasal (anterior ethmoidal) nerve and the anterior ethmoidal artery and vein.

ethmoidal c., posterior. A bony channel extending from the region of the frontal-ethmoidal suture in the orbit to the anterior cranial fossa and transmitting the posterior ethmoidal artery and vein and the nerve of Luschka.

external c's. of Sondermann. Collector channels.

Ferrein's c. A channel formed by the margins of the closed eyelids, which conveys tears to the lacrimal puncta.

c. of Fontana. The spaces of Fontana collectively.

Hannover's c. A circular channel about the equator of the crystalline lens between the anterior and posterior leaves of the zonule of Zinn that contains aqueous humor and zonular fibers. It is sometimes incorrectly called the *canal of Petit,* which is between the zonule of Zinn and the vitreous humor.

hyaloid c. A channel in the vitreous humor, between the optic disk and the postlenticular space of Berger, which harbors the hyaloid artery. This artery normally disappears prior to birth. Syn., *central canal; Cloquet's canal; Stilling's canal; tractus hyaloideus.* **persistent h.c.** A conspicuous hyaloid canal seen with the ophthalmoscope as a gray tubular cord, which may contain a persistent hyaloid artery.

infraorbital c. A bony channel beginning at the infraorbital groove in the floor of the orbit and leading to the infraorbital foramen of the maxillary bone below the orbital margin. It harbors the nerve and artery of the same name. Syn., *suborbital canal.*

inner c's. of Sondermann. Endothelial lined passageways that drain aqueous humor from the trabecular spaces adjacent to the canal of Schlemm; they are believed to empty into this canal.

lacrimal c. Nasolacrimal canal.

nasolacrimal c. A bony passage beginning at the fossa for the lacrimal sac in the anterior, medial portion of the orbit and ending at the inferior meatus of the nasal cavity. It contains the nasolacrimal duct for tear drainage. Syn., *lacrimal canal.*

optic c. A bony channel from the middle cranial fossa to the optic foramen in the small wing of the sphenoid bone, transmitting the optic nerve and the ophthalmic artery.

orbital c., posterior internal. Posterior ethmoidal canal. *Obs.*

c. of Petit. A circular space between the posterior leaf of the zonule of Zinn and the anterior surface of the vitreous humor, located peripheral to the retrolenticular space of Berger.

pterygoid c. A canal in the sphenoid bone for the vidian nerve.

von Recklinghausen's c's. Artifacts in stained corneal sections originally thought to be spaces between the lamellae of the corneal stroma.

c. of Schlemm. An annular vessel located just peripheral to and concentric with the posterior corneoscleral junction, anterior to the scleral spur, which receives aqueous humor from the meshwork of the angle of the anterior chamber and transmits it to the aqueous veins, deep scleral plexus, and efferent ciliary veins. It may bifurcate and unite again, has no proper wall of its own, and is lined with endothelium. Syn., *venous circle of Leber; sinus circularis iridis; scleral sinus of Rochon-Duvigneaud; sinus venosus sclerae.*

scleral c. The channel between the optic nerve and the choroid plus the deep one third of the sclera, bordered by the border tissue of Elschnig and the periphery of the lamina cribrosa.

c. of Stilling. Hyaloid canal.

suborbital c. Infraorbital canal. *Rare.*

supraciliary c. A small bony channel in the frontal bone containing and transmitting a nutrient artery, diploic vein, and a nerve of Kobelt to the frontal sinus.

supraorbital c. A short passage in the frontal bone related to the supraorbital foramen or notch, transmitting the supraorbital nerve and vessels.

zygomatic c. A bony channel, transmitting the zygomatic nerve, which begins at the zygomatic foramen and bifurcates into the zygomaticofacial and zygomaticotemporal canals.

◆

canaliculitis (kan"ah-lik"u-li'tis). Inflammation of a canaliculus.

canaliculodacryocystostomy (kan"-ah-lik'u-lo-dak"re-o-sis-tos'to-me). Surgical correction for a congenitally blocked tear duct in which the closed segment is excised and the open end is joined to the lacrimal sac.

canaliculotomy (kan"ah-lik-ūl-ot'o-me). Slitting of the lacrimal punctum and canaliculus, especially for the relief of epiphora.

canaliculus, lacrimal (kan"ah-lik'u-lus). A membranous duct for tear drainage, leading from a lacrimal punctum at the eyelid margin and ending at the sinus of Maier or common canaliculus, or ending directly at the lacrimal sac. Each superior and inferior canaliculus has a vertical portion, an ampulla or dilated portion, and a horizontal portion.

cancellation, selective. Cancellation or suppression of monocularly observed objects in particular directions or areas within a binocular field.

candela (kan'deh-lah). The unit of luminous intensity in the CIE photometric system. It is $1/60$ of the luminous intensity of 1 cm² of a blackbody radiator at the temperature of solidification of platinum. The term is intended by the CIE to be used in place of *candle, international candle,* and *new candle.* Symbol cd.

candle. A former unit of luminous intensity now replaced by *candela.* It was a specified fraction of the average intensity of a group of 45 carbon filament lamps preserved at the United States Bureau of Standards.

Hefner c. The Hefner-Kerze, abbreviated HK, a unit of luminous intensity approximately equal to 0.9 candela, formerly used in Germany and Austria.

international c. The unit of luminous intensity prior to January 1, 1948, now replaced by *candela*. By international agreement, it was the luminous intensity of the flame of a standard spermaceti candle of prescribed construction burning under prescribed conditions.

meter c. A unit of illumination equal to one lumen per square meter. Originally, the normal incident illumination intensity produced by one candle at a distance of one meter. Syn., *lux*.

millimeter meter c. The retinal illumination produced by a magnesium oxide surface which is receiving one meter candle of illumination and is viewed through a pupil one square millimeter in area.

new c. The term formerly used instead of candela to emphasize the difference from candle. Syn., *candela*.

standard c. The secondary standard formerly used to determine the unit of luminous intensity. Weighing ¹/₆ lb, made of sperm wax to certain specifications, and burning 120 grains of wax per hour, the standard candle has a luminous intensity of one candle.

candlepower. Luminous intensity expressed in *candelas*.

apparent c. A term used in connection with extended sources of light (as distinguished from concentrated sources) and which must be specified as valid only at a definite distance. It is the candlepower of a point source which would produce the same illumination at a specified distance as is actually produced by the extended source.

beam c. A term of somewhat indefinite concept; usually referring to light from a lamp which has been concentrated in a narrow angle for spotlight or searchlight purposes. It is the maximum candlepower in the center of the beam and should be specified as having been measured at a certain distance because the source does not act as a point.

horizontal c. The average candlepower in the horizontal plane passing through the geometrical center of the luminous volume of the source (axis of symmetry assumed vertical).

spherical c. The average candlepower of a light source in all directions in space. It is equal to the total luminous flux, in lumens, divided by 4π.

candoluminescence (kan'do-lu"mih-nes'ens). The very white radiation exhibited by the combined incandescence and fluorescence of certain heated materials such as cerium and thorium as, for example, in a Welsbach gas mantle.

Cantelli's sign (kahn-tel'ēz). Doll's head phenomenon.

canthal (kan'thal). Relating to the angles at the lateral and medial junctions of the eyelids.

canthectomy (kan-thek'to-me). Surgical removal of tissue at the junction of the upper and lower eyelids.

canthitis (kan-thi'tis). Inflammation of the eyelids in the region of the canthus.

cantholysis (kan-thol'is-is). Surgical division of a canthus of the eye.

canthoplasty (kan'tho-plas"te). Plastic surgery at a canthus of the eye.

canthorrhaphy (kan-thōr'ah-fe). Suturing at an outer canthus to shorten the palpebral fissure.

canthotomy (kan-thot'o-me). Surgical division of a canthus, usually the outer.

canthus (kan'thus). The angle formed at the nasal or temporal junction of the upper and lower eyelids. Syn., *palpebral angle*.

Cantonnet's (kan'ton-āz) **diploscope; test.** See under the nouns.

cap, corneal. Optic cap.

cap, optic. The anterior central area of the cornea within which the meridional curvature is maximum and relatively constant, not varying more than an arbitrary magnitude, such as 0.25 D. Syn., *corneal cap*.

capacity, rectifying. The influence of past experience on the interpretation of sensory stimuli such that the stimuli are modified by memories and the final percept does not correspond with the immediate stimuli, but conforms with past experience.

Capgras syndrome. Phantom double syndrome. See under *syndrome*.

capillarosis, retinal. Small, yellowish-white, irregularly shaped and variously sized retinal deposits presumed to be localized necrotic lesions associated with the deep retinal capillary plexus, perhaps the residue of small hemorrhages or microaneurysms.

capsula (kap'su-lah). A capsule.

c. adiposa bulbi. Cellular fat tissue within the orbit which fills the spaces between other orbital structures.

c. bulbi. Tenon's capsule.

c. fibrosa. Sclera.

c. lentis. Capsule of the crystalline lens.

c. perilenticularis fibrosa. A condensation of the anterior surface of the primary vitreous which surrounds the posterior surface of the embryonic crystalline lens and contains terminal capillaries of the hyaloid artery. The tunica vasculosa lentis is derived from this structure.

capsule. 1. A structure enclosing an organ or a part. 2. A layer of white matter in the cerebrum.

adipose c. Capsula adiposa bulbi.

Bonnet's c. 1. Tenon's capsule. 2. That portion of Tenon's capsule posterior to the points where the rectus muscles pierce it.

crystalline lens c. The noncellular outer covering of the crystalline lens, secreted by the embryonic anterior and posterior epithelium, which receives the fibers of the zonule of Zinn and the hyaloideocapsular ligaments from the vitreous humor. Since the embryonic posterior epithelium disappears, the anterior epithelium forms the capsule for a longer period, resulting in a thicker anterior capsule than posterior. Syn., *capsula lentis; hyaline capsule.*

c. of the eyeball. Tenon's capsule.

hyaline c. Capsule of the crystalline lens.

hyaloid c. Internal limiting layer of the retina. *Obs.*

internal c. White matter between the thalamus or caudate nucleus and the lenticular nucleus of the forebrain which contains sensory and motor tracts, including the optic radiations.

lens c. Capsule of the crystalline lens.

ocular c. Tenon's capsule.

optic c. Developmental tissue that forms the sclera.

perilenticular c. Concentric fibrils from the cone-shaped projections of the embryonic lens plate that are said to form the anterior limiting membrane of the vitreous and the base of the vitreous.

Tenon's c. The fibrous membrane surrounding the sclera which sends trabeculae to it and to the extra-ocular muscles. It is continuous with the dura mater of the optic nerve, episclera, and bulbar conjunctiva at the limbus. Syn., *capsula bulbi; Bonnet's capsule; capsule of the eyeball; ocular capsule; vaginal coat; bulbar fascia.*

capsulectomy (kap″su-lek′to-me). Surgical removal of a capsule, as of the crystalline lens.

capsulitis (kap″su-li′tis). So-called inflammation of the capsule of the crystalline lens.

capsulociliary (kap″su-lo-sil′e-er″e). Pertaining to the crystalline lens capsule, the zonule of Zinn, and the ciliary body epithelium.

capsulolenticular (kap″su-lo-len-tik′u-lar). Pertaining to the crystalline lens and its capsule.

capsulopupillary (kap″su-lo-pu′-pih-ler″e). Pertaining to the crystalline lens capsule and the pupil of the iris.

capsulotomy (kap-su-lot′o-me). The incision of a capsule, such as that of the crystalline lens in cataract operations.

caput medusae. The tortuous irregular circle of anastamoses of dilated anterior ciliary veins appearing with absolute glaucoma.

carbachol (kar′bah-kol, -kal). Carbaminoylcholine.

carbaminoylcholine (kar-bam″in-o-il-ko′lin). A chloride salt which is a cholinergic parasympathetic stimulant and, when instilled into the eye in diluted solution, acts as a powerful miotic. See also *Carcholin* and *Doryl*. Syn., *carbachol.*

carcel (kar-sel′). A French photometric unit equal to 9½ candlepower. It is the light produced by a carcel lamp burning 42 gm of oil an hour with a flame 40 mm high. *Obs.*

Carcholin (kar′ko-lin). A trade name for a powdered form of carbaminoylcholine used in the preparation of ophthalmic solutions and ointments.

carcinoma (kar-sih-no′mah). A malignant tumor of epithelium which typically spreads via lymphatic vessels, but which may also spread via blood vessels.

cards, fusion. Cards used for testing and training fusion, usually in connection with a stereoscope or an amblyoscope. The term is often applied to sets which include cards for simultaneous binocular vision, stereopsis, and the like.

card, test. See *chart.*

carmine (kar′min, -mīn). A rich, purplish-red, intermediate between red and magenta; an extraspectral color corresponding to a mixture of long wavelength red and short wavelength blue or violet; the complement of a green of wavelength approximately 520 mμ.

Carmona y Valle's theory (kar-mōn'ah e vah'yes). See under *theory*.

carotene, beta (kar'o-tēn). A yellow photopigment synthesized by plants, a carotenoid of the formula $C_{40}H_{56}$, its chemical derivatives being found in photosensitive parts of plants, Euglena-like flagellates, and as vitamin A_1 and A_2 in the outer segments of visual cells.

carotenoids (kah-rot'eh-noids). Fat-soluble, highly unsaturated pigmented organic chemicals, varying in color from red to yellow, which act as photochemical and photosensitive agents in plants and animals.

Carter's test (kar'terz). See under *test*.

Cartesian ovals (kar-te'zhan, -te'zih-an). Aplanatic refractive surfaces named after René Descartes, who first investigated these surfaces.

cartilage (kar'tih-lij). A solid, white, tough, connective tissue consisting of a homogenous, translucent, intercellular substance in which are scattered nucleated cells lying in spaces called lacunae.

palpebral c. An incorrect term for the tarsal plates of the eyelids which actually contain no cartilage.

scleral c. Hyaline cartilage found in the inner portion of the posterior sclera in certain animal groups, e.g., nonbony fish, frogs, reptiles, birds, and Monotreme mammals, having nonspherical eyes or eyes not otherwise protected by skeletal structures.

tarsal c. An incorrect term for the tarsal plates of the eyelids.

caruncle, lacrimal (kar'ung-kl). A pink, fleshy mound of relatively isolated skin in the lacrimal lake at the medial canthus area adjacent to the plica semilunaris.

caruncle, supernumerary (kar'ung-kl). A raised mass having all the structural characteristics of the normal lacrimal caruncle except that it is not isolated from the eyelid, being situated at the inner margin of the upper or lower eyelid; occurring as a rare congenital anomaly in addition to the normal caruncle.

◆
CASE

case. 1. A particular instance of a visual condition or of a disease. 2. A container and/or its contents.

accommodative c. Any of several types of cases said to represent or result from deficient, anomalous, or abnormal accommodation, especially in relation to convergence, e.g., one having a high AC/A ratio.

convergence c. Any of several types of cases said to represent or result from deficient, anomalous, or abnormal convergence, especially in relation to accommodation, e.g., one having a low AC/A ratio.

degenerated c. *Optometric Extension Program:* A case said to have developed characteristic visual test responses from prolonged exposure to a visual demand to the extent that removal of the demand is in itself inadequate to alleviate the visual problem.

disorganized c. *Optometric Extension Program:* A case whose compensations to an existing visual problem are not considered to be habitually fixed, and, hence, are readily adjustable to changes in lens prescription. Syn., *nonimbedded case.*

imbedded c. Organized case.

nonimbedded c. Disorganized case.

organized c. *Optometric Extension Program:* A case considered to have made habitually fixed compensations to an existing visual problem; hence, the case is highly unresponsive to changes in lens prescription and/or visual training. Syn., *imbedded case.*

reversal c. *Optometric Extension Program:* A case considered to have maintained a prolonged inhibition of a particular function so that when the inhibition is released, an excessive reverse action occurs.

trial c. A set of trial lenses and supporting rack or container used for refracting the eye.

c. type. *Optometric Extension Program:* In general, any of several groups into which cases have been classified for diagnostic purposes, with the concept that all cases falling into a particular case type would respond to a common therapy or to common therapeutic principles. The classifying criteria are frequently other than the type of lenses needed for best distance visual acuity. **c.t. A.** *Optometric Exten-*

sion Program: Those cases in which static retinoscopy (No. 4), base-in prism to break and recover at 20 ft (No. 11), phoria at 16 in. through the subjective finding (No. 13B), and base-in prism to break and recover at 16 in. (No. 17B) are concomitantly and quantitatively below the population mean. Also called "toxic interference case." Case type A is held to be characteristic of patients having systemic disturbances of non-visual origin. **c.t. B₁** *Optometric Extension Program:* A case type characterized by the base-out prism finding to break and recover at 16 in. (No. 16B) falling below the population mean, or similar standard. A few cases showing No. 16B "low" are classified as case type C (q.v.) on the basis of additional criteria, but in general No. 16B low is characteristic of case type B₁, also called the "accommodative problem" type of case. This syndrome is held by the Optometric Extension Program to be indicative of a need for extra convex lens power for both distant and near-point work. However, the basic therapeutic principle for this case type may be qualified as indicated by additional criteria. These additional criteria have been systematized by the Optometric Extension Program into subcase types called "degenerations" of the basic type. Two systems of identifying these degenerations have arisen. One of these labels the basic syndrome B₁-1 with the successive degenerations terminating in B₁-7. The other system starts with the basic syndrome labeled B₁-Simple and terminates in B₁-6. The latter system of notation is utilized in the material on this subject which follows. **c.t. B₁-Simple.** *Optometric Extension Program:* A case type in which the following findings are concomitantly equal to, or in excess of, the population mean (or similar standard): dynamic retinoscopy (No. 5), base-out prism to break and recover at 20 ft (No. 10), base-in prism to break and recover at 16 in. (No. 17B), dissociated cross-cylinder finding at 16 in. (No. 14A), base-out prism to blur-out at 16 in. (No. 16A), plus to blur-out at 16 in. (No. 21), and minus to first blur on reading material at 13 in. (No. 19). At the same time the following findings are concomitantly below the population mean (or similar standard): base-in prism to break and recover at 20 ft (No. 11), base-out prism to break and recover at 16 in. (No. 16B), phoria at 16 in. through the dissociated

cross-cylinder finding (No. 15A), base-in prism to blur-out at 16 in. (No. 20). This syndrome is said to be characteristic of those B₁ cases most readily amenable to convex lens therapy for both distant and near-point work. **c.t. B₁-1.** *Optometric Extension Program:* The first degeneration of the basic type characterized by the No. 14A finding dropping below its expected value. Other finding relationships of the basic type remain unchanged. This syndrome is said to indicate a lowering of the acceptance of convex lenses at the near point, below the tolerance of the B₁-Simple. **c.t. B₁-2.** *Optometric Extension Program:* The second degeneration of the basic type characterized by a rise of the No. 15A finding above its expected value, with the other finding relationships of the B₁-1 remaining constant. This case typing is said to show a further decrease in the ability to accept extra convex lens power for use at the near point. **c.t. B₁-3.** *Optometric Extension Program:* The third degeneration of the basic type characterized by some change (any change) in the relationships of the No. 16A, No. 17A, No. 20, and No. 21 findings from those expected in the B₁-Simple case, with the other relationships of the B₁-2 remaining constant, said to indicate increasing resistance to convex lens therapy from that of the B₁-2. Visual training procedures to increase convex lens acceptance may accordingly be necessary. **c.t. B₁-4.** *Optometric Extension Program:* The fourth degeneration of the basic B₁ type characterized by the dropping of the No. 19 finding below its expected value of 5 diopters. Cases falling in this type are said to show still greater resistance to convex lens application than the B₁-3's, with the increased likelihood that the patient will need visual training before the desired extra convex lens power can be tolerated. **c.t. B₁-5.** *Optometric Extension Program:* The fifth degeneration of the basic type characterized by the falling of the No. 10 finding below its expected value. This syndrome is said to indicate that the amount of convex lens power prescribed for both distant and near point work be held to a minimum. Visual training is considered to be required in many instances. **c.t. B₁-6.** *Optometric Extension Program:* The sixth degeneration of the basic type characterized by the No. 5 finding falling below its expected value. This syndrome is said to indicate that the amount of convex lens power prescribed for both distant and near point work be held to a minimum. Visual training is almost always required. Those cases in which the No. 5, the No. 10, and the No. 16B are concomitantly below their expected value are to be considered carefully for possible assignment to the C case type category (q.v.). **c.t. B_2.** *Optometric Extension Program:* A case type characterized by the base-in prism finding to break and recover at 16 in. (No. 17B) falling below the population mean, or similar standard. The B_2 case differs from the B_1 case type in that in the former the No. 16B finding is above its expected value and the No. 17B finding is below its expected value. This reversal of these two findings is said to be characteristic of an increased demand for extra convex lens power for near point work and a reduction in convex lens power for distant work. Also called the *Intensified Near-Point Problem* type of case. The B_2 case type has been subdivided into six degenerations from the basic type in a manner similar to the B_1. **c.t. B_2-Simple.** *Optometric Extension Program:* A case type with all finding relationships identical to the B_1-Simple (q.v.) except that the No. 16B and the No. 17B findings are reversed. The therapeutic significance of the B_2-Simple differs from that of the B_1-Simple in that the former is said to call more insistently for an increase in convex lens power at the near point than does the latter, while at the same time calling for a decrease in convex lens power at the far point. **c.t. B_2-1.** *Optometric Extension Program:* The B_2 counterpart of the B_1-1 with the No. 16B and No. 17B of the latter transposed. The B_2-1 calls for the same type of modification of the basic B_2 therapy as does the B_1-1 of the basic B_1 therapy. **c.t. B_2-2.** *Optometric Extension Program:* The B_2 counterpart of the B_1-2 with the No. 16B and No. 17B of the latter reversed. The B_2-2 calls for the same modification of the basic B_2 therapy as does the B_1-2 of the basic B_1 therapy. **c.t. B_2-3.** *Optometric Extension Program:* The B_2 counterpart of the B_1-3 with the No. 16B and No. 17B of the latter reversed. The B_2-3 calls for the same modification of the basic B_2 therapy as does the B_1-3 of the basic B_1 therapy. **c.t. B_2-4.** *Optometric Extension Program:* The B_2 counterpart of the B_1-4 with the No. 16B and No. 17B of the

latter reversed. The B_2-4 calls for the same modification of the basic B_2 therapy as does the B_1-4 of the basic B_1 therapy. **c.t. B_2-5.** *Optometric Extension Program:* The B_2 counterpart of the B_1-5 with the No. 16B and No. 17B of the latter reversed. The B_2-5 calls for the same modification of the basic B_2 therapy as does the B_1-5 of the basic B_1 therapy. **c.t. B_2-6.** *Optometric Extension Program:* The B_2 counterpart of the B_1-6 with the No. 16B and No. 17B of the latter reversed. The B_2-6 calls for the same modification of the basic B_2 therapy as does the B_1-6 of the basic B_1 therapy. Since No. 17B rather than No. 16B is below its expected value, the B_2-6 can never be classified as a C type case. **c.t. B_3.** *Optometric Extension Program:* Originally said to be characterized by the No. 5, No. 9, and No. 14A being above their expected values concomitantly with No. 10 and No. 16B low. Since it was not characterized by a distinctive therapy, this classification has fallen into disuse, and cases formerly included in it are now classified as B_1-5's. Also known as *Undeveloped Type, Accommodative Problem. Obs.* **c.t. C.** *Optometric Extension Program:* Those cases with the No. 5, No. 10, and No. 16B below their expected values (see *case type B_1-6*), in which, through the use of additional criteria, it is decided that the patient is not amenable to convex lenses, even through visual training. Also known as *Adductive Problem.* Formerly called case type C_1 before the dropping of the categories of C_2 and C_3 (q.v.). **c.t. C_1.** *Optometric Extension Program:* Same as case type C (q.v.). Originally devised to provide a label distinctive from C_2 and C_3. Since these latter categories have fallen into disuse, the C_1 label has been simplified to C. *Obs.* **c.t. C_2.** *Optometric Extension Program:* Originally said to be characterized by both the syndrome of the C case (No. 5, No. 10, and No. 16B low) and the syndrome of the A case (No. 4, No. 11, No. 13B, and No. 17B low). Since such cases were handled as A cases, no distinctive therapy resulted, and the classification was discarded eventually through disuse. Also called *Adductive Problem, Toxic Type. Obs.* **c.t. C_3.** *Optometric Extension Program:* Originally said to be characterized by No. 5, No. 10, No. 16B, and No. 19 concomitantly below their expected values. Also known as *Adductive Problem with Presbyopia.* Since this type of case is said to accept convex lenses for near point work and can thus be handled as a B₁-5 case type, the C₃ was not characterized by a distinctive therapy and fell into disuse. *Obs.*

◆

Caspar's opacity (kas′parz). See under *opacity*.

cast. A lay term for strabismus.

casting. A positive model of the anterior segment of the eye, for use in the preparation of a contact lens, made by filling the negative model or mold of the eye with a mastic which hardens to artificial stone.

cat. Abbreviation for *cataract*.

catacaustic (kat″ah-kaws′tik). A caustic resulting from reflected light or produced by a reflecting optical surface or system.

catacleisis (kat″ah-kli′sis). Adhesive or spasmodic closure of the eyelids.

catadioptric (kat″ah-di-op′trik). Employing both reflecting and refracting optical systems.

catamysis (kat″ah-mi′sis). Closure of the eyelids.

cataphoria (kat″ah-fo′re-ah). 1. A tendency of the visual axes of both eyes to deviate below the horizontal plane of the head in the absence of a stimulus eliciting fixation attention. 2. Rarely, hypophoria.
 double c. 1. Cataphoria. 2. Double hypophoria.

◆

CATARACT

cataract (kat′ah-rakt). Partial or complete loss of transparency of the crystalline lens or its capsule; an opacity of the crystalline lens or its capsule.
 aculeiform c. Spear cataract.
 adherent c. A lenticular opacity in which the lens capsule is attached or adherent to the iris. Syn., *cataracta accreta*.
 adolescent c. A lenticular opacity which develops during youth.
 aftercataract. Secondary cataract.
 amber c. A mature senile cataract characterized by an amber-colored opacity. See also *black cataract*.
 annular c. Disk-shaped cataract.
 anterior axial embryonic c. A common congenital anomaly which does not affect vision, characterized by the presence of several small white dots in the region of the anterior Y-suture.

anterior capsular c. A small, white, well-defined, centrally located opacity of the anterior lens capsule occurring in early life as a congenital anomaly or due to a perforating ulcer of the cornea.
 anterior polar c. A lenticular opacity situated at the anterior pole of the lens which affects the lens substance and capsule or, rarely, the capsule only. It is either congenital or the result of a perforating corneal ulcer.
 anterior pyramidal c. A type of anterior polar cataract shaped like a pyramid with the apex pointing anteriorly.
 arborescent c. A lenticular opacity which has the appearance of branching lines.
 aridosiliculose c. Siliculose cataract.
 aridosiliquate c. Silibulose cataract.
 atopic c. A lenticular opacity associated with atopic allergic dermatitis, usually bilateral and subcapsular, and appearing in either of two typical forms, as a radiating star-shaped opacity or as a dense, white, irregularly shaped plaque.
 axial c. A lenticular opacity situated along the anteroposterior axis of the crystalline lens.
 axial fusiform c. A congenital central lenticular opacity elongated anteroposteriorly and touching upon both poles of the lens. Syn., *fusiform cataract*.
 axillary c. Spindle cataract.
 bipolar c. Cataract involving both the anterior and the posterior poles of the crystalline lens.
 black c. A mature senile cataract in which the lens has a black appearance. In the earlier sclerosing stages, the lens changes in color from yellow to amber (amber cataract) or gray (gray cataract), to reddish-brown, or, in a few cases, to black. Syn., *cataract nigra*.
 blood c. A blood clot anterior to the lens which obstructs the pupil, hence not actually a cataract. Syn., *sanguineous cataract*.
 blue c. Blue dot cataract.
 blue dot c. A developmental anomaly of the crystalline lens, found so frequently in adults as almost to be considered physiological, consisting of numerous small opacities in the adult cortex and nucleus seen only by oblique

illumination as fine blue-white dots. Syn., *blue cataract; cerulean cataract; dotted cataract; punctate cataract; cataracta cerulea.*

bony c. Cataracta ossea.

bottle maker's c. Glass blower's cataract.

brown c. A mature, senile cataract characterized by a brown-colored opacity. See also *black cataract.* Syn., *cataracta brunescens.*

brown saucer-shaped c. A usually bilateral deposit of mucopolysaccharides in a zone around the embryonic nucleus found in eyes which have been affected with interstitial keratitis and syphilitic choroiditis, of congenital origin but usually not noticed before the fifth decade of life.

cachectic c. Binocular, rapidly maturing, lenticular opacities found associated with weakness and emaciation due to either acute toxic illness or starvation.

calcareous c. Chalky cataract.

capsular c. An opacity affecting the crystalline lens capsule only.

capsulolenticular c. An opacity involving both the capsule and the substance of the crystalline lens.

caseous c. Cheesy cataract.

cavitation c. A transient and reversible opacity in the deeper layers of the cortex of the crystalline lens, around the nucleus, consisting of a thick cloud of air bubbles which results from irradiation with low frequency ultrasonic waves of high intensity. Cf. *thermal cataract.*

central c. An opacity of the central area of the crystalline lens.

central pulverulent c. A rare type of nonprogressive, usually bilateral, centrally located, variably sized, lenticular opacity occurring with a familial tendency and composed of a group of small, discrete, white dots, each of which may be surrounded by a halo. Ophthalmoscopically it appears as a sharply defined, circular disk which blocks the ordinary pupil, and with the slit lamp is seen to be in the fetal or embryonic nucleus. Syn., *Coppock cataract; discoid cataract; Doyne's cataract; Nettleship's cataract.*

cerulean c. Blue dot cataract.

chalky c. A hypermature cataract characterized by the presence of lime salt deposits. Syn., *calcareous cataract.*

cheesy c. A hypermature cataract in which the degenerated tissue has a cheesy appearance. Syn., *caseous cataract.*

cholesterin c. A hypermature cataract characterized by the presence of deposits of cholesterin.

choroidal c. A complicated cataract which follows inflammatory or degenerative processes in the posterior segment of the eye, the most frequent causes being high myopia and primary pigmentary degeneration of the retina.

complete c. An opacity which involves the entire crystalline lens.

complicated c. A lenticular opacity which accompanies or appears secondary to other intraocular disease. It is characterized initially by a polychromatic iridescence and a localized hazy opacity in the posterior subcapsular, usually polar, region. The opacity progresses, takes on a rosette shape, and continues to spread axially and peripherally to involve the entire lens. Syn., *cataracta complicata.*

concussion c. A type of traumatic cataract which results from an explosion or other form of concussion.

congenital c. A lenticular opacity present at birth.

contusion c. A type of traumatic cataract resulting from a bruising wound to the eyeball.

Coppock c. An old name for *central pulverulent cataract* (q.v.), from the Coppock family in which the anomaly was studied by Nettleship and Ogilvie.

coralliform c. A hereditary, congenital crystalline cataract occurring in the axial region of the lens, particularly in the fetal nucleus, in either of two forms. One radiates anteroposteriorly and is composed of amorphous, tubular, or discoid opacities. The other is made of masses of rectangular or rhomboid crystals lying in clusters.

coronary c. A series of opacities in a crown or ring formation at the periphery of the crystalline lens, the extreme periphery remaining clear; developmental in origin and common in occurrence. The opacities are usually club-shaped, with the rounded end pointing toward the center.

cortical c. A cataract in which the opacity lies in the cortex of the crystalline lens. According to the nature and position of the opacity, a number of types such as *cuneiform* and *cupuliform* are differentiated.

cretinous c. Lenticular opacity associated with cretinism.

crystalline c. Cataract characterized by random deposits of crystals in the axial region. They tend to be bilateral and hereditary, may impede vision if extensive, and are of various shapes but usually coralliform or needle-shaped.

cuneiform c. The most typical form of senile cortical cataract in which the opacities run from the periphery toward the center of the lens like spokes on a wheel.

cupuliform c. A form of senile cortical cataract consisting of many minute, yellow-appearing opacities lying in the posterior layers of the cortex directly beneath the capsule.

cystic c. Morgagnian cataract.

degenerative c. Any opacity of the normally developed crystalline lens which results from a degenerative change. One of the two major classifications of cataract (the other being *developmental cataract)* which includes senile cataracts, radiation cataracts, and others.

dermatogenous c. A lenticular opacity associated with general skin disease.

developmental c. A lenticular opacity due to interference with normal development of the crystalline lens. The cause may be heredity, malnutrition, or inflammation. One of the two major types of cataract, the other being *degenerative cataract.*

diabetic c. A rapidly forming bilateral cataract associated with diabetes mellitus. The senile form does not vary from the nondiabetic senile form, but the cataract in the young diabetic is typically the snowflake cataract.

dilacerated c. A type of juvenile cataract characterized by a delicate fretted structure, single or multiple, usually associated with some other type of opacity.

dinitrophenol c. A lenticular opacity due to the ingestion of dinitrophenol (DNP), a drug sometimes taken to reduce body weight.

disciform c. A type of congenital or developmental cataract consisting of a ring-shaped band opacity surrounding a central clear area.

discoid c. Cataracta centralis pulverulenta.

disk-shaped c. A congenital or developmental defect, usually bilateral, in which the lens nucleus is absent and is represented by a thin opaque membrane. A ring of lens fibers, of normal thickness, encircles this membrane, imparting to the lens the appearance of a lifebuoy, or in section that of a dumbbell. The surrounding lens fibers may be partially or completely opaque except at the extreme periphery, where they may remain clear. Syn., *annular cataract; lifebuoy cataract; umbilicated cataract.*

dotted c. Blue dot cataract.

Doyne's c. Cataracta centralis pulverulenta.

dry-shelled c. Siliculose cataract.

electric c. Cataract resulting from electric shock. Syn., *fulguration cataract.*

endocrine c. A discretely localized cataract attributed to anomalies of the endocrine glands such as hypoparathyroidism. See *focal cataract.*

ergot c. Cataract due to ergot poisoning caused by the eating of rye cereals contaminated by a fungus. Syn., *cataracta raphanica.*

false c. False lenticonus.

fasciculiform c. Spear cataract.

fibrinous c. A condition in which exudate resulting from severe iridocyclitis is deposited on the lens capsule and obscures vision. A type of complicated cataract.

fibrous tissue c. Pseudophakia fibrosa.

filiform c. A cataract of unknown etiology in which the entire crystalline lens is occupied by interlacing opaque filaments interspersed by numerous water-clefts, described by Bückler as occurring in a son and a daughter of consanguineous parents.

fissured c. A cataract resulting from senile changes consisting of clear radial clefts occurring most frequently in the cortex, just underneath the capsule, but occasionally in the adult nucleus. Later, as cataractous changes develop, they become filled with debris and fatty droplets and eventually become opaque.

fleck c. Minute white stationary subcapsular nonprogressive flecks associated with remnants of the primitive vascular system, on the anterior capsule with those of the pupillary membrane, on the pre-equatorial capsule with those of the capsulo-pupillary membrane, and, rarely, on the posterior capsule with those of the hyaloid artery. They do not affect vision.

floriform c. A type of developmental or congenital cataract in which the opacity takes the form of petals of a flower. Syn., *Koby's cataract.*

fluid c. A hypermature cataract which has degenerated into a milky fluid. Syn., *lacteal cataract; milky cataract.*

focal c. A degenerative cataract localized to a discrete area and usually associated with anomalies of the endocrine glands.

foliaform c. Rosette-shaped cataract.

frosted c. Spear cataract.

fulguration c. Electric cataract.

fusiform c. Axial fusiform cataract.

galactosemic c. Cataract associated with galactosemia, a congenital disturbance of galactose metabolism. The opacities are bilateral and appear during the first three months of life. With prompt diagnosis and treatment, the prognosis for regression is good.

general c. A lenticular opacity of both lens cortex and nucleus. Syn., *mixed cataract.*

glass blower's c. A posterior cortical lens opacity found in glass blowers or steel puddlers and due to long exposure to intense heat and light. Syn., *bottle maker's cataract; heat-ray cataract.*

glaucomatous c. A type of complicated cataract occurring as a sequela of glaucoma.

gray c. A mature senile cataract characterized by a gray-colored opacity. See also *black cataract.*

green c. A green-gray pupil in advanced glaucoma, due to partial loss of transparency of the media; not a true cataract.

grumous c. An opacity due to hemorrhage into the cornea, aqueous, or vitreous; not a true cataract. *Obs.* Syn., *cataracta cruenta.*

gypseous c. A hypermature, white-appearing, lenticular opacity.

hard c. Cataract in which the lens nucleus has become hard, such as a nuclear cataract. Syn., *sclerocataracta.*

heat-ray c. Cataract due to long exposure to high temperatures. Syn., *glass blower's cataract.*

hedger's c. A corneal opacity due to a perforating wound caused by a thorn; so named because of its frequency in persons who trim hedges; not a true cataract. *Obs.*

heterochromic c. A complicated cataract secondary to heterochromic cyclitis.

hook-shaped c. An irregular form of stationary opacity in the axial region of the crystalline lens in which a ring of hook-shaped figures lies in a plane between the fetal and infantile nuclei. Syn., *internuclear uncinate cataract.*

hyaloid c. An opacity in the anterior portion of the vitreous; not a true cataract. *Obs.*

hypermature c. The fourth stage in the development of senile cataract, in which the lens becomes either dehydrated and flattened or liquid and soft. See also *incipient, immature,* and *mature cataract.* Syn., *overripe cataract.*

hypocalcemic c. Numerous small, white, punctate, discrete opacities associated with hypocalcemia in both the anterior and posterior cortex of the crystalline lens in layers separated by a clear zone, occasionally aggregated into elongated larger flakes or interspersed with angular iridescent crystals.

immature c. The second stage in the development of senile cataract, during which the lens absorbs fluid and swells considerably. See also *incipient, mature,* and *hypermature cataract.* Syn., *unripe cataract.*

incipient c. The first stage of senile cataract development which usually begins with the appearance of streaks similar to the spokes of a wheel or with an increased density of the nucleus. There is little loss of vision and frequently the cataract does not progress beyond this stage. See also *immature, mature,* and *hypermature cataract.*

infantile c. A lenticular opacity present in an infant or very young child.

infrared c. Cataract due to excessive exposure to infrared radiation.

internuclear uncinate c. Hook-shaped cataract.

intumescent c. A cataract characterized by an absorption of water and, consequently, a swollen lens.

irradiation c. A cataract caused by exposure to radium or x-ray radiation. It is sometimes synonymous with radiational cataract and, hence, due to overexposure to any form of radiant energy.

juvenile c. A congenital or developmental defect of the crystalline lens.

Koby's c. Floriform cataract.

lacteal c. A hypermature senile cataract in which both the cortex and the nucleus have degenerated into a milky fluid. Syn., *cataracta lactea*.

lamellar c. Zonular cataract.

lenticular c. An opacity which appears in the crystalline lens but not in the capsule.

lifebuoy c. Disk-shaped cataract.

lightning c. 1. Cataract found in persons who have been struck by lightning. 2. A cataract attributed to a person's having observed flashes of lightning.

massage c. A cataract resulting from massage of the crystalline lens as may occur from dislocation of the lens into the anterior chamber to come into repeated contact with the cornea.

mature c. The third stage in the development of senile cataract. The lens has lost the fluid which was taken on in the preceding stage, has become completely opaque, and may be easily separated from the capsule. See also *incipient, immature,* and *hypermature cataract.* Syn., *ripe cataract.*

membranous c. A congenital condition in which the substance of the crystalline lens is absorbed, leaving the lens capsule collapsed upon itself in the form of a gray or chalky white membrane. The absorption may be complete at birth or become complete after birth. Syn., *pseudoaphakia.*

milky c. Fluid cataract.

mixed c. General cataract.

Mongolian c. A lenticular opacity associated with Mongolian idiocy.

Morgagnian c. A cataract in which the cortex has degenerated into a milky white fluid with the nucleus

usually degenerated and at the bottom of the capsule. Syn., *cystic cataract.*

myotonic c. A cataract secondary to myotonic dystrophy and characterized by fine dustlike punctate opacities localized just beneath the capsule.

naphthalinic c. Cataract caused by the ingestion of naphthalene.

needle-shaped c. Spear cataract.

Nettleship's c. Cataracta centralis pulverulenta.

neutron c. Cataract due to neutron radiation from atomic explosion, characterized initially by posterior cortical opacities which may progress to involve the entire lens cortex.

nodiform c. A trauma-induced cataract consisting of dense, round, and discrete subepithelial opacities with a layered structure similar to an anterior polar cataract.

nuclear c. An opacity of the central nucleus of the crystalline lens. Syn., *central cataract.*

overripe c. Hypermature cataract.

partial c. An opacity of only part of the crystalline lens.

perinuclear c. An opacity around the nucleus of the crystalline lens.

peripheral c. An opacity in the periphery, or away from the center, of the crystalline lens.

pigmented c. A type of traumatic cataract characterized by a deposition on the crystalline lens of pigment detached from the iris. See also *Vossius ring cataract.*

pisciform c. Rare congenital opacities in the axial region of the lens, characteristically curved, wider and rounder at one end and narrow and pointed at the other, simulating the shape of a fish.

poikilodermic c. Cataract occurring in association with the skin condition of poikiloderma.

polar c. An opacity at either pole of the crystalline lens. See also *anterior polar cataract; posterior polar cataract.*

posterior capsular c. A congenital anomaly in which the posterior capsule is affected.

posterior cortical c. Any lenticular opacity beginning in the posterior cortex, such as *radiational cataract.*

posterior polar c. An opacity at

the posterior pole of the crystalline lens, usually due to remnants of the hyaloid artery or of the posterior fibrovascular sheath of the lens (not a true cataract). A true cataract sometimes develops as a result of degenerative changes of the lens fibers in this region.

primary c. A lenticular opacity not associated with any other ocular or general disease.

progressive c. A lenticular opacity which has passed, or will pass if not arrested, through the immature, mature, and hypermature stages.

punctate c. A cataract consisting of numerous small, discrete, dotlike opacities scattered throughout the crystalline lens.

pupillary c. A congenital iris defect in which the pupil is not formed; not a true cataract.

pyramidal c. An anterior polar cataract, conoidal in shape with the apex pointing forward. Sometimes this name is given to a congenital anterior polar cataract which protrudes into the anterior chamber as a laminated prominence.

radiating subcapsular c. Rosette-shaped cataract.

radiational c. An opacity of the crystalline lens resulting from overexposure to any form of radiant energy. Wavelengths between 8,000 and 15,000 Å are believed to be particularly harmful. Such cataracts usually begin in the posterior cortex, occasionally in the anterior cortex, or in both simultaneously.

reduplicated c. A type of congenital anterior polar cataract characterized by an opaque area in the capsular region and another in the cortex, with a clear layer of lens substance between.

ripe c. Mature cataract.

rosette-shaped c. A star-shaped or leaf-shaped lenticular opacity resulting from trauma. Syn., *foliaform cataract; radiating subcapsular cataract.*

rubella c. Congenital cataract in which the mother has been infected with German measles during the first three months of pregnancy. It is more often bilateral and occurs either as a dense, pearly white, central opacity with a clear periphery, or as a total opacity.

sanguineous c. Blood cataract.

secondary c. An opacity of the lens capsule after the crystalline lens has been removed by an extracapsular operation. Syn., *after-cataract.*

sedimentary c. A soft cataract, the denser parts of which have moved downward, due to gravity.

senile c. A lenticular opacity in older persons. This is the most frequently seen type of cataract and its etiology presumably differs from those of others, such as *congenital, traumatic,* etc. The opacity is usually nuclear.

shrunken fibrous tissue c. A congenital posterior polar cataract in which fibrous tissue has invaded the lens substance, leaving the lens filled with shrunken, degenerated, fibrocellular material.

siliculose c. A cataract characterized by absorption and atrophy of the crystalline lens and calcareous deposit in the capsule. Syn., *aridosiliculose cataract; aridosiliquate cataract; dry-shelled cataract; siliquose cataract.*

siliquose c. Siliculose cataract.

snowflake c. 1. A familial, infantile, cortical cataract characterized by grayish or whitish flakelike opacities of irregular outline. The condition may be progressive and may occur in conjunction with stellate cataract. Syn., *cataracta nivea.* 2. A cataract characterized by numerous blue-white flakelike opacities. It is usually associated with severe diabetes and is the typical cataract in young diabetics.

soft c. Cataract in which the crystalline lens is of soft consistency and milky appearance, typified by congenital or juvenile cataract in which the lens nucleus has not hardened.

solar c. A cataract due to absorption of radiant energy from the sun. Wavelengths between 8,000 and 15,000 Å are believed to be particularly harmful.

spear c. A hereditary, congenital crystalline cataract in the axial region of the lens consisting of branching needle-shaped opacities, randomly arranged, and variously reported to be situated in the embryonic, fetal, or adult nucleus. Syn., *aculeiform cataract; fasciculiform cataract; frosted cataract; needle-shaped cataract; Vogt's cataract.*

spindle c. A spindle-shaped, lenticular opacity extending in an anteroposterior direction. Syn., *axillary cataract.*

spirochetiform c. An irregular form of stationary opacity in the axial region of the crystalline lens composed of many short wavy lines in the posterior nucleus.

spurious c. An opacity caused by adhesion of extraneous substance to the capsule of the crystalline lens, usually remnants of the hyaloid artery if on the posterior capsule, or of the pupillary membrane if on the anterior capsule; not a true cataract. Syn., *cataracta spuria.*

stationary c. A lenticular opacity which has not become more extensive over a considerable period of time.

stellate c. Sutural cataract.

steroid c. Cataract attributed to prolonged use of corticosteroids, characterized by discrete granular opacities in the posterior subcapsular polar region.

subcapsular c. A lenticular opacity situated beneath the capsule of the crystalline lens.

sunflower c. A sunflower-shaped opacity of the crystalline lens consequent upon the presence of copper, as in hepatolenticular degeneration. Syn., *chalcosis lentis.*

sutural c. An opacity developing about the time of birth and affecting the Y-shaped sutures of the fetal nucleus. Syn., *stellate cataract; triradiate cataract.*

syndermatotic c. Cataract appearing in association with diseases of the skin.

tetany c. Cataract occurring in association with tetany, typically zonular when congenital or infantile, and subcapsular when occurring spontaneously in later life or following parathyroid damage or removal. Syn., *cataracta parathyropiva.*

thermal c. A dense white permanent opacity of the crystalline lens which develops from the heat generated by irradiation with ultrasonic waves of high frequency and intensity. Cf. *cavitation cataract.*

total c. A cataract involving the entire lens substance.

toxic c. A lenticular opacity in individuals who have been exposed to certain drugs, such as paradichlorobenzene or dinitrophenol. See also *dinitrophenol cataract.*

traumatic c. The general term for any lenticular opacity resulting from injury to the crystalline lens, its capsule, or the eyeball itself. Traumatic is sometimes used when the wound is perforating; contusion, when nonperforating; and concussion, when resulting from an explosion.

tremulous c. A cataract associated with tremulous movement of the crystalline lens and iris upon the movement of the eyeball. Syn., *vacillating cataract.*

triradiate c. Sutural cataract.

true c. Lenticular cataract as opposed to other disorders such as *blood cataract* or *fibrinous cataract.*

ultrasonic c. Cataract resulting from irradiation with ultrasonic waves. See *cavitation cataract* and *thermal cataract.*

umbilicated c. Disk-shaped cataract.

unripe c. Immature cataract.

vacillating c. Tremulous cataract.

vesicular c. A rare form of congenital cataract characterized by a few vesiclelike opacities scattered throughout the lens substance.

Vogt's c. Spear cataract.

Vossius ring c. A rare type of traumatic cataract consisting of an annulus 3 or 4 mm in diameter at the center of the crystalline lens, believed to be composed of pigment from the posterior iris. Syn., *Vossius ring opacity; Vossius lenticular ring.*

x-ray c. A lenticular opacity due to prolonged exposure to roentgen rays.

zonular c. A lenticular opacity affecting one layer only, with clear lens substance on either side of the opaque zone or the lamella. Syn., *lamellar cataract.*

◆

CATARACTA

cataracta (kat″ah-rak′tah). Cataract.

c. accreta. The condition in which lens capsule and iris are adherent due to an iridocyclitic inflammation. Syn., *adherent cataract.*

c. acquisita. Any noncongenital lens opacity.

c. adiposa. Pseudophakia lipomatosa.

c. adnata. Congenital cataract.

c. adventitia. Any noncongenital, crystalline lens opacity.

c. arborescens. Arborescent cataract.

c. axialis. Axial cataract.

c. brunescens. Brown cataract.

c. centralis lentis. Nuclear cataract.

c. centralis pulverulenta. Central pulverulent cataract.

c. cerulea. Blue dot cataract.

c. complicata. Complicated cataract.

c. confirmata. Mature cataract.

c. congenita membranacea. A congenital membranous cataract.

c. congenita vasculosa. A congenital condition in which the crystalline lens has been invaded and replaced by vascularized mesodermal tissue.

c. consecutiva. Secondary cataract.

c. coronaria. Coronary cataract.

c. cruenta. Grumous cataract.

c. dermatogenes. Dermatogenous cataract.

c. disseminata subcapsularis glaucomatosa. Small, multiple, discrete, stationary subcapsular opacities that appear in the pupillary area subsequent to an attack of acute glaucoma or other occurrence of raised intraocular pressure as a result of iridocyclitis or a contusion.

c. elastica. Tremulous cataract.

c. fibrosa. Pseudophakia fibrosa.

c. fusca. A mature senile cataract in which the lens has a reddish-brown appearance.

c. gelatinosa. Soft cataract.

c. glauca. Green cataract.

c. glaucomatosa acuta. A cataract characterized by multiple, circumscribed, white spots beneath the anterior lens capsule. These are very white during an attack of glaucoma and less intense and more transparent when the intraocular pressure is reduced.

c. lactea. Lacteal cataract.

c. membranacea accreta. An aftercataract due to adherence of the anterior to the posterior capsule.

c. migrans. An opaque, dislocated, crystalline lens.

c. mollis. Soft cataract.

c. neurodermatica. Most common form of dermatogenous cataract.

c. nigra. Black cataract.

c. nivea. Snowflake cataract.

c. ossea. 1. Pseudophakia ossea. 2. A condition characterized by scar tissue and ossification of the crystalline lens. Syn., *bony cataract.*

c. parathyropiva. Tetany cataract.

c. raphanica. Ergot cataract.

c. scabrosa. Soft cataract.

c. spuria. Spurious cataract.

c. syndermotica. Dermatogenous cataract.

c. tenax. Hard cataract.

c. zonularis pulverulenta. Central pulverulent cataract.

◆

cataractous (kat″ah-rak′tus). Cataractlike; affected with cataract.

catarrh (kah-tahr′). Inflammation of a mucous membrane, accompanied by a mucus discharge.

　atropine c. Atropine conjunctivitis.

　dry c. Conjunctival hyperemia not consequent upon the presence of microorganisms. It is often caused by local irritants, may accompany nasal catarrh or hay fever, and may be associated with uncorrected errors of refraction.

　follicular c. Conjunctival folliculosis.

　Fruehjahr's c. Vernal conjunctivitis.

　Saemisch c. Vernal conjunctivitis.

　spring c. Vernal conjunctivitis.

　vernal c. Vernal conjunctivitis.

catatropia (kat″ah-tro′pe-ah). 1. A strabismus characterized by the downward deviation of either eye while the other fixates. Syn., *alternating* or *double hypotropia.* 2. Alternating or double hypophoria.

cathetometer (kath″eh-tom′eh-ter). A vertically adjustable horizontal telescope to measure small differences of height, as of columns of mercury.

cathodoluminescence (kath″o-do-lu″mih-nes′ens). Light resulting from bombardment by electrons.

catophoria (kat″o-fo′re-ah). Cataphoria.

catopter (kă-top′ter). A reflecting optical instrument; a mirror.

catoptric (kă-top′trik). Relating to a mirror or to reflected light; made by, or based on, reflection.

catoptrics (kă-top′triks). The branch of optics dealing with the behavior of light when it is reflected.

catoptry (kă-top′tre). The unit of reflective power of mirrors. A mirror that will reflect parallel rays of light to a point of focus at a distance of 1 m from the mirror has a unit of reflective power of 1 catoptry.

catotropia (kat"o-tro'pe-ah). Catatropia.

Cauchy dispersion formula. See under *formula.*

caustic (kaws'tik). The focal concentration of light in the caustic surface of a bundle of converging light rays.

cave, Meckel's. A cavity housing the Gasserian ganglion and located between the two layers of the dura mater near the apex of the petrous portion of the temporal bone. Syn., *Meckel's cavity; Meckel's space.*

caverns, Schnabel's. Schnabel's spaces.

cavity, Meckel's. Meckel's cave.

cavum lenticuli (ka'vum len-tik'u-li). A small fluid-filled vesicle located between the annular pad and crystalline lens in the eyes of some birds and reptiles; a remnant of the embryonic lens vesicle.

Cazenave's disease (kahz-nahvz'). Pemphigus foliaceus.

cc. Abbreviation for *concave; cum correctione (with correction)* usually expressed as c̄c; *cubic centimeter; comfort cable (temple).*

CCOC. See *Council on Clinical Optometric Care (AOA).*

CCR. Ceiling cavity ratio.

C/D. Cup to disk (optic) ratio.

cd. Abbreviation for *candela.*

cecity (se'sih-te). Blindness. *Obs.*

cecutiency (se-ku'shen-se). Partial blindness or a tendency toward blindness.

cecutient (se-ku'shent). 1. Partially sighted. 2. Having a tendency toward blindness.

cedmatophthalmia (sed-mat"of-thal'me-ah). Inflammation of the eye secondary to rheumatism or gout.

◆

CELL

cell. 1. Any of the minute masses of protoplasm containing a nucleus which make up organized tissue. 2. A rim or socket in a trial frame or an optical instrument into which a lens is mounted. 3. A compartment or small hollow receptacle.

absorption c., Pfund's. A device for measuring light absorption of gases and vapors consisting of a chamber containing the absorptive gas

or vapor, at each end of which is a pair of centrally perforated and internally reflecting concave mirrors of equal curvature separated by their focal length on a common axis, whence a beam of light entering the chamber in focus at one of the mirror perforations reflects successively at each mirror, thereby traversing the length of the chamber three times, and exits in focus at the perforation of the other mirror.

absorption c., White's. An optical system used to measure the light absorption of gases or vapors in which three converging mirrors increase the optical path by eight times the length of the system.

amacrine c. 1. A neuron with cell body in the inner nuclear layer of the retina whose nerve fibers synapse with ganglion cells and centripetal bipolar cells. 2. A centrifugal bipolar cell which sends an ascending fiber (axon) to synapse with cone feet and possibly with rod spherules and receives impulses from centripetal bipolar cells, ganglion cells, and efferent fibers of the optic nerve. 3. A neuron without an axon. Proper staining has revealed an axon in most amacrines. **knotty a.c.** An amacrine cell, identified by Polyak, having its body deep in the inner nuclear layer and dendritic processes arborizing throughout the inner molecular layer; its synaptic relations are obscure. **tasselled a.c.** An amacrine cell, identified by Polyak, having its cell body deep in the inner nuclear layer and dendritic processes which arborize laterally immediately upon entering the inner molecular layer; its synaptic relations are obscure.

associational c's. 1. Neurons completely in the brain or the spinal cord which functionally synapse with other neurons. 2. Cells in the retina which synapse with retinal cells of the visual pathway, such as horizontal cells, amacrine cells, and centrifugal bipolar cells.

barrier-layer c. Photovoltaic cell.

basal c's., corneal. The row of corneal epithelial cells adjacent to the basement membrane. Having rounded outer surfaces and flat inner surfaces, they undergo mitosis and are sloughed at the surface about a week after their origin.

Betz's c's. Giant pyramidal neurons located in the voluntary motor areas of the frontal cortex, with their cell bodies in layer 5 and their axons entering the corticobulbar and corticospinal tracts. They are the upper motor neurons that are under voluntary control when skeletal muscle, such as an extraocular muscle, is willfully contracted.

bipolar retinal c's. 1. Neurons whose cell bodies lie in the inner nuclear layer of the retina and connect rods or cones with the ganglionic cells. They are of two types: monosynaptic, connecting only a single cone to a single ganglion cell; and polysynaptic, connecting rods and/or cones to a ganglion cell. Both types are termed centripetal. 2. Neurons which receive impulses from efferent axons in the optic nerve and from ganglion cells and relay them to the visual cells. This type is termed centrifugal. **brush b.r.c's.** Diffuse bipolar retinal cells characterized by a single main dendritic expansion which terminates in a series of brushlike filaments of equal length in the inner zone of the outer plexiform layer, and by an axon that synapses only with dendritic processes of ganglion cells and not with their cell bodies. **diffuse b.r.c's.** Bipolar retinal cells that synapse with several rod or cone cells or with both; polysynaptic retinal bipolar cells. Cf. *midget bipolar retinal cells.* **flat-top b.r.c's.** Diffuse bipolar retinal cells characterized by a single dendritic expansion which terminates in undulating lateral branches in the inner zone of the outer plexiform layer, and by an axon that synapses only with dendritic processes of ganglion cells and not with their cell bodies. **midget b.r.c's.** Bipolar retinal cells characterized by a small cell body and thin, short, closely grouped dendritic ramifications which are smallest in the foveal area. They are monosynaptic in the central area, connecting one cone cell to one midget ganglion cell. Cf. *diffuse bipolar retinal cells.* **mop b.r.c's.** Diffuse bipolar retinal cells characterized by a dendritic process which repetitively divides into a moplike group of terminal branches, synapsing with both cone and rod cells, and an axon which synapses mainly with cell bodies of ganglion cells, although some branches do synapse with dendrites.

Cajal's c. Astrocyte.

clump c's of Koganei. Large, deeply pigmented, rounded cells commonly found in the normal stroma of the mammalian iris near the pupillary border and iris root. Traditionally considered of neuroepithelial origin, they now are suggested by recent electron microscopic studies to be macrophages containing melanin granules.

cone c. 1. A type of photoreceptor cell in the retina, consisting of an outer and an inner member in the layer of rods and cones, a nucleus in the outer nuclear layer, and a cone fiber and cone foot in the outer plexiform layer. It synapses with a bipolar cell and is involved in color vision, high visual acuity, and photopic vision. There are about 6 or 7 million in each retina, the greatest proportion of which are located in the macular area. The cell is long, thin, and somewhat rodlike in the area of the fovea centralis, becoming shorter and more conical toward the periphery. 2. The cone proper, consisting of the outer and inner members only.

corneal c. A specific form of fibroblast which has processes continuous with those of other corneal cells in the stroma of the cornea. Syn., *corneal corpuscle.*

dark c. of the corneal epithelium. Secretory cell of the corneal epithelium.

Dogiel's c. A ganglion cell of the retina, the cell body of which is located in the inner zone of the inner nuclear layer instead of in the ganglion cell layer.

ganglion c. 1. A retinal cell whose dendrites synapse with axons of bipolar and other cells in the inner plexiform layer and whose axons compose the nerve fiber layer from which they pass to the optic nerve to synapse in the lateral geniculate body, the pretectal area, or the superior colliculus. Its nucleus lies in the ganglion cell layer and both monosynaptic and polysynaptic types are found. 2. A large neuron in the central nervous system or in the sensory ganglia. **diffuse g.c.** A ganglion cell of the retina that synapses with numerous bipolar cells of all types; a polysynaptic ganglion cell. **garland g.c.** A diffuse ganglion cell characterized by a medium-sized body and by a few dendrites having thin, wavy, very long branches. **giant g.c.** A very large diffuse ganglion cell resembling the parasol or garland ganglion cell found in the periphery of the retina.

midget g.c. A ganglion cell primarily located in the central area and characterized by a small body and a single dendritic process terminating in a series of closely grouped small branches which synapse with a single midget bipolar retinal cell. However, other synapses do occur with diffuse bipolar retinal cells. **parasol g.c.** A medium- to large-sized diffuse ganglion cell characterized by an approximately spherical body and single or multiple dendrites which repetitively divide into an umbrellalike formation. **shrub g.c.** A diffuse ganglion cell characterized by a small body and two or three dendrites in a shrublike formation. **small diffuse g.c.** A diffuse ganglion cell characterized by a small body and long filamentous dendritic branches that spread horizontally or obliquely.

globular c's of Elschnig.
Elschnig bodies.

goblet c. A unicellular, mucin-producing gland located in a mucous membrane, such as the epithelium of the conjunctiva, intestine, or respiratory tract.

Golgi spider c. A small neuroglial or supporting cell with numerous processes in the vicinity of the ganglion cell layer of the retina. These cells are most numerous near the optic disk.

horizontal c. A neuron with a cell body in the inner nuclear layer of the retina which has dendrites connecting to one or to a few cone feet in the outer plexiform layer and an axon which synapses with a distant group of cone feet and rod spherules in the outer plexiform layer. Another type may also send a descending process into the inner plexiform layer.

Kerr c. A glass-walled cell containing two condenser plates in nitrobenzene, or other isotropic fluid, which becomes birefringent when subjected to an electrical field. See also *electrooptic shutter*.

Langerhans' c's. In the eye,
star-shaped cells located between the cells of the corneal epithelium.

Leber's c's. Large macrophages containing necrotic material; found in material expressed from trachoma follicles.

Mueller's c's. Neuroglial cells in
the retina with nuclei in the inner nuclear layer and with fibers extending between the external and internal limiting layers and forming a dense network of interlacing trabeculae in the innermost layers. They are supportive to the retinal neurons and participate in their metabolism by storing glycogen and oxidative enzymes.

photoconductive c. A photoelectric cell containing a material, the electrical resistance of which varies as a function of the intensity of the light which falls upon it.

photoelectric c. A device for detecting and measuring light, such as a photoconductive cell, or photovoltaic cell.

photoemissive c. Photoelectric cell.

photomultiplier c. Photomultiplier.

photovoltaic c. A photocell consisting essentially of three layers, a thin semitransparent metal film (cathode), a semiconductor, and a supporting metal base plate. Incident light passes through the metal film into the semiconductor, and electrons are released, creating an electrical current which may be measured by an attached meter. It is commonly used in photographic exposure meters and portable illumination meters. Syn., *barrier-layer cell*.

Photronic c. Trade name for a type of photovoltaic cell.

prickle c. In the eye, protoplasmic processes which link the cells of the corneal epithelium.

pyramidal c's. of Meynert.
Cells originating in the area striata and to a lesser extent in the parastriate area, whose axons enter the optic radiations, reach the superior colliculi, and make connections with nuclei that supply skeletal muscles. Syn., *solitary cells of Meynert*.

Remak's c's. Lemmocytes.

rod c. 1. A type of photoreceptor cell in the retina, consisting of an outer and an inner member in the layer of rods and cones, an outer rod fiber and cell body in the outer nuclear layer, and an inner rod fiber and end bulb in the outer plexiform layer. It synapses with a bipolar cell, contains rhodopsin in its outer member, and is involved in scotopic vision and detection of movement. About 130 million such cells exist in a human retina, exclusive of an area 300 to 400 microns in diameter, the fovea centralis. 2. The rod proper, consisting of the outer and inner member. **green r.c.** A rod cell in the frog retina having a mesopic spectral sensitivity curve with a maximum in the blue region (400 to 440 mμ) instead of at about 500 mμ, the usual rod maximum. Such cells constitute 8% to 10% of the rods in the frog retina.

secretory c. of the corneal epithelium. A glandlike cell sparsely distributed on the basement membrane of the cornea, which supplies the membrane with secretory material. Syn., *dark cell of the corneal epithelium.*

solitary c's. of Meynert. The pyramidal cells of Meynert.

spider c. Astrocyte.

star c. A star-shaped cell; one with many filaments extending from the cell body in all directions. The term is particularly applied to a neuroglial cell of this description.

surface c's. of the cornea. Flat squamous cells which constitute the superficial layer of the corneal epithelium.

umbrella c. Wing cell of the cornea.

visual c's. 1. The rod and cone cells of the retina. 2. Any of the neuroepithelial cells of the retina.

wing c's. of the cornea. The umbrella-shaped cells located between the basal columnar cells and the superficial squamous cells of the corneal epithelium. Syn., *umbrella cell.*

◆

cellulitis, orbital (sel"u-li'tis). Inflammation of the connective or cellular tissue of the orbit, usually caused by nasal accessory sinus disease, especially ethmoidal, but may be from dental infection, dacryocystitis, etc. It is usually characterized by pain, swelling, edema of the eyelid and conjunctiva, impaired mobility of the eyeball, and proptosis and may be unilateral or bilateral, mild or severe, acute or chronic. Syn., *orbital phlegmon.*

cellulosa choroideae (sel"u-lo'sah koroi'de-e). The suprachoroidal layer of the choroid.

cellulose acetate butyrate. A semirigid plastic used to manufacture contact lenses, said to have some degree of gas permeability and a lower wetting angle than PMMA. Abbreviated *CAB.*

Celor lens system. Gauss objective lens. See under *lens.*

cement, optical. Any of several transparent adhesive substances, such as

Canada balsam and certain thermosetting resins, used to join optical surfaces.

cement substance. See under *substance.*

◆

CENTER

center. 1. A collection of nerve cell bodies in the brain or spinal cord concerned with a particular function. 2. The middle point of a body or surface.

c's of accommodation. Brain centers subserving accommodation, consisting of higher, or cortical, centers, thought by some to be occipital, and paired lower centers in the Edinger-Westphal nuclei which relay impulses to the ciliary ganglia.

blinking c. 1. A center controlling voluntary blinking, located in the precentral gyrus of the frontal lobe. 2. A center involved in the dazzle reflex, probably located in the superior colliculus. 3. A center involved in the menace reflex, located in the occipital lobe. 4. Two facial motor nuclei in the pons.

boxing c. In the boxing method of frame specification, the point at the center of the rectangle that encloses the lens.

ciliospinal c. A collection of preganglionic sympathetic cell bodies in the lateral gray matter of cervical segments 7 and 8 and thoracic segments 1, 2, and 3 of the spinal cord. Their axons synapse in the superior cervical ganglion and supply the dilator of the pupil. Syn., *pupillo-dilatator center.*

c. of collineation. The point associated with a thin lens or a single refracting surface which is the center of perspective of object space and image space. It is the optical center of the thin lens or the center of the single refracting surface.

convergence c. 1. The portions of the paired oculomotor nuclei which control the medial rectus muscles. 2. A presumed, unknown, higher brain center, area, or complex which subserves the function of convergence and/or controls the paired oculomotor nuclei which control the medial rectus muscles.

c. of curvature. The intersection of two perpendiculars to an arc of a circle or a spherical surface.

datum c. The midpoint of the datum line.

distance c. 1. The intersection of the line of sight and the spectacle lens when the eye is in a straight-forward position or in any position otherwise defined to represent the eyes viewing a distant object. 2. The optical center or other point of reference of the portion of a multifocal lens used for distance seeing.

fusion c. An area assumed to exist in the cortex and in which sensory fusion is said to occur. This concept was introduced by Worth to account for the apparent absence of fusion or a "fusion sense" in some strabismic individuals. The assumption was made that the center was lacking or had failed to develop properly.

geometrical c. 1. In an ophthalmic lens, the point of intersection of the horizontal and vertical meridians which mutually bisect each other. 2. The point midway between the two vertical tangents and midway between the two horizontal tangents of the edges of a lens.

Hitzig's c's. Frontal eye fields.

mechanical c. The center of rotation of a lens former. In the boxing method, it is identical with the boxing center.

motor c. for fusion. An area assumed to be located in the cortex, on or near Brodmann's area 19, which controls the motor adjustment of the extraocular muscles to facilitate fusion.

oculogyric c. The portion of Brodmann's area 8 found in the middle frontal gyrus which is involved in voluntary eye movements.

optic c's. Visual centers.

optical c. 1. That point on the optical axis of a lens through which a ray of light, or its projection, passes when its paths before and after refraction by the lens are in the same direction. 2. That point on the surface of a lens where the optical axis intersects the surface.

pattern c. In the boxing method, the point at the center of the rectangle that encloses the lens former. It is identical with the mechanical center.

pontile c. A postulated collection of neuron cell bodies serving as a supranuclear center for yoke movements of the eyes to left or right.

c. of projection. A reference point from which objects in space are subjectively localized or projected;

usually considered to lie about midway between, and slightly posterior to, the centers of rotation of the two eyes.

pupillo-constrictor c. A center located in the region of the third nerve nucleus, usually considered to be the Edinger-Westphal nuclei, which gives origin to pre-ganglionic parasympathetic fibers for the constrictor pupillae and ciliary muscles of the eye.

pupillo-dilatator c. Ciliospinal center.

c. of rotation. The point about which the eye rotates. It varies slightly with the direction of gaze, being fixed neither with respect to the eye nor to the head, and is approximated by the intersection of the lines of sight for different directions of gaze. Cf. *sighting intersect*. **Mueller's c. of r.** The geometric center of the sclera considered as a sphere. **Volkmann's c. of r.** The point of intersection of the lines of sight in different positions of gaze. Syn., *sighting intersect*.

sighting c. A schematic point, said to be fixed with respect to the head, representing the point of intersection of the extensions of the line of sight for various directions of fixation.

visual c's. Centers of the brain concerned with vision. **basal v.c's.** Lower visual centers. **cortical v.c's.** Higher visual centers. **higher v.c's.** 1. Cortical centers or regions said to subserve the sensory visual pathways, such as the visual sensory area or the area striata and the parastriate and peristriate visual associational areas. 2. Cortical centers or regions said to subserve the oculomotor functions, such as the frontal and occipital eye fields and the higher occipital centers for convergence and accommodation. Syn., *cortical visual centers*. **lower v.c's.** Areas in which the ganglionic axons of the optic nerve terminate or synapse, namely: the lateral geniculate bodies which relay to the ipsilateral occipital cortex in the region of the calcarine fissure; the superior colliculi of the midbrain which relay to lower motor neurons supplying skeletal muscle; and the pretectal nuclei or areas which relay to both Edinger-Westphal nuclei for parasympathetic innervation of the sphincter pupillae muscle when light is flashed into an eye. Although some authorities list the pulvinar of the thalamus, it is doubtful if any ganglionic axons terminate here. Syn., basal visual centers; subcortical visual centers. **subcortical v.c.'s.** Lower visual centers.

visual c. of the cornea. The point of intersection of the line of sight with the cornea.

winking c. A center controlling voluntary winking, probably located in the prefrontal convolution of the cortex, which sends impulses via the motor nuclei of the facial nerves to stimulate the orbicularis oculi muscle of one eye while inhibiting that of the other.

◆

centering (sen'ter-ing). 1. Placing a lens so that its optical axis coincides with the mechanical axis of an instrument. 2. In ophthalmic lenses, placing the lens so that the line of sight will coincide with its optical axis. 3. Placing or mounting a lens so that its optical axis, optical center, or other point of reference coincides with the mechanical axis of a jig, as in a lens edging machine. 4. *Optometric Extension Program:* The total process by which a given stimulus in space is selected for special attention and localization. 5. Repositioning a corneal contact lens on the cornea after dislodgement onto the sclera.

centrad (sen'trad). A unit of ophthalmic prism power equal to $^1/_{100}$ of a radian and symbolized by an inverted delta (∇). See also *arc centune method.*

centrage (sen'trāj). The condition in which the centers of curvature of all the refracting and reflecting surfaces of an optical system lie on a single straight line.

centraphose (sen'trah-fōz). A sensation of darkness originating in the visual centers of the brain.

Centre d'Etude des Sciences Optiques Appliquées. A school in Brussels founded by the Union Nationale des Optometristes et Opticiens de Belgique circa 1955 for the training of optician-optometrist practitioners in both French and Flemish. Syn., *Studie Centrum der Toegepaste Optische Wetenschappen.*

centroid, spectral. A computed effective average wavelength of light emerging from a light filtering system, obtained by dividing the sum of the products of wavelength, incidence energy, transmission, and luminosity of each wavelength by the sum of the products of incidence energy, transmission, and luminosity of each wavelength.

Centrometer (sen-trom'eh-ter). An instrument with caliper points which can be inserted in the eyewire grooves of a spectacle frame to measure the distance between the nasal edges and the distance between the temporal edges of the eyewire grooves in accordance with the boxing system of dimensions.

Centrophore (sen'tro-fōr). An instrument devised by Bangerter for improving central fixation, subsequent to other pleoptic treatment, consisting essentially of a rotating spiral containing fixation letters at its center.

centrophose (sen'tro-fōz). A sensation of light originating in the visual centers of the brain.

centroptics (sen-trop'tiks). An orthoptic technique to improve central fixation and eliminate suppression in amblyopia ex anopsia by means of the *Centroscope.*

Centroscope (sen'tro-skōp). An instrument for successively producing vertical and horizontal afterimages, both in the same eye or alternately in each eye, and consisting essentially of a long luminous filament lamp in a light tight box having a viewing slit with a small red filter at its center to serve as a fixation point.

CEOSA. See *Centre d'Etude des Sciences Optiques Appliquées.*

cephalocele (sef'ah-lo-sēl", se-fal'-). 1. A hernia of the contents of the cranium. 2. A cyst at the root of the nose that extends into the orbit or eyebrow.

cephalopsin (sef-ah-lop'sin). A red photopigment found in the retina of the squid and other invertebrates and having absorptive characteristics similar to those of rhodopsin.

ceratitis (ser-ah-ti'tis). Keratitis.

cerato- (ser'ah-to-). See *kerato-.*

cerebro-ocular (ser"e-bro-ok'u-lar). Pertaining to the brain and eye.

cerebroscope (ser-e'bro-skōp). The ophthalmoscope when used to diagnose brain disease by examination of the eyeground.

cerebroscopy (ser-e-bros'ko-pe). The diagnosing of brain disease by examining the fundus with an ophthalmoscope.

Cestan's (ses-tanz') **sign; syndrome.** See under the nouns.

Cestan-Chenais syndrome (ses-tan'-shen-a'). See under *syndrome.*

cff. Abbreviation for *critical flicker frequency* or *critical fusion frequency.*

Chagas' disease (chag′as). See under *disease.*

chain, diagnostic. *Optometric Extension Program:* An arrangement of clinical findings into high and low groups as compared to accepted norms. Characteristic patterns are considered diagnostic of specific visual problems.

chain, pathological. *Optometric Extension Program:* A diagnostic chain considered to indicate a visual problem due to pathological anomalies.

chain, physiological. *Optometric Extension Program:* A diagnostic chain considered to indicate a visual problem due to physiological anomalies.

chair, Bárány's. A chair in which a subject may be rotated rapidly and stopped suddenly, used to demonstrate and test for the presence or absence, direction, and degree of labyrinthine nystagmus.

chalazion (kă-la′ze-on, shah-la′-). A chronic inflammatory granuloma primarily resulting from the retention of the secretion of a Meibomian gland in the tarsus of an eyelid. Typically, it begins as a hard, painless tumor, increases slowly in size and bursts eventually on the conjunctival surface. However, it may be absorbed and disappear, remain of constant size, or suppurate on secondary infection. Syn., *Meibomian cyst; tarsal cyst.*

chalcitis (kal-si′tis). Chalcosis.

chalcosis (kal-ko′sis). A deposit of particles of copper in the tissues, particularly of the eye. Syn., *chalcitis; chalkitis.*

    c. corneae. Copper deposition in the cornea, occurring in metal workers or after prolonged copper treatment for trachoma. The typical appearance in the cornea is of a brilliantly pigmented ring in the deep layers around the limbus.

    c. lentis. Sunflower cataract.

    ocular c. Inflammation of the tissues of the eye due to the effects of copper, characteristically seen in workers of this metal.

    c. retinae. Deposits of copper in the retina due to diffusion from a foreign body in the posterior segment of the eye. They typically appear as shiny lustrous flecks located around the main arteries and veins.

chalkitis (kal-ki′tis). Chalcosis.

chamber. A compartment; an enclosed space or cavity.

    anterior c. The space in the eye, filled with aqueous humor, bounded anteriorly by the cornea and a small portion of the sclera and posteriorly by a small portion of the ciliary body, the iris, and that portion of the crystalline lens which presents through the pupil.

    aqueous c. The space in the eye, anterior to the zonule of Zinn and the crystalline lens, filled with aqueous humor and divided into anterior and posterior chambers by the iris.

    c's. of the eye. The anterior and posterior chambers, containing aqueous humor, and the vitreous chamber containing the vitreous humor.

    Poster hydrometric c. Trade name for a wet-cell.

    posterior c. The space in the eye delimited by the posterior surface of the iris, the ciliary processes and the valleys between them, the zonule of Zinn, and the anterior surface of the crystalline lens; more extensively, it is also said to include the canal of Hanover, the canal of Petit, and the retrolental space of Berger.

    vitreous c. The space within the ocular globe taken up by the vitreous humor, bounded by the retina, ciliary body, canal of Petit, and the retrolental space of Berger.

Chambre Syndicate Nationale des Adaptateurs d'Optique de Contact. A French national association of contact lens fitters.

chamfer (cham′fer). A slight bevel on the edge of a rimless spectacle lens to prevent chipping. Syn., *safety bevel.*

Chandler's syndrome (chan′dlerz). See under *syndrome.*

channels, collector. Small vessels which transmit aqueous humor from the canal of Schlemm primarily to the deep scleral plexus of veins. Syn., *external canals of Sondermann; outlets of Ascher.*

Charcot's (shar′kōz) **disease; triad.** See under the nouns.

Charlin's syndrome (shar-lanz′). See under *syndrome.*

Charpentier's (shar-pan-tyāz′) **bands; illusion; law; method.** See under the nouns.

◆

CHART

chart. A sheet of paper, cardboard, etc., which contains test targets, a graphical representation, or tabulated information.

chart   [103]   *chart*

Allen c. A set of nine cards on one of which is a 13 mm Snellen E and on each of the others an acuity test character of approximately equal difficulty depicting very familiar objects for testing preschool children. The acuity is represented in the form of a fraction as the maximum resolvable distance in meters divided by nine, the distance at which the E subtends five minutes.

Amsler c's. A set of charts for detecting and measuring defects in the central visual field, each consisting of a black background on which is printed, in white, a 10 cm square containing various patterns, such as a grid of 5 mm squares, parallel lines, or a central grid of 2.5 mm squares in a grid of 5 mm squares. A dot in the center of the pattern is fixated at a distance of 30 cm from the eye, and a defect is demonstrated by the absence or irregularities of the lines. Syn., *Amsler grids*.

AO H-R-R c's. AO H-R-R plates.

arrow test c. A chart for subjectively determining the principal meridians of ocular astigmatism by means of an arrowlike pattern which may be rotated until the symmetrically arranged cuneiform lines or "feathers" appear equally clear or sharp.

astigmatic c. Any chart designed to determine the amount and axis of astigmatism. It usually consists of a series of radially arranged black lines.

Bailey-Lovie c. An acuity chart designed at the National Vision Research Institute of Australia to comply with the British acuity standards, with letter sizes ranging from 20/200 to 20/10 in 14 rows of 5 letters each with those of each successively smaller row approximately four-fifths the size of the next larger letters. The letters in each row are selected from 10 letters, DE-FHNPRUVZ, said to be of approximately equal legibility. (See Fig. 5.)

Bannon-Raubitschek c. Paraboline chart.

Beach test c. A visual acuity test chart, consisting of letters, Landolt broken rings, and Maltese crosses of various sizes.

Becker's c. An astigmatism test chart consisting of sets of three parallel

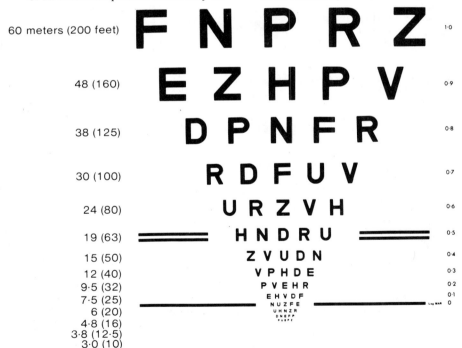

60 meters (200 feet)	F N P R Z	1·0
48 (160)	E Z H P V	0·9
38 (125)	D P N F R	0·8
30 (100)	R D F U V	0·7
24 (80)	U R Z V H	0·6
19 (63)	H N D R U	0·5
15 (50)	Z V U D N	0·4
12 (40)	V P H D E	0·3
9·5 (32)	P V E H R	0·2
7·5 (25)	E H V D F	0·1
6 (20)	N U Z F E	Log MAR 0
4·8 (16)	U H N Z R	
3·8 (12·5)	D N F F P	
3·0 (10)	P U E F Z	

Fig. 5 Bailey-Lovie Distance Acuity Chart. (From I. L. Bailey, School of Optometry, University of California at Berkeley, 1979; copyright © 1975, National Vision Research Institute of Australia)

chart   [104]   *chart*

lines, each oriented in a different meridian.

Berens c. 1. A test chart with numbers, crosses, words, and tumbling Es, of various sizes, used for testing accommodation and near visual acuity. 2. A visual acuity chart containing tumbling Es and colored targets in the form of objects familiar to small children, scaled according to Snellen notation. 3. A chart for testing subnormal vision ranging from 20/500 to 20/40, containing large pictures and smaller tumbling Es on one side and large tumbling Es and smaller pictures on the other.

Betts's reading readiness c's. A series of stereoscope slides for determining reading rate and comprehension.

Boettcher c. A chart consisting of a series of geometrical figures for testing visual acuity.

Borish nearpoint c. A vectographic card presenting on the front side three grids for crossed cylinder testing and a diamond-shaped target for phoria testing, and on the back side three reduced Snellen charts, a target for vergence testing, and a fixation disparity test pattern.

Boström's c's. Boström's plates.

Boström-Kugelberg c's. Boström-Kugelberg plates.

clock dial c. An astigmatism test chart consisting of 12 sets of lines radially oriented to correspond with the positions of the hours on a clock face.

color c. 1. A chromaticity diagram. 2. A systematic arrangement of color samples mounted for convenient reference.

Cowan c. A visual acuity test chart with letters so constructed that the spaces within each letter subtend the same angles as the bars, stems, and arms of the letter.

Dennett c. A visual acuity test chart with differences in size of the various letters of the alphabet for any given test distance, so as to compensate for differences in inherent readability of the individual letters.

Duane's accommodation c. A test chart for determining the near point of accommodation, consisting of a card engraved with a single line, 0.2 mm wide and 3 mm long, at its center. The test card is brought toward the eyes until it appears blurred or doubled.

Dvorine animated fusion c's. A series of colored, line drawing stereograms designed to train fusion and fusional vergence. Some contain a rotatable disk on which are printed a series of pictures, one of which is exposed at a time through an aperture in the stereogram as the disk is turned.

Dvorine's color vision c's. Dvorine's plates.

Eastman c. A circular test target for subjective determination of the axis and amount of astigmatic correction, consisting of eight radially extending black test stripes, each having a width of one minute subtense at 6 meters and bordered on both sides by half as wide white stripes and surrounded throughout its corresponding 45° sector of the target by parallel, alternate, narrow black and white stripes of equal width which are too narrow to be resolved at a distance of 6 meters and hence appear as a uniform gray field. The test pattern and background are designed to have equal areas of black and white to result in equal average reflectance. Below the threshold of acuity the test stripes merge imperceptibly into the background instead of appearing blurred. Syn., *Eastman-Guth chart.*

Edmond's picture c. A chart consisting of pictures of familiar objects for testing visual acuity of illiterates and children.

Elleman c. A rotatable chart for astigmatism measurement consisting of five radially arranged single lines, or of five radially arranged paired parallel lines, separated by angles of 72°, to be adjusted (rotated) for the fogged eye so that the two lines, or two pairs of lines, adjacent to the most distinct line or pair of lines are balanced for clarity, whereupon cylindrical lenses are then placed in front of the eye with axes parallel to the most distinct line until all five lines or pairs of lines are equally distinct.

Ewing c. A visual acuity test chart for illiterates, in which the basic test pattern consists of three parallel bars separated by the width of a single bar, with variously located discontinuities or gaps in the middle bar, each gap having the dimension of a bar width.

fan dial c. A chart or test pattern consisting of a semicircle of radially oriented lines (hence resembling a fan), used for determining the presence or

chart [105] *chart*

the amount and meridional orientation of astigmatism. Syn., *sunburst chart.*

Feinbloom c. A thirteen page, spiral-bound book for measuring subnormal acuity, having test numerals instead of letters ranging in 18 sizes which subtend 5 minutes in roughly geometric progression from 700 ft (213 m) to 20 ft (6.1 m).

Flom c's. A series of 21 acuity charts, each providing a 5% gradation of optotype size and consisting of a square pattern of 17 equal-sized Snellen Es and eight Landolt rings randomly oriented, with 16 of the Es along the edges and one in the center, with the eight rings symmetrically arranged as a square around the central E, and with the space between each two optotypes equaling the size of the optotype. The scoring is done in terms of only the Landolt rings. Also called *psychometric chart of Flom.*

Foucault c. Groups of alternate black and white bars spaced at various pre-calculated distances, employed as a resolution test object. Syn., *Foucault grating.*

Fridenberg's c. A visual acuity test chart for illiterates, consisting of groups of dots or squares in various numbers separated by distances equal to their dimensions. The test consists of counting the number of dots or squares in each group. Syn., *stigmometric chart.*

Friedenwald c. An astigmatism test chart consisting of radially oriented lines upon a gray ground. The lines not corresponding to the axis of astigmatism become less visible than if on a white ground.

Gould's c. A chart for measuring visual acuity in which the test objects or letters are white and the background black.

Green's c. Any of a series of commercially available wall cabinet test charts with opaque test characters on a transilluminated field, astigmatic dial, and various other incidental test chart features.

Grow c. A visual acuity test chart consisting of a block of letters which can be masked for presenting in columns or rows to eliminate memorization.

Guibor c. A chart for determining visual acuity at a 14 in. test distance consisting of 10 graduated lines, each line containing the letter E oriented in various positions. A panel containing a small window slides over each line, exposing one letter at a time. The lines are designated in terms of Jaeger and Snellen visual acuity and in percentage of visual efficiency.

Guillery c. A visual acuity test chart consisting of a series of disks or dots of graduated sizes, each eccentrically located in a separated square. The test consists of identifying the location of the disk in each square.

Guth c. See *Eastman chart.*

Haitz c's. Charts designed for use in plotting central visual field defects with a stereoscope.

Hardy-Rand-Rittler c's. AO H-R-R plates.

Heppel muscle c. A test chart consisting of a central light source around which a pointer is pivoted and calibrated to show the distance and direction of displacement of a second image of the light source seen under dissociation when different colored lenses are placed in front of the two eyes.

Hertel's c's. Hertel's plates.

Highman c. A visual field testing chart for use monocularly at 30 cm consisting of a 16 cm vertically by 22 cm horizontally elliptical pattern of low contrast gray 2.5 x 2.5 mm quadrille rulings on cream colored paper with a 5 mm red fixation spot at the center and an 8 mm black spot offset 7.5 cm laterally on the major axis so as to become invisible on the observer's blind spot when held at the proper distance from the eye. The visual field is explored by noting the integrity of the peripherally observed quadrille rulings in the various areas.

Hutchinson's c. A chart to test visual acuity at near and intermediate distances in the fitting of trifocals.

illiterate E c. A visual acuity test chart employing a graduated series of the Snellen letter E oriented in various directions for identification.

industrial motor field c. A chart for plotting the diplopia field and computing the binocular vision factor in the visual efficiency formula.

international c. Landolt's broken ring chart.

Ishihara c's. Ishihara plates.

*iso-*color c. A chromaticity chart divided into zones such that all stimuli represented by points lying within a given zone will appear identical when

chart [106] *chart*

their brightnesses are equal. In dichromatism, the zones are strips extending from one side to the other of the chromaticity diagram, converging to the red corner of the diagram in protanopia and being approximately parallel to the long wavelength side of the diagram in deuteranopia.

Jaeger c. A chart for testing visual acuity at given reading distances, consisting of words and phrases in various sizes of ordinary printer's type.

Javal's N c. A stereogram designed to overcome horror fusionis by presenting to one eye a vertical column of round spots and to the other a horizontal row, making it impossible to avoid superimposition of at least two spots.

Jessen's lighted letter c. A chart with words variously transilluminated by red, green, and polarized light and seen on a black or opaque background, intended especially for refractive testing of contact lens wearers.

Keeler c. A chart for testing visual acuity at a 25 cm distance, containing capital letters, Landolt rings, and isolated words.

kindergarten test c. A visual acuity test chart consisting of designs

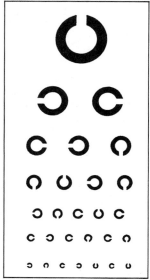

Fig. 6 Landolt's broken ring chart. (From Lyle and Jackson, *Practical Orthoptics in the Treatment of Squint*, 4th ed. New York: Blakiston, 1955; copyright© 1955; used with permission of McGraw-Hill Book Co.)

familiar to young children and conforming, insofar as practicable, to the principle of design of the Snellen test letters.

Lancaster c. 1. A Snellen letter test chart in which each successive row of letters is 25% larger, e.g., 20/20, 20/25, 20/31.25, etc. 2. A chart for determining the axis and amount of astigmatism.

Lancaster-Regan c. An astigmatism test chart employing both a fixed set of radiating lines and a rotatable cross.

Landolt's broken ring c. A visual acuity test chart employing a graduated series of incomplete rings with radial thickness and gaps equal to one fifth of their outer diameters. (Fig. 6.) The test consists of identifying the radial orientation of the gap. Syn., *International chart; Landolt's C chart.*

Lebensohn c. 1. A chart for testing visual acuity at 14 inches, containing on one side a miniature Snellen chart in letters and numbers, a small cross for the binocular crossed cylinder test, a line of music, and a test for accommodation in which the near point is determined by the sudden appearance of a third line between two others, and, on the other side, words in point type small letters in English and Spanish, a duochrome test, and a column of crosses to be counted by illiterates. 2. A chart employing the principle of the Grow chart.

Lutes near point c's. A set of three slides, each containing targets for vision testing at near, and a holder which attaches to the phoropter rod. The holder has a central aperture to expose only the desired target.

Maddox tangent scale c. Maddox cross.

Maddox V c. A test chart for determining the axis of astigmatism, consisting of a fan dial and a V which is moved along the circumference of the dial to the region of the radiating line seen blackest or most distinct. The position in this region in which both limbs of the V appear equally black or clear indicates the axis of the correcting cylindrical lens.

Marano c. A chart for testing astigmatism, consisting of one or more transilluminated or luminous radially arranged lines on an opaque or dark background, each line composed of a series of small alternately red and green

chart [107] *chart*

rectangles which, when seen out-of-focus, appear as a resultant yellow line. The axis and power of the astigmatism are determined by rotation of the two-colored line and the application of cylindrical lenses until the line is seen correctly in all meridians.

Newton's color c. Newton's color circle.

object c. A visual acuity test chart for illiterates, consisting of objects instead of letters.

orthops c. A subjective sight-testing chart, designed by Laurance, which includes a fan dial, Snellen test letters, and a red and green tangent scale.

Paraboline c. A rotatable test target with the parabolic curves of the Raubitschek chart in combination with a pair of broken, dashed lines of equal length, one along the axis of the funnel-form pattern and the other bisecting the axis perpendicularly. It is used for determining the axis and the amount of the astigmatic correction. Syn., *Bannon-Raubitschek chart.*

Pray's astigmatic c. A chart for estimating the axis of astigmatism, consisting of letters constructed of short hatched lines in a specific meridian, the lines for each letter being oriented in a different meridian.

pseudoisochromatic c. A color vision test chart with varicolored dots composing both the pattern to be observed and the background, the colored dots being so arranged as to make the pattern unrecognizable to one who confuses certain colors.

Rabkin's c's. A set of twenty pseudoisochromatic plates designed by Rabkin to detect color vision abnormalities and to classify them according to type and severity of deficiency.

Raubitschek c. A rotatable test target with two parabolic curves symmetrically arranged in a funnel-form pattern with the less curved ends forming the almost parallel small end of the funnel and the more curved ends diverging approximately 90° from each other. It is used for determining the axis and the amount of the astigmatic correction. See also *Raubitschek test.*

Reber's c. A chart for determining the visual acuity of very young children and illiterates, consisting of simple pictures of familiar objects.

resolution c. A pattern of alternate, equally wide, black and white lines in groups differing in line width and orientation to test the resolving power of an optical system.

von Reuss's color c. A color vision test chart consisting of colored letters printed on a colored background.

Robinson Cohen c. A commercially available instrument and projector slide for use with a projector in vision testing, its principal feature being a pair of rotating crossed lines projected in a field of red for astigmatic determination. See also *Robinson Cohen test.*

Seitz c. A chart for testing visual acuity of children and illiterates, consisting of pictures of animals and inanimate objects.

Sheard c. A phoria and vergence testing chart having on one side a small black dot followed by "Read these words letter by letter" and on the reverse side a vertical row of letters arranged to read "Keep this row of letters single."

sine wave c. A test chart consisting of several series of black-on-white lines the luminance of which in cross section varies as a sine wave function and each series of which differs in number of lines per unit of linear dimension.

Slataper c. A test chart with a short, fine line on one side and a pair of short, fine, parallel lines separated by the width of one line on the other side. The chart is moved away from the eye until the pair of lines can be resolved and then toward the eye until the single line blurs. These two positions together provide an indication of the amplitude of accommodation.

Sloan c's. 1. Two visual acuity test charts, one used at 20 feet and the other at 16 inches, each consisting of a set of ten capital letters graded in equal logarithmic steps and selected to be of comparable difficulty to each other and to the Landolt ring. 2. A set of nine reading cards providing samples of continuous text, used in the testing of subnormal vision to determine the magnification required to read newsprint. The letters range in size from a designation of 1.0 m to 10.0 m, 1.0 m approximating newsprint and subtending a visual angle of 5 minutes at 1 meter.

Snellen's c. A visual acuity test chart made up of Snellen test type.

chart [108] *chiasmometer*

stigmometric c. Fridenberg's chart.

Stilling's c's. Stilling's plates.

Stimson c's. 1. A series of charts for evaluating near visual acuity and for detecting central scotomata and malingering in persons with reduced visual acuity. Each chart contains groups of three disks, two neutral gray and one of concentric black and white circles of equal width and of varying angular subtense. 2. A reduced Snellen chart for determining visual acuity at a 35 mm test distance in persons with subnormal vision. 3. A chart of words all composed of the same seven letters, used to evaluate visual acuity and/or the efficacy of an optical aid at near, in persons with subnormal vision.

Streidinger c. A visual acuity test chart consisting of sets of dots notated with the distance at which they should be counted.

sunburst c. Fan dial chart.

Swann-Cole c's. A series of haploscope cards for determining the quality of fusion and stereoscopic vision.

Thomas' c. An astigmatic test chart consisting of a revolving cross, each arm of which contains three parallel lines.

Thorington c. A visual acuity test chart containing yellow Gothic letters on a black ground, so constructed as to subtend an angle of 4 minutes at specified test distances.

Vari-Test c. A reversible chart for near vision testing containing, on one side, an aperture exposing various test targets printed on a rotating disk, and on the other side, reading material of different type sizes for near and intermediate distances. It may be attached to a phoropter rod or be hand held.

Velhagen's c's. Velhagen's plates.

Verhoeff c. An astigmatic test chart consisting of a pair of rotating disks, one containing a series of concentric circles and 24 uniformly spaced radial lines, and the other a series of concentric squares with two lines transecting at right angles.

Walker's c. A chart for recording both perimeter and tangent screen findings with large radial dimension scales centrally, to permit greater detail, and successively smaller dimensional

scales peripherally, whence the 0°–10° interval is twice the 80°–90° interval.

Wallace c. A visual acuity test chart consisting of Gothic letters which subtend an angle of 4 minutes at specified test distances.

◆

chassis (chas'e). The metal eyewires and bridge of a browline frame.

Chauvel's box. See under *box.*

Chavasse (shah-vahz'). **lens; occluder; theory.** See under the nouns.

Chédiak-Higashi syndrome (cheh'-de-ak-hih-gash'e). See under *syndrome.*

cheiroscope (ki'ro-skōp). A haploscopic instrument designed for presenting a line drawing to the view of one eye to be projected visually and traced by means of a pencil or a crayon in the field of view of the other eye; a kind of binocular camera lucida.

chemiluminescence (kem"ih-lu"mih-nes'ens). The emission of light by a substance after excitation by chemical action.

chemosis (ke-mo'sis). Severe edema of the conjunctiva, least marked in the tarsal region.

chessboard of Helmholtz. A checkered pattern distorted into a nonrectilinear pattern as though stretched from the four corners, so designed that when viewed at a theoretically predetermined distance from the eye, the pattern will appear rectilinear. It was devised by Helmholtz to demonstrate subjectively the nonrectilinearity of peripheral vision.

Chevalier lens (shev-ahl'ya). See under *lens.*

chiaro-oscuro (kih-ah"ro-o-sku'ro). Chiaroscura.

chiaroscura (kih-ah"ro-sku'rah). The creation of apparent differences in distance in a two-dimensional picture through the use of shading.

chiasm, optic (ki'azm). A structure of nervous tissue formed by the junction and partial decussation of the optic nerves in the region above the pituitary body. The nasal fibers of each optic nerve decussate and enter the contralateral optic tract. Syn., *chiasma opticum.*

chiasma opticum (ki-az'mah op'tih-kum). Optic chiasm.

chiasmometer (ki"as-mom'eh-ter). An instrument designed by Landolt to measure the distance between the centers of rotation of the eyes. Two slits, each seen monocularly, are separated until they appear to be individually aligned with a single slit midway between the plane of the two slits and the eyes.

chiastometer (ki″as-tom′eh-ter). Chiasmometer.

chiastopic fusion (ki-as-top′ik). See under *fusion.*

Chievitz layer (che′witz). See under *layer.*

chionablepsia (ki″o-nah-blep′se-ah). Snow blindness.

chionablepsy (ki″o-nah-blep′se). Snow blindness.

chipping. The breaking away of excess glass with a special tool, for the purpose of roughly shaping a lens.

chiroscope (ki′ro-skop). Cheiroscope.

chloasma (klo-az′mah). A skin discoloration due to pigmentary hypertrophy, occurring in patches of various sizes and shapes, usually light brown, but they may be yellow or black.

chlorobutanol (klo″ro bu′tah-nol). A substituted alcohol used as a preservative in eye drops.

chlorolabe (klo′ro-lāb). The name proposed by W. A. H. Rushton for a retinal photopigment having its maximum absorption or maximum spectral sensitivity in the midspectral (green) region.

chloroma (klo-ro′mah). Multiple neoplasms usually occurring in or about the bones of the orbit; typically green in color and accompanied by a blood picture of leukemia.

chlorophane (klo′ro-fān). A yellowish-green pigment in the retinal cones of some animals but not of man.

chloropia (klo-ro′pe-ah). Chloropsia.

chloropsia (klo-rop′se-ah). A condition in which objects appear green, as may occur in digitalis poisoning; green vision.

choline (ko′lēn; kol′ēn, ko′lin, kol′in). A compound, $C_5H_{15}NO_2$, included in the vitamin B complex. It affects fat metabolism, helping to prevent fatty livers and "deficiency" hemorrhages in the eyes and kidneys and to develop appetite and growth. When used as a drug, it has an effect similar to that of parasympathetic stimulation.

chondrodystrophia calcificans congenita punctata (kon″dro-distro′fe-ah kal-sif′ih-kanz kon-jen′ih-tah punk-tah′tah). Stippled epiphyses.

chondrodystrophia fetalis hypo-

plastica (kon″dro-dis-tro′fe-ah fetal′is hi″po-plas′tih-kah). Stippled epiphyses.

chondrodystrophy, congenital calcareous (kon″dro-dis′tro-fe). Stippled epiphyses.

chopper, optical. A device which interrupts a beam of light at short regular intervals.

chorea, Huntington's. Huntington's disease. See under *disease.*

choriocapillaris (ko″re-o-kap″ih-la′ris). A layer of the choroid between the lamina vitrea and Sattler's layer, consisting of a network of capillaries which supplies the outer 5 layers of the retina. The network is densest at the macula. Syn., *entochoroidea.*

choriocele (ko′re-o-sēl). A protrusion or hernia of the choroid.

choriodialysis (ko″re-o-di-al′ih-sis). A surgical procedure for the drainage of subretinal fluid in retinal detachment in which the sclera is opened and separated from the choroid, and then the choroid is perforated.

chorioid (ko′re-oid). Choroid. (The etymologically more nearly correct spelling, *chorioid,* is becoming obsolete.)

choriopathy (ko″re-op′ah-the). 1. A morbid condition or disease of the choroid. 2. Noninflammatory disease of the choroid as distinguished from *choroiditis.*

central angioneurotic c. A detachment of the retina in the macular area due to transudates from the choriocapillaris which accumulate behind the pigment epithelium or between the pigment epithelium and retina. When the fluid is situated between the pigment epithelium and the retina, it appears as a circumscribed, elevated, darkened area; when situated behind the pigment epithelium, it may simulate the appearance of a malignant melanoma of the choroid. Subjective symptoms may be reduced vision, micropsia, and metamorphopsia. The visual fields may reveal a central scotoma, often larger for blue than for red or white, which tends to be permanent. However, there may be an acquired hypermetropia with relatively good central vision.

central serous c. Central angiospastic chorioretinopathy.

chorioretinal (ko″re-o-ret′ih-nal). Pertaining to or involving the choroid and retina.

chorioretinitis (ko"re-o-ret"ih-ni'tis). Simultaneous inflammation of the choroid and retina.

c. adhesiva of Krückman. A subacute chorioretinitis with destruction of the membrane of Bruch and resultant infiltration of fibrous tissue into the retina, so that the retina and choroid ultimately adhere into one continuous fibrous scar.

c. centralis serosa. Central angiospastic chorioretinopathy.

congenital syphilitic c. Chorioretinitis appearing in infancy in association with congenital syphilis and occurring in several classified clinical forms. Type 1. Small reddish-yellow spots interspersed with pigment giving the fundus a salt and pepper appearance. Type 2. Large, round, confluent pigment patches in the periphery of the fundus together with patches of atrophic choroid. Type 3. Round, grayish or yellowish spots, extending from the periphery to the posterior pole, which may become confluent into stalactite shape formations. Pigmentation develops later and has a reticular appearance. Type 4. Atrophy of the retina and optic nerve with sclerotic choroidal vessels visible, small and large clumps or branching deposits of pigment resembling retinitis pigmentosa.

diffuse syphilitic c. Chorioretinitis appearing typically in the second stage of syphilis, characterized initially by dense dustlike vitreous opacities, retinal edema, and blurring of the margins of the optic disk without involvement of the nerve head itself. Exudates which may be few or numerous are sometimes found, especially around the macula, the veins are slightly engorged, the arteries normal, and the vessels may become sheathed. In the later stages the vessels are attenuated, the optic disk yellowish, the choroidal vessels sclerosed appearing white and readily visible, and atrophy of the pigment epithelium results in migration of pigment into small or large irregular deposits. The macular area may be spared with preservation of central vision.

c. proliferans. Chorioretinitis sclopetaria.

c. sclopetaria. A term originally introduced into the German literature to identify the choroidal and retinal trauma due to the concussive impact of a bullet entering the orbital area but not penetrating the globe. Syn., *chorioretinitis proliferans*.

c. striata. Chorioretinal helicoid peripapillary degeneration.

toxoplasmic c. Chorioretinitis caused by infection with the protozoan parasite *Toxoplasma*, occurring in congenital or acquired forms. It is typically bilateral and appears as deep, heavily pigmented, necrotic lesions affecting both macular and peripheral areas. There is extensive connective tissue proliferation from the lesions, the retina surrounding the lesions remains normal, and a secondary optic atrophy may occur.

chorioretinopathy (ko"re-o-ret"ih-nop'ah-the). 1. A morbid condition or disease of the choroid and retina. 2. Noninflammatory disease of the choroid and retina as distinguished from *chorioretinitis*.

central angiospastic c. A disease similar to central angiospastic retinopathy but more severe due to added involvement of the neighboring choroid. The elevation of the macular region is more pronounced, visual acuity is considerably reduced, proliferation of the pigment epithelium occurs in early stages, the refraction may become more hypermetropic, and the lesion is more diffusely distributed and contains silvery, irregularly shaped figures. The disease is recurring and prognosis is less favorable. It is attributed to coexisting extravasations from the retinal and choroidal vessels and may lead to circumscribed retinal detachment. Syn., *chorioretinitis centralis serosa; central serous chorioretinopathy; central serous choroiditis; Kitihara's disease; Masuda's disease.*

central serous c. Central angiospastic chorioretinopathy.

choroid (ko'roid). The portion of the vascular tunic or uvea posterior to the ciliary body; the middle coat of the eye lying between the retina and sclera. It is composed of 5 main layers, the suprachoroid, Haller's layer, Sattler's layer, the choriocapillaris, and the lamina vitrea; its primary function is to nourish the retina. Syn., *chorioid; choroidea.*

detached c. A separation of the choroid from the sclera, usually caused by traction from within or by accumulation of fluid in the perichoroidal space.

choroidal (ko-roi'dal). Pertaining to the choroid.

choroidal cleft; fissure. Fetal fissure.

choroidea (ko-roi'de-ah). Choroid.

choroideremia (ko"roi-der-e'me-ah). A sex-linked hereditary degeneration of the pigment epithelium and choroid, usually detected in early life but may be present at birth. In males it is progressive, commences with pigment degeneration, providing a salt and pepper appearance to the peripheral fundus, and advances to complete atrophy with exposure of the white sclera. The earliest symptom is night blindness followed by constriction of the visual fields and eventual total blindness. In the female carrier it is benign and nonprogressive, with no visual complaints, and with the fundus having the salt and pepper appearance. Syn., *progressive choroidal atrophy; progressive tapetochoroidal atrophy; progressive tapetochoroidal dystrophy.*

◆

CHOROIDITIS

choroiditis (ko-roid-i'tis). Inflammation of the choroid.

acute diffuse serous c. 1. A type of diffuse exudative choroiditis of sudden onset in adults, characterized by a diffuse, yellowish, edematous lesion of the entire fundus, retinal detachment, later retinal reattachment, and good prognosis for the return of vision lost during the disease process. 2. Harada's disease.

c. aerata. Chorioretinal helicoid peripapillary degeneration.

albuminuric c. Choroidal changes associated with advanced nephritis.

anterior c. Choroiditis limited to the anterior portion of the globe and, hence, to the periphery of the fundus.

areolar c. Choroiditis in which the first lesion occurs at the macula, with later lesions appearing at increasing distances from it. Unlike other types of choroiditis, the single spots are initially pigmented, and depigmentation follows, proceeding from the center outward. Syn., *Förster's choroiditis, Förster's disease.*

central c. Choroiditis in the region of the macula. Syn., *macular choroiditis.*

central serous c. Central angiospastic chorioretinopathy.

circumpapillary c. Choroiditis near or around the optic disk.

circumscribed c. Exudative choroiditis in which the lesion occurs in one or more clearly defined patches, differentiated from *disseminated* and *diffuse choroiditis.*

conglomerate c. A rare form of choroiditis found in tubercular individuals, characterized by the presence of a conglomerate tubercle as a single irregular mass.

deep c. Choroiditis with lesions deep in the choroid.

diffuse c. Exudative choroiditis in which the lesion is large and diffuse, the result of the coalescing of numerous small, exudative plaques, as differentiated from *circumscribed* and *disseminated choroiditis.*

disseminated c. Exudative choroiditis with numerous isolated, inflammatory foci covering the fundus, as differentiated from *circumscribed* and *diffuse choroiditis.*

Doyne's familial honeycombed c. A primary familial degeneration of the choroid characterized by many colloid deposits in a ring-shaped formation in the area around the macula. In the late stages there is complete degeneration in the central region.

equatorial c. Paving-stone degeneration of the retina.

exudative c. Choroiditis in the exudative or active stage, a result of endogenous infection. The pathology consists of an inflammatory mononuclear infiltration followed by an atrophic stage with scarring and pigmentation in the destroyed spaces. The three major subdivisions are *diffuse, disseminated,* and *circumscribed choroiditis.*

Förster's c. Areolar choroiditis.

geographic c. Serpiginous choroiditis.

c. guttata senilis. Colloid bodies in the macular region; not a true choroiditis, but a degenerative change. Syn., *Hutchinson-Tay choroiditis; Tay's choroiditis; Tay's central guttate choroiditis.*

guttate c. A degenerative disorder characterized by the universal distribution of hyaline bodies or colloid excrescences beneath the retina.

histoplasmic c. Choroiditis due to infection with the fungus *Histoplasma capsulatum,* characterized by isolated, round, yellow-white nodules, of about ⅓ to ½ disk diameter in size, and diagnosed by specific tests for histoplasmosis.

Hutchinson-Tay c. Choroiditis guttata senilis.

c. hyperplastica of Schöbl. A subacute choroiditis with destruction of the lamina vitrea and resultant infiltration of fibrous tissue into the retina and vitreous.

Jensen's c. Jensen's disease.

juvenile exudative macular c. Juvenile disciform degeneration of the macula. See under *degeneration, disciform.*

juxtapapillary c. Jensen's disease.

macular c. Central choroiditis.

miliary c. Tuberculosis of the choroid associated with miliary tuberculosis, typically characterized by the presence of multiple, small, round, ill-defined, yellowish spots scattered over the fundus.

myopic c. 1. Chronic inflammation of the choroid attributed to myopia. 2. Degenerative choroidal changes accompanying myopia of high degree.

nonsuppurative c. Exudative choroiditis.

c. proliferans. A sequel of an inflammatory retinal detachment consisting of profuse and dense scar tissue appearing as flat white subretinal strands.

purulent c. Suppurative choroiditis.

senile macular exudative c. Senile disciform degeneration of the macula. See under *degeneration, disciform.*

septic c. of Friedenwald. A rare type of bilateral granulomatous uveitis occurring at a late stage of septicemia.

c. serosa. Glaucoma.

serpiginous c. A suddenly developing, slowly resolving and recurring disease of the choroid of unknown etiology which begins as a gray, well-defined lesion at the level of the pigment epithelium, eventually destroying the epithelium and resulting in choroidal atrophy. Syn., *geographic choroiditis.*

superficial c. Choroiditis in which the lesions are located superficially in the choroid.

suppurative c. Choroiditis ac-companied by the formation of pus. Syn., *purulent choroiditis.*

syphilitic c. Choroiditis attributable to the presence of syphilis.

Tay's c. Choroiditis guttata senilis.

tuberculous c. Choroiditis attributable to the presence of tuberculosis.

◆

choroidocyclitis (ko-roi″do-sik-li′tis, -si-kli′tis). Inflammation involving both the choroid and the ciliary body.

choroido-iritis (ko-roi″do-i-ri′tis). Inflammation involving both the choroid and the iris.

choroidopathy (ko-roid-op′ah-the). A morbid or diseased condition of the choroid, not necessarily inflammatory. Cf. *choroiditis.*

choroidoretinitis (ko-roi″do-ret-ih-ni′tis). Inflammation involving both the choroid and the retina. Syn., *chorioretinitis.*

choroidoscopy (ko″roi-dos′ko-pe). Examination of the choroid, usually performed by transilluminating the eye and observing the fundus with an uniluminated ophthalmoscope.

choroidosis (ko″roi-do′sis). Noninflammatory degeneration of the choroid.

choroidotomy (ko″roi-dot′o-me). Surgical incision of the choroid.

Choyce implant (chois). See under *implant.*

Choyce Mark VIII lens. See under *lens.*

Christian's disease (kris′chanz). Schüller-Christian-Hand disease.

Christian's syndrome (kris′chanz). Schüller-Christian-Hand syndrome.

Christiansen filter (kris′chan-sen). See under *filter.*

chroma (kro′mah). 1. The dimension of the Munsell system of color which corresponds most closely to saturation. 2. Saturation; hue content. 3. Chromatic color. A visual quality manifesting hue and saturation.

chromaesthesia (kro″mah-es-the′ze-ah). Chromesthesia.

chromaphotometer (kro″mah-fo-tom′-eh-ter). Chromophotometer.

chromaphotometry (kro″mah-fo-tom′-eh-tre). Chromophotometry.

chromascope (kro′mah-skōp). Chromoscope.

chromasia (kro-ma′zhuh, -ze-uh). The

coloring of an optical image, due to chromatic aberration in the optical system.

chromastereopsis (kro"mah-ste"re-op'sis). Chromostereopsis.

chromatelopia (kro"mat-el-o'pe-ah). Chromatelopsia.

chromatelopsia (kro"mah-tel-op'se-ah). Color blindness; defective perception of colors. One of a number of rarely used or obsolete terms denoting defective color vision, such as *chromotelopia, chromatodysopia, chromatometablepsia, chromatopseudopsis, chromatopseudoblepsia, dyschromatopia, dyschromatopsia.*

chromatelopsis (kro"mah-tel-op'sis). Chromatelopsia.

chromatherapy (kro"mah-ther'ah-pe). Treatment of disease by means of colored light; the real or supposed effects of such treatment. Syn., *chromotherapy.*

chromatic (kro-mat'ik). 1. Possessing the visual attribute of hue; colored; hued. 2. Perceptibly different in quality from a neutral gray of the same brightness value. 3. Pertaining to color or colors or to light from different regions of the visible spectrum.

    c. audition. A form of synesthesia in which a subjective sensation of color is caused by sound, or the reverse (phonopsia). See also *chromesthesia.*

    c. contrast. See under *contrast.*

    c. dispersion. See under *dispersion.*

    c. fading. The phenomenon of the sequence of colored afterimages which follows fixation of a white or a white object. Syn., *flight of colors.*

chromaticity (kro"mah-tih'sih-te). 1. The color quality of a stimulus defined by its trichromatic (CIE) specification or by specification of its dominant (or complementary) wavelength and purity. 2. Quality, as distinguished from quantity, of light. 3. The color quality of a stimulus, without reference to the luminance, as defined by two of the trichromatic coefficients (chromaticity co-ordinates) of the standard CIE coordinate system (usually x and y).

chromaticness (kro-mat'ik-nes). The attributes of chromatic color sensation, *hue* and *saturation* collectively, as distinguished from *intensity.*

chromatics (kro-mat'iks). The science of color; that part of optics which treats of

the properties of color. Syn., *chromatology.*

chromatism (kro'mah-tizm). 1. Chromatic aberration. 2. Color manifested in an optical image as a result of chromatic aberration.

    lateral c. Lateral chromatic aberration.

    longitudinal c. Longitudinal chromatic aberration.

chromatoblast (kro-mat'o-blast"). A cell that produces or synthesizes a pigment, such as melanin or a sensitizing visual pigment.

chromatodysopia (kro"mah-to-dis-o'pe-ah). Color blindness. See also *chromatelopsia.*

chromatogenous (kro"mah-toj'enus). Producing color; causing pigmentation.

chromatology (kro"mah-tol'o-je). Chromatics.

chromatometablepsia (kro"mah-to-met"ah-blep'se-ah). Color blindness. See also *chromatelopsia.*

chromatometer (kro"mah-tom'eh-ter). Chromometer.

chromatometry (kro"mah-tom'eh-tre). Chromometry.

chromatophobia (kro"mah-to-fo'be-ah). 1. A morbid aversion to colors or to a particular color, e.g., erythrophobia, a hysterical fear of red. 2. An abnormal sensitivity of the eye to certain colors, resulting in a marked aversion to a particular color, e.g., the erythrophobia or intolerance to red which sometimes occurs after cataract operation. 3. Resistance to stains on the part of cells and tissues; the quality of staining poorly or not at all. Syn., *chromophobia.*

chromatophorotropin (kro"mah-to-for"o-tro'pin). A hormone which regulates concentration or dispersion of pigment in the retina or other pigment-containing structures.

chromatophotometer (kro"mah-to-fo-tom'eh-ter). Chromophotometer.

chromatopseudoblepsia (kro"mah-to-su"do-blep'se-ah). Color blindness. See also *chromatelopsia.*

chromatopseudopsis (kro"mah-to-su-dop'sis). Color blindness. See also *chromatelopsia.*

chromatopsia (kro"mah-top'se-ah). Colored vision; an abnormal condition in which all objects appear in a particular color or tinged with that color. The various chromatopsias are designated according to the color seen, as xanthopsia (yellow vision), erythropsia (red vision), chloropsia (green vision), and cyanopsia (blue vision). Colored vision may occur as an accompanying symptom in various illnesses and diseases, after cataract operation, and following prolonged exposure to dazzling light. Syn, *chromopia; chromopsia; chromopsy; chroopsia.*

toxic c. Colored vision induced by certain toxic drugs, infections, or certain diseases.

chromatopsy (kro'mah-top-se). Chromatopsia.

chromatoptometer (kro"mah-top-tom'eh-ter). Chromometer.

chromatoptometry (kro"mah-top-tom'eh-tre). Chromometry.

chromatoscope (kro-mat'o-skōp"). 1. Chromoscope. 2. A reflecting telescope for studying the scintillations of stars. Part of it may be rotated eccentrically to produce the image of a star as a ring instead of as a point.

chromatoscopy (kro"mah-tos'ko-pe). Chromoscopy.

chromatoskiameter (kro"mah-to-ski-am'eh-ter). A type of chromometer employing colored shadows.

chromatrope (kro'mah-trōp). 1. A device, usually used as a lantern slide, consisting of transparent colored disks with radiating designs, so arranged that by rotating them in opposite directions, one in front of the other, a kaleidoscopic effect is produced. 2. A disk so painted with different colors that when it is rotated on its central axis, streams of color appear to flow to or from the center.

chrome orthoptics (krōm or-thop'-tiks). See under *orthoptics.*

chromesthesia (krōm-es-the'ze-ah). 1. A form of synesthesia in which colors are seen when certain sounds are heard or when certain smells or tastes are sensed. 2. The association of colors with various words, sounds, names, phrases, tastes, smells, or tactile sensations. 3. A condition in which another sensation, such as taste or smell, is excited by the perception of color. 4. The color sense.

chromheteropia (krōm"het-er-o'pe-ah). Heterochromia iridis.

chromic (kro'mik). 1. Pertaining to, having, or related to, color. 2. Of or pertaining to chromium.

chrominance (kro'min-ans). In color vision technology, the colorimetric difference between a color sample and a reference standard, usually achromatic, of the same luminance, and usually expressed as the product of the chromaticity difference and the luminance.

chromodacryorrhea (kro"mo-dak"re-o-re'ah). The discharge of tears containing blood.

chromometer (kro-mom'eh-ter). An instrument or scale for doing chromometry. Syn., *chromatometer; chromatoptometer; chromoptometer.*

chromometry (kro-mom'eh-tre). Measurement (or testing) of color or color perception by matching or mixing procedures, or by direct measurement. Cf. *chromophotometry; chromoscopy; colorimetry.* Syn., *chromatometry; chromatoptometry.*

chromophane (kro'mo-fān). A retinal pigment; the coloring matter of the fat globules found in the retinal cones of birds.

chromophobia (kro"mo-fo'be-ah). Chromatophobia.

chromophose (kro'mo-fōz). A subjective sensation of color.

chromophotometer (kro'mo-fo-tom'-eh-ter). An instrument for doing chromophotometry.

chromophotometry (kro"mo-fo-tom'-eh-tre). Photometry of colors and colored light sources.

chromopia (kro-mo'pe-ah). Chromatopsia.

chromopsia (kro-mop'se-ah). Chromatopsia.

chromopsy (kro-mop'se). Chromatopsia.

chromoptometer (kro"mop-tom'eh-ter). Chromometer.

chromoretinography (kro"mo-ret'ih-nog"rah-fe). Color photography of the fundus of the eye.

chromoscope (kro'mo-skōp). An instrument or scale for doing chromoscopy.

chromoscopy (kro-mos'ko-pe). The observation, demonstration, or testing of color phenomena and color performances related to characteristics of color perception or to the optical properties of colored lights or pigments. Cf. *chromometry; chromophotometry; colorimetry.*

chromostereopsis (kro"mo-ster-e-op'sis). Stereopsis resulting from differential prismatic effects in the eyes for different wavelengths of light when the pupils are eccentric with respect to the optical axes, whence, binocularly, a red object will normally appear closer than an equally distant green object. The effect may be eliminated, reversed, or accentuated by the proper placing of artificial pupils before the eyes.

chromostroboscope (kro"mo-stro'bo-skōp). A stroboscopic or kinetoscopic device employing color as an essential feature, or one used to demonstrate persistence of vision for various colors.

chromotalopsia (kro"mo-tah-lop'se-ah). Chromatelopsia.

chromotherapy (kro"mo-ther'ah-pe). Chromatherapy.

chromotrope (kro'mo-trōp). Chromatrope.

chronaxia (kro-nak'se-ah). Chronaxie.

chronaxie (kro'nak-se). The index of sensitivity of a tissue to electrical stimulation. It is the minimum time required to produce an effect with a constant current twice the rheobase.

chronaxy (kro'nak-se). Chronaxie.

chronoscope (kron'o-skōp). An instrument for measuring the duration of extremely short-lived exposures or flashes, utilizing a rapidly rotating mirror which projects the flash in an arc, the length or displacement of which corresponds to its duration.

chroopsia (kro-op'se-ah). Chromatopsia.

chrysiasis (krih-si'ah-sis). The permanent deposition of gold in the tissue following repeated parenteral administration of gold salts.

    c. corneae. Chrysiasis of the subepithelial tissue of the cornea.

    ocular c. Chrysiasis of the conjunctiva and/or cornea.

chrysopsin (kris-op'sin). A photosensitive pigment, "visual gold," found in the retinae of some deep sea fishes, of golden color because of high absorption of short wavelengths of light and relatively high reflectance of longer wavelengths.

chrysosis (kris-o'sis). Chrysiasis.

chuck. A device for centering and holding the lens in an edger or grinding machine.

Chvostek's sign (vos'teks). See under *sign.*

chymotrypsin, *alpha* (ki"mo-trip'sin). A proteolytic enzyme used in the procedure of zonulolysis to facilitate surgical removal of the crystalline lens. It is also used in the treatment of keratitis

and corneal ulcers and in certain affections of the conjunctiva or sclera.

Ciaccio's gland (chah'chōz). See under *gland.*

Cibis test. See under *test.*

CIE. See *Commission Internationale de l'Eclairage.*

cilia (sil'e-ah). 1. The eyelashes. 2. Minute, lashlike processes.

ciliariscope (sil"e-ar'ih-skōp, si"le-). An instrument composed of a prism attached to an ophthalmoscope for examining the ciliary body of the eye.

ciliarotomy (sil"e-ar-ot'o-me). Surgical division of the ciliary zone in the treatment of glaucoma.

ciliary (sil'e-er"e). Pertaining to the eyelashes, the ciliary body, or to any hairlike processes.

ciliary body; canal; corona; folds; ganglion; injection; muscle; processes. See under the nouns.

ciliectomy (sil"e-ek'to-me). 1. Surgical removal of part of the ciliary body. 2. Surgical removal of part of a margin of an eyelid containing the roots of the eyelashes.

ciliogenesis (sil"e-o-jen'e-sis). The development and regeneration of eyelashes.

ciliometer (sih"le-om'eh-ter). Cilometer.

cilioretinal (sil"e-o-ret'ih-nal). 1. Pertaining to both the ciliary body and the retina. 2. Pertaining to an arterial branch of the circle of Haller, which enters the retina on the temporal side of the optic disk; rarely to a vein that drains the macular region, emptying into a choroidal vein.

cilioscleral (sil"e-o-skle'ral). Pertaining to both the ciliary body and the sclera.

ciliosis (sil"e-o'sis). Cillosis.

ciliospinal (sil"e-o-spi'nal). Pertaining to the ciliospinal center.

ciliotomy (sil-e-ot'o-me). Surgical section of the ciliary nerves.

cilium (sil'e-um). 1. An eyelash. 2. A minute, hairlike process.

    c. inversum. A rare congenital anomaly in which an eyelash grows inward into the skin of the eyelid.

cillo (sil'o). Cillosis.

cillosis (sil-o'sis). Spasmodic twitching of the eyelids. Syn., *ciliosis; cillo.*

cilometer (sih-lom'eh-ter). An accommodation measuring instrument employing the Badal optometer system.

cinching (sinch'ing). Surgical dividing of an extraocular muscle tendon into several strands around which a cable of threads is wound and pulled taut, effecting a shortening of the tendon.

cinclisis (sin'klih-sis). Rapid winking.

Cinefro bifocal contact lens (sin'eh-fro). See under *lens, contact, bifocal.*

CIP. Abbreviation for *corneal indentation pulse.*

◆

CIRCLE

circle. 1. A closed curved line, all points of which are equidistant from a point within called the center. 2. A circular anastomosis of arteries or veins.

arterial c. of the canal of Schlemm. An incomplete circle of arterioles which embraces the canal of Schlemm over most of its extent and which is derived from the anterior ciliary arteries.

Berry's c's. Circles, used as a stereopsis test, which provide varying degrees of retinal disparity.

blur c. A cross section of a bundle of focused rays originating from a point source. Syn., *circle of confusion; diffusion circle; circle of dispersion.*

color c. A system of hues represented on a circle; the spectral colors in their original order arranged on a circle, with the purple hues connecting the extremes of the visible spectrum; a horizontal section of the color solid. Syn., *hue circle.* **Farnsworth double c.c.** A double-color circle in which the inner circle is a Munsell color circle modified to 85 hues and the outer is a circle showing the corresponding dominant spectral wavelengths. **Helmholtz' c.c.** A color chart with saturated colors on the circumference of a circle and with white in the center. The transitions from white to any saturated color at a point on the circumference of the circle lie along the radius drawn to this point. Syn., *Helmholtz' color table.* **Hering's c.c.** A psychologic color circle represented by an oval on two concentric circles such that it is tangent to the inner circle in the vertical meridian and to the outer circle in the horizontal meridian. The four crescent-shaped areas are labeled red and green at the top and bottom, respectively, and blue and yellow at the left and right, respectively, and the thickness of each crescent at any given meridian indicates the relative intensities of the primary ingredients in each color. The colors on opposite sides of the circle cannot be blended, while adjacent colors can be blended to form mixed hues. **Munsell c.c.** A color circle consisting of an orderly arrangement of 100 hues of constant Munsell value and chroma based on a just noticeable hue difference scale. **Newton's c.c.** A schema for mixing colors, consisting of Newton's colors arranged about a circle subtending distances proportional to the musical intervals of the octave, with white (gray) at the center. Syn., *Newton's color table.* **Ostwald c.c.** A diagram based on Hering's color circle divided into 24 numbered hues, based on eight principal color regions each divided into three sections. The eight principal color regions are derived from four primal colors and four in-between blends. Ostwald also published a similar color circle with 100 hue divisions. **psychologic c.c.** An orderly arrangement of the primal colors and their blends in a circle to demonstrate the continuous variation in hue from red to yellow to green to blue to red. **Southall's double c.c.** A pair of concentric circles with hues designated on the inner circle and the corresponding spectral wavelengths of the hues on the outer circle which is incomplete because purples are not present in the spectrum.

c. of confusion. Blur circle.

corresponding c. of sensation. Panum's area.

diffusion c. Blur circle.

direction c's. The circles on the spherical field of fixation that pass through the occipital point. There are two sets of direction circles, i.e., the set that lies in a horizontal plane perpendicular to the vertical xz plane and the set that lies in a vertical plane perpendicular to the horizontal xy plane. The projection of each set of direction circles onto a plane perpendicular to the primary direction forms two families of hyperbolic arcs, the curves of which intersect orthogonally. (Helmholtz)

c. of dispersion. Blur circle.

greater arterial c. of the iris. A vascular circle, formed by anastomoses of 7 anterior ciliary arteries and 2 long posterior ciliary arteries, located about the root of the iris in the ciliary body. It supplies the ciliary body, anterior choroid, and the lesser arterial circle of the iris. Syn., *annulus iridis major; circulus arteriosus iridis major.*

c. of Haller. An arterial circle about the optic nerve within the sclera, formed by anastomoses of a few short posterior ciliary arteries. Branches pass to the optic nerve, the pia mater, the optic nerve head, and the neighboring choroid and retina. The cilioretinal artery, when present, arises from it. Syn., *circle of Zinn; vascular circle of the optic nerve; Zinn's corona.*

c. of Hovius. A network of veins in most mammals, other than man, located in the sclera posterior to the corneoscleral margin, which drains aqueous humor into the vortex veins. Syn., *circulus venosus hovii; Hovius' plexus; Leber's venous plexus.*

hue c. Color circle.

primary isogonal c. The circle passing through the point of fixation and the centers of rotation of the two eyes. The plane of the circle contains the two visual axes and the two horizontal retinal meridians. See also *Vieth-Mueller circle, longitudinal horopter,* and *monoscopter.*

secondary isogonal c. A circle passing through the centers of rotation of the two eyes and through any indirect point of view which lies above or below the point of fixation at a distance equal to that of the point of fixation, this distance being measured from the midpoint of the line connecting the centers of rotation. For a given fixation distance there is an infinite number of secondary isogonal circles, the plane of each containing only indirect visual lines.

c. of least aberration. Circle of least confusion.

c. of least chromatic aberration. The circular image of a point source of heterochromatic light when the receiving screen lies approximately midway between the focal images of the extreme red and blue rays.

c. of least confusion. 1. The circular section found intermediate between the two line images of the bundle of rays forming Sturm's conoid. 2. The smallest cross section of a circular (non-astigmatic) bundle of rays. Syn., *circle of least aberration; circle of least diffusion.*

c. of least diffusion. Circle of least confusion.

Leber's venous c. Canal of Schlemm.

lesser arterial c. of the iris. An incomplete vascular circle formed by arterio-venous anastomoses in the region of the collarette, near the pupillary margin of the iris. It receives blood from the greater arterial circle of the iris and supplies the pupillary zone of the iris. Syn., *annulus iridis minor; minor vascular circle; circulus arteriosus iridis minor.*

lymphatic c. of Teichmann. Terminal lymphatic loops encircling the cornea, in the region of the limbus, which drain into the radial vessels of Teichmann.

Minsky's c's. A series of circles on clinical record cards for pictorially recording eye lesions, each circle representing one of a series of planes from the cornea to the retina. The circles are lettered *C* for *cornea, AC* for *anterior chamber, I* for *iris, L* for *lens, V* for *vitreous,* and *R* for *retina.* The layers are further divided, there being, e.g., 5 corneal layers labeled from C-1 to C-5. A lesion of the epithelial layer would be depicted in the circle labeled C-1.

minor vascular c. Lesser arterial circle of the iris.

Mueller's horopter c. Vieth-Mueller horopter.

optical c. In physics, a graduated circle fitted with the necessary appliances for illustrating the laws of refraction and reflection or, when accurately constructed, for measuring interfacial angles, refractive indices, etc.

parhelic c. A luminous horizontal circle or halo at the solar level in a cirrus clouded sky. Syn., *parhelic ring.*

Ramsden c. The exit pupil of a telescope or microscope seen as a bright disk of light floating in the air near the eyepiece, or focused on a white paper held near the eyepiece, when the instrument is pointed toward an extended bright surface.

Rowland's c. In a concave mirror diffraction grating, the locus of points where the spectrum is in focus.

Thompson's c's. An apparatus for producing motion afterimages; an apparatus for creating the illusion of motion in a stationary object after previous exposure to a stimulus in motion, similar to Plateau's spiral.

vascular c. of the optic nerve. Circle of Haller.

venous c. of Leber. Canal of Schlemm.

Verhoeff's c. A visual acuity test object consisting of two concentric rings of 1 minute of arc width separated by a space of the same width when viewed at a specified distance. Syn., *Verhoeff's rings.*

Vieth-Mueller c. Vieth-Mueller horopter.

c. of Willis. An arterial ring surrounding the optic chiasm and hypothalamus, formed by the basilar, posterior cerebral, posterior communicating, internal carotid, anterior cerebral, and anterior communicating arteries.

c. of Zinn. Circle of Haller.

◆

circulus (ser'ku-lus). Circle.

c. arteriosus halleri. Circle of Haller.

c. arteriosus iridis major. Greater arterial circle of the iris.

c. arteriosus iridis minor. Lesser arterial circle of the iris.

c. arteriosus nervi optici. Circle of Haller.

c. senilis. An arcus senilis which completely surrounds the cornea.

c. vasculosus nervi optici. Circle of Haller.

c. venosus hovii. Circle of Hovius.

c. zinii. Circle of Haller.

circumbulbar (ser"kum-bul'bar). 1. Situated around the eyeball. 2. Situated around the hindbrain part of the brain stem.

circumcorneal (ser"kum-kōr'ne-al). Surrounding the cornea, as in circumcorneal injection.

circumlental (ser"kum-len'tal). Surrounding the crystalline lens at the equator, as does the canal of Hannover between the leaves of the zonule of Zinn.

circumocular (ser"kum-ok'u-lar). Surrounding the eyeball. Syn., *circumbulbar.*

circumorbital (ser"kum-ōr'bih-tal). Surrounding the bony orbit.

circumpapillary (ser"kum-pap'ih-ler"e). Surrounding the optic disk.

cirsophthalmia (ser"sof-thal'me-ah). 1. Conjunctivitis in which the vessels are in a varicose condition. 2. Corneal staphyloma in which the surface of the cornea and sclera have a bluish varicose appearance.

cis-retinene (sis-ret'ih-nēn). See *retinaldehyde.*

cistern, chiasmatic (sis'tern). A subarachnoid space between the pituitary body and the optic chiasm. Syn., *cisterna basalis.*

cisterna basalis (sis-tern'ah ba-sal'is). Chiasmatic cistern.

clarity, visual. The overall subjective impression that a scene or display is distinct in detail and perceptually satisfying.

Clason acuity meter (cla'son). See under *meter.*

Claude's syndrome (klodz). See under *syndrome.*

Claude Bernard's syndrome (klod ber-narz'). See *syndrome, Bernard's.*

cleaner, ultrasonic. A cleaner containing liquid vibrated at ultrasonic frequency to remove dirt particles from lenses, frames, etc., immersed in it.

clearness. A perceptual attribute of transparent and translucent materials, the opposite of *milkiness* or *cloudiness.* The quality of being clear, sharp, without blur.

cleft. A crevice, groove, or fissure.

choroidal c. Fetal fissure.

ciliary c. 1. In the avian eye, an opening between ciliary processes which provides passageway between the anterior and posterior chambers. 2. A triangular space between the outer scleral portion and the inner uveal portion of the anterior ciliary body in the region of the angle of the anterior chamber of lower animals such as rodents. In man and other primates it is replaced by tissue leaving only a remnant. Syn., *ciliary sinus.*

corneal c. The groove of the sclera into which the cornea fits.

fetal c. Fetal fissure.

Fuchs' c. A narrow space, seen at about the fifth fetal month, between the pupillary region of the iris and the pupillary membrane prior to its atrophy.

clinic. A place and organization for the examination, diagnosis, study, and treatment of physical and mental disorders.

clinical. 1. Pertaining to findings of a routine examination as opposed to findings obtained under controlled conditions for specific research purposes. 2. Pertaining to the observation of the symptoms and course of a disease. 3. Pertaining to a clinic.

clinometer (kli-nom'eh-ter). An apparatus for measuring ocular torsion.

Duane's c. An instrument for studying torsional movements of the eye.

clinoscope, Stevens' (kli'no-skōp). An instrument for measuring cyclophoria, consisting essentially of two tubes nearly 20 in. long, each mounted so that it may be rotated about its longitudinal axis.

clip, Halberg. A trade name for a plastic device with cells for holding trial lenses which is clipped over the lens of a pair of spectacles.

clip-on. A lightweight frame without temples, for holding auxiliary lenses, which can be attached to regular spectacles by means of wire hooks. Syn., *fit-on; fit-over.*

clip-over. Clip-on.

clivus (kli'vus). The gently curved wall of the fovea.

CLMA. See *Contact Lens Manufacturers Association.*

clock, lens. Lens measure.

clock, Luer's. A cylindro-spherometer.

Cloquet's canal (klo-kāz'). See under *canal.*

closure. A perception of a single large unit rather than a number of apparently unrelated parts; collective configuration.

closure, visual. 1. Perception of an incomplete object as if it were complete. 2. Perception of an incompletely seen object as if it were complete, as, for example, a horizontal line traversing the blind spot of Mariotte.

clouding, central corneal. A superficial diffuse edema of the cornea, usually circular, and associated with the wearing of contact lenses which either bear on the central epithelium or entrap tear fluid in this area. It is most easily seen without magnification with sclerotic scatter illumination from the beam of a slit lamp, appearing as a dull, gray area surrounded by clear cornea.

club, Landolt. A sclerally directed dendrite of a retinal bipolar cell which passes between the bodies of rods and cones to terminate in the vicinity of the external limiting membrane; of unknown synaptic relations and function.

clue, fusion. In a pair of haploscopic stimulus targets, the elements of the pattern which are presented to one eye only for the purpose of confirming that the eye is being used during binocular testing or training. Syn., *control.*

cm. Abbreviation for *centimeter.*

coagulation, light (ko-ag"u-la'shun). Photocoagulation.

coat. 1. A layer of substance covering another. 2. A membrane covering or lining a part or an organ.

fibrous c. of eyeball. The cornea and sclera together.

nervous c. of eyeball. The retina.

uveal c. The vascular coat of the eyeball.

vaginal c. Tenon's capsule.

vascular c. of eyeball. The uvea, consisting of the choroid, ciliary body, and iris.

coating, lens. A thin deposit of a metallic salt, such as magnesium fluoride, about one fourth as thick as a wavelength of light, applied to the surfaces of a lens to reduce, by interference, the amount of light reflected, and, if combined with a coloring ingredient, to reduce light transmission also.

Coats' (kōts) **disease; retinitis; rings.** See under the nouns.

cocaine (ko-kān', ko'kān, ko'kuh-ēn). An alkaloid derivative from coca leaves used as a local anesthetic, mydriatic, and narcotic. Its hydrochloride stimulates peripheral sympathetic nerve endings in the iris and causes moderate dilatation of the pupil with little effect on the ciliary muscle and hence on accommodation.

Cochet's test (ko-shāz'). See under *test.*

Cochet-Bonnet esthesiometer (ko'-sha-bo-na'). See under *esthesiometer.*

Cockayne's (kok'ānz) **disease; syndrome.** See under *syndrome.*

Coddington lens (kod'ing-tun). See under *lens.*

◆

COEFFICIENT

coefficient (ko"e-fish'ent). A number or a letter symbol which denotes any of a group of numbers. The coefficient or number may denote or express any of the following: (1) the amount by which a mathematical expression is to be multiplied; (2) the amount of change or the amount of effect due to change; (3) the amount or degree of a quality possessed; (4) a ratio.

c. of absorption. The fraction of the incident intensity absorbed per unit thickness of a transmitting medium.

c. of attenuation. The reduction of collimated radiant flux normally traversing an infinitesimal layer of an absorbing and slightly diffusing medium divided by the product of the incident flux and the thickness of the layer.

chroma-brilliance c. The ratio of the number of units of chromatic valence to the number of units of brightness in a sample visual stimulus.

dichromatic c's. The relative intensities of the components (primary colors) of a two-color mixture required by a dichromat to match a sample color.

c. of facility of aqueous outflow. The change in tonometric scale readings during prolonged tonometry in terms of units of intraocular fluid expelled, divided by units of pressure change and time; expressed by the ratio:

$$C = \frac{\Delta V}{T[average\ P_t - (P_0 + \Delta P_v)]}$$

in which

C = coefficient of the facility of aqueous outflow

ΔV = intraocular fluid expelled

T = time

P_t = intraocular pressure during tonometry

P_0 = intraocular pressure just prior to tonometry

ΔP_v = pressure change in the episcleral veins (approx. 1.25 mm Hg)

The P_0 values are those of the 1955 conversion scale for the Schiötz tonometer.

Fresnel's dragging c. A coefficient dealing with relative motion of ether and light waves. It is expressed as a fraction $1 - \frac{1}{n^2}$, where n is the index of refraction. *Obs.*

Friedenwald's c. A numerical quantity representing the resistance of the ocular coats to distension, determined by Friedenwald by taking two readings with the Schiötz tonometer, each with a different weight, and relating these measurements to the volume changes produced by these weights. A high value indicates a more rigid coat and a low value a more pliable one.

c. of light extinction. The relative amount or percentage of incident light of a given wavelength absorbed by a 1% solution of a substance in a layer 1 cm thick.

luminosity c. The constants by which the color mixture data for any color must be multiplied so that the sum of the three products is equal to the luminance of the color. Syn., *visibility coefficient.*

c. of ocular rigidity. A numerical value mathematically derived from two tonometric readings with different weights and said to represent the resistance of the ocular coats to distension, used in calculating intraocular pressure. Syn., *coefficient of scleral rigidity.*

c. of reflection. The ratio of reflected flux to incident flux. Syn., *reflectance.*

c. of refraction. Index of refraction. *Obs.*

scattering c. The proportion of light scattered per unit thickness of the transmitting medium.

c. of scleral rigidity. Coefficient of ocular rigidity.

transmission c. The fractional portion of incident energy transmitted per unit thickness of the transmitting medium.

trichromatic c's. Chromaticity coordinates.

c. of utilization. The ratio of luminous flux (lumens) received on the work plane to the rated lumens emitted by the lamps.

visibility c. Luminosity coefficient.

◆

coelostat (se'lo-stat). A clock-driven mirror which rotates about an axis parallel to the plane of the mirror and to the axis of the earth in synchrony with the earth's rotation so that the reflected image of a star outside of the solar system remains fixed with respect to a terrestrial point of reference.

Cogan's (ko'ganz) **corneal dystrophy; implant; lid twitch sign; syndrome.** See under the nouns.

Cogan-Kinsey theory (ko'gan kin'se). See *theory, osmotic pump.*

coherence (ko-hēr'ens). 1. A property of electromagnetic radiation from a source in which all the propagated energy is in phase, the maxima and minima of all waves being coincident; the energy being propagated from each point at the emitter is in phase with every other point. 2. In fiber optics, a point to point relationship between the two ends of the fiber bundle.

lateral c. Phase synchronism across a wavefront. Syn., *spatial coherence.*

longitudinal c. Temporal stability of phase in succeeding wavefronts of a wave train. Syn., *temporal coherence.*

spatial c. Lateral coherence.

temporal c. Longitudinal coherence.

Cohn's (kōnz) **test; theory.** See under the nouns.

COIT. See *Current Optometric Information and Terminology.*

Colenbrander's formula (ko'len-brand"erz). See under *formula.*

collar. That part of a rimless spectacle mounting which fits against the edge of the lens and to which the straps are attached. Syn., *shoe.*

collarette (kol"er-et'). The line of junction between the pupillary zone and the ciliary zone on the anterior surface of the iris. In the normal iris, it is an irregular circular line lying about 1.5 mm from the pupillary border.

collective configuration. 1. The perception of a complete pattern, although parts of it are absent in the immediate stimulus, as in perceiving a straight line unbroken when it traverses the blind spot. 2. The tendency to perceive a complex pattern as a whole rather than as an assembly of its parts.

collectors. Very small ducts which transmit aqueous humor from the canal of Schlemm to the deep scleral plexus.

collector, cosine. A device which effectively summates the cosines of the angles of incidence of light falling on a flat surface, such as a slab of opal glass, which transmits light approximately in proportion to the cosine of the angle of incidence.

College of Optometrists in Vision Development. An American association of optometrists founded in 1971 by the merger of three prior associations to promote interest in developmental aspects of vision, orthoptics, visual training, and children's vision, and to certify optometrists skilled in the specialty.

Collet's sign (kol-lets'). See under *sign.*

colliculus, inferior (kŏ-lik'u-lus). Either of the lower paired eminences of the dorsal midbrain, acting as relay centers for auditory reflexes.

colliculus, superior (kŏ-lik'u-lus). Either of the upper paired eminences of the dorsal midbrain, located near the pineal body, acting as relay centers for visual reflexes that affect skeletal muscle.

Collier's (kol'e-erz) **sphenoidal palsy; sign.** See under the nouns.

collimate (kol'ih-māt). 1. To render a bundle of rays parallel. 2. To adjust an optical instrument so that its mechanical and optical axes are coincident or parallel.

collimator (kol'ih-ma"tor). A device for producing parallel rays of light. Usually, an achromatic objective with a point source of light at one of its focal points.

collineation (kŏ-lin"e-a'shun). A point to point geometric correspondence between object and image space of an optical system.

central c. A method, by geometric construction, of locating images produced by the refraction of paraxial rays at a single spherical surface or through an infinitely thin lens.

Collins-Franceschetti-Zwahlen syndrome (kahl'inz-fran"ses-chet'-e-zwah'len). Mandibulofacial dysostosis. See under *dysostosis.*

Collins' glands; theory. See under the nouns.

collyria (kŏ-lir'e-ah). The plural of collyrium.

collyrium (kŏ-lir'e-um). An eyewash or a lotion for the eyes.

colmascope (kol'mah-skōp). An instrument which uses transmitted polarized light for determining stress and strain in glass.

colmatage (kall'med-idge). A surgical procedure for retinal detachment in which triple rows of cauterizations are made underneath a conjunctival flap dissected up from the limbus.

◆

COLOBOMA

coloboma (kol"o-bo'mah). 1. A congenital anomaly in which a portion of a structure of the eye (or eyelid) is absent. The majority are due to incomplete closure of the fetal fissure and are located inferiorly (typical coloboma). 2. Any defect in which a portion of a structure of an eye (or eyelid) is absent. It may be congenital, pathologic, or operative.

atypical c. A coloboma not located inferiorly in any part of the eye or not due to incomplete closure of the fetal fissure.

bridge c. A coloboma in which isolated areas of the fetal fissure fuse to form a bridge of tissue across the defect.

c. of the choroid. A congenital absence of choroidal tissue in a portion of the fundus of the eye, typically located inferiorly and due to incomplete closure of the fetal fissure. The retina in the corresponding area is also absent, resulting in a scotoma in the visual field. The ophthalmoscopic picture is of a white area of exposed sclera with a sharply defined pigmented border.

c. of the ciliary body. A congenital absence of tissue of the ciliary body which typically appears as an anterior indentation with a characteristic hyperplasia of the adjacent ciliary processes, forming large polypoid masses. The ciliary muscle is absent and the pigmented epithelium is incomplete in the region of the defect.

complete c. 1. A coloboma caused by failure of closure of the fetal fissure along its entire length, thus involving the iris, ciliary body, choroid, retina, and optic disk. 2. A coloboma in which there is a local absence of both ectodermal and mesodermal layers.

c. of the eyelid. A congenital notch or cleft in the upper or lower eyelid margin.

Fuchs' c. A congenital crescentic colobomatous defect of the choroid at the lower margin of the optic disk.

c. of the fundus. A congenital absence of retinal and choroidal tissue in a portion of the fundus of the eye, typically located inferiorly and due to incomplete closure of the fetal fissure. The ophthalmoscopic picture is of a white area of exposed sclera with a sharply defined pigmented border. **bridge c. of the f.** A coloboma of the fundus which is divided into two or more sections by a strip of apparently normal tissue.

incomplete c. 1. Partial coloboma. 2. Coloboma in which there is a local absence of either the mesodermal or the ectodermal layer.

c. of the iris. A congenital notch or cleft in the iris. It may be total, partial, simple, complete, incomplete, or notch coloboma. **bridge c. of the i.** Coloboma of the iris in which mesodermal tissue derived from the pupillary membrane stretches across the defect. **complete c. of the i.** Coloboma of the iris in which both mesodermal and ectodermal layers are absent. Cf. *incomplete*

coloboma of the iris. **incomplete c. of the i.** Coloboma of the iris in which either the mesodermal or the ectodermal layer is absent. Cf. *complete coloboma of the iris.* Syn., *pseudocoloboma.* **notch c. of the i.** A partial coloboma of the iris at the pupillary margin. It occurs typically in the lower sector of the iris and may be multiple. **partial c. of the i.** Coloboma of the iris not involving a whole sector up to the ciliary border. It may be in one of three forms: (1) a notch in the pupillary margin; (2) a hole in the iris substance (pseudopolycoria); (3) a peripheral defect near the ciliary margin (iridodiastasis). **simple c. of the i.** Coloboma occurring only in the iris in the presence of a normally closed fetal fissure. **total c. of the i.** Coloboma of the iris involving an entire sector of the iris up to the ciliary border.

c. of the lens. A congenital notch or cleft at the margin of the crystalline lens, usually downward and with an associated defect of the zonule of Zinn in the same region.

macular c. A congenital defect in which there is an absence of choroidal tissue in the macular area.

notch c. A partial coloboma of the iris at the pupillary margin. It occurs typically in the lower sector of the iris and may be multiple.

c. of the optic disk. A coloboma of the optic nerve head which may be part of a complete coloboma, be associated with coloboma of the fundus, or be limited to the region of the optic disk when only the proximal end of the fetal fissure fails to close. Ophthalmoscopically, it appears as a white area, usually considerably larger than the normal optic disk.

c. of the optic nerve. A congenital defect in the formation of the optic nerve or its sheaths which characteristically appears as a craterlike excavation at the optic disk, surrounded by a hyperplasia of the adjacent retina.

c. palpebrale. A congenital notch or cleft of an eyelid at its margin.

partial c. A coloboma caused by failure of closure of part of the fetal fissure, thus involving only the iris, ciliary body, choroid, optic disk, or retina, but not all.

peripapillary c. Congenital failure of choroidal and retinal development immediately around a normal optic nerve.

c. of the retina. A congenital notch or cleft of the retina, usually located inferiorly.

simple c. A coloboma occurring only in the iris in the presence of a normally closed fetal fissure.

total c. A coloboma of the iris involving an entire sector of the iris up to the ciliary border.

typical c. A coloboma due to an incomplete closure of the fetal cleft and located inferiorly.

c. of the vitreous. A congenital indentation or separation of the vitreous body by persistent mesodermal tissue in the vitreous chamber. The ectodermal vitreous body is actually intact.

◆

COLOR

color. 1. A sensory or perceptual component of visual experience, characterized by the attributes of *hue, brightness,* and *saturation,* and usually arising from, or in response to, stimulation of the retina by radiation of wavelengths between about 380 and 760 mμ. Sensory components, such as white, gray, and black, which have neither hue nor saturation, are sometimes included with colors. Variously synonymous with *hue, tint,* or *shade.* 2. A stimulus or a visual object which evokes a chromatic response.

accidental c. A color percept resulting from an immediate pre-exposure to a nonneutral stimulus, as an afterimage effect.

achromatic c. Sensory or perceptual components possessing a brightness level but no hue or saturation. The achromatic colors are white, gray, and black.

c. amnesia. See under *amnesia.*

antagonistic c. Any of the colors paired in the Hering theory of color vision.

aperture c. A color perceived as filling an aperture. It may be seen close to the plane of the aperture or at some indefinite distance behind it. It is filmy and soft in character and is contrasted with a surface color, which is hard in appearance and exactly localized in space.

c. blend. See under *blend.*

c. blindness. See under *blindness.*

body c. Color perceived in an object by the reflection of light after it has penetrated the object a certain distance and has undergone selective absorption. The same color would thus be seen upon transmission of light through the substance of the object. It should be distinguished from *surface color.*

bulky c. Spatial color.

catoptrical c's. Iridescent colors. *Obs.*

c. chart. See under *chart.*

chromatic c. Color perceptions possessing hue and saturation in addition to the attribute of *brightness,* as red, green, blue, or yellow. Cf. *achromatic color.*

c. circle. See under *circle.*

complementary c's. 1. Any pair of colors in which the direct perception of one produces an afterimage of the other. 2. Any pair of colors in which the direct perception of one produces simultaneous contrast of the other. 3. Two colors which, when additively mixed, produce light gray or white. 4. Two colors which, when subtractively mixed, produce black or gray.

compound c's. Color sensations produced by additively mixing two or more primary colors, as, for example, purple or orange.

c. cone. A type of color solid.

confusion c. A color which appears the same as another color to a person who is color blind.

c. contrast. See under *contrast.*

cool c. A color said to give a psychological feeling of coolness, quietness, or lack of activity, as, for example, green or blue.

c. cycle. Color circle.

dark c. A color of relatively low brightness level. This may exist for any hue, depending on its luminance in relation to its background.

c. disk. See under *disk.*

c. equations. See under *equation.*

equilibrium c. A spectral hue which does not change with variations in intensity. See also *Bezold-Brücke phenomenon.*

equiluminous c's. Colors varying in chromaticity but not in luminance.

extraspectral c. A color, such as purple, which cannot be produced by any one wavelength of the spectrum.

Fechner's c's. Colored rings seen on a rotating disk which is marked out into black and white sectors.

c. fields. See under *field, visual.*

film c. A color seen as indefinitely localized and not belonging to any particular surface or object, as the color seen in the spectroscope.

c. flight. See under *flight.*

full c. A color sample in the Ostwald or Ridgway system which has maximum purity for a particular hue. See also *Ostwald semichrome.*

fundamental c's. 1. Any set of three colors of light, e.g., red, green, and blue, from which all other color sensations can be produced by additive mixing. Syn., *primary colors.* 2. The colors which subjectively seem pure, i.e., not psychologically composed of other colors. These are red, green, blue, and yellow. Syn., *primal colors.*

c. fusion. See under *fusion.*

glowing c. A color seen as an attribute of a glowing body. (David Katz)

hard c. 1. Color seen as an attribute of a hard or firm surface. 2. Certain colors classified by artists and psychologists as inherently hard or firm in appearance, as, for example, red or yellow. Cf. *soft color.*

harmonic c. One of a pair of complementary colors.

illuminant c. Color seen as glowing or as a light source either by virtue of its being an attribute of a light source, as in a neon light, or by possessing a high reflectance in relation to its background.

illumination c. A color seen as belonging to illumination distributed in space, as blue light flooding a stage.

impure c. Any color produced by a mixture of two or more wavelengths; opposite of *monochromatic color.*

induced c. A color appearing in a portion of the visual field, produced by simultaneous contrast from a neighboring portion of the field. Syn., *resulting color.*

inducing c. A color stimulus which induces or produces a color effect in the surrounding region of the visual field by simultaneous contrast.

c. induction. See under *induction.*

invariable c. Stable color.

iridescent c's. Rainbowlike colors produced by interference, as exhibited by soap bubbles or mother-of-pearl.

isomeric c's. Colors of identical spectrophotometric composition and tristimulus values. Syn., *isomeric pair.*

isovalent c's. In the Ostwald system, color of differing hue but having the same proportions of black and white content.

located c. A color in a mode of appearance which makes the stimulus object appear to be finitely located in space, as, for example, bulky or filmy.

luminous c's. A color having the appearance of being a light source. Syn., *illuminant color.*

luster c. A composite color which has the appearance of a color being situated behind and shining through another color, or a color in which bright areas seem to shift upon the surface.

c. matching. See under *matching.*

memory c. The color of an object as retained in one's memory.

metallic c. A color produced by selective reflection from semipolished metallic surfaces, or having the appearance of such colors, e.g., bronze.

metameric c's. Colors of different spectrophotometric composition which appear the same under given conditions. Syn., *metamers; metameric pair.*

mirrored c. Color having the appearance of being reflected in a mirror.

c. mixer. See under *mixer.*

c. mixing. Any process of combining two or more color stimuli, additively or subtractively, so as to produce a single resultant color, as by mixing pigments, superimposing colored lights, or presenting colored surfaces in rapid succession. **additive c.m.** The mixing of colors by summation of the wavelength composition of two or more color stimuli. **binocular c.m.** The subjective mixing of two color stimuli by viewing one color stimulus with one eye and another color stimulus with the corresponding retinal area of the other eye. **subtractive c.m.** The mixing of colors by subtraction of the wavelength composition of one color stimulus from that of another color stimulus, as in pigment mixing or in placing a selectively absorbing filter in front of a color stimulus.

c. mixture. See under *mixture.*

monochromatic c. A color produced by a single wavelength or by a narrow band of wavelengths of the spectrum.

Munsell c's. A series of about one thousand standard color samples, each designated by a letter-number system. The series represents various combinations of hue, saturation, and brightness and includes variations of brightness of the achromatic colors which have neither hue nor saturation.

neutral c. A color which has neither hue nor saturation, but which varies from other such colors in brightness only, as, for example, gray, black, or white.

Newton's c's. Seven principal colors (red, orange, yellow, green, blue, indigo, and violet) designated by Newton in his division of the visible spectrum into seven intervals of widths proportional to the intervals in the musical scale.

nonspectral c. Color or hue which cannot be matched by monochromatic light. Syn., *extraspectral hue; purple.*

object c. 1. The color of light transmitted or reflected by an object illuminated by a standard light source such as illuminant A, B, or C. 2. A color perceived as an inherent attribute of an object resulting from characteristics of the object, and of the surround, viewing direction, and color adaptation of the eye.

Ostwald c's. A series of several hundred chromatic and achromatic color samples, designated by a letter-number system.

pale c. A color possessing a low degree of saturation.

pastel c. A color of low saturation and high lightness or brightness; a color containing a high proportion of white.

plane c. A color perception unassociated with any system of orientation or localization in space and, hence, regarded as the end result of complete color reduction. (David Katz) **plane transparent c.** A plane color which appears transparent, such as that of colored glass. (David Katz)

primal c's. Four colors which psychologically do not contain component sensations of any other colors or of each other. They are red, green, blue, and yellow. Syn., *fundamental colors; psychological primary colors.*

primary c's. Any set of three colors of light, e.g., red, green, and blue, from which all other color sensations can be produced by additive mixing. Syn., *fundamental colors.*

prismatic c's. The colors produced from white light as it is reduced to its component parts by the dispersing action of a prism. They are often listed as red, orange, yellow, green, blue, indigo, and violet. (Newton)

pure c. 1. A color stimulus which approaches the condition for maximum saturation. 2. Monochromatic color.

c. pyramid. A type of color solid.

reacting c. A color which by simultaneous contrast is altered to another color (induced color) from the effects of the inducing color.

reduced c. 1. Aperture color. 2. Plane color.

c. reduction. See under *reduction.*

reflected c. Color seen as though reflected from a perceived object.

resulting c. Induced color.

Ridgway c's. An early system of 1,115 combinations of hue, saturation, and brightness, varying in approximately equal just-noticeable-difference steps.

saturated c. A color of any given hue at its maximum possible degree of saturation.

secondary c. 1. A color produced by additive mixing of primary colors. 2. Any color not identified as a primary color.

c. sense. See under *sense.*

c. shadows. See under *shadow.*

soft c. 1. Any color stimulus appearing soft in texture. 2. Certain colors classified by artists and psychologists as inherently soft in appearance, as, for example, blue or green. Cf. *hard color.*

c. solid. See under *solid.*

spatial c. A color perceived in three dimensions, as having a space-filling attribute, or as being solid, such as is seen in colored liquids and transparent fogs. (David Katz) Syn., *bulky color; volume color.*

spectral c's. The colors visible in the spectrum.

c. spindle. A type of color solid.

stable c. Any hue which does not change with variations in brightness or with variations in the area of the retina stimulated. Syn., *invariable color.*

c. stereoscopy. See under *stereoscopy.*

strong c. A color of high saturation.

subjective c. The sensation of color derived from stimulation other than with chromatic stimuli, as may occur from intermittent exposure at low frequencies to achromatic stimuli or from exposure to dazzling lights. **binocular s.c.** Chromatic responses to intermittent achromatic stimuli (about 40 cycles per sec.) which are observed binocularly but not monocularly.

c. surface. See under *surface*.

surface c. A color perceived as belonging to the surface of an object and in the same plane. **artificial s.c.** A color perceptually projected on the surface of an object to which it does not physically belong. **transparent s.c.** A color perceived in a two-dimensional manner and possessing the property of transparency, whereby other objects can be seen through it.

c. table. See under *table*.

c. temperature. See under *temperature*.

tertiary c. A color with spectral composition more complex than a secondary color, i.e., consisting of more than the three primary wavelengths.

c. threshold. Chromatic threshold.

c. triangle. See under *triangle*.

true c. 1. The sensation of a hue as interpreted by an individual with normal color vision. 2. The color of an object as seen under ordinary conditions in normal diffuse daylight by the light-adapted eye. (David Katz)

unique c. A color which cannot be described in terms of any other color. Red, yellow, blue, green, white, black, and gray are considered to be the seven unique colors. Syn., *unitary color*.

unitary c. Unique color.

volume c. Spatial color.

warm c. A color said to give a psychological effect of warmth, as, for example, red or yellow.

weak c. A color of low saturation.

c. weakness. See under *weakness*.

c. zones. See under *zone*.

◆

colorant. Anything, such as a pigment, dye, or filter, that can induce, produce, or modify the color of something else.

colorimeter (kul″or-im′eh-ter). A color-matching device used to designate an unknown colored stimulus by matching it with a known colored stimulus; a color comparator.

Abney's c. A colorimeter in which colors used in matching are isolated by three slits placed in the plane of a spectrum. The luminances of the components are varied by altering the widths of the slits. Syn., *Abney's sensitometer*.

Ives's c. A type of anomaloscope in which the colors used in matching are obtained from light passing through three adjustable slits for controlling the relative intensities of light through blue, green, and red glass filters.

Meisling's c. A type of colorimeter in which the colors used in matching are produced by passing light through a system consisting of six quartz plates, of varying thickness, placed between two Nicol prisms. Any color used is specified in terms of the thickness of quartz plate and the angle between the Nicol prisms.

monochromatic c. A colorimeter calibrated to designate a particular color mixture in terms of the wavelength of monochromatic light which will produce the same hue sensation.

photoelectric c. A device employing a photoelectric detector to measure three quantities related by linear combination to the tri-stimulus values of any sample. Such devices usually employ either a single photocell and three color filters, or three separate photocells. Syn., *photocolorimeter*.

trichromatic c. A colorimeter calibrated to designate any particular hue in terms of the relative proportions of the three primary colors of light, red, green, and blue, whose mixture gives the same hue sensation.

Wright's c. A type of anomaloscope in which the colors used in matching are obtained by dispersing prisms and are focused directly into the observer's eye instead of projected onto a screen.

colorimetry (kul″or-im′eh-tre). The quantitative evaluation of color either in terms of such attributes as hue, saturation, and brightness or as equivalents or matches of fixed or known standards. Cf. *chromometry*; *chromophotometry*; *chromoscopy*.

direct c. Colorimetry in which the color of the sample is matched by varying combinations of known color stimuli, either visually or with light-sensitive instruments.

indirect c. Designation of a color in terms of colorimetric specifications computed from known color data.

colorless. Without color or chroma. The achromatic colors, white, gray, and black, are said to be "colors without color" since they lack hue and saturation. When white, gray, and black are considered as colors, then only transparent substances, such as water, are without color.

colytropia (ko"le-tro'pe-ah). A tropia due to paralytic or mechanical causes; nonconcomitant strabismus.

coma (ko'mah). An oblique monochromatic aberration of an optical system in which the image of a point off the optical axis appears comet-shaped, with the tail pointing toward the axis. It is a result of unequal magnification in different zones of the system and can be corrected by the sine condition or, if in Seidel's formulae, by S_1 and $S_2 = 0$.

negative c. Coma in which the magnification for the central rays is greater than that for the peripheral rays.

positive c. Coma in which the magnification for the peripheral rays is greater than that for the central rays.

Comberg (kōm'berg) **contact lens; method.** See under the nouns.

comedo (kōm'e-do, ko-me'do). A plug of dried sebaceous material retained in an excretory duct of the skin, commonly called a blackhead.

comitance (kom'ih-tans). Concomitance.

comitancy (kom'ih-tan"se). Concomitance.

comitant (kom'ih-tant). Concomitant.

comma (ko'mah). A term used by Duke-Elder for coma.

Commission Internationale de l'Eclairage. An international organization devoted to studying and advancing the art and science of illumination. It is variously referred to as CIE, or ICI from the English translation, International Commission on Illumination. Its membership is made up of national committees representing individual countries, and a limited number of local representatives from countries where there are no national committees. Individuals are members of the national committees and not of the CIE.

commissure (kom'ih-shūr). 1. The point or line of union between two parts, as that of the eyelids. 2. A band of nerve fibers connecting corresponding structures in the two sides of the brain or spinal cord.

arcuate c. Commissure of von Gudden.

basal c. Meynert's commissure.

c. of Ganser. The most dorsal of the three supraoptic commissures; its composition is not fully known. It originates in part in the globus pallidus of the lentiform nucleus, conducts fibers to the ventromedial hypothalamic nuclei, and probably connects the hypothalamic regions of the two sides. Syn., *basal commissure; superior commissure; anterior hypothalamic decussation.*

c. of von Gudden. A commissure connecting the medial geniculate body and inferior colliculus of one side to the opposite side by means of the medial portions of the optic tracts and the optic chiasm. In man, such fibers are lacking, but some authorities still use this term for the same region of the human brain. Syn., *arcuate commissure; ventral supraoptic decussation.*

inferior c. Postoptic commissure.

lid c., lateral. 1. The juncture of the upper and lower eyelids at the lateral canthus. 2. Loosely, the lateral canthus.

lid c., medial. 1. The juncture of the upper and lower eyelids in the region of the medial canthus. 2. Loosely, the medial canthus.

Meynert's c. The largest of the three supraoptic commissures; it lies underneath the commissure of Ganser and is considered to be composed in part of fibers originating in the globus pallidus and ending in the lateral hypothalamic region and in part of autonomic fibers which leave the visual pathway to reach the supraoptic and tuberal nuclei. Syn., *superior commissure; dorsal supraoptic decussation.*

optic c. 1. Optic chiasm. 2. The nerve fibers from the left occipital lobe to the right occipital lobe which some authorities believe help to account for sparing of the macula.

posterior c. Myelinated nerve fibers connecting the opposite sides of the posterior parts of the diencephalon and of the superior colliculi. Some pupillary pathway fibers from the pretectal areas pass through to reach the contralateral Edinger-Westphal nucleus.

postoptic c. Nerve fibers connecting the left and right hypothalami via the floor of the third ventricle adjacent to the optic chiasm. Syn., *inferior commissure.*

superior c. Meynert's commissure.

supraoptic c's. In mammals, three fine bundles of transverse nerve fibers which cross dorsal to the optic chiasm, the commissures of *von Gudden, Meynert,* and *Ganser* (q.v.).

commotio retinae (ko-mo'she-o reh'-tih-ne). An edematous condition of the retina, particularly in the macular area, due to trauma. Syn., *Berlin's disease; Berlin's edema.*

comparator (kom-par'ah-tor). Any of several optical devices for the inspection of quality and the measurement of dimensions of an object by comparison to a standard or to a set of specifications, as, for example, a measuring magnifier used for contact lenses.

compensation. 1. The effect produced by rolling eye movements opposite to the direction of head movement to maintain stability of the visual field. 2. The effect of visual adaptation to varying levels of illumination. 3. The effect of amblyopia or suppression, when normal binocular vision is difficult to maintain. 4. The effect of head turning, or tilting, in strabismus or hyperphoria. 5. The effect of bifocal segment decentration to eliminate prismatic imbalances resulting from the distance prescription.

Bechterew's c. Compensation for the head and eye deviations which follow unilateral labyrinthectomy, such that removal of, or injury to, the other labyrinth gives rise to head and eye deviations as if the first labyrinth were intact. The head and eyes are deviated toward the operated side and a jerky nystagmus occurs with the slow phase toward this same side.

prism c. The equalization or neutralization, totally or in part, of prismatic effects at specified points of spectacle lenses by means of decentration,

segment selection, or bicentric grinding.

compensator (kom'pen-sa"tor). A crystal plate of variable thickness used to produce or analyze elliptically polarized light.

Babinet c. A pair of quartz prisms arranged in sequence with axes perpendicular, for use in the study of elliptically polarized light phenomena.

Soleil c. A Babinet compensator adapted by means of a third prism to produce the same phase difference throughout a large field.

complement. One of a pair of two colors which, when mixed additively, produce white or gray, e.g., blue-green is the complement of red.

component, direct illumination. That portion of the illumination on a task received directly from the luminaires. Abbreviation *DIC.*

Compton effect (komp'tun). See under *effect.*

Compumatic Computer. A commercial name for a device for determining the back surface curvatures and optical zone diameter for the corneal contact lens which will provide a lacrimal layer of uniform thickness for a cornea of known curvatures. The data are obtained by matching graphic representations of lens curvatures to those of the cornea.

comus (ko'mus). A crescent-shaped, yellowish area seen near the optic disk in some high myopes.

con. Abbreviation for *convergence.*

concave (kon'kāv). Having a curved, depressed surface, as the inside of a sphere; opposed to *convex.*

concavoconcave (kon-ka"vo-kon'kāv). Having concave surfaces on both sides, as a double concave lens.

concavoconvex (kon-ka"vo-kon'veks). Having a concave surface on one side and a convex surface on the other.

concentric (kon-sen'trik). Having a common center of curvature or symmetry.

concept, Traquair's. The three dimensional representation of the visual field as an "island of vision in a sea of blindness" in which the field of vision is represented radially in degrees at the base while the altitude is plotted on a log scale as the ratios of threshold target diameters to their respective test distances, giving a central pinnacle corresponding to the point of fixation, a deep pit for the blind spot, and rapidly declining slopes toward the periphery.

concession, visual. Adaptive loss of a visual skill.

conclination (kon″klin-a′shun). Intorsion.

concomitance (kon-kom′ih-tans). The condition in which the two eyes move as a unit, maintaining a constant or relatively constant angular relationship between the lines of sight for all directions of gaze, usually indicating absence of paresis or paralysis of the extraocular muscles. Syn., *comitance; comitancy; concomitancy.*

secondary c. Concomitance following a period of noncomitance due to contracture and other compensating mechanisms.

concomitancy (kon-kom′ih-tan″se). Concomitance.

concomitant (kon-kom′ih-tant). Pertaining to or having concomitance. Syn., *comitant.*

concretions, conjunctiva (kon-kre′-shunz). Minute, hard, yellow masses found in the palpebral conjunctivae of elderly people, or following chronic conjunctivitis, composed of the products of cellular degeneration retained in the depressions and tubular recesses in the conjunctiva; incorrectly called *lithiasis conjunctivae.*

condenser (kon-den′ser). A large aperture, short focus lens or optical system used in microscopes and projectors, by means of which large angle cones of light are collected from a small source, transilluminating the whole object to be viewed or projected, and made to pass through the lens system. Syn., *condensing lens.*

Abbe c. A substage microscope condenser consisting of a doublet with high numerical aperture.

cardioid c. A condenser used in dark field microscopy which permits only light that has been diffracted or dispersed by the specimen to enter the microscope.

dark field c. A condenser used in dark field microscopy that forms a hollow cone-shaped beam of light with its focal point in the plane of the specimen.

lacemaker's c. An invention of the early seventeenth century, consisting essentially of four glass spheres filled with water to concentrate the light from a candle flame upon four small areas for four different workers. It was also used by engravers, jewelers, cobblers, etc.

condition. 1. A state essential to the appearance or occurrence of something else. 2. A mode or a state of being.

Abbe's c. Sine condition.

Airy's c. Tangent condition.

Gauss's c. A condition fulfilled by an optical system in which chromatic aberration is corrected for two colors.

isoplanasie c. Isoplanatism.

Petzval's c. A condition met by Petzval's formula necessary to eliminate curvature of the field in an optical system.

sine c. The condition for eliminating distortion which is met when the magnification ratio in the various zones of a lens or optical system is equal to a constant representing the ratio of object to image size. Syn., *Abbe's condition.*

tangent c. The optical condition in which the ratio of the tangents of the angles of the emergent and incident rays with the optical axis is constant. This condition must be met in order for the optical system to be free from distortion. Syn., *Airy's condition.*

cone. 1. A solid body, with a circular base, tapering to a point. 2. A cone cell.

color c. A type of color solid.

crystalline c. A cone-shaped, light-collecting structure lying just beneath the corneal facet in an ommatidium of the compound eye of arthropods. Syn., *lens cone.*

double c's. Cones of the retina which sometimes occur in pairs in many fish, amphibians, birds, and marsupials, but are absent in higher mammals. They consist of a chief cone to which is attached an accessory cone. Syn., *twin cones.*

c. fiber. See under *fiber.*

c. foot. See under *foot.*

c. granule. See under *granule.*

lens c. Crystalline cone.

c. of light. A cone-shaped bundle of light rays defined by a point source (as the apex) and an entrance pupil of an optical system or eye (as the base), or a similar bundle defined by a point image and an exit pupil.

muscle c. Muscular funnel.

c. pedicle. Cone foot.

c. proper. The outer and inner members of a cone cell; a cone cell in the restricted sense.

retinal c. A cone cell.

Roger's c. A glass cone which, when held in front of the eye, distorts a test source into a circle of light, hence, useful as a dissociation device in heterophoria determination.

Steinheil c. An optical element, used in some telescopic spectacles, consisting of a solid truncated cone of glass, convex at the base, and concave at the opposite surface, with the concave surface having the shorter radius of curvature.

twin c's. Double cones.

Tyndall c. The luminous cone-shaped path of a beam of light as it passes through a medium containing minute light-scattering particles.

visual c. 1. The subtense of an area of regard with its apex at the nodal point of the reduced eye, considered as a cone. 2. The subtense of the entrance pupil of the eye with its apex at the point of regard, considered as a cone.

configuration. Form, pattern, structure, or Gestalt; an integrated whole, not a mere summation of units or parts.

confluence. The perceptual effect in which separate figures in space are perceived as a total single impression, as demonstrated by the Mueller-Lyer visual illusion.

confocal (kon-fo'kal). Having a common focus.

conformer. A device placed in the conjunctival sac to preserve the shape of the fornices after enucleation or evisceration, prior to insertion of an artificial eye. Syn., *stint.*

confusion. The common localization of two objects in space while perceptually aware of their physical separation, occurring especially in strabismus.

conjunctiva (kon"junk-ti'vah). A mucous membrane extending from the eyelid margin to the corneal limbus, forming the posterior layer of the eyelids (palpebral conjunctiva) and the anterior layer of the eyeball.

c. adnata. Bulbar conjunctiva.

c. arida. Xerosis of the conjunctiva.

bulbar c. The portion of the conjuctiva between the fornix and the cornea proper, hence, the scleral and limbal conjunctivae. Some also include the corneal epithelium as part of the bulbar conjunctiva. Syn., *conjunctiva adnata; ocular conjunctiva.*

corneal c. The stratified squamous epithelium of the cornea and, according to comparative anatomists, also Bowman's membrane and the outer portion of the stroma.

fornix c. The loose, free conjunctiva connecting the palpebral with the bulbar conjunctiva. Syn., *cul-de-sac; retrotarsal fold.*

limbal c. The portion of the bulbar conjunctiva in the region of the limbus which is fused with the episclera and Tenon's capsule.

marginal c. The portion of the palpebral conjunctiva extending from the eyelid margin to the tarsal conjunctiva.

ocular c. The conjunctiva on the anterior portion of the eyeball including the scleral, the limbal, and, by many, the corneal conjunctiva. Syn., *bulbar conjunctiva.*

orbital c. The portion of the palpebral conjunctiva between the tarsal conjunctiva and the fornix.

palpebral c. The portion of the conjunctiva on the posterior surface of the eyelids consisting of the marginal, the tarsal, and the orbital conjunctivae.

scleral c. The portion of the bulbar conjunctiva on the sclera that is easily lifted by forceps, thus excluding the limbal conjunctiva.

tarsal c. The portion of the palpebral conjunctiva between the marginal and the orbital conjunctivae.

conjunctival (kon"junk-ti'-val). Pertaining to the conjunctiva.

conjunctivitides (kon-junk"tih-vit'-ih-dēz). The plural for conjunctivitis; therefore, collectively, the various forms of conjunctivitis.

◆

CONJUNCTIVITIS

conjunctivitis (kon-junk"tih-vi'tis). Inflammation of the conjunctiva.

acne rosacea c. Inflammation of the conjunctiva, occasionally occurring with acne rosacea of the skin of the face, manifested in either of two forms: (1) a diffuse hyperemia characterized by an engorgement of the vessels of the tarsal and ocular conjunctiva; (2) a nodular form characterized by small, gray, highly vascularized nodules usually near the limbus on the interpalpebral area.

actinic c. Conjunctivitis resulting from exposure to ultraviolet rays, as from acetylene torches, therapeutic lamps, or klieg lights. Syn., *actinic ophthalmia.*

acute c., simple. Acute catarrhal conjunctivitis.

agricultural c. Conjunctivitis observed in farm districts, characterized by enormously swollen eyelids, lymph node involvement, superficial necrosis of the skin of the eyelids, and a conjunctival pseudomembrane. The condition may possibly be caused by a large Gram-positive anaerobic bacillus.

allergic c. Inflammation of the conjunctiva caused by hypersensitivity of the tissues to various allergens, not by a local organismal infection.

angular c. Subacute or chronic bilateral inflammation of the conjunctiva caused by the diplobacillus of Morax-Axenfeld, characterized by hyperemia in the area of the canthi, especially the outer, and extending into the skin at these regions. The discharge is grayish yellow, stringy, never abundant, adheres to the lashes, and accumulates especially at the angles. Syn., *diplobacillary conjunctivitis; Morax-Axenfeld conjunctivitis.*

arc-flash c. Actinic conjunctivitis caused by electric welding.

c. arida. Xerosis of the conjunctiva.

c. artefacta. Inflammation of the conjunctiva due to an irritant being purposely rubbed into the eye by a malingerer or by a hysterical or mentally unbalanced person.

artificial silk c. Inflammation of the conjunctiva common to workers in the artificial silk industry, probably caused by the acids used.

atopic c. Allergic conjunctivitis in persons with a familial history of hypersensitivity. It is of rapid onset and due to airborne substances such as dust or pollens, or to the ingestion of certain foods.

atropine c. Follicular inflammation of the conjunctiva from continued use of atropine in the eye.

bacillary dysentery c. Metastatic inflammation of the conjunctiva occurring in association with bacillary dysentery and urethritis; characterized by hyperemia and no discharge.

Beal's c. See *conjunctivitis, follicular, acute (of Beal).*

blennorrheal c. Gonococcal conjunctivitis.

calcareous c. Lithiasis conjunctivitis.

c. calcificans. Lithiasis conjunctivitis.

catarrhal c. Inflammation of the conjunctiva associated with cold or catarrhal irritation and marked by hyperemia and mucoid discharge, occurring in either acute, subacute, or chronic form. Syn., *blennophthalmia; catarrhal ophthalmia.* **acute c.c.** Acute, infectious inflammation of the conjunctiva associated with cold or catarrhal irritation and characterized by a bright red hyperemia (most intense near the fornices), swelling, loss of translucency, and a mucoid or mucopurulent discharge. Syn., *simple acute conjunctivitis; mucopurulent conjunctivitis.* **chronic c.c.** A mild, chronic inflammation of the conjunctiva with a slight hyperemia and mucoid discharge. Commonly, a sequel to acute catarrhal conjunctivitis, but may be due to a constant irritative element such as dust, glare, ingrowing lashes, exposure from ectropion, exophthalmos, or eyestrain.

c. catarrhalis aestiva. Vernal conjunctivitis.

chemical c. Inflammation of the conjunctiva due to exposure to chemical irritants.

contagious c., acute. Acute contagious inflammation of the conjunctiva caused by Koch-Weeks bacillus or pneumococcus infection. The disease starts approximately 36 hours after infection, with a feeling of smarting, is followed by all the symptoms of an acute catarrhal conjunctivitis, and intense hyperemia with a profuse mucopurulent discharge is typical. It occurs mainly in the spring, occasionally in the fall. Syn., *acute epidemic conjunctivitis; Koch-Weeks conjunctivitis; pink eye.*

c. corneae. Inflammatory edema in the corneal epithelium with pain and photophobia occurring in association with acute catarrhal conjunctivitis.

croupous c. Pseudomembranous conjunctivitis.

diphtheritic c. Membranous conjunctivitis caused by the Klebs-Loeffler bacillus. **diphtheritic catarrhal c.** A rare inflammation of the conjunctiva, usually found in the newborn, characterized by hyperemia of the conjunctiva and the skin of the eyelids and by a sticky yellow discharge which accumulates at the inner canthus and forms threads and flakes in the lower fornix. There is an associated rhinitis and swollen preauricular glands. The positive diagnosis is the presence of the Klebs-Loeffler bacillus, although the pneumococcus and staphylococcus may also be present.

diplobacillary c. Angular conjunctivitis.

eczematous c. Phlyctenular conjunctivitis.

Egyptian c. Trachoma.

epidemic c. Acute contagious conjunctivitis. **acute e.c.** Acute contagious conjunctivitis.

estival c. Vernal conjunctivitis.

exanthematous c. An infectious inflammation of the conjunctiva associated with an eruptive disease, as measles or scarlet fever, the symptoms usually being that of an acute catarrhal conjunctivitis.

flash c. Actinic conjunctivitis due to exposure to a high tension electric spark or arc, as from a welder's torch.

follicular c. Inflammation of the conjunctiva characterized by the formation of follicles, caused by chemical, toxic, or bacterial irritation. **acute f.c.** An acute epidemic mucopurulent inflammation of the conjunctiva characterized by the appearance of small, round or oval, pinkish, translucent follicles, usually in the lower fornix, occasionally in the upper. It may easily be misdiagnosed as trachoma. **acute f.c. of Beal.** A form of acute conjunctivitis characterized by rapid onset, swelling of the preauricular glands, mild symptoms, and rapid and complete recovery. Syn., *Greeley's conjunctivitis.* **Axenfeld's f.c.** Conjunctivitis characterized by small discrete follicles especially in the fornices and having a prolonged benign course to complete resolution. Commonly occurring in epidemics, it mainly affects children. Syn., *orphans' conjunctivitis.* **chronic f.c.** A low grade catarrhal inflammation of the conjunctiva characterized by small, discrete follicles appearing especially in the lower fornix. **toxic f.c.** Acute follicular conjunctivitis.

giant papillary c. "Giant cobblestone" appearance of the inside of the upper eyelid, resembling vernal conjunctivitis, resulting from wearing either hard or soft contact lenses.

gonococcal c. A severe and acute inflammation of the conjunctiva caused by the gonococcus, characterized by a beefy-red, edematous, greatly swollen conjunctiva, swollen eyelids, and profuse purulent discharge. It is usually unilateral at onset, and corneal involvement may result in loss of the eye. It may occur in adults from self-contamination (gonorrheal ophthalmia) or in the newborn from passing through the birth canal of an infected mother (ophthalmia neonatorum). **endogenous g.c.** Metastatic inflammation of the conjunctiva occurring bilaterally in association with a generalized gonococcal infection. Symptoms are those of an acute catarrhal conjunctivitis. Syn., *epibulbar gonorrheal subconjunctivitis.*

gouty c. Chronic inflammation of the conjunctiva without infection, characterized by hyperemia, scanty discharge, itching and burning of the eyelids, and a foreign body sensation. Syn., *hot eye.*

granular c. Trachoma.

c. granulosa syphilitica. A follicular conjunctivitis accompanying the skin eruption in the secondary stage of syphilis. Syn., *pseudogranular conjunctival syphilis.*

Greeley's c. Acute follicular conjunctivitis of Beal.

herpetic c. Infection of the conjunctiva with the herpes virus which usually appears in an acute follicular form in association with preauricular lymphadenopathy.

c. ichthyotoxica. Acute, chemotic inflammation of the conjunctiva occurring in fishermen, caused by the blood of eels.

inclusion c. Follicular inflammation of the conjunctiva, caused by a filter-passing virus, characterized by slight discharge and extensive hyperemia and differentiated from trachoma by its slow onset, benign course, and the absence of corneal complications. The infantile form is called *inclusion blennorrhea* and the adult *swimming pool conjunctivitis.*

infective granulomatous c. Parinaud's conjunctivitis.

influenzal c. A rare form of conjunctival inflammation usually associated with influenza epidemics. Generally, the symptoms are of a chronic catarrhal conjunctivitis, although they last only about ten days.

interstitial c. Any type of conjunctival inflammation which involves the deeper connective tissue as well as the epithelial tissue.

klieg (or kleig) c. Actinic conjunctivitis caused by excessive exposure to klieg lights.

Koch-Weeks c. Acute contagious conjunctivitis.

lacrimal c. A chronic inflammation of the conjunctiva caused by infection and obstruction of the lacrimal passages.

larval c. Inflammation of the conjunctiva caused by the presence of larvae in the conjunctival sac.

leprous c. An inflammation of the conjunctiva occurring in leprotics which may manifest itself in either of two forms: (1) anesthetic, in which the nerve supply to the cornea, conjunctiva, and eyelids is affected, causing loss of nutritional control, failure or diminution of the flow of tears, and exposure of the cornea and conjunctiva resulting in a diffuse catarrhal conjunctivitis with papillary hypertrophy; (2) nodular, in which nodules, either in crops or singly, appear on the conjunctiva.

leptotrichous c. Parinaud's conjunctivitis.

ligneous c. A rare form of pseudomembranous or sometimes membranous conjunctivitis originating in childhood and persisting for months or years and associated with the massive development of granulomatous tissue. It is of unknown etiology and more common in females than males.

lithiasis c. A condition of the palpebral conjunctiva marked by the presence of minute, hard, yellow spots, consisting of products of cellular degeneration contained in Henle's glands or in glands of new formation. Only rarely are there calcareous deposits. Syn., *calcareous conjunctivitis; conjunctivitis calcificans; conjunctivitis petrificans; uratic conjunctivitis; lithiasis conjunctivae.*

lymphatic c. Phlyctenular conjunctivitis.

c. medicamentosa. An inflammation of the conjunctiva caused by the application of medicine in the eye.

c. meibomiana. A chronic inflammation of the Meibomian glands and adjacent conjunctiva, characterized by a swollen tarsal plate and a frothy seborrheic secretion.

membranous c. A severe inflammation of the conjunctiva caused, typically, by the Klebs-Loeffler bacillus, less commonly by the streptococcus or the pneumococcus, characterized by the formation of a grayish-yellow infiltrating membrane which cannot be removed without leaving a raw, bleeding surface. The membrane may occur in plaques or may involve the entire conjunctiva and is caused by the deposition of a profuse fibrinous exudate from the cul-de-sac on and into the epithelium. The preauricular glands are swollen and the eyelids are red, swollen, painful, and acquire a characteristic boardlike hardness. The usual results are a coagulative necrosis and subsequent cicatrization of the involved areas.

meningococcal c. An acute metastatic inflammation which infrequently accompanies epidemic meningitis, usually catarrhal in nature and benign.

microbilallergic c. Allergic conjunctivitis due to hypersensitivity to products of such microorganisms as bacteria, fungi, or parasites.

molluscum c. Inflammation of the conjunctiva due to molluscum contagiosum.

Morax-Axenfeld c. Angular conjunctivitis.

mucopurulent c. Acute catarrhal conjunctivitis.

necrotic infectious c. A unilateral suppurative necrotic inflammation of the conjunctiva characterized by small, scattered, elevated, white spots in the fornices and palpebral portions and by an associated swelling of the preauricular, parotid, and submaxillary glands on the affected side. Syn., *Pascheff's conjunctivitis.*

Newcastle disease c. An acute follicular conjunctivitis, usually unilateral and of short duration, associated with preauricular adenopathy, due to a virus transmitted from fowls.

nodular c. An inflammation of the conjunctiva caused by irritation from the hairs of caterpillars or certain plants which have entered the cul-de-sac, characterized by nodules resembling those found in tuberculosis. Frequently associated are iridocyclitis and hypopyon. Syn., *pseudotubercular conjunctivitis; caterpillar hair ophthalmia; ophthalmia nodosa; pseudotrachoma.*

orphans' c. Axenfeld's follicular conjunctivitis.

papillary c. An inflammation of the conjunctiva characterized by the appearance of papillae in the palpebral portion. Syn., *pseudofollicular conjunctivitis.*

c. papulosa. Granular syphilitic conjunctivitis.

Parinaud's c. An inflammation of the conjunctiva, usually unilateral, by a leptothrix infection and characterized by large polypoid granulations and swelling of the preauricular, parotid, submaxillary, and cervical glands. Syn., *infective granulomatous conjunctivitis; leptotrichous conjunctivitis.*

Pascheff's c. Necrotic infectious conjunctivitis.

c. petrificans. Lithiasis conjunctivitis.

phlyctenular c. A circumscribed inflammation of the bulbar conjunctiva characterized by the formation of one or more small elevations surrounded by a reddened area and due to allergic reaction to endogenous toxin. Syn., *eczematous conjunctivitis; lymphatic conjunctivitis; scrofulous conjunctivitis; eczematous ophthalmia; phlyctenular ophthalmia; scrofulous ophthalmia; strumous ophthalmia.*

plastic c. Pseudomembranous conjunctivitis.

pneumococcal c. Acute contagious conjunctivitis caused by pneumococcal infection.

prairie c. A chronic inflammation of the conjunctiva characterized by the appearance of white spots on the palpebral conjunctiva.

pseudofollicular c. Papillary conjunctivitis.

pseudomembranous c. Any inflammation of the conjunctiva characterized by the appearance upon, but not within, the conjunctiva of a coagulated fibrinous network which may be peeled off, leaving the epithelium intact. It may be due to infection, chemical irritants, or the wound-healing process. It is relatively rare and may be acute, subacute, chronic or recurrent, or circumscribed. Syn., *croupous conjunctivitis; plastic conjunctivitis.*

pseudotubercular c. Nodular conjunctivitis.

purulent c. 1. Any inflammation of the conjunctiva containing or forming pus. Syn., *purulent ophthalmia.* 2. Gonococcal conjunctivitis.

rheumy c. A chronic catarrhal conjunctivitis occurring in the aged and in alcoholics in which the eyes are watery and the lower eyelids sag.

rosacea c. Acne rosacea conjunctivitis.

Samoan c. An acute, purulent inflammation of the conjunctiva, endemic to the Samoan Islands, diagnosed by the presence in the discharge of a diplococcus similar to the gonococcus. Severe pains, marked photophobia, and a profuse purulent discharge are present, and corneal complications are common.

Sanyal c. Unilateral conjunctivitis due to actinomycetic infection apparently from direct contact with dirt, characterized by a velvety chemotic appearance of the conjunctiva without lymphatic involvement and with spontaneous clearing in about 8 to 10 weeks.

scrofulous c. Phlyctenular conjunctivitis.

serous c. Acute inflammation characteristic of certain viral infections and consisting of intense hyperemia of conjunctival and episcleral vessels with edema of the bulbar conjunctiva without a gross discharge.

shipyard c. Epidemic keratoconjunctivitis.

c. sicca. An inflammation of the conjunctiva usually accompanying keratitis sicca. See also *keratoconjunctivitis sicca.*

snow c. Actinic conjunctivitis caused by excessive solar glare from snow.

spring c. Vernal conjunctivitis.

squirrel plague c. Tularemic conjunctivitis.

superficial c. Any type of conjunctival inflammation which involves only the epithelial tissue and not the deeper connective tissue.

swimming pool c. The adult form of inclusion conjunctivitis.

syphilitic c. A general term for any inflammation of the conjunctiva accompanying syphilis. **granular s.c.** An inflammation of the conjunctiva occurring in the secondary stage of syphilis, characterized by diffuse, rose-red, follicularlike formations on the tarsal conjunctiva of one or both eyelids, especially the upper. It may be accompanied by pannus and involvement of the preauricular glands. Syn., *conjunctivitis papulosa; syphilitic pseudotrachoma.* **simple s.c.** An inflammation of the conjunctiva frequently occurring early in the secondary stage of syphilis, usually characterized by violent injection and chemosis and accompanied by other secondary manifestations of syphilis elsewhere in the skin and mucous membranes.

trachomatous c. Trachoma.

traumatic c. An inflammation of the conjunctiva caused by the action of irritant substances, such as dust, acids, vapors, or by excessive rubbing or by foreign bodies.

tuberculous c. An inflammation of the conjunctiva, caused by either a primary or a secondary infection with the tubercle bacillus, occurring generally in two forms: ulcerative, characterized by small miliary ulcers; or hyperplastic, characterized by yellow or gray subconjunctival nodules.

tularemic c. An infectious inflammation of the conjunctiva due to the bacterium *Pasteurella tularensis,* transmitted to human beings from rabbits or other rodents, characterized by chemosis, small yellow necrotic ulcers, and involvement of the preauricular, parotid, cervical, and submaxillary glands. Syn., *conjunctivitis tularensis.*

tularensis c. Tularemic conjunctivitis.

uratic c. Lithiasis conjunctivitis.

vaccinic c. An inflammation of the conjunctiva caused by accidental inoculation with smallpox vaccine, characterized by ulcers, usually in the palpebral portion, which are covered with a thick, gray, adherent membrane. The eyelids are red and greatly swollen, and, usually, the preauricular and postauricular glands are involved.

varicellic c. An inflammation of the conjunctiva which infrequently accompanies chickenpox, characterized by small pustules which may develop into ulcers with swollen, dark-red margins.

variolic c. A mild, catarrhal inflammation of the conjunctiva frequently accompanying smallpox and developing about the fifth day. Pustules rarely occur.

vernal c. A chronic, bilateral inflammation of the conjunctiva, of unknown etiology, which recurs seasonally during warm weather. It may take two forms: (1) the palpebral, characterized by hard, flattened papillae, separated by furrows, having a cobblestone appearance in the upper palpebral portion, with both upper and lower palpebral portions of a bluish-white color; (2) the bulbar or limbal, characterized by gelatinous-appearing nodules, sometimes slightly pigmented (Tranta's dots), adjacent to the limbus. The inflammation is accompanied by photophobia and intense itching. Syn., *Fruehjahr's catarrh; Saemisch catarrh; vernal catarrh; estival conjunctivitis; spring conjunctivitis; spring ophthalmia.*

verrucose c. Conjunctivitis resulting from prolonged infection by a wart on the margin of the eyelid, of a subacute nature with little discharge, and usually characterized by a smooth conjunctival surface.

welder's c. Actinic conjunctivitis caused by glare from acetylene or electric welding torches.

Widmark's c. An acute catarrhal inflammation of the conjunctiva, of unknown etiology, characterized by congestion and epithelial loss in the lower bulbar and tarsal portions.

◆

conjunctivoanstrostomy (kon-junk"-tiv-o"an-stros'to-me). A surgical procedure for the treatment of epiphora in which an opening is made from the inferior conjunctival cul-de-sac into the maxillary sinus.

conjunctivochalasis (kon-junk"tiv-o"kah-lah'sis). An abnormal fold in the conjunctiva of the lower fornix.

conjunctivoma (kon-junk"tiv-o'mah). A tumor of conjunctival tissue occurring on the eyelid.

conjunctivoplasty (kon"junk-tiv'o-plas"te, -ti'vo-plas"te). Plastic surgery of the conjunctiva.

Con-Lish method (kon'lish). See under *method.*

conoid of Sturm (ko'noid). The astigmatic bundle of rays between the two mutually perpendicular focal line images of a point source. Cf. *interval of Sturm.*

conomyoidin (ko"no-mi-oi'din, -mi'oidin). Contractile protoplasmic material in the cones of the retina which reacts to light stimuli.

conophthalmus (kōn"of-thal'mus). Corneal staphyloma.

conoscope (kōn'ah-skōp). A wide-angle polarizing microscope used for observation of interference figures and related phenomena of crystal plates, especially for determining axial angles. Syn., *hodoscope.*

Conradi's syndrome (kon'rah-dēz). Stippled epiphyses.

consensual (kon-sen'shu-al). Excited by reflex stimulation; especially, the contraction of the contralateral pupil when the retina of only one eye is stimulated.

constancy. The relative apparent stability or lack of perceived change of certain object properties, despite a change in the stimulus characteristics which initiated the perception.

brightness c. A perceptual phenomenon wherein the perceived or subjectively attributed brightness of an object or a surface tends to remain fixed at a pre-perceived or attributed brightness level, rather than in direct ratio with the actual brightness, e.g., a piece of intensely illuminated coal may continue to seem black though actually brighter than an adjacent sheet of dimly illuminated white paper. Syn., *lightness constancy.*

c. of clear vision. See *li test.*

color c. The relative apparent stability or lack of perceived change of the color of an object, despite a change in the spectral composition of incident light, or of adjacent surfaces, or of other related stimulus factors.

distance c. The relative lack of change in the perceived size of an object as a function of the viewing distance.

form c. Shape constancy.

lightness c. Synonymous with *brightness constancy,* but preferred by some on the theory that the phenomenon is based on relative light reflectance, rather than on an attribute of brightness perception.

shape c. The relative apparent stability or lack of perceived change in the shape of an object, despite a change in the direction or angle of view.

size c. The relative apparent stability or lack of perceived change in the size of an object, despite a change in viewing distance, actual size, or other related stimulus factors.

constant. 1. Anything invariable, remaining unaltered, or not subject to change. 2. A magnitude or numerical quantity which retains the same value throughout an investigation, or during a stage of an investigation.

Abbe's c. Nu (ν) value.

Cotton-Mouton c. In the Cotton-Mouton effect, the birefringence constant that, when multiplied by path

length and the square of the magnetic field strength, yields the phase difference between the ordinary and the extraordinary rays.

Kerr c. A measure of the Kerr electro-optic effect equal to the difference between the indices of refraction for the ordinary and the extraordinary rays divided by the light wavelength and by the square of the electric field strength.

optic c's. of the eye. Numerical values or measurements said or assumed to represent the optical dimensions and refractive properties of a typical or specially defined eye. Classic tables of such values include those of Helmholtz, Tscherning, Gullstrand, and others.

Planck's c. The universal constant for electromagnetic energy, equal to 6.624×10^{-27} erg sec.

Stefan-Boltzmann c. The energy radiated per unit area per unit time by a blackbody divided by the fourth power of the blackbody's temperature; equal to $(5.6696 \pm 0.0010) \times 10^{-8}$ (watts) (meter)$^{-2}$ (degrees Kelvin)$^{-4}$.

Verdet c. The angle of rotation of plane-polarized light in a magnetized substance divided by the product of the length of the light path in the substance and the magnetic field strength, a constant in the equation of the Faraday effect.

zonal c. A factor varying with zone size, by which the mean candlepower emitted by a source of light in a given angular zone is multiplied to obtain the lumens in the zone.

constringence, optical (kon-strin'-jens). The ν (nu) value of optical glass; the reciprocal of the dispersive power of the glass, denoted by the Greek letter ν.

$$\nu = \frac{N_D - 1}{N_F - N_C},$$

where N_D, N_F, and N_C are the refractive indices of the glass for the D, F, and C lines of the spectrum.

construction, Rousseau. The graphical transposition of the radial dimensions of a curve which is plotted on half of a polar coordinate system to ordinate dimensions on a rectilinear coordinate system for which the abscissa values are the sines of the corresponding polar angle values from 0° to 180°. When this transposition is applied to a luminous flux distribution curve of a lamp with symmetrical flux distribution, the mean ordinate value on the transposed scale is the mean spherical candle-power of the lamp.

Con-Ta-Chek. An ophthalmometer attachment for measuring the curvature of a contact lens, containing a chamber filled with fluid on which the lens floats and a front surface mirror, inclined at 45°, which reflects the surface being measured into the instrument.

Contact Lens Manufacturers Association. An association of manufacturers of contact lenses organized in Chicago, Illinois, in 1963.

contact, optical. The effective optical elimination of the space between two optical surfaces, or the effective elimination of optical surfaces, usually accomplished by filling the intervening space with a substance of the same refractive index as that of one or both of the media whose surfaces bound that space.

contactology (kon-tact-ol′o-je). (*Infrequent*) The science and practice of contact lens fitting.

Contactometer (kon″tak-tom′eh-ter). An ophthalmometer attachment for holding contact lenses during measurement of their surface curvatures and having one or more auxiliary reflecting surfaces of known curvatures for immediate calibration.

Contascope (kon′tah-skōp). An instrument for inspecting edge profiles and thickness, curvature characteristics, and surface integrity of contact lenses, consisting essentially of a light source, a stage for holding lenses, and a 20× optical system.

content, black. The difference between unity and the higher of the two reflectance values in the Ostwald system of specifying surface colors.

content, full color. The higher of the two reflectance values minus the lower in the Ostwald system of specifying surface colors.

content, white. The lower of the two reflectance values in the Ostwald system of specifying surface colors.

continuance (kon-tin′u-ans). The tendency to follow a linear pattern in the same direction and movement, despite conflicting interruptions by other linear patterns, as the tending to see a straight line in its continuation throughout a pattern. It may also apply to gradation of hues where the eye moves along the direction of the gradation.

contracture (kon-trak′tūr). 1. The temporary inability of a muscle to relax

fully. 2. The state of rigidity of a contracted muscle. 3. Used incorrectly, a muscle in tetanus.

contraocular (kon″trah-ok′u-lar). Pertaining to the opposite eye.

contrast. The manifestation or perception of difference between two compared stimuli.

　　apparent c. The contrast of an object with its background as viewed from a specific direction and through a given distance of atmosphere which attenuates and/or scatters light.

　　binocular c. Induction effects on judgments, or sensitivity of an eye, produced by stimulation of the other eye.

　　border c. The enhanced contrast seen near the border between two juxtaposed fields. Syn., *marginal contrast.*

　　brightness c. 1. Luminance contrast. 2. Enhanced difference in the brightness of two fields owing to their proximity, juxtaposition, successive stimulation, or other related stimulus factors influencing brightness perception. Syn., *luminosity contrast.*

　　chromatic c. Color contrast.

　　color c. 1. The manifestation or perception of difference in color saturation or hue. 2. The enhanced contrast in the color (saturation or hue) of two stimuli owing to their proximity, juxtaposition, successive stimulation, or other related factors influencing color perception. 3. The change in hue or saturation of a color as a result of the proximity to, juxtaposition with, or successive stimulation by another color.

　　curvature c. A presumed perceptual attribute or phenomenon said to account for certain geometrical illusions involving curves.

　　depth c. Contrast between surfaces at different distances or depth levels.

　　edge c. See *acutance.*

　　c. illusion. See under *illusion.*

　　inherent c. The actual contrast of an object with its background in a specific direction when it is unaltered by atmospheric attenuation or scatter or by the presence of a glare source in the field of view.

　　luminance c. The ratio or other numerical representation of the difference in luminance between two stimulus fields or surfaces. Syn., *brightness contrast.*

　　luminosity c. Brightness contrast.

marginal c. Border contrast.

phase c. Contrast produced in phase microscopy by translating into intensity differences the phase differences produced by unequal optical path lengths in a thin uniform section made up of elements having different indices of refraction.

c. phenomenon. See under *phenomenon*.

physical c. The relationship between the luminances of an object and its immediate background, equal to $\Delta B/B$, where ΔB is the luminance difference between the object and its background, and B is the luminance of the background.

physiological c. The relationship between the apparent or subjective brightness of two objects which are seen either at the same time (simultaneous contrast) or sequentially (successive contrast) against backgrounds which may or may not be identical.

simultaneous c. Contrast manifested or induced on simultaneous presentation of two stimulus fields.

successive c. Contrast manifested or induced on successive presentation of stimuli.

surface c. Contrast in brightness or color of two surfaces, usually juxtaposed.

control. 1. In a pair of haploscopic stimulus targets, the elements of the pattern which are presented to one eye only for the purpose of confirming that the eye is being used during binocular testing or training. Syn., *fusion clue*. 2. The portion of an experiment which is used to check or compare the results of another portion which involves some additional factor under investigation.

Controlled Reader. An instrument for training reading skills, by controlling the span and duration of fixation, consisting essentially of a 35 mm film strip projector, providing a left to right presentation of groups of words at a rate of up to 1,000 words per minute.

contusio bulbi (kon-tu′ze-o bul′bi). Blunt injury of the eyeball.

conus (ko′nus). 1. A cone. 2. A large, circular, white patch around the optic disk due to the exposing of the sclera as a result of degenerative change or congenital abnormality in the choroid and retina. 3. Posterior staphyloma.

distraction c. A myopic crescent located adjacent to the temporal margin of the optic disk.

Fuchs' c. A small, crescentic, white area adjacent to the inferior edge of the optic disk.

myopic c. Conus due to degenerative changes associated with myopia.

opticohyaloid c. A rare congenital formation on the optic disk which extends into the vitreous.

c. papillaris. A pigmented, vascularized, conical protrusion from the optic nerve head into the vitreous of reptiles, functioning to nourish the inner layers of the retina.

supertraction c. A gray or yellowish ring at the nasal margin of the optic disk, sometimes occurring in myopic eyes, due to displacement of the retina over the optic disk.

conv. Abbreviation for *convergence*.

converge (kon-verj′). To tend toward a point. Visually, to turn the lines of sight inward toward each other. Optically, to turn light toward a point or focus.

◆

CONVERGENCE

convergence (kon-ver′jens). 1. The turning inward of the lines of sight toward each other. 2. The directional property of a bundle of light rays turned or bent toward a real image point; to be distinguished from the divergence property of a bundle of rays emanating from a point source.

accommodative c. Convergence changes physiologically induced by, related to, or associated with changes in accommodation, clinically measured by changes in phorias or changes in the convergence limits of clear, single, binocular vision with changes in accommodation. See also *convergence accommodation; gradient; AC/A ratio.* Syn., *associative convergence*.

active position of c. The state of convergence of the eyes during normal binocular fixation of a single object. Syn., *fixation position of convergence*.

amplitude of c. See under *amplitude*.

associative c. Accommodative convergence.

asymmetric c. Convergence of the eyes toward a point outside the plane perpendicular to and bisecting the interocular base line.

center of c. See under *center*.

directional c. Proximal convergence.

dynamic c. Convergence as a physiological function in the maintenance of bifoveal fixation, distinguished from *static convergence*. Cf. *fusional convergence; supplementary convergence.*

c. excess. 1. Esotropia or high esophoria in near vision in association with a relatively orthophoric condition in distance vision, a relatively high increase in convergence being associated with an increase in accommodation. 2. The condition of esophoria or esotropia in near vision, esophoria or esotropia in distance vision being considered *divergence insufficiency*. 3. A condition in which esophoria or esotropia is greater at near than at distance.

far point of c. The point of intersection of the lines of sight when the eyes are in the position of maximum divergence or minimum convergence.

fixation position of c. The active position of convergence.

fusional c. Convergence induced by fusion stimuli without a manifest change in accommodation. **fusional amplitude of c.** See under *amplitude*. **fusional reserve c.** 1. The amount of available fusional convergence in excess of that required to overcome the heterophoria. 2. Relative convergence. **fusional supplementary c.** Supplementary convergence.

inhibition of c. See under *inhibition*.

initial c. The fusional convergence effecting a change from the phoria position to that of single binocular fixation of a distant object.

c. insufficiency. 1. Exotropia or high exophoria in near vision in association with a relatively orthophoric condition in distance vision, a relatively low increase in convergence being associated with an increase in accommodation. 2. The condition of exophoria or exotropia in near vision, exophoria or exotropia in distance vision being considered *divergence excess*. 3. A condition in which esophoria or esotropia is greater at far than at near. 4. Inability to converge the eyes to the average or normal near point of convergence. **absolute c.i.** A limitation of total convergence ability to less than 30°. (Duke-Elder) **relative c.i.** A limitation of total convergence ability to less than three times the amount of convergence habitually required. (Duke-Elder)

lag of c. 1. Physiological exophoria. 2. A tendency or manifestation of convergence to be less than the amount necessary for single binocular vision, as indicated by an exophoria.

near point of c. The point of intersection of the lines of sight when the eyes are in the position of maximum convergence. Syn., *punctum convergens basalis*. **absolute n.p. of c.** The point of intersection of the lines of sight when the eyes are converged maximally. **relative n.p. of c.** The point of intersection of the lines of sight when

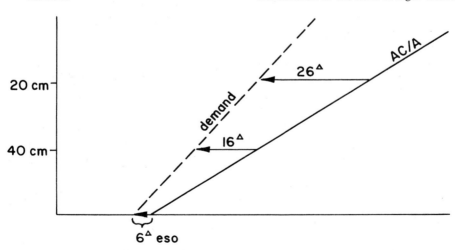

Fig. 7 Graphical illustration of convergence excess. (From J. R. Griffin, *Binocular Anomalies*. Chicago: Professional Press, 1976)

the eyes are in the position of maximum convergence with accommodation fixed at a given level.

negative c. 1. Divergence. 2. Convergence measured in the negative or divergent direction from a given reference position of the eyes as, for example, the straight-forward position or the position corresponding to the fusional demand. **negative fusional c.** 1. Fusional divergence. 2. Fusional convergence measured from the phoria position of the eyes to the prism base-in limit of clear, single, binocular vision. **negative fusional reserve c.** Fusional divergence in excess of that required to overcome the existing esophoria, clinically measured from the fusional demand point to the prism base-in limit of clear, single, binocular vision. Syn., *negative fusional reserve.* **negative relative c.** Relative convergence measured negatively or in a divergent direction from the convergence position corresponding to the normal fusional demand. Clinically, the base-in prism range of clear, single, binocular vision. Syn., *negative relative reserve convergence; negative reserve convergence.* **negative relative reserve c.** Negative relative convergence. **negative reserve c.** Negative relative convergence.

c. paralysis. See under *paralysis.*

passive position of c. The relative position of the two eyes under dissociation.

perverted c. A convergence faculty regarded as a function of anomalous retinal correspondence and said to be responsible for maintaining a convergent strabismus persisting over many years.

positive c. Convergence measured in a positive or increasing direction from a given reference position of the eyes. **positive fusional c.** Fusional convergence clinically measured in a positive or increasing direction from the phoria position of the eyes to the base-out prism limit of clear, single, binocular vision. **positive fusional reserve c.** Fusional convergence in excess of that required to overcome the existing exophoria, clinically measured from the fusional demand point to the prism base-out limit of clear, single, binocular vision. Syn.,*positive fusional reserve.* **positive relative c.** Relative convergence measured positively or in a convergent direction from the position corresponding to the normal fu-

sional demand. Clinically, the base-out prism range of clear, single, binocular vision. Syn., *positive relative reserve convergence; positive reserve convergence.* **positive relative reserve c.** Positive relative convergence. **positive reserve c.** Positive relative convergence.

posture of c. The state of convergence of the eyes for a given set of stimulus conditions, distinguished from convergence as a movement or response.

proximal c. 1. Convergence response attributed to the awareness or impression of nearness of a fixation object. Syn., *directional convergence; psychic convergence.* 2. The convergence of two lines toward their optical vanishing point in a perspective view, as represented in the retina or in the graphic correlate of the retinal image.

psychic c. Proximal convergence.

range of c. The linearly specified distance between the far and near points of convergence.

reflex c. Any convergence response regarded as a part of a reflex action, as distinguished from *voluntary convergence.*

relative c. Fusional convergence measured and specified with reference to the position of the eyes corresponding to the normal fusional demand for the given testing distance. Clinically, the base-out and/or base-in fusion range to the limits of clear, single, binocular vision.

reserve c. 1. Fusional convergence in excess of the amount needed for normal binocular fixation, clinically measured by the amount of base-in or base-out prism which can be overcome without blur or diplopia. 2. Convergence ability in excess of the amount needed for normal binocular fixation, clinically measured by determining the near point of convergence.

static c. The state of convergence, or divergence, of the lines of sight when the eyes are said to be at rest, as in the absence of stimuli to accommodation and convergence in clinical phoria testing.

supplementary c. Fusional convergence which is used to compensate for the heterophoria in binocular fixation, hence, quantitatively equal to the heterophoria itself in persons with normal binocular vision.

tonal c. Tonic convergence.

tonic c. The continuous convergence response maintained by the extraocular muscle tonus, hence absent in paralysis and in death, and diminished during sleep or narcosis; the amount of convergence in effect when fixating a distant object with accommodational and fusional impulses absent. Syn., *tonal convergence*.

voluntary c. Convergence produced volitionally, as distinguished from *reflex convergence*.

◆

Convergence Trainer. An instrument devised by Bangerter for improving convergence facility, consisting essentially of a chin rest fixed to one end of a rod on which targets slide to approach the eyes. The targets are either letters presented in rapid succession or a rotating spiral.

convergent (kon-ver'jent). Characterized by, associated with, or related to convergence.

convergiometer (kon-ver"je-om'eh-ter). An instrument for measuring phorias.

conversion, color (kon-ver'shun). Any perceived change in the characteristics of a color as a result of change in the viewing conditions.

convex (kon'veks). Having a curved, elevated surface, as the outside of a sphere.

convexoconcave (kon-vek"so-kon'kāv). Having a convex surface on one side and a concave surface on the other.

convexoconvex (kon-vek"so-kon'veks). Having convex surfaces on both sides, as a double convex lens.

Cooke lens. See under *lens*.

co-ordinate. In plotting or graphic representation, one of a system of magnitudes used to fix the position of a point, a line, or a plane.

chromaticity c's. The ratios of each of the tristimulus values to the sum of the three. Symbols: x, y, z. Syn., *trichromatic coefficients*.

coordination, hand-eye. A relationship between visual and kinesthetic clues, resulting in accurate, manual, spatial localization.

Coordinator (ko-ōr'din-a"tor). An instrument for diagnosis and treatment of eccentric fixation designed by Cüppers and consisting essentially of a rotating transilluminated Polaroid filter which, when viewed through a blue filter, produces Haidinger's brushes localized in relation to a fixation point mounted on the instrument.

Copeland lens (kōp'land). See under *lens*.

copiopia (kop"e-o'pe-ah). Fatigue of vision; asthenopia.

copiopsia (kop"e-op'se-ah). Copiopia.

COPT. See *Current Optometric Procedural Terminology*.

coquille (ko-kēl'). A deep, curved, blown or molded, glass lens commonly used in inexpensive sunglasses.

Cords' (kōrdz) **hypothesis; test.** See under the nouns.

core- (kōr'e). A combining form meaning the pupil.

coreclisis (kōr"e-kli'sis). Obliteration of the pupil.

corectasis (kōr-ek'tah-sis). A pathological dilatation of the pupil.

corectomedialysis (ko-rek"to-me-di-al'is-is). Excision of a small portion of the iris at its junction with the ciliary body to form an artificial pupil.

corectomy (kōr-ek'to-me). Any surgical cutting operation on the iris at the pupil.

corectopia (kōr-ek-to'pe-ah). A condition in which the pupil is not in the center of the iris. Syn., *ectopia pupillae*.

coredialysis (ko"re-di-al'is-is). Iridodialysis.

corediastasis (ko"re-di-as'tah-sis). A dilated state of the pupil.

corediastole (ko"re-di-as'to-le). Dilatation of the pupil.

coreitis (ko"re-i'tis). Keratitis.

corelysis (ko-rel'is-is). Surgical detachment of adhesions of the iris to the capsule of the crystalline lens or to the cornea.

coremetamorphosis (kōr"e-met"ah-mōr'fo-sis). The condition of an irregularly shaped pupil.

coremorphosis (kōr"e-mōr-fo'sis, -mōr'-fo-sis). Surgical formation of an artificial pupil.

corenclisis (kōr"en-kli'sis). Iridencleisis.

coreometer (ko"re-om'eh-ter). An apparatus for measuring the size of the pupil of the eye. Syn., *pupillometer*.

coreometry (ko"re-om'eh-tre). Measurement of the size of the pupil of the eye.

coreoplasty (ko"re-o-plas'te). Coreplasty.

coreplasty (ko're-plas"te). Plastic surgery of the iris, usually for the formation of an artificial pupil.

corestenoma (ko"re-ste-no'mah). An anatomical partial closure of the pupil.

c. congenitum. A congenital partial closure of the pupil caused by outgrowths from the sphincter margins. These usually meet but leave several small openings.

coretomedialysis (ko"re-to-me"di-al'is-is). Corectomedialysis.

coretomy (ko-ret'o-me). Corectomy.

Coriolis effect (ko-re-o'lis). See under *effect.*

cornea (kōr'ne-ah). The transparent anterior portion of the fibrous coat of the eye consisting of five layers, stratified squamous epithelium, Bowman's membrane, stroma, Descemet's membrane, and endothelium (mesenchymal epithelium), and serving as the first refracting medium of the eye. It is structurally continuous with the sclera, is avascular, receiving its nourishment by permeation through spaces between the lamellae, and is innervated by the ophthalmic division of the trigeminal nerve via the ciliary nerves and those of the surrounding conjunctiva which together form plexuses.

black c. Black deposits appearing in the cornea after prolonged use of adrenalin drops, varying in size from a small perilimbal spot to black discoloration of the entire corneal surface.

conical c. A cornea abnormally conoid in shape. Syn., *keratoconus.*

decentration of c. A condition in which the optical center of the cornea is not located at its geometric center.

ectasia of c. Corneal staphyloma.

c. farinata. A senile change, occurring bilaterally, in which the corneal stroma is marked with fine dustlike opacities, usually visible only with high magnification. Syn., *Vogt's floury cornea.*

c. globosa. Megalocornea.

c. guttata. Dystrophy of the endothelial cells of the cornea, characterized in its earliest stages by large black spherules and a golden hue on the posterior surface visible by indirect illumination. In later stages the posterior surface takes on a bronzed appearance. It is bilateral, though one eye may be affected more than the other, and vision is eventually reduced. Syn., *endothelial corneal dystrophy.*

c. opaca. Sclera.

c. plana. A congenital condition in which the cornea is flatter than normal.

sugar-loaf c. Keratoconus.

c. urica. Keratitis urica.

c. verticillata. Vortex corneal dystrophy.

Vogt's floury c. Cornea farinata.

Corneagram (kōr'ne-ah-gram). Trade name of a photograph of the corneal profile produced by the Corneopter Corneagraph.

corneal (kōr'ne-al). Pertaining to the cornea.

corneal allotransplant; autotransplant; bedewing; cap; basal cells; corpuscle; deturgescence; dystrophy; ectasia; facet; graft; image; lacunae; lens; mesothelium; radius; reflex; transplantation; ulcer. See under the nouns.

Cornealometer (kōr"ne-al-om'eh-ter). A type of ophthalmometer mounted to traverse an arc centered on the observed eye while the eye is fixating a stationary target, thus permitting direct readings of corneal curvature at any portion of the corneal surface.

corneascope (kōr'ne-ah-skōp"). An illuminating binocular loupe for viewing the cornea.

corneitis (kōr"ne-i'tis). Keratitis.

corneoblepharon (kōr"ne-o-blef'ah-ron). Adhesion of the eyelid to the cornea.

corneo-iritis (kōr"ne-o-i-ri'tis). Inflammation involving both the cornea and the iris.

Corneopter Corneagraph (kōr-ne-op'ter). Trade name of a camera which records the profile of the cornea in segments for direct matching with comparison curves of a Corneopter Simulator.

Corneopter Simulator (kōr-ne-op'ter). Trade name of an instrument for measuring the curvature of a photographed corneal profile, consisting essentially of a low power microscope with a revolving template of comparison arcs of known curvature.

corneosclera (kōr"ne-o-skle'rah). The sclera and the cornea when considered as forming one coat of the eyeball.

corneosclerectomy (kōr"ne-o-skle-rek'to-me). A surgical procedure for glaucoma in which trephining is performed at the superior corneolimbal junction into the anterior chamber under a conjunctival flap, followed by an iridectomy at the trephine hole.

Cornsweet (kōrn'swēt) **edge illusion; effect.** See under the nouns.

Cornu (kōr-nu') **prism; spiral.** See under the nouns.

Cornu-Jellet prism (kōr-nu'-jeh-la'). See under *prism*.

corocleisis (kōr″o-kli'sis). Coreclisis.

coroclisis (kōr″o-kli'sis). Coreclisis.

corodialysis (ko″ro-di-al'is-is). Iridodialysis.

corodiastasis (ko″ro-di-as'tah-sis). Corediastasis.

corona (ko-ro'nah). A crown or crownlike structure.

　　c. ciliaris. The ciliary processes considered as a single structure. Syn., *pars plicata.*

　　ciliary c. A large number of thin lines of light extending radially through the halo observed around a small bright light viewed in a dark room.

　　c. conjunctivae. The portion of the conjunctiva surrounding the cornea.

　　c. palpebrarum. The tarsus of the eyelid.

　　c. radiata. White matter containing fibers which pass to and from the internal capsule in the forebrain and which begin or end in the cerebral cortex, the optic radiations being in its posterior portion.

　　Zinn's c. Circle of Haller.

coroparelcysis (ko″ro-par-el'sih-sis). An operation to correct for partial opacity of the cornea, in which the pupil is drawn aside to bring it in line with a more transparent portion of the cornea.

corophthisis (ko-rof'thi-sis). Permanent contraction of the pupil resulting from an atrophy-producing disease of the eye.

coroplasty (ko'ro-plas″te). Coreplasty.

coroscopy (ko-ros'ko-pe). Retinoscopy.

corotomy (ko-rot'o-me). Corectomy.

corpora (kōr'po-rah). The plural of corpus.

　　c. amylacea. Amyloid bodies.

　　c. geniculata. The paired geniculate bodies in the diencephalon of the forebrain. Only the external geniculate bodies are visually important, serving as a relay center between the optic tract and the optic radiations.

c. nigra. Cystic protrusions of the pigmented retinal layers around the pupillary margin, characteristic of certain hoofed animals.

　　c. quadrigemina, anterior. The paired superior colliculi in the tectum of the midbrain. As a lower visual center they receive ganglionic axons from the retina and reflexly connect with lower motor neurons that control skeletal muscles.

　　c. quadrigemina, posterior. The paired inferior colliculi in the tectum of the midbrain which act as a relay center for reflex movements of the eyes in relation to sound.

corpus (kōr'pus). A relatively solid structure forming a part of an organ.

　　c. adiposum orbitae. The mass of fatty tissue in the orbit filling the interstices between the eyeball, the optic nerve, the extraocular muscles, the blood vessels, the nerves, and the lacrimal gland.

　　c. callosum. The great transverse commissure connecting the cerebral hemispheres consisting of a broad, arched band of white matter lying at the bottom of the longitudinal fissure. Its thickened posterior extremity, the splenium, is thought to be concerned with integration of opposite halves of the visual field and with the transmission of visual learning from one hemisphere to the other.

　　c. ciliare. Ciliary body.

　　c. ciliare choroideae. The iris and ciliary body, the term "choroideae" being used to mean "of the uvea." *Obs.*

　　c. ciliare hyaloideae. The vitreous humor in the region between the crystalline lens and the ora serrata. *Obs.*

　　c. ciliare retinae. The inner posterior portion of the ciliary body derived from the optic cup; it consists of a two-layered epithelium and the internal limiting membrane; the pars ciliaris retinae of present-day usage.

　　c. geniculatum. Geniculate body.

　　c. vitreum. Vitreous humor.

corpuscle (kōr'pus-l). 1. A small mass or body. 2. A sensory nerve end bulb. 3. A cell, especially that of the blood or the lymph.

　　conjunctival c. A tactile nerve ending of the conjunctiva.

　　corneal c. One of a number of fixed cells of connective tissue found between the lamellae of the substantia propria of the cornea. Each corpuscle is a flattened cell with a large flattened nucleus and branching processes which communicate with nearby corpuscles. Syn., *Toynbee's corpuscle; Virchow's corpuscle; keratocyte.*

Dogiel's c. A sensory end organ, somewhat resembling Krause's end bulbs, found in the mucous membranes of the eyes, the nose, the mouth, and the genitals.

c's. of Donders. Cytoblasts of Henle.

hyaloid c. A vestige of the hyaloid artery remaining as a small white plaque just nasal to the posterior pole of the crystalline lens.

Krause's c's. Specialized end organs or nerve endings, ovoid in shape, acting as cold receptors. Primarily sensitive to decrements in temperature, they are found superficially in the skin and in large numbers in the mucous membranes of the mouth, nose, eyes, and genitals. Syn., *end bulbs of Krause.*

sclerotic c's. Connective tissue cells found in the lymph spaces of the sclera.

Toynbee's c. Corneal corpuscle.

Virchow's c. Corneal corpuscle.

corradiation (ko-ra″de-a′shun). Radiation to or from one point or focus.

Correct-Eye-Graph. A picture designed to be used in the Correct-Eye-Scope for cheiroscopic drawing.

Correct-Eye-Scope. A trade name for a Brewster type stereoscope mounted on an adjustable stand, so designed that it may also be used as a cheiroscope.

correction. A term applied to a lens prescription used to rectify a refractive error, a muscular imbalance of the eyes, or both.

Corrector. A visual training instrument designed by Bangerter to establish correct spatial localization, centric fixation, and normal visual acuity, in the treatment of amblyopia ex anopsia. It consists essentially of insulated line drawings on a metal plate which are traced with a hand-held metal stylus. Contact of the stylus with the metal plate completes an electric circuit, causing a light to flash or a buzzer to sound, which signifies that the stylus is off target.

corrector, Maksutov. A thick meniscus lens having spherical surfaces of equal radii placed before a spherical mirror to correct for spherical aberration.

corrector, Schmidt. Schmidt plate.

◆

CORRESPONDENCE

correspondence. The state of being in accord or harmony; the relation or adaptation of things to each other.

motor c. The coordinated relationship of the extraocular muscle functions obtaining concomitant movements and bifoveal fixation. **secondary m.c.** The coordinated relationship of the extraocular muscle functions obtaining concomitant movements in strabismus. (Chavasse)

secondary proprioceptive c. The condition in which the supposed proprioceptive impulses resulting from heterotropia are either suppressed (inhibitory) or altered (exhibitory). (Chavasse) **exhibitory s.p.c.** The condition in which the supposed proprioceptive impulses resulting from heterotropia are interpreted by the mind as though the anomalous associated area of the deviating eye were a true fovea. (Chavasse) **inhibitory s.p.c.** The condition in which the supposed proprioceptive impulses resulting from heterotropia are inhibited. (Chavasse)

retinal c. The faculty of vision which gives rise to the unitary percept of a binocularly seen object or of a pair of objects viewed individually and separately by the two eyes, when the respective retinal images stimulate retinal receptors functioning co-ordinately to subserve this faculty. These receptors have common lines of direction and, thus, images stimulating them are interpreted as arising from the same direction or point in space. **abnormal r.c.** Anomalous retinal correspondence. **anomalous r.c.** A type of retinal correspondence, occurring frequently in strabismus, in which the foveae of the two eyes do not give rise to common visual directionalization, the fovea of one eye functioning directionally with an extrafoveal area of the other eye. Syn., *abnormal retinal correspondence; secondary retinal correspondence.* **anomalous (anatomical) r.c.** Anomalous retinal correspondence attributable to anatomical anomalies of the sensory mechanism, hence innate. **anomalous (asymmetrical) r.c.** Anomalous retinal correspondence in which the angle of anomaly is different when the right eye is fixating than when the left eye is fixating. (Chavasse) **anomalous (functional) r.c.** Anomalous retinal correspondence learned or acquired as a functional response. **anomalous (harmonious) r.c.** A type of anomalous retinal correspondence in which the angle of anomaly is equal to the objective angle of strabismus. **anomalous (inharmonious) r.c.** Unharmonious anomalous retinal correspondence. **anomalous (negative) r.c.** Anomalous retinal correspondence in which the impulses from the retina of the deviating eye are inhibited. (Chavasse) **anomalous (negative central) r.c.** Anomalous retinal correspondence in which there is inhibition of impulses from both the macula and the anomalous associated area of the deviating eye. (Chavasse) **anomalous (negative macular) r.c.** Anomalous retinal correspondence in which there is an inhibition of impulses from the macula of the deviating eye. (Chavasse) **anomalous (negative macular and positive pseudomacular) r.c.** Anomalous retinal correspondence in which there is an inhibition of impulses from the macula of the deviating eye and in which the impulses from the anomalous associated area of the deviating eye are interpreted as though originating in the macula. (Chavasse) **anomalous (negative subtotal) r.c.** Anomalous retinal correspondence in which the inhibition of the impulses from the macula is so slight (subtotal) that the subject can shift from anomalous correspondence to normal correspondence at will. (Chavasse) **anomalous (non-harmonious) r.c.** Unharmonious anomalous retinal correspondence. **anomalous (paradoxical) r.c.** A type of anomalous retinal correspondence in which either the subjective angle of strabismus or the angle of anomaly exceeds the objective angle of strabismus. It is often manifested after corrective surgery in a strabismic in whom anomalous retinal correspondence previously existed. **anomalous (paradoxical) r.c., type I.** A type of anomalous retinal correspondence in which the angle of anomaly (A) is greater than the objective angle of deviation (H), e.g., H equal to 15 prism diopters of exotropia and A equal to 20 prism diopters. Formula A=H-S with esotropia noted as positive and exotropia as negative. **anomalous (paradoxical) r.c., type II.** A type of anomalous retinal correspondence in which

the subjective angle of deviation (S) is greater than the objective angle of deviation (H) and the angle of anomaly (A) has a directional value opposite to either H or S, e.g., H equal to +15 prism diopters of esotropia, S equal to +20 prism diopters of esotropia, and A equal to −5 prism diopters. **anomalous (positive) r.c.** Anomalous retinal correspondence in which impulses from an anomalous associated area of the deviating eye are interpreted as though they originated at its fovea. **anomalous (suppression) r.c.** Anomalous retinal correspondence characterized by a suppression of one or the other of the two ocular images stimulating anomalously corresponding receptors, noted especially in clinical attempts to determine the subjective angle of strabismus. **anomalous (symmetrical) r.c.** Anomalous retinal correspondence in which the angle of anomaly is the same with either eye fixating. (Chavasse) **anomalous (unharmonious) r.c.** A type of anomalous retinal correspondence in which the subjective angle of strabismus is less than the objective angle of strabismus but, in magnitude, lies between the objective angle and zero. Hence, the angle of anomaly is not equal to the objective angle. Syn., *inharmonious anomalous retinal correspondence; nonharmonious anomalous retinal correspondence.* **normal r.c.** Retinal correspondence in which the two foveae and other binocularly paired extrafoveal receptor areas, having similar relative retinal localization with respect to the foveae, co-ordinate functionally as corresponding receptors to give rise to a unitary percept. Thus, the foveae of the two eyes have common lines of direction or a common local sign. Syn., *primary retinal correspondence.* **primary r.c.** Normal retinal correspondence. **secondary r.c.** Anomalous retinal correspondence, usually induced by surgical change of the angle of strabismus, differing from a previous anomalous correspondence. (Chavasse) See also *paradoxical anomalous retinal correspondence.*

sensory c., secondary. Anomalous retinal correspondence. (Chavasse)

◆

cortex (kŏr′teks). The outer or superficial part of an organ, situated beneath the capsule.

calcarine c. The superficial gray matter above and below the calcarine fissure. Syn., *Brodmann's area 17; area striata; visuo-sensory area.*

c. of crystalline lens. The portion of the crystalline lens surrounding the nucleus and bounded anteriorly by the epithelium and posteriorly by the capsule. It contains lens fibers and amorphous, intercellular substance.

occipital c. The superficial gray matter on the posterior lobe of each cerebral hemisphere, composing Brodmann's areas 17, 18, and 19. It is thought to contain, also, centers for reflex fixation, pursuit movements, accommodation, convergence, and, probably, pupil size.

retinal c. The retina when considered as an extended portion of the cerebral cortex.

visual c. Area striata.

visuo-motor c. Parastriate area.

visuo-psychic c. Peristriate area.

visuo-sensory c. Area striata.

cortical (kōr'te-kal). Pertaining to the cortex of an organ.

coruscation (kōr"us-ka'shun). The subjective sensation of flashes of light.

Cotton effect. Circular dichroism.

Cotton-Mouton (kot'un moo'tun) **constant; effect.** See under the nouns.

couching (kowch'ing). Surgical displacement of the crystalline lens.

Council on Clinical Optometric Care (AOA). A commission created in 1967 and appointed by the American Optometric Association to survey and accredit clinics providing optometric services.

counter, photon. A device for the measurement of light at very low intensities by counting the number of photons incident upon its receiving surface per unit time.

countersink. A concave cavity formed on a lens blank into which the segment button is fitted and fused in the manufacture of a multifocal lens.

COVD. See *College of Optometrists in Vision Development.*

Cowan chart (kow'an). See under *chart.*

Cowen's sign (ko'wenz). See under *sign.*

Craig Reader. See under *reader.*

Craik's blindness (krāks). See under *blindness.*

Cramer's theory (kra'merz). See under *theory.*

Crampton's muscle (kramp'tunz). See under *muscle.*

craniostenosis (kra"ne-o-ste-no'sis). Any congenital malformation of the cranium in which an abnormally shallow orbital cavity is present. In all, the embryonic or infantile type of orbit is retained.

Créde's method (kra-dāz'). See under *method.*

creep. Uneven flow during the process of polymerization of material for plastic lenses, causing a wavy internal stress.

Creix-Levy syndrome. See under *syndrome.*

crescent. A sickle-shaped structure, like a moon in the first quarter.

choroidal c. A mottled, lightly pigmented patch of exposed choroid around the optic disk, visible because the pigment epithelium of the retina stops short of the disk.

inverse c. A myopic crescent extending toward the nasal side of the optic disk. Syn., *myopia inversa.*

myopic c. A crescentic white patch, usually situated temporally about the optic disk, due to myopic degenerative change of the choroid and retina, allowing the sclera to become visible.

supertraction c. A gray or yellowish ring at the nasal margin of the optic disk, sometimes occurring in myopic eyes, due to pulling of the retina over the optic disk.

crest. A projection or ridge, especially on a bone.

anterior lacrimal c. A ridge on the maxillary bone which borders the fossa for the lacrimal sac.

posterior lacrimal c. A ridge on the lacrimal bone which borders the fossa for the lacrimal sac.

temporal c. A ridge that begins near the upper lateral orbital margin on the frontal bone and is continuous with the temporal lines on the parietal bone.

Creté's prism (kra-tāz'). See under *prism.*

CRF. Contrast rendition factor.

cribbing. The breaking or chipping of excess glass from an uncut lens or lens blank.

cribra orbitalia (krib'rah ōr-bih-tah'le-ah). Spongy-appearing bone in the orbital roof, especially in the region of the fossa for the lacrimal gland, containing small apertures through which pass veins from the orbital diploë.

cribriform plate (krib're-fōrm). See under *plate.*

Crichton-Browne sign (kri'ton brown). See under *sign.*

crisis. 1. The turning point of a disease, for better or for worse. 2. A sudden, striking change, or intensification, of a disease.

glaucomatocyclitic c. Recurring mild cyclitis associated with open angle glaucoma, usually limited to one and the same eye. Typically, pain is mild, the pupil is dilated, few keratic precipitates are present, vision is near normal, tension is elevated to 40 mm Hg or higher, recovery is spontaneous in two weeks or less, and prognosis is good despite repeated attacks. Syn., *Posner-Schlossman syndrome.*

ocular c. A sudden attack of intense pain in the eyes accompanied by photophobia, lacrimation, and sometimes blurring of vision.

oculogyric c. A condition occurring in epidemic encephalitis in which the eyes are fixed in one position for minutes or hours.

Pel's c. A sudden attack of intense ocular pain, lacrimation, and photophobia, occurring in tabes dorsalis. Syn., *Pel's syndrome.*

Crisp-Stine test. See under *test.*

criteria, Flom's. A five level list of criteria for the functional cure of strabismus, cured, almost cured, moderately improved, slightly improved, and not improved. Cured indicates clear, comfortable, single, binocular vision at all fixation distances, a normal range of motor fusion, stereopsis, strabismus not more than one percent of the time providing diplopia occurs, and the wearing of only small amounts of prism. The requirements for the other four levels are less stringent.

criteria, Sarver's. A set of five clinical criteria for the selection of patients for whom the Soflens is indicated: one to six diopters of myopia; less than a half diopter of residual astigmatism; visual acuity of 0.8 or better with a Soflens; good lens centration; and adequate lens movement with versions and blinking.

criterion. Clinically, a formula, a standard rule of thumb, or a syndrome serving as a basis for diagnosis, prognosis, or prescription.

balance plus and minus c. The criterion based on the assumption that asthenopia is not attributable to muscular imbalance when the positive and negative relative accommodation ranges are equal.

Judd c. A means of rating the diagnostic efficiency of a pseudoisochromatic plate, based on its misclassification of normal and of color-deficient subjects by the formula $Q_n + Q_d$, Q_n being the proportion of normal who fail the plate and Q_d the proportion of color-deficient who pass it.

Percival c. The criterion based on the assumption that asthenopia is not attributable to muscular imbalance when the convergence demand or stimulus is in the middle third of the total fusional convergence range. (Incorrectly referred to as Percival criteria.)

Rayleigh c. Two images are said to be just resolved when the central maximum in the diffraction pattern of one of the images is located at the first minimum in the diffraction pattern of the other.

Sheard c. The criterion based on the assumption that asthenopia is not attributable to muscular imbalance when the degree of heterophoria is less than half the opposing fusional convergence in reserve. (Incorrectly referred to as Sheard criteria.)

Sloan-Green c. A means of rating the diagnostic efficiency of a pseudoisochromatic plate, based on its misclassification of normal and of color-deficient subjects by the formula $(Q_n)^2 + (Q_d)^2$, Q_n being the proportion of normal who fail the plate and Q_d the proportion of color-deficient who pass it.

Strehl c. Strehl definition.

critical flicker frequency. See under *frequency.*

crocodile shagreen. See under *degeneration.*

Crookes' (krooks) **adaptometer; glass; radiometer.** See under the nouns.

Cross's (kros'ez) **method; stereoscope.** See under the nouns.

cross. A figure, mark, or structure formed by two intersecting straight limbs.

Maddox c. A scale for measuring vertical and lateral phorias or tropias, consisting of a graduated vertical line and a graduated horizontal line, in the form of a cross, and a light source placed at the point of intersection. Syn., *Maddox tangent scale chart; Maddox tangent scale.*

optical c. 1. A diagrammatic scheme for charting the axes and dioptric powers of the principal meridians of ophthalmic lenses, consisting of two lines crossing each other at right angles and oriented to represent the principal meridians. Each line is notated at one end with the degree and at the other end with the dioptric power. 2. The intersecting lines in the center of an optical protractor.

cross-disparity. A variation, found in Helmholtz' writings, of Hering's crossed disparity, and understood by him to represent any retinal disparity producing perception of stereopsis.

crossed cylinders. Crossed cylinder lens.

cross-eyed. The popular term for esotropic.

cross-hairs. A reticle of thin threads or wires stretched at right angles in the focal plane of the eyepiece of an optical instrument, for purposes of localization and focusing adjustments.

crossing, A-V. Arteriovenous crossing, referring to the crossing of arteries over veins, or vice versa, in the eyeground. See also *A-V nicking.*

cross-polarized. Pertaining to media with polarizing planes perpendicular to each other.

Crouzon's disease (kroo-zonz'). Hereditary craniofacial dysostosis.

crowding. Crowding phenomenon.

Crowe's sign (krōz). See under *sign.*

Cruise stereoscope (krōōz). See under *stereoscope.*

crus cerebri (krus ser'e-bri). Cerebral peduncles.

crutch, ptosis. A spectacle frame attachment to support and elevate a ptotic eyelid. Syn., *ptosis prop.*

Cruveilhier's valve (kroo-vāl-yāz'). Plica lacrimalis.

cryoextraction (kri"o-eks-trak'shun). Intracapsular cataract extraction in which the lens is removed by a refrigerated instrument to which it adheres by freezing. Syn., *cryoprehensile extraction.*

cryoextractor (kri'o-eks-trak'tor). An instrument containing a refrigerant, used in cryoextraction. Syn., *cryophake.*

cryopexy (kri-o-peks'e). For retinal detachment, the fixing of retina to choroid by localized freezing at the scleral surface.

cryophake (kri'o-fāk). Cryoextractor.

crypt. 1. A small pitlike depression. 2. A glandular cavity.

conjunctival c's. Glands of Henle.

c's. of Fuchs. Pitlike depressions, located near the collarette of the iris, serving as passageways for aqueous fluid. At these crypts the anterior endothelium and the anterior limiting layer are meager.

c's. of iris. The crypts of Fuchs and also similar, but smaller, pits located near the root of the iris.

cryptophthalmia (krip"tof-thal'me-ah). Cryptophthalmos.

cryptophthalmos (krip"tof-thal'mos). A congenital anomaly in which the eyelids are totally absent, with skin passing continuously from the forehead over a malformed or rudimentary eye, onto the cheek. The cornea and the conjunctiva are usually replaced by vascularized fibrous tissue adherent to the skin. Syn., *cryptophthalmia; cryptophthalmus.*

cryptophthalmus (krip"tof-thal'mus). Cryptophthalmos.

crys. Abbreviation for *crystalline lens.*

crystal. A body having natural external plane faces and formed by a three-dimensional array of atoms, ions, or molecules, which is built up by some fundamental unit of structure which repeats regularly and indefinitely in the three dimensions.

anistropic c. A crystal that exhibits different optical properties for light traveling through it in different directions; a crystal exhibiting double refraction.

biaxial c. A doubly refracting crystal that has two directions in which plane-polarized waves of light travel with the same velocity and without change in their state of polarization. In these two directions it acts as an isotropic crystal, in all other directions as an anisotropic crystal.

dichroic c. A doubly refracting crystal that unequally absorbs the ordinary and extraordinary rays, thereby producing linearly polarized light.

herapathite c. A synthetic dichroic crystal of iodoquinine sulfate which transmits one linearly polarized beam and absorbs the other; discovered by and named after W. B. Herapath, it served as the basis for the original Polaroid material.

isotropic c. A crystal the optical

properties of which are identical in all directions.

left-handed c. An optically active crystal that rotates the plane of vibration of plane-polarized light in a counterclockwise direction as viewed by an observer looking toward the oncoming light.

negative c. A uniaxial anisotropic crystal in which the extraordinary ray is refracted away from the optic axis of the crystal.

optically active c. A crystal that rotates the plane of vibration of plane-polarized light that passes through it.

positive c. A uniaxial anisotropic crystal in which the extraordinary ray is refracted toward the optic axis of the crystal.

right-handed c. An optically active crystal that rotates the plane of vibration of plane-polarized light in a clockwise direction as viewed by an observer looking toward the oncoming light.

uniaxial c. A doubly refracting crystal in which there is one direction along which the two sets of refracted waves travel with the same velocity and without change in polarization. In this direction it acts as an isotropic crystal, in all other directions as an anisotropic crystal. **negative u.c.** A uniaxial crystal in which the index of refraction for the extraordinary ray is less than the index of refraction for the ordinary ray. **positive u.c.** A uniaxial crystal in which the index of refraction for the extraordinary ray is greater than the index of refraction for the ordinary ray.

crystalline, alpha. One of the three soluble protein fractions and antigens found in the crystalline lens and classified according to their precipitating properties, the other two being *beta* and *gamma crystalline.*

crystalline, beta. One of the three soluble protein fractions and antigens found in the crystalline lens and classified according to their precipitating characteristics, the other two being *alpha* and *gamma crystalline.*

crystalline, gamma. One of the three soluble protein fractions and antigens found in the crystalline lens and classified according to their precipitating characteristics, the other two being *alpha* and *beta crystalline.*

crystallitis (kris″tal-i′tis). Phacitis.

crystalloiditis (kris″tal-oi-di′tis). Phacitis.

crystalloluminescence (kris″tal-o-lu″mih-nes′ens). The emission of light by certain substances while they are crystallizing.

cube. A body of six equal square sides.

von Hornbostel c. A striking form of optical illusion named for the German psychologist. It consists of a skeleton wire cube which, when observed monocularly under proper conditions, will reverse as does the Necker cube. When perceived as reversed, rotations or tilting of the cube produce a visual perception of movement opposite to that felt by the hand moving it.

Inouye's c's. Two cubes, one containing Landolt C's of various sizes, the other Snellen E's of various sizes, used to train fixation by centering the doughnut-shaped negative afterimage on the test target, after stimulating the peripheral retina with bright light.

Lummer-Brodhun c. An optical device used in photometry consisting of two 45° by 90° prisms, one of which has on its hypotenuse face a convex spherical surface, except for a small central region which is flat and placed in apposition to the hypotenuse face of the other prism. Light normally incident from two comparison sources enters the cube from perpendicular directions. The light incident on the prism having the spherical face will pass undeviated through the central flat region to form a disk of light, and light entering the prism having the flat hypotenuse will be totally reflected and deviated 90° in the peripheral region where the air space is present, to form an annulus of light surrounding the disk.

Necker c. A two-dimensional perspective drawing of the outlines of a cube, which, upon steady fixation, appears to turn inside out, or to reverse perspective periodically.

Cuignet's (ke-ēn-yāz′) **method; test.** See under the nouns.

cul-de-sac (kul′duh-sak′). The fornix of the conjunctiva.

cullet (kul′et, -it). Leftover glass from previous melts which is added to the raw materials of a new batch in the manufacture of optical glass.

cum correctione. With correction, abbreviated c̄c.

cuneus (ku'ne-us). The portion of the medial surface of an occipital lobe above the calcarine fissure, containing the upper halves of both the higher visual centers and the visual association centers.

cup. A bowl-shaped drinking vessel, or any similar shaped structure.

cartilaginous c. A supporting structure of hyaline cartilage located in the sclera of the posterior hemispherical segment of the eyes of some birds.

glaucomatous c. A deep depression of the optic disk, seen in glaucoma and characterized by steep or overhanging walls over which the central retinal vessels may bend sharply to reappear faintly at the bottom of the depression.

ocular c. Optic cup.

optic c. A two-layered, cuplike structure, formed by invagination of the distal wall of the optic vesicle, which commences at about the fourth week of embryonic life and gives origin to the retina, the inner surfaces of the ciliary body and the iris, and the intrinsic muscles of the iris. Syn., *secondary optic vesicle.*

perilimbal suction c. A plastic, funnel-shaped device used in glaucoma testing to close the aqueous outflow channels for evaluating aqueous flow and out-flow resistance. The narrow end is joined to a suction pump, and a flange of 15 mm radius of curvature at its wide end is placed around the limbus. See also *perilimbal suction cup test.*

physiological c. A funnel-shaped depression at or near the center of the optic disk where the central retinal vessels leave or enter the retina; a normal physiological depression lined by the meniscus of Kuhnt.

Cüpper's (ke'perz) **afterimage method; test; theory.** See under the nouns.

curl. The portion of a riding bow temple which wraps around the base of the pinna.

current. A stream or flow of fluid, electricity, or gas in a certain direction, or the rate of such flow.

action c. The flow of electrons as a result of active portions of a tissue or cell being electrically negative to resting portions.

optic nerve c. An action current traveling in the optic nerve.

photoelectric c. A nerve current initiated by stimulation of receptors in the retina by wavelengths of the visible spectrum.

retinal c. A current in the retina initiated through stimulation of receptors by light waves. The stimulated cells are electronegative to the nerve fiber layer or optic nerve and form the basis for the electroretinogram.

Current Optometric Information and Terminology. A glossary of terms published by the American Optometric Association as a guide toward uniform and comprehensive interpretation of conditions commonly seen in the practice of optometry, with emphasis on etiology, symptoms, diagnostic criteria, complications, recommendations, and synonyms.

Current Optometric Procedural Terminology. A booklet published by the American Optometric Association to describe, classify, and codify conventional and special diagnostic, treatment, and material services involved in optometric care, especially to facilitate contracting with, and reimbursement by, third party agencies.

curvature. The act of curving or the state of being curved; a bending from a rectilinear direction.

c. contrast. See under *contrast.*

c. of the field. An aberration of refractive and reflective optics wherein a curved image surface results from a plane object, due to each object point being a different distance from the refracting or reflecting surface.

c. of the image. Curvature of the field.

◆

CURVE

curve. 1. A bending or deviation without finite angles from a straight course; that which is bent or flexed. 2. A line, usually curved, representing graphically a variable element.

absorption c. A graphical representation of absorption as a function of some other factor, i.e., wavelength, temperature, or ion concentration.

base c. 1. In ophthalmic lenses, the standard or reference surface in a lens or series of lenses, classified by (varying) manufacturing nomenclature as having a given base curve. 2. In a toric surface, the curve of least power.

3. In multifocal lenses, the spherical curve on the segment side. 4. In single vision spherical ophthalmic lenses, the curve of the surface of lesser curvature. 5. In contact lenses, the curve of the posterior surface in the area corresponding to the optical zone.

blend c. A curved surface of narrow width on the posterior surface of a contact lens, designed to reduce the sharpness at the junction between two curves of unlike radii, usually produced by polishing with a tool having an intermediate radius. Syn., *transitional curve.*

Broca-Sulzer c. A curve showing changes in perceived brightness of light of constant illuminance with varied durations of flash, maximum values being obtained for intermediate durations.

caustic c. In optics, the cusp-tipped curve described by the intersections of consecutively adjacent pairs of rays in a longitudinal section through the axis of a bundle of converging rays, whence all rays in the section are tangent to the curve. If formed by reflection, it is termed *catacaustic*, by refraction, *diacaustic*.

cold c. In dichromatic vision, the sensation curve representing the color-mixing primary in the short (blue) wavelength region of the spectrum.

color c's., Maxwell's. The set of three curves representing the relative amounts of Maxwell's three primary colors needed to match visually each of the spectrum colors. Syn., *Maxwell's sensation curves.*

color mixture c. Curves representing the relative amounts of primary color required to match each part of the spectrum.

color valence c's., Hering's. Two interlacing curves, showing the variation in effectivity of spectral wavelengths in producing the sensations of (a) red and green, (b) blue and yellow. Relative valences for red and for yellow are shown above the zero axis, those for green and for blue below, to indicate that red and green are opponent pairs of colors, as are blue and yellow. Syn., *Hering valence diagram.*

corrected c. See *lens, corrected curve.*

countersink c. The spherical concave curve ground into the surface of a lens blank to which a segment will be fused in the manufacture of a multifocal lens.

cross c. The curve of greatest power of a toric surface, i.e., that lying in the meridian 90° from the base curve.

dichromatic coefficient c. A graphical representation, as a function of wavelength, of the proportions of suitable primary colors in a two-color mixture required by a dichromat to match a sample color.

dominator c., photopic. Granit's term for a spectral sensitivity curve, obtained by recording electrical responses of optic nerve fibers and ganglion cells, the maximum of which is about 555 mμ. The curve is characteristic of light-adapted eyes having cone receptors. See also *dominator-modulator theory.*

dominator c., scotopic. Granit's term for a spectral sensitivity curve, obtained by recording electrical responses of optic nerve fibers and ganglion cells, the shape and maximum of which correspond closely to the absorption curve of visual purple, and said to be characteristic of dark-adapted eyes having rod receptors. See also *dominator-modulator theory.*

equal energy c. The spectral luminous efficiency curve, so named from the assumption that it is the luminous response curve of a hypothetical source with equal energy at all wavelengths.

fixation disparity (forced vergence) c. The locus of points plotted for the magnitude and direction of fixation disparity, under varying conditions of forced vergence starting from a fixed accommodation and convergence stimulus level.

fundamental c. Base curve.

fundamental response c's. A set of three curves derived to represent the spectral sensitivity functions of the three types of receptors responsible for color vision, their maxima corresponding to about 435, 540, and 565 mμ.

hue discrimination c. A graphic representation of the ability to discriminate differences in hue throughout the spectrum. Usually the wavelength difference threshold is plotted against wavelength. Syn., *sensibility for relative hue curve.*

learning c. The curve obtained by plotting a measure of success in some task as the ordinate and the amount of practice (trial number) as the abscissa. Syn., *practice curve.*

light distribution c. A curve showing the variation of luminous intensity of a lamp or a luminaire with the angle of emission.

logistic c. An exponential curve used to describe the growth of various biological populations.

luminosity c. Spectral luminous efficiency curve. **photopic l.c.** Photopic spectral luminous efficiency curve. **relative l.c.** Photopic spectral luminous efficiency curve. **scotopic l.c.** Scotopic spectral luminous efficiency curve.

meter c. An arc of curvature having a radius of one meter; a basic unit in geometrical optics.

modulator c's. Granit's term for narrow spectral sensitivity curves derived from recordings of electrical activity of retinal ganglion cells and optic nerve fibers and considered by him to subserve the mechanism of color vision. See also *theory, Granit's.*

Ostwalt c. The lower half of the Tscherning ellipse representing the front surface curvature values providing minimum oblique astigmatism in ophthalmic lenses of various power.

persistency c. The curve obtained by plotting as ordinates the duration of sensation, measured by critical flicker frequency techniques, for different wavelengths plotted as abscissae.

Petzval c. The curved image field of an optical system corrected for oblique astigmatism.

photosensitivity c. Spectral luminous efficiency curve.

practice c. Learning curve.

primary c. The curve of the central posterior surface of a contact lens is the area corresponding to the optical zone. Syn., *base curve.*

radiometric c. A curve showing radiant energy emitted by a given source at various wavelengths.

recovery c. A curve representing any of several aspects of recovery in retinal sensitivity of the eye following pre-exposure to an adapting stimulus of a given intensity.

secondary c. The curve on the posterior surface of a contact lens adjacent and peripheral to, and of longer radius than, the base curve.

sensation c's. Curves representing the amount of luminous energy from each of three selected primary colors required in an additive mixture to match each part of an equal energy spectrum. **equal area s.c's.** Sensation curves for three primaries, red, blue, and green, in which the ordinates of two of the curves have been multiplied by factors making the enclosed areas of all three curves equal. **fundamental color s.c's.** Sensation curves based on the three primary colors with actual luminosity values plotted against wavelength. **Maxwell's s.c's.** Maxwell's color curves.

sensibility for relative hue c. Hue discrimination curve.

spectral luminous efficiency c. A plot of spectral luminous efficiency values against wavelength. It usually pertains to photopic vision unless otherwise stated and indicates the relative capacity of radiant energy of various wavelengths to produce visual sensation. Syn., *luminosity curve; visibility curve.* **photopic s.l.e.c.** A plot of spectral luminous efficiency values for photopic vision against wavelength, with unity at wavelength of maximum luminous efficacy (555 nanometers). Syn., *photopic luminosity curve; relative luminosity curve; relative visibility curve.* **scotopic s.l.e.c.** A plot of spectral luminous efficiency values for scotopic vision against wavelength, with unity at wavelength of maximum luminous efficacy (approximately 507 nanometers). Syn., *scotopic luminosity curve.*

spectral sensitivity c. A graph of sensitivity (usually the reciprocal of stimulus energy required to produce a threshold response) as a function of spectral wavelength or, less frequently, of spectral wave number or frequency. Often synonymous with *luminosity curve,* but usually restricted to threshold measurements rather than suprathreshold matches.

spectral transmission c. A curve showing the transmission of radiant energy of a filter at different wavelengths.

spectrophotometric c. A graphic representation of spectral transmittance, reflectance, absorbance, or relative spectral emittance as a function of wavelength.

spectroradiometric c. A graph of radiant energy versus wavelength, for a given radiant source.

tertiary c. The curve on the posterior surface of a contact lens adjacent and peripheral to, and of longer radius than, the secondary curve.

tonographic c. A graphic representation of the continuous changes in tonometer readings recorded during tonography.

transitional c. 1. Blend curve. 2. The curve of the intermediate zone between the corneal and scleral portions of a scleral contact lens.

transmission c. A curve formed by plotting the transmission factor against wavelength.

Tscherning c. Tscherning ellipse.

visibility c. Spectral luminous efficiency curve. **relative v.c.** Photopic spectral luminous efficiency curve.

warm c. In dichromatic vision, the sensation curve representing the color-mixing primary in the long (red) wavelength region of the spectrum.

wavelength discrimination c. A curve representing the change in wavelength required at a given wavelength to elicit a just noticeable difference in hue.

◆   *

Cushing's loop (koŏsh'ingz). Meyer's loop.

Cushing's syndrome (koosh'ingz). Chiasmal syndrome.

cushion, Soemmering's. Soemmering's ring.

Cushion lock. A trade name for a rimless spectacle mounting in which the shoes and straps are lined with a thin strip of rubber where they contact the lens.

Cutler's implant (kut'lerz). See under *implant.*

cutoff. In the manufacture of certain fused multifocal lenses, the portion of the button having the same index of refraction as the blank, and, hence, blending with the blank after fusing.

cutter. A machine for cutting ophthalmic lenses to desired sizes and shapes.

cutting line. See under *line.*

cx. Abbreviation for *convex.*

cyan (si'an). A bluish color normally corresponding to that produced by radiant energy of wavelength 494 mμ.

cyanocobalamin (si-an-o-ko-bal'ah-min). A vitamin which is the antianemia factor of liver considered necessary for the normal maturation of erythrocytes and used in the treatment of pernicious anemia. A deficiency of this

and of other of the B vitamins may be a factor in nutritional amblyopia. Syn., *vitamin B$_{12}$.*

cyanolabe (si-an'o-lāb). The name proposed by W. A. H. Rushton for a blue-sensitive retinal photopigment, the existence of which is theoretical and has not yet been detected experimentally.

cyanometer (si-an-om'eh-ter). An instrument for measuring blueness, as of the sky.

cyanophose (si-an'o-fōz, si'an-o-fōz"). A subjective sensation of blue light or color.

cyanopia (si-ah-no'pe-ah). A perversion of vision in which all objects appear blue. It may be a temporary condition following cataract extraction or may occur rarely with diseases of the retina or the choroid. Syn., *blue vision.*

cyanopsia (si-ah-nop'se-ah). Cyanopia.

cyanopsin (si"ah-nop'sin). A photosensitive synthesized carotenoid protein with an absorption maximum at 620 mμ and considered to have a spectral sensitivity similar to that of cone receptor cells of some animals.

cyanosis (si"ah-no'sis). A bluish discoloration of the skin and mucous membranes, due to insufficient oxygenation of the blood.

c. bulbi. Bluish discoloration of the sclera in cyanosis.

c. of retina. A condition characterized by marked engorgement and tortuosity of the retinal veins, with a purplish coloration of the fundus, and occasional hemorrhages. It is part of a general cyanosis and is usually associated with congenital heart disease.

cycle. A complete course or round of regularly recurring events or phenomena with a return to the original state.

color c. Color circle.

duty c. Pulse-to-cycle fraction.

Kühne c. The serial photoproducts formed in the breakdown and recomposition of visual purple, as depicted graphically by Kühne. The components of the cycle include *rhodopsin, visual yellow,* and *visual white.*

Lythgoe c. The serial photoproducts formed in the breakdown and recomposition of visual purple, as depicted graphically by Lythgoe. The components of the cycle include *rhodopsin, transient orange, indicator yellow,* and *visual white.*

Wald c. The serial photoproducts formed in the breakdown and recomposition of visual purple, as depicted graphically by Wald. The photoproducts include retinene and protein, and vitamin A and protein.

cyclectomy (si-klek'to-me, sik-lek'-). Excision of a portion of the ciliary body.

cyclicotomy (si"kle-kot'o-me, sik"le-). Cyclotomy.

cyclitis (si-kli'tis, sik-li'-). Inflammation of the ciliary body, usually accompanied by an inflammation of the iris (iridocyclitis). It occurs in three forms, plastic, purulent, and serous, and is characterized by circumcorneal injection fading toward the fornix (ciliary flush), normal intraocular tension, marked tenderness, dimming of vision, keratic precipitates, photophobia, lacrimation, and sometimes hypopyon.

annularis exudativa pseudotumorosa c. A circular detachment of the choroid in the anterior periphery which often follows iridocyclitis and may be combined with a detachment of the retina. Due to its color and solid appearance it can resemble a tumor such as a malignant melanoma.

herpetic c. Inflammation of the ciliary body associated with herpes zoster of the cornea.

heterochromic c. of Fuchs. Complicated heterochromia.

plastic c. A severe inflammation of the ciliary body characterized by a copious plastic exudate, rich in fibrin, which accumulates in the anterior and posterior chambers and in the vitreous. The exudate may become organized and eventually consolidate into fibrous tissue and terminate in phthisis bulbi.

pure c. Inflammation of the ciliary body without an accompanying iritis.

purulent c. An acute inflammation of the ciliary body accompanied by a profuse discharge of pus. It usually involves the entire uveal tract constituting endophthalmitis.

serous c. An inflammation of the ciliary body characterized by a relatively fluid exudate which travels into the anterior and posterior chambers and vitreous. Keratic precipitates are present on the posterior cornea, the iris, and sometimes the lens capsule, and aqueous flare is visible with the slit lamp.

sympathetic c. An inflammation of the ciliary body associated with sympathetic ophthalmia.

traumatic c. An inflammation of the ciliary body following ocular contusion.

cycloanemization (si"klo-an"e-mi-za'-shun). Surgical obliteration of the long ciliary arteries in the treatment of glaucoma.

cycloaniseikonia (si"klo-an"ih-si-ko'ne-ah). Aniseikonia in which a difference in image size exists in oblique meridians of the two eyes but at perpendicular axes, e.g., right eye 1% axis 45°, left eye 1% axis 135°.

cycloceratitis (si"klo-ser"ah-ti'tis). Cyclokeratitis.

cyclochoroiditis (si"klo-ko"roid-i'tis, sik"lo-). An inflammation of both the ciliary body and the choroid.

cyclocryotherapy (si"klo-kri"o-ther'ah-pe). Local freezing of the ciliary body, used in the treatment of glaucoma.

cyclodamia (si"klo-da'me-ah). A noncycloplegic method of refraction employing a fogging technique for relaxing accommodation, especially one employing excessive amount of convex sphere to determine acuity-reduction gradients from which the refractive error may be estimated by extrapolation.

cyclodeviation (si"klo-de"ve-a'shun). 1. Cyclotropia or cyclophoria. 2. A rotation or rotary displacement of the eye about an anteroposterior axis.

cyclodialysis (si"klo-di-al'is-is). The operation, to reduce the intraocular pressure in glaucoma, which involves the detachment of the ciliary body from the sclera to form a communication between the suprachoroidal space and the anterior chamber.

cyclodiathermy (si"klo-di'ah-ther-me). A procedure for the treatment of glaucoma in which a portion of the ciliary body is destroyed by the heat generated from a high frequency alternating electric current passed through the tissue. The resulting decrease in aqueous humor production lowers the intraocular pressure.

cycloduction (si"klo-duk'shun). 1. Disjunctive torsional movements of the eyes to maintain single binocular vision, measured clinically by rotating oppositely a pair of straight lines, each seen by only one eye, until the limit of fusion is reached. 2. Cyclorotation.

cycloelectrolysis (si"klo-e-lek"trol'ih-sis). A procedure for the treatment of glaucoma in which a portion of the ciliary body is destroyed by the chemical action caused by a low frequency direct electric current passed through the tissue. The resulting decrease in aqueous humor production lowers the intraocular pressure.

cyclofusion (si"klo-fu'zhun). The relative rotation of the two eyes around their respective anteroposterior axes, in response to a cyclofusional stimulus, i.e., in response to retinal images meridionally disoriented, so as to necessitate the relative rotation of the eyes about their anteroposterior axes, to stimulate corresponding retinal areas.

cyclogoniotomy (si"klo-go-ne-ot'o-me). A surgical procedure for producing cyclodialysis, in which the ciliary body is cut from its attachment at the scleral spur under gonioscopic control.

cyclography, impedance (si-klog'rah-fe). The passing of a small high frequency alternating current across the ciliary muscle during accommodation and recording the changes of impedance.

Cyclogyl (si'klo-jil"). A trade name for *cyclopentolate hydrochloride.*

cyclokeratitis (si"klo-ker"ah-ti'tis). Inflammation of both the ciliary body and the cornea.

cycloparesis (si"klo-pah-re'sis, -par'e-sis). A weakened condition of the ciliary muscle.

cyclopentolate hydrochloride (si"-klo-pen'to-lāt hi"dro-klo'rīd). A parasympatholytic drug used in 0.5%, 1.0%, and 2.0% solutions as a short-acting mydriatic and cycloplegic.

cyclophoria (si"klo-fo're-ah). The relative orientation of the two eyes about their respective lines of sight in the absence of cyclofusional stimuli, specified in terms of the deviation of the corresponding retinal meridians from parallelism.

    anatomical c. Cyclophoria attributable to anomalies or variations in anatomical structure, usually involving the extraocular muscles.

    asymmetrical c. Cyclophoria characterized by unequal cyclorotary deviations of the two eyes from a common reference plane, such as the median plane of the head or the perpendicular bisector of the interocular base line.

    essential c. Cyclophoria attributable to anomalies or variations in

anatomical or muscular structure or function. Syn., *static cyclophoria.*

    intrinsic c. Cyclophoria inherently related to muscular anomalies, not related secondarily to innervation of convergence or other auxiliary functions.

    minus c. Cyclophoria characterized by downward divergence of the corresponding vertical retinal meridians. Syn., *incyclophoria.*

    myologic c. Cyclophoria attributable to anomalies or variations in muscular structure or function.

    optical c. 1. Refractive cyclophoria. 2. Cyclophoria acquired through prolonged corrective torsion in compensation for meridional distortions due to uncorrected oblique astigmatism or to the prolonged wearing of oblique correcting cylinders.

    paretic c. Cyclophoria attributable to paresis, especially of the extraocular muscles.

    plus c. Cyclophoria characterized by upward divergence of the corresponding vertical retinal meridians. Syn., *excyclophoria.*

    refractive c. Apparent cyclophoria resulting from meridional differences in the refracting power of an ophthalmic lens being worn while the measurement is made. Syn., *optical cyclophoria.*

    static c. Essential cyclophoria.

    symmetrical c. Cyclophoria characterized by equal cyclorotary deviations of the two eyes from a common reference plane, such as the median plane of the head or the perpendicular bisector of the interocular base line.

cyclophorometer (si"klo-fo-rom'eh-ter). An instrument for measuring cyclophoria.

cyclopia (si-klo'pe-ah). Elements of the two eyes fused into one median eye in the center of the forehead of a fetal monster. Syn., *synophthalmia; synopsia.*

cycloplegia (si"klo-ple'je-ah). Paralysis of the ciliary muscle and the power of accommodation, usually accompanied by a dilated pupil. It may be pathological, or artificially induced.

cycloplegic (si"klo-ple'jik). 1. Pertaining to cycloplegia. 2. A drug which causes cycloplegia.

cycloposition (si"klo-po-zish'un). The position of the eye with reference to its rotation around an anteroposterior axis.

cyclops (si'klops). A developmental monster characterized by having only one eye.

cyclorotation (si"klo-ro-ta'shun). A wheel-like rotation of the eye around an anteroposterior axis. Syn., *torsion*.

cyclospasm (si'klo-spazm"). A spasm of the ciliary muscle.

cyclostasis (si"klo-sta'sis). The static position the covered eye assumes if it deviates in an incyclo- or excyclodirection during a cover test. (Lancaster)

cyclotomy (si-klot'o-me). Surgical incision of the ciliary body, usually for the relief of glaucoma. Syn., *cyclicotomy*.

cyclotonic (si"klo-ton'ik). A state of constant accommodation such as may occur with the administration of an anticholinesterase agent; the opposite of *cycloplegia*.

cyclotorsion (si"klo-tōr'shun). A wheel-like rotation of an eye around an anteroposterior axis. Syn., *torsion*.

cyclotropia (si"klo-tro'pe-ah). A strabismic condition in which there is a meridional deviation around the anteroposterior axis of one eye with respect to the other.

cyclovergence (si"klo-ver'jens). A relative wheel-like rotation of the eyes around their respective anteroposterior axes, so that their vertical retinal meridians converge above (incyclovergence) or below (excyclovergence).

cycloversion (si"klo-ver'zhun). The meridional rotation of both eyes in the same direction around the anteroposterior axes.

   negative c. Levocycloversion.

   positive c. Dextrocycloversion.

cyl. Abbreviation for *cylinder* or *cylindrical*.

cylicotomy (sil"e-kot'o-me). Cyclotomy.

cylinder. 1. A surface traced by one side of a rectangle rotated around the parallel side as the axis, or a body of such form. 2. Cylindrical lens.

   dielectric c. A cylinder of dielectric material such as glass, quartz, or optical plastic used in fiber optic devices.

   rough c. Semifinished cylinder.

   semifinished c. A glass lens blank with one surface unfinished and the other ground and polished into cylindrical or toric form. Syn., *rough cylinder*.

cylinder-prism. A lens which combines cylinder power with prism power.

cylindroma (sil"in-dro'mah). An epithelioma occurring in a benign form which affects the skin of the head or upper chest, and in a malignant form which affects mucous membranes. The malignant form is a type of carcinoma and is one of the most common of the tumors affecting the lacrimal gland.

cylindro-spherometer (sih-lin"dro-sfe-rom'eh-ter). An instrument for determining lens power or curvature in any given meridian by the sagittal depth method, which employs three aligned contact points, the center one of which controls an indicator needle on a calibrated dial face. Syn., *lens clock; Luer's clock; lens measure*.

cyst. A sac, especially one having a distinct membrane and containing fluid or semisolid matter.

   Blessig's c's. Cystic spaces in the peripheral retina, near the ora serrata, first described by Blessig. See also *degeneration, cystic of retina*.

   dermoid c. See *dermoid*.

   Meibomian c. A chalazion.

   prepapillary hyaloid c's. Single or multiple grayish bodies, anterior to the optic disk, representing cystic formations of hyaloid remnants, typically small and round and lying close to the disk, but may be elongated and project into the vitreous humor.

   tarsal c. A chalazion.

   vitelline c. of the macula. Vitelline disk of the macula.

cysticercus subretinalis (sis"tih-ser'kus sub-ret"ih-nal'is). A parasitic infection beneath the retina which leads to retinal detachment and vitreous opacities.

cysticerkosis, ocular (sis"tih-ser-kō'sis). Infection of the eye with the larval stage of *Taenia solium*, the pork tapeworm, or *Taenia saginata*, the beef tapeworm, which may result in an acute ocular inflammation.

cystinosis (sis"tin-o'sis). An inborn defect in which the renal tubules are defective and in which there is a disturbance of amino acid metabolism resulting in the deposition of cystine crystals in various tissue. In the eye, the crystals are found in the anterior corneal stroma and the superficial layers of the conjunctiva, giving the pathognomonic appearance of a myriad of scintillating, polychromatic, fine, refractile bodies.

cystitomy (sis-tit'o-me). Surgical incision of the capsule of the crystalline lens. Syn., *capsulotomy*.

cytoblasts of Henle (si'to-blasts). Cells of unknown origin and function in the peripheral portion of the vitreous body, situated close to the retina and more numerous near the pars plana. Syn., *corpuscles of Donders*.

Czermak's (chār'mahks) **experiment; phosphene.** See under the nouns.

D

D. Abbreviation for *diopter*.

Daae's color table (da'ēz). See under *table*.

dacrocystitis (dak"ro-sis-ti'tis). Dacryocystitis.

dacry- (dak're). See *dacryo-*.

dacryadenoscirrhus (dak"re-ad-e-no-skir'us). A hardened tumor of the lacrimal gland.

dacryagog (dak're-ah-gog"). Dacryagogue.

dacryagogatresia (dak"re-ag"o-ga-tre'-ze-ah, dak"re-ah-gog"ah-). A closure or an obstruction of a tear duct.

dacryagogue (dak're-ah-gog"). 1. Inducing a flow of tears. 2. A substance which induces a flow of tears.

dacrycystalgia (dak"re-sis-tal'je-ah). Pain localized in a lacrimal sac.

dacryelcosis (dak"re-el-ko'sis). Dacryohelcosis.

dacryhemorrhysis (dak"re-hem"o-ri'-sis). Dacryohemorrhea.

dacryma (dak're-mah"). Fluid secretion of the lacrimal gland; a tear.

dacryo- (dak're-o). A combining form denoting relationship to tears or to the lacrimal apparatus.

dacryoadenalgia (dak"re-o-ad"e-nal'je-ah). Pain localized in a lacrimal gland.

dacryoadenectomy (dak"re-o-ad"e-nek'to-me). Surgical removal of a lacrimal gland.

dacryoadenitis (dak"re-o-ad"e-ni'tis). Inflammation of a lacrimal gland.

dacryoblennorrhea (dak"re-o-blen"o-re'ah). A chronic mucus discharge from a lacrimal sac.

dacryocanaliculitis (dak"re-o-kan"al-ik"u-li'tis). Inflammation of a lacrimal canal.

dacryocele (dak're-o-sēl). A pathologic swelling of a lacrimal sac.

dacryocyst (dak're-o-sist"). A lacrimal sac. *Obs.*

dacryocystalgia (dak"re-o-sis-tal'je-ah). Dacrycystalgia.

dacryocystectasia (dak"re-o-sis-tek-ta'ze-ah). A dilation of a lacrimal sac.

dacryocystectomy (dak"re-o-sis-tek'to-me). Surgical removal of a part of a lacrimal sac.

dacryocystenosis (dak"re-o-sis"ten-o'sis). Dacryocystostenosis.

dacryocystitis (dak"re-o-sis-ti'tis). Inflammation of a lacrimal sac.

    blennorrheal d. A suppurative inflammation of a lacrimal sac. Syn., *dacryocystoblennorrhea*.

    catarrhal d. A chronic catarrhal inflammation of the lacrimal sac usually due to an obstruction in the nasolacrimal duct.

    phlegmonous d. Inflammation of the lacrimal sac and the surrounding soft tissues.

dacryocystoblennorrhea (dak"re-o-sis"to-blen"o-re'ah). Blennorrheal dacryocystitis.

dacryocystocele (dak"re-o-sis'to-sēl). A swelling or protrusion of the lacrimal sac. Syn., *dacryocele*.

dacryocystogram (dak"re-o-sis'to-gram). An x-ray photograph of the lacrimal apparatus of the eye, made visible by radiopaque dyes.

dacryocystography (dak"re-o-sis-tog'rah-fe). Radiography of the lacrimal drainage apparatus of the eye, made visible by radiopaque dyes.

dacryocystoptosis (dak"re-o-sis"top-to'sis). A downward displacement or prolapse of a lacrimal sac.

dacryocystorhinostenosis (dak"re-o-sis"to-ri"-no-ste-no'sis). Constriction of the nasolacrimal duct.

dacryocystorhinostomy (dak"re-o-sis"to-ri-no'sto-me). An operation to restore the flow of tears into the nose from the lacrimal sac when the nasolacrimal duct does not function.

dacryocystorhinotomy (dak"re-o-sis"to-ri-not'o-me). Dacryorhinocystotomy.

dacryocystostenosis (dak"re-o-sis"to-ste-no'sis). Narrowing of a lacrimal sac.

dacryocystostomy (dak"re-o-sis-tos'to-me). Incision of a lacrimal sac, usually to promote drainage.

dacryocystotomy (dak"re-o-sis-tot'o-me). Incision of a lacrimal sac.

dacryogenic (dak"re-o-jen'ik). Causing a flow of tears.

dacryohelcosis (dak"re-o-hel-ko'sis). Ulceration of the lacrimal duct or of the lacrimal sac.

dacryohaemorrhoea (dak"re-o-hem"o-re'ah). Dacryohemorrhea.

dacryohemorrhea (dak"re-o-hem"o-re'ah). The discharge of bloody tears or of blood from the lacrimal sac.

dacryohemorrhysis (dak"re-o-hem"o-re'sis). Bloody tears. Syn,. *lacrimae cruentae.*

dacryolin (dak're-o-lin). An albuminous material found in tears.

dacryolite (dak're-o-līt"). Dacryolith.

dacryolith (dak're-o-lith"). A calcareous concretion in the lacrimal apparatus.

dacryolithiasis (dak"re-o-lih-thi'ah-sis). The presence or the formation of calcareous concretions in the lacrimal apparatus.

dacryoma (dak"re-o'mah). 1. A tumor of the lacrimal apparatus. 2. A blockage of a lacrimal punctum, producing swelling.

dacryon (dak're-on). A cranial point located at the junction of the lacrimo-maxillary, frontolacrimal, and frontomaxillary sutures.

dacryopericystitis (dak"re-o-per"e-sis-ti'tis). Inflammation of the tissues adjacent to the lacrimal sac, usually secondary to a purulent dacryocystitis.

dacryops (dak're-ops). 1. A watery condition of the eye. 2. A cyst of a tear duct of the lacrimal gland.

dacryoptosis (dak"re-op-to'sis). Dacryocystoptosis.

dacryopyorrhea (dak"re-o-pi-o-re'ah). A discharge of tears containing pus.

dacryopyosis (dak"re-o-pi-o'sis). Suppuration of the lacrimal passages.

dacryorhinocystotomy (dak"re-o-ri"no-sis-tot'o-me). The passing of a probe through the lacrimal sac into the nasal cavity.

dacryorrhea (dak"re-o-re'ah). An abnormally profuse flow of tears.

dacryosolen (dak're-o-so"len). A lacrimal canal or duct.

dacryosolenitis (dak"re-o-so"le-ni'tis). Inflammation of a lacrimal canal or duct.

dacryostenosis (dak"re-o-ste-no'sis). A narrowing or a stricture of a lacrimal duct.

dacryosyrinx (dak"re-o-si'rinks, -sir'-inks). 1. A lacrimal fistula. 2. A syringe used to irrigate lacrimal ducts.

dacryrrhea (dak-rir'e-ah). Dacryorrhea.

dadeleum (de-de'le-um). A stroboscopic apparatus devised by Horner.

daedeleum (de-de'le-um). Dadeleum.

Dalén's spots (da'lenz). See under *spot.*

Dalén-Fuchs nodule (da'len-fūks). See under *nodule.*

Dallos contact lens (dal'os). See under *lens.*

Dalrymple's (dal'rim-pelz) **disease; sign.** See under the nouns.

Daltonism (dawl'ton-izm). Color blindness. So named because John Dalton (1766-1844), who was partially color blind, published a description of his condition.

Dandy-Walker syndrome (dan'de-wok'er). Atresia of the foramen of Magendie syndrome. See under *syndrome.*

Daniel's spirals. See under *spiral.*

Dannheim (dan'hīm) **implant; lens.** See under *lens.*

dark. *(adj.)* 1. Pertaining to a color embodying a content of blackness induced by a brighter surround. 2. Pertaining to an area or a space devoid, or partially devoid, of light.

dark. *(n.)* An absence, or gross insufficiency, of light, usually connoting a percept of blackness.

darkness. The state or quality of being dark.

    total d. 1. Complete absence of

light. 2. A luminance level below the human absolute threshold.

Darkschewitsch's (dark-sha'vich-ez) **nucleus; tract.** See under the nouns.

Dartnall's theory (dart'nalz). See under *theory*.

Davidson's reflex (da'vid-sunz). See under *reflex*.

Dawes limit. See under *limit*.

daylight. A mixture of sunlight and skylight.

 artificial d. 1. Illumination produced by a source of artificial or controlled light matching the color quality of daylight obtained under standard conditions. 2. Illumination produced by a standard light source having a color temperature approximating expressed daylight conditions, such as CIE Illuminant C.

 natural d. Light or illumination as received from the sun and sky combined without filtering, directional selection, or selective reflection. It varies in spectral character with the time of day, atmospheric conditions, or season of the year. Cf. *sunlight; skylight.*

dazzle. 1. To obscure or confuse vision by exposure to excessive or extraneous light, or moving lights. 2. To stimulate the peripheral retina with intense light while shielding the central retina, a procedure used in the pleoptic treatment of amblyopia ex anopsia to render the central area relatively more receptive to fixation stimuli.

DBC. Abbreviation for *distance between centers.*

DBL. Abbreviation for *distance between lenses.*

dcc. Abbreviation for *double concave*, as applied to an ophthalmic lens.

DCLP. Diploma in Contact Lens Practice (British Optical Association).

dcx. Abbreviation for *double convex*, as applied to an ophthalmic lens.

dd. Abbreviation for *disk diameter* of the optic nerve head.

dec. Abbreviation for *decenter* or *decentration*, as applied to ophthalmic lenses.

de Carle bifocal contact lens (deh-karl'). See under *lens, contact, bifocal.*

decenter. To displace, in the fabrication or the design of an ophthalmic lens, the optical center with respect to the geometric center or to some other mechanical point of reference.

decentration. The process of decentering, the decentered condition, or the amount of decentering. See also *decenter.*

 stereoscopic d. The relative, horizontal displacement between pairs of reference points in the two monocularly seen halves of a stereogram, vectogram, or other stereoscopic target, so as to produce retinal disparity.

declination (dek"lih-na'shun). In a plane perpendicular to an anteroposterior axis of the eye or of an optical instrument, the angle between two meridians of reference, one of which may be the horizontal, the vertical, or an anatomically or functionally designated meridian, and the other a measured or experimentally determined meridian the orientation of which is attributable to ocular torsion or is otherwise induced by viewing plane or lens distortions. Variously called *declination error*, it may be designated either as an angle or in terms of instrumental adjustment units necessary to correct it, as in eikonometry.

declinator (dek'lih-na"tor). An instrument for measuring the torsion of the eyeball or the declination of the ocular meridians. Syn., *declinometer.*

declinograph (de-kli'no-graf). A recording declinator.

declinometer (dek"lih-nom'eh-ter). Declinator.

decoding (de-kōd'ing). The process of translating responses to electro-chemical sensory stimuli so that they may be perceived and comprehended, as in reading.

decoding, visual. Comprehension of pictures and printed words.

decoloration (de"kul-or-a'shun). 1. Lack or loss of color. 2. Bleaching or removal of color.

decolorize (de-kul'or-īz). To bleach; to remove color.

decomposition. The division or breaking down of a substance into its component parts, as in the decomposition of rhodopsin by light, or the dispersion of light by a prism or a grating.

decompression, orbital. Surgical relief of pressure behind the eyeball, as in exophthalmus, by the removal of bone from the orbit.

decussation (de-kus-a'shun). A crossing over, especially of nerve fibers crossing the midsagittal plane of the central nervous system and connecting with structures on the opposite side.

anterior hypothalamic d. Ganser's commissure.

dorsal supraoptic d. Meynert's commissure.

dorsal tegmental d. Fountain decussation of Meynert.

fountain d. of Meynert. The crossing over of nerve fibers from cells of the gray matter of the superior colliculi which, after decussation, connect with oculomotor nuclei. Syn., *dorsal tegmental decussation.*

optic d. In the visual pathway, the crossing over of the nerve fibers originating in the two nasal retinae to the opposite optic tracts; the optic chiasm.

ventral supraoptic d. Commissure of von Gudden.

defect. The absence, failure, or imperfection of a part or an organ.

arteriovenous crossing d. Any deviation of the crossings of retinal vessels from normal, as in A-V nicking.

hemianopic d. A blind area comprising approximately one half of the field of vision of one or both eyes and bounded by either horizontal or vertical diameters of the field.

optical d. Any physical or mechanical defect of an optical system that prevents the clear formation of an image, as in ametropia of the eye or aberrations of a lens system.

sector d. of visual field. A blind portion of the visual field, roughly or exactly defined by two radii of the field, extending to and continuous with the peripheral limit.

definition. 1. The sharpness of imagery produced by an optical system. 2. In the eye, the maximum ability to discriminate between two points. See also *visual resolution; resolving power.*

Strehl d. A criterion proposed by K. Strehl (1902) for evaluation of the imaging quality of optical systems. The ratio of the maximum intensity in the central part of a point-image formed by an actual optical system, to the corresponding intensity in the point-image formed by an aberration-free system of the same aperture and focal length. Syn., *Strehl criterion; Strehl intensity ratio.*

degeneratio (de-jen"er-a'she-o). Degeneration.

d. cristallinea cornea hereditaria. Crystalline corneal dystrophy.

d. hyaloideoretinalis. Vitreoretinal degeneration.

d. punctata albescens. Retinitis punctata albescens.

d. sine pigmento. Retinitis pigmentosa sine pigmento.

d. spherularis elaioides. A progressive bilateral condition occurring in old people wherein droplets resembling oil appear under the corneal epithelium near the limbus, starting nasally and temporally and progressing upward and downward and then axially to possible interference with visual acuity.

◆

DEGENERATION

degeneration. Deterioration of an organ or a tissue resulting in diminished vitality, either by chemical change or by infiltration of abnormal matter.

band-shaped d. of cornea. See under *dystrophy.*

cavernous d. The depression of the central area of the optic nerve head by the coalescence of the small, empty spaces left by degenerated nerve fibers in glaucoma.

circinate d. Retinitis circinata.

cobblestone d. of the retina. Paving-stone degeneration of the retina.

colloid d. of retina. A degenerative disease involving the deposition of masses of hyaline material (drusen) on Bruch's membrane. It may occur under three sets of circumstances: (1) as a senile change commonly found in persons over 60 years of age, less frequently found in persons under this age; (2) as a degeneration secondary to certain vascular, inflammatory, or neoplastic diseases of the retina or the choroid; and (3) in association with heredodegenerative diseases of the retina, such as retinitis pigmentosa or Doyne's familial honeycombed choroiditis.

crocodile shagreen d. of cornea, deep. A very rare degeneration of Descemet's membrane of the cornea occurring in the axial region and giving the appearance of crocodile leather.

crocodile shagreen d. of cornea, superficial. A rare degeneration of Bowman's membrane of the cornea characterized by a thin, central, disklike opacity, traversed by dark streaks attributed to tears in Bowman's membrane, and resembling crocodile leather.

crystalline d. of cornea. See under *dystrophy*.

cystic d. of the macula. A localized macular degeneration, resulting in edema and the formation of cystic spaces in the central area of the retina, which lead to a macular depression or to a complete macular hole. The etiology may be traumatic, toxic, or circulatory. Syn., *macular vesicular edema; honeycombed macula.*

cystic d. of the retina. A secondary degeneration of the retina of varied etiology in which gaps are formed within the tissue, usually at the macula or at the periphery, due to disintegration of neural elements. It usually arises in the outer and inner nuclear layers, rarely in other layers, and may be a cause of retinal detachment. Syn., *cystic retinal disease; Iwanoff's cystic edema.*

disciform d. of the macula, juvenile. A degeneration of the macula characterized by a subretinal exudative-type mass, probably caused by an extravasation, mainly of serum, between Bruch's membrane and the pigmentary epithelium, due to vascular disturbance in the choriocapillaris. It occurs in persons 20 to 40 years of age and is similar to a senile disciform degeneration of the macula, being differentiated by visual resolution, leaving little impairment of vision. Syn., *juvenile exudative macular choroiditis.*

disciform d. of the macula, senile. A rare disease characterized in the early stages either by a central subretinal hemorrhage or by a central grayish-white opacity, either varying in size from that of the optic disk to several times larger. Later the retina in the affected area becomes thickened into a sharply defined, raised mound, grayish-yellow in color, which projects for several diopters. The retinal vessels pass over the mound and may be seen to anastomose with choroidal vessels in the region of the lesion. Superficial and deep hemorrhages are present at the margin of the lesion and patches of exudate surround it. Other senile degenerative changes of the retina are usually present. The condition is permanent and central vision is completely or almost completely lost. It is attributed to transudation of plasma or blood from the choriocapillaris through a perforation in Bruch's membrane which, with reactive tissue formation, is organized into a fibroplastic mass. Syn., *senile macular exudative choroiditis; Kuhnt-Junius disease; disciform retinitis; exudative senile macular retinitis; central disk-shaped retinopathy.*

granular d. of the cornea. Granular corneal dystrophy.

Haab's d. 1. Latticelike corneal dystrophy. 2. Senile macular degeneration of Haab. 3. Traumatic macular degeneration of Haab.

helicoid peripapillary chorioretinal d. Hereditary optic atrophy occurring in either a congenital or an adult form and characterized by a peripapillary chorioretinal atrophy with winglike radial extensions that have no relation to, or involvement of, the retinal vessels. So called by its ophthalmoscopic picture resembling an aeroplane propeller (helix). Syn., *choroiditis aerata; circumpapillary dysgenesis of the pigment epithelium; chorioretinitis striata.*

hepatolenticular d. Wilson's disease.

hyaloideoretinal d. Vitreoretinal degeneration.

lattice d. of the cornea. Lattice-like corneal dystrophy.

lattice d. of the retina. A thinning of the retina, at or anterior to the equator, resulting in a sharply demarcated circumferentially oriented lesion characterized by an arborizing network of fine white lines with some pigmentation. Usually it is bilateral, occurs in the superior temporal quadrant, and may progress to the formation of round holes and tears along the posterior margin of the lesion and to retinal detachment.

Leber's retinal d. A disease of the retina characterized by numerous sharply defined microaneurysms in a slightly elevated area of the fundus, considered to be an early stage of Coats's disease. Syn., *Leber's disease.*

lenticular progressive d. Wilson's disease.

macular congenital d. A bilateral congenital degeneration of the macula unaccompanied by other degenerative changes. Syn., *Best's disease.*

marginal d. of the cornea. Peripheral corneal ectasia.

microfibrillar d. of the vitreous. Nodular interlacing filaments in front of fibrillar diaphanous membranes visible with the slit lamp in myopic or senile degeneration of the vitreous.

myopic choroidal d. Posterior polar degeneration of the choroid occurring with malignant myopia.

palisade d. of the retina. Latticelike corneal dystrophy.

paravenous retinal d. Pigmented paravenous retinochoroidal atrophy.

paving-stone d. of the retina. A thinning and depigmentation of the retina typically located between the ora serrata and the equator and characterized by small, discrete, yellow-white areas which may have pigmented borders and may coalesce to form band-shaped lesions. It is of unknown etiology and may lead to detachment of the retina. Syn., *peripheral chorioretinal atrophy; equatorial choroiditis; cobblestone degeneration of the retina; punched-out chorioretinal degeneration.*

polymorphous d. of the cornea, deep. Hereditary deep corneal dystrophy.

punched-out chorioretinal d. Paving-stone degeneration of the retina.

reticular d. of the cornea. Latticelike corneal dystrophy.

Salzmann's nodular d. Salzmann's corneal dystrophy.

senile macular d. of Haab. Macular degeneration in the aged characterized by fine pigmentary stippling which becomes denser as the disease progresses. It is attributed to arteriosclerosis of the choriocapillaris. Beginning unilaterally, it almost invariably becomes bilateral.

snail-track d. of the retina. Sharply demarcated bands of white, crinkled, or frost-like lesions of the retina localized in the equatorial region, often associated with vitreous degeneration and high myopia.

Sorsby's inflammatory d. of the macula. A dominant hereditary bilateral degeneration of the macula characterized initially by edema, hemorrhages, and exudates which progress to pigmented scar formation. In the later stages the peripheral choroidal vessels become exposed and sclerosed and eventually atrophy, leaving an exposed pigmented sclera. Typically, onset is at about age 40 with progression spreading over a 30-year period.

Stargardt's macular d. Stargardt's disease.

tapetoretinal d. A primary degeneration of the pigment epithelium layer of the retina, as occurs in retinitis pigmentosa, retinitis punctata albescens, etc.

traumatic macular d. of Haab. Degeneration of the macula following severe concussion or electric shock, characterized by pigmentary changes ranging from fine stippling to dense mottling or a heavily pigmented ring. Initially, the central area appears redder than normal, and small hemorrhages may be present. Syn., *traumatic macular atrophy; central traumatic retinitis.*

vitelline macular d. A hereditary macular degeneration occurring congenitally or in early life and characterized by reddish-orange lesions having the appearance of egg yolk.

vitreoretinal d. A rare familial condition characterized by a clear vitreous, except for preretinal filaments and veils which have been loosened from the retina, a dense hyaloid membrane which is perforated and detached, and masses of peripheral retinal pigmentation interspersed with areas of depigmentation. The visual fields are restricted, and detachment of the retina, cataract, optic atrophy, glaucoma, and atrophy of the iris, retina, and choroid are common complications. Syn., *hyaloideoretinal degeneration; Wagner's disease.*

Vogt's mosaic d. A rare degeneration of the cornea characterized by a central, thin, disklike opacity traversed by a mosaic of dark streaks and having the appearance of crocodile skin. It occurs in either of two forms, one affecting Bowman's membrane, the other Descemet's membrane.

◆

degrees of fusion. See under *fusion*.

de Haan. See *Haan*.

de Hertogh. See *Hertogh*.

dehiscence, retinal (de-his'ens). A tearing of the retina from its attachment at the ora serrata. Syn., *dialysis retinae; retinal disinsertion; retinodialysis*.

Déjerine-Klumpke syndrome (deh"-zher-ēn' klump'ke). Lower radicular syndrome. See under *syndrome*.

Déjerine-Sottas disease (deh"zher-ēn'sot'tahz). Hypertrophic neuritis. See under *neuritis*.

Delaborne prism (del'ah-bōrn). Dove prism. See under *prism*.

Delacato Stereo-Reader (del-ah-kat'o). See under *Stereo-Reader*.

delacrimation (de"lak-re-ma'shun). An abnormally excessive flow of tears.

Delboeuf (del-buf') **disk; visual illusion.** See under the nouns.

Della Casa adaptometer. See under *adaptometer*.

dellen (del'en). Transient ellipsoid depressions, hence "dells," in the cornea close to the limbus, most often temporally; about 1.5 x 2.0 mm in size with their longest axes parallel to the limbus and sharply delimited, each with a steep wall on the corneal apex side and a flatter, slanting border on the limbus side, occurring most frequently within one or two weeks subsequent to strabismus surgery but also following swelling of the limbus (in episcleritis, angioma, etc.), after cataract surgery, cocaine administration, paralytic lagophthalmus, and in the elderly. Syn., *Fuchs' dimples*.

delos (de'los). The ratio of the greatest distance at which an object of given dimension can be discerned for a given value of field luminance to the greatest distance at which the same object can be discerned under best field luminance conditions. (P. Moon and D. E. Spencer)

delta (δ, Δ)(del'tah). The Greek letter used as a symbol for (1) *delta movement* (δ); (2) *prism diopter* (Δ); (3) a small increment (Δ); (4) the inverted delta (∇) is used to represent *centrad;* (5) *angle of declination* (δ).

delta-filcon A. The nonproprietary name of a hydrophilic material of which contact lenses are made.

demecarium (dem"e-ka're-um). A very potent, topically applied, anticholinesterase drug used for prolonged effect in the treatment of open angle glaucoma; the generic name for *Humorsol*.

demonstrator, halo. A light diffusing device held before the eye for looking at a bright light to simulate and demonstrate the halo seen in glaucoma.

Demours membrane (da-mūrz'). Descemet's membrane.

deneutralization (de-nu"tral-ih-za'-shun). A procedure for treatment of suppression and/or amblyopia, usually consisting of stimulation of the suppressing eye with strong light or a bright target, to induce simultaneous perception. See also *neutralization*.

Dennett's (den'its) **chart; method.** See under the nouns.

densitometer (den"sih-tom'eh-ter). An instrument for measuring optical density.

densitometry, retinal (den"sih-tom'eh-tre). A technique for studying visual pigments in the living eye consisting of measuring with a detector the fraction of light from a beam of monochromatic light shone into the eye and reflected by the epithelium posterior to the retina before and after bleaching the pigments with a bright source.

density. 1. The state or quality of being dense as opposed to rarity. 2. Quantity per unit area or volume. 3. The measure of the degree of opaqueness. 4. The measure of the degree of retardation of the speed of transmission.

luminous d. The quantity of light per unit volume, expressed in lumen-hours per cubic centimeter of the radiating substance.

luminous flux d. Luminous flux emitted or incident per unit area of surface. Cf. *luminous emittance* and *illumination*.

optical d. 1. The property possessed by bodies or by substances of resisting the speed of light. When compared to that of air or vacuum as a standard, it is termed the *index of refraction*. 2. The light-absorbing property of a translucent medium, usually expressed as the logarithm of the reciprocal of transmittance. Syn., *absorbance*.

photographic film d. The logarithm of the ratio of incident to transmitted light. Cf. *opacity.*

radiant d. Radiant energy per unit volume, expressed in ergs per cubic centimeter of the radiating substance.

radiant flux d. Radiant flux emitted or incident on a surface, expressed in watts per unit area. Cf. *radiant emittance* and *irradiance.*

reflection d. The logarithm to base ten of the reciprocal of the reflectance.

deorsumduction (de-ōr″sum-duk′-shun). Infraduction.

deorsumvergence (de-ōr″sum-ver′-jens). Infravergence.

deorsumversion (de-ōr″sum-ver′zhun). Infraversion.

deplumation (de″plu-ma′shun). Loss of the eyelashes. *Obs.*

depolarization (de-po″lar-ih-za′shun). The process or act of depolarizing.

depolarize (de-po′lar-īz″). 1. To deprive of polarity; to reduce to an unpolarized condition. 2. Occasionally, to change the direction of the polarization of light.

depolarizer (de-po′lar-i″zer). A reflecting or transmitting medium which depolarizes.

deposits, mutton-fat. Small masses of exudate which adhere to the posterior surface of the cornea, consisting of mononuclear leucocytes, fibrin, and serum, often found in iridocyclitis, especially of the tubercular types. Syn., *mutton-fat keratic precipitates.*

depression. Downward rotation of the line of sight.

depressor. A muscle which depresses; most frequently, the inferior rectus muscle; less frequently, the superior oblique muscle.

d. oculi. 1. Inferior rectus muscle. 2. The superior oblique muscle when used synergistically with the inferior rectus.

deprimens oculi (dep′re-menz ok′ule). Inferior rectus muscle.

depth. 1. The perceived or actual, relative or absolute, difference in the distance of points in the visual field. 2. An attribute of color associated with increased saturation and decreased brightness.

d. criteria. The visual clues by which an individual determines the relative or absolute difference in the distance of points in the visual field.

They may be monocular, such as motion parallax, geometrical perspective, or binocular, such as convergence and stereopsis.

d. of field. The variation in the object distance of a lens or an optical system which can be tolerated without incurring an objectionable lack of sharpness in focus. The greatest distance through which an object point can be moved and still produce a satisfactory image.

d. of focus. The variation in image distance of a lens or of an optical system which can be tolerated without incurring an objectionable lack of sharpness in focus. Without objectionable blurring of the image, it is the greatest distance through which the image can be moved with relation to the image screen or receptoral surface, or the greatest distance through which the image screen or receptoral surface can be moved.

d. perception. See under *perception.*

sagittal d. The height or depth of a segment of a circle or a sphere; on an arc, AB, it is the perpendicular distance from the center of the chord, AB, to the arc. Thus, in the case of a planoconvex lens, the sagittal depth of the curved surface is the same as the center thickness of the lens, if the lens is ground to a knife edge. Syn., *sagitta.*

vertex d. The distance between the posterior pole (apex of the posterior concavity) of an ophthalmic lens and the plane containing the posterior edge of the lens.

depthoscope (dep′tho-skōp). An instrument for testing or training depth perception, consisting essentially of a rectangular, interiorly illuminated box, about one half meter in length, containing movable targets. The subject views from one end of the box and adjusts the targets until they appear equidistant.

Derby's stereoscope (der′bēz). See under *stereoscope.*

deresolution (de″rez-o-lu′shun). The process, or the result of, deresolving.

deresolve (de-re-solv′). To modify an image so as to make it more difficult to resolve.

dermatitis herpetiformis (der″mah-ti′tis her-pet″e-fōrm′is). A recurring, inflammatory disease of the skin of unknown etiology, characterized by erythematous, papular, pustular, or vesicular lesions which tend to group and are accompanied by itching and burning. The conjunctiva is frequently affected with vesicles, erosions, pseudomembranous formations, xerosis, and keratinization which may lead to symblepharon and result in exposure keratitis. Syn., *Duhring's disease.*

dermatitis, spectacle (der″mah-ti′tis). A contact dermatitis due to sensitivity to the metal or the plastic materials in a spectacle frame or mounting.

dermatoconjunctivitis (der″mah-to-kon-junk″tih-vi′tis). Inflammation of the skin and the palpebral conjunctiva near the eyelid margins.

    allergic d. Inflammation of the conjunctiva and eczema of the eyelids due to an allergic reaction to local contact with such agents as drugs, cosmetics, or chemicals. The allergic response is delayed, occurring 24 to 48 hours after contact.

dermato-ophthalmitis (der″mah-to-of″thal-mi′tis). Inflammation of the skin of the margin of the eyelid and of the cornea, the conjunctiva, or other anterior portions of the eye.

dermatopsia (der″mah-top′se-ah). Sensitivity to light in cells in the outer layer of some lower animals and subserving phototropic responses.

dermochalasis (der″mo-kal′ah-sis). Epiblepharon.

dermoid (der′moid). 1. A benign mixed tumor, usually congenital, containing teeth, hairs, skin glands, fibrous tissue, and other skin elements, rarely found in the limbal region of the eye and orbit. Syn., *dermoid cyst.* 2. Resembling skin.

dermolipoma (der″mo-lip-o′mah). A congenital, benign tumor, occurring in and under the bulbar conjunctiva at the external canthus as a fatty herniation covered by thick epidermal epithelium which may contain hair.

Descartes' (da-karts′) **law; ovals; ray.** See under the nouns.

Descemet's membrane (des-eh-māz′). See under *membrane.*

descemetitis (des″eh-meh-ti′tis). An apparent or a pseudo-inflammation of Descemet's membrane.

descemetocele (des-eh-met′o-sēl). A forward bulging of Descemet's membrane through a weakened or an absent corneal stroma, as a result of trauma or a deep corneal ulcer. Syn., *keratocele.*

Desmarre's law (da-marz′). See under *law.*

desmosomes (dez′mo-sōmz). Attachment bodies between cells, such as in the corneal epithelium, which possibly allow tonofibrils to pass from cell to cell and which can degenerate to allow cells to migrate to cover a denuded area.

desumvergence (de″sum-ver′jens). Infravergence.

detachment of retina. See *retina, detached.*

detachment of vitreous. See *vitreous, detached.*

deturgescence, corneal (de″ter-jes′ens). The state of relative dehydration maintained by the normal intact cornea which enables it to remain transparent.

deutan (du-tan′). One having deuteranomaly or deuteranopia; a deuteranomal or a deuteranope. Syn., *deuteranoid.*

deutanolabe (du′tan-o-lāb). A presumed anomalous pigment in the green cones of deuteranomals similar to normal chlorolabe but with the peak of its sensitivity curve shifted toward that of erythrolabe.

deuteranoid (du′ter-an-oid″). 1. One having deuteranomaly or deuteranopia; a deuteranomal or a deuteranope. Syn., *deutan.* 2. Of, pertaining to, or having the characteristics of deuteranopia or deuteranomaly.

deuteranomal (du″ter-an′o-mal). One having deuteranomaly.

deuteranomalopia (du″ter-ah-nom″ah-lo′pe-ah). Deuteranomaly.

deuteranomaly (du″ter-ah-nom′ah-le). A form of anomalous trichromatism in which an abnormally large proportion of green is required in a mixture of red and green light to match a given yellow. In the green to red region of the spectrum, hue discrimination is poor, and colors appear relatively more desaturated to the deuteranomal than they do to the normal trichromat, leading to confusion of light tints or of very dark shades of these colors. The degree of the defect covers a range from nearly normal to nearly deuteranopic. A sex-linked hereditary defect, it is the most common of all color vision deficiencies, occurring in about 5% of all males and 0.25% of all females. Syn., *deuteranomalopia; partial deuteranopia; deuteranomalous trichromatism; deuteranomalous vision; green-weakness.*

deuteranope (du′ter-an-ōp″). One having deuteranopia; a green-blind dichromat.

deuteranopia (du"ter-ah-no'pe-ah). A form of dichromatism in which relative spectral luminosity does not differ noticeably from normal, but in which all colors can be matched by mixtures of only two primary colors, one from the long wavelength portion of the spectrum (yellow, orange, or red), the other from the short wavelength portion (blue or violet). A neutral point (colorless or white) occurs at a wavelength of about 497 mμ, and it is in this region that hue discrimination is best. Light of shorter wavelengths appears blue; of longer wavelengths, yellow, with saturation increasing toward the ends of the spectrum. Thus, red, orange, yellow, and green cannot be differentiated when their brightness and saturations are made equal. Similarly, blue, violet, and blue-purple differ only in brightness and saturation, but not in hue. It is a sex-linked hereditary defect and occurs in about 1% of all males and only rarely in females. Syn., *green blindness; deuteranopic vision.*

anomalous d. A form of defective red-green color vision, with essentially normal relative spectral luminosity, in which the range of mixtures of red and green to match a given yellow, although principally of the deuteranomalous variety (requiring abnormally large proportions of green), is very much greater than the range of acceptable mixtures in deuteranomaly, yet not so great as the range in deuteranopia. A pure red (and, less frequently, a pure green) cannot be matched to yellow, and the normal observer's match (which is acceptable in deuteranopia) may be rejected. Disputed as representing a distinct type of defective color vision, it is also referred to as *deviant deuteranopia, incomplete deuteranopia,* or *extreme deuteranomaly.*

partial d. Deuteranomaly.

deuteranopic (du"ter-ah-nop'ik). Pertaining to or having deuteranopia.

◆

DEVIATION

deviation. 1. A departure from an expected or a normal course of behavior. 2. A turning without change of vergence of a beam of light by an optical device or an optical system. In this sense, the concept of "deviation of light" is often used to account for a lateral difference in position between a real object and its virtual image as seen in an optical system. 3. A movement of one or both eyes, singly or jointly, from the median line, or from the original direction of fixation. 4. In strabismus, the departure of the foveal line of sight of one eye from the point of fixation. 5. In diplopia, the apparent difference in the position of the two images. 6. The departure of a value from a given point of reference.

basic d. The fusion-free position of the eyes present in the straightforward position, with fixation at infinity and with natural or artificial emmetropia, i.e., accommodation at the zero level.

concomitant d. A strabismic deviation which is approximately constant for all directions of gaze; a characteristic of nonparalytic strabismus. The separation of double images resulting from such a deviation will remain relatively constant regardless of the direction of fixation.

conjugate d. The joint and approximately equal excursions of the two eyes, usually found as a physiological movement in certain conjugate palsies, in which there is inability to fixate objects in certain portions of the visual field. The term has been subdivided by certain writers into *parallel conjugate deviation, convergent deviation,* and *divergent deviation,* q.v. **parallel c.d.** The type of conjugate deviation in which both eyes move in equal amounts and in the same direction, found in the physiological form only when the gaze is shifted from one object to another equidistant object, or when the gaze pursues an object which moves at a constant distance. It is found in the pathological form when both eyes fail, in equal amounts and in the same direction, to fixate the object of regard. The gaze is often retained on the object by a compensating rotation or tilt of the head.

convergent d. 1. That type of conjugate deviation in which both eyes move nasally in equal amounts, demonstrated in the physiological form when the gaze is shifted from a distant to a near object on the median line. 2. Esotropia. 3. A nasalward turning of the occluded eye in the cover test.

divergent d. 1. That type of conjugate deviation in which both eyes move temporally in equal amounts, found in the physiological form when the gaze is shifted from an object on the median line to a farther object on the same line. 2. Exotropia. 3. A temporalward turning of the occluded eye in the cover test.

Hering-Hillebrand d. The deviation of the equidistant line of the horopter (often called the *frontoparallel plane*) from the Vieth-Mueller circle.

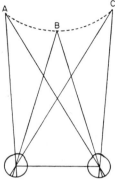

Fig. 8 Hering-Hillebrand deviation. Fixation point B beyond two meters. (From H. W. Gibson, *Textbook of Orthoptics*. Kent, England: Hatton Press, 1955)

latent d. 1. The deviation of an eye during occlusion, as in a cover test in a case of heterophoria. 2. The potential deviation in heterophoria or in intermittent or periodic strabismus.

lateral d. An inclusive term denoting either convergent deviation or divergent deviation of the occluded eye in the cover test or in strabismus.

manifest d. A deviation actually present and observable, as in strabismus.

minimum d. The least change of direction of a bundle of light rays from its original path by a prism. This condition occurs when the angle of incidence is equal to the angle of emergence. See also *angle of minimum deviation*.

nonconcomitant d. A strabismic deviation which varies with the direction of gaze; a characteristic of paralytic strabismus. The separation of double images resulting from such a deviation will vary with the direction of fixation.

nonparalytic d. A concomitant deviation not attributable to paralysis or paresis of the extaocular muscles.

paralytic d. A nonconcomitant deviation attributable to paralysis or paresis of one or more of the extraocular muscles.

primary d. The deviation, in strabismus, of the nonfixating eye from the point of fixation when the normally fixating eye fixates.

secondary d. The deviation, in strabismus, of the normally fixating eye from the point of fixation when the normally deviating eye is made to fixate.

skew d. A spasmodic, disjunctive, binocular deviation in which the eyes move in equal amounts in opposite directions, usually vertically. See also *Magendie-Hertwig sign*.

strabismic d. The deviation of the nonfixating eye from the point of fixation in strabismus.

vertical d. 1. That type of conjugate deviation in which both eyes move vertically in equal amounts, found in the physiological form when the gaze is shifted from an object on the median line to another object above or below it. 2. The type of deviation found in strabismus in which the deviating eye is turned upward or downward with respect to the fixating eye. 3. An upward or a downward turning of the occluded eye in the cover test. **dissociated v.d.** Double hyperphoria.

◆

Devic's disease (dev′iks). Neuromyelitis optica.

device, Berson. An image-intensifying, night vision instrument adapted for use by persons with night blindness.

device, R-C. A lens system which is attached to the lens stop of a lensometer for the measurement of the base curve of a contact lens. It consists essentially of a standard lens of known curvature and thickness, and of an index of refraction equal to that of the contact lens to be measured. The contact lens is held to the standard lens by the surface tension of a thin film of fluid the index of refraction of which is the same as that of both lenses, thus neutralizing the refractive power of the front surface of the contact lens. Through provided tables, the reading of the lensometer and the thickness of the contact lens will indicate the radius of curvature of the base curve.

devioception (de′ve-o-sep″shun). Proprioception said to be derived from the deviating eye in strabismus.

deviograph, Aves's (de've-o-graf"). An instrument designed to permit the strabismic patient to record the apparent position of an object, presented in front of one eye, by a stylus seen only with the other eye. It consists of a chart holder set at 33 cm from the patient's eyes, a target of 8 circles set in a rectangle calculated to include an area of the visual field subtending an angle of 20° laterally and 16° vertically, and the necessary chin and head rests, lens wells, and septum.

deviometer (de"ve-om'eh-ter). A device for measuring ocular deviation in strabismus.

Owen's d. A deviometer consisting essentially of a chin and head rest, a movable target, a prism bar, and an occluder.

Smukler's d. An instrument of hard plastic material shaped to the contours of the lower orbital region of the face and on which two slender vertical bars are laterally adjustable on a millimeter scale to be aligned sequentially with either the internal or external limbus of the deviating eye, first while it is deviating and then while it is fixating a distant object monocularly. Each millimeter represents 4.5° of strabismus.

Worth's d. A deviometer consisting of a series of fixation points on a graduated horizontal scale, to be fixated by one eye, and a fixed source of light over which the corneal reflex of the deviating eye is observed. The fixating eye is made to fixate successive points on the scale until the corneal reflex on the deviating eye is centered.

dextroclination (deks"tro-klin-a'shun). Rotation of the top of the vertical meridian of an eye toward the right; intorsion of the left eye or extorsion of the right eye. Syn., *dextrocycloduction; dextrotorsion.*

dextrocular (deks-trok'u-lar). Pertaining to the right eye, or to the condition of dextrocularity.

dextrocularity (deks"trok-u-lar'ih-te). A condition in which better vision exists in the right eye, or in which the right eye is dominant.

dextrocycloduction (deks"tro-si"klo-duk'shun). Dextroclination.

dextrocycloversion (deks"tro-si"klo-ver'zhun). Rotation of the top of the vertical meridians of both eyes toward the subject's right. Syn., *positive cycloversion.*

dextroduction (deks"tro-duk'shun). Rotation of an eye toward the right.

dextrogyration (deks"tro-ji-ra'shun). A turning to the right; motion, especially rotatory, to the right; said of eye movements and of the plane of polarization.

dextrophoria (deks"tro-fo're-ah). A phoria in which the nonfixating eye turns toward the right.

dextrorotatory (deks"tro-ro'tah-to"re). 1. Turning of the plane of polarization toward the observer's right (looking against the oncoming light). 2. Bending rays of light toward the right. 3. Pertaining to dextroclination.

dextrotorsion (deks"tro-tor'shun). Dextroclination.

dextroversion (deks"tro-ver'zhun). Conjugate rotation of both lines of sight to the right.

DFP. An abbreviation for the organic phosphate, di-isopropyl fluorophosphate, a powerful inhibitor of cholinesterase which in solution produces marked and prolonged miosis. It is used in the treatment of glaucoma and esotropia.

DGF. Discomfort glare factor.

DGR. Discomfort glare rating.

diacaustic (di"ah-kaws'tik). Denoting or pertaining to the *caustic curve* formed by refracted rays, as opposed to *catacaustic*, which denotes the caustic curve caused by reflected rays.

diactinic (di"ak-tin'ik). Having the property of transmitting actinic rays.

diagnosis. 1. The art or act of determining or distinguishing a disease. 2. In refraction, the determination of the refractive, muscular, or functional origin of the sources of visual discomfort or difficulty.

diagnostic chain. See under *chain.*

diagram. A chart or a graphic drawing demonstrating relative values, distributions, or relation of parts to the whole.

Adams' chromatic value d. A nonlinear transformation of the CIE chromaticity diagram designed by Adams to provide greater uniformity in spacing of colors in relation to their perceived differences.

chromaticity d. A plane diagram, usually triangular, formed by plotting one of the three trichromatic coefficients against another, thus constituting a graphical representation of stimulus characteristics derived from *diagram* [170] *diastereotest*

color-mixture data. The colorimetric primaries are represented at the corners, and all other combinations of dominant wavelength and colorimetric purity are represented by points within the diagram. The most commonly used diagram at present, the CIE (x, y) diagram is essentially a right triangle plotted in rectangular co-ordinates (actually, a projection onto the x, y plane of an equilateral triangle whose corners lie on the $x, y,$ and z axes of a three-dimensional co-ordinate system), representing hypothetical primaries and the entire chromaticity gamut of the CIE standard observer. Another well known diagram is the Maxwell color triangle, plotted with oblique co-ordinates, having real primaries represented at the corners, thereby excluding portions of the chromaticity gamut for the normal observer. Syn., *color chart; color diagram; color table.*

color d. Chromaticity diagram.

Hering valence d. Hering's color valence curves.

isocandela d. A coordinate plot of one or more isocandela lines representing the locus or loci of directions in space around a source of light for which the candlepower is of a given value or of a series of given values.

isofootcandle d. Isolux diagram.

isolux d. A series of lines for various illumination values plotted on any appropriate coordinates, each representing the locus of points on a surface for which illumination is of equal value. Syn., *isofootcandle diagram.*

Rousseau d. Rousseau construction.

Tschermak's d. A modification of Hering's color valence curves in which the individual curves have bell-shaped forms. It includes photopic and scotopic white valence (luminosity) curves in addition to the valence curves for red and green, blue and yellow.

dial, astigmatic. A chart or a pattern used for determining the presence or the amount and meridional orientation of astigmatism.

dial, fan. See *chart, fan dial.*

dial, sunburst. See *chart, fan dial.*

dialysis retinae (di-al'ih-sis ret'ih-ne). A tearing of the retina from its attachment at the ora serrata and the optic disk. Syn., *retinal dehiscence; retinal disinsertion; retinodialysis.*

diameter, disk. See under *disk.*

diameter, optical. The diameter of the optical zone of a contact lens.

Diamox (di'ah-moks). A trade name for acetazolamide.

diaphanometer (di"af-ah-nom'eh-ter). An instrument for measuring the transparency of substances such as gases or liquids.

diaphanoscope (di-af'ah-no-skōp, di"ah-fan'o-). An instrument for viewing a body cavity or tissue by transillumination.

diaphanoscopy (di"af-ah-nos'ko-pe). Examination with a diaphanoscope.

diaphragm (di'ah-fram). 1. A dividing membrane, a thin partition, or a septum. 2. A perforated plate or screen serving to limit the aperture or field of view of a lens or optical system; a stop.

condensing d. A diaphragm with an aperture containing lenses for the purpose of rendering the emergent light rays parallel or, in some cases, convergent.

iris d. A diaphragm with a central aperture of variable diameter, usually controlled by an annular arrangement of thin, movable plates or leaves whose medial edges intersect to approximate a circle.

lacrimal d. The posterior portion of the medial palpebral ligament and the lateral lacrimal fascia which act together to facilitate tear drainage in the lacrimal apparatus.

diaphragma sellae (di-ah-frag'mah sel'i). A circular layer of dura mater which forms the roof of the fossa for the pituitary body and is pierced by the stalk of the pituitary gland. Its posterior part usually lies below the optic chiasm.

diascope (di'ah-skōp). 1. (med.) A glass plate held against the skin through which one can observe changes in the underlying tissue. 2. Any device which provides or permits a transilluminated, transparent, or skiagraphic view of an object.

diasporometer (di"ah-spo-rom'eh-ter). 1. An instrument for measuring light scattering or dispersion. 2. A rotary prism, especially when used in a range-finder to measure angular deviation of images from coincidence.

diastereotest (di"ah-ster'e-o"-test). A hand-held test, ordinarily a modified flashlight, for determining the presence or absence of stereopsis in which the subject is asked to identify the nearest of three identical opaque disks, one of which is mounted slightly forward from a transilluminated diffusing surface, while the other two are directly in contact with the surface. Stereopsis threshold determinations may also be made with the same instrument by varying the test distance.

DIC. Direct illumination component.

dichoptic (di-kop'tik). 1. Having paired compound eyes, the borders of which are separated from each other. Cf. *holoptic.* 2. With each of a pair of eyes having a separate and independent view.

dichroic (di-kro'ik). Exhibiting, or pertaining to, dichroism.

dichroism (di'kro-izm). 1. The property of producing two different colors; associated with different directions of transmission of light, different directions of viewing, different thicknesses or concentrations of the transmitting substance, differences between color of transmitted and reflected light, etc. 2. The property of unequal absorption of the ordinary and extraordinary rays by certain doubly refracting substances.

circular d. The unequal absorption of two circularly polarized waves. Syn., *Cotton effect.*

linear d. The property of unequal absorption of two linearly polarized beams by certain doubly refracting substances.

dichromasia (di"kro-ma'zhuh, -ze-ah). Dichromatism.

dichromasy (di-kro'mah-se). Dichromatism.

dichromat (di'kro-mat). One having dichromatism; a protanope, a deuteranope, a tritanope, or a tetartanope.

dichromatic (di"kro-mat'ik). Pertaining to or having dichromatism.

dichromatism (di-kro'mah-tizm). 1. A form of defective color vision requiring only two primary colors, mixed in various proportions, to match all other colors. The spectrum is seen as comprised of only two regions of different hue separated by an achromatic band. Dichromatism may occur as *protanopia, deuteranopia, tritanopia,* or some irregular form such as *tetartanopia.* Syn., *partial color blindness; dichromasia; dichromasy; dichromatopsia; dichromatic vision.* 2. Dichroism.

anomalous d. Color vision deficiency approaching dichromatism, although all colors cannot be matched by mixtures of only two primary colors.

Since three primaries are required to match some colors, the condition is actually an extreme form of anomalous trichromatism, although hue discrimination is generally so poor that the condition more closely resembles dichromatism. See also *anomalous deuteranopia.*

dichromatopsia (di-kro"mah-top'se-ah). Dichromatism.

dicoria (di-ko're-ah). Two pupils in one eye. Syn., *diplocoria.*

dictyoma (dik"te-o'mah). Diktyoma.

Dieffenbach's theory (de'fen-bahks). See under *theory.*

Dietzel-Roelofs phenomenon. See under *phenomenon.*

difference. 1. The measure, state, or quality of being dissimilar or unlike. 2. That by which one thing is distinguished from another; a distinction.

just noticeable d. The smallest difference between two stimuli that, for a given individual, gives rise to a perceived difference in sensation. Abbreviation *jnd.* Syn., *differential limen; differential threshold.*

lens size d. The vertical subtracted from the horizontal dimension of a rectangle the sides of which are tangent to the apex of the bevel at the top, bottom, and sides of a spectacle lens.

light d. Brightness difference threshold.

d. in magnification, chromatic. The size difference of images formed by two different wavelengths of light in a system with chromatic aberration.

path d. The difference in length of the paths of light rays in passing through different parts of an optical system, as the difference in length of the paths of light rays in passing through the margin and the center of a lens.

phase d. The difference in the position and character of the wave of an oscillatory motion at two instances. In a wave motion, when two points on the wave have the same displacement and direction, they are said to be in phase. In a representation of the wave as a sine function, the wave repeats itself every 2 pi radians (360°); thus, any two points 360° apart will be in phase.

difficulty, dissociation. Crowding phenomenon.

difficulty, separation. Crowding phenomenon.

diffraction (dih-frak'shun). The tendency of light to deviate from a straight line path in an isotropic medium. In complete wavefronts, this tendency is canceled through mutual effects of the neighboring points on the wavefront. At the edge of a wavefront, as when a wavefront passes by an edge or through a slit, the canceling effects are eliminated on one side and the wavefront at that point bends in the direction of the removed portion of the wavefront.

   d. figure. Diffraction pattern.

   Fraunhofer d. Fraunhofer's diffraction phenomenon.

   Fresnel d. Fresnel's diffraction phenomenon.

   d. grating. See under *grating.*

   d. pattern. See under *pattern.*

   Poisson d. Diffraction of light by a circular or spherical obstacle in the path of a light source, producing a bright spot in the center of the shadow having the same intensity as if no obstacle were present.

diffrangible (dih-fran'jih-bl). Capable of being diffracted.

diffuser, cosine (dih-fūz'er). A diffusely reflecting surface or transmitting layer which reflects or transmits in accordance with Lambert's cosine law. Syn., *lambertian diffuser; lambertian surface.*

diffuser, lambertian (dih-fūz'er). Cosine diffuser.

diffusion (dih-fu'zhun). 1. The scattering of light in passing through a heterogeneous medium by a series of reflections. 2. The scattering of light by irregular reflection at a surface.

   d. circle. Blur circle.

   d. image. See under *image.*

   perfect d. The distribution of emitted or reflected light in accordance with Lambert's cosine law.

Dighton-Adair syndrome (di'tun-ah-dār'). Van der Hoeve's syndrome.

diktyoma (dik"te-o'mah). An epithelial tumor of the pars ciliaris retinae which has the structure of an embryonic retina. It usually occurs in the young, developing slowly as a white flat lesion from the ciliary body and growing over the iris, the anterior surface of the crystalline lens, and the posterior surface of the cornea.

dilator iridis (di-la'tor ir'id-is). The dilator pupillae muscle.

dilator pupillae (di-la'tor pu'pih-le). The dilator pupillae muscle.

dim. Having relatively low brightness; the opposite of *bright.*

dimefilcon. The nonproprietary name of a hydrophilic material of which contact lenses are made.

Dimitri's syndrome (dih-me'trēz). Sturge-Weber syndrome.

Dimmer's (dim'erz) **nummular keratitis; latticelike corneal dystrophy.** See under the nouns.

dimness. The state or quality of being dim; the subjective attribute of any light sensation giving rise to the percept of relatively low luminous intensity. Cf. *brightness.*

dimples, corneal. Fuchs' dimples.

dimples, Fuchs'. Transient, superficial, dimplelike excavations on the cornea near the limbus, occurring as a senile change or due to interference with, or obliteration of, limbal vessels as may follow episcleral inflammation or cataract surgery. Syn., *dellen.*

dimpling. A cluster of small, round, discrete, concave depressions on the surface of the cornea, filled with air bubbles, sometimes found in association with the wearing of a corneal contact lens. It is associated with regions of entrapped tear fluid or with air bubbles entering beneath the edge of a lens which flares away from the cornea during blink.

diode, light emitting. A crystal acting as having an anode and a cathode and serving as a light source when proper voltage is applied. Abbreviation *LED.*

dionin (di'o-nin). A derivative of morphine used in the eye as an analgesic in cases of iritis, iridocyclitis, or keratitis.

diopsimeter (di"op-sim'eh-ter). An instrument for measuring the extent of the visual field.

diopter (di-op'ter). 1. A unit proposed by Monoyer to designate the refractive power of a lens or an optical system, the number of diopters of power being equal to the reciprocal of the focal length in meters; thus, a 1 D lens has a focal length of 1 m. 2. A unit of curvature, the number of diopters of curvature being equal to the reciprocal of the radius of curvature in meters. 3. An archaic optical instrument for measuring altitude.

   prism d. A unit proposed by Prentice to specify the amount of deviation of light by an ophthalmic prism, the number of prism diopters being equal to 100 times the tangent of the angle of deviation. Thus, a prism of 1 prism diopter will deviate light 1 cm at a distance of 1 m. It is represented by the exponential symbol Δ. Syn., *tangent centune.* See also *Prentice's method.*

diopto-eikonometer (di"to-i'kon-om'eh-ter). An instrument designed to measure refractive power and magnification properties of ophthalmic lenses.

dioptometer (di"op-tom'eh-ter). An instrument used in the measurement of ocular refraction; an optometer.

dioptometry (di"op-tom'eh-tre). The measurement of ocular refraction by means of the dioptometer.

dioptoscopy (di"op-tos'ko-pe). Dioptroscopy.

dioptre (di-op'ter). Diopter.

dioptric (di-op'trik). 1. Of the nature of, or pertaining to, the diopter. 2. Pertaining to the refraction of light by transmission, as distinguished from *catoptric.*

dioptrics (di-op'triks). That branch of optics which deals with the refraction of light by transparent media.

dioptrometer (di"op-trom'eh-ter). Dioptometer.

dioptrometry (di"op-trom'eh-tre). Dioptometry.

dioptroscopy (di"op-tros'ko-pe). The measurement of the refraction of the eye by means of the ophthalmoscope.

dioptry (di-op'tre). Diopter.

dip. Abbreviation for *diplopia.*

diplegia, cerebral (di-ple'je-ah). Little's disease.

diplegia, congenital facial (di-ple'je-ah). Moebius' syndrome.

Dipl. Opt. Optical Diploma (Association of Opticians, Ireland).

diplocoria (dip"lo-ko're-ah). The condition of an iris having two pupils.

diplometer (dih-plom'eh-ter, dip"lo-me'ter). An instrument designed to measure the distance between the two images in diplopia.

diplomometer (dip"lo-mom'eh-ter). Diplometer.

◆

DIPLOPIA

diplopia (dip-lo'pe-ah). The condition in which a single object, or the haploscopically presented equivalent of a single object, is perceived as two objects rather than as one; double vision.

binocular d. Diplopia in which one image is seen by one eye and the other image is seen by the other eye.

crossed d. Heteronymous diplopia.

direct d. Homonymous diplopia.

distal d. Physiological diplopia for objects beyond the point of binocular fixation.

dynamic d. The movement of diplopic images toward or away from each other as binocular fixation varies from one distance to another.

heterolocal d. Heterotopic diplopia.

heteronymous d. Diplopia in which the image seen by the right eye is to the left of the image seen by the left eye. Syn., *crossed diplopia.*

heterotopic d. Diplopia in which one object (or point) is seen in two directions at once, hence in two places at once, as distinguished from *homotopic diplopia.* Syn., *heterolocal diplopia.*

homolocal d. Homotopic diplopia.

homonymous d. Diplopia in which the image seen by the right eye is to the right of the image seen by the left eye. Syn., *uncrossed diplopia.*

homotopic d. In binocular vision, the perceiving of two different objects (or points) in one direction, as if superimposed or coincident in one place in space, as distinguished from *heterotopic diplopia.* Syn., *homolocal diplopia.*

horizontal d. Diplopia in which the two images appear at the same level.

incongruous d. Diplopia in which the two images do not conform to the laws of projection, for example, an exotrope experiencing homonymous diplopia. Syn., *paradoxical diplopia.*

insuperable d. Intractable diplopia.

intractable d. Binocular diplopia that cannot be eliminated by optical superimposition of the two perceived images of a single object or by the suppression of one. Syn., *insuperable diplopia; horror fusionis.*

introspective d. Physiological diplopia.

maculomacular d. A term employed by Worth to represent a form of diplopia present in strabismus, in which the image of a nonfixated object is not on the macula of either eye, resulting in a rivalry between the two maculae for fixation.

maculopseudomacular d. A term employed by Worth to represent a form of diplopia present in strabismus, in which the image of the object of regard is on the macula of the fixating eye and on a nonmacular area of the deviating eye.

monocular d. Diplopia identified with one eye only. It may be induced with a double prism, or it may occur either as a result of double imagery due to an optical defect in the eye, or as a result of simultaneous use of normal and anomalous retinal correspondence.

paradoxical d. 1. A form of diplopia present in individuals with anomalous retinal correspondence in which diplopic images do not conform to the laws of projection of normal retinal correspondence; for example, an esotrope experiencing heteronymous diplopia. Syn., *incongruous diplopia.* 2. A form of diplopia sometimes found in paralysis of the vertical rectus muscles. The diplopia occurs in the area of the visual field where the action of the affected muscle is least, that is, opposite in direction to the main field of action of the muscle.

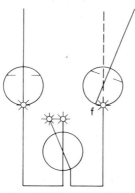

Fig. 9 Pathological diplopia with illustration of cyclopean projection. (From J. R. Griffin, *Binocular Anomalies.* Chicago: Professional Press, 1976)

pathological d. 1. Any diplopia resulting from a pathologic or anomalous condition of the visual mechanism, as in diplocoria, subluxation of the crystalline lens, or certain conditions of cataract. 2. Diplopia caused by the deviation of one eye in strabismus when the image of the fixated object falls on a nonmacular area of the deviating eye. Differentiated from *physiological diplopia.* (See Fig. 9.)

physiological d. Diplopia occurring in normal binocular vision for nonfixated objects whose images stimulate disparate points on the retinae outside of Panum's areas. (See Fig. 10.)

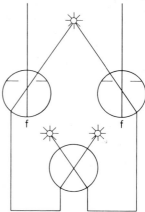

Fig. 10 Physiological diplopia with illustration of cyclopean projection. (From J. R. Griffin, *Binocular Anomalies.* Chicago: Professional Press, 1976)

postoperative d. Diplopia occurring as a postsurgical symptom, as that following an extraocular muscle operation for strabismus.

proximal d. Physiological diplopia for objects nearer than the point of binocular fixation.

stereoscopic d. Physiological diplopia.

temporal d. Homonymous diplopia.

uncrossed d. Homonymous diplopia.

vertical d. Diplopia in which the two images do not lie at the same elevation in the visual field.

◆

diplopiaphobia (dip-lo"pe-ah-fo'be-ah). An aversion to diplopia.

diplopiometer (dip"lo-pe-om'eh-ter). An instrument for measuring the distance between the two images in diplopia.

diploscope (dip'lo-skōp). Any of several instruments which test or train fusion or determine phorias and tropias.

Cantonnet's d. An instrument designed by Cantonnet for determining and measuring phorias or tropias. It consists of a tube fitted into the center of a plate perpendicular to the tube, a thin, transparent arrow indicator in the opening of the tube, two vertical slits in the plate, one on each side of the tube 60 mm from the arrow, and holes at 1 cm intervals lateral to each slit. The slits are marked zero and the holes are consecutively numbered. The instrument is used by placing the tube before one eye and directing it horizontally toward a light source. The hole to which the arrow appears to point indicates the type and approximate extent of the phoria or the tropia.

Rémy d. A diploscope consisting essentially of a bar with a target at one end which is viewed from the other end. Interposed between the target and the observer is a perforated screen through which letters on the target are seen.

direction. 1. The line or course in space in which an object is moving, aimed to move, or pointing. 2. The characteristic which differentiates two or more straight lines radiating from a common point.

absolute d. The direction of an object or an image with respect to a specified point of reference identified with the subject or subject's eye.

egocentric d. The perceived direction of an object or an image from a subjective point of reference thought of as the visual self; an absolute direction.

d. of gaze, cardinal. The direction of gaze in the major field of action of any of the six extraocular muscles. There are six commonly recognized cardinal directions; right, left, left superiorly, right superiorly, left inferiorly, and right inferiorly.

motor d. The direction of an object from an observer, determined by the innervation to the extraocular muscles in moving the eyes to assume fixation of the object.

objective d. The direction of an object in space in relation to an observer, as physically determined; to be distinguished from *subjective direction*.

oculocentric d. The direction associated with a particular retinal point or area. It is independent of eye position and always maintains a fixed relationship to other oculocentric directions in that eye. It is a relative direction which contributes to the absolute direction (egocentric direction).

homologous o.d.'s Directions from each eye as a center which are expressed as an angular measurement from the line of sight and which are identical for the two eyes. Thus, stimulation of corre-

sponding retinal (or cortical) points arouses a percept for each eye, the two percepts lying in homologous oculocentric directions.

principal vibration d. The direction of wave vibration of planepolarized light, as of either the ordinary or the extraordinary ray in double refraction.

relative d. The direction of an object or an image, or the direction associated with a retinal point or area, which is evaluated relative to the direction of another object, image, or retinal point or area. See also *oculocentric direction*.

subjective d. The absolute or relative direction of an object or an image as perceived in the visual space of a subject; to be distinguished from *objective direction*.

visual d. Relative direction in subjective visual space associated with a given retinal receptor element. The subjective correlate of the line of direction. See also *oculocentric direction*. **principal v.d.** The straight-ahead visual direction subjectively associated with the point of fixation, hence functionally associated with the center of the fovea, and serving as a direction of reference in relation to which all other visual directions are experienced.

directionality. The visual perceptual ability to project the internal awareness of the two sides of the body into extrapersonal space. Cf. *laterality*.

disability, reading. Reading retardation in which achievement is significantly below the normal expectancy for the mental age. Generally a one-year retardation is considered significant in the primary grades.

disaggregation (dis″ag-re-ga′shun). In hysteria, the inability to integrate or co-ordinate visual perception with other sensory perceptions.

disassociation of the eyes (dis″ah-so″se-a′shun). The suspension of fusion in binocular vision, as may be accomplished by elimination of fusion stimuli. Syn., *dissociation*.

disc. See *disk*.

discharge. 1. A secretion, usually morbid. 2. An electrical manifestation in nerve tissue, particularly the transient electrical potentials in the axon (nerve fiber). In vivo, this is originated by the nerve cell body in the form of a series or train of nerve impulses and conducted along the fiber. In laboratory experiments, the discharge is often recorded from a nerve trunk consisting of a bundle of nerve fibers.

ganglion cell d. The discharge of the ganglion cells which constitute the final layer of the retina and whose axons make up the fibers of the optic nerve. This output of nerve impulses has been studied to determine the possible reorganization and elaboration of the initial discharge pattern of the sense cells themselves.

maintained d. On response.

off d. Off response.

on d. On response.

on-off d. On-off response.

optic nerve d. The electrical activity recorded from the optic nerve. The record is a picture of the temporal pattern of the discharge of impulses in the many fibers of the optic nerve. It is thus an over-all record.

X-type d. On response.

Y-type d. On-off response.

Z-type d. Off response.

dischromatopsia (dis″kro-mah-top′se-ah). Dyschromatopsia.

dischromatopsy (dis-kro′mah-top″se). Dyschromatopsia.

discission (dih-sish′un, -sizh′un). A surgical procedure for either soft cataract, in which the lens capsule is punctured to allow absorption of the lens substance, or aftercataract, in which capsular remnants in the pupillary area are cut. Syn., *needling.*

disclination (dis″klin-a′shun). Extorsion.

discoria (dis-ko′re-ah). Dyscoria.

discrimination. 1. The aspect of sensory response in which one feature of the stimulus is compared to another, that is, one area may be perceived as equal to, greater than, or less than another in brightness, area, linear dimension, hue, saturation, or orientation. 2. The principle of a response bearing some quantitative or qualitative relation to the stimulus and, thus, becoming less or different as the stimulus is physically reduced or changed and becoming greater or different as the stimulus is increased or otherwise changed. 3. The actual process of discriminating as described in definitions 1 and 2.

brightness d. Discrimination of the achromatic quality of color, usually specified in terms of energy or photometric units producing just noticeable differences in brightness.

color d. Discrimination of any of the several attributes of color, such as hue, saturation, or brightness, or of any combination of attributes of color, such as may be represented by linear distances on a color diagram or in a color solid.

figure-ground d. The perceptual differentiation of figure and ground.

form d. Discrimination of differences of shape or pattern of a two-dimensional visual stimulus.

hue d. Discrimination of the hue attribute of color. It is often measured by the wavelength change producing a just noticeable difference and, in this case, is synonymous with wavelength discrimination.

saturation d. Discrimination of the saturation attribute of color, usually measured by the number of barely distinguishable steps observable for a given hue.

spatial d. Discrimination involving any of several spatial attributes, such as separation or resolution of two objects, direction, orientation, or geometric pattern.

two point d. The ability to experience two points as two. This term is applied most generally in cutaneous stimulation, but may refer also to two points of light. When either the contact or the visual stimuli are placed very close to each other, they tend to be experienced as a single area, rather than as two points.

utrocular d. The ability to judge which eye is perceiving.

visual d. The aspect of sensory response in which the stimulus features compared are perceived visually.

discus opticus (dis′kus op′tih-kus). Optic disk.

◆

DISEASE

disease. An alteration of the state of the body, or of any of its organs or parts, which interrupts or disturbs the performance of the vital functions or of the mind; a specific type of such alteration, especially one having particular causes or symptoms. For diseases not listed, see under *syndrome.*

Addison's d. A systemic disease, usually fatal, due to hypofunction of the cortical portion of the adrenal gland, characterized by bronzed pigmentation of the skin, general weakness, low blood pressure, severe anemia, and digestive disturbances. Eye symptoms include enophthalmos and bronzed pigmentation of the skin of the eyelids.

Aland d. Forsius-Eriksson syndrome.

Albers-Schönberg d. A rare anomaly of osteogenesis, of hereditary tendency, in which the bones become dense, sclerosed, and marblelike. It frequently affects the orbit and maxillary bone, resulting in progressive proptosis of the eyeball and optic atrophy. Syn., *osteopetrosis.*

Albright's d. Polyostotic fibrous dysplasia (q.v.) when associated with precocious puberty; primarily affecting girls.

Barlow's d. An acute systemic disease, often referred to as infantile scurvy, due to a deficiency of vitamin C and characterized by general weakness, spongy gums, a tendency to mucocutaneous hemorrhages, night blindness, and, rarely, retinal hemorrhages.

Basedow's d. Exophthalmic goiter.

Batten-Mayou d. The juvenile form of amaurotic family idiocy in which there is a widespread lipoid degeneration of the ganglion cells of the central nervous system and retina. It usually appears between the ages of 5 and 10, and defective vision is often the earliest symptom. This is followed by progressive mental deterioration, spasticity, epileptiform convulsions, disturbance of speech, blindness, and death between the ages of 14 and 18. The ophthalmoscopic picture varies, but characteristically the macula is pigmented, the optic disk is pale, the retinal vessels are narrowed, and in the later stages the peripheral retina is usually mottled with pigment. Syn., *neuronal ceroid lipofuscinosis; Spielmeyer-Stock disease; Vogt-Spielmeyer disease.*

Bayle's d. In the insane, progressive general paralysis, including ocular structures.

Bechterew's d. Ankylosing spondylitis.

Begbie's d. Exophthalmic goiter, together with localized hysterical choreaform muscular twitchings.

Behçet's d. Aphthous ulcers in the mouth and on the genitalia, lesions of the conjunctiva and cornea, and iridocyclitis with hypopyon, tending to recur at intervals of from 1 to 2 months, with blindness usually resulting after 15 to 20 years. It primarily affects males under the age of 40. Uveitis and optic atrophy may be accompanying complications. Syn., *hypopyon recidivans; iridocyclitis recidivans purulenta; iridocyclitis septica; ophthalmia lenta.*

Behr's d. Macular degeneration in the adult at about the age of 20, believed to be caused by a primary degeneration of the tapetoretinal type.

Benson's d. Asteroid hyalosis.

Berlin's d. Commotio retinae.

Besnier-Boeck d. Sarcoidosis.

Besnier-Boeck-Schaumann d. Sarcoidosis.

Best's d. Hereditary degeneration of the macula, occurring congenitally or during the first few years of life, but occasionally reported with onset in adulthood, and characterized by a round or oval, egg-yolk-like, delimited lesion (*vitelline disk*) on or adjacent to the macula, varying in size from one-half to 4 disk diameters, which eventually absorbs leaving a permanent atrophic, sometimes pigmented area. Syn., *vitelline corneal dystrophy; infantile heredomacular dystrophy.*

Biedl's d. An inherited disturbance of functions of some of the endocrine glands, e.g., the pituitary and/or other hypothalamic structures. The disease has physical and mental manifestations and is more commonly known as the *Laurence-Moon-Biedl syndrome.* The chief characteristics are obesity (of the "girdle" type), hypogenitalism, polydactyly or syndactyly, and mental retardation. The eyegrounds show a characteristic pigmentary degeneration of the retina.

Bielschowsky-Jansky d. The late infantile form of amaurotic family idiocy.

van Bogaert's d. Subacute sclerosing panencephalitis.

Bourneville's d. A rare congenital disease in which the essential pathology is the appearance of multiple tumors in the cerebrum and in other organs, such as the heart or the kidneys. It has a multitude of clinical symptoms, of which three are more or less characteristic, namely, mental deficiency, epilepsy, and adenoma sebaceum. The eyegrounds often show pathognomic tumor formations around the optic disk which are glistening gray and mulberry-like in structure. Syn., *epiloia; tuberous sclerosis.*

Bowen's d. Intraepithelial epithelioma affecting the skin and sometimes the mucous membranes. It may involve the cornea or the conjunctiva as a diffuse, slightly elevated, vascularized, gelatinous-appearing lesion, usually in the limbal region.

Brooke's d. Cystic adenoid epithelioma. See under *epithelioma.*

Buerger's d. A vascular disease, chiefly affecting young adult males, resulting in occlusion of arteries and veins, which impairs circulation, especially in the extremities. Ocular manifestations are recurrent hemorrhages in the retina and into the vitreous which are usually peripheral and spare the macula. The condition may partially clear up, but more often various complications supervene, such as glaucoma or retinitis proliferans, with detachment of the retina. Syn., *thromboangiitis obliterans.*

Bürger-Grütz d. Essential familial hyperlipemia.

Caffey's d. Infantile cortical hyperostosis. See under *hyperostosis.*

Cazenave's d. Pemphigus foliaceus.

Chagas' d. Infection with *Trypanosoma cruzi*, usually occurring in children. It is generally unilateral, and edema of the eyelids and conjunctiva is common. Dacryoadenitis may occur, but the infection rarely spreads to the eyeball or to the orbit.

Charcot's d. Multiple sclerosis. See also *Charcot's triad.*

Christian's d. Schüller-Christian-Hand disease.

Coats's d. Retinitis, typically occurring in young, apparently healthy males, characterized by large elevated masses of yellowish exudate, generally lying underneath the retinal vessels, chiefly in the posterior region near the optic disk or the macula. Multiple small aneurysms, present at the ends of the vessels, may burst to form hemorrhages, and the vessels often show caliber differences, sheathing, looping, and nodule formations. In the later stages, large retinal hemorrhages and retinal detachment may occur. Syn., *Coats's retinitis; retinitis exudativa externa; retinitis hemorrhagica externa; massive exudative retinitis.*

Cockayne's d. A progressive disease considered hereditary, commencing in the second year of life and characterized by dermatitis, mental retardation, dwarfism, maxillary prognathism, large hands and feet, prominent ears, carious teeth, microcephaly, loss of hearing, loss of fatty tissue in the face, optic atrophy, pigmentary degeneration of the retina of the salt and pepper type primarily in the macular area, and cataracts. Syn., *Cockayne's syndrome.*

Crouzon's d. Hereditary cranio-facial dysostosis.

cystic retinal d. Cystic degeneration of the retina.

Dalrymple's d. Inflammation of the cornea and the ciliary body.

Déjerine-Sottas d. Hypertrophic neuritis. See under *neuritis.*

Devic's d. Neuromyelitis optica.

Duhring's d. Dermatitis herpetiformis.

Eales's d. Recurrent hemorrhages in the retina and the vitreous, found mainly in apparently healthy young males. The etiology may be latent tuberculosis. Syn., *angiopathia retinalis juvenilis; primary retinal perivasculitis.*

Eddowes' d. The familial condition of osteogenesis imperfecta associated with blue sclerae. Syn., *Lobstein's disease.*

Ehlers-Danlos d. Meekrin-Ehlers-Danlos syndrome.

Erb's d. Myasthenia gravis.

Erb-Goldflam d. Myasthenia gravis.

Fabry's d. A recessive, sex-linked, hereditary, metabolic disease in which glycolipid is deposited in the tissues of the body. It is characterized by small purple skin lesions in the region of the thighs, navel, buttocks and genitalia, especially in males, but usually absent in females. Typical ocular signs include: periorbital and retinal edema, tortuosity of the conjunctival and retinal blood vessels, filmy opacities of the corneal epithelium which radiate from the central cornea, and branching, spokelike, posterior capsular cataracts. Syn., *angiokeratoma corporis diffusum.*

Fanconi's d. Simple recessive familial aplastic anemia appearing in children ages 5 to 7 and characterized by spots of brown pigmentation on the skin, microcephalia, genital hypoplasia, tendon hyperreflexia, convergent strabismus, sometimes band keratopathy, and, rarely, bilateral severe microphthalmos.

Flajani's d. Exophthalmic goiter.

Förster's d. A localized choroiditis starting at the macula and gradually developing other patches peripherally. At first the spots are uniformly black, but later become depigmented in the center so that they appear as dark circles with white interiors. Syn., *areolar choroiditis.*

Friedreich's d. A hereditary progressive degeneration of various nerve tracts, particularly the spinocerebellar and corticospinal tracts, the posterior columns, and the posterior roots, occurring in childhood. The clinical symptoms are general impairment of coordination of movement, nystagmus, loss of tendon reflexes, and occasionally ptosis and external ophthalmoplegia. Syn., *Friedreich's spinal ataxia.*

Fuchs' d. Gyrate atrophy of choroid and retina. See under *atrophy.*

Gaucher's d. A lipoid degeneration, often occurring in members of the same family, believed due to a congenital defect in metabolism, in which the cerebroside kerasin is deposited in the reticuloendothelial cells of the spleen, the liver, the lymph nodes, and bone marrow. The spleen and the liver are enlarged, and there is pronounced microcytic anemia. In infants, the brain is involved; the findings are similar to those of amaurotic idiocy, and it is invariably fatal. In adults, it is chronic, the nervous system is not affected, the conjunctiva is brownish and may have a wedge-shaped thickening with the base near the limbus. Syn., *cerebroside lipoidosis.*

Gerlier's d. An epidemic disease, found in Switzerland and Japan, characterized by vertigo, ptosis, ophthalmoplegia, restricted visual fields, and dimness of vision. It is seasonal, beginning in the spring and lasting until fall, and is considered to be of infectious origin. Syn., *epidemic paralyzing vertigo.*

von Graefe's d. Progressive paralysis of all the ocular muscles.

Graves's d. Hyperthyroidism characterized by increased pulse rate, tremors, anxiety, loss of weight and sometimes diarrhea. Early eye signs are those of von Graefe, Dalrymple, Stellwag, Moebius, and Gifford, q.v.

Exophthalmos may be an accompanying eye sign. Typically, it occurs between the ages of 15 and 50 and predominantly affects females. Syn., *Basedow's disease; Flajani's disease; March's disease; Parry's disease; Stokes's disease; thyrotoxic goiter; thyrotoxicosis.*

Hand's d. Schüller-Christian-Hand disease.

Harada's d. A disease characterized by bilateral, acute, diffuse, exudative choroiditis, retinal detachment, headache, loss of appetite, nausea, vomiting, and sometimes temporary vitiligo, poliosis, and deafness. The retinae may reattach and the visual acuity improve. The disease is of undetermined etiology, but is thought to be due to a virus infection and probably synonymous with *Vogt-Koyanagi syndrome.*

Hebra's d. Erythema multiforme exudativum.

Heerfordt's d. Uveoparotitis.

hepatolenticular d. A group of diseases, having in common degeneration of the liver and the lenticular nucleus, and characterized by attacks of jaundice, followed by difficulty in speaking, swallowing, and mastication. Eye symptoms include pigmentation of the cornea, which appears as a colored ring (red, yellow, or gray-green) on the posterior surface of the cornea (Kayser-Fleischer ring) and, occasionally, night blindness.

von Hippel's d. A rare, unilateral or bilateral disease, sometimes familial, in which hemangiomata occur in the retina, characterized opthalmoscopically in the initial stage by one or more round or oval, elevated, reddish nodules, usually in the periphery, to each of which course from the optic disk an enormously dilated and tortuous artery and companion vein. Dense white exudates appear later and are followed by retinal detachment, iridocyclitis, glaucoma, and cataract. The course is slowly progressive, and many years may pass from the onset of the tumor to the complete loss of vision. Syn., *angiomatosis of the retina; Lagleyze-von Hippel disease; hemangioblastosis retinae; von Hippel's hemangiomatosis.*

von Hippel-Lindau d. Hemangioma of the retina associated with angiomatous cysts in the cerebellum, medulla, or spinal cord and similar cystic or angiomatous tumors in the pancreas, the liver, the kidneys, or other organs. See also *von Hippel's disease.* Syn., *angioblastomatosis; angiogliomatosis; retinocerebral angiomatosis.*

Huntington's d. A hereditary condition (autosomal dominant) characterized by vertical gaze palsy, strabismus, personality changes, and involuntary choreiform movements in the face, neck, and upper extremities. Its onset is usually in the fourth to sixth decades and is due to degenerative changes in the caudate and lenticular nuclei in the cerebral cortex. Syn., *Huntington's chorea.*

Hurler's d. An autosomal recessive congenital disease named after a German pediatrician, Gertrude Hurler, who first described it as *lipochondrodystrophy*, characterized by dwarfism, crookedness of the spine, short fingers, stiff joints, mental deficiency, large thickened eyelids, convergent strabismus, and increasing cloudiness of the cornea. It is characterized chemically by extensive chondroitin sulfate B and heparitin sulfate in urine and tissues. Syn., *dysostosis multiplex; gargoylism; mucopolysaccharidosis I; Hurler's syndrome.*

Hutchinson's d. Tay's choroiditis.

Jansky-Bielschowsky d. The late infantile form of amaurotic family idiocy.

Jensen's d. A localized choroiditis neighboring the optic disk which causes a sector-shaped defect in the visual field, characteristically extending farther toward the periphery than the actual lesion. The scotoma may reach the periphery and is sometimes found only in the periphery. The lesion is attributed to blockage of the deep vessels and consequent destruction of the neuroepithelium; because of its location the disease has been called *choroiditis juxtapapillaris.* The overlying retina may be involved only slightly, or it may be affected so very seriously that some have labeled it *retinochoroiditis juxtapapillaris.* Syn., *Jensen's choroiditis; Jensen's retinitis; juxtapapillary retinitis.*

Johnson-Stevens d. Stevens-Johnson syndrome. See under *syndrome.*

Kalischer's d. Sturge-Weber disease.

Kaposi's d. Xeroderma pigmentosum.

Kayser's d. A systemic disease, the clinical manifestations of which include pigmentation of the skin of the body, greenish discoloration of the cornea, and intention tremor; usually associated with enlargement of the spleen and cirrhosis of the liver.

Kitihara's d. Central angiospastic chorioretinopathy.

Kuhnt-Junius d. Senile disciform degeneration of the macula. See under *degeneration.*

Lafora's d. A rare autosomal recessive hereditary derangement of carbohydrate metabolism in the form of a glyco-protein-acid mucopolysaccharide dystrophy commencing in late childhood with myoclonus and epilipsy and terminating in amaurosis, pseudobulbar palsy, dementia, and tetraplegia. Basophilic deposits (Lafora bodies) in the central nervous system, retina, and other organs are characteristic.

Lagleyze-von Hippel d. Von Hippel's disease.

Lauber's d. Fundus albipunctatus.

Leber's d. 1. A relatively rare disease occurring about the age of 20 in individuals who are otherwise apparently healthy; characterized by bilateral optic atrophy generally leading to marked bilateral reduction of vision. It is considered a sex-linked, recessive condition although it is reported that the disease is transmitted by the sisters of an affected male rather than being transmitted by his daughters. There may be some degree of visual improvement after the disease has run its course, and occasionally complete restoration of vision. 2. Leber's retinal degeneration. Syn., *dysgenesis neuroepithelialis retinae.*

Leiner's d. Generalized exfoliative dermatitis including the skin of the eyelids, corneal ulcers, diminished corneal sensitivity, and, possibly, symblepharon. This condition occurring in adults is known as *Wilson-Broca disease.*

Lindau's d. Angiomatosis of the central nervous system. See also *von Hippel's disease.*

Lindau-von Hippel d. Von Hippel-Lindau disease.

Little's d. Congenital bilateral paralysis and rigidity or spasticity of the arms and legs, mental deficiency, and ocular signs which may include strabismus, optic atrophy, nystagmus, or cataract. Syn., *cerebral diplegia; congenital spastic paralysis.*

Lobstein's d. Eddowes' disease.

Malherbe's d. Benign calcifying epithelioma of the eyelid occurring usually in young adults and more commonly in females. The lesion may appear to be malignant histologically but it does not metastasize.

Manz's d. Retinitis proliferans.

March's d. Exophthalmic goiter.

Marie's d. A hereditary cerebellar ataxia in which palsies of the extraocular muscles, internal ophthalmoplegia, and optic atrophy are common, while nystagmus is rare. The onset is usually between the ages of 20 and 40, and it is slowly progressive, resulting in mental deterioration and helplessness. Syn., *Marie's cerebellar ataxia; Nonne-Marie syndrome.*

Masuda's d. Central angiospastic chorioretinopathy.

Ménière's d. Ménière's syndrome.

Mikulicz's d. A chronic, bilateral, noninflammatory, symmetrical enlargement of the lacrimal and the salivary glands, especially of the parotid and the submaxillary, with an associated swelling and drooping of the eyelids and a marked narrowing of the palpebral fissures, occurring in association with other disease, such as reticulosis, tuberculosis, sarcoidosis, and syphilis.

Minamata d. Organic mercurial poisoning from eating contaminated fish, named after Minamata Bay, Japan, and characterized by visual field constriction, dysarthria, tremors, ataxia, salivation, sweating, and mental changes.

Moebius' d. Congenital paralysis of the sixth and seventh cranial nerves. The former involves the external rectus muscles, the latter involves the muscles of the face, giving it a masklike appearance. The internal recti may show slight weakness in lateral movements, but the function of convergence is intact.

Morquio's d. A familial, autosomal disease characterized by dwarfism, flexion deformities, large head, and widely spaced orbits; an appearance similar to that of Hurler's disease except that mentality is normal and corneal changes are not as pronounced. Syn., *Brailsford syndrome; mucopolysaccharidosis IV.*

Newcastle d. A virus disease of fowls which may be transmitted to man and cause an acute follicular conjunctivitis and enlargement of the preauricular nodes. It is usually unilateral and of short duration.

Niemann's d. Niemann-Pick disease.

Niemann-Pick d. A widespread, hereditary, lipoid degeneration, sometimes familial, affecting the reticuloendothelial and parenchymatous cells of the body, including the ganglion cell layer and the nuclear layer of the retina, usually affecting female Jewish infants. There is extreme enlargement of the liver and spleen, causing an enlarged abdomen, severe anemia, enlargement and hardening of the lymph nodes, usually a brownish pigmentation of the skin, and frequently a cherry-red spot at the macula surrounded by a white edematous area (as that found in Tay-Sachs disease). It usually commences between 3 and 6 months of age and terminates in death by the age of 2. It is differentiated from Tay-Sachs and Gaucher's diseases by its widespread involvement, gross enlargement of the liver and the spleen, and by the appearance of foam cells containing the lipids lecithin and sphingomyelin (phosphatides) in the affected organs. Syn., *essential lipoid histiocytosis; lipoid spleno-hepatomegaly.*

Nonne-Milroy-Meige d. A rare hereditary dysplasia of the lymphatics, resulting in lymphedema and hyperplasia of the subcutaneous tissue, which chiefly affects the lower extremities and may produce elephantiasis. It may be congenital or may appear as late as puberty. Ocular involvement may include conjunctival edema, blepharoptosis, buphthalmos, and strabismus.

Norrie's d. Congenital bilateral pseudotumor of the retina with recessive x-chromosomal inheritance. In the first few months of life the eyes appear of normal size with transparent corneae and crystalline lenses, behind which are dense retrolental membranes. With advancing age the corneae become opaque, the crystalline lenses cataractous, and the eyeballs become wasted and shrunken. Blindness is present from birth, and deafness and mental retardation are frequently present. Syn., *atrophia bulborum hereditaria.*

Oguchi's d. A form of congenital and hereditary night blindness, occurring mainly in Japan, in which visual acuity, visual fields, and the color sense are usually normal. The fundus has a grayish-white appearance, usually limited to the region of the papilla and the macula, but may extend to the periphery. After the eyes have been occluded for several hours, the fundi show a normal appearance.

Ohara's d. Oculoglandular tularemia. See under *tularemia.*

Osler-Vaquez d. Vaquez' disease.

Paget's d. A hereditary systemic disorder of the skeletal system accompanied by a variety of ocular symptoms, the most common being retinal arteriosclerosis and central choroidal sclerosis. Other symptoms include brown corneal opacities, optic atrophy, retinitis pigmentosa, exophthalmos, or angioid streaks. Syn., *osteitis deformans.*

Pappataci's d. Sandfly fever. See under *fever.*

Parry's d. Exophthalmic goiter.

Pick's d. A form of retinitis seen in cases of advanced anemia and other wasting diseases and characterized by the appearance of multiple hemorrhages, exudates, and, occasionally, a macular "star." There is a progressive atrophy of the nerve fibers and extensive lipoid degeneration of the retinal substance. The cause is probably a toxic factor added to the anemia. Syn., *retinitis cachecticorum.*

pulseless d. A disease characterized by the absence of palpable arterial pulsation in the arms, the carotid arteries, and the superficial temporal arteries. Arteriovenous anastomoses occur around the optic nerve head, and the carotid sinus is hypersensitive. Other signs may include cataract, absence of detectable blood pressure in the arms, slight enophthalmos, mydriasis, atrophy of the iris, retinal hemorrhages, dilated retinal vessels, and retinal detachment. Retinal and optic atrophy appear at a late stage. It usually commences during or after puberty, especially in females, is due to gradual occlusion of the aortic arch and its branches, and prognosis is poor. Syn., *brachycephalic arteritis; Takayasu's disease; Takayasu-Ohnishi disease; thrombo-obliterative aortic arch disease; aortic arch syndrome; Martorell's syndrome; pulseless syndrome.*

Purtscher's d. Angiopathy of the retina following severe skull trauma or compression injuries to the body, characterized by numerous large, white, blurred patches closely associated with the retinal veins and sometimes covering them, located in the area of the disk or the macula. Hemorrhages and retinal edema are usually present, and the retinal vessels may be dilated. The condition is usually transient and recovery complete. Syn., *angiopathia retinae traumatica of Purtscher; angiopathica traumatica of Purtscher; traumatic liporrhagia retinalis; traumatic lymphorrhagia retinalis; Purtcher's traumatic angiopathic retinopathy; retinal teletraumatism.*

Quincke's d. Angioneurotic edema.

Raynaud's d. A primary vascular disorder causing local and recurring interruption of the arterial circulation through the distal parts of the extremities. The principal eye manifestation is a spasm of the retinal vessels which, if it involves the central artery of the retina, causes almost complete loss of vision. The fundus picture resembles that seen in an embolus of the central retinal artery, namely, a cherry-red spot in the macula surrounded by a large white, opaque area. Sometimes there is a localized, complete anemia due to obliteration of the choroidal vessels which leads to destructive retinal lesions.

von Recklinghausen's d. A congenital disorder affecting various parts and organs of the body, characterized by the formation of multiple tumors, especially along the cranial and peripheral nerves but also involving the sympathetic system. There is pigmentation of the skin, small nodular growths often appear on the chest and extremities, and a tumor growth may be present in any of the structures of the eye or adnexa. Syn., *neurofibromatosis.*

Reiter's d. A systemic disease characterized by a triad of clinical manifestation: urethritis, conjunctivitis, and arthritis. The conjunctivitis is purulent and involves both eyes; keratitis and iritis may occur as complications.

Rendu-Osler d. A simple dominant hereditary disease, affecting both sexes equally, characterized by multiple telangiectases and hemorrhages of the skin and mucous membranes, including the conjunctiva. Similar vascular defects may occur in the retina. It usually does not become fully developed until late adolescent or adult life, but may occur in infancy or at birth. Syn., *hereditary hemorrhagic angiomatosis; hereditary hemorrhagic telangiectasia.*

Rieger's d. A dominant hereditary developmental anomaly of the cornea, iris, and the angle of the anterior chamber. It is characterized by a grayish-white translucent band opacity at the periphery of the cornea on its posterior surface, hypoplastic changes of the anterior stromal layer of the iris, and the presence of fibers connecting the iris and posterior cornea at the angle of the anterior chamber. Syn., *Rieger's anomaly; mesodermal dysgenesis of the cornea and iris; Rieger's syndrome.*

Robles d. Onchocerciasis.

Romberg's d. Progressive atrophy of all structures of one side of the face, including skin, subcutaneous tissue, muscle, and bone. Of undetermined etiology, it frequently commences in the orbital region, resulting in thin eyelids, a sunken and retracted eyeball, whitening and/or loss of eyelashes, and sometimes anhidrosis. Syn., *facial hermiatrophy; Romberg's syndrome.*

Roth's d. A mild and benign condition of septic retinitis, usually associated with systemic infections, especially endocarditis, probably caused by an endotheliotoxin of relatively low virulence. There are round or oval white spots in the retina, usually near the disk, frequently surrounded by a hemorrhagic area so that the latter appears as if it had a white center (Roth's spots). Syn., *Roth's retinitis; retinitis septica of Roth.*

Rothmund's d. A rare, recessive, heredofamilial disease, occurring in early childhood, characterized by an atrophic, tightly stretched skin showing patches of depigmentation and

hyperpigmentation, and telangiectasies, hypogonadism, and rapidly developing cataracts composed of discrete opacities.

Sachs' d. The infantile form of amaurotic family idiocy named after an American neurologist, Bernard Parnay Sachs (1858-1944); also known as Tay-Sachs disease because Tay later described the characteristic cherry-red spot in the macula. See *Tay-Sachs disease.*

St. Clair's d. A large group of eye diseases, of varied etiology and seriousness, generally classed under ophthalmia.

Sanders' d. Epidemic keratoconjunctivitis, first fully described by James Sanders, an English physician (1777-1843).

Schaumann's d. Sarcoidosis.

Schilder's d. A disease occurring mainly in infancy and childhood, characterized by massive demyelination of nerve fibers in the subcortical regions of the cerebrum and the cerebellum, resulting in apathy, convulsions, blindness, deafness, and spastic paralysis. Histological examination of the optic nerve may fail to reveal a single myelin sheath, the sheaths being replaced by dense glial tissue.

Schüller-Christian-Hand d. A lipoid degeneration affecting membraneous bones and other tissues, occurring primarily in male children, and characterized by exophthalmos, diabetes insipidus, and deposits of xanthomatous cells in the bones, especially of the skull. Other symptoms may include deafness, impairment of the sense of taste, ophthalmoplegia, xanthomatous tumors of the eylids, bronze pigmentation of the skin, optic atrophy, and nystagmus. Syn., *cranio-hypophysial xanthomatosis; diabetic exophthalmic dysostosis; dysostosis hypophysaria; lipoid granulomatosis.*

sickle-cell d. A hereditary anemia, affecting Negro and other dark-skinned peoples, in which the erythrocytes become sickle-shaped due to a defect in the hemoglobin molecule. Ocular manifestations include: retinal neovascularization, microaneurysms, hemorrhages and exudates, angioid streaks, papilledema, cataract, conjunctival telangiectasis and hemorrhage, glaucoma, and extraocular palsies. Syn., *Dresbach syndrome; Herrick syndrome; sickle-cell anemia.*

Silverman-Caffey d. Infantile cortical hyperostosis. See under *hyperostosis*.

Spielmeyer-Stock d. Batten-Mayou disease.

Spielmeyer-Vogt d. Batten-Mayou disease.

Stargardt's d. A heredofamilial, bilateral, macular degeneration occurring at puberty and not associated with degenerative changes in the central nervous system and not accompanied by any mental symptoms. Syn., *Stargardt's macular degeneration; Stargardt's foveal dystrophy.*

Steinert's d. Myotonic dystrophy.

Stevens-Johnson d. Stevens-Johnson syndrome.

Still's d. Juvenile polyarthritis.

Stokes's d. Exophthalmic goiter.

Strümpell-Lorrain d. Familial spasmodic paraplegia.

Strümpell-Marie d. Ankylosing spondylitis.

Sturge-Weber d. Malformation of the small vessels in various areas of the body, particularly of the skin, the brain, the pia mater, and the eye, characterized by cerebral symptoms, vascular nevi, epileptic convulsions, glaucoma, and calcification in the cortex of the brain. All of these changes are present in the complete syndrome, but each may occur alone. Syn., *nevoid amentia; encephalocutaneous angiomatosis; encephalotrigeminal angiomatosis; meningocutaneous angiomatosis; Kalischer's disease.*

Takayasu's d. Pulseless disease.

Tay's d. A senile colloid or hyaline degeneration of the choroid in the macular area, characterized ophthalmoscopically by small, oval, yellowish-white spots arranged around the macula. Syn., *choroiditis guttata senilis; Tay's choroiditis.*

Tay-Sachs d. The infantile form of amaurotic family idiocy in which there is widespread lipoid degeneration of the ganglion cells of the nervous system and the retina, confined principally in the latter to the ganglion cell layer. It primarily affects Jewish infants between 4 and 8 months of age, is of familial tendency, and is characterized by listlessness, flaccid muscles, rapid loss of vision, frequently progressing to blindness, mental deterior-

ation, marked loss of weight, convulsions, and ophthalmoscopically by a cherry-red spot at the macula surrounded by a white area, due to edema and lipoid deposits, and pallor of the optic disk. The disease terminates in death, usually by the age of 2, and is differentiated from Niemann-Pick disease in that the liver and spleen are not enlarged, the nervous system is the primary site of involvement, and the affected cells contain a phosphorus-free lipoid.

Thompson's d. A congenital variation of Leber's disease.

Thomsen's d. A familial disease, characterized by delayed relaxation of the voluntary muscles but without wasting or atrophy, which commences during early life and is often associated with some mental defectiveness. The only definitely known ocular involvement is that a sudden closure of the eyelid may be followed by inability to open the eyes for several seconds. Lens changes similar to those always seen in myotonic dystrophy occur rarely in this condition. Syn., *myotonia congenita.*

thrombo-obliterative aortic arch d. Pulseless disease.

Türk's d. Duane's retraction syndrome. See under *syndrome*.

Urbach-Wiethe d. Lipid proteinosis.

Vaquez' d. A disease of the blood-forming system, characterized by an enormous increase in the erythrocytes. The uveal vessels, especially the veins, are greatly dilated and are dark in color, so much so that the choroid may be thickened to several times its normal size. The color of the iris changes from a blue to a reddish-brown, and there may be an associated degeneration and scattering of the iris pigment. Syn., *Osler-Vaquez disease; erythremia; polycythemia rubra vera.*

Vogt-Spielmeyer d. Batten-Mayou disease.

Wagner's d. Vitreoretinal degeneration.

Weil's d. A spirochete infection (*spirochetosis icterohemorrhagica*) characterized by jaundice, splenomegaly, hepatitis, and hemorrhages in almost every organ of the body. The eye involvement is occasionally iridocyclitis, usually associated with conjunctivitis. Syn., *leptospirosis.*

Wernicke's d. A disease characterized by bilateral, external ophthalmoplegia, prostration, delirium, excitement or stupor, and sometimes nystagmus, ptosis, pupillary abnormalities, and slight internal ophthalmoplegia, considered due to acute thiamine deficiency. Syn., *superior hemorrhagic polioencephalitis; Wernicke's syndrome.*

Wilson's d. A systemic disease of unknown etiology, characterized by degenerative changes in the lenticular nucleus and a mixed type of cirrhosis of the liver. General clinical symptoms are impairment of voluntary motion with rigidity, contractures, tremors, and chorealike movements. A prominent eye symptom is the appearance of a Kayser-Fleischer ring. Syn., *hepatolenticular degeneration; lenticular progressive degeneration; psuedosclerosis of Westphal.*

Wilson-Broca d. Generalized exfoliative dermatitis including the skin of the eyelids, diminished corneal sensitivity and subsequent ulceration, and, possibly, symblepharon. This condition occurring in infancy is known as *Leiner's disease.* Syn., *erythroderma exfoliativa.*

Zinsser-Thomson d. Rothmund syndrome.

◆

disinhibitor. The third in a hypothetical series of three retinal neurons in parallel which have inhibitory effects on each other by their adjacency, the third being considered as a disinhibitor by reason of its inhibiting the inhibiting effect of the second on the first.

disinsertion, retinal (dis"in-ser'shun). A detachment of the retina at the ora serrata. Syn., *dialysis retinae; retinal dehiscence; retinodialysis.*

◆

DISK

disk (also spelled disc). A circular or round flat structure.

Airy's d. The bright central disk, surrounded by concentric light and dark rings, in a diffraction pattern formed by plane waves from a point source passing through a circular aperture. Syn., *diffraction disk.*

anangioid d. An optic disk without blood vessels, due to congenital defects in vascularization.

Benham's d. Benham's top.

Brücke d. A rotating disk of several alternately white and black sectors on which is concentrically placed a smaller disk of the same whiteness as the peripheral white sectors to demonstrate the *Brücke-Bartley effect.*

choked d. Noninflammatory edema of the optic nerve head, due to intracranial pressure. As observed ophthalmoscopically, the optic disk appears raised above the level of the retina and its margins are blurred. Accompanying changes are dilation, tortuosity, and engorgement of the retinal veins, with retinal edema most pronounced in the area of the disk. Syn., *papilledema.*

color d. A disk composed of sectors of different colors which, when rapidly rotated, blend perceptually into a single color.

color d's., Walker's. Visual field test objects consisting of a thin rodlike handle, at each end of which is mounted a circular disk oriented at right angles to the disk at the opposite end. On each side of each disk is a different color; only one of the four colors is visible at a given time.

cupped d. An exaggerated depression of the optic disk, being larger and more basin-shaped than the normal physiological cup; commonly present in advanced glaucoma.

Delboeuf d. A device for determining the relationship of different brightnesses by the method of equal sensation intervals. It usually contains three concentric sectored rings which, when rapidly rotated, present three values of gray, the intermediate one of which is adjusted by the observer to appear midway between the brightness of the other two.

d. diameter. A unit of measurement equal to the diameter of the optic disk as seen with the ophthalmoscope, used for localizing retinal lesions, etc., in terms of the number of disk diameters away from the optic disk or other point of reference.

diffraction d. Airy's disk.

dragged d. An optic disk which appears to be displaced nasally from its normal position due to the temporal displacement of the retina and the emerging retinal vessels, caused by traction of temporal scar tissue formation in partially resolved retrolental fibroplasia.

Inouye's d. A home training device consisting of a flat, black, round metal disk, with a small central fixation dot, attached to a lamp to shield the macular area and provide light stimulation only to the peripheral retina. The resulting doughnut-shaped after-image is used in fixation training by centering it around a fixation target.

magic d. Stroboscopic disk.

Martius d. A color disk for determining the neutral brightness or gray-value of colors. A ring of the color being studied is placed on the disk between a central and a peripheral gray, each of which may be varied from black to white. The grays are adjusted until they are no longer darkened or lightened by the contrast-inducing action near the borders adjacent to the colored ring. When so adjusted, the brightness or the grayness of the variable rings is equal to the neutral brightness or gray-value of the color.

Mason's pupil d. An opaque disk with a movable slide containing several openings of different sizes which can be centered in front of the pupil in the trial frame, thus serving as an artificial pupil.

Masson d. A white disk with small, black, circularly sectioned sectors arranged in concentric order and of different sizes, used in determinations of brightness difference thresholds. When the disk is rapidly rotated, a series of neutral gray rings are seen, the brightness of each ring depending on the circumferential size of the black sectors composing the ring.

Maxwell's d. A color disk in which two or more differently colored disks are cut along a single radius and fitted together to overlap in any desired ratio of exposure.

Newton's d. A disk containing the seven colors of the spectrum which, when rotated rapidly, appears white or gray.

opaque d. A round opaque disk mounted in a trial lens rim and used in a trial frame as an occluder.

optic d. The portion of the optic nerve, seen in the fundus with the ophthalmoscope, which is formed by the meeting of all the retinal nerve fibers. It is insensitive to light, corresponds to the physiological blind spot, is pinkish in color, due to its many capillaries, and, normally, has a central depression, the physiological cup, often spelled *optic disc*. Syn., *optic papilla*.

phase d. Phase plate.

pinhole d. An opaque disk mounted in a trial lens rim and containing a small (usually 2 mm or less) perforation. It is frequently used to determine the maximum attainable visual acuity.

Placido's d. A form of keratoscope; a circular disk marked with concentric black and white rings and having a central opening through which the examiner observes the reflected image of the disk on the patient's cornea. It is used to determine the curvature characteristics of the anterior surface of the cornea.

Ramsden d. The exit pupil of a telescope.

Rekoss' d. A device consisting of two revolvable disks which may be turned independently about a common axis, each with a series of lenses of differing focal lengths mounted in openings around the periphery. By turning either disk, any one lens or combination of two lenses may be utilized. This device has found wide application in the construction of modern ophthalmoscopes and refracting units.

Scheiner's d. An opaque disk containing two small pinholes spaced to fall within the diameter of the pupil, used in demonstrations and investigations of the function of accommodation and of the refractive status of the eye.

Sherrington's d. A disk on which are constructed two narrow concentric rings, a semicircle of each of which is blue, with the other semicircle of each black. The smaller blue semicircle and the larger black semicircle are in the half of the disk having a yellow color or background, while the smaller black semicircle and the larger blue semicircle are in the other half of the disk having a black color or background. Although each ring is half black and half blue, the outer ring shows flicker at a higher rate of rotation.

stenopaic d. 1. An opaque disk mounted in a trial lens rim and containing a narrow opening or slit aperture, used in detecting and measuring astigmatism of the eye. Syn., *stenopaic slit*. 2. A pinhole disk.

straboscopic d. A lens or a disk used in visual testing to distort objects viewed through it.

stroboscopic d. 1. A disk with

alternate open and closed sectors which, when revolving, gives successive instantaneous views of a moving object or a series of pictures. 2. A disk carrying a series of pictures showing the successive phases of a motion or a scene, as for use in the stroboscope.

vitelline d. of the macula. A round or oval, well delimited, lesion covering the macula, or immediately adjacent to it, varying in size from one-half to four disk diameters and of a pale or reddish-yellow color; an anomaly found in Best's disease. Syn., *vitelline cyst of the macula.*

Volkmann's d's. A pair of disks with a circle and a single radius drawn on each which, when viewed haploscopically, can be rotated so that the radial lines appear as a single diameter, thus indicating the angle between the apparently parallel meridians of the two eyes.

◆

dislocation of the lens. A displacement of the crystalline lens from its normal position. Syn., *subluxation of the lens.*

Disontegrator (dih-son'teh-gra"tor). A trade name for a device which generates ultrasonic waves and transmits them through a tank containing a solution, for the purpose of cleaning small objects such as contact lenses.

disorder, iatrogenic. A condition involving adverse effects induced by a physician in the care of his patient.

disorganization, visual. *Optometric Extension Program:* A syndrome of refractive findings held to be characteristic of one who will adjust readily to changes in lens prescription, especially to increases in convex lens power.

disparation (dis"pah-ra'shun). 1. The apparent separation of the two images during diplopia. 2. Retinal disparity.

crossed d. Heteronymous diplopia.

uncrossed d. Homonymous diplopia.

disparator (dis'pah-ra"ter). A Brewster-type stereoscope with an attachment which introduces a continuous variation in the separation of corresponding points on split stereograms as the targets are moved from the infinity position to a near point position, so as to maintain a relatively constant relationship between accommodation and convergence stimuli. Syn., *stereodisparator.*

disparity (dis-par'ih-te). The state or condition of being distinct in respect to quality or character; inequality; dissimilarity.

conjugate d. The normal disparity or difference in the size or the location of the retinal images in the two eyes, created by asymmetrical convergence.

crossed d. 1. Retinal disparity induced by an object nearer than the longitudinal horopter. (Hering) 2. Separation of diplopic images in which the right eye image is seen to the left of the left eye image.

disjugate d. The normal disparity or difference in the size or location of any pair of extrafoveal images of a single object not on the longitudinal horopter. This creates the condition of physiological diplopia.

fixation d. A condition in which the images of a bifixated object do not stimulate exactly corresponding retinal points, but still fall within Panum's areas, the object thus being seen singly. It may be considered to be a slight over- or underconvergence, or vertical misalignment, of the eyes. Syn., *retinal slip.* **negative f.d.** A small relative divergence or underconvergence of the eyes while maintaining single binocular vision for the point of fixation. Syn., *exodisparity.* **positive f.d.** A small relative overconvergence of the eyes while maintaining single binocular vision for the point of fixation. Syn., *esodisparity.*

position d. Overconvergence or underconvergence of the eyes while fusion is maintained. The same as fixation disparity, but applicable also to the case where only peripheral stimuli are presented for fusion, i.e., when no central or foveal target for fixation is present.

retinal d. 1. Failure of the two retinal images of an object in the field of vision to fall on corresponding retinal points, as is obtained, for example, when the object lies outside the horopter, or when a pair of haploscopically viewed patterns are not identical. 2. Incongruities in anatomical and physiological aspects of the two retinae, such as lack of conformity of the various corresponding retinal elements, lack of confluence of the perceptual and anatomical vertical and horizontal meridians of each eye, and the difference in space values of the temporal and the nasal segments of each eye.

uncrossed d. 1. Retinal disparity induced by an object beyond the longitudinal horopter. (Hering) 2. Separation of diplopic images in which the right eye image is seen to the right of the left eye image.

dispenser, ophthalmic. One who supplies and adapts prescribed ophthalmic products or appliances to the patient.

dispersion (dis-per'shun). 1. The act or state of being broken apart, scattered, or separated. 2. Chromatic dispersion. 3. *Statistics:* The variation of the scores or measures of a given sampling from one another or from some designated point, such as the mean.

angular d. The angular separation of the component rays of a pencil of light on passing through a refractive medium whose sides are not parallel to each other.

anomalous d. Dispersion produced by prisms of certain refractive media so that the spectral colors are not in their usual order. Such media are characterized by a high absorption band within the visible spectrum, a rapidly increasing index of refraction as the absorption band is approached from the red end, and a rapidly decreasing index as the band is approached from the blue end. Syn., *inverse dispersion.*

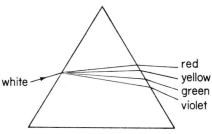

Fig. 11 Chromatic dispersion by a prism. (From *Vision and Visual Perception,* ed. by C. H. Graham. New York: John Wiley and Sons, 1965)

chromatic d. The splitting of a beam of white light into its component wavelengths or colors, as with a prism or a diffraction grating. (See Fig. 11.)

false internal d. In a medium, the internal scattering or refraction of light due to innumerable minute foreign particles, slight changes in struc-

ture, tiny fractures, etc., causing the medium to appear cloudy and self-luminous.

inverse d. Anomalous dispersion.

irrational d. Dispersion that is not a simple function of wavelength, occurring characteristically in a spectrum produced by a prism, in which the spectrum produced by one prism cannot be exactly reproduced by a prism of another substance.

linear d. The difference in distance to the red and blue image planes of an optical system.

mean d. The partial dispersion for the Fraunhofer C and F lines of the spectrum, designated by $(n_F - n_C)$, where n_F is the index of refraction for the wavelength of light of the F line (486.1 mμ), and n_C is the index for the C line (656.3 mμ).

normal d. Dispersion proportional to the wavelengths of the components of the light; the type of dispersion produced by a diffraction grating.

partial d. The difference in the index of refraction of a medium for two given wavelengths, especially wavelengths corresponding to prominent Fraunhofer lines.

prismatic d. The separation of white light into its component colors by passing through a prism.

reciprocal d. The reciprocal of the dispersive power of an optical medium, usually called the *nu (ν) value,* and represented by the formula:

$$\nu = \frac{n_D - 1}{n_F - n_C}$$

where $n_D, n_F,$ and n_C represent the indices of refraction for three Fraunhofer lines corresponding to yellow, blue, and red, respectively. It is used in designing achromatic lenses, where the higher the nu value, the less the chromatic aberration.

relative d. The ratio of the mean dispersion to the mean deviation for a substance, usually termed *dispersive power* and designated by the formula:

$$\text{dispersive power} = \frac{n_F - n_C}{n_D - 1}$$

where $n_F, n_C,$ and n_D are the indices of refraction for three Fraunhofer lines corresponding to blue, red, and yellow wavelengths, respectively. The higher the dispersive power, the more chromatic aberration a lens will have.

residual d. The chromatic aberration remaining in an optical system which has been rendered achromatic for two or more wavelengths.

rotatory d. The differential rotation of the plane of polarization of different wavelengths by an optically active substance. The amount of rotation differs with the wavelength of light and is approximately proportional to the inverse square of the wavelength.

true internal d. Fluorescence.

dissector, image. In fibers optics, a bundle of fibers which spatially rearranges the points in an image.

disseminated sclerosis (dih-sem″ih-na″ted skle-ro′sis). Multiple sclerosis.

dissimilation (dih-sim″ih-la′shun). According to the Hering theory of color vision, the breaking down of the three primary substances in the retina by red, yellow, and white light; the reverse of *assimilation.*

dissimulation (dis″sim-u-la′shun). Malingering.

dissociation. The elimination of stimulus to fusion, usually by occlusion of one eye, gross distortion of the image seen by one eye, or by excessive displacement of the image seen by one eye.

Gestalt d. An inability to see things as a whole; the inability of an individual to conceptualize a totality.

sensory d. The absence of fusion because of a visual sensory pathway defect.

dissolve. See *view, dissolving.*

◆

DISTANCE

distance. The measure of space between two points of reference.

abathic d. The viewing distance at which the apparent frontoparallel plane, which varies in curvature with fixation distance, coincides with an actual frontoparallel plane.

d. between centers. 1. In the boxing method of frame specification, the distance between the boxing centers of the spectacle frame. Abbreviation DBC. Syn., *frame center distance.* 2. The distance between the geometric centers of a spectacle frame. Abbreviation DBC. Syn., *frame center distance.* 3. The distance between the optical centers of lenses mounted in a spectacle frame.

d. between lenses. 1. The shortest distance between the nasal edges of a pair of lenses; separation of the vertical tangents of lenses at the bridge. 2. Separation of lenses at the datum line. 3. Designation of the bridge width. Abbreviation DBL.

centration d. *British:* The distance between major reference points of lenses mounted in a spectacle frame.

conjugate d's. The object distance and the image distance with respect to an optical system.

d. of distinct vision. An arbitrary projection distance used in the conventional formula for determining the magnifying power of an optical instrument, usually taken as 10 in. or 25 cm.

egoriginal d. The distance of an object from the ego or self.

equivalent d. Reduced distance.

eyewire d. The distance, along the line of sight, between the vertex of the cornea and the plane of the spectacle frame eyewire, with the eyes in the straightforward position.

focal d. The distance from an optical surface to a principal focal point, along the optical axis. In a compound optical system, it is the distance from a principal plane to the corresponding principal focal point, along the optical axis. Syn., *focal length.* **anterior f.d.** Primary focal distance. **back f.d.** Posterior vertex focal distance. **conjugate f.d's.** In a single surface optical system, the distances of conjugate focal points from the optical surface, along the optical axis. In a compound optical system, the distances of conjugate focal points from the respective principal planes. **front f.d.** Anterior vertex focal distance. **posterior f.d.** Secondary focal distance. **primary f.d.** The distance from an optical surface to the primary principal focal point, along the optical axis. In a compound optical system, it is the distance from the primary principal plane to the primary principal focal point, along the optical axis. Syn., *anterior focal distance; anterior principal focal distance; primary principal focal distance; anterior focal length; primary focal length.* **principal (anterior) f.d.** Primary focal distance. **principal (posterior) f.d.** Secondary focal distance. **principal (primary) f.d.** Primary focal distance. **principal (secondary) f.d.** Secondary focal distance. **secondary f.d.** The distance from an optical surface to the secondary principal focal point, along the optical axis. In a compound optical system, the distance from the secondary principal plane to the secondary principal focal point, along the optical axis. Syn., *posterior focal distance; posterior principal focal distance; secondary principal focal distance; posterior focal length; secondary focal length.* **vertex (anterior) f.d.** In an optical system or lens, the distance along the optical axis from the anterior optical surface (first surface to the left) to the primary principal focal point. Syn., *front focal distance; anterior vertex focal length.* **vertex (posterior) f.d.** In an optical system or a lens, the distance along the optical axis from the posterior optical surface (last surface to the right) to the secondary principal focal point. Syn., *back focal distance; posterior vertex focal length.*

frame center d. Distance between centers.

homologous d. The lateral distance between two corresponding objects in a stereogram.

hyperfocal d. The shortest distance for which a photographic lens may be focused to permit satisfactory image definition of an object at infinity.

hyperplastic d. The perceived distance of an image, especially from an optical instrument, when it is greater than the actual physical distance of the object.

hypoplastic d. The perceived distance of an image, especially from an optical instrument, when it is less than the actual physical distance of the object.

image d. The distance from the optical surface to the image. In a compound optical system, the distance from the secondary principal plane to the image. Symbol u'. **extrafocal i.d.** The distance of an image formed by an optical system from the secondary focal point of the system. **reduced i.d.** The image distance divided by the index of refraction of the medium in which the image lies, the reciprocal being the reduced image vergence.

infinite d. The distance from which light emanates to strike an optical surface with parallel rays. In vision testing, it is usually considered to approximate 20 ft, or 6 m.

interocular d. 1. The distance between the centers of rotation of the eyes; the length of the base line. 2. The distance between the optical centers of the two eye-pieces of a binocular instrument.

interpupillary d. The distance between the centers of the pupils of the eyes. Unless otherwise specified, it refers to the distance when the eyes are fixed at infinity. Abbreviation PD. Syn., *pupillary distance.*

d. motivator. Stereomotivator.

object d. In optics, the distance from the optical surface to the object. In compound optical systems, it is expressed as the distance from the primary principal plane to the object. Symbol u. **extrafocal o.d.** The distance of an object from the primary focal point of an optical system. **reduced o.d.** The object distance divided by the index of refraction of the medium in which the object lies. The reciprocal of this quantity is known as the reduced object vergence.

optical center d. The distance between the optical centers of a pair of mounted spectacle lenses without prescribed prism or with prescribed prism neutralized.

orthoplastic d. The perceived distance of an image, especially from an optical instrument, when it is equal to the actual physical distance of the object.

pupillary d. Interpupillary distance.

reduced d. The distance between any two points in an optical medium, divided by the index of refraction of the medium. It represents the distance that light would travel in the medium in the same time that it would travel the distance between the two points in air. Syn., *equivalent distance; reduced separation.*

sighting center d. The distance between the sighting center and the point of intersection of the line of sight with the anterior surface of the cornea.

stop d. The distance between the back vertex of a spectacle lens and the center of rotation of the eye, the latter being considered the field stop of the motile eye.

vertex d. 1. The distance, along the line of sight, from the posterior surface of a spectacle lens to the apex of the cornea, with the eye in the straightforward position. 2. The distance, along the line of sight, from the plane containing the center of the edge of a spectacle lens to the apex of the cornea, with the eye in a straightforward position.

working d. 1. In retinoscopy, the distance from the plane of the correcting lenses to the peephole of the retinoscope. 2. The distance at which the patient desires or is required to read or perform other essential functions. 3. In the use of microscopes and other optical devices, the distance from the objective lens to the object viewed.

◆

distichia (dis-tik′e-ah). Distichiasis.

distichiasis (dis-tih-ki′ah-sis). An anomalous condition in which there are two rows of eyelashes, one being normal, the other being on the inner lid border and turning in against the eye. The Meibomian glands are absent when this condition is present. Syn., *distichia.*

Distinguished Service Foundation of Optometry. An organization sponsoring optometric research; established in 1927 and incorporated in 1931 in Washington, D.C.

distometer (dis-tom′eh-ter). A device for determining the distance between the back surface of a spectacle lens and the apex of the cornea.

distortion. 1. An aberration as a result of unequal magnification of object points not on the optical axis of a lens system. 2. Any change in which the image does not conform to the shape of the object, such as when viewed through a cylindrical lens.

    anamorphic d. Distortion in which magnification varies in different meridians, the directions of maximum and minimum magnifications being at right angles.

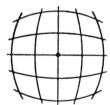

Fig. 12 Barrel-shaped distortion. (From Jenkins and White, *Fundamentals of Optics*, 3d ed. New York: McGraw-Hill, 1957; copyright © 1957; used with permission of McGraw-Hill Book Co.)

    barrel-shaped d. Distortion resulting from decreasing magnification with increasing distance of object points from the axis of an optical system. As a result of this distortion, the corners of the image of a square would be closer to the center than expected, with a resulting barrel-shaped appearance. (Fig. 12.) Syn., *positive distortion.*

    Keystone d. The trapezoidal image formation of a rectangular object such as may be effected by the obliquely upward projection of a picture of a vertical screen.

    negative d. Pincushion distortion.

    perspective d. Perceptual distortion resulting from viewing a photograph from a position other than one at which the angular subtenses of points in the photograph are identical with the angular subtenses of points in the scene as viewed by the camera.

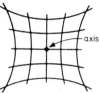

Fig. 13 Pincushion distortion. (From Jenkins and White, *Fundamentals of Optics*, 3d ed. New York: McGraw-Hill, 1957; copyright © 1957; used with permission of McGraw-Hill Book Co.)

    pincushion d. Distortion resulting from increasing magnification with increasing distance of object points from the axis of an optical system. As a result of this distortion, the corners of the image of a square would be farther from the center than expected, with a resulting pincushion appearance. (See Fig. 13.) Syn., *negative distortion.*

    positive d. Barrel-shaped distortion.

    prism d. Differential magnification or differential displacement of objects in the field of view seen through a thin prism, resulting essentially in straight lines appearing curved.

    radial d. Variation of image magnification along a radius from the center of the image field to a point in its periphery, e.g., *barrel-shaped* and *pincushion distortion.*

    stereoscopic d. A distorted perception of depth in a stereogram due to the incongruence or incompatibility of the separation of the optical components of the stereo camera and that of the optics of the binocular viewing system.

    tangential d. In a poorly collimated optical system the tangential displacement of the image of an eccentrically located object point.

distribution. The arrangement in space or time of things of any kind; the arrangement of values in a collection of data.

light d., asymmetrical. Light distribution from a luminaire or a lamp, in which the distribution is not the same in all vertical planes.

light d., symmetrical. Light distribution from a luminaire or a lamp, in which the distribution is substantially the same in all vertical planes.

divergence (di-ver'jens). 1. Binocularly, a deviation or a relative movement of the lines of sight of the two eyes outward from parallelism, so that the lines of sight intersect behind the eyes, or from some other relative position of reference, so that the lines of sight intersect at a greater distance in front of the eyes or a lesser distance behind; negative convergence. 2. Monocularly, a deviation or a movement of the line of sight of an eye outward from a straightforward or other position of reference. 3. The directional property of a bundle of light rays, as when emanating from a point source; to be distinguished from the convergence property of a bundle of rays directed toward a real image point.

consecutive d. Exotropia occurring in a previously esotropic individual and attributed to development of marked amblyopia ex anopsia with a resultant loss of convergence function. Syn., *secondary divergence.*

d. excess. 1. Exotropia or high exophoria in distant vision associated with normal fixation in near vision. 2. Exophoria or exotropia in distant vision, exophoria or exotropia at near being considered as convergence insufficiency. 3. Exophoria or exotropia greater at distance than at near.

fusional d. Lateral divergence of the lines of sight of the two eyes in response to fusion stimuli, such as may be induced clinically by base-in prisms.

d. insufficiency. 1. Esotropia or high esophoria in distant vision associated with normal fixation in near vision. 2. Esophoria or esotropia in distant vision, esophoria or esotropia at near being considered convergence excess. 3. Esophoria or esotropia greater at distance than at near.

d. paralysis. See under *paralysis.*

secondary d. Consecutive divergence.

vertical d. Vertical deviation or relative vertical movement of the lines of sight of the two eyes from parallelism. **dissociated v.d.** Double hyperphoria. **negative v.d.** Vertical divergence in which the left eye deviates upward in relation to the right. **positive v.d.** Vertical divergence in which the right eye deviates upward in relation to the left.

Dixon's mirror telescope (dik'sunz). See under *telescope.*

Dixon Mann's sign (dik'sun manz'). Mann's sign.

DL. Abbreviation for *difference limen.*

D.O. Diploma in Ophthalmology (United Kingdom).

Dobson's test (dob'sunz). See under *test.*

Dogiel's (do-zhe-elz') **cell; corpuscle.** See under the nouns.

dolichostenomelia (dol"ih-ko-sten"o-me'le-ah). Arachnodactyly.

doll's eye sign. Doll's head phenomenon. See under *phenomenon.*

Döllinger's (del'ing-erz) **membrane; ring.** See under the nouns.

Dollond's objective (dōl'ondz). See under *objective.*

Dolman's test (dōl'manz). See under *test.*

Doman-Delacato theory. See under *theory.*

dominance. The fact or state of having the prevailing or controlling influence.

cerebral phi movement d. A visual dominance demonstrated by the perception of apparent movement in either the left half or the right half of the visual field, in a test situation in which the center light of three lights is constantly fixated, either monocularly or binocularly, and the center light is flashed alternatingly with the two side lights. The two side lights may be two actual lights or, with binocular fixation, they may be diplopic images of a single light situated either nearer or farther from the subject than the fixated light. This visual dominance is attributed to a superiority of one half of the visual cortex over the other half.

crossed d. A condition in which the dominant eye and dominant hand are on opposite sides; right-handed and left-eyed, or vice versa.

eye d. Ocular dominance.

ocular d. 1. The superiority of one eye over the other in some perceptual or motor task. The term is usually applied to those superiorities in function which are not based on a difference in visual acuity between the two eyes, or on a dysfunction of the neuromuscular apparatus of one of the eyes. 2. Sighting ocular dominance. **alternating o.d.** Mixed ocular dominance. **directional o.d.** Ocular dominance of the eye with which one ascertains the direction of a point with reference to the self as the center of subjective space. **mixed o.d.** A condition in which one eye is dominant in one function and the other eye is dominant in another function. Syn., *alternating ocular dominance.* **motor o.d.** Ocular dominance based on a superiority of the neuromuscular apparatus of one eye over that of the other; said to be demonstrated by various sighting dominance tests, by the convergence test for ocular dominance, and by other motor tests. **perceptual o.d.** Ocular dominance based on a sensory superiority of one eye over the other rather than on a motor difference between the two eyes. Types of perceptual ocular dominance include rivalry ocular dominance and the dominance demonstrated by the chromatic test. **pseudosensory o.d.** An apparent ocular dominance resulting from a difference in visual acuity between the two eyes. **rivalry o.d.** A perceptual ocular dominance in which the stimulus presented to one eye is perceived for a significantly greater percentage of the time than the stimulus simultaneously presented to the other eye, when rivalry is induced by a difference in the two stimuli. **sighting o.d.** A type of motor ocular dominance in which the same eye is usually or always used in visual tasks requiring unilateral sighting. It is best demonstrated by tests made with the manoptoscope or the V-Scope in which a subject is not aware that he is being required to sight with only one eye. See also *preferred eye.*

visual d. 1. Ocular dominance. 2. A superiority of one member of a paired part of the visual mechanism over the other member of the pair. For example, a dominance of the left half of the visual cortex over the right half. See also *visual laterality.*

dominator, photopic. Granit's term for a retinal element exhibiting spectral sensitivity for a wide spectral band with a maximum corresponding to that of the light-adapted retina containing cones. See also *dominator-modulator theory.*

dominator, scotopic. Granit's term for a retinal element exhibiting spectral sensitivity for a wide spectral band with a maximum corresponding to the dark-adapted retina or to the absorption curve of visual purple. See also *dominator-modulator theory.*

D.O.M.S. Diploma in Ophthalmic Medicine and Surgery (United Kingdom). dom).

Donders' (don'derz) **painful accommodation; corpuscles; experiment; reduced eye; glaucoma; law; line; method; wire optometer; patterns; rings; table; test; theories.** See under the nouns.

Doppler effect (dop'ler). See under *effect.*

D. Opt. Diploma in Ophthalmics (Institute of Optical Science).

dorsalis nasi (dōr-sa'lis na'zi). The nasal artery.

dorsum sellae (dōr'sum sel'i). A plate of bone which forms the posterior boundary of the sella turcica.

D. Orth. Diploma in Orthoptics (British Optical Association).

Doryl (do'ril). A trade name for carbaminoylcholine.

D.O.S. Abbreviation for Doctor of Ocular Science or Doctor of Optometric Science.

dot. 1. A small spot or a small round mark, such as may be made with a pen or a pencil. 2. Anything small and comparatively like a speck.

creek d's. Gunn's dots.

Gunn's d's. Small, white or yellowish nonpathological dots sometimes observed in the eyegrounds, usually in clusters. Syn., *creek dots.*

Mittendorf's d. A white dot seen, with the biomicroscope, 1 or 2 mm nasal to the posterior pole of the crystalline lens. It appears to rest on the posterior lens surface and to serve as a place of attachment for one or several corkscrewlike white threads, remnants of the tunica vasculosa lentis, which hang down and float freely in the vitreous.

Nettleship's d's. Numerous small white dots in the peripheral retina, described by Nettleship, and said to be associated with familial pigment changes and night blindness.

Tay's d's. Yellowish colloid bodies occurring in or near the central region of the retina in Tay's choroiditis.

Trantas' d's. Small white dots in the limbal conjunctiva, described by Trantas, and said to be associated with vernal conjunctivitis.

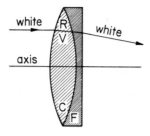

Fig. 14 Achromatic doublet. (From Jenkins and White, *Fundamentals of Optics*, 3d ed. New York: McGraw-Hill, 1957; copyright © 1957; used with permission of McGraw-Hill Book Co.)

doublet (dub'let). A fixed combination of two lenses, as in a telescope objective or a microscope eyepiece.

achromatic d. A combination of two lenses, usually a crown positive and a flint negative, which corrects for chromatic aberration. (See Fig. 14.)

orthoscopic d. A combination of two identical lenses with a stop midway between them, correcting for spherical aberration with respect to the entrance and exit pupils. This system is relatively free of distortion. Syn., *orthoscopic lenses; rectilinear lens.*

separated d. An achromatic optical system employing two thin lenses made of the same glass and separated by a distance equal to half the sum of their focal lengths.

Troutman's air space d. A plastic anterior chamber implant consisting of a biconvex lens and a biconcave lens, separated by an air space, used in uniocular aphakia to correct ametropia and minimize aniseikonia.

Wollaston's d. A simple microscope consisting of a combination of two separated planoconvex lenses whose plane faces are both turned toward the object. The focal lengths of the lenses are in the ratio of 1:3, the stronger lens being the one nearer the object.

douzième (dōō-zyem'). A unit for designating lens thickness, equal to $1/12$ of a ligne, or approximately 0.19 mm. *Obs.*

Dove prism. See under *prism.*

Down's syndrome (downz). See under *syndrome.*

Doyne's (doinz) **cataract; choroiditis; guttate iritis; occluder.** See under the nouns.

Draeger tonometer (dra'ger). See under *tonometer.*

Draper's law (dra'perz). See under *law.*

Dresbach syndrome (dres'bahk). Sickle-cell disease. See under *disease.*

drifts. Slow, smooth, ocular fixation movements of greater amplitude than microsaccades.

drill, lens. A machine with a revolving point, usually a diamond, used to bore holes in lenses to be fitted to rimless mountings.

Driver's test. See under *test.*

driving, alpha. Photic driving.

driving, photic. The stimulation of the eye with a flashing light at frequencies which induce an alteration in the normal alpha rhythm, as evidenced in electroencephalographic recordings of brain waves from the occipital cortex. Syn., *alpha driving.*

drop. 1. In a spectacle lens, the distance of the geometrical or mechanical center below the mounting line. 2. In a spectacle lens, the difference between the distance of the mounting line below the top of the lens and the distance of the mounting line above the bottom of the lens. *Rare.*

drops. A popular name for any solution instilled into the eyes.

dropsy, subchoroidal (drop'se). An accumulation of fluid between the retina and the choroid.

dropsy, subsclerotic (drop'se). An accumulation of fluid between the choroid and the sclera.

droxifilcon. The nonproprietary name of a hydrophilic material of which contact lenses are made.

Druault's (dru'altz) **marginal bundle; theory.** See under the nouns.

drum, optokinetic. Optokinetoscope.

drusen (dru'sen). Small, sharply defined, circular, yellow or white dots lying below the level of the retinal vessels, either discrete or coalesced into larger masses, located throughout the fundus but tending to collect in the region of the macula, around the optic disk, or in the periphery. They may occur in adolescence, but generally do not appear until middle age or later, consist of hyaline material on the lamina vitrea of the choroid, are considered to be formed by secretions of cells of the pigment epithelium due to degenerative changes, and usually do not interfere with vision. Syn., *colloid bodies; hyaline bodies.*

d. of the optic disk. Sharply defined, white or yellow masses of hyaline material on the optic disk, which may protrude over the disk margin and project into the vitreous in grapelike clusters. They are attributed to degenerative changes in the glial cells and may become calcified.

Drysdale (drīz′dāl) **method; principle.** See under *method.*

DSFO. See *Distinguished Service Foundation of Optometry.*

Duane's (du-ānz′) **chart; clinometer; field; phenomenon; rule; screen; syndrome; table; test; theory.** See under the nouns.

Duane-White syndrome (du-ān′-hwīt). See under *syndrome.*

duct. A tube or channel for conveying fluid.

lacrimal d. 1. Each of about a dozen ducts that receive the secretion of both lobes of a lacrimal gland and empty into the lateral superior fornix; one may empty into the lateral inferior fornix. 2. Incorrectly, the lacrimal canaliculus leading from the lacrimal punctum toward the lacrimal sac, or the nasolacrimal duct emptying into the inferior meatus of the nose.

nasolacrimal d. A membranous tube within the bony nasolacrimal canal, connecting the lacrimal sac to the inferior meatus of the nose, for the drainage of tears. This distal portion of the lacrimal apparatus has a mucous membrane lined by pseudostratified columnar epithelium with some goblet cells. Less accurately, the nasal duct.

tear d. 1. Nasolacrimal duct. 2. One of the dozen or so ducts of the lacrimal gland.

duction (duk′shun). 1. Under monocular conditions, the movement of an eye by the extraocular muscles. 2. The movement, or the test for movement, of the two eyes in opposite directions to maintain fusion through prisms, at a fixed testing distance; more correctly termed a *vergence.*

compensating d. Vergence used to overcome existing heterophoria.

jump d. A rapid change in convergence to maintain fusion induced by an instantaneous change in base-in or base-out prism effect; more correctly termed *jump vergence.*

lateral d. The movement, or the test for movement, of the two eyes in opposite directions to maintain fusion through base-in or base-out prism effect, at a fixed testing distance; more correctly termed *induced convergence* or *divergence.*

vertical d. The movement of the two eyes in opposite directions to maintain fusion through base-up or base-down prism effect at a fixed testing distance; more correctly termed *induced supravergence* or *infravergence.*

ductus nasolacrimalis (duk′tus na″zo-lak″rih-mah′lis). Nasolacrimal duct.

Duddell's membrane (dud′elz). Descemet's membrane.

Duhring's disease (dūr′ingz). Dermatitis herpetiformis.

Duke-Elder lamp (dūk-el′der). See under *lamp.*

Dunnington-Berke test. See under *test.*

duochroism (du″o-kro′izm). The property of showing a different shade or hue by reflected light than by transmitted light.

duplicatio supercilii (du-plih-kah′te-o). A rare condition consisting of two rows of eyebrows, one above the other, separated by a clear area.

dura mater (du′rah ma′ter). The outermost tough member of the three meninges covering the brain, the spinal cord, and the optic nerve. At the optic foramen it divides into two layers, the outer becoming continuous with the periorbita the inner forming the dural covering of the optic nerve and becoming continuous with the sclera.

dural sheath (du′ral shēth). Dura mater.

duration of fixation. 1. The time interval between saccadic movements of the eyes, especially while reading. 2. The time of exposure of a tachistoscope.

Durham tonometer. See under *tonometer.*

Dutemps and Cestan sign (du-tahn′-ses-tan′). See under *sign.*

Dvorine's (dvor′ēnz) **charts; plates; stereograms; pseudoisochromatic test.** See under the nouns.

Dx. Diagnosis.

dynamometer (di″nah-mom′eh-ter). 1. An instrument for estimating the magnifying power of lenses. 2. Landolt's ophthalmodynamometer. 3. An instrument for measuring and training relative convergence.

Dynascope (di″nah-skōp′). A small, manually controlled instrument, handheld before the right eye, containing a pair of articulated plane mirrors which may be synchronously rotated to alter the direction of incident light. Light entering the front opening of the instrument is reflected by the first mirror onto the second mirror, which in turn reflects the light through the rear peephole. It is used for fusion and vergence training, and three-dimensional viewing. Syn., *Dynamic Stereoscope; Engelmann Stereoscope.*

dysadaptation (dis-ad″ap-ta′shun). Lack of, or defective, adjustment of the visual mechanism to variations in light intensity.

dysanagnosia (dis-an″ag-no′se-ah). A form of dyslexia in which there is an inability to recognize certain words.

dysantigraphia (dis-an″tih-graf′e-ah, -gra′fe-ah). The inability to copy writing although the words can be seen.

dysaptation (dis″ap-ta′shun). Dysadaptation.

dysautonomia (dis-aw″to-no′me-ah). Riley-Day syndrome.

dyschromasia (dis″kro-ma′ze-ah). Dyschromatopsia.

dyschromatope (dis-kro′mah-tōp″). One having dyschromatopsia.

dyschromatopia (dis″kro-mah-to′pe-ah). Dyschromatopsia.

dyschromatopsia (dis″kro-mah-top′se-ah). Imperfect discrimination of colors; incomplete or partial color blindness. See also *chromatelopsia.* Syn., *dyschromasia.*

dyscoria (dis-ko′re-ah). Abnormality in the shape of the pupil.

dyscrania, neuro-endocrine (dis-krān′e-ah). Pigmentary dystrophy of the retina with optic atrophy, associated with dystrophia adiposo-genitalis, cranial deformity, usually oxycephaly, and imbecility. Syn., *osteo-neuro-endocrine dysplasia.*

dyserethesia (dis″er-e-the′ze-ah). A reduced sensibility to stimuli.

dysgenesis, circumpapillary, of the pigment epithelium. Helicoid peripapillary chorioretinal degeneration.

dysgenesis, mesodermal, of the

cornea and iris (dis-jen′eh-sis). Rieger's disease.

dysgenesis neuro-epithelialis retinae (dis-jen′eh-sis). Leber's disease.

dyskeratosis (dis″ker-ah-to′sis). A disturbance in normal keratinization, resulting, in the eye, in hornification of the epithelial layer of the cornea or conjunctiva.

   benign intraepithelial d. A hereditary dyskeratosis of the conjunctiva, resembling a pterygium, and of the mouth, resembling leukoplakia. The eye lesions may spread to cover the cornea and cause blindness.

dyslexia (dis-lek′se-ah). Partial alexia in which letters but not words may be read, or in which words may be read but not understood.

   dyseidetic d. Lack of ability to perceive whole words or similar configurations as unitary symbols or gestalts.

   dysphoneidetic d. Combined dyseidetic and dysphonetic dyslexia.

   dysphonetic d. Lack of ability to identify visual symbols, particularly letters and words, with sounds.

dysmegalopsia (dis″meg-ah-lop′se-ah). A condition in which the perceptual size of objects is abnormal, termed *micropsia* when smaller, and *macropsia* when larger.

dysmetropsia (dis″met-rop′se-ah). The inability to evaluate properly the measure or size of perceived objects; macropsia or micropsia.

dysmorphia, cervico-oculo-facial (dis-mor′fe-ah). Cervico-oculo-acoustic syndrome.

dysmorphia, mandibulo-oculofacial (dis-mor′fe-ah). A prominent nose "parrot-beak" giving a bird-like appearance to the face, marked hypoplasia of the mandible, and congenital cataract often with microcornea and microphthalmos. Syn., *Hallermann-Streit syndrome.*

dysmorphopsia (dis″mōr-fop′se-ah). A disturbance or anomaly of form visualization.

dysnomia (dis-no′me-ah). Anomia.

Dyson interferometer (di′sun). See under *interferometer.*

dysopia (dis-o′pe-ah). Dysopsia

dysopsia (dis-op′se-ah). Defective or uncomfortable vision.

dysostosis (dis″os-to′sis). Defective bone formation.

craniofacial d., hereditary. A developmental cranial deformity characterized by a knoblike protuberance on the frontal bone, a hooked nose, protruding lower jaw and teeth, divergent strabismus, wide separation and proptosis of the eyes, and optic atrophy. It is familial and is fully developed in the first few months of life. Syn., *Crouzon's disease.*

diabetic exophthalmic d. Schüller-Christian-Hand disease.

d. hypophysaria. Schüller-Christian-Hand disease.

mandibulofacial d. A rare congenital anomaly characterized by antimongoloid oblique palpebral fissures, coloboma of the lower eyelids (sometimes upper), hypoplasia of the facial bones, especially malar and mandible, malformations of the external ears and sometimes middle and inner ears, an abnormally large mouth with high palate and abnormal dentition, fistulae between the mouth and the ears, and tongue-shaped projections of the hairline onto the cheek. Syn., *Franceschetti syndrome; Franceschetti-Zwahlen syndrome; Treacher Collins syndrome.*

d. multiplex. Hurler's disease.

dysphotia (dis-fo'te-ah). Myopia. *Obs.*

dysplasia (dis-pla'se-ah). Abnormal tissue development or growth occurring subsequent to the appearance of the primordial cells.

encephalo-ophthalmic d. Bilateral congenital dysplasia of ocular tissue including the retina, choroid, and optic nerve, and of the central nervous system. The retina is detached and bunched into a mass fused with remnants of the tunica vasculosa lentis. Retinal hemorrhages are frequent and atrophy and gliosis are widespread. Associated ocular anomalies may include microphthalmus, colobomata, cataract, and glaucoma. Neurological symptoms include microcephalus or hydrocephalus and mental deficiency. Skeletal deformities and systemic anomalies may also be present. Syn., *retinal dysplasia; Krause's syndrome.*

d. epiphysialis punctata. Stippled epiphyses.

iridocorneal mesodermal d. Axenfeld's syndrome.

macular d. 1. A congenital defect of the macula lutea usually attributed to intrauterine choroiditis and which shows pigmentation or abnormality of the retinal vessels. 2. A rare congenital condition in which the macula lutea is absent.

oculo-auricular d. Goldenhar's syndrome.

oculodentodigital d. Dysplasia of the extremities, such as campodactyly, syndactyly and polydactyly, of the teeth, and of the eyes, such as microphthalmus and coloboma. Syn., *Meyer-Schwickerath-Weyers syndrome; oculodentodigital syndrome.*

oculovertebral d. A congenital syndrome consisting of malformations of the spine and ribs, unilateral dysplasia of the maxilla resulting in facial asymmetry and dental malocclusion, and unilateral microphthalmos, anophthalmos, or cryptophthalmos. Syn., *oculovertebral syndrome; Weyers-Thier syndrome.*

osteo-neuro-endocrine d. Neuro-endocrine dyscrania.

periosteal d. Osteogenesis imperfecta.

polyostotic fibrous d. A developmental skeletal anomaly characterized by replacement of the cancellous bone and marrow by solid fibrous tissue with a resulting widening of the affected bones. Endocrine dysfunction and skin pigmentation may occur. Involvement of the cranium may produce proptosis, papilledema, and optic atrophy. Syn., *disseminated osteitis fibrosa; fibrous osteodystrophy.*

posterior marginal d. of the cornea. Embryotoxon.

retinal d. 1. Any abnormal differentiation of retinal tissue occurring subsequent to the appearance of the primordial cells. 2. Encephalo-ophthalmic dysplasia.

septo-optic d. Hypoplasia of the optic disk, poor vision, nystagmus, and bitemporal loss of the visual fields due to a congenital agenesis of the septum pellucidum, a cerebral anomaly.

dystrophia (dis-tro'fe-ah). Dystrophy.

d. adiposa corneae. A primary fatty degeneration of the cornea occurring physiologically as an arcus senilis. Only rarely is it pathological, affecting either the central or the peripheral area. Syn., *steatosis corneae; xanthomatosis corneae.*

d. adiposogenitalis. Froehlich's syndrome.

d. annularis. Ring-shaped corneal dystrophy.

d. calcarea corneae. A rare primary degeneration of the cornea in which deposits of calcium phosphate occur in its superficial layers.

d. corneae granulosa. Granular corneal dystrophy.

d. corneae maculosa. Macular corneal dystrophy.

d. corneae reticulata. Latticelike corneal dystrophy.

d. endothelialis corneae. Cornea guttata.

d. epithelialis corneae. Epithelial corneal dystrophy of Fuchs.

d. filiformis profunda corneae. A degeneration of the cornea characterized by fine, wavy, threadlike opacities deep in the stroma, just anterior to Descemet's membrane.

d. marginalis cristallinea. Scintillating punctate opacities in the superficial layers of the corneal stroma in the limbal region. Syn., *Bietti's marginal crystalline corneal dystrophy.*

d. mesodermalis congenita hyperplastica. Marchesani's syndrome.

d. mesodermalis congenita hypoplastica. Arachnodactyly.

d. punctiformis profunda corneae. Deep punctiform corneal dystrophy.

d. uratica corneae. Keratitis urica.

d. urica. Keratitis urica.

◆

DYSTROPHY

dystrophy (dis'tro-fe). 1. Faulty or defective nutrition. 2. Abnormal or defective development. 3. Degeneration.

adiposogenital d. Froehlich's syndrome.

albipunctate d., progressive. Retinitis punctata albescens which progresses with increasing diminution of the visual fields, loss of central vision, night blindness, and some optic atrophy. Cf. *fundus albipunctatus.*

albipunctate d., stationary. Fundus albipunctatus.

Batten's myotonic d. Myotonic dystrophy.

corneal d. Defective nutrition, abnormal development, or degeneration of the cornea. **annular c.d.** Ring-shaped corneal dystrophy. **band-shaped c.d.** A degeneration of the cornea characterized by the slow development of a horizontal gray band in the central area, first appearing as a slight turbidity at the level of Bowman's membrane in which are pathognomonic, small, dark, round holes. The most common form is secondary to iridocyclitis, a less common form is primary and occurs in the apparently normal eyes of the elderly, and the rarest form occurs in children, most of whom have rheumatism associated with a chronic iritis. It may also follow trauma due to exposure to irritants. Syn., *zonular corneal dystrophy; keratitis petrificans; band keratopathy; zonular keratopathy.* **band-shaped nodular c.d.** Bietti's nodular corneal dystrophy. **Bietti's marginal crystalline c.d.** Dystrophia marginalis cristallinea. **Bietti's nodular c.d.** A degeneration of the cornea characterized by elevated nodular opacities distributed in a horizontal band-shaped area within the palpebral fissure, usually bilateral and mainly found in hot arid regions. Syn., *band-shaped nodular corneal dystrophy.* **Braley's polymorphic c.d.** A rare, familial, bilateral dystrophy characterized by numerous, variously sized, irregular yellow masses in deep retinal layers around the macular zone, sometimes in a confluent ring less dense in the center than in the surrounding retina, and with a pigmented lesion at the fovea. **Bückler's annular c.d.** A rare dominant progressive degeneration of the corneal epithelium and Bowman's membrane, commencing in childhood and characterized by thin, irregularly shaped, threadlike grayish opacities which gradually merge and obscure vision. The condition occurs in episodes accompanied by pain, subsides at puberty, and reappears about two decades later in association with ulcers. Syn., *Bückler's type IV corneal dystrophy.* **Bückler's type I c.d.** Granular corneal dystrophy. **Bückler's type II c.d.** Macular corneal dystrophy. **Bückler's type III c.d.** Latticelike corneal dystrophy. **Bückler's type IV c.d.** Bückler's annular corneal dystrophy. **Cogan's epithelial microcystic c.d.** A nonhereditary bilateral corneal dystrophy occurring in adults and characterized by variously shaped, grayish-white corneal epithelial cysts seen with retroillumination and which appear "putty-like" grayish-yellow with focal illumination. Symptoms are minimal and vision is unaffected unless the lesions are clustered in the pupillary zone. **crumblike c.d.** Granular corneal dystrophy. **crystalline c.d.** A dominant, inherited, bilateral and symmetrical degeneration of the cornea occurring early in life and characterized by numerous fine needlelike opacities in the anterior stroma, often forming a central ring pattern. Syn., *Schnyder's corneal dystrophy.* **deep filiform c.d.** Dystrophia filiformis profunda corneae. **deep punctiform c.d.** A hereditary, bilateral, corneal dystrophy, described by Pillat, characterized by deep, grayish to bluish, fine punctate and short linear opacities in the central area, surrounded by a clear normal zone, and numerous, short, glassy, radial lines at the limbus peripheral to the clear area. **Dimmer's c.d.** Latticelike corneal dystrophy. **ectatic marginal c.d.** Peripheral corneal ectasia. **endothelial c.d.** Cornea guttata. **epithelial c.d. of Fuchs.** A degeneration of the cornea first described by Fuchs as an epithelial dystrophy, but later found to be dependent on a prior endothelial dystrophy. It occurs most commonly in females past the age of 50, the epithelial changes start with an edema consisting of vesicles which later become opacities, and after an extremely slow course, the cornea becomes opaque and insensitive. **epithelial diffuse c.d.** A dominant familial degeneration of the corneal epithelium commencing in infancy and involving Bowman's membrane in the later stages. Repeated acute attacks leave scars and lead to reduced visual acuity. **epithelial juvenile c.d. of Kraupa.** A degeneration of the cornea occurring early in life and involving the surface epithelium and, to a lesser extent, the corneal stroma. **Fehr's spotted c.d.** Macular corneal dystrophy. **fingerprint c.d.** A corneal dystrophy characterized by concentric contoured lines in the epithelium, resembling a fingerprint, thought to be secondary to splitting of superficial layers of Bowman's membrane and a stage in the development of Cogan's epithelial microcystic corneal dystrophy. Fingerprint c.d. occurs equally in men and women, is more common in older age groups, and is usually asymptomatic. **fleck c.d.** François' speckled corneal dystrophy. **Fleischer's whorl-like c.d.** Vortex corneal dystrophy. **François' cloudy**

central c.d. A rare, inherited, familial, bilateral dystrophy of the corneal stroma characterized by numerous, small, grayish, snowflakelike opacities, primarily occurring in the pupillary area and the deep layers. It is unaccompanied by pain or inflammation, is essentially nonprogressive, and vision remains unimpaired. **François' speckled c.d.** An autosomal, dominantly inherited, bilateral degeneration of the corneal stroma characterized by diffusely scattered dot opacities. It is either congenital or occurs in early life, is benign and nonprogressive, and vision is unimpaired. **Fuchs' c.d.** See *dystrophy, corneal, epithelial of Fuchs.* **granular c.d.** A dominant inherited degeneration of the cornea with onset usually at about 5 years of age, in which, initially, small, superficial, and deep, white dots occur in the center of the cornea or form radiating lines from the corneal center. The lesions gradually increase in size and have irregular shapes and patterns. Vision is at most only mildly affected. Syn., *Bückler's type I corneal dystrophy; crumblike corneal dystrophy; Groenouw's nodular type I corneal dystrophy.* **Groenouw's macular type II c.d.** Macular corneal dystrophy. **Groenouw's nodular type I c.d.** Granular corneal dystrophy. **Haab-Dimmer c.d.** Latticelike corneal dystrophy. **hereditary, deep c.d.** A rare, autosomal, dominantly inherited, bilateral degeneration of the cornea characterized by vesicularlike areas surrounded by gray polymorphous opacities in the corneal endothelium, in Descemet's membrane, and occasionally in the deep stroma. It is either congenital or occurs early in life, remains limited to the posterior cornea, and is essentially nonprogressive. Syn., *posterior polymorphous corneal dystrophy; polymorphous deep degeneration of the cornea.* **Koby's c.d.** A bilateral progressive degeneration of the corneal epithelium with formation of linear fissures in Bowman's membrane, occurring in middle-aged, healthy persons without inflammation or discomfort. A faint opalescence bounded by a line of relief appears in the central region of the cornea, the underlying stroma is hazy, and vision deteriorates progressively. **Kraupa's epithelial c.d.** See *dystrophy, corneal epithelial juvenile of Kraupa.* **latticelike c.d.** A slowly progressive, dominant, familial degeneration of the superficial stroma of the cornea, beginning occasionally in infancy but usually at puberty, characterized by the deposit of fine lines of hyalinelike material in a cobweb, star-shaped, or crisscross formation. The lines increase in number and thickness into a diffuse opacification in later life, with vision mildly or severly affected. Syn., *Haab's degeneration; lattice degeneration of the cornea; reticular degeneration of the cornea; Bückler's type III corneal dystrophy; Dimmer's corneal dystrophy; reticular corneal dystrophy; lattice keratitis; reticular keratitis.* **lipid c.d.** Any of several corneal dystrophies in which lipoid deposits are found in the cornea. **macular c.d.** A recessive familial degeneration initially affecting Bowman's membrane and then the surface epithelium and stroma. It commences in the first decade of life as a diffuse subepithelial opacification, with patches of greater density, and gradually increases in intensity, especially centrally, until, about the age of 30, little vision remains. Syn., *Bückler's type II corneal dystrophy; Groenouw's macular type II corneal dystrophy; Fehr's spotted corneal dystrophy.* **Maeder-Danis deep filiform c.d.** A corneal dystrophy seen in association with keratoconus in which the deep layers of the corneal stroma, just anterior to Descemet's membrane, contain bilateral opacities in corkscrew-shaped filaments. **marginal c.d.** Arcus senilis. **Meesmann's c.d.** A dominant, hereditary, bilateral dystrophy involving only the corneal epithelium. It commences at about 18 months of age, with gradual progression, and is characterized by numerous small punctate opacities regularly distributed throughout the epithelium. **nodular c.d.** Granular corneal dystrophy. **Pillat's parenchymatous c.d.** Dystrophic corneal changes observed in two sisters, consisting of punctate opacities of varying size in the middle and deeper layers of the stroma appearing blue-gray in direct illumination and transparent on retro-illumination. Between the opacities the stroma was clear and at the periphery of the cornea at the limbus, and separate from the central changes, were numerous glasslike lines, about 0.75 mm in length, in the anterior layers of the cornea. **posterior polymorphous c.d.** Deep hereditary corneal dystrophy. **Reis-Bückler's ringlike c.d.** Bückler's annular corneal dystrophy. **reticular c.d.** Latticelike corneal dystrophy. **reticular pigmentary of Sjögren c.d.** An autosomal recessive familial corneal dystrophy characterized by a net-shaped or reticular pigmentation extending over the posterior pole of the fundus and a pigmented ring around the macula. **ring-shaped c.d.** A bilateral, annular or ring-shaped degeneration, possibly dominant familial, affecting Bowman's membrane. The onset is early, acute attacks are frequent, and eventually poor vision results. In the late stage, the cornea has a moplike appearance. Syn., *dystrophia annularis; annular corneal dystrophy.* **Salzmann's c.d.** An early hypertrophic and later degenerative change in the superficial corneal tissues, occurring in persons previously affected with phlyctenular keratitis. It is rare, noninflammatory, slowly progressive, and is characterized by the presence of several bluish-white nodules on the surface of the cornea. It is nonfamilial, usually unilateral, mainly affects females, and may appear at any age. **Schnyder's c.d.** Crystalline corneal dystrophy. **spotted c.d.** Macular corneal dystrophy. **Terrien's marginal c.d.** Peripheral corneal ectasia. See under *ectasia, corneal.* **total c.d.** Degeneration of the cornea involving all of its layers. **uric c.d.** A rare corneal dystrophy commencing near the limbus and progressing centrally, characterized by the deposition of uric acid crystals in the stroma and epithelium. It is accompanied by corneal vascularization and frequently by recurring ulcers and anterior uveitis. Syn., *keratitis urica.* **vitelline c.d.** Best's disease. **vortex c.d.** A rare, dominantly inherited, corneal dystrophy involving the superficial layers of the cornea and characterized by small brownish opacities on Bowman's membrane, arranged in a whirlpool-shaped line formation radiating out from the center of the cornea. Syn., *cornea verticillata; Fleischer's whorl-like corneal dystrophy; whorl-shaped opacity.* **Waardenburg-Jonkers c.d.** A dominant hereditary corneal dystrophy appearing at about the end of the first year of life as acute eye irritation associated with minute snow-flakelike spots in the corneal stroma which later spread to Bowman's membrane and the epithelium. Vision is mildly affected. **zonular c.d.** Band-shaped corneal dystrophy.

cranio-carpo-tarsal d. A congenital condition characterized by clubfoot, flat face with long upper lip and small mouth, ulnar deviation of the hands, enophthalmos, epicanthus, hypertelorism, and strabismus. Intelligence is normal. Syn., *Freeman-Sheldon syndrome.*

dermo-chondro-corneal d. A dystrophy due to a disturbance in the metabolism of polysaccharides and characterized by deformities of the hands commencing between the ages of 1 and 2, of the feet about the age of 5, xanthomata of the skin also about age 5, and bilateral corneal dystrophy, consisting of superficial and central opacities, appearing about age 8 or 9. The face spine, and cranium are unaffected and intelligence is normal. Syn., *François' dermo-chondro-corneal dystrophy; osteochondral-dermal-corneal dystrophy.*

François' dermo-chondro-corneal d. Dermo-chondro-corneal dystrophy.

heredomacular d., infantile. Best's disease.

hyaloideoretinal d. Vitreoretinal degeneration.

Laurence-Moon-Biedl d. Laurence-Moon-Biedl syndrome.

myotonic d. A heredofamilial disease characterized by a selective atrophy of muscles with lessened power to relax after contraction, baldness, atrophy of the gonads, premature senility, mental enfeeblement, and such ocular manifestations as fine punctate subcapsular lenticular opacities, low intraocular pressure, ptosis, enophthalmos, and occasionally lagophthalmos or blepharoconjunctivitis. Syn., *Batten's myotonic dystrophy; Batten-Steinert syndrome; Steinert's disease.*

oculopharyngeal d. Weakness of the orbicularis oculi muscles and of the pharyngeal muscles causing dysphagia, occurring in conjunction with hereditary external ophthalmoplegia.

osteochondral-dermal-corneal d. Dermo-chondro-corneal dystrophy.

polyvisceral d. Dystrophy characterized by low blood calcium and high blood phosphate. Clinical findings include stunted growth, thick skin, teeth and nail anomalies, abnormal thirst, polyurea, blue sclerae and cataracts. Syn., *Martin-Albright syndrome.*

progressive tapetochoroidal d. Choroideremia.

reticular d. of the retina. A rare progressive dystrophy of the pigment epithelium of the retina, characterized initially by the accumulation of pigment at the fovea; progresses to the formation of a cecocentral network of black pigmented lines with enlarged black spots at their junctions. In the later stages the network gradually disintegrates and fades, and small white areas appear in the deep retina. It is either congenital or occurs in early childhood and may be accompanied by deafmutism.

retinal d., primary pigmentary. Retinitis pigmentosa.

senile macular d. Macular degeneration occurring in the aged without apparent clinical cause and characterized by fine pigmentary stippling which becomes denser as the disease progresses, with a corresponding loss in vision. It typically commences unilaterally and eventually becomes bilateral.

Sorsby's macular d. A rare dominantly inherited dystrophy of the macula which is typically progressive and, in the elderly, is sometimes indistinguishable from senile macular degeneration. Vision is but slightly affected in childhood, except for color vision anomalies, but is significantly reduced in adult life.

Stargardt's foveal d. Stargardt's disease.

tapetoretinal d. Tapetoretinal degeneration.

vitreoretinal d. Vitreoretinal degeneration.

◆

dysversion of the optic disk (dis-ver'-zhun). An apparent tilting of the plane of the optic nerve head away from its normally more tangential position, usually bilateral and probably due to anomalous insertion of the optic stalk into the optic vesicle.

E. Abbreviation for *emmetropia* or *esophoria.*

E. Symbol for (1) *illumination;* (2) *coefficient of ocular rigidity.*

E$_s$. Equivalent sphere illumination.

Eales's disease (ēlz'es). See under *disease.*

Eames test (ēmz). See under *test.*

earthlight. Sunlight reflected from the earth that faintly illuminates the dark part of the moon, best seen during the moon's crescent phases. Syn., *earthshine.*

Eastman chart (ēst'man). See under *chart.*

Ebbecke's theory (eb'ek-ēz). See under *theory.*

Ebbinghaus' (eb'ing-hows) **figure; visual illusion; law.** See under the nouns.

ecblepharos (ek-blef'ah-rōs). A prosthesis mounted on the posterior side of a spectacle frame to simulate the appearance of an eye, usually consisting of a metal piece on which an eye and the surrounding structures are painted.

eccanthus (ek-kan'thus). A fleshy growth at the angle of the eyelids.

ecchymosis of the conjunctiva (ek"-ih-mo'sis). An extravasation of blood under the bulbar conjunctiva; a subconjunctival hemorrhage.

ecchymosis of the eyelid (ek"ih-mo'-sis). An extravasation of blood into the loose areolar tissue of the eyelid, or the resulting discoloration of the skin. Syn., *black eye; suggilation of the eyelid.*

eccle rest (ek'l rest). A cork or zylonite pad attachable to the underside of a saddle bridge to distribute the weight of the frame over a larger area.

ECG. Abbreviation for *electrocorticogram.*

echelette (esh-eh-let'). A diffraction grating designed by R. W. Wood for the production of infrared spectra, made by ruling parallel V-shaped grooves in a polished metal plate.

echelle (esh-el'). A diffraction grating with a facet width of several hundred microns, hence intermediate between the narrow grooved grating with only a few microns and the echelon grating with thousands.

echelon (esh'eh-lon). A type of diffraction grating consisting of a number of rectangular blocks of glass all cut from a single planeparallel plate of optical glass and arranged in the form of a flight of steps, each step forming a line of the grating.

echinophthalmia (e-kin"of-thal'me-ah). Inflammation of the eyelid margins with an accompanying bristlelike appearance of the lashes. *Obs.*

echogram, ocular. A recording of the reflection of ultrasonic waves from the structures of the eye, used to detect and locate intraocular tumors and to determine distances between intraocular structures.

echography, orbital (eh-kog'grah-fe). Orbital ultrasonography.

echondroma (ek"on-dro'mah). A rare tumor of the eyelid occurring, usually, in the tarsal plate.

echophotony (ek"o-fot'o-ne). The association of certain colors with certain sounds.

echothiophate iodide (ek"o-thi'o-fāt). An anticholinesterase drug with a long duration of action (1-4 weeks) following a 10-45 minute onset; used for the treatment of primary open angle glaucoma and accommodative esotropia. The generic name for *Phospholine Iodide.*

l'Ecole d'Optique Lunettier de Lille. An ophthalmic optics school in Lille, France.

l'Ecole Supérieure Libre d'Optometrie. An optometry school at Bures-Sur-Yvette, France.

ectasia (ek-ta′se-ah). Dilatation, or distention, of a hollow organ or a tubular vessel.

    corneal e. A forward bulging of the cornea as a result of intraocular pressure against corneal tissue which has been weakened by trauma, ulceration, atrophy, or inflammation. **peripheral c.e.** Ectasia of the peripheral cornea resulting from idiopathic progressive degeneration of the marginal corneal tissue. The condition commences with an opacity resembling an arcus senilis, except that the clear zone between it and the sclera is vascularized. A gutterlike furrow appears in this area and is followed by the ectasia. Syn., *senile marginal atrophy; ectatic marginal corneal dystrophy; Terrien's marginal corneal dystrophy; peripheral furrow keratitis.*

    scleral e. A bulging or distention of the sclera which may be total, as in buphthalmos, or partial, as in staphyloma. **peripapillary s.e.** An ectasia of the peripapillary sclera resulting in an ophthalmoscopic picture of a deeply recessed optic disk.

ectiris (ek-ti′ris). The anterior endothelium of the iris.

ectochoroidea (ek″to-ko-roid′e-ah). The outer layer of the choroid; the suprachoroid.

ectocornea (ek″to-kŏr′ne-ah). The anterior epithelium of the cornea.

ectodermosis erosiva pluriorificialis (ek″to-der-mo′sis). Stevens-Johnson syndrome.

ectopia (ek-to′pe-ah). Malposition or displacement of a part.

    e. lentis. Displacement, subluxation, or malposition of the crystalline lens.

    e. maculae. Malposition of the macula, either congenital or acquired, and possibly resulting in reduced acuity, metamorphopsia, or strabismus.

    e. oculi. Displacement or malposition of the eyeball in the orbit.

    e. pupillae. A marked displacement of the pupil from its normal position. Syn., *corectopia.*

    e. tarsi. A congenital ectopia in which the tarsus is separated from the rest of the eyelid.

ectorbital (ekt′ŏr-bih″tal). Situated upon or pertaining to the temporal portion of the orbit.

ectoretina (ek″to-ret′ih-nah). The pigment epithelium of the retina.

ectropion (ek-tro′pe-on). A rolling or turning outward (eversion) as of the margin of an eyelid. Syn., *reflexio palpebrarum.*

    atonic e. Ectropion due to loss of muscular tone, particularly of the orbicularis oculi muscle. Loss of skin tone may also contribute to the eversion.

    cicatricial e. Ectropion due to scar tissue on the margins or the surrounding surfaces of the eyelids.

    e. luxurians. Ectropion sarcomatosum.

    mechanical e. Ectropion due to pressure from behind the eyelid. It may occur from a markedly thickened conjunctiva, as in trachoma, from tumors, or from an enlarged eyeball (buphthalmos).

    paralytic e. Ectropion of the lower eyelid, due to facial paralysis involving the orbicularis oculi muscle.

    e. of the pigment layer. Spreading of the pigment layer from the posterior iris surface around the pupillary margin to the anterior iris surface, usually after postinflammatory atrophy.

    e. sarcomatosum. A sequela to senile ectropion in which the conjunctiva, due to exposure, hypertrophies and produces granulation-like masses which accentuate the original ectropion. Syn., *ectropion luxurians.*

    senile e. In the aged, ectropion of the lower eyelid due to atrophic changes in the eyelid structure, especially in the orbicularis oculi muscle and the lateral palpebral ligament.

    spastic e. Ectropion due to contraction of the orbicularis oculi muscle together with other conditions, such as a swollen or thickened conjunctiva, staphyloma of the cornea, or a prominent or bulging eyeball. It may occur in either the upper or the lower eyelid, or in both.

    e. uveae. A turning of the pigment epithelium of the posterior iris over the pupillary margin to the anterior surface, seen as a narrow black rim of the pupil or, if extending further, as a black sector of the iris. It may occur as a congenital anomaly, or pathologically as in glaucoma or atrophy of the iris.

ectropium (ek-tro'pe-um). Ectropion.

Eddowes' (ed'ōz) **disease; syndrome.** See under the nouns.

edema (e-de'mah). An excessive amount of fluid, either intracellular or intercellular, in the tissues of the body or in body cavities.

    angioneurotic e. A generalized, probably hereditary allergic reaction characterized by noninflammatory swelling of subcutaneous tissues and mucous membranes, with marked predilection for the face, especially the eyelids and lips, and for the viscera. It may subside in hours or remain for days, and may recur either frequently or infrequently. In the eye, it may affect the cornea, conjunctiva, or uvea. Syn., *Quincke's disease.*

    Berlin's e. Commotio retinae.

    cilio-choroidal e. Fluid accumulation in the choroid and ciliary body especially in the perichoroidal space; usually termed *detached choroid.*

    Iwanoff's cystic e. Cystic degeneration of the retina.

    macular vesicular e. Cystic degeneration of the macula.

    preretinal e. of Guist. Central angiospastic retinopathy.

edge. 1. The border of circumferential surface of an ophthalmic lens, usually cut, ground, or polished parallel to the lens axis for mounting in a rimless frame, or to a bevel or roof-shaped surface for insertion in an eyewire or a plastic frame. 2. To grind the periphery of a lens to a desired shape and profile.

    refracting e. The line of intersection of the two surface planes of a prism.

Edge-Cote. Trade name for a coating applied to the circumferential surface of a minus spectacle lens, usually of a color that blends with the frame eyewire to make its edge thickness less conspicuous.

edger. A machine with a rotating, wet, abrasive stone for grinding the margins of an ophthalmic lens to a desired shape.

edging. The process of forming a lens to exact size and shape and of putting on

the type of edge required for a particular mounting after it has been roughly cut to size and shape.

Edinger-Westphal nucleus (ed'ing-er-vest'fal). See under *nucleus.*

edipism (ed'ih-pizm). Intentional self-inflicted injury to the eye.

Edmond's chart (ed'mundz). See under *chart.*

Edridge-Green (ed'rij-grēn') **lamp; test; theory.** See under the nouns.

edrophonium (ed"ro-fo'ne-um). An anticholinesterase agent having a very short duration of action, therefore useful as a diagnostic agent in myasthenia gravis but not for therapy. The generic name for *Tensilon.*

EDTA. Ethylenediamine tetraacetate.

Edward syndrome (ed'wahrd). Trisomy 18 syndrome. See under *syndrome.*

EEG. Abbreviation for *electroencephalogram.*

◆

EFFECT

effect. The consequence or result of an action.

    Abney's e. Abney's phenomenon.

    autokinetic e. Autokinetic visual illusion.

    Ball e. The desaturation of an intermittent train of monochromatic light of short wavelength.

    Bezold-Brücke e. Bezold-Brücke phenomenon.

    Broca-Sulzer e. A change in perceived brightness of light of constant illumination with varied durations of flash, maximum values being obtained for intermediate durations. Syn., *Broca-Sulzer phenomenon.*

    Brücke-Bartley e. The increased brightness of intermittent stimulation (illumination) over continuous illumination of the same intensity. The Brücke effect proper is the effect gained by using a revolving disk with dark and light sectors and comparing it to a solid surface similar to the light sector. The Bartley effect proper is produced by using a motionless surface intermittently illuminated and comparing it to a continuously illuminated one. See also *brightness enhancement.*

    chartreuse e. A phenomenon of dichroism occurring in a liquid under varying conditions of volume or concentration. The name is derived from the chartreuse liqueur which appears deep ruby red in the flagon and brilliant emerald green when poured into a glass.

Compton e. The acquisition of energy and momentum by an electron at rest when a photon of energy collides with it. The photon flies off in a direction different from that of incidence and with a loss of energy. The energy imparted to the electron plus the energy lost by the photon equals the energy of the incident photon. The effect is demonstrated experimentally with x-rays or γ-rays and is considered to be evidence for the existence of photons.

Coriolis e. Disintegration of visual and other perceptual reference in space resulting from stimulation with acceleration in one set of semicircular canals with deceleration in another set and virtual disintegration of sensory perception and motor performance.

Cornsweet e. Cornsweet edge illusion.

Cotton e. Circular dichroism.

Cotton-Mouton magneto-optic e. The creation of double refraction in certain liquids when situated in a magnetic field.

crumple e., of tears. A shimmering "wet-silk" appearance of innumerable horizontal folds of the corneal tear film surface seen under the broad beam of a slit lamp while the eyelids are closing.

dimming e. An enhancement or a recovery of either a chromatic or an achromatic afterimage when the field upon which the afterimage is projected is reduced in intensity.

Doppler e. A change in the frequency of waves, as of sound or light, which occurs when the distance between the source and an observer is changing. The wave frequency increases with decreasing distance and decreases with increasing distance; e.g., as a star recedes from or approaches the earth, its color is shifted toward red or violet, respectively.

end e. In a series of chromatic samples of the same dominant wavelength and luminance arranged on a neutral background in order of purity, the appearance of the end sample, the purest, being more saturated than it would be if followed by a still purer sample.

Faraday's e. The rotation of the plane of vibration of plane-polarized light as it passes through glass which has been made optically active by subjection to a strong magnetic field.

geometric size e. A rotatory displacement of the frontal plane horopter around the point of fixation, away from the eye whose ocular image is larger in the horizontal meridian, as in real or induced aniseikonia.

Heinrich's e. The attribute of tridimensionality in monocular space perception resulting from the fact that with any given accommodation every object in space has a characteristic retinal image form unlike that obtained for any other position in space.

Helmholtz-Kohlrausch e. A lack of linear additivity in direct comparison, heterochromatic photometry, as manifested, for example, in a mixture of a red and green, each of which has been matched to a standard white, being judged less white than a white equal to twice the luminance of the original standard. Syn., *Kohlrausch effect; Kohlrausch phenomenon.*

Helson-Judd e. For a given light adaptation level, objects having reflectances above that level arouse responses which tend to take on the hue produced by the illuminant, objects having reflectances below that level arouse responses that tend to take on the hue of the afterimage complementary, and objects of low purity relative to the weighted mean chromaticity of the field and having reflectances about equal to that of the adaptation level tend to appear as neutral or achromatic.

Hoefer e. With a fixated object, *F*, a second laterally adjustable object, *P*, in the same apparent frontoparallel plane, and a third object, *R*, beyond the frontoparallel plane and on the line of sight of one eye, *L*, but not visible to that eye, the object *P* must be more displaced laterally to make *R* and *P* and *F* and *R* appear to subtend the same angle with respect to the other eye when one eye, *L*, is occluded, than when both eyes are open.

Hubble e. Red shift.

induced size e. A rotation of the frontal plane horopter around the point of fixation toward the eye whose ocular image is larger in the vertical meridian. The effect is as if the horizontal meridian of the other ocular image were larger.

jack-in-the-box e. Jack-in-the-box phenomenon.

Kerr electro-optic e. The creation of double refraction in certain isotropic substances when situated in a strong electric field so that they behave optically as a uniaxial crystal with the optic axis parallel to the field direction. Syn., *electro-optical birefringence.*

Kohlrausch e. Helmholtz-Kohlrausch effect.

Köllner e. The initial momentary appearance of a bipartite color field when a white surface is viewed through two different color filters, one before the right eye and the other before the left. The field to the right of the fixation point is of the color of the right filter, and the field to the left of the fixation point is of the color of the left filter. The effect is attributed to a fleeting binasal hemianopsia and is followed immediately by binocular rivalry or fusion.

Liebmann e. Loss of clarity and fading of a colored figure into its neutral background when the figure and ground are equally luminous and fixation is constant on the figure. Syn., *Liebmann phenomenon.*

Mach-Dvořák e. Mach-Dvořák phenomenon.

Mandelbaum e. The tendency to focus the eye on resolvable contours in an intervening transparent surface or plane while viewing a distant object.

Marx e. Decrease of the energy of a photoelectric emission resulting from simultaneous incidence of radiation of lower frequency than that causing the emission.

McCollough e. A visual aftereffect of color related to the orientation of colored lines or edges, whereby a grid of vertical black lines is seen to have a different colored background than a grid of horizontal black lines, following pre-exposure to vertical lines of one color and to horizontal lines of another color.

moiré e. Moiré pattern.

O'Brien e. O'Brien edge illusion.

off e. Off response.

on e. On response.

on-off e. On-off response.

photochemical e. A chemical change of a substance as a result of exposure to light, as in bleaching of the visual purple.

photoconductive e. An increase in electrical conductivity due to a change in resistance produced by absorption of radiation.

photoelectric e. The emission of electrons from a cathode plate as the result of incident light.

pincushion e. Pincushion distortion.

pleated drape e. of tears. The formation of "rolls" of oil just below the upper eyelid margin while the lid is being lowered.

practice e. The effect of repetition on a perceptual or motor function. The nature and magnitude of the effect depends not only on the number of repetitions but also on the attitude and motivation of the subject, as well as the manner in which it is done.

prismatic e. The bending of a ray of light by a prism or as though by a prism; the prismatic equivalent of the bending of a ray of light traversing a lens peripheral to the optical center.

Pulfrich e. The apparently ellipsoid or circular excursion of a pendulum actually swinging in a plane perpendicular to the direction of view when a light-absorbing filter is placed in front of one eye. Syn., *Pulfrich stereophenomenon.*

Purkinje's e. Purkinje's phenomenon.

Raman e. In certain substances, the occurrence of scattered light of wavelength differing slightly from that of the incident light. It differs from fluorescence in that the incident wavelength exhibiting the effect does not correspond to an absorption line or band of the substance, the intensity of the scattered light is much less, and the wavelength of the scattered light shifts with the wavelength of the incident light.

Roenne's e. Roenne's phenomenon.

rolled scum e. of tears. A rolled collection of tear solids and oil in the form of a small, raised, horizontal line extending across the corneal surface at approximately the level of the lower pupillary margin after the eyelids are opened.

spreading e. of Bezold. The appearance of a spot of color as being darker when surrounded by a black rim, and of being lighter when surrounded by a white rim. The black rim creates an apparent increase in saturation and the white rim an apparent decrease, an effect opposite to that expected on the basis of simultaneous contrast.

Stark e. The broadening and splitting of emission lines in a gaseous spectrum when subjected to a strong electric field.

Stiles-Crawford e. 1. *Of the first kind:* the difference in stimulus effectiveness (brightness) of two pencils of light incident on the same retinal point, one passing through the center of the pupil and the other passing through an eccentric part of the pupil, the central pencil producing a more intense response. 2. *Of the second kind:* the difference in perceived hue and saturation of two pencils of light of the same wavelength incident on the same retinal point, one passing through the center of the pupil and the other passing through an eccentric part of the pupil, the eccentric pencil appearing desaturated and shifted in hue slightly toward the red end of the spectrum, except for wavelengths near 526 mμ, which appear more saturated and shifted slightly toward the blue end of the spectrum.

Talbot e. The experience of continuous light from a rapidly intermittent source, but of an intensity equivalent to that produced if the total amount of light were equally distributed in time; the phenomenon giving rise to Talbot's law.

theta e. The apparent circulating movement of a spot of light seen through a red filter around the same spot seen by the other eye through a rotating prism.

Thomson e. A failure of two very small areas of the central visual field, which are matched precisely in hue for yellow wavelengths, to match either longer or shorter wavelengths. This effect is said to present evidence for the cluster hypothesis.

Thouless e. Underestimation of the extent of rotation of a target by approximately half of the actual amount.

trace e's. The effects, left by a perception or an experience, which influence and modify the nature of a later perception or experience. Memory consists of the organization of trace effects. Learning consists of the influence of trace effects upon later perceptual and motor activities.

Troxler's e. Troxler's phenomenon.

Tyndall e. Scattering of light by small particles suspended in a liquid or a gas, thus rendering the particles visible. Syn., *Tyndall phenomenon.*

Voigt e. Magnetic double refraction.

Zeeman e. The splitting of each line in a spectrum into three or more when the source is placed in a powerful magnetic field.

Zuber e. The increase of duration of the fixation pause between saccades associated with increase of reading information to be processed.

◆

effectivity. The curvature of a wavefront at a given point of reference with respect to an optical system. For example, an ophthalmic lens may be said to produce a wavefront with a given effectivity at the cornea. Cf. *effective power.*

efferent (ef'er-ent). Carrying away from a main structure or organ, as a motor neuron carrying impulses away from the central nervous system.

efficacy (ef'ih-kah-se). The power to produce an effect.

luminous e. of a light source. The quotient of the total luminous flux emitted by the source to the total power input to the source. In the case of an electric lamp, efficacy is expressed in lumens per watt.

luminous e. of radiant flux. The quotient of total luminous flux divided by total radiant flux, expressed in lumens per watt. **spectral l.e. of r.f.** The quotient of the luminous flux at a given wavelength divided by the radiant flux at that wavelength, expressed in lumens per watt. Syn., *luminosity factor; visibility factor.*

efficiency. 1. The ability or capacity to produce desired results or to perform an action; competency. 2. The ratio of the output of energy or work, as from a machine or a storage battery, to the input of energy.

e. of a light source. The ratio of the total luminous flux to the total power input, expressed in lumens per watt.

luminaire e. The ratio of luminous flux (lumens) emitted by a luminaire to that emitted by the lamp or lamps used therein.

luminous e. Luminous efficacy of radiant flux. See under *efficacy.*

quantum e. A ratio indicating the number of molecules which will react per quantum of light energy absorbed, provided the quantum energy is sufficient to activate the molecule or molecules concerned. The ratio may be less than, equal to, or greater than unity.

spectral luminous e., photopic. Spectral luminous efficiency of radiant flux obtained with photopic vision; identical to the Y values of the spectral tristimulus values adopted by the CIE in 1931.

spectral luminous e. of radiant flux. The ratio of the luminous efficacy for a given wavelength to the value at the wavelength of maximum luminous efficacy. Syn., *relative luminosity factor; relative visibility factor; relative luminosity.*

spectral luminous e., scotopic. Spectral luminous efficiency of radiant flux obtained by dark-adapted observers.

visual e. 1. The ability to perform visual tasks easily and comfortably. 2. A rating used in computing compensation for ocular injuries, based on a formula adopted by the American Medical Association and incorporating certain measurable functions of central acuity, field vision, and ocular motility. 3. The Snellen acuity fraction expressed in per cent. **industrial v.e.** A rating based on any of several scales, tables, or formulas adopted for computing or specifying visual competence or adequateness for industrial employment or for determining compensation in case of ocular injury. See also *visual efficiency.*

Egger's line (eg'erz). See under *line.*

egilops (e'jih-lops). An abscess at the inner canthus.

egocenter (e"go-sen'ter). A point of reference in, or identified with, the self, usually between the eyes, in relation to which absolute judgments of distance and direction of external objects are made.

Ehlers-Danlos syndrome (a'lerz-dan'los). Meekrin-Ehlers-Danlos syndrome.

Ehrlich-Türk line (ār'lik-tĕrk). Line of Türk.

eiconometer (i"ko-nom'eh-ter). Eikonometer.

eidetic imagery (i-det'ik im'ij-re). See under *imagery.*

eidetiker (i-det'ih-ker). One having the ability of eidetic imagery.

eidoptometry (i"dop-tom'eh-tre). The measurement of the acuteness of form vision.

eikonometer (i"ko-nom'eh-ter). 1. Any instrument used for measuring aniseikonia. 2. *Iconometer*, q.v.

space e. An instrument, designed for the measurement of aniseikonia, using a target, the parts of which are seen three-dimensionally in space. Introduction of magnification by means of adjustable optical systems causes the spatial relationship of the target elements to change.

standard e. An instrument designed for the measurement of aniseikonia and using a direct comparison target viewed through Polaroid plates so that some of the detail in the target is seen by both eyes, some by the right eye only, and some by the left eye only.

eikonometry (i"ko-nom'eh-tre). The measurement of aniseikonia.

Einstein (īn'stīn) **shift; theory.** See under the nouns.

EIRG. Abbreviation for *internal electroretinogram.*

EKP. Epikeratoprosthesis.

elastosis dystrophica (e"las-to'sis dis-trof'ih-kah). A degeneration of the membrane of Bruch resulting in angioid streaks. Syn., *Touraine syndrome; Touraine's systemic elastorrhexia.*

electrocorticogram (e-lek"tro-kōr'tih-ko"gram). A graphic recording of the changes in electrical potential associated with the activity of the cerebral cortex, obtained by applying electrodes directly to the surface of the cortex and plotting voltage against time.

electrocortigography (e-lek"tro-kōr"tih-gog'raf-e). The production and study of the electrocorticogram.

electrodiaphake (e-lek"tro-di'ah-fāk). A diathermic instrument for removing the crystalline lens.

electroencephalogram (e-lek"tro-en-sef'ah-lo-gram). A graphic recording of the changes in electrical potential associated with the activity of the cerebral cortex, made with the electroencephalograph by means of electrodes applied either to the scalp or to the surface of the cortex, or placed within neural tissue of the brain; voltage is plotted against time. Abbreviation EEG.

electroencephalograph (e-lek"tro-en-sef'ah-lo-graf). An instrument for performing electroencephalography, i.e., for making electroencephalograms.

electroencephalography (e-lek″tro-en-sef-ah-log′rah-fe). The production and study of the electroencephalogram.

electrokeratoplasty (e-lek″tro-ker′ah-to-plas″te). Thermokeratoplasty in which the heat is generated by placing electrodes at the corneal periphery and passing a small amount of current through the cornea.

electroluminescence (e-lek″tro-lu″-mih-nes′ens). The emission of light from a high-frequency discharge through a gas, or from application of alternating current to a layer of phosphor.

electromyogram (e-lek″tro-mi′o-gram). The recorded electrical change in potential difference associated with muscular activity.

electromyography (e-lek″tro-mi-og′-rah-fe). The recording and study of the electromyogram.

Electronic Orthoptor. Trade name of an instrument which monocularly and intermittently provides a small bright yellow spot of light on the macula as a treatment for amblyopia and two alternately flashing red lights for anti-suppression training.

electronystagmogram (e-lek″tro-nis-tag′mo-gram). An electro-oculogram which graphically depicts ocular movements in nystagmus.

electronystagmography (e-lek″tro-nis-tag-mog′rah-fe). The electrical recording of ocular movements in nystagmus. Abbreviated ENG.

　　vector e. Electronystagmography in which recordings are made simultaneously in more than one meridian in order to localize the positions of the eye by vector analysis.

electro-occipitogram, evoked (e-lek″tro-ok-sip′ih-to″gram). A graphic record of changes in electrical potential, as measured by two midline scalp electrodes at the occiput when the eye is stimulated by light which is computer regulated to be of different frequency than the alpha rhythm. Failure to record indicates blindness in the area of the retina stimulated by light. Abbreviation EVOG.

electro-oculogram (e-lek″tro-ok′u-lo-gram). A record of eye position made by recording, during eye movement, the difference in electrical potential between two electrodes placed on the skin at either side of the eye. The potential difference is a function of eye position and changes in the potential difference are due to changes in alignment of the resting potential of the eye in reference to the electrodes. Abbreviated EOG. Syn., *electro-ophthalmogram.*

electro-oculography (e-lek″tro-ok″u-log′rah-fe). The production and study of the electro-oculogram. Syn., *electro-ophthalmography.*

　　vector e. Electro-oculography in which recordings are made simultaneously in more than one meridian in order to localize the position of the eye by vector analysis.

electro-ophthalmogram (e-lek″tro-of-thal′mo-gram). Electro-oculogram.

electro-ophthalmography (e-lek″tro-of″-thal-mog′rah-fe). Electro-oculography.

electro-optics (e-lek″tro-op′tiks). Various light phenomena wherein changes are brought about by strong electric fields.

electroperimetry (e-lek″tro-per-im′eh-tre). Objective determination of the integrity of the visual field by recording changes in the electrical potential, as measured by two midline scalp electrodes at the occiput when the eye is stimulated by light which is computer regulated to be of different frequency than the alpha rhythm. Failure to record an evoked occipital potential indicates blindness for the retinal area stimulated.

electrophotoluminescence (e-lek″-tro-fo″to-lu-mih-nes′ens). Photoluminescence modified by means of an electrical input.

electroretinogram (e-lek″tro-ret′ih-no-gram). The electrical effect (action potential) recorded from the surface of the eyeball and originated by a pulse of light. It is usually recorded as a monophasic or a diphasic wave, but may be more complex. Abbreviated ERG. See also *E retina; I retina.*

　　internal e. A record of the electrical activity for a restricted region of the retina in response to a light stimulus near a retinal electrode at the level of the bipolar cells. The waveform is similar to that of the electroretinogram but of reverse polarity.

electroretinography (e-lek″tro-ret″ih-nog′rah-fe). The production and study of the electroretinogram.

flicker e. Electroretinography in which the electroretinogram is elicited by a flickering light stimulus.

internal e. The production and study of the internal electroretinogram.

element, retinal. 1. *Anatomy:* One of the many anatomical elements of the retina, such as rods, cones, bipolar cells, amacrines, or Mueller's fibers; more usually used in connection with a rod or a cone. 2. An element of direction apparently associated with, or emanating from, some point on the retina. Each element or point is considered to have its own "local sign," direction in space, or visual direction.

elephantiasis neuromatosa (el"eh-fan-ti'ah-sis nu"ro-mah-to'sah). Neurofibromatosis of the eyelid. See also *von Recklinghausen's disease.*

elephantiasis oculi (el"eh-fan-ti'ah-sis ok'u-li). 1. Enlargement and protrusion of the eyelids due to lymphatic obstruction. 2. Extreme exophthalmia. *Obs.*

elevator. 1. A muscle which raises an eyelid. 2. A muscle which rotates the eye upward.

Elleman chart (el'eh-man). See under *chart.*

Elliot's (el'e-ots) **scotometer; sign.** See under the nouns.

ellipse (ē-lips'). A smooth symmetrical oval, each point of which has a constant sum of distances from two fixed points within it.

aniseikonic e. An elliptical diagram representing the aniseikonic ratio in all meridians.

Tscherning e. A graphical curve resulting from the plotting of front surface powers against total lens powers in best-form lenses, i.e., those forms which reduce marginal astigmatism and field curvature to a minimum. **Ostwalt branch of T.e.** The lower portion of the Tscherning ellipse used in the designing of so-called corrected curve lenses. **Wollaston branch of T.e.** The upper portion of the Tscherning ellipse.

ellipsoid, Fresnel's. The representation of the wavefront originating from a point source located within a birefringent substance as an ellipsoid for which the semiaxes are proportional to the principal indices of refraction of the substance.

ellipsoid, visual cell. The refractile outer portion of the inner member of a rod or cone cell located between the myoid and the outer member. It contains mitochondria for metabolic activity.

Ellis stereoscope; visual designs test. See under the nouns.

Elschnig (elsh'nig) **bodies; globular cells; physiologic excavation; limiting membrane; pearls; spots; syndrome; tissue.** See under the nouns.

em. Abbreviation for *emmetropia.*

embolism, retinal (em'bo-lizm). The blocking of a retinal artery or arteriole by an embolus which may result in atrophy and blindness of the portion of the retina affected. Obstruction of the central retinal artery presents a characteristic ophthalmoscopic picture in which all arteries are constricted and the fundus is milky white except for a cherry-red spot at the macula. Central vision may be spared when a cilioretinal artery is present.

embolus (em'bo-lus). A bit of foreign matter which enters the blood stream at one point and is carried until it is lodged or impacted in an artery and obstructs it. It may be a blood clot, an air bubble, fat or other tissue, or clumps of bacteria.

embryotoxon (em"bre-o-tok'son). A ring opacity of the periphery of the cornea, situated in its deep layers, distinguished from an arcus senilis in that it appears to be continuous with the sclera, having no clear zone at the limbus. It is a developmental anomaly due to an adhesion of the lamina capsulo-pupillaris to the cornea. Syn., *posterior marginal dysplasia of the cornea; postcorneal ring.*

anterior e. Arcus juvenilis.

posterior e. Embryotoxon.

emergence, grazing. The emergence of a refracted ray from a more dense to a less dense optical medium, such that it travels along the interface between the two media. It constitutes the limiting value of the angle of refraction.

emissivity (em"is-iv'ih-te). The ratio of the energy radiated by a nonblackbody at any temperature to that radiated by a blackbody at the same temperature.

spectral e. Emissivity for a specific wavelength.

total e. Emissivity at all wavelengths.

luminous e. Luminous exitance.

radiant e. Luminous exitance.

Emmert's law (em′erts). See under *law.*

emmetrope (em′e-trōp). One having emmetropia.

emmetropia (em″e-tro′pe-ah). A visual condition identified by the location of the conjugate focus of the retina at infinity when accommodation is said to be relaxed; thus, the retina lies in the plane of the posterior principal focus of the dioptric system of the static eye. In emmetropia, an infinitely distant fixated object is imaged sharply on the retina without inducing an accommodative response.

emmetropic (em″e-trop′ik). Pertaining to or having emmetropia.

emmetropization (em″ē-tro″pih-za′-shun). A process presumed to be operative in producing a greater frequency of occurrence of emmetropia and near emmetropia than would be expected in terms of chance distribution, as may be explained by postulating that a mechanism co-ordinates the formation and development of the various components of the human eye which contribute to the total refractive power.

emphysema (em″fi-se′mah, -ze′mah). The abnormal presence of air or gas in the body tissues, as may occur in the eyelids through a fracture of the lamina papyracea of the ethmoid bone.

empiricism (em-pir′is-izm). 1. Generally, a theory that certain aspects of behavior or knowledge are dependent on accumulated experience or learning and are not innate. 2. The concept that spatial localization is a learned process based on experience and is not innate. Cf. *nativism.* 3. Empirical method or practice.

encanthis (en-kan′this). 1. A small neoplasm or tumor in the inner canthus of the eye. 2. A simple inflammatory hypertrophy of the lacrimal caruncle.

encanthoschisis (en-kan″tho-skih′sis). Formation of a caruncle in two parts, or its division by a horizontal furrow.

encephalitis periaxialis diffusa (en″-sef-ah-li′tis per″ih-aks-e-al′is dih-fu′sah). Schilder's disease.

encephalocele, orbital (en-sef′ah-lo-sēl″). A protrusion of a portion of the cerebral substance into the orbit, usually causing exophthalmos and lateral displacement of the eyeball.

encephalomyelitis optica (en-sef′ah-lo-mi″el-i′tis op′tih-kah). Neuromyelitis optica.

encephalopathy, infantile subacute necrotizing. Leigh syndrome.

encephalopsy (en-sef′ah-lop″se). The association of certain colors with certain flavors, numbers, words, etc.

encoding (en-kōd′ing). The sum of the abilities required to express ideas in words or gestures, as in spelling.

encyclophoria (en″si-klo-fo′re-ah). Incyclophoria.

encyclotropia (en″si-klo-tro′pe-ah). Incyclotropia.

encyclovergence (en″si-klo-ver′jens). Incyclovergence.

end bulb. See under *bulb.*

end foot. The end of a cone cell, shaped like a pedicle, which synapses with a bipolar cell dendrite in the outer molecular layer of the retina. Syn., *cone foot; cone pedicle.*

end knob. The end of a rod cell of the retina, located in the outer molecular layer of the retina, which synapses with bipolar and horizontal cells. Syn., *end bulb; rod spherule.*

endophlebitis, retinal (en″do-fle-bi′-tis). Venous thrombosis involving the retinal venules.

endophthalmitis (en-dof′thal-mi′tis). Inflammation of the tissues of the internal structures of the eye. Syn., *entophthalmia.*

   e. phacoallergica. Endophthalmitis phacoanaphylactica.

   e. phacoanaphylactica. Inflammation of the uveal tract occurring after extracapsular cataract extraction or a needling operation, presumed to be an allergic reaction to one's own liberated lenticular proteins. Syn., *endophthalmitis phacoallergica; endophthalmitis phacogenetica.*

   e. phacogenetica. Endophthalmitis phacoanaphylactica.

   phacotoxic e. Endophthalmitis attributed to the toxic effect of liberated crystalline lens material, as that from a hypermature cataract.

   suppurative e. Purulent inflammation of the uveal tract; a purulent uveitis.

endothelioma (en″do-the″le-o′mah). A malignant tumor derived from endothelium of the vascular system or the lining cells of body cavities. Reticulo-endothelial cells and cells of the tunica adventitia of vessels are claimed by some to yield endotheliomas.

endpiece. The part at the temporal end of a spectacle frame or mounting which contains the pivot for the temple.

energy. 1. The capacity for performing work. 2. Inherent power; the capacity of acting to produce an effect.

infrared e. Electromagnetic or radiant energy of wavelengths just longer than that which will ordinarily stimulate the eye, extending from approximately 760 mμ through several octaves of longer wavelengths.

luminous e. Visible radiant energy; light.

radiant e. Energy traveling in the form of electromagnetic waves considered as to its physical qualities and not as to its sensation-producing effect on the eye. It is measured in units of energy such as ergs or joules. **spectral r.e.** Radiant energy with respect to a specified wavelength or narrow wavelength interval. **visible r.e.** Radiant energy capable of eliciting the sensation of light when received on the retina, corresponding approximately to the wavelength range of 380 to 760 mμ.

spectral e. The radiant energy of the spectrum referring either to the visible spectrum only or to the total electromagnetic spectrum.

ultraviolet e. Electromagnetic or radiant energy of wavelengths just shorter than that which will ordinarily stimulate the eye, extending from approximately 380 mμ through several octaves of shorter wavelengths.

Engel fundus lens (eng'el). See under *lens.*

Engelmann (eng'el-man) **Stereoscope; Bar Trainer.** See under the nouns.

Engström's accessory outer segment (eng'stremz). See under *segment.*

enhancement, brightness. 1. The increase in brightness resulting from making a stimulus intermittent. The rate of intermittency must lie materially below the critical flicker frequency and the photic pulses must not be feeble or enhancement will not occur. See also *Brücke-Bartley effect.* 2. The apparent increase of brightness of a surface when surrounded by a dark area as compared to when it is surrounded by a light area.

maximum brightness e. Maximum increase in the brightness of a target or other area intermittently illuminated, over one continuously illuminated. Under some conditions a maximum occurs when the stimulus rate is in the neighborhood of 8 to 10 pulses per sec., dropping with either higher or lower pulse frequencies. Under other conditions, enhancement increases continuously as pulse frequency decreases until the resulting flashes are so widely separated as not to be compared in brightness with continuous light.

enhancement, contrast. The apparent increase of brightness of a surface when it is surrounded by a dark area as compared to when it is surrounded by a light area.

Enoch's theory (e'noks). See under *theory.*

EOG. Abbreviation for *electro-oculogram.*

enophthalmia (en"of-thal'me-ah). Enophthalmos.

enophthalmos (en"of-thal'mos). Recession of the eyeball into the orbit.

enophthalmus (en"of-thal'mus). Enophthalmos.

enorthotrope (en-ōr'tho-trōp"). A form of zoetrope.

Enroth's sign (en'roths). See under *sign.*

enstrophe (en'stro-fe). Inversion of the eyelid margins.

entiris (en-ti'ris). The posterior pigment epithelium of the iris.

entochoroidea (en"to-ko-roi'de-ah). Choriocapillaris.

entocornea (en"to-kōr'ne-ah). 1. Descemet's membrane. 2. The posterior endothelium of the cornea.

entophthalmia (ent"of-thal'me-ah). Endophthalmitis.

entoptic (ent-op'tik). Arising from within the eye, pertaining especially to certain phenomena related to the optical or sensory effects of internal structures perceived illusorily, as in the external field of vision. Classic examples include muscae volitantes, Haidinger's brushes, and phosphene.

entoptoscope (en-top'to-skōp). 1. An instrument for examining the media of the eyes to determine their transparency. 2. An instrument providing a grossly out-of-focus retinal image of a small light source so as to make shadows of intraocular objects in the light path subjectively apparent.

entoptoscopy (ent"op-tos'ko-pe). The observation of the interior of the eye for determining transparency of the ocular media.

entorbital (ent-ōr'bih-tal). Pertaining to the inner portion of the orbit.

entoretina (en"to-ret'ih-nah). The inner five layers and the internal limiting membrane of the retina.

entrance port; pupil; window. See under the nouns.

entropion (en-tro'pe-on). A rolling or turning inward (inversion) of the margin of an eyelid. Syn., *blepharelosis.*

 cicatricial e. Entropion due to scar tissue and subsequent contraction of the tarsus and conjunctiva.

 contraction e. Entropion due to, or occurring with, contraction of the palpebral portion of the orbicularis oculi muscle.

 mechanical e. Entropion due to lack of support to the eyelid, such as may occur in enophthalmos or lack of orbital fat.

 organic e. Mechanical entropion.

 senile e. Entropion occurring in the aged, usually due to loose, atrophied, and inelastic skin of the eyelids, together with normal tone of the palpebral portion of the orbicularis oculi muscle and a deep-set eye.

 spastic e. Entropion due to spasm of the palpebral portion of the orbicularis oculi muscle.

 superciliary e. A turning inward of the cilia of the eyebrow toward the eye; of pathological, traumatic, or congenital origin.

entropium (en-tro'pe-um). Entropion.

enucleate (e-nu'kle-āt). To remove a whole tumor or an entire organ, as in the removal of the eye from its socket.

enucleation (e-nu"kle-a'shun). The removal of a whole tumor or an entire organ, as in the removal of the eye from its socket.

EOG. Abbreviation for *electro-oculogram.*

EOL. See *l'Ecole d'Optique Lunettier de Lille.*

EOS. European Optometric Society. See *Societé d'Optometrie d'Europe.*

epaulet (eh-pah'let). A pannus consisting of a dense invasion of blood vessels at the limbus, raising the epithelium in a gelatinous pink mass to resemble an epaulet following a destructive lesion near the margin of the cornea.

ependyma (ep-en'dih-mah). Neuroglial-like cells lining the cavity of the neural tube of the central nervous system and bounding the cerebrospinal fluid of the canals and the ventricles. Visual cells are thought to develop from the ependyma of the embryo.

ephedrine (eh-fed'rin). A pharmaceutical agent that when applied topically for mydriasis is thought to have a direct stimulatory effect on both alpha and beta receptors as well as indirectly causing the release of norepinephrine from postganglionic nerve endings.

epiblepharon (ep"ih-blef'ah-ron). A rare developmental anomaly in which a fold of skin overlaps the eyelid margin, pressing the eyelashes inward. Syn., *dermochalasis.*

epibulbar (ep"ih-bul'bar). Situated on the eyeball. Syn., *epiocular.*

epicanthus (ep"ih-kan'thus). A fold of skin partially covering the inner canthus, the caruncle, and the plica semilunaris. It is normal in the fetus, in some infants, and in Mongolians and other peoples characterized by low nasal bridges.

 e. inversus. A condition in which a fold of skin from the lower eyelid runs crescentically upward, meeting the upper eyelid at the inner canthus. It is associated with a congenital ptosis.

 e. lateralis. An acquired condition in which a fold of skin rides over the outer canthus.

 oblique e. The oblique median eye fold characteristic of Mongolian races. Syn., *Mongoloid fold.*

 e. palpebralis Epicanthus in which the fold of skin originates above the tarsal fold of the upper eyelid.

 e. supraciliaris. Epicanthus in which the fold of skin originates from the region of the eyebrows.

 e. tarsalis. Epicanthus in which the fold originates from the skin of the tarsal fold of the upper eyelid.

epicauma (ep"ih-kaw'mah). Any superficial burn or ulcer of the eye.

epichoroid (ep"ih-ko'roid). The outer layer of the choroid adjacent to the sclera. Syn., *lamina fusca; suprachoroid.*

epicorneoscleritis (ep"ih-kor"ne-o-skle-ri'tis). Superficial inflammation of the cornea and the sclera.

epidermolysis bullosa (ep"e-der-mol'is-is bul'o-sah). A disease of the skin, usually hereditary, characterized by the development of vesicles and bullae on irritation or slight trauma of the skin. Vesicles resembling phlyctenules may appear in the conjunctiva and, when recurrent, may lead to superficial symblepharon. Affection of the conjunctiva is frequently accompanied by the corneal complications of blebs and ulcers.

epidiascope (ep″ih-di′ah-skōp″). An optical instrument for projecting opaque pictures onto a screen; an opaque projector.

epikeratoprosthesis. (ep-ih-ker″ah-to-pros-the′sis). A plastic (methyl methacrylate) lens similar to a corneal contact lens which is bonded by adhesive to Bowman's membrane after surgical removal of the corneal epithelium. Abbreviation EKP.

epilation (ep″ih-la′shun). The removal of hair by the roots, as in the removal of misdirected eyelashes.

epilepsy, photogenic (ep′ih-lep″se). Epilepsy precipitated by intermittent light stimulation.

epiloia (ep-ih-loi′ah). Bourneville's disease.

epinephrine (ep′ih-nef′rin). A hormone of the adrenal medulla which, when instilled in the eye in dilute solution, constricts the conjunctival vessels, dilates the pupil by stimulating the sympathetic nerve endings of the dilator pupillae muscle, and reduces intraocular pressure. It is used to control conjunctival hemorrhages, to reduce conjunctival congestion, and to release recent iritic adhesions. It is also of value in acute glaucoma. Syn., *adrenalin.*

epiocular (ep″e-ok″u-lar). Epibulbar.

epipephysitis (ep″ih-pef′ih-si′tis). Conjunctivitis.

epiphora (e-pif′o-rah). An overflow of tears onto the cheek caused by excessive lacrimation, by obstruction of the lacrimal ducts, or by ectropion.

epiphysis cerebri (e-pif′ih-sis ser′-e-bri). The pineal body in the forebrain which, in some low vertebrates, represents a median eye.

episclera (ep″ih-skle′rah). A loose structure of fibrous and elastic connective tissue on the outer surface of the sclera. It contains a large number of small blood vessels in contrast to the sclera proper, which is almost avascular.

episcleral (ep″ih-skle′ral). 1. Located on the outer surface of the sclera. 2. Pertaining to the episclera.

episcleritis (ep″ih-skle-ri′tis). Inflammation of the episclera and/or the outer layers of the sclera itself.

e. fugax. Episcleritis periodica fugax. **partial e.f.** Episcleritis periodica fugax.

e. multinodularis. A condition in which numerous nodules appear in the episcleral and conjunctival tissues and are associated with itching, discharge, hyperemia, and possibly iritis. The nodules are fleeting, consist of small mononuclear cells and eosinophils, and are associated with rheumatoid arthritis.

nodular e. An inflammation of the episclera characterized by the appearance of localized purplish nodules, round or oval in shape and very sensitive to touch. The nodules are firmly attached to the sclera, but the conjunctiva moves freely over them. It occurs in adults, is benign, chronic, recurrent, of obscure etiology, and is differentiated from a phlyctenule by the mobility of the overlying conjunctiva.

e. periodica fugax. A transient and recurrent inflammation of a portion of the episclera, lasting from a few hours to a few days. It persistently recurs in different areas in the same eye or in the other eye, is fiery red, is sometimes painful, and usually does not affect vision or have serious sequelae. Syn., *episcleritis fugax; partial episcleritis fugax.*

e. rosacea. A rare inflammation of the episclera characterized by the appearance of transient, recurring, highly vascularized, small, gray nodules.

episclerotitis (ep″ih-skle″ro-ti′tis). Episcleritis.

episcotister (ep″ih-sko-tis′ter). A sectored disk which may be rotated in front of a light source to produce flashes of light. It is used in the study of the critical flicker frequency.

epitarsus (ep″ih-tar′sus). A congenital anomaly consisting of apronlike folds of conjunctiva attached to the inner tarsal surface of the eyelid. The edges of the folds are sufficiently free that a probe may be passed beneath. Syn., *congenital pterygium.*

epithelioma (ep″ih-the″le-o′mah). A tumor derived from epithelium, such as a cancer of the skin, or rarely, of a mucous membrane.

cystic adenoid of Brooke e. Familial, dominant, sebaceous adenomas of the face or eyelids characterized by multiple, small, symmetrical tumors of a reddish-yellow color resembling pearls. A benign proliferation of the basal cells, usually in connection with the hair follicles. Syn., *Brooke's disease.*

Fuchs' e. A benign neoplasm appearing as a brown pigmented mass up to 5 mm in size, oval or round in shape, usually on the ridge of a ciliary process or in a valley between, and ordinarily noted only in histological examination but occasionally seen gonioscopically.

epitheliopathy, acute posterior multifocal placoid pigment (ep"-ih-the"le-op'ah-the). Multiple, flat, yellow-white lesions in the retinal pigment epithelium at the posterior pole appearing suddenly and resolving spontaneously, leaving irregularity to the pigment epithelium and minimal damage to the choroid or retina; visual acuity returns after several weeks.

epsilon [ε] (ep'sih-lon). The Greek letter used as the symbol for (1) the *angle epsilon;* (2) the *dispersive power* of a light transmitting medium; (3) the *angle of deviation* of a refracted ray of light.

Epstein's (ep'stīnz) **implant; lens; symptom.** See under the nouns.

equate. In color vision, to combine colors to equal another color sensation.

equation. An expression of equality between two magnitudes.

color e's. Equations representing the proportions of the primary colors needed in additive color mixing to match a particular hue.

Fresnel's e. Fresnel's formula.

Luckiesh-Guth e. An empirical equation describing the relationship between the BCD value of the brightness of the source, the separations of the source from the subject's line of sight, the solid angle of subtense of the source, and the field brightness.

Rayleigh e. The proportion of red (usually 670 nm) and green (usually 535 nm) required in a mixture to match a given yellow (usually 589 nm). It is used as a test to differentiate certain types of deficient color vision.

equator. A circle or a circular line which divides the surface of a body into two equal and symmetrical parts.

e. of crystalline lens. The outer zonular margin of the crystalline lens, lying in a vertical plane.

e. of the eye, anatomical. The circumference of the eye representing a locus of points equidistant from the anterior and the posterior poles.

e. of the eye, functional. A diagrammatic circle joining the arc of contact of the lateral rectus muscle (4 mm behind the anatomical equator) and the arc of contact of the medial rectus muscle (4 mm in front of the anatomical equator). It serves as a guide in strabismic surgery.

e. of the eye, geometrical. The circumference of the eye in a plane perpendicular to and bisecting the anterior-posterior axis.

equilibrium, photochemical. The level of light or dark adaptation for which the rate of synthesis is equal to the rate of breakdown in the Wald cycle.

equivalent. That which is equal in value, force, significance, weight, worth, or size.

spherical e. 1. A spherical lens whose focal point coincides with the circle of least confusion of a given spherocyclindrical lens. 2. A lens differing in form from another lens, but including the same optical focal length from the posterior principal plane to the posterior principal focus; more correctly described as *equivalent power*. A single lens whose effective power is equal to the sum total effective power of a combination of lenses.

spherocylinder e. 1. A single lens or a combination of lenses with an effective power equivalent to that of a given combination of spheres and cylinders. 2. Any of the series of formulas obtained by transposition of the formula for a given spherocylinder combination.

Erb's disease; method. See under the nouns.

erector. An erecting prism.

ERG. Abbreviation for *electroretinogram.*

Erggelet's retrolental space (er'geh-letz). See under *space, retrolental.*

ergograph (er'go-graf). An instrument for recording the value of work done by muscular contractions, primarily used in studies of muscular fatigue. The extent and duration of muscular contractions are recorded on a kymograph attached to the apparatus.

ophthalmic e. An instrument for studying fatigue of convergence and/or accommodation, consisting essentially of a movable target carrier which repeatedly approaches the eye of the observer and is connected to a kymograph for recording.

ergophthalmology (erg-of"thal-mol'o-je). The biotechnological branch of ophthalmology.

erisiphake (er-is'e-fãk). Erysiphake.

erisophake (er-is'o-fãk). Erysiphake.

ERP. Early receptor potential.

error. The failure to achieve, or a deviation from, the right course or standard; a departure from truth or accuracy; a mistake.

alley e. The difference between the parallel and distance type of Blumenfeld alleys.

declination e. The apparent fore or aft deviation of vertical lines, specified in degrees, induced by oblique meridional magnification lenses or oblique meridional aniseikonia.

horopter e. Hering-Hillebrand deviation.

image shell e. The dioptric difference between the Petzval surface of a point-focal lens and the far point sphere of the eye, or near point sphere when appropriate, for a given oblique pencil of rays. Syn., *marginal spherical error.*

marginal spherical e. Image shell error.

mean oblique e. The mean dioptric power of a spherical lens for a given oblique ray minus its back vertex power.

oblique astigmatic e. The tangential dioptric vertex power of a spherical lens minus its sagittal dioptric vertex power for a given oblique ray.

e. of refraction of the eye. The dioptric power of the correcting lens which, together with the dioptric system of the eye, converges parallel rays to focus on the retina, with accommodation fully relaxed. See also *ametropia.*

skew e. In a right angle reflecting prism, an error due to the edge of the 90° apex not being perpendicular to the long side of the hypotenuse face.

erysipelas (er"ih-sip'eh-las, -lus). An acute, spreading, febrile disease characterized by inflammation of the skin, subcutaneous tissues, and mucous membranes, due to infection of the lymph spaces of the corium and underlying parts by *Streptococcus erysipelatis* (*S. pyogenes*). When the eye is involved, there is great swelling and redness, the eyelids are swollen shut, and this may be followed by abscess of the eyelids and sloughing of the skin. If the disease extends into the orbit, it may cause orbital cellulitis, thrombosis of retinal veins, optic neuritis, or optic atrophy.

erysiphake (er-is'ih-fãk). A surgical instrument for the removal of a cataractous crystalline lens by suction. See also *phacoerisis.*

erythema (er"ih-the'mah). Redness of the skin occurring in variably sized and shaped patches.

e. bullosum. Erythema vesiculosum.

e. circinata. Erythema exudativum multiforme in which the patches are ring-shaped.

e. exudativum multiforme. An eruption of the skin or the mucous membranes characterized by red patches of various shapes and associated with an edematous exudate. In the conjunctiva it may appear in three forms: mild catarrhal conjunctivitis, purulent conjunctivitis, or severe pseudomembranous conjunctivitis. Syn., *Grignolo syndrome; Hebra's disease.*

e. nodosum. An eruption of the skin or the mucous membranes characterized by large nodular swellings, dark purple in the center and brighter red at the periphery. Occasionally, the subconjunctival tissues are affected with the appearance in the palpebral fissure of an edematous area containing vesicles or nodules.

e. purpuricum. Erythema exudativum multiforme in which the patches are blood-stained.

e. vesiculosum. Erythema exudativum multiforme in which blisters are formed due to excessive exudation. Syn., erythema bullosum.

erythremia (er"e-thre'me-ah). Vaquez' disease.

erythrochloropia (e-rith"ro-klo-ro'pe-ah). A form of deficient color vision in which red and green are the only colors correctly perceived.

erythrochloropsia (e-rith'ro-klo-rop'-se-ah). Erythrochloropia.

erythrochloropy (e-rith"ro-klor'o-pe). Erythrochloropia.

erythroderma exfoliativa (eh-rith"-ro-der'mah eks-fo'le-ah"tiv-ah). Wilson-Brocq disease.

erythrolabe (e-rith'ro-lãb). The name proposed by W. A. H. Rushton for a retinal photopigment more sensitive to long wavelength (red) radiation than are other retinal photopigments, although its maximum absorption and spectral sensitivity appear to be in the yellow-green, or perhaps the orange, portion of the spectrum rather than in the red.

erythrophane (e-rith'ro-fān). A red pigment found in the retinal receptor cells of some animals, but not of man.

erythrophobia (e-rith"ro-fo'be-ah). A fear of, or an aversion to, the color red.

erythrophose (e-rith'ro-fōz). A subjective sensation of red light or color.

erythropia (er"e-thro'pe-ah). Erythropsia.

erythropsia (er"e-throp'se-ah). A condition in which all objects are seen tinged with red. It may appear after overexposure to bright light, as in snow blindness, or following cataract extraction. Syn., *red vision.*

erythropsin (er"e-throp'sin). Rhodopsin.

escorcin (es-kōr'sin). A chemical compound which in solution imparts a red color to lesions of the cornea or the conjunctiva and is used for their observation.

eserine (es'er-in). A chemical compound used as a parasympathetic stimulant which, when instilled in the eye, constricts the pupil. Syn., *physostigmine.*

ESI. Equivalent sphere illumination.

ESO. See *l'Ecole Supérieure Libre d'Optometrie.*

esocataphoria (es"o-kat"ah-fo're-ah). The combined conditions of esophoria and cataphoria, the eyes tending to turn down and in.

esodeviation (es"o-de"ve-a'shun, e"so-). The deviation of the line of sight of the nonfixating eye from the point of fixation of the other eye, in esophoria with dissociation, or in esotropia.

esodisparity (es"o-dis-par'ih-te, e"so-). Fixation disparity in which the eyes overconverge slightly while single binocular vision is maintained for the point of fixation. Syn., *positive fixation disparity.*

esophoria (es"o-fo're-ah, e"so-). The inward turning, or the amount of inward turning, of the two eyes relative to each other as manifested in the absence of a fusion stimulus, or when fusion is made impossible, such that the lines of sight cross at a point in front of and nearer to the eyes than a given point of reference, this point of reference usually being the point of binocular fixation prior to the phoria test or, more arbitrarily, at an infinite distance.

accommodative e. The manifestation of esophoria, or of that portion of total esophoria, resulting from accommodative convergence.

anatomical e. The manifestation of esophoria, or of that portion of total esophoria, attributable to structural (anatomical) anomalies or variations.

basic e. Esophoria which is approximately the same at both far and near fixation distances.

convergence excess e. Esophoria of greater degree at a near than at a far fixation distance.

divergence insufficiency e. See *divergence, insufficiency.*

innervational e. The manifestation of esophoria, or of that portion of total esophoria, attributable to hypertonicity of the extraocular musculature subserving convergence. Syn., *tonic esophoria.*

intrinsic e. Esophoria attributable to primary structural, myologic, or neurological anomalies as distinguished from pseudoesophoria attributable to spurious manifestations of accommodative convergence.

monofixational e. See *phoria, monofixational.*

physiological e. Oversufficiency of accommodative convergence producing increased esophoria or decreased exophoria as the fixation object is brought nearer. It occurs when the AC/A ratio is greater than six.

relative e. 1. The amount by which the exophoria at near is less than the physiological exophoria, or the amount of esophoria at near plus the amount of the physiological exophoria. 2. The distance esophoria regarded as a finding different from the absolute value that would be obtained with tonic convergence eliminated. 3. The amount of esophoria expressed in relation to given test conditions and given points of reference for purposes of quantitative specification.

tonic e. Esophoria attributable to excess or anomalous tonicity of the extraocular musculature. Syn., *innervational esophoria.*

esophoric (es"o-fōr'ik, e"so-). Pertaining to or manifesting esophoria.

esostasis (es"o-sta'sis). An inward deviation of the eye from a straightforward position when all fixation stimuli and voluntary influences are eliminated.

esotrope (e-so-trōp', es-o-trōp'). One affected with convergent strabismus.

hyperkinetic e. An esotrope showing small to moderate hyperopia, normal amplitude of accommodation, extremely variable esotropia, unstable fusion, and personal instability, according to Costenbader.

hypoaccommodative e. Hypokinetic esotrope.

hypokinetic e. An esotrope with a high AC/A ratio presumed to be due to an unexplained weak accommodative mechanism. Syn., *hypoaccommodative esotrope.*

esotropia (es"o-tro'pe-ah, e"so-). Convergent strabismus.

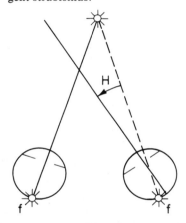

Fig. 15 Esotropia of the right eye at near. The objective angle of deviation is represented by the letter *H*. (From J. R. Griffin, *Binocular Anomalies.* Chicago: Professional Press, 1976)

basic e. Esotropia having approximately the same magnitude at both far and near fixation distances.

convergence excess e. Esotropia of greater degree at a near than at a far fixation distance.

divergence insufficiency e. See *divergence, insufficiency.*

esotropic (es"o-trop'ik, e"so-). Pertaining to or manifesting esotropia.

Espildora-Luque syndrome. See under *syndrome.*

esthesiometer (es-the"ze-om'eh-ter). An instrument for determining sensibility, especially one for tactile sensation.

Boberg-Ans e. Boberg-Ans corneal sensibilitometer.

Cochet-Bonnet e. A device used to evaluate corneal sensitivity consisting essentially of a nylon thread, 0.0113 mm^2 in section, mounted in a handle so that its length may be varied, and calibrated in milligrams of weight necessary to bend a given length of the thread when pressed against the cornea. The criterion is the greatest thread length which causes a just noticeable sensation of pain.

Schirmer's e. A device used to evaluate corneal sensitivity consisting essentially of a small plastic disk attached to one end of a wire, the other end being connected to a spring mechanism giving readings in milligrams of force.

ET. Constant esotropia at far.

ET'. Constant esotropia at near.

eta [η] (e'tah, a'tah). The Greek letter used as a symbol for the *angle of relative binocular parallax* or the *angle of stereopsis.*

etafilcon A. The nonproprietary name of a hydrophilic material of which contact lenses are made.

etalon (et'ah-lon). Two parallel, optically plane, glass plates partially silvered on their inner surfaces and mounted at a fixed distance from each other, which produce circular interference fringes of high resolution in the light transmitted after it undergoes multiple reflections in the air space between the two plates.

Fabry-Pérot e. A Fabry-Pérot interferometer whose plate separation is fixed.

ethmoiditis (eth"moid-i'tis). Inflammation of the ethmoid sinuses or of the ethmoid bone.

ethylenediamine tetraacetate (eth"ih-lēn-di'ah-men). A chelating agent having high affinity for certain metals; used topically on the cornea to remove calcium deposits and also as an anti-bacterial agent in certain ophthalmic preparations. Abbreviation EDTA.

eucatropine (u-kat'ro-pēn, -pin). Euphthalmine.

euchromatopsia (u-kro"mah-top'se-ah). Normal color perception.

euchromatopsy (u-kro'mah-top"se). Euchromatopsia.

eucone (u'kōn). A separate refractive body called a crystalline cone, in the ommatidia of compound eyes in arthropods. It lies between the cornea and the retinal elements.

euphausiopsin (u"fah-u"sih-op'sin). A pigment of the vitamin A$_1$ group with a maximum absorption of 462 mμ, found in the photochemical system of the eyes of the shrimplike euphausiid crustaceans.

euphoropsia (u"fo-rop'se-ah). Comfortable or good vision; the absence of visual discomfort.

euphthalmine (ūf-thal'min). A derivative of eucaine which acts as a mydriatic of brief duration. Syn., *eucatropine.*

European Optometric Society. See *Societé d'Optometrie d'Europe.*

euryblepharon (u"re-blef'ah-ron). Large eyelids.

euryopia (u"re-o'pe-ah). Abnormally wide palpebral fissures.

euryphotic (u"ref-o'tik). Having the ability to see in any of a wide range of illumination intensities.

euscope (u'skōp). An instrument for projecting an enlarged image from a compound microscope on a screen.

euthyphoria (u"the-fo're-ah). The absence of anaphoria or cataphoria, hence a tendency of the lines of sight to remain horizontal.

Euthyscope (u'the-skōp). An instrument used in treating amblyopia, consisting essentially of an ophthalmoscope containing a small opaque disk, in the center of the condensing lens, subtending a nonilluminated area of either 3° or 5°. The shadow is directed onto the macula, and the surrounding retinal area is illuminated with a 30° cone of intense light, rendering the macula relatively more sensitive for a short period.

evagination, optic (e-vaj"e-na'shun). The diverticulum in the forebrain of the embryo, from which the eyecup is developed.

Evans' test (ev'anz). See under *test.*

eversion of the eyelid (e-ver'zhun). The folding back of the eyelid on itself.

evisceration of the eye (e-vis"er-a'shun). Surgical removal of the inner contents of the eye, the sclera being left intact.

evisceration of the orbit (e-vis"er-a'shun). Surgical removal of the contents of the orbit including its periosteum.

evisceroneurotomy (e-vis"er-o-nu-rot'o-me). Evisceration of the eye with a resection of the optic nerve.

EVOG. Abbreviation for *evoked electro-occipitogram.*

evulsio nervi optici (e-vul'se-o ner'vi op'tih-ki). Traumatic evulsion of the optic nerve from the eyeball.

Ewald's law (a'vahlts). See under *law.*

Ewing chart (u'ing). See under *chart.*

excavatio papillae nervi optici (eks"kah-va'she-o pah-pil'e ner'vi op'-tih-ki). The physiological cup of the optic nerve head.

excavation. The act or process of forming a cavity or hollow, or the cavity or hollow itself.

   atrophic e. A pathological cupping of the optic papilla due to atrophy of the optic nerve fibers.

   glaucomatous e. Glaucomatous cup.

   e. of the optic disk. A physiological or pathological depression in the central area of the optic nerve head.

   physiologic e. A funnel-shaped depression at or near the center of the optic disk where the central retinal vessels leave or enter the retina; a normal physiological depression lined by the meniscus of Kuhnt. Syn., *physiological cup.* **Elschnig's p.e. types.** A classification of normal optic nerve head excavations into five types: Type I: Funnel-form. A small craterlike depression slightly lighter in color than the rest of the disk, located lateral to the central artery which rises in the center of the disk and branches on its surface. The central vein is formed at the apex of the funnel. Type II: Cylindric-form. The medial wall is steeper than the lateral, the lamina cribrosa is usually visible, the vessels are nasal, the central artery bifurcates on the disk surface, and the central vein is formed at the apex. Type III: Dish-form. The lamina cribrosa is very visible, the vessels are nasal, the central artery bifurcates on the floor or wall, and the central vein is formed within the excavation. Type IV: Gradually sloping lateral wall, as though derived from Type II or III by a bending outward of the lateral wall of the entrance canal. The lamina cribrosa is visible and conus formation is almost always present. Type V: Atypical form occurring in developmental anomalies such as coloboma of the choroid at the border of the optic nerve head. The excavation is almost always directed toward the greatest width of the usually associated conus formation.

excess, convergence. See under *convergence.*

excursion. 1. The path of movement of an eye in following a moving target. 2. Any movement of the eye.

excyclofusion (ek"si-klo-fu'zhun). The relative rotation of the two eyes around their respective anteroposterior axes in response to a cyclofusional stimulus, such that the upward extensions of their vertical meridians rotate templeward.

excyclophoria (ek″si-klo-fo′re-ah). The turning, or the amount of turning, of the two eyes relative to each other about their respective anteroposterior axes or lines of sight as manifested in the absence of a fusion stimulus, or when fusion is made impossible, such that their respective vertical meridians of reference diverge from each other superiorly and converge inferiorly. Syn., *plus cyclophoria*.

excyclotropia (ek″si-klo-tro′pe-ah). The turning, or the amount of turning, of the two eyes relative to each other about their respective anteroposterior axes or lines of sight so that their respective vertical meridians of reference diverge from each other superiorly and converge inferiorly. It is the same as excyclophoria except that the condition is continuous and unrelated to the presence or the absence of a fusion stimulus.

excyclovergence (ek″si-klo-ver′jens). The turning, or the amount of turning, of the two eyes with respect to each other about their respective anteroposterior axes so as to diverge the upward extensions of the vertical meridians of reference.

exenteration of the orbit (eks-en″ter-a′shun). Surgical removal of the orbital contents.

exit port; pupil; window. See under the nouns.

exitance, luminous. The density of luminous flux leaving a surface, usually expressed in lumens per unit area of the surface. Syn., *luminous emittance*. Symbol, *M*.

exitance, radiant. Luminous exitance.

Exner's theory (eks′nerz). See under *theory*.

exocataphoria (eks″o-kat″ah-fo′re-ah). Exophoria combined with cataphoria.

exocone (ek′so-kōn). A transparent ingrowth of the cornea which replaces the refractive crystalline cone in the ommatidia of compound eyes of arthropods.

exodeviation (eks″o-de″ve-a′shun). The deviation of the line of sight of the nonfixating eye from the point of fixation of the fixating eye, in exophoria with dissociation, or in exotropia.

exodisparity (eks″o-dis-par′ih-te). Fixa-

tion disparity in which the eyes underconverge slightly while single binocular vision is maintained for the point of fixation. Syn., *negative fixation disparity*.

exophoria (eks″o-fo′re-ah). The divergent turning, or the amount of divergent turning, of the two eyes relative to each other as manifested in the absence of a fusion stimulus, or when fusion is made impossible, such that the lines of sight cross at a point behind the eyes or at a point in front of the eyes beyond a given point of reference, this point of reference usually being the point of binocular fixation prior to the phoria test or, more arbitrarily, at an infinite distance.

accommodative e. The manifestation of exophoria, or that portion of the total exophoria, resulting from lack of accommodative convergence or from failure of accommodation with the concomitant lack of accommodative convergence in a testing situation in which a given amount of accommodation is a part of the test condition.

anatomical e. The manifestation of exophoria, or that portion of the total exophoria, attributable to structural (anatomical) anomalies or variance.

basic e. Exophoria which is approximately the same at both far and near fixation distances.

convergence insufficiency e. See *convergence, insufficiency*.

divergence excess e. See *divergence, excess*.

innervational e. The manifestation of exophoria, or that portion of the total exophoria, attributable to hypotonicity or lack of normal tonicity of the extraocular musculature subserving convergence.

intrinsic e. Exophoria attributable to primary structural, myologic, or neurological anomalies as distinguished from pseudoexophoria attributable to spurious manifestations, or failures of manifestation, of accommodative convergence.

monofixational e. See *phoria, monofixational*.

physiological e. 1. The mean exophoria at near for a given population and a given test procedure, usually considered to be about 5^Δ or 6^Δ exophoria for a 40 cm distance. 2. The near phoria minus the distance phoria when exophoria is assigned positive value, and esophoria negative. 3. The portion of the exophoria in a near test corresponding to the amount of exophoria at distance.

relative e. 1. The amount of exophoria at near in excess of the physiological exophoria. 2. The distance exophoria regarded as a finding different from the absolute value that would be obtained with tonic convergence eliminated. 3. The phoria at near minus the phoria at distance, when exophoria is assigned positive value and esophoria negative value. 4. The amount of exophoria expressed in relation to given test conditions and given points of reference for purposes of quantitative specification.

exophoric (eks"o-fōr'ik). Pertaining to or manifesting exophoria.

exophthalmia (eks"of-thal'me-ah). Exophthalmos.

e. cachectica. Exophthalmic goiter.

e. fungosa. A late stage of retinoblastoma, in which the neoplasm perforates the cornea and protrudes from it.

exophthalmic (eks"of-thal'mik). Characterized by, or pertaining to, exophthalmos.

exophthalmic goiter; ophthalmoplegia. See under the nouns.

exophthalmometer (eks"of-thal-mom'-eh-ter). An instrument for measuring the degree of exophthalmos. Syn., *ophthalmostatometer; proptometer; protometer.*

exophthalmometry (eks"of-thal-mom'-eh-tre). The measurement of the degree of exophthalmos with the exophthalmometer. Syn., *ophthalmostatometry.*

exophthalmos (eks"of-thal'mos). An abnormal protrusion or proptosis of the eyeball from the orbit. Syn., *protrusio bulbi.*

endocrine e. Exophthalmos attributed to malfunction of the thyroid gland, the pituitary gland, or both. Syn., *hormonal exophthalmos.*

hormonal e. Endocrine exophthalmos.

intermittent e. An abnormal intermittent protrusion of the eyeball due to varicose veins in the orbit. Any condition which leads to stasis of blood in the head area, such as bending over or coughing, may cause this to occur if varicose veins are present.

malignant e. Exophthalmos,

usually bilateral and marked, accompanied by severe edema of the eyelids, conjunctiva, and orbital fat and connective tissue; inflammation, degeneration, and increase in size of the extraocular muscles; and ophthalmoplegia. Although it may occur in association with either hyperthroidism, hypothyroidism (as after thyroidectomy), or with a normal thyroid state, it has been considered by some to be an advanced or severe form of Graves's disease but more recently is attributed to overactivity of the anterior lobe of the pituitary gland and especially that of the thyrotrophic hormone. Typically occurring in middle age, it affects males and females equally except after thyroidectomy, in which case it affects males more frequently than females. The course and prognosis vary, with a tendency toward self-limitation. Syn., *progressive exophthalmos; thyrotropic exophthalmos; exophthalmic ophthalmoplegia.*

paralytic e. Exophthalmos caused by partial or total paralysis of the extrinsic muscles of the eye.

progressive e. Malignant exophthalmos.

pulsating e. Exophthalmos characterized by a pulsation of the eyeball which is synchronous with the heart beat, usually due to traumatic rupture of the internal carotid artery into the cavernous sinus.

thyrotoxic e. Exophthalmos present typically in hyperthyroidism; one of the early manifestations of exophthalmic goiter.

thyrotropic e. Malignant exophthalmos.

traumatic e. Exophthalmos resulting from injury involving scar tissue formation, hemorrhage in the orbit, callus formation of fractured bones, etc.

exophthalmus (eks"of-thal'mus). Exophthalmos.

exorbitism (eks-ōr'bit-izm). Exophthalmos.

exotrope ek-so-trōp). One affected with divergent strabismus.

exotropia (eks"o-tro'pe-ah). Divergent strabismus.

basic e. Exotropia having approximately the same magnitude at both far and near fixation distances.

convergence insufficiency e. See *convergence, insufficiency.*

◆
EXPERIMENT

experiment. A trial, test, procedure, or special observation to discover some unknown effect or principle, to confirm or disprove a hypothesis or theory, or to illustrate a known truth.

alley e. the experiment producing the Blumenfeld alleys.

Baumgardt-Segal e. The alternate presentation of two visual stimuli consisting of concentric circular spots of light of different size. When the spots are presented for 10 milliseconds each, with a 10 millisecond interval between, the large spot is seen with a brighter center. When the interval is increased to 50 milliseconds, a ring of light is seen with a black area the size of the small spot in the center.

Bidwell's e. The producing of the perception of the complement of a color stimulus, instead of the real color, by viewing it through an opening in a rotating disk which consists of three

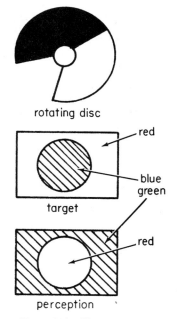

rotating disc

target

perception

Fig. 16 Bidwell's experiment.

sectors, one black, one white, and one cut away to form the opening. The disk is rotated to present the stimuli in the sequence: black, color, and white.

Blackowski's e. An experiment in brightness discrimination, in which a small white disk is surrounded by a larger annular area, the differential brightness limen between the two decreasing as the area of the annulus increases. That this is due to a shift in contours rather than an increase in area was shown by Fry and Bartley in a later experiment.

colored shadow e. The induction of a colored shadow by interposing an opaque object between a colored light source and a luminous white surface, the color of the shadow appearing complementary to the colored source although objectively achromatic.

Czermak's e. The observation of the apparent motion of an object, such as a thread, moved across a pinhole through which the eye is fixating a luminous surface, the pinhole being nearer the eye than the point of focus of the eye. When the object is between the eye and the pinhole, the apparent motion is opposite the real movement; when beyond the pinhole, the apparent motion is the same as the real movement.

Donders' e. The demonstration and/or measurement of relative convergence by the reading of print through prisms.

dropping e. Hering's dropping experiment.

Flechner's cloud e. The observation that a just noticeable difference in brightness of two adjacent cloud areas is still perceptible when viewed through a neutral filter which reduces the brightness of each proportionally.

Fizeau's e. The measurement of the velocity of light by the interval of interruption of light by means of a rotating toothed wheel, before and after traversing a long optical path reflected upon itself.

flicker e. Sherrington's flicker experiment.

Foucault's e. The measurement of the speed of light by the interval between reflections in a rotating plane mirror, before and after traversing a long optical path reflected upon itself.

Fresnel's biprism e. An experiment to produce interference fringes, without relying upon diffraction, by the use of Fresnel's biprism.

Fresnel's mirror e. A method of demonstrating interference by the use of a doubling mirror which splits incident light into two overlapping beams.

Hensen-Völckers e. A demonstration of the action of the ciliary muscle in accommodation by inserting needles through the sclera into the ciliary muscle. Stimulation of the muscle causes a backward movement of the free ends of the needles, indicating a forward movement of their points.

Hering's dropping e. A demonstration or test of depth perception, in which small beads viewed through a tubular aperture are dropped in front of or behind fine wires and are judged to be in front of or behind the plane of the wires.

Kravkov's e. A study of the relative effects of irradiation and brightness discrimination on visual acuity by determining the minimal separation of two black bars necessary for the perception of two when the brightness of the surround and the width of the bars are varied.

Lie's e. An experiment that sought to distinguish between the perceptions of brightness and lightness of neutral surfaces.

Lloyd's e. Lloyd's method.

Mariotte's e. An experiment demonstrating the existence of the physiological blind spot of the eye. The eye fixates a cross on a card which also contains a spot to the templeward side of the cross. The card is moved to and from the eye, and at a certain distance the spot will not be seen.

Meyer's e. A method of demonstrating simultaneous contrast. A narrow strip of gray paper is placed on a larger colored field, and the whole is covered with white tissue paper through which the gray strip appears as a complementary color to the surrounding field.

Molyneux e. An experiment suggested by Molyneux which consists of the showing of various objects to an adult, blind from birth but with vision just restored, to determine if the objects can be identified without tactile clues.

von Noorden-Burian e. The determination of blanking time and perception time in normal and amblyopic eyes, found to be longer in the latter.

partition e. An experiment demonstrating the asymmetry of the two halves of the retina in which an individual, with constant monocular fixation, subjectively bisects a horizontal line. Underestimation of the temporal half of the line is termed *Kundt's monocular asymmetry*, while the reverse is termed *Münsterberg's monocular asymmetry*.

Ragona Scina e. A demonstration of color contrast in which an observer looks through a colored glass placed midway between two touching white screens set at right angles to each other, such that he sees, by reflection in the glass, one screen superimposed on the other. A black spot on the reflected screen will appear to be the same color as the glass, and one on the directly viewed screen will appear as its complement.

reversal e. The observation that a pin moved across a pinhole through which the eye is fixating appears to move in the opposite direction, providing the pinhole is nearer the eye than the point of focus and the pin is nearer than the pinhole.

Sachs's needle e. A demonstration of the action of the ciliary muscle in accommodation by inserting needles in the ciliary muscle of an eye through the sclera at varying distances from the equator of the eyeball. When the muscle contracts, the needle protruding from a certain portion remains motionless, the protruded part of the needle in front of this portion moves forward, and the needle farther back moves backward.

Scheiner's e. A demonstration of the dioptric changes occurring during accommodation by observing a small object through a pair of laterally

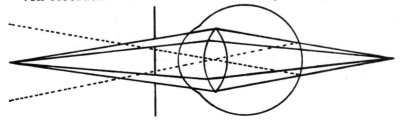

Fig. 17 Scheiner's experiment.

separated pinholes confined within the area of the pupil. The object appears double at all distances from the eye except the distance for which the eye is in focus. (See Fig. 17.)

Sherrington's flicker e. An experiment to investigate binocular fusion of uniocular sensations produced by flickering lights with precisely controlled dark and light intervals, presented to each eye in a variety of sequences and frequencies and compared to summation effects obtained for both stimuli in one eye.

side-window e. A demonstration of binocular contrast in which the observer stands in profile to a window or other bright source so that one eye is strongly transilluminated from the side while the other eye is shaded. White objects will now appear greenish to the illuminated eye, reddish to the other eye.

Stratton's e. An experiment in which, by means of an optical inverting system, the visual directions are completely reversed for one eye for a long period of time, the other eye being occluded. Stratton learned to reach for an object which was visually to his right by moving his hand to his left. This learning, however, did not change the reversed perception of the location of objects in space.

Wundt's e. An experiment to determine the relative effects of accommodation and convergence on the judgment of distance.

Young's e. The first experiment to produce interference fringes performed by Thomas Young in 1802. Two coherent beams of light, produced by passing light from a pinhole in one screen through two pinholes in a second screen, come together to form interference fringes on a third screen.

◆

exposure, light. The product of illuminance and its duration, expressed in lux-seconds. Formerly *quantity of illumination.* Cf. *quantity of light.*

exteriorization (eks-te"re-or-ih-za'-shun). A form of perception in which an object viewed monocularly appears as though seen through an opaque body placed in front of the other eye. The *hole-in-the-hand test* is an example.

external rectus (eks-ter'nal rek'tus). See under *muscle.*

extorsion (eks-tōr'shun). 1. The real, or

apparent, turning of the two eyes relative to each other about their respective anteroposterior axes so that their respective vertical meridians of reference diverge from each other superiorly and converge inferiorly. 2. The real or apparent turning of an eye about an anteroposterior axis so that the upward extension of its vertical meridian of reference deviates temporally from the true vertical. Syn., *disclination.*

extort (eks-tōrt'). To turn toward a position of extorsion or away from a position of intorsion.

extraction (eks-trak'shun). The act or process of pulling or drawing out.

aspiration e. Surgical removal of congenital or other soft cataracts in which an incision is made into the anterior capsule of the crystalline lens and the lens mass evacuated by suction.

combined e. Surgical removal of a cataractous crystalline lens, together with iridectomy.

cryoprehensile e. Cryoextraction.

extracapsular e. Surgical removal of a cataractous crystalline lens by incising the anterior capsule of the lens and expressing the opaque lens.

intracapsular e. Surgical removal of a cataractous crystalline lens, together with its capsule.

linear e. Surgical treatment of soft or traumatic cataract in which an incision is made into the anterior capsule of the crystalline lens and the lens mass evacuated through the corneal wound by pressure or irrigation.

simple e. Surgical removal of a cataractous crystalline lens, without iridectomy.

extraocular (eks"trah-ok'u-lar). External to or outside of the eye.

extrarectus (eks"trah-rek'tus). External rectus muscle.

extravisual (eks"trah-vizh'u-al). Other than visual; outside of the field of vision, or beyond the visible spectrum.

◆

EYE

eye. The organ of vision. In humans, it is a spheroid body approximately 1 in. in diameter, with the segment of a smaller sphere, the cornea, in front. It occurs in pairs, one in each of the bony orbits of the skull, and consists of an external coat of fibrous sclera and transparent

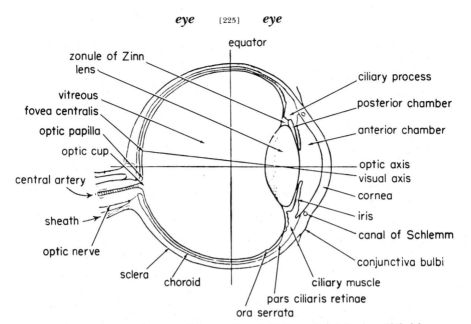

equator

zonule of Zinn
lens

vitreous
fovea centralis
optic papilla
optic cup
central artery
sheath
optic nerve
sclera
choroid

ciliary process
posterior chamber
anterior chamber
optic axis
visual axis
cornea
iris
canal of Schlemm
conjunctiva bulbi
ciliary muscle
pars ciliaris retinae
ora serrata

Fig. 18 Schematic cross section of the eye. (From A. E. Town, *Ophthalmology*. Philadelphia: Lea and Febiger, 1951)

cornea; a middle vascular coat, the uvea, composed of the iris, the ciliary body, and the choroid; and an internal nervous coat, the retina, which includes the sensory receptors for light. Within, it contains the anterior, the posterior, and the vitreous chambers, the aqueous humor, the vitreous body, the crystalline lens, the zonule of Zinn, and the intraocular portion of the optic nerve. Six extraocular muscles control its movements. Broader definitions sometimes include the conjunctiva, Tenon's capsule, and associated appendages.

acone e. A compound eye found in certain arthropods in which the region of each ommatidium normally containing the crystalline cone is cellular and nonrefractive.

aggregate e. A group of closely packed ocelli which resembles a compound eye, but differs in that each ocellus remains anatomically and functionally independent.

amaurotic cat's e. See under *amaurotic*.

aphakic e. An eye in which the crystalline lens is not present. See also *aphakia*.

apotropaic e. An amulet symbolic of an eye which purportedly averts or turns aside evil.

appendages of e. The ocular adnexa, consisting of the eyelids, the eyebrows, the conjunctiva, lacrimal apparatus, Tenon's capsule, and the extrinsic ocular muscles. Some authorities omit the latter two.

apposition e. The typical compound eye in which both the crystalline cone and the retinule of each ommatidium is ensheathed by pigment cells so that light striking the corneal facet cannot reach or stimulate neighboring ommatidia. Hence, light from one corneal facet is incident upon only one rhabdome. Cf. *superposition eye*.

artificial e. A prosthesis made of glass, plastic, or similar material which simulates the anterior portion of an eye. It is placed in the socket after enucleation or evisceration or over the remnants of a nonfunctioning eye for cosmetic purposes. **custom a.e.** An artificial eye expressly made to fit a patient's orbit. It is usually hand painted if made of plastic or has a handmade iris if made of glass. **semicustom a.e.** An artificial eye especially made to fit the patient's orbit but having a stock iris. **stock a.e.** Any one of an assortment of ready-made artificial eyes from which a selection is made to fit a patient.

biunial e. Cyclopean eye.

black e. Ecchymosis of the eyelid.

blear e. An irritated or a watery-appearing eye.

bung e. A permanent swelling of the upper eyelid in association with onchocerciasis.

cerebral e. The eye of a vertebrate which has its retina derived from the forebrain via an optic cup and not from the surface ectoderm as in many invertebrates.

chameleon e. Pronounced proptosis with downward, or downward and lateral, displacement of the eyeball, usually accompanied by impaired motility, chemosis, and eyelid edema, and resulting from an intraorbital tumor or invasion of the orbit by a tumor.

compound e. The eye of arthropods, such as insects, which consists of a grouping of structurally and functionally associated elements, ommatidia, whose surfaces collectively form a mosaic-patterned segment of a sphere.

congenital cystic e. A congenital cyst in the space normally occupied by the eyeball due to failure of the primary optic vesicle to involute.

controlling e. Predominant eye.

crossed e's. Convergent strabismus.

cupulate e. A type of simple eye composed of a group of contiguous light-sensitive epithelial cells which have invaginated to form a cup-shaped depression.

cyclopean e. An imaginary mental eye located between the two real eyes which serves as a center for directionalization. It represents a composite hypothetical visual perception area for the two eyes, with a macula, a center of rotation, a nodal point, and a principal point, all lying in a straight line in a medially located reference plane of the head. Syn., *biunial eye; mental eye.* **bimacular c.e.** The cyclopean eye in subjects with anomalous retinal correspondence. The apparent direction of a bifoveally perceived object differs for the right and the left eyes. This difference in direction can be represented by assuming that the imaginary cyclopean eye has two maculae instead of one. **macular c.e.** The cyclopean eye in subjects with normal retinal correspondence.

dark-adapted e. An eye which has been sufficiently exposed to decreased illumination to bring about the chemical and physiologic changes necessary for maximum sensitivity to light. Such changes include dilation of the pupillary aperture, regeneration and advancement of rhodopsin in the rods of the retina, and dependence on peripheral retinal stimulation. See also *duplicity theory; scotopic vision.*

deviating e. The nonfixating eye in strabismus or under phoria testing conditions.

directing e. The dominant eye as established by criteria which are presumed to determine which eye primarily subserves the perception of direction or the function of guiding the orientation of the subject.

dominant e. 1. The eye that is dominant when ocular dominance exists. 2. The fixating eye in unilateral strabismus.

emmetropic e. An eye having the condition of emmetropia.

equidominant e's. Eyes equally dominant or failing to show dominance in reference to a specific type of ocular dominance.

eucone e. The typical compound eye of arthropods in which each ommatidium has a surface cuticular lenslike formation (corneal facet) and an underlying crystalline cone.

exciting e. In sympathetic ophthalmia, the eye which is originally injured and which seems to serve as a source of inflammation for the other eye. The term, *sympathogenic,* has also been suggested for this eye. Syn., *primary eye.*

exocone e. A compound eye found in certain arthropods in which the region of each ommatidium normally containing the crystalline cone is, instead, a conelike invagination of the surface corneal facet.

fixating e. 1. In strabismus, the eye which is directed toward the object of regard. 2. In cases of diplopia, natural or induced by testing devices, the eye which serves to locate correctly the object of regard in space; the eye which receives stimulation from the object at the fovea; the eye which serves as the organ of reference for the cyclopean eye. 3. The eye used for viewing through monocular instruments or small single apertures.

flat e. A type of simple eye composed of a few contiguous light-sensitive epithelial cells which, together, form a surface plaque.

e. fold. See under *fold.*

following e. In strabismus, the deviating eye.

gas e. An eye characterized by inflammation and photophobia and found among attendants of natural gas pumping stations.

hare's e. Lagophthalmos.

hop e. An eye with conjunctivitis caused by irritation from the hairs of the hop plant.

hot e. Jonathan Hutchinson's name for gouty conjunctivitis.

hyper e. An eye situated higher than its fellow in relation to an assumed horizontal plane of reference defined by one or another structural feature of the body, head, or face.

klieg e. An eye with conjunctivitis, photophobia, lacrimation, and edema, caused by exposure to the intense illumination from klieg lights.

lead e. 1. In strabismus, the fixating eye. 2. Predominant eye.

light-adapted e. An eye which has been sufficiently exposed to bright illumination to bring about the necessary physiological and photochemical changes for photopic or daylight vision. These changes include decreasing the pupil aperture, bleaching and retraction of the rhodopsin, and concentration on cone rather than rod vision. Color sensitivity is generally assumed to be associated with the light-adapted eye. See also *duplicity theory; photopic vision.*

master e. Dominant eye.

e. memory. Visual memory.

mental e. Cyclopean eye.

monochromatic e. An eye which perceives only one color.

optic constants of the e. See under *constant.*

phakic e. An eye in which the crystalline lens is present.

pineal e. A rudimentary median eye appearing in some lower forms of animal life.

pink e. 1. Acute contagious conjunctivitis. 2. (Vet. Med.) In livestock, infectious keratitis.

predominant e. The eye considered to control visual perception in binocular vison; to be differentiated from the sighting eye in sighting ocular dominance. Syn., *controlling eye; lead eye.*

preferred e. 1. The eye usually or always selected when unilateral viewing is required by some visual task. The term is best applicable when the subject is aware that only one eye can be used, as in the use of a monocular microscope. See also *sighting dominance.* 2. The eye which fixates the greater percentage of the time in alternating strabismus.

primary e. Exciting eye.

pseudocone e. A compound eye found in certain insects in which the ommatidium has a fluid substance instead of a crystalline cone.

reduced e. A mathematical concept (model) of the optical system of the eye as if it were a single ideal refracting surface with only one nodal point, principal point, and index of refraction. **Donders' r.e.** A simplified concept of the optical constants of the eye in which the refracting portions are represented as a single spherical surface of which the radius of curvature is 5.73 mm, the index of refraction is 1.336, the refractive surface is 1.35 mm behind the cornea, and the nodal point lies 7.08 mm posterior to the cornea. Its anterior focal distance is 17.054 mm, and its posterior focal distance is 22.78 mm, both measured from the refracting surface of the reduced eye. **Gullstrand's r.e.** A reduced eye which has a radius of curvature of 5.7 mm, an index of refraction of 1.33, and a length of 22.8 mm. **Listing's r.e.** A reduced eye which has a radius of curvature of 5.1248 mm, an index of refraction of 1.35, and a length of 20.0 mm.

reform e., Snellen's. An artificial eye consisting of two convexoconcave laminae with an air space between them.

schematic e. 1. A diagrammatic representation of the optical system of an ideal normal eye based on a careful analysis of the dioptric systems of a number of emmetropic eyes. It includes constants for curvature, indices of refraction, and distances between the optical elements. 2. A simplified mechanical model of the human eye having a single refracting lens, a pupillary aperture, and a representation of the retina, used in the practice of retinoscopy and ophthalmoscopy. 3. An eye model, usually simplified and enlarged, to show the mechanical, optical, and anatomical features of the eye. **Fisher's s.e.** A model eye designed with a single refracting lens, a variable pupillary aperture, and a means of varying the distance from the lens to the surface representing the retina, used for practice in ophthalmoscopy and retinoscopy. **Gullstrand's s.e.** A representative or schematic eye computed from the average of a large number of human eye measurements by Allvar Gullstrand (1862-1930). Gullstrand gave values for the position of the principal, nodal, and focal points and thus defined the eye as an optical instrument. **simplified s.e.** An approximation based on the schematic eye, in which calculations are carried out to fewer decimal places, and certain small values are considered negligible.

secondary e. Sympathizing eye.

shell e. An artificial eye consisting of a single thin layer. Cf. *Snellen's reform eye.*

e. shield. 1. A covering for the eye to protect it from light, infection, or injury. 2. An occluder.

shipyard e. Epidemic keratoconjunctivitis.

sighting e. The dominant eye in sighting ocular dominance.

simple e. An ocellus.

squinting e. The deviating eye in strabismus.

subdominant e. The eye considered to subserve the fellow (predominant) eye in binocular vision.

superposition e. A compound eye found in some nocturnal insects in which, in the dark-adapted state, the pigment is concentrated around the crystalline cones, leaving the retinules without insulation, so that light from several corneal facets may pass through several retinules to converge upon a single rhabdome. Cf. *apposition eye.*

sympathizing e. In sympathetic ophthalmia, the uninjured eye which is affected by an inflammation of the uveal tract following injury to the exciting eye. Syn., *secondary eye.*

trichromatic e. An eye with normal trichromatic color vision.

vesicular e. The most advanced type of simple eye composed of a group of contiguous light-sensitive epithelial cells which have invaginated to form a closed subepithelial globe.

◆

eyeball. The globe or ball of the eye.

congenital cystic e. A large, bulging, tumorlike orbital mass existing from birth, due to failure of the optic vesicle to invaginate.

luxated e. An eyeball displaced

forward from its normal position in the orbit.

eyebright (also eye-bright, eiebright, and eie-bright). Any of several herbs of the genus Euphrasia, a popular 17th-century remedy for many eye ailments, used both topically and internally.

eyebrow. 1. An appendage of the eye located in the region of the superciliary ridge of the frontal bone and consisting of skin with hairs (supercilia), subcutaneous tissue, three skeletal muscles, areolar connective tissue, and the cranial periosteum (pericranium). 2. The row of hairs (supercilia) between the upper eyelid and the forehead. Syn., *supercilium.*

eyecells. Postoperative shields made of black cup-shaped porcelain that fit over the eyelids.

Eye Conservation Week. See *Save Your Vision Week.*

eyecup. 1. The optic cup of the early embryo which gives rise to the retina and the inner portions of the ciliary body and the iris. 2. A vessel which may be filled with fluid and fitted to the orbital aperture to bathe or treat the area of the conjunctival sac.

eyecurrent. 1. The electrical effect that is recorded as the electroretinogram (ERG). 2. The "current of rest," or the resting potential in the eye; an electrical potential from the eye when no light is involved, sometimes recorded when the eye is rendered neurally inactive. The effect is then due simply to ionic differences across membranes. The cornea is positive to the back of the eye.

eyedness. Ocular dominance.

eyeglass. 1. A monocle. 2. The eyepiece, or the ocular, of an optical instrument.

eyeglasses. 1. A pair of ophthalmic lenses together with the frame or the mounting; spectacles. 2. A pair of ophthalmic lenses supported in a frame or a mounting that is held on the nose by spring pressure without the aid of temples, as in a pince-nez or oxford.

eyeground. The fundus of the eye as seen with the ophthalmoscope.

eyelash. A cilium growing on the margin of the eyelid.

eyelens. The lens nearest the observer's eye in an eyepiece.

eyelids. A pair of protective coverings of the eye, consisting of a lower eyelid extending upward from the cheek and an upper eyelid extending downward from the eyebrow and more movable, due to the action of a levator muscle. Each eyelid consists of the following layers: skin, subcutaneous connective tissue, orbicularis oculi muscle, submuscular connective tissue, a fibrous layer made up of a tarsus with sebum-producing Meibomian glands and an orbital septum attached to the orbital margin, a smooth muscle of Mueller, and the palpebral conjunctiva.

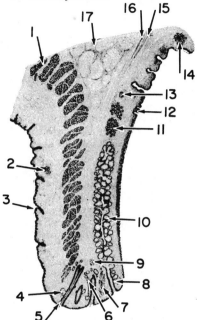

Fig. 19 Section through the upper eyelid. (1) Orbicularis oculi muscle. (2) Sweat gland. (3) Hair follicle. (4) Gland of Zeis. (5) Cilium. (6) Gland of Moll. (7) Pars ciliaris muscle. (8) Muscle of Riolan. (9) Inferior arterial arcade. (10) Meibomian gland. (11) Gland of Wolfring. (12) Conjunctival crypts. (13) Superior arterial arcade. (14) Gland of Krause. (15) Mueller's superior palpebral muscle. (16) Levator palpebrae superioris muscle. (17) Fat. (From S. Duke-Elder, *Textbook of Ophthalmology*, vol. V. London: Henry Kimpton, 1952)

fused e. 1. The normal epithelial joining of the eyelid folds present from about the ninth week until the seventh or eighth month of fetal life. 2. A congenital anomaly in which the eyelids remain joined. Syn., *ankyloblepharon.*

granulated eyelid. A lay term for chronic blepharitis, characterized by scaly desquamation.

third eyelid. Nictitating membrane.

tucked eyelid. A retraction of the upper eyelid, usually associated with ophthalmoplegia and occurring in lesions of the upper brain stem in the region of the posterior commissure.

eyepiece. The lens or a combination of lenses in a telescope, microscope, or other optical instrument to which the human eye is applied in order to view the image formed by the objective system. Syn., *eye lens; ocular.*

Abbe's e. An orthoscopic eyepiece consisting of a triplet field lens and a planoconvex eye lens, designed to have a chromatic difference of magnification opposite to that of the objective and having a shorter focal length for red light than for blue light.

autocollimating e. Gauss eyepiece.

compensating e. An eyepiece in a lens system compensating for spherical or longitudinal aberration of the objective.

filar e. An eyepiece with fine threads imaged across the field of view to measure image size.

Gauss's e. An eyepiece in which the cross hairs or reticle can be illuminated from the side to serve as an object for an autocollimating telescope, as in a spectroscope. Syn., *autocollimating eyepiece.*

Huygens' e. An eyepiece, the most common on microscopes, designed by Huygens, a Dutch physicist (1629-1695), consisting of two planoconvex lenses, the convex side of each being directed toward the objective lens system. The first lens, the field lens, usually has a focal length three times that of the eye lens, and the separation is twice the focal length of the eye lens.

Kellner e. A modification of the Ramsden eyepiece, widely used in high power telescopes, gunsights, and, commonly, in prism binoculars, designed to reduce the amount of lateral chromatic aberration. The eye lens is an achromatic doublet made of dense barium crown glass and light flint glass.

measuring e. Micrometer eyepiece.

micrometer e. An eyepiece having a ruled or filar scale in its focal plane so as to coincide with the objective image and facilitate measurement of its dimensions. Syn., *measuring eye-piece.*

negative e. An eyepiece in which a real image is formed between its lenses.

orthoscopic e. An eyepiece especially corrected for distortion, usually consisting of a triple field lens and a single eye lens, providing a wide field of view and high magnification; it is used on telescopes and range finders.

positive e. An eyepiece in which a real image is formed outside the eyepiece and which can be used as a magnifier.

Ramsden e. An eyepiece designed by Ramsden, an English optician, consisting of two planoconvex lenses, the convex side of each facing the other within the eyepiece. The lenses are often equal in focal length and separated by three fourths the focal length of either.

simple e. An eyepiece consisting of a single lens.

symmetrical e. An eyepiece consisting of two similar lenses, usually two symmetrical achromatic doublets, used primarily in telescopic sights on guns where the eye must be a distance from the eyepiece.

terrestrial e. An eyepiece which contains an erecting system in addition to its usual eyepiece lenses.

wide-field e. An eyepiece designed to give a wide field of view, as an orthoscopic eyepiece.

eyepoint. 1. The point in an optical system where a given point of reference of the observer's eye, such as the entrance pupil of the eye, should be placed; the exit pupil of a viewing system, e.g., of a telescope. 2. A reference point within the eye used in specifying angular magnification or distortion of an ophthalmic prism; usually the entrance pupil of the eye, the center of rotation of the eye, or a theoretical point that assumes that both the entrance pupil and the center of rotation are coincident.

eyesight. The sense of seeing; vision.

eyesize. The dimension of the eyewire of a spectacle frame. There are various methods of determining this dimension. It is specified by the Standards Committee of the American Optometric Association and the Technical Committee of the Optical Manufacturers Association as "the width of eye, length between vertical tangents to the ends of lens, 'boxed' length."

Eye-Span Trainer. A trade name for a manually operated tachistoscope used in flash recognition training of numbers, words, or phrases.

eyespot. A light-sensitive pigmented spot, found in unicellular organisms and in other invertebrates, which serves in phototaxis. Syn., *stigma.*

eyestrain. Discomfort or fatigue associated with the eyes or the use of the eyes and attributed to uncorrected errors of refraction, ocular muscle anomalies, prolonged use of the eyes, etc.

eye-vesicle (i-ves'i-k'l). Optic vesicle. *Obs.*

eyewash. Any fluid medication or cleanser applied to the eye. Syn., *collyrium.*

eyewire. The portion of a spectacle frame that conforms to the periphery of a lens and thereby retains the lens. It may be grooved to fit a beveled lens edge, or round (wire or nylon thread) to fit a grooved lens edge.

F. Symbol for (1) *rate of aqueous outflow;* (2) *visual field;* (3) *focal power.*

f. Symbol for *focal length.*

f number. See under *number.*

F.A.A.O. Fellow of the American Academy of Optometry.

Fabry's disease (fah-brēz'). See under *disease.*

Fabry-Pérot (fah-bre'peh-ro') **etalon; filter; fringes; interferometer.** See under the nouns.

face tilt. A forward or a backward tilt of the head, especially as a postural symptom of an extraocular muscle paresis or paralysis.

face turn. Head rotation.

facet, corneal. 1. A small dip, or fossa, on the outer surface of the cornea, resulting from failure of the floor of an ulcer to fill in with tissue. 2. The surface lenslike structure, superficial to the crystalline cone, in the ommatidium of the compound eye of arthropods.

facial hemiatrophy (fa'shal at'ro-fe). Romberg's disease.

facial hemiplegia, alternate (fa'shal hem"ih-ple'je-ah). Millard-Gubler syndrome.

F.A.C.L.P. Fellow of the Association of Contact Lens Practitioners.

◆

FACTOR

factor. 1. One of the circumstances, elements, or constituents contributing to produce a result. 2. Any of the quantities or elements that form a product when multiplied together; a quantity by which a magnitude must be divided or multiplied to express it in other terms. 3. A desirable or essential nutritional element. 4. A gene.

absorption f. 1. Absorptance. 2. In glass manufacture, the ingredient serving to make the glass absorptive.

allowance f. The factored out quantity in a polynomial ophthalmic lens formula which represents the difference between the sum of the two surface powers and the back vertex power.

contrast rendition f. The ratio of visual task contrast with a given lighting environment to that obtained with sphere illumination. Abbreviation *CRF.*

daylight f. The ratio of the daylight illumination at a given point of reference inside a building to the simultaneous illumination on a small horizontal exterior area exposed to the whole sky but excluding direct rays from the sun.

discomfort glare f. The numerical assessment of the capacity of a single source of brightness, such as a luminaire, in a given visual environment for producing discomfort. Abbreviation *DGF.* Cf. *discomfort glare rating.*

discrimination f. The reciprocal, $B/\Delta B$, of the differential threshold in brightness discrimination, where ΔB equals the difference in luminance between the two parts of the test field and B equals the luminance of one of them. Syn., *discrimination index.*

field f. In lighting practice, the factor by which a threshold or standard derived in a research laboratory should be multiplied to make it applicable to environmental conditions or requirements in the field.

fitting f. Wrap factor.

glow f. The number of lumens emitted by fluorescent material per milliwatt of incident black light.

inclination f. Obliquity factor.

lighting effectiveness f. The ratio of equivalent sphere illumination to ordinary measured or calculated illumination. Abbreviation *LEF*.

luminance f. Radiance factor.

luminosity f. Spectral luminous efficacy of radiant flux. See under *efficacy*. **relative l.f.** Spectral luminous efficiency of radiant flux. See under *efficiency*.

obliquity f. In Huygens' wave theory of light propagation the variation of the amplitude of the disturbance of a secondary wave initiated at an element of the original wave surface, due to the angle between the normals to the original and secondary wavefronts. Syn., *obliquity function; inclination factor*.

radiance f. The ratio of the radiance in a given direction and at a given point on the surface of a non-self-radiating body to that of a perfect reflecting or transmitting diffuser identically irradiated. Syn., *luminance factor*.

reduction f. The ratio of the mean spherical candlepower of a source of light to its mean horizontal candlepower. Syn., *spherical reduction factor*.

reflection f. The ratio of flux reflected from a surface to that incident on it. Syn., *reflectance*. **diffuse r.f.** The ratio of flux diffusely reflected from a surface to that incident on it. Syn., *diffuse reflectance*. **specular r.f.** The ratio of flux regularly reflected from a surface to that incident on it. Syn., *specular reflectance*. **total r.f.** The ratio of flux reflected both diffusely and regularly from a surface to that incident on it. Syn., *total reflectance*.

room utilization f. The ratio of the luminous flux received on the workplane to that emitted by the luminaires.

shape f. The factored out quantity in a polynomial lens formula which contains the thickness and curvature symbols.

transient adaptation f. A mathematical index of the relative visibility of a task in a given lighting installation for which typical patterns of eye movement introduce transient exposures to varying luminances in comparison with the same task visibility obtained during steady fixation while adapted to a uniform reference lighting condition; usually expressed as 1-K log R where K is a constant and R is the ratio of the luminance contrast of the former task to that of the latter at equal visibility levels. Abbreviation *TAF*.

transmission f. The ratio of radiant flux transmitted through a body to that incident on it. Syn., *transmittance*.

visibility f. 1. Spectral luminous efficacy of radiant flux. See under *efficacy*. 2. A coefficient obtained by any of several procedures or formulas to represent the extent to which glare affects visual acuity or brightness discrimination. **relative v.f.** Spectral luminous efficiency of radiant flux. See under *efficiency*.

wrap f. The ratio of the back central optic radius of an undistorted hydrated contact lens to the back central optic radius of the lens when it is on the eye. Syn., *fitting factor*.

◆

faculty, fusion. 1. The ability to perceive with the two eyes a single, integrated, fused image of a pair of haploscopically presented objects or an object viewed binocularly, especially when characterized by the associated ability to maintain single, fused imagery through a finite range of changes in convergence stimulus. 2. The ability to perceive continuously uniform light when the stimulus is intermittent. *Rare*.

critical f. f. The ability to appreciate intermittent visual stimulation as continuous when it reaches a certain frequency.

F.A.D.O. Fellow of the Association of Dispensing Opticians.

FAHRE. See *Federation of Associations of Health Regulatory Boards*.

faisceau isthmique (fa-so' is'mēk). Druault's marginal bundle.

fallacia optica (fah-la'shih-ah op'tih-kah). A visual illusion or a visual hallucination.

Falls-Kurtesz syndrome (fals-kur'-tez). See under *syndrome*.

fan dial. See under *chart, fan dial*.

fan, macular. Deposits of lipid material in Henle's fiber layer in an incomplete star formation radiating out from the macula in a previously edematous area. See also *macular star*.

Fanconi's disease (fan-kŏn'ēz). See under *disease*.

Fanconi-Türler syndrome (fan-kŏn'e-tēr'ler). See under *syndrome*.

fantascope (fan'tah-skōp). Phenakistoscope.

fantasy. Imagination; the mental creation of nonexistent objects or images, or the so-created mental image itself.

far point (farpoint) of accommodation; convergence; fusion. See under the nouns.

Faraday's (far'ah-dāz) **birefringence; effect.** See under the nouns.

Farnsworth (fahrns'worth) **color circle; test.** See under the nouns.

Farnsworth-Munsell test (fahrns'-worth-mun-sel'). See under *test*.

farsighted. Hypermetropic.

farsightedness. Hypermetropia.

fascia (fash'e-ah). A layer or sheet of connective tissue covering, insheathing, partitioning, supporting, or binding together structures or internal parts of the body.

    bulbar f. Tenon's capsule.

    lacrimal f. The periosteum which encloses the lacrimal sac.

    orbital f. A general term for all the fibrous membranes within the orbit, including the periorbita, the orbital septum, Tenon's capsule, intermuscular membranes, check ligaments, and others.

    palpebral f. Septum orbitale.

    tarso-orbital f. Septum orbitale.

    f. of Tenon. Tenon's capsule.

fasciculus, anterior accessory, of Bochenek (fah-sik'u-lus). Anterior accessory optic tract of Bochenek.

fasciculus, medial longitudinal (fah-sik'u-lus). Medial longitudinal bundle.

fat, orbital. Fatty tissue which fills the interstices in the orbit in the regions of the optic nerve, the muscles, the lacrimal gland, the vessels, and the nerves.

fata morgana (fa'tah mōr-gah'nah). A mirage named for Morgan le Fay that creates fantastic mountains, cliffs, columns, or castles as images of relatively flat objects.

fatigue. The condition of organs or cells in which the power or capacity to respond to stimulation is decreased or lost, due to excessive activity.

    color f. 1. Chromatic adaptation, usually of such long duration or high intensity that all or most of the color has perceptually disappeared from the response. The observer perceives only a colorless, gray, or brown adapting light or stimulus surface. Perception of other colors, particularly colors complementary to the adapting color, may be heightened. 2. An excessively rapid perceptual fading of steadily observed colors.

    retinal f. 1. The condition attributed to the retina when the sensory end result is impoverished as, for example, when a small, peripherally located target initially seen, disappears after continued fixation of another target. 2. A condition postulated to explain negative afterimages, successive contrast, etc. Under the most recent view of fatigue and impairment, fatigue seems to be an ill-chosen term.

    visual f. 1. A condition of improper or reduced function considered to accrue from the use of the eyes. It has been of concern as to where this fatigue takes place, whether in the eye, somewhere along the optic pathway, or elsewhere in the central nervous system. In the common view, there is no single set of signs or symptoms that indicates visual fatigue. Actually, some of the symptoms and signs pertain to nonvisual parts of the body. 2. A state of inadequacy of the individual attributable to the use of the visual apparatus. Under this view, visual fatigue, just as any other fatigue, pertains to the person as a whole, and differs from other forms primarily in the kind of task under which it develops. This view makes a distinction between fatigue and tissue impairment, and thus bypasses the need for distinguishing between mental and physical fatigue, except for the mode of production of the end result, fatigue itself.

favus (fa'vus, fah'vus). A skin disease due to a fungus infection, characterized by the presence of round, yellow, saucer-shaped crusts having a peculiar mousy odor. It mainly affects the scalp but may occur on the eyelids. Syn., *tinea favosa*.

FB. Foreign body.

F.B.O.A. Fellow of the British Optical Association.

FCR. Floor cavity ratio.

FDA. Food and Drug Administration.

feather. A feather-shaped defect in glass or other transparent materials which may be due to inhomogeneity, folds, or clusters of fine bubbles.

Fechner's (fek'nerz) **colors; experiment; fraction; law; paradox.** See under the nouns.

Fechner-Helmholtz law (fek'ner-helm'hōltz). Law of coefficients.

Federation of Associations of Health Regulatory Boards. An organization founded in 1973 to facilitate exchanges of information relative to problems, procedures and policies involved in examining, licensing, registering, and regulating health professionals and in accrediting health profession schools and colleges and continuing education programs.

Federation of Manufacturing Opticians. A British national trade association of the ophthalmic optical manufacturing industry founded in 1917 and consisting of eight constituent trade associations.

Federazione Nazionale Titolari Esercizi Ottica Optometrica e Ottica in Genere. A national Italian organization of optician-optometrists and owners and employees of optical and ophthalmic optical retail establishments, founded in Rome in 1956 and serving to represent the trade and professional interests of its members.

FEDEROTTICA. See *Federazione Nazionale Titolari Esercizi Ottica Optometrica e Ottica in Genere.*

feeble-mindedness. 1. Mental inferiority or deficiency which is subdivided into three groups: *idiocy, imbecility,* and *moronity.* 2. Moronity.

Fehr's spotted corneal dystrophy (ferz). Macular corneal dystrophy.

Feinbloom (fin'blūm) **chart; contact lens.** See under the nouns.

Feincone contact lens (fin'kōn). See under *lens, contact.*

Feldman's adaptometer. See under *adaptometer.*

feldspar (feld'spar). Fluorite.

Felty syndrome (fel'te). See under *syndrome.*

fentoscopy (fen-tos'ko-pe). Observation, with the unaided eye, of the passage of the beam of a slit lamp through ocular structures.

Féréol-Graux's ocular palsy (fa-ra-ōl'grawz). See under *palsy.*

Fermat's (fer-māz') **law; principle.** See under the nouns.

Ferree-Rand axometer (fer'e-rand). See under *axometer.*

Ferrein's canal (fer'inz). See under *canal.*

Ferry-Porter law (fer'e-pōr'ter). See under *law.*

FERV. See *Foundation for Education and Research in Vision.*

Fery prism (fer'e). See under *prism.*

fever, pharyngoconjunctival. A triad of fever, pharyngitis, and acute follicular conjunctivitis caused by a virus infection, usually type 3 adenovirus. All three components are not always present, but the conjunctivitis is usually the chief complaint, lasting from a few days to a few weeks and always ending in full recovery. It is usually transmitted through swimming pools and mainly affects children.

fever, sandfly. Conjunctivitis, occasional neuritis, and systemic chills and fever; a viral disease transmitted by the sandfly *Phlebotomus papatasii.* Syn., *Pappataci's disease.*

fever, uveoparotid. Uveoparotitis.

◆

FIBER

fiber. A filament or a threadlike structure.

 arcuate f's. The portion of the ganglionic axons in the nerve fiber layer of the retina which are temporal to the optic disk, and exclusive of the papillomacular bundle, traveling above and below this bundle in an arcuate course.

 f. basket of Schultze. Fine extensions of the external limiting layer of the retina, or of the fibers of Mueller as some claim, which surround the inner members of the rods and the cones.

 cilio-equatorial f's. The fibers of the suspensory ligament of the crystalline lens, originating in the area of the ciliary processes and inserting into the lens capsule at the equator.

 cilioposterior f's. The fibers of the suspensory ligament of the crystalline lens, originating in the region of the ciliary processes and inserting into the posterior capsule of the lens, posterior to the equator.

 cone f. A fiberlike extension of the retinal cone cell extending from the cell body or nuclear region to the inner member and the cone foot.

corticobulbar f's. Axons of pyramidal cells located in the cerebral cortex which enter the contralateral corticobulbar tract and synapse in the motor nuclei of cranial nerves located in the brain stem. See also *corticobulbar tract.*

f's of Gratiolet. Axons in the optic radiations which leave the lateral geniculate body and end in the area striata.

f's of Henle. Long S-shaped rod and cone fibers in the region of the macula lutea which enter the outer molecular layer of the retina and collectively form the fiber layer of Henle.

interretinal f's. Axons that supposedly leave one retina, enter the optic nerve, cross over in the chiasm, and enter the contralateral optic nerve and retina; commissural fibers between the two retinae.

f's of Landolt. Processes of dendrites of cone bipolar neurons of the retina of certain fishes, amphibians, reptiles, and birds, which continue outward to the external limiting membrane.

lens f. An elongated protoplasmic unit, usually hexagonal in section, which is derived from an epithelial cell just within the capsule of the crystalline lens, and is attached to an anterior and to a posterior suture. **primary l.f's.** Fibers of the crystalline lens derived embryonically by the elongation of the posterior epithelium of the lens to fill in the cavity of the lens vesicle, present in the embryonic portion of the nucleus of the adult. **secondary l.f's.** Hexagonal fibers of the crystalline lens, formed at the periphery of the equator of the lens by the posterior portion of the anterior epithelium, which surround the few primary fibers at the very center of the nucleus, are produced throughout life, and eventually lose their nuclei.

longitudinal f's. 1. Smooth muscle fibers, comprising Brücke's muscle, that attach to the scleral spur and uveal meshwork, course through the length of the ciliary body, and attach to the suprachoroid at the equator. 2. The temporal ganglionic axons from the retina that do not decussate but enter the ipsilateral optic tract. 3. Any fiber oriented along the length of the structure of which it is a part.

medullated nerve f's. 1. Nerve fibers, axons, or dendrites which have myelin or fatty sheaths. 2. Ophthalmoscopically observable, anomalously medullated, ganglionic axons in the vicinity of the optic disk. Syn., *opaque nerve fibers.*

Meynert's f's. Axons in the tectobulbar tracts which leave the superior colliculus, synapse in the motor nuclei, and supply the extrinsic muscles of the eye.

Monakow's f's. Efferent pupillary fibers for the direct or consensual light reflexes. *Obs.*

Mueller's f's. Fibers of neuroglia in the retina, extending between the external and internal limiting layers, filling in the space between the conducting neurons and forming a dense network of interlacing trabeculae in the innermost layers. They are supportive to the retinal neurons and participate in their metabolism by storing glycogen and oxidative enzymes.

opaque nerve f's. Medullated nerve fibers.

orbiculoanterior f's. Fibers of the suspensory ligament of the crystalline lens that originate from the smoother posterior part of the ciliary body, just anterior to the ora serrata, and insert into the capsule of the lens, just anterior to the equator.

orbiculociliary f's. Accessory fibers of the suspensory ligament of the crystalline lens that run from the smoother posterior portion of the ciliary body to the ciliary processes, preventing the latter from moving forward.

orbiculoposterior f's. Fibers of the suspensory ligament of the crystalline lens which originate in the posterior smooth portion of the ciliary body and insert into the lens capsule just posterior to its equator.

papillomacular f's. Ganglionic axons from the macular region of the retina which comprise the papillomacular bundle in the nerve fiber layer and which enter the temporal portion of the optic disk and travel in the central portion of the optic nerve.

pupillary f's. 1. Ganglionic axons in the optic nerve that leave the optic tract via a brachium, reach the pretectal region anterior to the superior colliculus, and mediate the afferent impulses of the direct and consensual light pupillary constriction reflexes. 2. Fibers in the oculomotor nerve that synapse in the ciliary ganglion and mediate the efferent impulses of the direct and consensual light pupillary constriction reflexes.

retinomotor f's. 1. Efferent fibers in the optic nerves of lower vertebrates which supposedly control the movement of the outer members of the visual cells by contraction of the myoid elements or of the pigmented processes of the epithelium. If present in man, their function is unknown. 2. Efferent fibers that synapse with centrifugal bipolars of the retina and convey impulses to the cone feet.

Ritter's f's. Granulated fibrils located axially in inner rod segments.

rod f. A thin, delicate fiber extending from the inner member of a rod cell, through the external limiting membrane to the rod granule, and continuing to end in the outer molecular layer as a small end knob which is surrounded by the terminal arborizations of the bipolar cells.

Sappey's f's. Smooth muscle fibers found in check ligaments of the extrinsic eye muscles, near the orbital insertions of the ligaments.

sustentacular f's. The neuroglia or supporting cells of the retina, such as the fibers of Mueller, astrocytes, and others.

tectobulbar f's. Axons of neuron cell bodies, located in the superior and inferior colliculi of the midbrain, which enter the contralateral tectobulbar tract and synapse in the motor nuclei of cranial nerves located in the brain stem. See also *tectobulbar tract.*

trophic (in optic nerve) f's. Efferent fibers in the optic nerve that supposedly affect the nutrition of the retina. Such fibers have not been identified in humans.

visual f's. Axons from the ganglion cell layer of the retina that synapse in the lateral geniculate body and project back to the region of the calcarine fissure, conveying impulses for vision.

zonular f's. The noncellular fibers of the suspensory ligament of the crystalline lens which originate at the ciliary body and insert into the lens capsule near its equator. **capsular z.f's.** Fibers of the zonule of Zinn which insert into the capsule of the crystalline lens. **coronal z.f's.** Fibers of the zonule of Zinn which insert into the corona

ciliaris. **orbicular z.f's.** Fibers of the zonule of Zinn which insert into the pars plana.

◆

fiberscope (fi'ber-skōp). An optical device consisting essentially of a flexible bundle of transparent fibers which transmits an image, thus enabling the viewing of objects which cannot be seen directly, such as the interior of the stomach.

fibrodysplasia hyperelastica (fi"-bro-dis-pla'se-ah hi"per-e-las'tih-kah). Meekren-Ehlers-Danlos syndrome.

fibroma (fi-bro'mah). A benign tumor, primarily consisting of masses of white, fibrous, connective tissue, which commonly appears on the conjunctiva or the eyelid as a result of inflammation or trauma, and may also occur on the sclera, the cornea, the choroid, or the optic nerve.

f. molluscum. The neurofibroma of von Recklinghausen's disease; a diffuse proliferation of the Schwann cells of the peripheral nerves which may involve any part of the eye or the adnexa.

fibroplasia, retrolental. Retinopathy of prematurity.

fibrosis, massive retinal (fi-bro'sis) An elevated grayish-white mass of glial tissue protruding from the retina, due to the organization of a massive retinal hemorrhage. In the newborn, it is primarily attributed to obstetrical trauma and is located near the optic disk or macula. In the adult, the affected eye often shows evidence of endophthalmitis, and the mass is usually at the ora serrata. Syn., *retinal pseudotumor.*

fibrosis, musculo-fascial (fi-bro'sis) Ptosis, marked restriction of all eye movements, particularly of elevation, and absence of Bell's phenomenon as a result of a familial congenital general fibrosis of all the extrinsic ocular muscles with adhesions of Tenon's capsule to the eyeball.

fibrosis, preretinal macular (fi-bro'sis). A disease of unknown etiology occurring in the aged, presenting an ophthalmoscopic picture of a glinting reflex in the macular region. Small white exudates, venous anomalies, and hemorrhages may also be present. Usually unilateral, visual acuity is characteristically 20/50 or better, and the Amsler grid is generally distorted. Syn., primary retinal folds; preretinal membrane; macular pucker; cellophane retinopathy.

Fick's phenomenon; theory; tonometer. See under the nouns.

◆

FIELD

field. 1. An area, a region, or a space. 2. A range or sphere of activity.

curvature of the f. See under *curvature*.

depth of f. See under *depth*.

diagnostic action f. Any of six meridional directions of ocular rotation which correspond to principal planes of action of the six extraocular muscles and in which limitation of movement is most definitely diagnosed as a specific muscle paresis. Cf. *diagnostic position of gaze*.

diplopia f. The portion or regions of the field of fixation in which diplopia occurs, a clinical finding used in the differential diagnosis of extraocular muscle paresis or paralysis. **Duane's d.f.** A diplopia field plotted for various directions of gaze with a number of small, independently illuminated light sources in fixed positions on the test screen as fixation targets.

f. of excursion. Field of fixation.

f. of fixation. The total angular range of rotatory excursion of the eye, with the head fixed, represented by a plot of the limits of fixation on a tangent screen, or on a spherical surface concentric with the center of rotation of the eye. The approximate monocular limits specified from the straightforward position are: 45° outward, 50° inward, 35° upward, and 50° downward. Syn., *field of excursion; motor field; field of rotation*. **bifoveal f. of f.** The total angular range or limits of excursion of the eyes under conditions of binocular fixation, with the head fixed, usually represented on a field of fixation diagram or plot. **practical f. of f.** The field of fixation obtained with combined head and eye movements.

frontal adversive f. Brodmann's area 6, alpha beta.

frontal eye f. The posterior portion of the middle frontal gyrus of each frontal lobe, controlling voluntary contradirectional conjugate eye movements; Brodmann's area 8, alpha beta delta.

f. of full illumination. In an optical system, the angular subtense of the entrance port when the sides of the enclosing angle are extended to the edges of the entrance pupil on the same side of the optical axis.

induced f. In simultaneous contrast, the portion of the visual field acted on and modified by the *inducing field*.

inducing f. In simultaneous contrast, the portion of the visual field acting on and modifying another portion of the visual field, the *induced field*.

motor f. Field of fixation.

object f. Field of view.

occipital eye f. The reflex center in each occipital lobe, controlling pursuit and fixation ocular movements.

perceptual f., ambiocular. The region of space panoramically perceived in certain conditions of strabismus. See also *ambiocularity*.

perceptual f., binocular. The region of space binocularly perceived with normal retinal correspondence.

perceptual f., monocular. The region of space perceived by a single eye.

f. of phoria. In paralytic strabismus, the area in the field of fixation in which single binocular vision can be maintained. Cf. *field of tropia*.

receptive f. The area of the visual field within which a light stimulus can cause a change in the average firing rate of a single retinal ganglion cell.

receptor f. of optic nerve fiber. The retinal area whose visual receptors, via synapses with bipolar cells, are subserved by a single ganglion cell.

f. of regard. The portion of the visual field dominant in consciousness at any given time.

retinal f. That portion of the retina containing visual sense cells; the anatomical correlate of the visual field.

f. of rotation. Field of fixation.

sagittal f. The image surface formed by the sagittal foci of the points in an object surface perpendicular to the axis of the optical system.

schlieren f. The conjugate focal plane of the image plane for the objective lens of a schlieren optical system.

tilting f. A device used in demonstrating the effects of aniseikonia on spatial localization, usually consisting of a plane surface mounted on a universal pivot, on which objects designed to enhance stereoscopic clues are placed. When the observer sets the surface so that it appears level, the type and the amount of tilt indicate the kind and the degree of aniseikonia.

triangular f. of Wernicke.

The portion of the posterior part of the posterior limb of the internal capsule of the corpus striatum which contains the general sensation pathway and the auditory and optic radiations.

f. of tropia.

In paralytic strabismus, the area in the field of fixation in which single binocular vision is not possible. Cf. *field of phoria.*

f. of view.

1. The extent of the object plane visible through, or imaged by, an optical instrument. Syn., *absolute field of view.* 2. In an optical system, the angular subtense of the entrance port measured from the center of the entrance pupil. Cf. *field of full illumination; absolute field of view.* **absolute f. of v.** In an optical system, the angular subtense of the entrance port when the sides of the enclosing angle are extended to the edges of the entrance pupil on the opposite side of the optical axis. **apparent f. of v.** The angle subtended by the exit port of a visual aid at the center of the entrance pupil of the eye. **linear f. of v.** The extent of object space imaged by an optical system, expressed as a linear distance in the object plane. **real f. of v.** True field of view. **true f. of v.** The angle subtended at the center of the entrance pupil of the eye by that part of the object plane visible to the eye through a visual aid. Syn., *real field of view.*

visual f.

The area or extent of physical space visible to an eye in a given position. Its average extent is approximately 65° upward, 75° downward, 60° inward, and 95° outward, when the eye is in the straightforward position. **absolute v.f.** The visual field that would exist if the obstruction by the facial structures were eliminated so that the entire retina could be stimulated. It can be determined by using successively different positions of fixation other than the straightforward position. Cf. *relative visual field.* Syn., *maximum visual field; physiologic visual field.* **accordion v.f.** A visual field associated with hysteria and showing contraction in successively measured, alternate meridians so that the border of the plot looks like folds in a bellows. **anatomic v.f.** Relative visual field.

antagonistic v.f. Visual fields of the two eyes which cannot be integrated binocularly into a single composite percept, such as the two fields of vision normally seen by a strabismic individual, or those resulting from a pair of differing visual stimulus patterns presented haploscopically to the two eyes in a retinal rivalry test. **binocular v.f** 1. The combined visual field. 2. The common visual field. **central v.f.** The area of the visual field corresponding to the fovea or the macula. Syn., *direct visual field.* **color v.f.** The portion of the visual field within which color can be perceived, the field for any given color being smaller than, and roughly concentric with, the visual field for white. In order of size of largest to smallest, the clinically obtained color fields are yellow, blue, red, green. The field for each color varies greatly with variation in such factors as target size, saturation, brightness, and contrast. **interlacing of color v.f's.** The interlacing of the borders of the plotted visual fields for two or more test objects of different color. **overlapping of color v.f's.** The extension of the visual field for a given color beyond the border of the visual field of another color normally expected to be larger. **combined v.f.** The extent of the visual field viewed with binocular fixation, including the extreme temporal regions visible to one eye only. **common v.f.** The extent of the visual field viewed with both eyes simultaneously during binocular fixation, i.e., not including the temporal regions visible to one eye only. Its vertical dimension is the same as the monocular visual field and its horizontal dimension is approximately 120°. **congruent v.f.** Visual fields of the two eyes which have defects identical in size, shape, and position, so as to form a single defect of the binocular visual field. **cribriform v.f.** A visual field containing a number of isolated scotomata. **depressed v.f.** A visual field characterized by general or local reduction of sensitivity to stimuli within it. The isopters are smaller than normal or are missing, but an increase in intensity of the stimulation produces a field of normal extent. **direct v.f.** Central visual field. **dynamic v.f.** The composite of all visual fields, plotted for all possible positions of fixation, with the head fixed. Cf. *static visual field.* **exclusive left v.f.** The monocularly seen portion of the visual field to the left of the common visual field. **exclusive right v.f.** The monocularly seen portion of the visual field to the right of the common visual field. **exhaustion of Wilbrand v.f.** A visual field associated with neurasthenia and characterized by apparently continuous shrinkage in any meridian as it is being plotted and replotted. **fixation v.f.** Field of fixation. **flicker fusion frequency v.f.** A visual field plotted by determining the critical fusion frequencies throughout its extent and comparing these frequencies to known norms. **form v.f.** The portion of the visual field within which form or shape can be recognized, varying greatly with such factors as target size, shape, brightness, and contrast. **heteronymous v.f.** The nasal or temporal half of the visual field of one eye with reference to the nasal or temporal half, respectively, of the visual field of the other eye. **homonymous v.f.** The nasal or temporal half of the visual field of one eye with reference to the temporal or nasal half, respectively, of the visual field of the other eye. **hysterical v.f.** Any of several visual field patterns resulting from hysterical responses during the testing, often including such anomalous characteristics as spiraling borders, successive contractions of the borders with repeated testing, fixed borders unrelated to the test distance (tubular visual field), and the reversal of color field borders. **indirect v.f.** Peripheral visual field. **maximum v.f.** Absolute visual field. **monocular v.f.** The visual field of an eye in a given position, especially in the straightforward position. **motion v.f.** The area or extent of the visual field in which motion can be detected. **neurasthenic v.f.** Any of several visual field patterns associated with neurasthenia, usually characterized by continual changes as the field is being plotted. **oscillating v.f.** A visual field associated with hysteria and characterized by apparent concentric ring scotomata. The test target intermittently disappears and reappears as it is moved radially toward or away from the point of fixation. **overshot v.f.** A visual field in which there is a large scotomatous area approaching the macula, but not including it or its immediately adjacent area. **peripheral v.f.** The entire visual field exclusive of that corresponding to the fovea or the macula. Syn., *indirect visual field.* **physiologic v.f.** Absolute visual field. **recuperative extension v.f.**

of von Reuss. A visual field associated with hysteria and neurasthenia, characterized by a marked increase in the size of an originally small field, following a purposive rest, or in response to the exhortations of the examiner. **relative v.f.** The visual field plotted with the eye in the straightforward position and including as limitations the restrictions produced by the nose, the brows, and the cheeks. Cf. *absolute visual field.* Syn., *anatomic visual field.* **reversal of v.f.'s.** A deviation in the normal order of size of the color fields, e.g., the blue field being smaller than the red field. **shifting v.f. of Förster.** A visual field associated with hysteria or neurasthenia, characterized by a large displacement in its limits when plotted, first, from the invisible (continuing to the invisible in each meridian) and, second, by the same method in each meridian starting in the opposite direction. **spiral v.f.** A type of visual field pattern, usually attributed to neurasthenia or hysteria, in which there is a continuous progressive contraction as it is being plotted from meridian to meridian. A line connecting the limits of all the meridians has the shape of a spiral. **static v.f.** 1. The visual field obtained by measuring the luminance threshold at a series of fixed locations by varying the luminance of stationary targets of various sizes while the eye remains fixed in the straightforward position. 2. The visual field obtained with the eye fixed in the straightforward position. Cf. *dynamic visual field.* **surplus v.f.** The portion of the visual field in incomplete hemianopsia which remains unaffected and extends beyond the point of fixation into the affected side. **tubular v.f.** A visual field pattern usually attributed to hysteria or malingering, characterized by concentric contraction and constancy of diameter, irrespective of the testing distance. **uncinate v.f.** A visual field pattern resulting from baring of the superior portion of the blind spot of Mariotte. **uncinate (inverted) v.f.** A visual field pattern resulting from baring of the inferior portion of the blind spot of Mariotte.

◆

field-stop. An opaque aperture rim which limits the field of view in an optical system.

Fiessinger-Leroy-Reiter syndrome. Oculo-urethro-synovial syndrome.

Fiessinger-Rendu syndrome. Stevens-Johnson syndrome. See under *syndrome.*

Fieuzel glass (fu-zel′). See under *glass.*

figure. That part of, or pattern in, the perceived visual field which has the perceptual attribute of completeness or definitiveness of form, distinct from other portions of the field perceptually appreciated as ground.

ambiguous f. A pattern or a drawing so structured as to be open to more than one interpretation.

Baldwin's f. A diagram consisting of a dot midway between two laterally separated circles of unequal size, giving rise to the illusion that the dot is nearer the larger circle.

Bourdon's f. A drawing consisting of two wedge-shaped areas joined at their apices, whose upper borders form a common, continuous, straight line, giving the illusion that the upper straight line is curved.

diffraction f. Diffraction pattern.

Ebbinghaus' f. A drawing consisting of two equal lines or demarcated spaces, one filled with a series of intersecting lines or narrow bands and the other left undifferentiated, and giving the illusion that the "filled" line or space is longer.

fortification f's. Fortification spectrum.

Hering's f. Any of several drawings consisting of a pair of parallel straight lines, intersected or met by a series of radiating lines, and giving the illusion that the parallel lines are bowed toward or away from each other.

Höfler's f. A drawing consisting of two arcs of equal length and radius, placed one above the other, and giving the illusion that the arc nearer the centers of curvature is longer.

Mach's f. A line drawing depicting a half-opened book which, when viewed continuously, alternately appears to be open toward and away from the observer.

Mueller-Lyer f. A diagram consisting of two parallel lines of equal length, one having arrow-like appendages and the other having quill-like appendages at their ends, and giving the illusion that the lines are of unequal length.

Poggendorff's f. A line drawing consisting of a bandlike rectangular area overlaying a diagonal line and giving the illusion that the two visible portions of the line, one on each side of the band, are not parts of a continuous straight line.

Purkinje's f's. Entoptically observable patterns formed by the shadows of the blood vessels in the eye when light is projected obliquely or grossly out of focus onto the retina. Syn., *Purkinje's shadows.*

reversible f. A geometric figure or pattern having two or more possible interpretations which are simultaneously incompatible and involve apparent differences in orientation, dimensional relationships, or perceptual interchanges of figure and ground.

Schroeder's f. A line drawing consisting of alternately parallel, steplike, line formations extending from the upper corner of a parallelogram to the lower opposite corner. Upon continuous viewing, the perspective changes from a staircase viewed from above to a staircase viewed from below, or vice versa. Syn., *Schroeder's staircase.*

Stifel's f. A black disk containing a central white spot, used as a test target for locating the physiological blind spot of the eye.

Thiéry's f. A line drawing consisting of a rectangular box to which is attached the side and base of another such box. Upon constant fixation, the perspective changes so that it appears to be two solid boxes, or one box with an extra side and base attached.

Werner's f. A pair of targets, such as an annulus and a disk which would fit precisely inside of the annulus, which are in effect two portions of a single form and presented to the eye in the same centered location but one about 150 milliseconds later than the other, resulting in a perceptual suppression of part or all of the earlier exposed portion.

Wundt's f. A line drawing consisting of a pair of parallel straight lines crossed by lines radiating toward, and meeting, each other from two points, one on each side of the parallel lines, and giving the illusion that the parallel lines are bowed.

Zöllner's f. A line drawing consisting of long parallel lines, each crossed by a series of short diagonal lines which are parallel to each other, but which are angled opposite to those crossing the adjacent parallel lines, and giving rise to the illusion that the long parallel lines converge toward, or diverge from, each other. Syn., *Zöllner's lines.*

figure-ground. The basic two-part nature of the perceived visual field, providing for perceptual differentiation of figure and ground.

filaments, basal. Hairlike projections of a cone foot at the regions of synapse with bipolar or horizontal cells.

Filaria loa (fih-la're-ah lo'ah). Filaria oculi.

Filaria oculi (fih-la're-ah ok'u-li). A parasitic, threadlike worm from one to two inches long, found in West Africa, which inhabits the subcutaneous connective tissue of the body, traversing it freely. It is seen especially about the orbit and even under the conjunctiva, rarely reported in the vitreous chamber. Syn., *Loa loa; Filaria loa.*

filariasis, Bancroft's (fil"ah-ri'ah-sis). Elephantiasis of the eyelids, sometimes accompanied by iritis and retinal hemorrhages; seen principally in Australia and caused by the nematode parasite *Wuchereria bancroftii* transmitted by insect.

film, antireflection. A thin film of transparent material, such as magnesium fluoride, deposited on the surface of a lens which increases light transmission through the lens and reduces surface reflection. Syn., *lens coating.*

film, precorneal. The fluid covering the anterior surface of the cornea, approximately 10μ in thickness, which is composed of three sublayers, a superficial derived from the Meibomian glands, a middle derived from the lacrimal gland, and a deep mucoid derived from conjunctival glands. Syn., *lacrimal layer; tear layer.*

filoma (fih-lo'mah). A fibroma or benign connective tissue tumor of the sclera.

◆

FILTER

filter. A device or material which selectively or equally absorbs or transmits wavelengths of light.

   actinic f. 1. A filter which selectively transmits actinic radiations. 2. A filter which absorbs actinic radiations.

   birefringent f. A system of alternate quartz plates and polarizers for isolating a narrow spectral band of a few angstrom units. Syn., *polarization interference filter.*

   blue f. A filter which selectively transmits only blue light, either by selective absorption or by interference.

   blue-free f. Minus-blue filter.

   Christiansen f. A type of pass-band filter consisting of coarse particles of transparent solid immersed in a clear liquid which for the desired wavelength to be transmitted has the same index of refraction as the solid so that other wavelengths are reflected away from the beam path.

   cobalt blue f. A glass filter containing cobalt which transmits light primarily from the red and blue regions of the spectrum, absorbing the midspectral wavelengths.

   conversion f. A filter used to change the color temperature of a radiator.

   dichroic f. 1. A neutral filter or a color filter consisting of a doubly refracting medium which transmits only the ordinary or the extraordinary beam. 2. A light filter which permits only two colors to pass through. 3. A light filter which transmits a certain color when in a thin layer and a different color when in a thick layer.

   Fabry-Pérot f. A transmission interference filter consisting of an extremely thin solid transparent medium with plane and parallel faces coated by uniformly thin semitransparent metallic films.

   gradient f. An optical filter whose transmission varies across the face of the filter. Syn., *optical wedge.*

   green f. A filter which selectively transmits only green light, either by means of selective absorption, or by interference.

   green-free f. Minus-green filter.

   infrared f. 1. A filter which selectively transmits only infrared radiations. 2. A filter which does not transmit infrared radiations.

   interference f. A light filter which usually consists of five layers, two outside glass, two intermediate evaporated metal films, and one central evaporated layer of transparent material. Multiple reflections cause destructive interference for all but one (approximately) wavelength, resulting in an emergent beam of one color.

   lens/plate f. Absorption lens.

   minus-blue f. A filter which selectively absorbs blue light. Syn., *blue-free filter.*

minus-green f. A filter which selectively absorbs green light. Syn., *green-free filter.*

minus-red f. A filter which selectively absorbs red light. Syn., *red-free filter.*

neutral f. A filter which transmits all visible wavelengths in approximately equal but reduced amounts.

passband f. An optical filter which transmits a wavelength band or narrow range of wavelengths with maximum efficiency or a wavelength band within which the transmittance is high.

polarization interference f. Birefringent filter.

Polaroid f. A patented product, usually in sheet form, made from minute crystals of a dichroic material embedded in a plastic, which transmits only plane-polarized light.

red f. A filter which selectively transmits only red light.

red-free f. Minus-red filter.

Tscherning's f's. A series of neutral filters for determining the light threshold and light adaptation of the eye, each successive filter in the series having an absorption factor ten times that of the preceding filter.

ultraviolet f. A filter which selectively transmits only ultraviolet radiations.

wedge f. Gradient filter.

Wood's f. A glass filter containing nickel oxide which absorbs light of the visible spectrum and transmits ultraviolet radiation in the region near the visible spectrum. The light is used with certain dyes, such as fluorescein, to create fluorescence for diagnostic purposes, such as the detection of corneal abrasions or evaluation of the fit of contact lenses. Syn., *Wood's glass.*

Wratten f's. A series of commercially available gelatin color filters manufactured to catalogued specifications of transmission characteristics.

yellow f. A filter which selectively transmits only yellow light.

◆

Fincham's (fin'chamz) **coincidence optometer; theory.** See under the nouns.

Fincham-Sutcliffe scotometer (fin'cham-sut'clif). See under *scotometer.*

finding. Data derived from an observation, an examination, or a test; that which is found.

equilibrium f's. *Optometric Extension Program:* Four blur points, clinically determined at a 40 cm testing distance, representing the limits of positive and negative relative convergence and positive and negative relative accommodation.

gross f. In clinical testing, a direct numerical result or unmodified test score, usually implying that a net finding is to be computed from it.

net f. In clinical testing, a numerical result obtained by modifying the gross finding by some formula, rule, correction factor, or empirical allowance.

finger-piece. See under *frame.*

fining. The final lens surfacing process, prior to polishing, in which the smallest grain abrasive is used to smooth the surface.

Fink Near-Vision test. See under *test.*

F.I.O. Fellow of the Institute of Optometrists (Australia).

F.I.O. Sc. Fellow of the Institute of Ophthalmic Science.

firecrack. A shallow crack in or near the surface of a glass lens, due to overheating such as in grinding or polishing.

Firth test (furth). See under *test.*

Fisher's (fish'erz) **schematic eye; syndrome.** See under the nouns.

Fischer-Kuhnt spot (fish'er-koont). See under *spot.*

Fischer-Schweitzer test (fish'er-shvīt'ser). See under *test.*

fissure (fish'ūr). A cleft or a groove. In the brain, it applies to the deepest clefts. See also *groove* and *sulcus.*

calcarine f. The sulcus on the medial aspect of the occipital lobe, between the cuneus and lingual gyrus. Its anterior limb is in front of the parieto-occipital fissure, and the longer posterior limb extends back to the occipital pole region. Syn., *calcarine sulcus.*

central f. Fissure of Rolando.

choroidal f. Fetal fissure.

embryonic f. Fetal fissure.

fetal f. The incomplete portion or gap in the embryonic optic cup, ventrally, which normally disappears. If it remains, coloboma of the uveal tract occurs. Syn., *choroidal cleft; fetal cleft; choroidal fissure; embryonic fissure.*

f. of the optic cup. The fetal fissure in the inferior portion of the optic cup.

f. of the optic stalk. The fetal

fissure in the inferior portion of the optic stalk, continuous with that of the optic cup.

orbital f., inferior. An elongated opening in the orbit, bounded posteriorly by the great wing of the sphenoid bone and anteriorly by the maxillary and the palatine bones, through which pass the maxillary-infraorbital nerve junction, the zygomatic nerve, the infraorbital artery, and an anastomosis between the inferior ophthalmic vein and the pterygoid venous plexus. The fissure commences below and lateral to the optic foramen and runs anteriorly and temporally for approximately 20 mm. Syn., *sphenomaxillary fissure.*

orbital f., superior. An elongated opening in the orbit, between the wings of the sphenoid bone. The portion within the annulus of Zinn is the oculomotor foramen. The fissure transmits the abducens, the frontal, the lacrimal, the nasociliary, the oculomotor, and the trochlear nerves, the sympathetic root to the ciliary ganglion, the superior ophthalmic vein, and recurrent arteries. Syn., *sphenoidal fissure.*

palpebral f. The region between the upper and lower eyelid margins within which can be seen, when the lids are open, the caruncle, the semilunar fold, the iris, the cornea, the sclera, the conjunctival and episcleral vessels, and other structures. Syn., *rima palpebrarum.* **antimongoloid p.f.** A palpebral fissure which slants downward toward the external canthus.

f. of Rolando. The sulcus or groove between the frontal and parietal lobes of the cerebral cortex. Syn., *central fissure.*

sphenoidal f. Superior orbital fissure.

sphenomaxillary f. Inferior orbital fissure.

fistula (fis'tu-lah). An abnormal passage from one hollow structure of the body to another, or from a hollow structure to the surface, formed by an abscess, disease process, incomplete closure of a wound, or by a congenital anomaly.

corneal f. A fistula extending from the anterior chamber through the cornea to the exterior of the eye. It usually develops in a weakened corneal scar and is usually lined by adherent iridic tissue or by a downward growth of corneal epithelium.

lacrimal f. A fistula, extending from a lacrimal sac or duct to the skin, which may develop after a severe dacrocystitis.

fit. The quality or state of being of the proper dimensions; adjustment; preparedness; adaptedness.

chemical f. The selection of a compatible solution to be used as a fluid filler in scleral contact lenses. Factors believed to control acceptability are chemical composition, hydrogen ion concentration, and relative osmotic pressure.

finished f. The alteration of an approximately fitted contact lens, as to size and shape, to the desired fit.

optical f. The determination of the dioptric power required in a contact lens to correct a patient's refractive error.

physical f. The adaptation or selection of the dimensional elements of a contact lens to conform to the shape and the size of the eye, either by means of a molded impression of the eye or by trial-and-error fitting.

psychological f. The teaching of the techniques of inserting, removing, and caring for contact lenses and the implementing of the patient's confidence and motivation during the early stages of wear.

semifinished f. A stage in the mechanical fitting of a contact lens, prior to the finished fit, in which certain mechanical criteria of excellence of fit are met, but in which further alterations may be necessary to obtain maximum wearing comfort.

fit-on. Clip-on.

fit-over. Clip-over.

◆

FIXATION

fixation (fik-sa'shun). The process, condition, or act of directing the eye toward the object of regard, causing, in a normal eye, the image of the object to be centered on the fovea.

anomalous f. 1. Eccentric fixation. 2. The apparent fixation by the deviating eye in strabismus with anomalous retinal correspondence. See also *facultative eccentric fixation.* Syn., *abnormal fixation.*

bifoveal f. Fixation in which the images of the object of fixation simultaneously fall upon the foveae of both eyes. Syn., *binocular fixation.*

binocular f. Bifoveal fixation.

central f. Centric fixation.

centric f. Fixation in which the image of the object of fixation falls upon the center of the fovea. Syn., *central fixation*.

contralateral f. The fixation of objects in the left half of the visual field with the right eye and objects in the right half of the visual field with the left eye, as may occur especially in esotropia or in paralysis of the lateral rectus muscles.

f. disparity. See under *disparity*.

eccentric f. Fixation not employing the central foveal area. Syn., *anomalous fixation; false fixation; pseudomacular fixation*. **facultative e.f.** The apparent or functional fixation by the deviating eye in strabismus with anomalous retinal correspondence, in which the image of the object of fixation falls upon its anomalous associated area only under binocular conditions. Syn., *false associated fixation*. **obligatory e.f.** The apparent or functional fixation by the deviating eye in strabismus with anomalous retinal correspondence, in which the image of the object of fixation falls upon its anomalous associated area both under binocular conditions and when the normally fixating eye is occluded. **paradoxical e.f.** Eccentric fixation by the deviating eye in strabismus in which the retinal site used for fixation, under monocular conditions, is on the side of the fovea opposite to which the image of the object of fixation lies under binocular conditions, e.g., the temporal side in esotropia.

false f. Eccentric fixation.

false associated f. Facultative eccentric fixation.

field of f. See under *field*.

foveal f. Normal fixation in which the image of the object of fixation falls upon the fovea.

homolateral f. The fixation of objects in the right half of the visual field with the right eye and objects in the left half of the visual field with the left eye, as may occur especially in exotropia or in paralysis of the medial rectus muscles.

jump f. Saccadic fixation.

line of f. See under *line*.

lost f. 1. The absence of ability to fixate repeatedly or continuously with the same retinal area, normally the fovea, a condition associated with degeneration or destruction of the fovea or with amblyopia of high degree. 2. In reading, fixation which fails to provide or fails to be associated with adequate meaning of the words to be read, ordinarily resulting in a form of backtracking, termed *regression*.

monocular f. Fixation by one eye only, the vision in the other eye being absent, disregarded, suspended, or suppressed, as in conditions of monocular occlusion, monocular blindness, dissociation, or strabismus.

paradoxic f. Paradoxical eccentric fixation.

parafoveal f. Fixation utilizing a retinal area within the macula but not at the center of the fovea.

paramacular f. Fixation utilizing a retinal area near, but not within, the macula.

f. pause. The momentary cessation of eye movement occurring alternately with saccadic movement in reading or in a series of fixations by which an extended region is meaningfully scanned.

peripheral f. Fixation with a retinal area located in the peripheral retina, remote from the macular area.

persistent f. A prolonged staring fixation or fixation pause, ostensibly involuntary and often associated with hysteria, debilitation, fright, daydreaming, or paralysis of the extraocular muscles.

physiologic f. Normal centric fixation, the image of the fixated target stimulating the foveal center.

plane of f. See under *plane*.

point of f. See under *point*.

position of f. See under *position*.

pseudomacular f. Eccentric fixation. *Obs.*

pursuit f. 1. The continued fixation of a moving object, implying a dynamic movement of the eye, so as to keep the image of the object continuously on the fovea. 2. The repetitive fixation of a moving object, implying a series of corrective refixations, in response to the effort to keep the image of the object continuously on the fovea.

reflex f. Involuntary fixation such as may occur in response to peripheral retinal stimulation.

f. response. See under *response*.

f. response time. See *time*.

saccadic f. 1. A rapid change of fixation from one point in the visual field to another. More properly: *saccadic eye movement.* Syn., *jump fixation.* 2. The rapid phase of a nystagmoid cycle.

scanning f. A series of rapid fixations associated with an attempt to survey quickly the details of a view subtending a relatively large area of the visual field.

steady f. Continuous fixation of a nonmoving object for a given period of time.

f. time. See under *time.*

tracing f. A type of fixation occurring in response to an effort to move fixation along the path of a line drawing without the aid of a moving object, characterized by a series of saccadic movements.

voluntary f. Conscious and purposeful fixation as distinguished from reflex fixation.

wandering f. The absence of ability to fixate continuously with the same retinal area.

◆

Fizeau (fe-zo') **experiment; fringes; interferometer; method.** See under the nouns.

Flajani's disease (flah-jan'ēz). Exophthalmic goiter.

flakes, capsular. A type of congenital cataract consisting of white, oval or round, sharply circumscribed, dense opacities, up to 1 mm in size, which are usually multiple and are found on the anterior surface of the capsule of the crystalline lens.

flange, scleral. 1. The temporal spherical section of a Feincone contact lens. 2. The portion of a scleral type contact lens which covers the sclera.

flare. Light resulting from interreflection between refracting surfaces.

aqueous f. Tyndall's effect, or the scattering of light in a beam directed into the anterior chamber, occurring as a result of increased protein content of the aqueous humor, a sign of severe inflammation of the iris and/or the ciliary body.

flash. A very short exposure of light, or the associated visual experience.

green f. A momentary, brilliant, predominantly green appearance at the upper edge of the sun's disk as it disappears below or emerges above the horizon, due to optical properties of the earth's atmosphere.

Flash Reader. A trade name for a hand-operated tachistoscopic device used for brief exposure of reading material.

flat, optical. A disk of high quality quartz glass usually about 2 cm thick with at least one side ground and polished with a maximum deviation from flatness of less than 50 millimicra, used to check the contours of other approximately flat surfaces by the formation of interference light bands between two such surfaces placed in contact with each other.

Flatau's sign (flat-owz'). See under *sign.*

flattener, field. A fiber optics bundle with differential density of fibers to accomplish a flattening of the curved image field produced by an anastigmatic optical system.

flaw, Griffith. A flaw or crack of sufficient size to reduce total fracture resistance of a solid material, such as glass or metal, below that essential for its intended use.

Flechsig's (flek'sigz) **temporal knee; loop.** See under the nouns.

fleck, Förster-Fuchs. Fuchs' spot.

flecks, Michel's. Michel's spots.

Fleischer's (fli'sherz) **whirling corneal dystrophy; line; ring.** See under the nouns.

Fles's box (flez'ez). See under *box.*

Flexner-Wintersteiner rosettes (fleks'ner-vint"er-stīn'er). See under *rosettes.*

flicker. Variations in brightness or hue perceived upon stimulation by intermittent or temporally non-uniform light.

binocular f. Flicker produced by alternate photic stimulation of the two eyes.

brightness f. Flicker produced by intermittent variations in brightness or illuminance. Cf. *chromatic flicker.* Syn., *illumination flicker.*

chromatic f. Variations in saturation or hue, perceived on alternately intermittent stimulation by light of two different colors but of constant brightness. Cf. *brightness flicker.*

contrast f. Flicker induced into a constantly illuminated field by flicker in a neighboring field.

field f. Flicker induced or observed in a dark or a constantly illuminated field which surrounds a target varying in intensity. Cf. *spot flicker.*

f. frequency. See *frequency.*

illumination f. Brightness flicker.

marginal f. In critical fusion frequency experiments, the last trace of flicker observable in parts of the test field just before total fusion is obtained. Syn., *vestigial flicker.*

spot f. Flicker in the region of the field constituting the test target, as distinguished from the flicker in the visual field surrounding the target. Cf. *field flicker.*

vestigial f. Marginal flicker.

flicks. Rapid saccadic movements occurring after a latent period of 0.12 to 0.18 seconds with an amplitude of approximately 5 to 10 minutes of arc.

Flieringa-Bonaccolto ring (flēr'ing-ah-bon-ah-kōl'to). See under *ring.*

Flieringa-Legrand ring (flēr'ing-ah-le'grahnd). See under *ring.*

flight of colors. The temporal succession of colors observed in an afterimage of a bright source.

float. To appear to remain suspended in space, as in the case of those elements of a fused stereogram, a vectogram, or an anaglyph that exhibit stereoscopic parallax relative to the perceived plane of the stereogram, the vectogram, or the anaglyph.

floaters. In the normally transparent vitreous, deposits of various size, shape, consistency, refractive index, and motility, which may be of embryonic origin or acquired. If acquired, they may be an indication of degenerative changes of the retina or the vitreous humor. See also *muscae volitantes.*

flocculi (flok'u-li). Small, wool-like tufts or flakes.

cystic f. of the iris. Congenital, pigmented cysts occurring on the pupillary margin of the iris.

nodular f. of the iris. A congenital hyperplasia of the pigment epithelium of the iris resulting in grapelike clusters of small black nodules at the pupillary margin.

Flocks's pore tissue. Endothelial meshwork of Speakman.

Flom chart; criteria. See under the nouns.

Floropryl (flor'o-pril). A trade name for DFP in 0.10% solution dissolved in peanut oil.

Flouren's law (floo'ranz). See under *law.*

fluid. A substance, such as a liquid or a gas, which alters in shape in response to any force, however small.

aqueous f. Aqueous humor.

intraocular f. All the fluid within the eye with the exception of that contained within the blood vessels. It includes the aqueous humor, the vitreous humor, and the tissue fluids of the eye. **plasmoid i.f.** Intraocular fluid differing from the normal by more nearly approximating the composition of plasma, as may be produced by an increase in the permeability of the capillary walls following a sudden decrease in intraocular pressure, or due to a pathological process.

lacrimal f. The clear, salty, slightly alkaline fluid secreted by the lacrimal gland, constituting the major portion of the tear fluid.

Morgagnian f. 1. The amorphous material between the anterior epithelium of the crystalline lens and its anterior capsule. Syn., *Morgagni's humor; liquor Morgagni.* 2. A milky fluid consisting of the disintegrated cortex of the hypermature cataract and containing the nucleus of the crystalline lens.

vitreous f. Vitreous humor.

fluoren (floo'o-ren). A black light flux unit equal to one milliwatt of radiant energy in the wavelength range 320 to 400 nanometers.

fluoresce (floo-o-res'). To exhibit, produce, or undergo fluorescence.

fluorescein (floo″o-res'e-in). A fluorescent, yellowish-red crystalline compound, $C_{20}H_{12}O_5$, whose sodium salt is used in dilute solution as a dye in determining the fit of contact lenses or in the detection of corneal abrasions, ulcers, etc., the affected areas staining a yellow-green.

fluorescence (floo″o-res'ens). The property of emitting radiation as the result of, and only during, the absorption of radiation from some other source, the emitted radiation being of longer wavelength; also, the emitted radiation. Cf. *phosphorescence.*

resonance f. Resonance radiation.

fluorescent (floo″o-res'ent). Characterized by, having, exhibiting, or caused by fluorescence.

fluorite (floo'or-īt). A mineral composed of calcium fluoride and serving as a principal source of fluorine. It fluoresces under ultraviolet light and may phosphoresce upon heating or after exposure to ultraviolet light. It crystallizes in cubes or octahedrons and, in its clear colorless form of optical quality, is used for apochromatic lenses because of its low index of refraction and low dispersion. Syn., *feldspar.*

fluorochrome (floo"or-o-krōm'). Any of various fluorescent substances, such as sodium fluorescein.

fluorometry (floo"or-om'eh-tre). A method for estimating aqueous outflow in which the concentration of intravenously introduced fluorescein in the anterior chamber is determined at intervals by a slit lamp fluorometer and related to the concentration of fluorescein in the blood.

fluorophor (floo"or-o-fōr'). A substance which has the property of absorbing energy and releasing it again in the form of fluorescence.

Fluress. Trade name for a solution of 0.4% benoxinate combined with 0.25% sodium fluorescein, used for applanation tonometry.

flush, ciliary. A diffuse, rose-red coloration surrounding the cornea as a result of congestion of the branches of the anterior ciliary arteries, in cyclitis, iridocyclitis, or deep keratitis.

flux (fluks). The rate of flow of fluid or energy.

> **chromatic f's.** Radiant fluxes expressed in arbitrary energy units, in general different for the three primary colors, chosen to satisfy certain convenient relationships involving matches with other specified lights.

> **density f., luminous.** See under *density.*

> **luminous f.** The time rate of flow of light, usually designated in lumens.

> **radiant f.** The time rate of flow of radiant energy expressed in watts or ergs per second. **spectral r.f.** Radiant flux with respect to a specified wavelength or narrow wavelength interval.

FMO. See *Federation of Manufacturing Opticians.*

focal (fo'kal). Pertaining to or having a focus.

focal depth; distance; illumination; intercept; interval; length; line; plane; point; power; ratio. See under the nouns.

focimeter (fo-sim'eh-ter). A device for determining the vergence power of a lens.

focometer (fo-kom'eh-ter). An instrument for the determination of the vertex power of ophthalmic lenses; a variation of a focimeter.

◆

FOCUS

focus (fo'kus). 1. The point at which a pencil of rays or their prolongations can be made to meet after reflection or refraction. 2. To adjust the elements of an optical system to achieve sharp imagery. 3. The center, the principal site, or the starting point of a disease process.

> **anterior f.** Primary principal focus.

> **aplanatic f.** The image point for which an optical system is corrected for spherical aberration and at which all zones of the system produce images of equal size.

> **back f.** The secondary principal focal point of a lens or optical system located in reference to its distance from the posterior surface of the lens.

> **conjugate foci.** Two points in an optical system such that rays originating at one are focused at the other, and vice versa.

> **depth of f.** See under *depth.*

> **marginal f.** The point at which the nonparaxial rays or their prolongations meet after refraction or reflection by an optical system.

> **meridional f.** Tangential focus.

> **negative f.** Virtual focus.

> **paraxial f.** The point to which the central (paraxial) rays or their prolongations converge after refraction or reflection by an optical system.

> **posterior f.** Secondary principal focus.

> **primary f.** Primary principal focus.

> **primary f. in oblique astigmatism.** Tangential focus.

> **principal f.** 1. Either the anterior or the posterior principal focus of a lens or an optical system. 2. The virtual or real axial meeting point of rays, parallel to the optical axis on incidence, after reflection by a spherical surface. **anterior p.f.** Primary principal focus. **posterior p.f.** Secondary principal focus. **primary p.f.** The axial meeting point of incident rays which

become parallel after refraction by an optical system. Syn., *anterior focus; anterior principal focus; primary focus.*

secondary p.f. The axial meeting point of rays parallel to the optical axis on incidence, after refraction by a lens or an optical system. Syn., *posterior focus; posterior principal focus; secondary focus.*

radial f. Sagittal focus.

real f. The point at which a real image is formed by the meeting of convergent light rays.

sagittal f. The image formed by those rays contained in a sagittal (secondary) section of a homocentric bundle of rays obliquely incident on an optical system containing spherical surfaces. The sagittal (secondary) section is made up of two planes perpendicular to the tangential (primary) plane, one plane containing the incident rays, the other plane containing the emergent rays. The image of a point source will be a line perpendicular to the sagittal (secondary) section. Cf. *tangential focus.* Syn., *secondary focus in oblique astigmatism.*

secondary f. Secondary principal focus.

secondary f. in oblique astigmatism. Sagittal focus.

tangential f. The image formed by those rays contained in the tangential (primary) plane of a homocentric bundle of rays obliquely incident on an optical system containing spherical surfaces. The image of a point source will be a line perpendicular to the tangential (primary) plane. Cf., *sagittal focus.* Syn., *meridional focus; primary focus in oblique astigmatism.*

virtual f. The point at which a virtual image is formed by the intersection of the backward extensions of diverging light rays. Syn., *negative focus.*

◆

focusing (fo'kus-ing). Adjusting the elements of an optical system, or the position of the image surface or screen, in order to create or obtain a clear and sharply defined image, or to obtain a desired relationship between object distance and image distance.

Fodéré's sign (fod-a-rāz'). See *sign.*

fogging. The deliberate overcorrection of hypermetropia or the undercorrection of myopia for various purposes in the refraction of the eye. It is used in testing for astigmatism to reduce the tend-

ency of the eye to accommodate during the test.

Foix's syndrome (fwahz). See under *syndrome.*

fold. A doubling; a turning of a part upon itself; a layer or a thickness.

Arnold's f. A fold of mucous membrane found in the lacrimal sac.

ciliary f's. Small ridges in the furrows between the ciliary processes. Syn., *plica ciliaris.*

conjunctival f. The part of the conjunctiva which joins the bulbar and the palpebral portions of the conjunctiva but is unattached to the eyelid and the eyeball. Syn., *cul-de-sac; palpebral fold; retrotarsal fold; fornix of the conjunctiva.*

contraction f's of Schwalbe. Contraction furrows of Schwalbe.

Eskimo f. An eye fold resembling the Mongoloid fold but originating from the tarsal part of the upper eyelid.

eye f. An upper eyelid skin fold which hangs over and partially covers the eyelashes.

falciform f. A thickening in the cleft between the tendon of an extraocular muscle and the eyeball, formed by the fusion of the muscle sheath and Tenon's capsule. Syn., *pulley bar.*

Hasner's f. Plica lacrimalis.

Indian f. A temporal extension of the Mongoloid fold into the lower eyelid which tends to cover the lateral canthus and spread to the outer aspect of the lower eyelid; found in South American Indians.

lacrimal f. Plica lacrimalis.

f. of Lange. A forward projecting fold of the retina in the region of the ora serrata, in the eye of infants.

malar f. A vaguely defined furrow in the skin that runs downward and inward from the external canthus which, together with the nasojugal fold, indicates the junction of the tissue of the lower eyelid with that of the cheek.

median f. An uncommon type of eye fold which overhangs the medial part of the upper eyelid and leaves both canthi unobscured.

Mongoloid f. An eye fold which begins at the medial part of the upper eyelid and covers the lacrimal caruncle, or which, in its more complete form, obscures the lower edge of the upper eyelid from the external to the internal canthus. Syn., *oblique epicanthus; hemi-epicanthus.*

nasojugal f. A furrow in the skin extending inferiorly and laterally from the internal canthus which, together with the malar fold, indicates the junction of the tissue of the lower eyelid with that of the cheek.

Nordic f. An eye fold which begins at the medial part of the upper eyelid, laterally obscuring its margin and covering the external canthus.

orbital f. The loose protruding skin just above the upper tarsus of the eyelid, especially in the aged.

palpebral f. Conjunctival fold.

primary retinal f's. Preretinal macular fibrosis.

retinal f., congenital. Congenital retinal septum.

retrotarsal f. Conjunctival fold.

semilunar f. A fold of bulbar conjunctiva lateral to the caruncle in the region of the medial canthus and concentric with the limbus, representing a vestigial nictitating membrane or a rudimentary third eyelid.

structural f's of Schwalbe. Structural furrows of Schwalbe.

follicle (fol'ih-kl). 1. A small gland, crypt, or sac. 2. A small cavity or deep, narrow depression, as a hair follicle. 3. A small, localized aggregation of lymphocytes resembling a lymph node, occurring as a result of continued chronic irritation.

ciliary f's. Meibomian glands.

conjunctival f. A dense, localized, subepithelial infiltration of the conjunctiva by large, mononuclear lymphocyte, plasma, mast, and polymorphonuclear cells, occurring as the result of lymphatic tissue reaction to irritation and usually appearing as a small, round or oval, pinkish, translucent body.

palpebral f's. Meibomian glands.

school f's. Conjunctival folliculosis.

trachoma f's. Sac-like initial accumulations of lymphocytes in trachoma, with subsequent central zones of reticulo-endothelial cells which often degenerate and become necrotic.

folliculosis, conjunctival (fol-lik"u-lo'sis). A condition, frequently found in children, characterized by the presence of discrete follicles in the conjunctiva, mainly in the lower fornix. It is unaccompanied by inflammatory signs or secretions and runs a chronic, benign course with no sequelae. Syn., *follicular catarrh; school follicles.*

Foltz's valve (fōltz'ez). See under *valve.*

Fontana's (fon-tah'naz) **canal; spaces.** See under the nouns.

foot, cone. The end of a cone cell that synapses with a centripetal, horizontal, or centrifugal bipolar cell in the outer molecular layer of the retina. Syn., *end foot; cone pedicle.*

foot, end. Cone foot.

footcandle. A unit of illumination equal to uniformly distributed flux of 1 lumen per sq. ft. Symbol: fc. Other units and conversion factors:

1 *lux (lumen/m²)* = 0.0929 fc
1 *metercandle* = 0.0929 fc
1 *phot* = 929 fc

apparent f. Footlambert.

equivalent f. Footlambert.

footlambert. A unit of luminance equal to $1/\pi$ candela per sq. ft., or to the average luminance of a surface emitting or reflecting light at the rate of one lumen per sq. ft. The average luminance of any reflecting surface in footlamberts is the product of the illumination in footcandles and the reflectance of the surface. Symbol: fL. Other units and conversion factors:

1 *lambert* = 929 fL
1 *millilambert* = 0.929 fL
1 *stilb* (candela per cm²) = 2919 fL
1 *candela* per ft² = 3.142 fL
1 *candela* per in.² = 452fL
1 *nit* (candela per m²) = 0.2919 fL
1 *apostilb* = 0.0929 fL

Syn., *apparent footcandle; equivalent footcandle.*

foramen (fo-ra'men). A natural hole or perforation, especially one in a bone.

Arnold's f. Frontal foramen.

Bozzi's f. Macula lutea. *Obs.*

corneal f. Corneal interval.

ethmoidal f., anterior. An opening into the anterior ethmoidal canal located in the fronto-ethmoidal suture, or in the frontal bone, which permits the anterior ethmoidal vessels and the nasal nerve to leave the orbit.

ethmoidal f., posterior. An opening, a short distance behind the anterior ethmoidal foramen, which permits the posterior ethmoidal vessels and nerve (Luschka) to leave the orbit.

frontal f. An opening in the frontal bone, sometimes present just medial to the supraorbital foramen on the medial superior orbital margin, which transmits medial branches of the supraorbital nerve, vein, and artery. If the bone is incomplete below, it is termed a *frontal notch.* Syn., *Arnold's foramen.*

fronto-ethmoidal f. The anterior or posterior ethmoidal foramen.

infraorbital f. The anterior opening of the infraorbital canal, slightly below the lower orbital margin, which transmits the infraorbital vessels and nerve. Syn., *suborbital foramen.*

oculomotor f. That part of the superior orbital fissure, bounded by the annulus of Zinn, which transmits the sympathetic root of the ciliary ganglion and the nasociliary, oculomotor, and abducens nerves into the orbit.

optic f. The opening of the optic canal into the orbit, located in the small wing of the sphenoid bone, transmitting the optic nerve and the ophthalmic artery with its carotid plexus of sympathetic nerve fibers.

opticoscleral f. Posterior scleral foramen.

f. ovale. 1. The opening in the great wing of the sphenoid in the cranium which serves as the exit of the mandibular division of the fifth cranial nerve and of the masticator nerve. 2. The opening in the interatrial septum which allows fetal blood to enter the left atrium and bypass the pulmonary circuit.

f. rotundum. The opening in the great wing of the sphenoid bone in the cranium, which permits the maxillary division of the fifth cranial nerve to enter the pterygo-palatine fossa before reaching the inferior orbital fissure.

scleral f., anterior. Corneal interval.

scleral f., posterior. The passageway in the posterior sclera which transmits the optic nerve. Syn., *opticoscleral foramen.*

Soemmering's f. Macula lutea. *Obs.*

suborbital f. Infraorbital foramen.

supraorbital f. An opening in the frontal bone at the upper and slightly medial margin of the orbit, serving as the exit of the supraorbital vessels and nerve. If the bone is incomplete below, it is termed a *supraorbital notch.*

zygomatic f. An opening in the lateral, anterior portion of the orbit which transmits the zygomatic nerve and vessels. Occasionally, the zygomatic nerve divides within the orbit and, in this case, a zygomaticofacial and a zygomaticotemporal foramen are found instead.

forceps, Feincone radius (fŏr'seps). A plierlike instrument with contoured jaws which may be preheated for making peripheral shaping adjustments to plastic scleral contact lenses.

foriagraph (fo're-ah-graf"). Phoriagraph.

former, lens. A master pattern, usually of metal, used to guide and control the lens shape in lens cutting and edging machines. Syn., *lens pattern.*

◆

FORMULA

formula. 1. A principle or rule expressed in mathematical symbols. 2. A symbolic expression of the chemical composition of a substance. 3. A prescription.

Abney's f. The formula, $y = k\sqrt{x}$, for calculating the diameter (y) of the opening of a pinhole camera, in which k equals a constant 0.008 when x and y are in inches, or 0.01275 when x and y are in centimeters. x equals the distance of the pinhole from the plate.

airlight f. An equation expressing the relationship between the perceived luminance of a distant, black object and that of the background sky as the extinction coefficient of the intervening atmosphere.

apparent depth f. A formula giving the apparent depth of an object when seen through an interface separating two optical media of different indices of refraction.

Binkhorst's f. A formula based on the axial length of the eye, the distance of the anterior corneal surface from the implant, and the corneal curvature, to determine the power of an intraocular implant to replace the crystalline lens.

Brunswik f. See *ratio, Brunswik.*

Cauchy's dispersion f. For wavelengths in the visible range, the index of refraction of a gas is accurately calculated as a constant, plus a second constant, divided by the square of the wavelength.

Colenbrander's f. In subnormal vision, the dioptric power of the addition for reading ordinary newsprint is equal to the reciprocal of Snellen visual acuity, less one diopter, plus the normal reading addition.

cube root f. An expression, $A\sqrt[3]{I} = K$, intended to represent the interrelationship of the intensity (I) and the area (A) of the stimulus which produces a constant response (K).

displacement f. 1. A formula expressing the apparent lateral displacement of an object when seen obliquely through a plane-parallel plate. 2. Any formula expressing the relative position of an image as a function of the optical variables.

Fresnel's f. A formula for determining the loss of light by reflection in the case of perpendicular incidence on an interface between two transparent media. Expressed numerically, the reflection is equal to

$$\frac{(n_2 - n_1)^2}{(n_2 + n_1)^2}$$

n_1 being the index of refraction of the first medium and n_2 of the second.

Friedenwald's f. A formula devised by Friedenwald for calculating the intraocular pressure during tonometry (P_t) when employing the Schiötz tonometer: $P_t = \dfrac{W}{c_1 + c_2 R}$, where W = tonometer weight, R = tonometer scale reading, and c_1 and c_2 are constants.

van der Heijde f. A formula based on the corneal curvature and thickness, the implanted lens thickness, the anterior chamber depth, and the indices of refraction of the aqueous and implant, to determine the power of an intraocular implant to replace the crystalline lens.

Hofstetter's amplitude f. The formula, $A = 18.5 - 0.3Y$, in which A = average amplitude of accommodation and Y = age, based on a combined evaluation of Donders' and Duane's data and expressed with reference to the spectacle plane.

Hofstetter's practice appraisal f. The formula, $A = I + 0.11G$, for determining the median appraised value of an optometry practice in which A = appraised value, I = inventory value, and G = the sum of the gross incomes of the 24 preceding months.

Imbert-Fick f. In applanation tonometry, the relationship between intra-ocular pressure in mm Hg = P/sA; where P is the weight applied in grams, A is the area of the surface flattened, and s is the specific gravity of mercury.

Judd's f's. Empirical formulas to predict the hue, saturation, and brightness of achromatic or chromatic surfaces that are uniformly illuminated by chromatic light.

Kestenbaum's f. In subnormal vision, the dioptric power of the addition for reading ordinary newsprint (Jaeger 5) is numerically equal to the reciprocal of Snellen visual acuity.

Magnus f. An empirical formula for estimating the earning ability of a worker who has sustained an injury affecting his vision, employing scaled values for central visual acuity, the visual field, extraocular muscle function, and the class of occupation. Syn., *Magnus-Würdemann formula.*

Newton's f. A formula expressing the relationship between the focal lengths of an optical system and the object and image distances as measured from the respective focal points.

Percival's f. A formula to calculate the power of a spectacle lens which will have the same dioptric power effect on the eye for an object at near as a given spectacle lens has for an object at distance.

Petzval f. The formula, $n_1 f_1 + n_2 f_2 = 0$, expressing the condition for eliminating the curvature of a stigmatic image produced by a system of two thin lenses, in contact or separated, in which n = index of refraction and f = focal length. Syn., *Petzval's condition.*

Renier f. A formula to determine the compensated equivalent spherical power of an intraocular implant used to replace the crystalline lens:

$$C_e = (I_p - I_c) + R_a$$

where C_e = compensated spherical equivalent

I_p = intraocular power computed to the iris plane

I_c = calculated lens power from A-scan

R_a = actual spherical equivalent result.

Seidel f's. Five formulas expressing mathematically the 5 monochromatic aberrations of optical systems. The abberrations treated are (1) *spherical aberration;* (2) *coma;* (3) *oblique astigmatism;* (4) *curvature of the field;* (5) *distortion.*

Smith-Helmholtz f. The formula expressing Lagrange's law, q.v.

Snellen f. The formula, $V = d/D$, in which V represents a simple numerical expression for visual acuity, d the testing distance, and D the distance at which the smallest readable Snellen letter subtends an angle of 5 minutes. See also *Snellen fraction.*

thick lens f's. Formulas which apply to a combination of refracting surfaces centered on a common axis and in which Gaussian cardinal points are used instead of the vertices of the surfaces as reference points for specifying object and image distances.

Thompson f. A formula in four steps for finding the equivalent combination sphere Y and cylinder X of a pair of cylinders of powers A and B crossed at angle θ where ϕ is the angle that the resultant axis makes with the axis of A, as follows:

$$\frac{X}{\sin 2\theta} = \frac{A}{\sin 2(\theta-\phi)} = \frac{B}{\sin 2\phi} \quad (1)$$

$$X^2 = A^2 + B^2 + 2AB \cos 2\theta \quad (2)$$

$$\sin 2\phi = \frac{B}{X} \sin 2\theta \quad (3)$$

$$Y = \frac{A+B-X}{2} \quad (4)$$

thin lens f's. Formulas which apply to a combination of refracting surfaces centered on a common axis and in which the distances between the surfaces are ignored and the vertices of all the surfaces and the Gaussian cardinal points are assumed to coincide.

visual efficiency f. Any of several formulas using visual test scores as a basis for computing visual efficiency ratings, usually for purposes of compensation in occupational injury cases.

◆

fornix of the conjunctiva (fōr'niks). The part of the conjunctiva which joins the bulbar and the palpebral portions of the conjunctiva and which is unattached to the eyelid and the eyeball. Syn., *cul-de-sac; conjunctival fold; palpebral fold; retrotarsal fold.*

Förster's (fers'terz) **choroiditis; dis-** ease; shifting visual field; photometer; ring scotoma; theory; uveitis. See under the nouns.

Förster-Fuchs fleck (fers'ter-fooks). Fuchs' spot. See under *spot.*

fossa (fos'ah). A cavity, depression, or pit.

accessory f. of Rochon-Duvigneaud. The posterior portion of the fossa for the lacrimal gland, containing mostly orbital fat.

hyaloid f. The anterior concavity of the vitreous body located just posterior to the retrolental space. Syn., *lenticular fossa; patellar fossa.*

hypophyseal f. A deep central depression in the floor of the sella turcica containing the pituitary body. Syn., *pituitary fossa.*

f. for the inferior oblique muscle. A small depression on the maxillary bone, on the anterior medial floor of the orbit, just lateral to the upper end of the nasolacrimal canal, which is the point of origin of the inferior oblique muscle.

f. for the lacrimal gland. A large concavity of the frontal bone located in the upper wall of the orbit, lateral and posterior to the orbital margin, in which the orbital lobe of the lacrimal gland rests.

f. for the lacrimal sac. A broad vertical groove in the anterior medial wall of the orbit, formed by the frontal process of the superior maxillary bone and the lacrimal bone, and bounded by the anterior and posterior lacrimal crests. It is approximately 14 mm in height and 5 mm deep inferiorly, becoming gradually more shallow as it extends superiorly, and contains the lacrimal sac.

lenticular f. Hyaloid fossa.

f. orbitalis. Orbit.

patellar f. Hyaloid fossa.

pituitary f. Hypophyseal fossa.

pterygopalatine f. The concavity between the pterygoid process of the sphenoid bone and the palatine and maxillary bones. As the maxillary nerve leaves the foramen rotundum in the cranium, it enters this fossa and lies near the infraorbital artery, the pterygoid plexus, and the sphenopalatine ganglion. Syn., *sphenomaxillary fossa.*

sphenomaxillary f. Pterygopalatine fossa.

trochlear f. A small depression, posterior to the medial upper margin of the orbit in the frontal bone, which contains the pulley of the superior oblique muscle. Syn., *trochlear fovea*.

fossette (foh-set'). A small and deep ulcer of the cornea.

Foster-Kennedy syndrome (fos'ter-ken'eh-de). Kennedy's syndrome.

Foucault's (foo-kōz') **chart; experiment; patterns; prism; test.** See under the nouns.

Foundation for Education and Research in Vision. An American organization incorporated in 1956 by optometrists to raise funds for the support of education and research in the sciences and professions related to vision.

Fourier's (foo-ryāz') **analysis; integral; series; theory.** See under the nouns.

fovea (fo've-ah). A small depression or pit.

 f. centralis. An area approximately 1.5 mm in diameter within the macula lutea where the retina thins out greatly because of the oblique shifting of all layers except the pigment epithelium layer and the members of the visual cells. It includes the sloping walls of the fovea (clivus) and contains a few rods in its periphery. In its center (foveola) are the cones most adapted to yield high visual acuity, each cone being connected to only one ganglion cell.

 f. externa of Schäfer. The outer fovea.

 false f. 1. A nonfoveal region of the retina functionally associated with the fovea of the other eye in anomalous retinal correspondence. Syn., *anomalous associated area*. 2. A nonfoveal region of the retina used for fixation.

 inner f. Fovea centralis.

 f. lentis. Lens pit.

 outer f. An area in the retina, immediately external to the fovea centralis, where the external limiting membrane bulges slightly anteriorly due to the increased length of the slender outer and inner segments of the cones in this region. Syn., *fovea externa of Schäfer*.

 trochlear f. Trochlear fossa.

foveola (fo-ve-o'lah). The base or bottom of the fovea centralis, not including the clivus.

Foville's (fo-vēlz') **paralysis; syndrome.** See under the nouns.

FP. Abbreviation for *finger-piece*.

fraction. A part of the whole; the quotient of one expression divided by another.

 Fechner f. Weber's fraction.

 light-time f. Pulse-to-cycle fraction.

 on-time f. Pulse-to-cycle fraction.

 pulse-to-cycle f. In a repetitive, intermittent, light stimulus pattern, the light time divided by the total time of the light-dark cycle. Abbreviation PCF. Syn., *duty cycle; light-time fraction; on-time fraction; light-dark ratio*.

 Snellen f. An expression of visual acuity in the form of an unreduced fraction in which the numerator represents the testing distance, and the denominator represents the distance at which the smallest readable Snellen test type subtends an angle of 5 minutes.

 Weber's f. A constant, $\Delta R/R$, derived from Weber's law, in which ΔR = the change in stimulus which produces a just noticeable difference and R = the value of the original stimulus. When applied to the smallest perceptible difference in brightness between two adjacent illuminated fields, it is a constant of about 1% for all but very high or very low brightnesses.

fragilitas ossium (frah-jil'ih-tas os'e-um). Osteogenesis imperfecta.

frame. A structure for enclosing, containing, or supporting.

 browline f. A spectacle frame with a plastic upper portion to which are fitted metal eyewires to retain the lenses.

 eyeglass f. 1. A spectacle frame, without supporting temples, held by a spring or pinching grip at the root of the nose. Syn., *pince-nez*. 2. Any spectacle frame.

 finger-piece f. An eyeglass frame held in position by a pinching grip on the sides of the narrow part of the nose by means of pad arms under tension of small coil springs, with small levers protruding anteriorly which may be grasped between the thumb and forefinger to release the tension to mount, reset, or remove the spectacles.

 Ful-Vue f. A spectacle frame on which the endpieces are several millimeters higher than the datum line, so as not to obstruct the lateral view of the eyes.

 innerrim f. A spectacle frame on which the metal eyewires are embedded in plastic. Syn., *Windsor frame*.

Keeler Headband Trial F. An adjustable headband with a suspended trial frame designed for use with children and aphakics.

library f. A heavyweight spectacle frame, usually a plastic, suitable for reading lenses and characterized by straight or nearly straight temples to facilitate slipping the frame on or off the face.

Numont f. Numont mounting.

Ortho-Nez Spring Clamp Spectacle F. Trade name for an eyeglass frame designed for wear after rhinoplastic surgery, the essential feature being a pair of spring held oversized nose pads which provide pressure to counteract postoperative swelling of the tissues.

reversible f. A spectacle frame that presents either lens to either eye. It may have either an X-shaped bridge with straight temples, or an arc-shaped bridge with double-jointed endpieces.

rimless f. Rimless mounting.

rimway f. Rimway mounting.

shell f. Originally, a spectacle frame made from shell. In present usage, it includes all plastic spectacle frames.

spectacle f. A frame for supporting ophthalmic correcting lenses in front of the eyes. It rests on the nose and, usually, is supported by a pair of temples.

thermoplastic f. A spectacle frame made from any thermoplastic material, such as zylonite or Plexiglas.

trial f. A type of spectacle frame having variable adjustments for pupillary distance, temple length, bridge size, etc., and constructed to allow for the easy insertion and removal of trial lenses. It is commonly used in the refraction of the eyes.

Windsor f. Innerrim frame.

Franceschetti (fran"ses-chet'e) **sign; symptom; syndrome.** See under the nouns.

Franceschetti-Gernet syndrome (fran"ses-chet'e-gar'na). See under *syndrome.*

Franceschetti-Zwahlen syndrome (fran"ses-chet'e-zvah'len). Mandibulo-facial dysostosis.

François' (frahn-swahz') **corneal dystrophy; dermo-chondrocorneal dystrophy; syndrome.** See under the nouns.

Fränkel syndrome (freng'kel). Ocular contusion syndrome.

Frankl-Hochwart syndrome (frank'-l-hok'vart). Pineal-neurologic-ophthalmic syndrome. See under *syndrome.*

Franklin bifocal lens; Reader; spectacles. See under the nouns.

Fraunhofer's (frown'höf-erz) **diffraction grating; lines; diffraction phenomenon.** See under the nouns.

Frazer (fra'zer) **visual illusion; spiral.** See under the nouns.

Freeman Near Vision Unit. See under *unit.*

Freeman-Sheldon syndrome (fre'-man-shel'don). Craniocarpo-tarsal dystrophy. See under *dystrophy.*

Freidreich's (frēd'rīks) **spinal ataxia; disease; syndrome.** Freidreich's disease.

Frenzel (fren'zel) **goggles; nystagmus; spectacles.** See under the nouns.

frequency. 1. In harmonic motions, the number of cycles or vibrations per unit of time. 2. The number of occurrences of a given value or score falling into a specified class or population.

flicker f. The rate of intermittency, alteration, or variation of the presentation of photic stimulation to the eye, usually expressed in cycles per second. **critical f.f.** Critical fusion frequency. **fusion f.f.** Critical fusion frequency. **subfusional f.f.** Flicker frequency below that required to produce uniform sensation. Syn., *subfusional pulse frequency.*

fusion f. Critical fusion frequency. **critical f.f.** The rate of presentation of intermittent, alternate, or discontinuous photic stimuli that just gives rise to a fully uniform and continuous sensation obliterating the flicker. Syn., *critical flicker frequency; fusion frequency; fusion flicker frequency; flicker fusion threshold.*

f. of light wave. The rate of electromagnetic vibration of luminous flux. Designated v (nu), it is equal to the quotient of the velocity of light (c) divided by the wavelength (λ); thus, $v = c/\lambda$. The frequency of visible light ranges from approximately 4.3×10^{14} to 7.5×10^{14} per sec.

pulse f., subfusional. Subfusional flicker frequency.

Fresnel (fra-nel'). A unit of frequency equal to 10^{12} cycles per second.

Fresnel (fra'nel) **biprism; coefficient; diffraction; ellipsoid; equation; experiment; formula; integrals; law; lens; loss; mirrors; phenomenon; rhomb; zone.** See under the nouns.

Fresnel-Arago laws (fra'nel-ar'ah-go). See under *law.*

von Frey's hairs (fon-frīz'). See under *hairs.*

Fridenberg's (frid'en-bergz) **chart; test.** See under the nouns.

Frieberg's theory (fre'bergz). See under *theory.*

Friedenwald's (fre'den-walds) **chart; coefficient; formula.** See under the nouns.

Friedmann visual field analyzer (frēd'mahn). See under *analyzer.*

Friedreich's (frēd'rīks) **spinal ataxia; disease.** Freidreich's disease.

frill, iris. The line of junction of the ciliary zone and the pupillary zone of the iris. Syn., *collarette.*

frill, pigment. Pupillary ruff.

fringe. One of the dark or light bands produced by the diffraction or interference of light.

    Brewster's f's. White light fringes obtained by placing two Fabry-Pérot interferometers in series so as to create a path difference of zero.

    circular f's. 1. Alternate circular bands of light and dark produced by interference of light from two coherent extended sources, as in the Michelson interferometer when the mirrors are optically parallel to each other, or by interference with a thin plane-parallel film. 2. The Haidinger's fringes, or fringes of constant inclination, observed with a thick plane-parallel plate or with the Fabry-Pérot interferometer. 3. The rings of a diffraction pattern produced by plane waves passing through a small circular aperture, or by diffraction of plane waves by a circular obstacle.

    color f's. 1. A border of colors around images produced by a lens or an optical system not corrected for chromatic aberration. 2. Bands of color produced by interference or diffraction of white light.

    f's of constant inclination. Haidinger's fringes.

    f's of constant thickness. Interference fringes representing iso-thickness contours in thin films. Syn., *Fizeau fringes.*

    diffraction f's. A pattern of alternate dark and light bands produced by interference between the rays of diffracted light from a single narrow opening of finite width. The fringes occur, as with simple interference fringes, at points where the optical path differences of rays from points within the borders of the opening result in constructive or destructive interference, but the resultant pattern and the intensity distribution differ from the simple interference pattern in that the central band is very much brighter than other bands and its width is twice the separation of the minima (dark bands).

    f's. of equal inclination. Haidinger's fringes.

    Fabry-Pérot f's. The series of rings formed in a Fabry-Pérot interferometer by a monochromatic light source.

    Fizeau f's. Straight interference fringes of equal thickness. Cf. *Haidinger fringes.* Syn., *fringes of constant thickness.*

    Haidinger f's. Concentric circular interference fringes with diameters proportional to the square roots of the natural sequence of numbers. Cf. *Fizeau fringes.*

    interference f's. A pattern of alternate light and dark bands produced by destructive and constructive interference between the propagation waves of two or more superposed beams of light from a coherent source, occurring as a result of a difference in the optical lengths of the paths of two or more beams of light (usually monochromatic) from a single source.

    Landolt f. A black or very dark slightly curved fringe or streak dividing the otherwise less darkened field seen when viewing a very brilliant light source through a pair of Nicol prisms oriented with their principal planes at right angles to each other, corresponding to the locus of perfectly perpendicular vibrations.

    localized f's. Interference fringes observed with thin films or with the Michelson interferometer when the reflecting surfaces are not parallel to each other. Rays from a point on the source, reflected from the two surfaces and interfering to produce an interference fringe, are not parallel, but instead appear to diverge from a point near the surfaces. Hence, in order to observe the fringes clearly, the observer's eye must be focused approximately in the plane of the reflecting surfaces or in the plane in which the fringes appear to be localized. The fringes are usually nearly straight and parallel to the edge of the effective air wedge or film wedge between the reflecting surfaces.

moiré f's. Dark fringes produced when two diffraction gratings are placed in contact with each other such that the lines of the gratings intersect at a small angle.

white light f's. Interference fringes obtained in an interferometer when white light is used for the source, observed only when the path difference is of the order of a few wavelengths or less. In general, the central fringe is dark, while the other fringes have colored borders.

Froboese syndrome. Myelin neuromatosis.

Froehlich's syndrome (fra'liks). See under *syndrome.*

Froment's sign (fro-mahnz'). See under *sign.*

front. The part of a spectacle frame, Numont, or rimway mounting, exclusive of the temple, i.e., the bridge and the eyewires or rims.

Frostig test (fros'tig). See under *test.*

frothing. An aggregation of numerous minute air bubbles under a contact lens, frequently due to intermittent and excessive flaring of the edge of the lens from the cornea.

Fruehjahr's catarrh (fru'hahrz, fru'-yahrz). Vernal conjunctivitis.

Fry's (frīz) **frame gauge; method.** See under the nouns.

F.S.A.O. Fellow of the Scottish Association of Opticians.

F.S.M.C. Freeman of the Spectacle Makers Company, or, more formally, Freeman of the Worshipful Company of Spectacle Makers of London.

Fuchs' (fooks') **angle; optic atrophy; cleft; coloboma; conus; crypts; cyclitis; dimples; disease; corneal dystrophy; epithelioma; heterochromia; heterochromic iridocyclitis; superficial punctate keratitis; anterior pigment layer; lines of**

clearing; phenomenon; spot; spur; syndrome. See under the nouns.

Fuller-Albright syndrome (ful'er-awl'brīt). See under *syndrome.*

Ful-Vue (ful'vu). 1. See under *frame* and *mounting.* 2. A trade name for one of several types of bifocal lenses having a reading segment with a slightly curved upper border.

function. 1. The special action which any tissue, organ, or system of the body performs. 2. Any fact or quality so related to another that it is dependent on and varies with it. 3. Either of two magnitudes so related that to values of one there correspond values of the other.

color-matching f's. The energy fluxes of the three chosen primary wavelengths required to match the unit energy flux of a given monochromatic test wavelength.

contrast transfer f. See *optical transfer function.*

edge spread f. A mathematical description of the distribution of light across the optical image of an edge, i.e., across the image of an extended target having a sharp change in luminance, or a luminance distribution described by a step function.

frequency response f. See *optical transfer function.*

line spread f. A mathematical description of the distribution of light across the image of an infinitesimally narrow bright-line object.

luminosity f. The relative brightness-producing capacity of light of different wavelengths measured by the reciprocals of the amounts of radiant flux required at each wavelength region to produce the same brightness. Syn., *photopic visibility function.*

modulation transfer f. See *optical transfer function.*

obliquity f. Obliquity factor.

ocular rigidity f. A mathematical expression which relates intraocular pressure change to a change in intraocular volume, dP/dV, where P is the symbol for pressure and V is the symbol for volume.

optical transfer f. A mathematical expression of the relationship of the light distribution in an optical image to that in the object, hence an expression of the optical reproduction or optical transfer properties of the system, often in terms of the ratio of image contrast to object contrast as a function of spatial frequency (of a grating target), hence variously referred to as *contrast transfer function, modulation transfer function, frequency response function, spatial frequency transfer function, sinewave response function,* etc. It is the Fourier transform of the spread function (see *line spread function, point spread function, edge spread function*).

photopic visibility f. Luminosity function.

point spread f. A mathematical description of the distribution of light in a cross section of the image of an infinitesimally small, bright, point object, hence a description of the point-imaging characteristics of an optical system.

sine-wave response f. See *optical transfer function*.

spatial frequency f. See *optical transfer function*.

Westheimer f. See *Westheimer method*.

fundus (fun'dus). The base of the internal surface of a hollow organ; the part farthest removed or opposite the aperture.

albinotic f. An ocular fundus characterized by partial or complete lack of pigmentation of the retinal and choroidal layers. Ophthalmoscopically, the choroidal and the retinal vessels are clearly visible against a light orange-red background.

f. albipunctatus. An inherited tapetoretinal degeneration, either congenital or occurring in early life, and characterized by numerous white dots scattered throughout an otherwise normal fundus and accompanied by night blindness in about two thirds of the affected. It may be either unilateral or bilateral, visual acuity is unaffected, the visual fields are normal or but slightly restricted, and the condition is nonprogressive. Some differentiate it from the progressive retinitis punctata albescens and others believe the two are transitional forms of the same entity. Syn., *Lauber's disease; stationary albipunctate dystrophy*.

f. diabeticus. An ocular fundus prodromal sign of diabetic retinopathy consisting of uniform distention or turgescence of the larger veins and their main branches without other visible

evidence of diabetic retinopathy and with normal retinal function except for decreased electrical activity in the ERG and EOG.

f. flavimaculatus. A tapetoretinal degeneration with a familial tendency characterized by multiple, irregularly shaped, yellow or yellowish-white spots of uniform size lying deep in the retina around the posterior pole of the fundus and appearing from ages 10 to 25. The peripheral visual fields are normal, visual acuity may be poor, and the ERG is normal or subnormal.

f. of the lacrimal sac. The superior portion of the lacrimal sac formed by its cul-de-sac and bounded inferiorly by the sinus of Maier.

leopard f. An ocular fundus of mottled appearance as a result of retinitis pigmentosa.

ocular f. The concave interior of the eye, consisting of the retina, the choroid, the sclera, the optic disk, and blood vessels, seen by means of the ophthalmoscope.

f. oculi. Ocular fundus.

f. polycythemicus. The appearance of an ocular fundus associated with *Vaquez' disease*, q.v.

salt and pepper f. The finely pigmented ocular fundus characteristic of hereditary syphilis; it consists of innumerable, small, bluish pigmented spots between which lie depigmented yellowish-red spots.

shot silk f. An ocular fundus, sometimes seen in young persons, which has an opalescent or shimmering appearance, due to retinal reflections of light from the ophthalmoscope.

tesselated f. A nonpathological ocular fundus to which a deeply pigmented choroid gives the ophthalmoscopic appearance of dark, polygonal-shaped areas between the choroidal vessels, noted especially in the periphery. Syn., *tigroid fundus*.

tigroid f. Tesselated fundus.

Funduscope (fun'dus-skōp). An ophthalmoscope.

funnel, muscular (fun'el). The four rectus muscles of the eye considered as a structural unit and so designated because of their resemblance to a cone or a funnel as they diverge from their common origin at the apex of the orbit and extend forward to their insertions on the eyeball. Syn., *muscle cone*.

funnel, vascular (fun'el). Physiological cup.

Furmethide (fur'meth-id). Furfuryl trimethyl-ammonium iodide, a parasympathomimetic drug used in the eye, usually in 10% solution, as a miotic.

furrow. A groove or narrow channel.

circular f's. Depressions of the posterior surface of the iris, concentric with the pupil and crossing the radial structural furrows at regular intervals, caused by a local thinning of the pigment epithelium.

contraction f's of Schwalbe. Shallow furrows near the pupillary margin of the posterior surface of the iris, extending radially for about 1 mm and bending over the pupillary aperture, causing crenations on the pupillary margin. Syn., *contraction folds of Schwalbe.*

structural f's of Schwalbe. Shallow furrows on the posterior surface of the iris, extending from the region of the sphincter pupillae muscle and becoming continuous with the valleys between the ciliary processes. Syn., *structural folds of Schwalbe.*

fuscin (fus'in, fu'sin). The melanin-like pigment found as granules or needles in the cytoplasm of the pigment epithelium layer of the retina, especially that pigment near the visual cells.

Fuse's nucleus (fu'zez). See under *nucleus.*

◆

FUSION

fusion. The act or process of blending, uniting, or cohering.

amplitude of f. See under *amplitude.*

f. attraction. The stimulus value of a pair of binocularly coexisting, disparate, retinal images which evokes a motor fusion response.

f. aversion. Horror fusionis.

binocular f. Sensory fusion.

breadth of f. The combined range of convergence and divergence of the two eyes within which single binocular vision is maintained. Clinically, it is usually determined at a specific distance by the sum of the base-in and the base-out prism effects through which single binocular vision can be maintained.

f. cards. See under *card.*

f. center. See under *center.*

chiastopic f. Fusion obtained by voluntarily converging to fixate directly two fusible targets, laterally separated in space, such that the right eye directly fixates the left target and the left eye the right target. Cf. *orthopic fusion.*

f. clue. See under *clue.*

color f. 1. A type of sensory fusion wherein spectral stimulation which differs for the two eyes is combined or integrated into a unitary percept unlike either of the stimulating fields. 2. A unitary perception of color which bears no resemblance to any of the individual colors which form the composite. Cf. *color blend.*

critical f. Critical fusion frequency.

degrees of f. A classification by Worth of binocular vision into three divisions. First degree fusion: simultaneous, binocular perception of dissimilar objects which are projected in the same visual direction, as in the projection of a star seen by one eye into a circle seen by the other. Second degree fusion: single, simultaneous, binocular perception of identical, haploscopically viewed targets. Third degree fusion: stereopsis, requiring fusion of stereoscopic targets with a resultant third dimension percept.

f. faculty. See under *faculty.*

far point of f. The farthest distance at which single binocular vision is maintained. Hypothetically, it may be beyond infinity as measured by the maximum base-in prism effect through which single binocular vision can be maintained.

flat f. Sensory fusion in which the resultant percept is two-dimensional, that is, occupying a single plane, as may be induced by viewing a stereogram in a stereoscope in which the separation of all homologous points is identical.

foveal f. Sensory fusion in which only foveal images are considered.

f. frequency. See under *frequency.*

grades of f. An arbitrary division of fusional ability into four grades, determined with a white fixation target and a red lens before one eye. Grade A: immediate perception of one pink image. Grade B: immediate perception of one red and one white image, which subsequently merge into one pink image. Grade C: continuous perception of one red and one white image. Grade D:

continuous perception of one image only, which is either red or white.

macular f. Sensory fusion in which only macular images are considered.

motor f. The relative movements of the two eyes in response to disparate retinal stimuli, to obtain or maintain simultaneous stimulation of corresponding retinal areas, so that sensory fusion may occur.

near point of f. The nearest distance at which single binocular vision is maintained. It may be determined by the push-up test for convergence, or by the maximum base-out prism effect through which single binocular vision can be maintained.

orthopic f. Fusion obtained by voluntarily diverging to directly fixate two fusible targets, laterally separated in space, such that the right eye directly fixates the right target and the left eye the left. Cf. *chiastopic fusion.*

per cent of f. An arbitrary rating of fusional ability into percent, one such rating being based on the smallest diameter of colored circular targets which can be fused when viewed haploscopically.

peripheral f. Sensory fusion in which the images in the peripheral portions of the retinae are considered, excluding the maculae.

quality of f. The degree of ability to maintain single, simultaneous, binocular vision. See also *grades of fusion* and *percent of fusion.*

sensory f. 1. The process by which stimuli seen separately by the two eyes are combined, synthesized, or integrated into a unitary percept. Under normal binocular conditions, this occurs when corresponding retinal areas are stimulated by the same object, or objects of similar content. Syn., *binocular fusion.* 2. The combining of stimuli, presented intermittently or alternately, into a single constant sensation.

stereoscopic f. Sensory fusion of disparate retinal stimuli with a resultant third dimensional effect.

f. supplement. Fusional convergence.

temporal f. 1. The combining or integrating of stimuli presented intermittently or alternately at a specific temporal sequence into a single constant sensation. 2. Simulated sensory fusion presumed to occur as a result of the rapid alternating perception of the images of the two eyes in rapid alternating suppression.

torsional f. The component or type of motor fusion represented by torsional movements of the eyes.

◆

Fusion-Aider. Trade name of a lightweight visual therapy instrument consisting of an electrically driven, rotating, three-sectored disk hand-held in front of the eyes to interrupt at about 8 Hertz the vision of both eyes simultaneously. Variation of disk positions allows alternate occlusion of the eyes. Attachable red and green filters permit anaglyphic presentations. Cf. *Translid Binocular Interaction Trainer.*

fusional convergence; divergence; reserve. See under the nouns.

f-value. Focal ratio.

F.V.O.A. Fellow of the Victorian Optometrical Association (Australia).

Fyodorov lens. See under *lens.*

G

Galassi's (gah-lahs′ēz) **phenomenon; reflex.** Orbicularis pupillary reflex.

galeropia (gal″eh-ro′pe-ah). A pathological condition in which objects appear abnormally light and clear.

galeropsia (gal″eh-rop′se-ah). Galeropia.

Galezowski's strabismometer (gal-eh-zow′skēz). See under *strabismometer*.

Galilean (gal″ih-le′an) **spectacle; telescope.** See under the nouns.

galloxanthin (gal-o-zan′thin). A pigment, isolated by Wald from the retina of a chicken, thought to assist in differentiating spectral radiation by absorbing violet.

Galton bar (gawl′ton). See under *bar*.

galvanoluminescence (gal-vah-no-lu″-mih-nes′ens). Light emitted by the passage of an electrical current through an electrolyte in which an electrode of certain metals is immersed.

gamma [γ] (gam′ah). The Greek letter used as the symbol for (1) *angle gamma;* (2) *gamma movement.*

ganglion (gang′gle-un). An aggregation of nerve cell bodies located outside of the central nervous system.

accessory g. of Axenfeld. Episcleral ganglion.

cervical g., inferior. The lowest of three prominences of the paired sympathetic chains of vertebral ganglia in the region of the neck. Preganglionic and postganglionic nerve fibers synapse here, but the preganglionic axons relaying to the head pass through the synapse in the superior cervical ganglion.

cervical g., middle. The sec-
ond of three prominences of the paired sympathetic chains of vertebral ganglia in the region of the neck. Preganglionic axons relaying to the head pass directly through and synapse in the superior cervical ganglion.

cervical g., superior. The highest of three prominences of the paired sympathetic chains of vertebral ganglia in the region of the neck. It is the relay station for thoracic sympathetic preganglionic neurons that supply the smooth muscles and glands in the head and orbit, and its destruction results in Horner's syndrome.

ciliary g. A terminal parasympathetic ganglion located within the orbit between the lateral rectus muscle and the optic nerve. By way of its short motor root, it receives preganglionic axons which synapse in the ganglion with postganglionic neurons supplying the sphincter pupillae and ciliary muscles. By way of its sympathetic root, it receives vasomotor postganglionic axons supplying the eyeball. Its long sensory root carries general sensory dendrites originating in the eyeball, and some sympathetic postganglionic axons going to the dilator pupillae muscle. It gives rise to six to ten short ciliary nerves which double in number, prior to piercing the posterior sclera, and carry the afferent and postganglionic fibers. Syn., *lenticular ganglion; ophthalmic ganglion; optic ganglion; Schacher's ganglion.*

episcleral g. A collection of postganglionic cell bodies in a terminal parasympathetic ganglion located adjacent to a ciliary nerve or the optic nerve, in or near the posterior episclera. It is the site of synapses in the near pupillary reflex pathway to the sphincter pupillae muscle. Syn., *accessory ganglion of Axenfeld.*

Gasserian g. A ganglion on the sensory root of the trigeminal nerve, located on the petrous portion of the temporal bone, which contains the unipolar cell bodies of the afferent neurons and to which are connected the ophthalmic, the maxillary, and the mandibular nerves. Syn., *semilunar ganglion; trigeminal ganglion.*

lenticular g. Ciliary ganglion.

Meckel's g. The parasympathetic terminal nodule in the pterygopalatine fossa which receives the vidian nerve and connects with the maxillary nerve. Vasodilator and secretory fibers for the lacrimal gland from the facial nerve synapse here, and sympathetic postganglionic axons for the lacrimal gland and for Mueller's orbital muscle pass through. Syn., *sphenopalatine ganglion.*

Mueller's intraocular g. Collectively, a group of sympathetic-type multipolar cells near the arterioles of the choroid which are associated with plexuses derived from the ciliary nerves and are thought to be of vasomotor function and to participate in the control of intraocular pressure.

oculomotor g. 1. Schwalbe's term for the ciliary ganglion. 2. Tiny nodules on the oculomotor nerve.

ophthalmic g. Ciliary ganglion.

optic g. 1. Any one of several structures, such as the superior colliculus, the pretectal nucleus, or the lateral geniculate body, and, less likely, the pulvinar of the thalamus, considered as a primary or lower optical center. 2. The ciliary ganglion. 3. A cluster of cell bodies within the tuber cinereum of the diencephalon.

Schacher's g. Ciliary ganglion.

semilunar g. Gasserian ganglion.

sphenopalatine g. Meckel's ganglion.

thoracic g., superior. A ganglion on the sympathetic chain just below the inferior cervical ganglion, receiving preganglionic axons from the ciliospinal center of Budge which pass up the chain to the superior cervical ganglion, where they synapse with sympathetic neurons supplying the dilator pupillae muscle. It receives sympathetic fibers that originate in the upper thoracic cord and synapse in the superior cervical ganglion with neurons that supply the smooth muscles and glands in the head and the orbit. Syn., *first thoracic ganglion.*

trigeminal g. Gasserian ganglion.

Ganser's commissure (gahn'zerz). See under *commissure.*

Ganzfeld (gahnz'felt). (From German "Das homogene Ganzfeld.") A visual stimulus provision for research purposes consisting of completely homogeneous and formless luminance conditions throughout the visual field.

Garcin syndrome (gar'sin). See under *syndrome.*

gargoylism (gar'goil-izm). Hurler's disease.

Gasperini syndrome (gas-par-e'ne). See under *syndrome.*

Gasserian ganglion (gah-sēr'ih-an). See under *ganglion.*

Gát's schema (gahtz). See under *schema.*

Gaucher's disease (go-shāz'). See under *disease.*

gauge. An instrument for measuring dimension, curvature, or pressure, or for determining position.

douzième g. A caliper-type lens thickness gauge calibrated in douzièmes.

drop g. A device for determining the diameter of a contact lens, consisting essentially of a plate with a series of graduated apertures of various diameters. The smallest aperture through which the lens can pass indicates its diameter.

Duplex P-D g. An instrument for measuring the distance of the pupil of each eye from the center of the root of the nose, for the purpose of accurately positioning optical centers and/or bifocal segments of spectacle lenses. While the patient fixates successively the straight ahead images of his own eyes in a full-silvered mirror, the examiner notes the position of the root of the nose and each successively straightforward eye on a millimeter scale projected in the plane of the patient's pupils by a second (semisilvered) mirror.

Fry frame g. A device for measuring the dimensions of a spectacle frame according to the boxing method. It consists essentially of a ruled plastic plate, on which the frame is placed, and four single lines engraved on moveable transparent plastic strips, two vertical and two horizontal. Appropriate adjustment of the moveable lines indicates eyesize, DBL, major reference points, and multifocal segment positions.

interpupillary g. An instrument for measuring the distance between the centers of the pupils of the eyes.

lens g. Lens measure.

Livingston's binocular g. An instrument for determining the near point of either convergence or accommodation, consisting of a rule, 36 cm long, with a track down its center for a movable vertical target. The near points are determined by placing one end of the rule against the face and moving the target toward the eyes until it blurs or doubles.

Obrig Radius Dial G. A trade name for a device used for measuring the base curve of a contact lens, consisting essentially of a shaft having a central plunger which protrudes from a rounded surface on one end and connects to a dial on the other end. When placed against the lens surface, the extent of protrusion of the plunger determines sagittal depth, which is converted to radius of curvature in millimeters on the dial.

strap g. A metal disk with calibrated notches along its periphery for measuring the edge thickness of spectacle lenses at the point of insertion into the strap.

surfacing g. A flat template, or one of a series of templates, with an edge of known curvature for checking the curvature of the surface of a lens or lap by inspection of its goodness of fit in contact with the surface.

thickness g. 1. A caliper used to measure spectacle lens thickness, especially during surface grinding. It may be calibrated in $1/5$ mm or $1/10$ mm as units, the $1/5$ mm unit markings often being referred to as "points" in laboratory practice. 2. A device used to measure the center thickness of a contact lens, usually consisting of a stage on which the lens is centered while against the opposite surface of the lens is placed a spring-loaded plunger attached to a dial, usually calibrated in $1/10$ mm units.

V g. A bar with a tapering slot calibrated in $1/10$ mm units. The narrowest point in the slot into which a contact lens slides indicates its diameter.

Gaule's (gōltz) **pits; spots.** See under *spot*.

Gault's reflex (gōltz). Cochleopalpebral reflex.

Gauss's (gows'ez) **condition; eyepiece; lens; theory.** See under the nouns.

Gaussian (gows'zhun) **curve; frequency distribution; optical system; points.** See under the nouns.

Gaviola's caustic test (gav"e-o'laz). See under *test*.

gaze. 1. To fixate steadily or continuously. 2. The act or the condition of gazing.

direction of g. See under *direction*.

following g. See *illusion, following gaze*.

position of g. See under *position*.

geisoma (gi-so'mah). The eyebrows or the supraorbital ridges.

geison (gi'son). Geisoma.

Gelineau syndrome (zha-lih-no'). See under *syndrome*.

Gemminger's ossicle (jem'ing-erz). Os opticus.

General Optical Council. A representative corporate body created by Parliament (British) to carry out the provisions of the Opticians Act, 1958, which provides for the registration of optometrists and opticians and the regulation of certain related functions.

Generation II. Trade name for a pocket-size, night vision viewing instrument which intensifies the image luminance about 700 times, designed for persons with defective rod vision.

generator (jen'er-a-tor). A machine with cutting tools on arc-mounted jigs adjustable to selected curvilinear motions to grind lenses to desired thicknesses and surface curvatures.

Gennari's (jen-ah'rēz) **band; line; stria.** See under *line*.

genotype (jen'o-tīp). 1. A type determined by the common genetic characteristics of a group. 2. The hereditary characteristics of an organism, based on the genes which are postulated as occurring in its chromosomes.

Gerlach, muscle of (ger'lak). Anterior lacrimal muscle.

Gerlier's disease (zher-le-āz'). See under *disease.*

geromorphism (jer"o-mōr'fizm). A disease in which the skin becomes flaccid and wrinkled, resembling that of an aged person, occasionally affecting the upper eyelid and causing ptosis.

gerontopia (jer"on-to'pe-ah). Senopia.

gerontotoxon (jer-on"to-tok'son). Arcus senilis.

gerontoxon (jer"on-tok'son). Arcus senilis.

gerontoxon lentis (jer"on-tok'son len'tis). A surgical displacement of a cataractous crystalline lens in the aged.

Gershun tube (gur'shun). See under *tube.*

Gerstmann's syndrome (garst'manz). See under *syndrome.*

ghost. 1. A phantom; a faint shadowy semblance. 2. An unwanted secondary image, as may be formed by internal reflection in a lens or an optical system, irregularity of spacing in a diffraction grating, or incomplete polarization by a Polaroid filter.

　Bidwell's g. Second positive afterimage.

　Lyman's g's. Ghosts or faint line images produced by a diffraction grating having an error in the spacing of its lines involving two periods or a single short period.

　Rowland's g's. Ghost or faint line images appearing symmetrically in spacing and intensity about the principal maxima, produced by a diffraction grating having a single periodic error in the spacing of its lines.

　Swindle's g. An excessively long positive afterimage.

Gianelli's sign (jah-nel'lēz). Tournay's pupillary reflex.

Giantscope. A trade name for an ophthalmoscope.

Gibson's (gib'sunz) **method; theory.** See under the nouns.

Giessen test (ge'sen). See under *test.*

Gifford's (gif'ordz) **reflex; sign.** See under the nouns.

gigantophthalmos (ji-gant"of-thal'-mos). An anterior megalophthalmos in which the anterior segment of the eye is greatly enlarged.

Giles-Archer color perception unit (jīlz-ar'cher). See under *unit.*

Gillespie's syndrome (gih-les'pēz). See under *syndrome.*

Giraud-Teulon law. See under *law.*

girdle, limbus, of Vogt. A white, ragged-edged, subepithelial opacity of the cornea, located chiefly in the interpalpebral region and concentric with the limbus. It is differentiated into two types: in one the opacity is discontinuous, having gaps, and is separated from the limbus by a clear zone; in the other the opacity is unbroken, is continuous with the sclera, and has short projections extending toward the center of the cornea.

Gladstone-Dale law. See under *law.*

glabella (glah-bel'ah). 1. The region of the frontal bone between the eyebrows. 2. The skin, generally hairless, between the eyebrows.

gland. A cell or an organ which secretes or excretes a substance or substances.

　Baumgarten's g's. Conjunctival glands located nasally in the eyelids of some animals but not man.

　Bruch's g's. Lymph follicles in the conjunctiva of the eyelids.

　g's. of Ciaccio. Glands of Wolfring and Ciaccio.

　ciliary g's. 1. Invaginations of the pigmented epithelium of the ciliary body, especially in the pars plana, thought by some to secrete aqueous humor. 2. Glands of Moll.

　g's. of Collins. Ciliary body glands in the region of the ciliary processes, formed by folds of the outer pigmented cells of the epithelium and thought by some to secrete aqueous humor.

　conjunctival g. 1. Any gland, the duct of which empties into the conjunctiva, such as Meibomian, Krause, Wolfring and Ciaccio glands, or a goblet cell. Some include the lacrimal gland. 2. Any accessory lacrimal gland.

　g. of Harder. A mucosebaceous secreting gland in nonprimate vertebrates, found near the attachment of the nicitating membrane. It rapidly degenerates in the human fetal eye.

　g's. of Henle. Crypts of the palbebral conjunctiva between the tarsus and the fornix in both the upper and the lower eyelids, probably nonsecretory. Syn., *conjunctival crypts.*

　infraorbital g. An accessory lacrimal gland located in the lower outer fornix of the conjunctiva, which is permanent in lower vertebrates and degenerates in the fetus of higher primates.

g's. of Krause. Accessory lacrimal glands of the conjunctiva, most of which are located in the region of the superior fornix beneath the inferior lacrimal gland, with a few located just beneath the inferior fornix.

lacrimal g. A compound tubuloalveolar gland which is divided into an orbital and a palpebral portion by the lateral horn of the aponeurosis of the levator palpebrae superioris muscle. The orbital lobe rests in a fossa of the frontal bone located laterally in the orbital roof, its ducts joining those of the palpebral lobe to form about twelve ducts which empty into the superior lateral fornix, although occasionally one empties into the inferior lateral fornix. The lacrimal gland forms the lacrimal fluid portion of the tears, to which mucin and·sebum are added. Syn., *glandula orbitaria.* **accessory l.g.** Any of the conjunctival glands which secrete lacrimal fluid; the glands of Krause, or the glands of Wolfring and Ciaccio.

g's. of Manz. Tiny, epithelial, cell-filled diverticula in the limbal conjunctiva of some domestic animals. Their presence in man is not established.

Meibomian g's. A series of simple, branched, alveolar, sebaceous glands, located in the tarsi of the eyelids, whose ducts empty into the eyelid margins in line with and lateral to the lacrimal puncta. Syn., *tarsal glands; tarsoconjunctival glands.*

g. of Moll. A sweat gland located in the region of an eyelash.

Rosenmueller's g. The inferior or palpebral portion of the lacrimal gland.

tarsal g's. Meibomian glands.

tarsoconjunctival g's. Meibomian glands.

Waldeyer's g's. Modified sweat glands at the margin of the eyelid, near the border of the tarsus.

g's. of Wolfring and Ciaccio. Accessory lacrimal glands in the upper eyelid, located in the region of the superior border of the tarsus, which empty into the palpebral conjunctiva.

g's. of Zeis. Simple, branched, alveolar, sebum-forming glands attached directly to the follicles of the eyelashes.

glandula (glan'du-lah). A gland, especially a small gland.

g. concreta. The superior or orbital portion of the lacrimal gland.

g. lacrimalis. Lacrimal gland.

g. mucosa. Gland of Krause.

g. orbitaria. Lacrimal gland.

Glan-Foucault (glan-foo-ko') **polarizer; prism.** See under *prism.*

Glan-Thompson prism (glan-tom'-son). See under *prism.*

glare. Relatively bright light, or the dazzling sensation of relatively bright light, which produces unpleasantness or discomfort, or which interferes with optimal vision.

g. accompaniment. Any of the sensory or motor end results, aside from the awareness or sensation of glare, elicited by glareproducing stimuli, such as the reduced ability to distinguish objects.

blinding g. Scotomatic glare.

central g. Glare as a result of intense light on the foveal or macular area of the retina, as occurs when directly viewing a small, bright light source. Syn., *direct glare.*

dazzling g. One of the three classes of glare designated by Bell, Troland, and Verhoeff. It is glare produced by adventitious light scattered in the ocular media so as not to form part of the retinal image. Cf. *scotomatic glare; veiling glare.*

direct g. 1. Central glare. 2. Glare resulting from light sources or reflecting surfaces insufficiently shielded to prevent the direct entry of light into the observer's eye.

disability g. Glare which reduces visual performance and visibility, and may be accompanied by discomfort.

discomfort g. Glare which produces discomfort but does not necessarily interfere with visual performance or visibility.

eccentric g. Glare as a result of intense light falling on the peripheral retina. Syn., *indirect glare.*

indirect g. Eccentric glare.

reflected g. Glare resulting from specular reflections from polished or glossy surfaces.

scotomatic g. One of the three classes of glare designated by Bell, Troland, and Verhoeff. It is glare produced by light of sufficient intensity to reduce appreciably the sensitivity of the retina. Cf. *dazzling glare; veiling glare.* Syn., *blinding glare.*

total g. Glare in which excessive light falls on the whole retina.

veiling g. One of the three classes of glare designated by Bell, Troland, and Verhoeff. It is glare produced by excess light uniformly distributed over the visual field so as to cause reduced contrasts and, therefore, reduced visibility. Cf. *dazzling glare; scotomatic glare.*

glarometer (gla-rom'eh-ter). An instrument for measuring sensitivity to glare from the headlights of an approaching automobile.

◆

GLASS

glass. 1. A substance, ordinarily hard, brittle, and lustrous, produced by fusing sand (silica) with oxides of potassium or sodium and other ingredients, especially lead oxide, alumina, and lime. It is usually transparent, although it may be translucent, and even opaque, in certain forms. Special treatment of glass may cause it to change into tough fibers used in insulation and even in textiles. Glass may be produced in various colors by the addition of various chemicals. 2. A lens or a light filter.

absorption g. Glass which transmits only a portion of the light incident upon it, the remainder being absorbed and transformed into other forms of energy. The term is applied particularly to colored glass.

adhesive g. A contact lens.

alabaster g. A white, translucent glass used principally for vases, ornaments, and busts.

amethyst g. An absorptive glass, particularly useful in the absorption of ultraviolet rays inasmuch as it totally absorbs those below 3,000 Å. It is produced by the addition of manganese dioxide to the glass batch.

antique g. A glass in which bubbles, striae, etc., are intentionally introduced to produce a slight nonuniform diffusion.

Arundel g. A slightly pink, absorptive glass devised in 1872 by T. A. Wilson.

Bagolini's striated g. A lens on which fine parallel striations have been grooved. Visual acuity through the lens is only slightly or negligibly reduced, but a light source viewed through the lens appears as a streak of light oriented 90° from the striations (similar to a Maddox rod). Two such lenses mounted in front of the two eyes, with the striations oriented 90° apart, are used in the determination of suppression, anomalous correspondence, and possibly fixation disparity.

barium-crown g. A type of ophthalmic glass used primarily in bifocal segments. It has an index of refraction ranging between 1.570 and 1.616 depending on the ingredients, and a v value between 55.0 and 57.0.

barium-flint g. A type of ophthalmic glass used primarily in multifocal segments and containing barium oxide, silica, lead oxide, and other elements. Its index of refraction ranges approximately between 1.58 and 1.62, depending on the proportion of ingredients, and its v value approximately between 43.0 and 53.0.

blown g. Glass which has been blown to some predetermined form either by machine or by human breath. Glass blowing has been used in the manufacture of glass artificial eyes and glass contact lenses. Blown glass lenses are used in some inexpensive sunglasses.

cased g. A composite of two or more fused layers of different kinds of glass, usually one clear, transparent and another opal, opalescent, or colored.

cladding g. In fiber optics, the glass sheath of lower refractive index around the glass core of the fiber.

cobalt-blue g. A cobalt-containing glass known for its property of transmitting light primarily from the red and blue ends of the spectrum. When used in refraction as a bichromatic filter for testing ametropia, it is sometimes called a *cobalt lens.*

configurated g. A nontransparent, diffusing glass having a patterned surface, such as pebbled or stippled glass.

Crookes g. Any of a series of commercially available absorptive glasses, ranging from pale amethyst to brownish gray or smoke in its usual forms, but also available in sage green, developed by Sir William Crookes about 1910, in association with the Chance Brothers, of Birmingham, England. It possesses the property of absorbing a large proportion of infrared rays and practically all ultraviolet rays. The transmission curve for

Crookes A shows an over-all 10% reduction of light intensity in the visible range, with a sharp dip (up to 30% absorption) around the wavelength 5,800 Å. The transmission curve for Crookes 246 shows a reduction of light intensity in the visible range of more than 75%.

crown g. An optical, alkali-lime glass having a low dispersion (v value 52.2) relative to the index of refraction ($n = 1.523$), commonly used in ophthalmic lenses. The word crown originally referred to the heavy blob of glass at the center of a layer of glass spun on a flat surface by early glassmakers. Cf. *flint glass*.

didymium g. A glass containing didymium to absorb yellow light and hence used in lenses for protection in glass-blowing and other occupations involving excessive exposure to sodium flare.

enameled g. A diffusing glass surfaced with enamel.

euphos g. A yellow-green, absorptive glass which does not transmit wavelengths shorter than 4,000 Å developed in 1907 by Drs. Schauz and Stockhousen, of Dresden, Germany.

Fieuzel g. A yellow-green glass which absorbs a high percentage of both ultraviolet and infrared rays.

flea g. A popular magnifying glass described by Descartes consisting of a small plano convex lens mounted with its plane face toward the observer's eye and its convex face in contact with an orifice at the apical center of a concave mirror facing away from the observer, so that light from a distant source, such as the sun, would illuminate a small object, such as a flea, placed at the coincident focal planes of the lens and the mirror, making the object observable in magnification.

flint g. A lead-containing, optical glass having a high dispersion relative to its refractive index, as compared, e.g., to crown glass. It is softer and heavier than crown glass and is used in ophthalmic lenses required to be thin, and as bifocal segments in crown glass lenses. Its name is said to be derived from the Latin word for a very fine silica in the form of flints which the early glass-makers used in the attempt to obtain transparency. Syn., *thinflint glass*.

fluor crown g. An optical glass that contains fluorine and has a low refractive index of 1.5 or less.

ground g. Glass which has been surface ground with rough emery to make it translucent; especially used as an occluding lens.

Hallauer g. A smoky-green glass, produced in 1905 by Dr. O. Hallauer, of Switzerland, which absorbs ultraviolet radiations, totally absorbing those below 4,000 Å.

homogeneous g. A glass of uniform composition, as differentiated from cased glass, although striae or bubbles may still be present.

kalichrome g. A commercially available yellow glass which totally absorbs ultraviolet and large portions of the violet, blue, and infrared, hence, said to reduce blue haze effects; frequently prescribed for spectacles used by marksmen and skeet shooters.

magnifying g. A simple converging lens or lens system, usually held in the hand and relatively near the object viewed, for magnifying apparent size without inversion.

mat-surface g. A highly diffusing glass having an etched, ground, or sandblasted surface.

Motex g. A trade name for glass of the same construction as Triplex glass.

neophane g. A yellow glass containing neodymium oxide used for lenses in sunglasses and in windshields.

noviol g. A yellow, absorptive glass, similar in type and purpose to kalichrome glass.

objective g. Objective lens.

opal g. A nearly white or milky, translucent diffusing glass.

opalescent g. A form of opal glass having selective properties of transmission which result in an iridescent appearance of transmitted light.

ophthalmic g. Optical glass meeting the specific requirements for ophthalmic lenses.

optical g. A form of glass meeting the specific requirements for use in optical systems with respect to transparency, homogeneity, bubbles, inclusions, striae, cloudiness, strain, refractive index, dispersive power, and chemical and physical stability.

Pfund's gold-plated g. A type of laminated absorptive glass consisting of a Crookes A glass to absorb ultraviolet, a very thin layer of gold to reflect infrared while transmitting visible light, and a crown glass to protect the layer of gold.

photochromic g. Transparent glass which darkens on exposure to light of high intensity and clears with reduced intensity.

plate g. Fine rolled, ground, and polished sheet glass.

polarizing g. Polarizing occluder.

prismatic g. A lenslike unit or assembly of transparent optical glass, molded or otherwise preformed so that different areas of the transmitting surface each have a prescribed prismatic effect to deflect light in a desired direction, thus to accomplish a distribution or a concentration of light suitable for special illumination purposes. Examples include horizontal sidewalk windows for illuminating basements, various luminaires, and automobile headlamp lenses.

red g. A glass transmitting red light more or less exclusively. When used monocularly in binocular clinical tests and training procedures, it is sometimes called a *red lens.*

repeat g. A multiple-facet lens through which a single pattern may be viewed to be seen as an array of duplicate patterns, used by wallpaper and textile designers.

safety g. 1. Nonshatterable, laminated glass consisting of a layer of transparent plastic between two layers of glass, commonly used in automobiles and goggles. 2. Glass, case-hardened by heat or chemical treatment, used in goggles and ophthalmic lenses.

Salvoc g. A trade name for a glass of the same construction as Triplex glass.

smoke g. A smoke-colored, absorptive glass transmitting the visible wavelengths more or less uniformly. Available commercially in various degrees of absorptiveness, it is useful for controlling illumination and brightness intensities.

thinflint g. Flint glass.

transparent g. Glass through which objects can be seen clearly.

Triplex g. A trade name for a safety glass consisting of two layers of clear glass cemented together with a layer of cellulose acetate or zylonite. When broken, it cracks into fragments but does not splinter or fly.

Uviol g. Trade name of a glass highly transparent to ultraviolet radiation.

window g. Glass used for windowpanes, usually manufactured in sheets by a rolling process and differing in characteristics from optical glass.

Wood's g. Wood's filter.

◆

glasses. Spectacles.
glasses, field. Binoculars.

◆

GLAUCOMA

glaucoma (glaw-ko'mah). An ocular disease, occurring in many forms, having as its primary characteristic an unstable or a sustained increase in the intraocular pressure which the eye cannot withstand without damage to its structure or impairment of its function. The consequences of the increased pressure may be manifested in a variety of symptoms, depending upon type and severity, such as excavation of the optic disk, hardness of the eyeball, corneal anesthesia, reduced visual acuity, seeing of colored halos around lights, disturbed dark adaptation, visual field defects, and headaches.

absolute g. A final, hopeless stage of glaucoma in which vision is completely and permanently lost, intraocular pressure is increased, the optic disk is white and deeply excavated, and the pupil is usually widely dilated and immobile. Syn., *glaucoma consummatum.*

acute g. Acute congestive glaucoma.

air block g. A type of pupillary block glaucoma resulting from interruption or retardation of the flow of aqueous humor from the posterior to the anterior chamber by an air bubble, created by injection of air into the anterior chamber, following cataract extraction, goniopuncture, or cyclodialysis.

aphakic obstructive g. Glaucoma, following surgery for cataract, due to delayed re-formation of the anterior chamber.

apoplectic g. Hemorrhagic glaucoma.

auricular g. Glaucoma associated with increased intralabyrinthine pressure.

capsular g. Glaucoma due to clogging of the filtration angle with debris consisting of cellular flakes from exfoliation of the anterior lens capsule.

g. cerebri. A condition in which the diastolic pressure of the central retinal artery is increased while the intracranial pressure and that of the central retinal vein remain normal, causing prodromal glaucomatous symptoms, but without actual glaucoma.

closed angle g. Glaucoma in which the angle of the anterior chamber is blocked, such that aqueous humor cannot drain from the anterior chamber. It is usually associated with acute congestive glaucoma.

compensated g. Noncongestive glaucoma.

congenital g. Glaucoma caused by developmental anomalies in the region of the angle of the anterior chamber which present an obstruction to the drainage mechanism of the intraocular fluids. It usually results in a distended eyeball, an enlarged flattened cornea, a thinning of the sclera, a deep anterior chamber, and an excavation of the optic disk in the later stages. Syn., *buphthalmos; infantile glaucoma; hydrophthalmos.*

congestive g. Glaucoma characterized by obvious symptoms such as circumcorneal injection, corneal edema, or pain. It may occur either in a chronic or in an acute form and is a result of a relatively rapid increase in intraocular pressure. Syn., *incompensated glaucoma; inflammatory glaucoma; noncompensated glaucoma.* **acute c.g.** Glaucoma characterized by a sudden violent elevation of the intraocular pressure which produces an excruciating eye pain radiating to the face, jaw, and head, accompanied by rapid loss of vision, intense ocular congestion, and constitutional disturbances. Usually, the cornea is hazy, the anterior chamber is shallow, the pupil is dilated and immobile, and pronounced circumcorneal injection is present. The majority of cases have prodromal attacks of less severity preceding the acute· stage. Syn., *acute glaucoma; glaucoma evolutum.* **chronic c.g.** Congestive glaucoma with symptoms similar to, but milder in intensity and slower in progress than, the acute form.

g. consummatum. Absolute glaucoma.

corticosteroid g. A type of open angle glaucoma attributed to the prolonged local or systemic use of corticosteroids.

developmental g. Glaucoma attributed to an abnormality of development of the angle of the anterior chamber.

dilatation g. Glaucoma induced in a predisposed eye by the instillation of a mydriatic.

Donders' g. Noncongestive glaucoma in an advanced stage.

g. evolutum. Acute congestive glaucoma.

fulminating g. Acute congestive glaucoma rapidly followed by blindness.

hemolytic g. Glaucoma attributed to obstruction of the outflow channels by erythrocytic debris and macrophages following intraocular hemorrhage.

hemorrhagic g. Glaucoma associated with retinal hemorrhages. Syn., *apopletic glaucoma; thrombotic glaucoma.*

hypersecretion g. A type of open angle glaucoma attributed to an increased rate of aqueous humor secretion in the presence of a normal drainage mechanism.

hyposecretory g. A low tension glaucoma in which hyposecretion is associated with a decreased facility of outflow.

iatrogenic g. Glaucoma arising from the use of certain drugs, especially corticosteroids or mydriatics, and sometimes miotics or sulphanomides.

incompensated g. Congestive glaucoma.

infantile g. Congenital glaucoma.

inflammatory g. Congestive glaucoma.

intermittent g. Glaucoma secondary to a low grade cyclitis which has produced changes characteristic of glaucoma in the visual field and in the fundus, but without manifesting a continued raised intraocular pressure.

inverse g. Secondary glaucoma due to a dislocation of the crystalline lens into the anterior chamber, or to the protrusion of the rounded anterior surface of a microphakic or spherophakic lens into the anterior chamber. A miotic substance raises the intraocular pressure and a mydriatic substance lowers it. Syn., *paradoxical glaucoma.*

iris blocked g. Glaucoma in which the angle of the anterior chamber is closed by adhesions at the root of the iris, blocking the outflow of aqueous humor.

juvenile g. Glaucoma occurring in young persons, so named because of the ordinary association of glaucoma with advanced years.

low tension g. An ocular condition or disease which does not manifest an increased intraocular pressure on prolonged observation, but does manifest all other glaucomatous changes.

malignant g. A severe form of glaucoma which rapidly leads to blindness in spite of surgery or other treatment.

mydriatic g. Glaucoma induced by a mydriatic which, with dilation of the pupil, increases the thickness of the iris tissue to form a mechanical blockage of the angle of the anterior chamber. It typically occurs in an eye which is predisposed by having a shallow anterior chamber with a narrow angle.

narrow angle g. Glaucoma in which the angle of the anterior chamber is narrow. (See Fig. 20.)

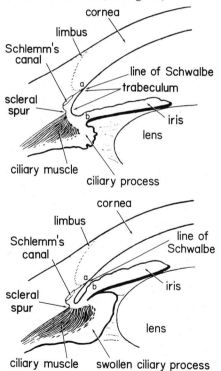

Fig. 20 *Top*, wide angle glaucoma showing normal filtration angle; *bottom*, narrow angle glaucoma showing blockage of the filtration angle. (From A. E. Town, *Ophthalmology*. Philadelphia: Lea and Febiger, 1951)

neovascular g. Glaucoma attributed to neovascularization involving the angle of the anterior chamber, as may occur in rubeosis iridis.

noncompensated g. Congestive glaucoma.

noncongestive g. A slowly, insidiously developing glaucoma in which subjective symptoms are minimal, and in which clinical signs of marked congestion are absent. If the disease is long standing, visual acuity is reduced, visual field defects are present, and the optic disk is excavated. Syn., *compensated glaucoma; noninflammatory glaucoma; quiet glaucoma; simple glaucoma.* **chronic n.g.** Noncongestive glaucoma.

noninflammatory g. Noncongestive glaucoma.

open angle g. Glaucoma in which the angle of the anterior chamber is open and free of obstruction. It is usually associated with noncongestive glaucoma.

paradoxical g. Inverse glaucoma.

phacogenic g. Phacolytic glaucoma.

phacolytic g. Glaucoma secondary to hypermature cataract and due to permeation of liquefied cortical material through the lens capsule into the anterior chamber, with subsequent absorption by large mononuclear cells which swell, plug the trabecular spaces at the angle of the anterior chamber, and prevent the adequate escape of aqueous humor. Syn., *phacogenic glaucoma.*

pigmentary g. Glaucoma associated with degeneration of the pigment epithelium of the iris and ciliary body, with marked deposition of pigment in the trabecular spaces at the filtration angle.

plethoric g. Glaucoma due to increased production of aqueous humor resulting from angiomatous changes in the ciliary body.

primary g. Glaucoma occurring without antecedent ocular disease in an otherwise apparently healthy eye.

pupillary block g. Glaucoma caused by interruption or retardation of the flow of aqueous humor from the posterior to the anterior chamber, due to the pupillary border being in contact with, or abnormally close to, the anterior capsule of the crystalline lens, or to the vitreous humor in aphakia. The resultant increased pressure in the posterior chamber causes the iris to bulge forward and block the filtration angle. It may occur as a primary glaucoma in narrow-angled eyes or be secondary to a swollen crystalline lens, posterior synechiae to the lens, lens dislocation, or posterior synechiae to the vitreous humor in aphakia.

quiet g. Noncongestive glaucoma.

secondary g. Glaucoma occurring as a result of a recognized preexisting ocular disease.

simple g. Noncongestive glaucoma.

sympathetic g. Glaucoma occuring in a formerly healthy eye following surgery on a glaucomatous eye.

thrombotic g. Hemorrhagic glaucoma.

trabecular g. Glaucoma due to blockage of the trabecular spaces at the angle of the anterior chamber, preventing adequate outflow of aqueous humor.

vitreous block g. A type of pupillary block glaucoma caused by adhesion of the iris to the hyaloid membrane of the vitreous humor in aphakia.

wide angle g. Glaucoma in which the angle of the anterior chamber is wide. (See Fig. 20.)

◆

glaucomatous (glaw-ko'mah-tus). Pertaining to or resulting from glaucoma.

glaucosis (glaw-ko'sis). Blindness resulting from glaucoma.

glaze. 1. To insert lenses into spectacle frames or mountings. 2. To overlay with a thin surface consisting of, or resembling, glass. 3. To make glossy.

Glazebrook (glāz'brook) **polarizer; prism.** See under *prism.*

glia, retinal perivascular (gli'ah). Cells of unknown function which surround the retinal capillaries with a loose network formed by their processes.

glial mantle, peripheral (gli'al man'-tl). See under *mantle.*

glioblastoma, retinal (gli"o-blas-to'mah). Retinoblastoma.

glioma (gli-o'mah). A tumor derived from neuroglial cells or their antecedents.

g. endophytum. Retinoblastoma endophytum.

g. exophytum. Retinoblastoma exophytum.

g. planum. Diffuse infiltrating retinoblastoma.

retinal g. Generally, a congenital, malignant tumor arising from retinal neuroblasts, as a retinoblastoma or neuroepithelioma. Specifically, a tumor arising from neuroglial elements of the retina, i.e., an astrocytoma, or "true" glioma.

glioneuroma (gli"o-nu-ro'mah). A benign tumor composed essentially of mature glial and neuronal elements, occurring in the central nervous system or retina.

glissade (glis'ād). A gliding movement of the eye lacking the velocity and trajectory characteristics of a saccade.

glitter. To gleam or shine with a brilliant and broken scintillating light.

globe (of eye). The eyeball.

globules, Morgagnian (glob'ūls). Drops of fluid which are formed in the spaces between lens fibers in early degenerative cataract. Syn., *Morgagnian spherules.*

glory. Appearance of concentric rings of colored light encircling an object or the head of a figure, especially as to suggest attributes of honor and splendor. Cf. *brocken specter.*

gloss. A shiny or lustrous appearance of a surface, as when much of the reflected light is specularly reflected.

glossiness. An attribute of the appearance of a surface dependent upon the type and the amount of reflection. Low glossiness is characteristic of rough diffusing surfaces and high glossiness of smooth surfaces that give a shiny or lustrous effect.

glossmeter (glos'me-ter). An instrument for determining the reflection factor of a surface or to determine the ratio of light regularly reflected from a surface to that diffusely reflected.

glossimeter (gloh-sim'eh-ter). Glossmeter.

glossy. Having the appearance of gloss.

glow. The perceived characteristic of a solid, self-luminous body in a relatively dark surround, as in the glow of an ember.

glycolacria (gli"ko-lak're-ah). An abnormally high concentration of glucose in tears, associated with hyperglycemia.

gobo. A mat or screen with a dark material covering used to shield a television or motion picture camera lens from unwanted light.

GOC. See *General Optical Council.*

Godtfredsen's syndrome (gōt'fred-senz). See under *syndrome.*

Goethe's theory (guh'tez). See under *theory.*

goggle 1. To stare with wide-open or bulging eyes. 2. To roll or bulge the eyes.

goggles. Spectacles, usually large, with auxiliary shields and padding, for protecting the eyes from wind, flying particles, intense light, and other external hazards. Some types may be worn over conventional corrective eye wear, and many types have a headband rather than temples.

> **diplopia g.** Goggle-type spectacles with lenses of different color, usually red and green, to produce dissociation of a fixated spot or light source.

> **underwater g.** Goggles with mounting frames which tightly fit the contour of the orbital rims to keep water out.

> **Frenzel g.** Frenzel spectacles.

goiter, exophthalmic (goi'ter). A systemic disease characterized by increased basal metabolism, exophthalmos, a tendency to increased appetite, loss of weight, vomiting, diarrhea, profuse sweating, tremors, increased pulse rate, and psychic disturbances. Signs associated with exophthalmic goiter are those of von Graefe, Dalrymple, Stellwag, Moebius, and Gifford, q.v. Syn., *Basedow's disease; Flajani's disease; Graves's disease; March's disease; Parry's disease; Stokes's disease; thyrotoxicosis.*

Goldenhar syndrome (gōld'en-har). See under *syndrome.*

Goldmann lens; tonometer. See under the nouns.

Goldmann-Weekers adaptometer. See under *adaptometer.*

GOMAC. See *Groupement des Opticiens du Marché Commun* (Association of Common Market Opticians).

goniolens, Troncoso (go'ne-o-lenz"). A hemispherical contact lens which fits beneath the eyelids, used in conjunction with a biomicroscope to view the filtration angle of the anterior chamber. Syn., *Troncoso contact lens.*

goniometer (go"ne-om'eh-ter). An instrument for measuring angles, such as those of crystals and prisms.

goniomyostomy (go"ne-o-mi-os'to-me). A cyclodialysis reinforced by interposing superior rectus muscle fibers, surgically inserted at a scleral incision anterior to the muscle attachment to the globe and pulled out through a second incision at the limbus.

goniophotography (go"ne-o-fo-tog'rah-fe). Photography of the angle of the anterior chamber of the eye.

goniophotometer (go"ne-o-fo-tom'eh-ter). Distribution photometer.

gonioplasty (go'ne-o-plas"te). A surgical procedure for glaucoma in which a plastic tube is implanted under the sclera to carry aqueous humor from the anterior chamber to subchoroidal and sub-Tenon's spaces.

gonioprism, Allen's (go'ne-o-prizm"). Allen's contact prism.

gonioprism, Allen-Thorpe (go'ne-o-prizm"). A prism in which the apex has been curved to fit against the cornea in gonioscopy. It is mounted on a handle held by the examiner, and all of its four sides are mirrored to afford an almost complete view of the filtration angle without its rotation.

goniopunciotomy (go"ne-o-punk"e-ot'-o-me). A surgical procedure for congenital glaucoma in which goniopuncture is combined with goniotomy.

goniopuncture (gon"ne-o-pungk'tūr). A surgical procedure for congenital glaucoma in which a puncture is made into the meshwork at the filtration angle, extending into the subconjunctival space, by means of a needle-knife inserted through the opposite limbus and carried across the anterior chamber, parallel to the iris. It is usually performed under the direct observation afforded by a gonioscope.

gonioscope (go'ne-o-skōp"). Any of several instruments, usually consisting of a biomicroscope used in conjunction with a prismatic contact lens, for viewing the filtration angle of the anterior chamber.

gonioscopy (go"ne-os'ko-pe). Observation of the filtration angle of the anterior chamber with the gonioscope.

> **direct image g.** Observation of the virtual, upright image of the filtration angle of the anterior chamber as formed by a gonioscopic lens and viewed with an ophthalmoscope or biomicroscope.

> **indirect image g.** Observation of the real, inverted, anteriorly located aerial image of the filtration angle of the anterior chamber as formed by a specially modified gonioscopic lens and viewed with an indirect ophthalmoscope.

goniosynechiae (go"ne-o-sih-nek'e-e). Adhesions of iritic tissue to corneal or scleral tissue at the angle of the anterior chamber, usually associated with closed angle glaucoma.

goniotomy (go"ne-ot'o-me). A surgical procedure for congenital glaucoma in which a sweeping incision is made in the meshwork at the filtration angle by means of a knife-needle inserted through the opposite limbus and carried across the anterior chamber parallel to the iris. It is usually performed under direct observation afforded by a special contact lens. Syn., *goniotrabeculotomy.*

goniotrabeculotomy (go"ne-o-trah-bek"u-lot'o-me). Goniotomy.

goniotripsy (go"ne-o-trip'se). A surgical procedure for congenital glaucoma, used when lack of corneal transparency interferes with direct observation of the angle of the anterior chamber. A specially designed straight-handled knife, with a flat blade rounded at its tip, is inserted through a corneal incision near the limbus into the angle of the anterior chamber adjacent to the incision, rotated about the axis of the handle, and then moved laterally so as to scrape the angle rather than incise it.

Goodenough-Harris Draw test. See under *test.*

goods, glazed. *Colloquial*: Ready-to-wear eyeglasses, including sunglasses, sold directly to the public as retail merchandise.

Gopalan syndrome. See under *syndrome.*

Goppert's (gop'ertz) **sign; syndrome.** See under the nouns.

Gorlin-Chaudhry-Moss syndrome. See under *syndrome.*

Göthlin's theory (guht'linz). See under *theory.*

Gougerot-Sjögren syndrome (gu-zher-o'-sye'gren). Sjögren's syndrome.

Gould's (gūldz) **chart; sign.** See under the nouns.

Gower's symptom (gow'erz). See under *symptom.*

Gower-Paton-Kennedy syndrome (gow'er-pat'en-ken'eh-de). Kennedy's syndrome.

GPOA. See *Guild of Prescription Opticians of America.*

gradation, Green's (gra-da'shun). A method for scaling the sizes of visual acuity test letters. Green proposed a series of 24 values bearing a constant ratio of 0.7937.

Gradenigo's syndrome (grah-den-e'-gōz). See under *syndrome.*

grades of fusion. See under *fusion.*

gradient. 1. The amount of change in phoria associated with a change of 1.0 D of lens power at a given target distance; hence, a measure of the AC/A ratio. The routine clinical test is usually made at 40 cm with the addition of 1.0 D of convex lens power. 2. A measurable, uniform change in rate or magnitude.

contrast g. The rate of change of illumination in the transition zone of a contrast border, a sharp border having a high gradient and a blurred border having a low gradient.

g. filter. See under *filter.*

intensity g. A uniform variation of light intensity or luminance over a surface.

g. test. See under *test.*

Gradle (gra'dl) **test; tonometer.** See under the nouns.

von Graefe's (fon gra'fēz) **disease; ophthalmoplegia; phenomenon; reaction; reflex; sign; spot; test; theory.** See under the nouns.

graft, corneal. Donor corneal tissue used in keratoplasty to replace removed opaque or diseased corneal tissue.

mushroom c.g. A mushroom-shaped corneal graft used in combined lamellar and penetrating keratoplasty, in which the superficial layers extend over most of the cornea, and the pedicle, which includes the posterior layers, is fitted into the central perforation.

Granit's theory (grah-nētz'). See under *theory.*

Granit-Harper law (grah-nēt'-hahr'-per). See under *law.*

granule (grā'nūl). A small grain or particle.

cone g. The nucleus within the cell body of a cone cell, located in the outer nuclear layer of the retina and staining differently than a rod granule.

rod g. A round, densely staining portion of the rod cell, composed of a nucleus surrounded by an attenuated layer of protoplasm, located in the outer nuclear layer of the retina, and attached on either side to a rod fiber.

granuloma (gran"u-lo'mah). A nodule or neoplasm consisting essentially of granulation tissue, occurring as a result of localized inflammation.

g. of the iris. A localized proliferation, within the iris, of inflammatory tissue containing lymphocytes. It is stimulated by the presence of a chronic irritative or infective agent such as an inorganic foreign body, tuberculosis, syphilis, actinomycosis, leprosy, or an attenuated form of pyogenic organism.

subconjunctival g. A firm, reddish, nonedematous, fleshy protrusion of the conjunctiva, forming a flat or rounded nodular mass 3.1 mm to 12.7 mm in extent, which may interfere with the closure of the eyelids.

Grassmann's laws (gras'manz). See under *law*.

Gratama's tubes (grah-tah'maz). See under *tube*.

graticule (grat'ih-kūl). A very small, transparent scale, gratelike pattern, or system of lines in the front focal plane of the eyepiece of an optical instrument, for direct observation of the apparent image size or position in the field of view. In binocular instruments, the two graticules may be designed to produce a stereo or distance scale for measuring object distance, as in range finding. Syn., *cross-hairs; reticle; reticule.*

Linksz g. A target used in conjunction with the Projectoscope for the detection and measurement of eccentric fixation, consisting of an open center, four-pointed, star-shaped pattern surrounded by two concentric circles subtending angles of three and five degrees. The star pattern is fixated, and the location of the shadows of it and the surrounding circles on the fundus, in reference to the foveal center, indicates the character of the fixation. (See Fig. 21.)

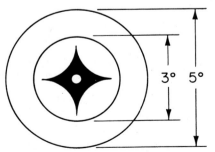

Fig. 21 Linksz star graticule used in the Projectoscope. (From J. R. Griffin, *Binocular Anomalies.* Chicago: Professional Press, 1976)

grating (grāt'ing). A lattice work of parallel bars or crossbars.

Arden g's. A set of seven plates each containing sinusoidal luminance grating patterns of varying contrast and fixed spatial frequency, as measured by the number of grating periods, or cycles, per degree of visual angle which are used for clinical testing of contrast sensitivity sometimes reduced in certain ocular disturbances though visual acuity is unaffected.

diffraction g. A system of close, equidistant and parallel grooves, slits, lines, or bars, such as lines ruled on a polished surface, used for producing spectra by diffraction. **amplitude d.g.** A diffraction grating which modulates the amplitude across the emergent wavefront leaving the phase essentially unchanged; usually one composed of alternate clear and opaque strips. **concave d.g.** A reflecting diffraction grating, ruled on a concave, spherical, metallic surface, which diffracts and focuses light simultaneously without auxiliary lenses. **echelette d.g.** A diffraction grating in which the grooves are cut with one side very steep and the other inclined at a small angle to the surface of the grating, so that most of the reflected light will go to the spectrum lying in the direction in which the light is reflected from the less inclined sides of the grooves, or most of the transmitted light will go to the spectrum lying in the direction in which the light is refracted by the prismatic effect of the grooves. **echelle d.g.** A type of diffraction grating having a facet width, usually of several hundred microns, between that of the few microns of a narrowgrooved diffraction grating and the thousands of microns of an echelon diffraction grating. **echelon d.g.** A diffraction grating of high resolving power, devised by Michelson, consisting of rectangular planeparallel plates of constant thickness stacked together with a constant offset of the edges, resembling a flight of stairs, each step forming a line of the grating. **filter d.g.** A plane grating blazed for the wavelength of the unwanted radiation, used as a reflectance filter, particularly in the far infrared. **Fraunhofer's d.g.** A diffraction grating consisting of regularly spaced, silver wires wound around two parallel screws. **phase d.g.** A diffraction grating which modulates the phase across the emergent wavefront, leaving the amplitude essentially unchanged; usually one composed of grooves. Most diffraction gratings are of this type. **piezoquartz d.g.** A quartz plate between two condenser plates which, when in an alternating electrical field, varies the index of refraction of the quartz differentially so that light transmitted parallel to the plates is retarded differentially and emerges to produce phase difference diffraction spectra. **plane d.g.** A diffraction grating that is ruled on a plane-parallel transmitting medium or on a plane-refracting surface. **reflection d.g.** A diffraction grating which diffracts light by reflection from a ruled, polished surface. **replica d.g.** A diffraction grating produced by making a cast of celluloid, collodion, etc., of a grating ruled on glass or metal. This cast is mounted on or between glass for protection. **Rowland's d.g.** The original concave diffraction grating. **transmission d.g.** A grating which diffracts light by transmission through a system of slits.

Foucault g. Foucault chart.

sinusoidal g. A grating target or pattern, usually black and white, in which the variations in luminous intensity across the grating lines conform to a sine wave function.

visual acuity g. 1. A diffraction grating producing bands of variable separation for measuring visual acuity. 2. A system of parallel lines or bars which can be presented to the eyes with variable separation or at different distances, in continuous motion perpendicular to the lines of sight, to induce optokinetic nystagmus. The moving pattern induces nystagmus as long as the lines are visually resolved. **Ives's v.a.g.** An apparatus consisting essentially of two transilluminated line gratings, which are rotated oppositively about a common axis corresponding to the line of sight of the viewing eye, to produce, when viewed from a distance in excess of that permitting resolution of the component gratings, a pattern of wide parallel lines of covarying width and separation; used for measuring visual acuity.

Gratiolet's (grah″te-o-lāz′) **fibers; optic radiations.** See under the nouns.

Graux ocular palsy (grawz). Féréol-Graux ocular palsy.

Graux-Féréol (graw-fa-ra-ōl) **ophthalmoplegia; paralysis.** Féréol-Graux ocular palsy.

Graves's disease (grāv-ez). See under *disease.*

gray. Any one of the series of colors said to be achromatic or without hue, ranging from white to black.

cool g. 1. A truly achromatic, neutral gray. 2. A neutral gray with a slight trace of green or blue.

cortical g. A median gray whose name is derived from the theory that gray is a primary color process due to activity in the cerebral cortex in the absence of retinal stimulation.

Hering g's. A set of fifty neutral gray papers ranging in lightness from extreme white to extreme black, in steps of equal, just noticeable difference units.

idioretinal g. The gray perceived by the dark-adapted eye in the total absence of light.

median g. A gray of lightness perceived as midway between the extremes of black and white.

retinal g. The gray perceived in the absence of visual stimulation, attributed to the normal, continuous, and spontaneous neuronal activity.

Gray oral reading test. See under *test.*

graybody. A thermal source of radiant energy or temperature radiation whose radiant flux at all wavelengths is less than that of a blackbody at the same temperature by a constant ratio. No known thermal source emits radiant flux in this manner throughout the ultraviolet, visible, and infrared regions. However, in the visible region, a carbon filament does so at a very nearly constant ratio and may be considered a practical approximation of a graybody. Syn., *incomplete radiator; nonselective radiator.*

grayout. Loss of peripheral vision due to positive gravitational acceleration, attributed to restriction of blood supply to the eye. It occurs at 4.1 ± 0.7 g to unprotected subjects seated upright. Cf. *blackout.*

Greeff's vesicles (grēfs). See under *vesicle.*

Greeley's conjunctivitis (gre′lēz). Acute follicular conjunctivitis of Beal. See under *conjunctivitis.*

green. 1. The hue attribute of visual sensations typically evoked by stimulation of the normal human eye with radiation of wavelengths approximately 515 mμ. 2. Any hue predominantly similar to that of a typical green. 3. One of the psychologically unique colors. 4. The complement of red-purple (magenta).

visual g. A green-colored pigment found in the retinal rod cells of frogs and some reptiles, having properties similar to those of visual purple in humans.

Green's chart. See under *chart.*

Greenough microscope (grēn'o). See under *microscope.*

green-weakness. Deuteranomaly.

Gregg syndrome. Rubella syndrome. See under *syndrome.*

Greig's (grēgz) **hypertelorism; syndrome.** See under the nouns.

grid. A network or pattern of perpendicularly intersecting lines.

Amsler g's. Amsler charts.

Haussmann multiple g. A pair of transilluminated, differentially rotatable, multiple stenopaic slits mounted one in front of the other so as to produce a grid pattern of variable dimensions according to the angle between the slits. It is used for testing subnormal visual acuity.

Hermann g. A grid of perpendicularly crossed white stripes in a black field, providing the qualitative appearance of darkened areas at the intersections, a contrast effect.

Javal's g. A form of bar reader consisting of five equally spaced parallel bars coupled together by two perpendicular bars and having a handle and two supporting legs.

Griffith flaw (grif'ith). See under *flaw.*

Griffith's sign (grif'iths). See under *sign.*

Grignolo syndrome. Erythema exudativum multiforme.

grinding, multiple. A lens-grinding procedure in which more than one lens is surfaced in the same operation.

Groenouw's corneal dystrophy (gru'nōz). See under *dystrophy, corneal.*

Grolman Fitting System. See under *system.*

Grönblad-Strandberg syndrome (grēn'blat-strand'berg). See under *syndrome.*

groove. A shallow furrow, channel, or linear depression. See also *fissure; sulcus.*

Blessig's g. The indentation of the embryonic and fetal eye, between the adult-forming retina and the blind part of the retina, which helps form the inner part of the ciliary body and iris; hence, the groove which becomes toward the ora serrata.

infraorbital g. A groove beneath the periorbita in the floor of the orbit, commencing at the inferior orbital fissure and extending anteriorly toward the infraorbital margin. It becomes roofed over to form the infraorbital canal, which dips beneath the margin to emerge anteriorly as the infraorbital foramen, and contains the infraorbital vein and artery. Syn., *infraorbital sulcus.*

lacrimal g. 1. The groove in the medial wall of the superior maxilla which forms a part of the nasolacrimal canal. 2. The fossa for the lacrimal sac.

Maddox g. A lens, named after E. E. Maddox, used in measuring heterophoria and heterotropia, and consisting of a long, narrow, concave, cylindrical groove which, when held in front of the eye, distorts a relatively distant light source into a long streak perpendicular to the axis of the groove.

optic g. A horizontal sulcus on the sphenoid bone, anterior to the pituitary fossa or sella turcica, leading from the regions of the paired optic canals. In about 5% of skulls, the optic chiasm rests in this groove, but in most it is posterior to it.

Stieda's g's. A series of shallow grooves separated by Stieda's plateaus and located in the palpebral conjunctiva, between the tarsus and the fornix.

supraorbital g. One of a few linear depressions on the frontal bone in the eyebrow region that leads into the supraorbital notch or foramen and to the notch or foramen of Arnold, if present. It contains a branch of a supraorbital nerve of a blood vessel.

zygomatic g. A groove on the lateral wall of the orbit which extends from the inferior orbital fissure to the zygomatic foramen and houses the zygomatic nerve and vessels.

Grotthus' law (grot'hus). Draper's law.

ground. 1. The relatively unstructured part of a figure-ground field. See also *background.* 2. The fundus, or the interior of the eye, as seen through the ophthalmoscope.

Groupement des Opticiens du Marché Commun. A committee of ophthalmic opticians, one from each member country of the European Economic Community (EEC), serving to represent the ophthalmic opticians and optometrists of their respective countries in negotiations with the EEC toward the formulation of proposals for implementing EEC directives.

Grow chart (gro). See under *chart.*

Gruber syndrome (groo'ber). Splanchnocystic dysencephaly. See under *dysencephaly*.

Gruner-Bertolotti syndrome. See under *syndrome*.

Grünert's spur (grēn'ertz). See under *spur*.

guard. The part of a spectacle frame or mounting designed to support the spectacles by resting against either side of the nose; a nose pad.

   g. arm. See under *arm*.

   offset g. A guard mounted behind the spectacle lens plane to position the spectacle frame or mounting farther away from the eye than usual.

Gubler's paralysis (goob'lerz). Millard-Gubler syndrome.

von Gudden's (fon gūd'enz) **commissure; posterior accessory optic tract; transverse peduncular tract.** See under the nouns.

Guiat's sign. See under *sign*.

Guibor (gwe'bōr) **chart; test.** See under the nouns.

Guild of Prescription Opticians of America. An association of independent dispensing opticians organized to serve the general vocational, educational, and representational objectives of the membership.

Guillery chart (ge'yur-e). See under *chart*.

Guist's preretinal edema (gīstz). Central angiospastic retinopathy.

Guist's sign (gīstz). See under *sign*.

Gullstrand's (gul'strandz) **reduced eye; schematic eye; law.** See under the nouns.

Gunn's (gunz) **dots; phenomenon; sign; syndrome.** See under the nouns.

Guth chart. See under *chart*.

Guy's (gīz) **color vision test.** See under *test*.

Guyton optometer (gi'tun). See under *optometer*.

gyrospasm (ji'ro-spazm). Spasmus nutans.

gyrus (ji'rus). A convoluted ridge between the sulci, or grooves, on the surface of the cerebral hemisphere.

   angular g. A sharply bent, cortical convolution about the posterior end of the superior temporal sulcus in the parietal lobe, included in visual associational Brodmann's area 19 and visual language areas.

   lingual g. The medial portion of the occipital lobe, below the calcarine fissure, containing the lower portions of the area striata and the visual associational areas.

H

H. 1. Abbreviation for *hypermetropia*. 2. Symbol for *irradiance*.

Haab's (hahbz) **degeneration; corneal dystrophy; band opacity; pupillometer; pupillary reflex; sign; striae.** See under the nouns.

de Haan's law (duh hahnz). See under *law*.

Haenel's sign (ha'nelz). See under *sign*.

Hague lamp (hāg). See under *lamp*.

Haidinger's (hi'ding-erz) **bands; brushes; fringes.** See under the nouns.

Haig's law. See under *law*.

hairs, von Frey. Hairs of various caliber and length used by von Frey to determine corneal sensitivity.

Haitz charts (hītz). See under *chart*.

halation (ha-la'shun). A spreading of light beyond its proper boundaries, such as may be reflected from the inner layers of the retina beyond the image border proper, and hence considered to be a cause of irradiation.

Halberg (hahl'burg) **clips; tonometer.** See under the nouns.

Hale telescope. See under *telescope*.

half eyes. A pair of glasses having lenses customarily for only the lower half of the field of view.

half-shade. A polarizing device, inserted in front of the polarizer of a polarimeter, which causes the transmitted light to vibrate in slightly different directions in the two halves of the sharply divided field of view. It is used to increase the accuracy of settings.

Hall's test (hawlz). See under *test*.

Hallauer glass (hal'ow-er). See under *glass*.

Halldén's (hawl-dānz') **method; test.** See under the nouns.

Haller's (hal'erz) **circle; layer; ratio; tunic.** See under the nouns.

Hallermann-Streif syndrome (hal'-er-man-strīf). Mandibulo-oculo-facial dysmorphia.

Hallgren syndrome (hawl'gren). See under *syndrome*.

hallucination, visual (hah-lu"sih-na'shun). Visual perception in the absence of a correlated physical stimulus. Cf. *illusion*.

    autoscopic v.h. A visual hallucination in which one has a vision of his own organs or body parts. See also *autoscopy def. 3*.

    cinematographic v.h. A formed visual hallucination consisting of a series of complex and integrated scenes.

    formed v.h. A visual hallucination consisting of a formed figure or scene.

    negative v.h. A form of functional blindness during which there is an inability to perceive objects in the visual field.

    positive v.h. A visual hallucination in which the subject "sees" an object where none exists, as distinguished from negative visual hallucination.

    unformed v.h. A visual hallucination without definite shape or form, as one merely of light or color.

hallucinosis, peduncular. A psychotic visual hallucination in which pleasant, highly colored, lilliputian figures are seen; said to be a diagnostic sign of suprapituitary tumor, but it may also occur under other conditions, particularly in senility.

halo. An annular flare of light surrounding a luminous body or image, occurring in optical imagery in varicolored patterns or as a brightness gradient, as a result of aberrations, internal reflections, diffraction, or scattering.

circumpapillary glaucomatous h. A ring of atrophy surrounding the optic disk in the later stages of simple glaucoma following degenerative change of the pigment epithelium, the pigment migrating into the retina and allowing the sclera to be seen through the atrophic ring.

glaucomatous h. 1. Entoptically visible colored rings around lights, due to diffraction of droplets of fluid in the corneal epithelium in the presence of corneal edema, in glaucoma. 2. A white, halo-like ring of exposed sclera around the optic disk, due to the degeneration and migration of the retinal pigment epithelium, in glaucoma.

lenticular h. Entoptically visible colored rings around a bright light source caused by the action of the radial fibers of the crystalline lens as a diffraction grating.

macular h. A glittering ring of reflected light sometimes seen around the macula during ophthalmoscopy.

senile peripapillary h. Senile circumpapillary choroidal atrophy.

halometer (ha-lom'eh-ter). An instrument for measuring ocular halos.

halometry (ha-lom'eh-tre). The measurement of halos.

Halsey Scope. An instrument utilizing the principle of moiré fringes used to determine the radii of curvatures of contact lenses.

Hamaker's satellite (ha'māk-erz). Second positive afterimage.

Hamilton slide (ham'il-tun). See under *slide.*

hamulus (ham'u-lus). 1. The inferior portion of the posterior lacrimal crest of the lacrimal bone which articulates with the maxillary bone at the superior end of the nasolacrimal canal. 2. Any hooked-shaped bony process, as on the pterygoid process of the sphenoid bone.

Hand's (handz) **disease; syndrome.** See under the nouns.

hand-eye coordination. See under *coordination.*

Hand-Eye Co-ordinator, Leavell. A Brewster type stereoscope with a clipboard attachment to hold targets for tracing.

Hanhart syndrome (han'hahrt). See under *syndrome.*

Hannover's canal (han'o-verz). See under *canal.*

haplopia (hap-lo'pe-ah). Single binocular vision, as opposed to binocular diplopia.

homolocal h. Normal single binocular vision in which the right and left ocular images of the same object are projected to the same spatial position. Cf. *heterotopic diplopia* and *homotopic diplopia.*

haploscope (hap'lo-skōp). An instrument for presenting separate fields of view to the two eyes so that they may be seen as one continuous, superimposed, integrated, or fused field, and hence useful for measuring or stimulating various binocular functions. Many specially designed experimental and clinical models provide for elaborate controls of the accommodation, convergence, and fusion stimuli, the color, brightness, and size of target and field, and stereo-producing disparity.

Hering h. A mirror haploscope designed by Hering and having the feature that the two fields of view are rotatable about separate vertical axes corresponding to the centers of rotation of the subject's eyes.

mirror h. A haploscope using mirrors to separate or displace the fields of view of the two eyes.

phase-difference h. A haploscope utilizing a pair of very rapidly rotating and alternately synchronized opaque sectored disks, one in front of each of the two eyes, and two additional similarly synchronized sectored disks to interrupt alternately the separate right and left eye views, thus providing independent but apparently continuous views to the two eyes.

haploscopic (hap-lo-skop'ik). Pertaining to or of a haploscope.

haptic. 1. The portion of a scleral contact lens which rests on the scleral conjunctiva; scleral flange. 2. Pertaining to a tactile-kinesthetic response, e.g., in writing, the arm moves while the fingers perceive the sensation of the pen or pencil.

Harada's (hah-rahd'az) **disease; syndrome.** See under the nouns.

Harder's gland (hahr'derz). See under *gland.*

Hardy-Rand-Rittler charts; plates; test. See under the nouns.

hare's eye (härz i). Lagophthalmus.

Harlan's test (hahr'lanz). See under *test.*

Harman's test (hahr'manz). See under *test.*

Harms's method. See under *method.*

Harrington tonometer (har'ing-tun). See under *tonometer.*

Harrington-Flocks (har'ing-tun-floks) **visual field screener; test.** See under the nouns.

Harris' syndrome; test; theory. See under the nouns.

Harting-Dove prism (hahrt'ing-duv). See under *prism.*

Hartline's stereoscope (hahrt'līnz). See under *stereoscope.*

Hartmann (hahrt'mahn) **screen; test.** See under the nouns.

Hartridge's theory (hahrt'rijz). See under *theory.*

Hasner's (hahs'nerz) **fold; theory; valve.** See under the nouns.

Hassall-Henle (has'al-hen'le) **bodies; warts.** See under the nouns.

Haussmann multiple grid (haus'-mahn). See under *grid.*

Hawkins trifocal lens (haw'kinz). See under *lens, trifocal.*

haze. 1. The spatial attribute of smokiness or dustiness which interferes, or seems to interfere, with clear vision. 2. A meteorological classification of atmospheric visibility conditions between thin fog and clear. 3. As applied to nearly perfect transparencies, especially plastics, the ratio of diffuse to total transmittance of a beam of light.

head. 1. The anterior or upper extremity of the animal body containing the brains, eyes, ears, nose, and mouth. 2. The front or foremost part of an object. 3. A part or attachment of an instrument or apparatus that performs a chief function.

    optic nerve h. Optic disk.

    photometer h. The portion of a photometer which presents to the eye the two surfaces between which a comparison of brightness is to be made. Syn., *photoped.*

    h. rotation. A deviation in position of the head about a vertical axis of reference and away from a straightforward position, especially as a clinical symptom. Cf. *head tilt; shoulder tipping.* Syn., *face turn; head turn.*

    schlieren h. The lens and/or mirror system in the schlieren system which focuses the light beam "through" the schlieren field and for which the first and second knife edges are approximately conjugate foci.

    h. tilt. 1. A deviation of the head from its upright position, especially as a clinical symptom. 2. A forward or a backward tilt of the head, as distinguished from *shoulder tipping.* Syn., *face tilt.*

    h. turn. Head rotation.

headache, ocular. A headache presumed to result from impaired function or organic disease of ocular structures or excessive use of the eyes.

Health Maintenance Organization. Any group of health professionals working together to provide a prepaid, comprehensive health care program, at a preset fee, for subscribing members.

hearing, color. A type of synesthesia in which certain sounds induce characteristic color sensations. Syn., *pseudochromesthesia.*

Hebra's disease (he'brahs). Erythema exudativum multiforme.

Hecht's theory (hekts). See under *theory.*

Hecht-Schlaer adaptometer. See under *adaptometer.*

Heerfordt's (hār'forts) **disease; syndrome.** See under the nouns.

hefilcon A. The nonproprietary name of a co-polymer of which contact lenses are made.

Heidenhain syndrome (hi'den-hīn). See under *syndrome.*

height, apparent. The angular subtense of an object at a given distance, especially at a distance from which viewed or photographed.

van der Heijde Biometer; formula. See under the nouns.

heiligenschein (hīl-ig'en-shīn). Halo; especially a diffuse white ring surrounding the shadow of a person's head cast on a dew-covered lawn by the sun. (In German, Heiligenschein.)

Heine (hīn'e) **contact lens; retraction.** See under the nouns.

Heinrich's effect (hīn'richz). See under *effect.*

helcoma (hel-ko'mah). A corneal ulcer.

heliometer (he"le-om'eh-ter). A split-lens telescope with adjustable image separation for measuring angular distances between stars or the diameter of the sun.

heliophobe (he'le-o-fōb). One who is neurotically afraid of being exposed to sunlight.

heliophobia (he"le-o-fo'be-ah). The neurotic fear of exposure to sunlight.

helioscope (he'le-o-skōp). An instrument, for example a telescope, with intensity reducing features to prevent injury to the eye when viewing the sun.

heliostat. A mirror automatically rotated in synchrony with the earth's movements so that sunlight is reflected constantly in a chosen direction.

Helmholtz' (helm'hōltz) **axes; chessboard; color circle; indicator; law; floating hearts phenomenon; stereogram; color table; ring target; telestereoscope; test; theories; color triangle.** See under the nouns.

Helmholtz-Kohlrausch effect (helm'hōltz-kōl'rowsh). See under *effect.*

Helson-Judd effect (hel'sun-jud). See under *effect.*

HEMA. Hydroxyethylmethacrylate.

hemachromatosis corneae (he"mah-kro-mah-to'sis kōr'ne-e, hem"ah-). Bloodstaining of the cornea.

hemangioblastosis retinae (he-man"-je-o-blas-to'sis ret'in-e). Von Hippel's disease.

hemangioma (he-man"je-o'mah). A tumor derived from blood vessels, usually as the result of aberrant development, but occasionally post-traumatic, ordinarily benign, and histologically consisting of endothelial-lined spaces containing red blood corpuscles, fibrinous coagula, or hyaline detritus. The stroma is cellular or fibrous and is richly vascular. There may be incorporation of other cellular elements, dependent upon the site of the tumor.

hemangiomatosis, von Hippel's (he-man"je-o-mah-to'sis). Von Hippel's disease.

hematoma, ocular (he"mah-to'mah). A tumorlike swelling due to sizable hemorrhage into the tissues of the eye.

hemeralope (hem'er-ah-lōp). One affected with hemeralopia.

hemeralopia (hem"er-ah-lo'pe-ah). A term used inconsistently to mean either *night blindness* or *day blindness;* synonymous or antonymous with *nyctalopia.*

hemiablepsia (hem"e-ah-blep'se-ah). Hemianopsia.

hemiachromatopsia (hem"e-ak-ro-mah-top'se-ah). Color blindness in one half of the visual field of one eye or of both eyes.

hemiakinesia, pupillary (hem"e-ah-kih-ne'se-ah). Constriction of the pupil in response to light stimulation of one half of the retina, and no pupillary response to light stimulation of the other half of the retina. Syn., *hemianopic pupillary paralysis.*

hemiamaurosis (hem"e-am"aw-ro'sis). Hemianopsia.

hemiamblyopia (hem"e-am"ble-o'pe-ah). Reduced vision in one half of the visual field of one or both eyes.

hemianopia (hem"e-an-o'pe-ah). Hemianopsia.

hemianopic (hem"e-an-op'ik). Pertaining to, or affected with, hemianopsia.

hemianopic pupillary paralysis. Pupillary hemiakinesia.

hemianopic pupillary reflex. See under *reflex.*

◆

HEMIANOPSIA

hemianopsia (hem"e-an-op'se-ah). Blindness in one half of the visual field of one or both eyes. Syn., *hemiablepsia; hemiamaurosis; hemianopia; hemiscotosis.* Cf. *hemiopia.*

absolute h. Hemianopsia in which the affected field is totally blind to all visual stimuli.

altitudinal h. Hemianopsia in either the upper or the lower half of the visual field of one or both eyes. Syn., *horizontal hemianopsia.* **crossed a.h.** Bilateral hemianopsia involving the upper half of the visual field of one eye and the lower half of the visual field of the other. **symmetrical a.h.** Bilateral hemianopsia involving either both upper halves or both lower halves of the visual fields.

bilateral h. Hemianopsia involving the visual fields of both eyes. Syn., *binocular hemianopsia.*

binasal h. Bilateral hemianopsia involving the nasal halves of the visual fields of both eyes. **crossed quadrant b.h.** Crossed binasal quadrantanopsia.

binocular h. Bilateral hemianopsia.

bitemporal h. Bilateral hemianopsia involving the temporal halves of the visual fields of both eyes. **crossed**

quadrant b.h. Crossed bitemporal quadrantanopsia.

h. bitemporalis fugax. Transient bitemporal hemianopsia sometimes associated with syphilis.

complete h. Hemianopsia involving a full half of the visual field.

congruous h. Homonymous hemianopsia in which the defects in the two visual fields are identical in size, shape, and position, so as to form a single defect of the binocular field.

crossed h. Altitudinal hemianopsia involving the upper half of the visual field of one eye and the lower half of the visual field of the other eye.

heteronymous h. Hemianopsia involving either both nasal halves or both temporal halves of the visual fields.

homonymous h. Hemianopsia involving the nasal half of the visual field of one eye and the temporal half of the visual field of the other eye. **left h.h.** Hemianopsia involving the temporal half of the visual field of the left eye and the nasal half of the visual field of the right eye. **right h.h.** Hemianopsia involving the nasal half of the visual field of the left eye and the temporal half of the visual field of the right eye.

horizontal h. Altitudinal hemianopsia.

incomplete h. Hemianopsia not involving a full half of the visual field.

incongruous h. Hemianopsia in which the defects in the two visual fields differ in size, shape, or position.

lateral h. Vertical hemianopsia.

nonscotomatous h. Hemianopsia in which there is no central scotoma in the early field changes.

quadrantic h. Quadrantanopsia.

relative h. 1. Hemianopsia involving a loss of vision for form or color but not for light. 2. Hemianopsia present only when stimuli are presented simultaneously to both halves of the visual field, as may occur following injury or disease to one visual sensory cortical area. See also *Oppenheim's test.*

scotomatous h. Hemianopsia in which a central scotoma is one of the early field changes.

transient h. Hemianopsia of temporary duration, due to angiospasm, hemorrhage, edema, etc.

unilateral h. Hemianopsia affecting the visual field of only one eye.

vertical h. Hemianopsia involving the lateral (nasal or temporal) half of the visual field of one or both eyes. Syn., *lateral hemianopsia.*

◆

hemianoptic (hem″e-an-op′tik). Pertaining to or affected with hemianopsia.

hemichromatopsia (hem″e-kro″mah-top′se-ah). Hemiachromatopsia.

hemicrania (hem-e-kra′ne-ah). An ache or a pain in one side of the head, as in migraine.

hemidyschromatopsia (hem″e-dis-kro-mah-top′se-ah). Dyschromatopsia in one half of the visual field of one or both eyes.

hemi-epicanthus (hem″e-ep-ih-kan′-thus). The oblique, median eye fold characteristic of Mongolian races. Syn., *Mongoloid fold.*

hemikinesimeter (hem″e-kin″e-sim′eh-ter). An instrument for detecting a hemianoptic pupillary reflex consisting essentially of a chin and forehead rest and two light sources to emit pencils of light of equal intensity into the eye from two different angles.

hemimacropsia (hem″e-mah-krop′se-ah). Macropsia in one half of the visual field.

hemimicropsia (hem″e-mi-krop′se-ah). Micropsia in one half of the visual field.

hemiopalgia (hem″e-op-al′je-ah). An ache or a pain in one side of the head and in one eye.

hemiopia (hem-e-o′pe-ah). Vision in only one half of the visual field of one or both eyes. Cf. *hemianopsia.*

hemiopic (hem-e-op′ik). Pertaining to, or affected with, hemiopia.

hemiplegia alternans facialis (hem″-e-ple′je-ah awl′ter-nans fa″she-al′is). Millard-Gubler syndrome.

hemiscotosis (hem″e-sko-to′sis). Hemianopsia.

hemophthalmia (he-mof-thal′me-ah). A hemorrhage within the eye.

hemophthalmitis, chronic. Recurrent hemorrhages from the anterior segment of the uvea as may occur in purpura and hemophilia, or subsequent to injury especially in the elderly. The hyphema stratifies, the newer layers being of brighter red, with uveitis and granulomatous inflammation being the typical sequelae.

hemophthalmos (he-mof-thal′mos). Hemophthalmia.

hemorrhage (hem'or-ij). An extravasation of blood from the vessels.

flame-shaped h. A radially striated hemorrhage in the inner layers of the retina, especially in the nerve fiber layer.

petechial h. A minute, punctate extravasation of blood.

preretinal h. A large extravasation of blood from the retinal vessels between the vitreous and the retina, characteristically shaped like a *D* with the straight edge or fluid level uppermost. Syn., *subhyaloid hemorrhage.*

subhyaloid h. Preretinal hemorrhage.

hemosiderosis bulbi (he"mo-sid-eh-ro'sis bul'bi). Deposits of iron-staining compounds, derived from the hemoglobin of the blood, in the ocular tissues following hemorrhage.

Henderson's theory (hen'der-sonz). See under *theory.*

Henkes electroretinography lens (henk'ēz). See under *lens.*

Henle's (hen'lēz) **bodies; cytoblasts; fibers; glands; layer; membrane; notch; stratum nerveum; warts.** See under the nouns.

Hennebert's syndrome (en-barz'). See under *syndrome.*

Henschen's theory (hen'shenz). See under *theory.*

Hensen-Völckers experiment (hen'sen-vel'kerz). See under *experiment.*

Hensy's sign (hen'sēz). Orbicularis sign. See under *sign.*

heptachromia (hep-tah-kro'me-ah). Normal color vision; perception of the total spectral scale of seven colors.

heptachromic (hep-tah-kro'mik). Having heptachromia, hence having normal color vision.

herapathite (her'ah-path"īt). A synthetic, dichroic, crystalline material which transmits one linearly polarized beam and absorbs the other; discovered by and named after W. B. Herapath, and served as the basis for the original Polaroid material.

Herbert's (her'berts) **pits; rosettes.** See under the nouns.

Hering's (her'ingz) **afterimage; color circle; color valence curves; valence diagram; experiment; figure; grays; haploscope; illusion; law; phenomenon; tests; theories; window.** See under the nouns.

Hering-Hillebrand (her'ing-hil'eh-brand) **deviation; horopter; phenomenon.** See under the nouns.

Hermann's grid (her'mahnz). See under *grid.*

hernia, iris (her'ne-ah). Protrusion of the iris through a corneal incision or wound, following surgery or trauma. Syn., *prolapse of the iris.*

herpes (her'pēz). An inflammatory disease of the skin or mucous membrane characterized by the formation of clusters of small vesicles.

h. corneae. Herpetic keratitis.

h. facialis. Herpes simplex of the face.

h. febrilis. See *herpes simplex.*

h. iridis. Herpetic iritis.

h. ophthalmicus. Herpes zoster ophthalmicus.

h. simplex. A superficial, epithelial, virus infection characterized by the presence of groups of small vesicles. It typically occurs on the borders of the lips, nostrils, or genitals and may occur on the eyelids, conjunctiva, cornea, or iris. See also *herpetic iritis; herpetic keratitis.*

h. zoster ophthalmicus, epidemic. A virus infection of the Gasserian ganglion and its nerve branches, characterized by discrete areas of vesiculation of the epithelium of the forehead, the nose, the eyelids, and the cornea, together with subepithelial infiltration. It is limited to one half of the face, with a sharp demarcation in the midline of the forehead and nose.

h. zoster ophthalmicus, symptomatic. A disease of the Gasserian ganglion and its nerve branches secondary to some infective, traumatic, or neoplastic disturbance, whose manifestations are identical to epidemic herpes zoster ophthalmicus.

von Herrenschwand syndrome. Sympathetic heterochromia.

Herrick syndrome (her'ik). Sickle-cell disease. See under *disease.*

Hersh palpebral traction contact lens (hursh). See under *lens, contact.*

Herschel prism (hur'shel). See under *prism.*

Hertel's chart: plates; test. See under the nouns.

de Hertogh's sign (dē-her'togz). See under *sign.*

Hertwig-Magendie (hert'vig-mah-zhan'de) **sign; syndrome.** Magendie-Hertwig sign. See under *sign*.

hertz. A unit of frequency equal to one cycle per second.

hesperanopia (hes"per-an-o'pe-ah). Night blindness.

Hess's (hes'ez) **afterimage; screen; theory.** See under the nouns.

Hess-Lancaster test (hes-lan'kas-ter). See under *test*.

Hesse's (hes'ēz) **organs; test.** See under the nouns.

heterocentric (het"er-o-sen'trik). Pertaining to light rays that do not meet at a common focal point; the opposite of *homocentric*.

heteroception (het"er-o-sep'shun). Proprioception said to be related to the heterophoria overcome during binocular fixation. (Chavasse; Lyle)

heterochromatic (het"er-o-kro-mat'ik). Pertaining to or having more than one color or hue.

heterochromatosis (het"er-o-kro-mahto'sis). Heterochromia.

heterochromia (het"er-o-kro'me-ah). A difference in the coloration of the parts of a structure or between two structures which are normally of the same coloration, as the iris or the irides. Syn., *heterochromatosis*.

    complicated h. A slow, chronic atrophy and depigmentation of the iris without associated inflammation or pain. The affected iris becomes thin, transparent, lighter in color than the other, and the usual iris markings are absent. It is frequently accompanied by cataract, corneal precipitates, vitreous opacities, and glaucoma. Syn., *heterochromic cyclitis of Fuchs*.

    h. of Fuchs. Complicated heterochromia.

    hyperchromic h. Inverse heterochromia.

    inverse h. Slow, chronic pigmentation of the iris resulting from trauma to the iris, or a resulting iritis, so that the iris becomes darker than its fellow although appearing otherwise normal. Syn., *hyperchromic heterochromia*.

    h. iridis. A diversity of color in different parts of the same iris. Syn., *chromheteropia*.

    h. iridum. A difference in the color of the two irides.

    neurogenic h. Changes in the color of the iris due to a lesion, paralytic or irritative, of the sympathetic nervous system.

    partial h. A coloration in one sector of the iris different from that in the remaining portions.

    simple h. Heterochromia characterized by difference in color between the two irides, or by zones of different color in one iris, and not attributed to pathology.

    sympathetic h. Heterochromia due to dysfunction of the sympathetic nerves which affect development of the iris and its pigment.

heterochromous (het"er-o-kro'mus). Pertaining to or affected with heterochromia.

heterokeratoplasty (het"er-o-ker'-ah-to-plas-te). The transplantation of corneal tissue from an animal to a human eye, or from one type of animal to another.

heterometropia (het"er-o-meh-tro'pe-ah). A condition in which the refractive errors of the two eyes differ. Syn., *anisometropia*.

heteronymous (het"er-on'ih-mus). 1. Pertaining to or designating crossed images of an object seen double, e.g., heteronymous diplopia. 2. Pertaining to or designating asymmetric halves of the visual fields, e.g., both temporal fields or both nasal fields.

heterophoralgia (het"er-o-fo-ral'je-ah). Asthenopia caused by heterophoria.

◆

HETEROPHORIA

heterophoria (het"er-o-fo're-ah). The tendency of the lines of sight to deviate from the relative positions necessary to maintain single binocular vision for a given distance of fixation, this tendency being identified by the occurrence of an actual deviation in the absence of an adequate stimulus to fusion, and occurring in variously designated forms according to the relative direction or orientation of the deviation, *as excyclophoria, incyclophoria, esophoria, exophoria, hyperphoria, hypophoria*.

    absolute h. Heterophoria present after one eye has been occluded for a period of time sufficient to eliminate factors associated with the use of binocular vision.

    accommodational h. Kinetic heterophoria.

    basic h. Heterophoria which is approximately the same at both far and near fixation distances.

    compensated h. The heterophoria demonstrable in the absence of fixation disparity, i.e., through the lenses, prisms, or other optical system which eliminates or neutralizes the manifestation of fixation disparity. Cf. *uncompensated heterophoria.*

decompensated h. Uncompensated heterophoria.

essential h. Heterophoria characterized by its structural, static, and permanent nature and not of accommodative origin. Cf. *symptomatic heterophoria.*

kinetic h. Heterophoria attributed to the reflex effect of accommodation on convergence, e.g., esophoria due to uncorrected hypermetropia. Cf. *neurogenic heterophoria; static heterophoria.* Syn., *accommodational heterophoria.*

neurogenic h. Heterophoria resulting from a faulty central nervous system innervational pattern to, or a mild paretic or spastic condition of, one or more of the extraocular muscles. Cf. *kinetic heterophoria; static heterophoria.*

relative h. 1. Relative exophoria or relative esophoria. 2. Heterophoria expressed in relation to given test conditions and given points of reference for purposes of quantitative specification.

static h. Heterophoria attributed to the anatomical structure of the eyes, orbits, extraocular muscles, and other adnexa. Cf. *kinetic heterophoria; neurogenic heterophoria.*

symptomatic h. Heterophoria characterized by its functional, dynamic, and variable nature. Cf. *essential heterophoria.*

uncompensated h. 1. The heterophoria or that portion of heterophoria which is presumed to induce, or manifest itself as, fixation disparity during sensory fusion. Cf. *compensated heterophoria.* 2. The condition in which a heterophore becomes a heterotrope. Syn., *decompensated heterophoria.*

◆

heterophoric (het″er-o-fo′rik). Pertaining to or affected with heterophoria.

heterophorometer, Bielschowsky's (het″er-o-fo-rom′eh-ter). A phorometer consisting of a fixation grid of vertical red lines with a green arrow above, all seen by one eye, while the other eye sees only the arrow, displaced and black, through a red filter and a dissociating prism.

heterophthalmia (het″er-of-thal′me-ah). A difference in the appearance of

the two eyes, as in heterochromia iridum.

heterophthalmos (het″er-of-thal′mos). Heterophthalmia.

heterophthalmus (het″er-of-thal′mus). Heterophthalmia.

heteropsia (het-er-op′se-ah). Unequal vision in the two eyes.

heteroptics (het-er-op′tiks). Visual hallucinations, illusions, perversions, or distortions.

heterorefraction (het″er-o-re-frak′-shun). The refraction of one's eyes by another person; the opposite of *autorefraction.*

heteroscope (het′er-o-skōp). An amblyoscope.

heterostereoscopy (het″er-o-ster″e-os′ko-pe). The viewing of a stereopsis-inducing pattern so as to perceive essentially the original scene, but not in true dimensional proportions. A type of distortion that may be induced, for example, by viewing a stereogram in a stereoscope different in focal length from that of the camera, by viewing a vectograph directly through Polaroid filters, or by making the lateral separation of the stereocamera lenses effectively different from that of the viewer's interpupillary distance. Cf. *orthostereoscopy.*

heterotopia, macular (het″er-o-to′pe-ah). Displacement of the macula from its normal location, relative to the optic disk, which may be congenital and accompanied by other anomalies, or the result of a pathological process such as the traction of scar formation in retrolental fibroplasia. It is evidenced by an abnormal angle lambda, which may give the appearance of strabismus when none is present.

heterotransplant, corneal (het″er-o-trans′plant). Transplantation of corneal tissue from one species to another. See also *allotransplant; autotransplant; homotransplant.*

heterotrichosis superciliorum (het″-er-o-trik-o′sis su″per-sil′e-ōr-um). Heterochromic eyebrows.

heterotrichous (het-er-ot′rih-kus). Having eyelashes that are irregular in shape, size, or distribution.

heterotropia (het″er-o-tro′pe-ah). Strabismus.

Hetzel (het′zel) **method; technique.** See under *method.*

Heubner's artery (hoyb′nerz). See under *artery.*

hexachromic (hek-sah-kro'mik). Pertaining to an individual who can perceive only six of the seven spectral colors, being unable to differentiate between violet and indigo.

Heyman's law (ha'manz). See under *law*.

Highman chart (hi'man). See under *chart*.

Hilding syndrome (hild'ing). Uveo-arthro-chondral syndrome. See under *syndrome*.

Hillebrand alley (hil'eh-brand). See under *alley*.

Hillebrand-Blumenfeld alleys (hil'-eh-brand-bloo'men-feld). Blumenfeld alleys.

von Hippel's disease (fon hip'elz). See under *disease*.

von Hippel-Lindau disease (fon hip'el-lin'dow). See under *disease*.

hippus (hip'us). Abnormal, rhythmic, irregular contraction and dilatation of the pupils. The oscillations occur within seconds, are of considerable excursion, reaching 2 mm or more, are bilateral, and are independent of illumination, convergence, or psychosensory stimuli.

   respiratory h. Contraction of the pupil during expiration, and dilation during inspiration.

Hirschberg's (hersh'bergz) **method; test.** See under the nouns.

His's marginal layer (his'ez). Marginal layer of the optic cup.

histamine (his'tah-min). An amine containing carbon, hydrogen, and nitrogen, which stimulates gastric secretion, dilates and increases the permeability of capillaries, and acts as a miotic on the eye.

histoplasmosis (his"to-plaz-mo'sis). A disease of the reticuloendothelial system caused by the fungus *Histoplasma capsulatum* and characterized by fever, anemia, and emaciation. Ocular signs include a clear media, disseminated scars around the optic disk due to circumpapillary choroiditis, and a typical pigment ring around the macula with detachment of the overlying sensory retina.

Hitzig's center (hit'zigz). Frontal eye field.

Hl. Abbreviation for *latent hypermetropia*.

Hm. Abbreviation for *manifest hypermetropia*.

HMO. See *Health Maintenance Organization*.

hodoscope. 1. Conoscope. 2. An instrument for path-tracing of high energy particles.

Hoefer effect (höf-er). See under *effect*.

van der Hoeve's (van der hövz) **scotoma; syndrome; theory.** See under the nouns.

van der Hoeve-Halbertsma-Waardenburg syndrome (van der höv hal'berts-mah-ward'en-burg). Waardenburg's syndrome.

Höfler's (hef'lerz) **figure; visual illusion.** See under the nouns.

Hofstetter's formulas (hof'stet-erz). See under formula.

hole in the macula. A condition in which the entire thickness of the retina, in the macular area, is lost as a result of trauma or degeneration, appearing ophthalmoscopically as a round, dark, red spot at the fovea. The edges are usually clearcut, and the hole has a depth of approximately 1.5 D.

Hollenhorst's plaques. See under *plaques*.

Holm's theory (hōmz). See under *theory*.

Holmes's stereoscope (hōmz'ez). See under *stereoscope*.

Holmes-Adie syndrome (hōmz-a'de). Adie's syndrome.

Holmgren test (hōlm'gren). See under *test*.

holocaine (hol'o-kān, ho'lo-). A proprietary brand of phenacaine, a synthetic alkaloid. The hydrochloride of para-diethoxyethenyldiphenylamidin, it occurs in the form of small, colorless, shiny crystals, or as a white powder, and is used as a local anesthetic in ophthalmic practice.

hologram (ho'lo-gram). A transparent photograph of interference patterns on light-sensitive film produced by an object when it is illuminated by, and reflects light to the film from, one beam of a coherent source, usually a laser, and the film receives light from another beam originating from the same source. Subsequent transillumination of the photograph by a coherent beam reconstructs an image of the original object in full dimension, seen as though the film were a window.

   absorption h. A hologram in which the radiant exposure results in increased absorption by the photographic emulsion. Cf. *phase hologram*.

   acoustical h. A hologram made with sound. Syn., *sonohologram;*

sonoptogram; sound hologram. See *acoustical holography.*

phase h. A hologram in which the radiant exposure results in change of refractive index of the photographic emulsion. Cf. *absorption hologram.*

sound h. Acoustical hologram.

holography (ho-log'rah-fe). The technique or process of producing a hologram.

acoustical h. A two stage process in which the diffraction pattern of an object irradiated by sound waves is biased, i.e., obliquely irradiated, by a coherent sound wave and recorded, such as on a photographic film, so that a realistic, three-dimensional visual image may be created when the recording or hologram is illuminated by a suitable coherent light source. Syn., *sonoholography; sonoptography; sound wave holography.*

color h. The generation of a three-dimensional image whose colors approximate those of the original object by means of three monochrome holograms providing primary colors with coordinated illumination by corresponding reference wavelengths.

sound wave h. Acoustical holography.

holophotal (hol"o-fōt'al). Pertaining to or having the features of a holophote.

holophote (hol'o-fōt). An optical system designed to direct essentially all the light emitted by a source in a single path or direction, as from the lamp of a lighthouse.

holoptic (hōl'op-tik). Having paired compound eyes the medial borders of which are contiguous. Cf. *dichoptic.*

holophotometer (hol"o-fo-tom'eh-ter). A photometer, equipped with mirrors, for the measuring and comparing of intensities of light emitted at various angles from a light source.

holotrichous (hol-ot'rih-kus). Normal positioning and spacing of the eyelashes.

Holt's method (hōltz). See under *method.*

Holth's method (hōlthz). Kinescopy.

Holtzer tape (hōlt'zer). See under *tape.*

homatropine (ho-mat'ro-pin). Oxytoluyl-tropeine, a mydriatic alkaloid obtained by the condensation of tropine and mandelic acid, used in solution as a cycloplegic. It is milder in effect than atropine.

homocentric (ho-mo-sen'trik). Pertaining to light rays that meet at a common focal point; the opposite of *heterocentric.*

homofocal (ho-mo-fo'kal). Pertaining to light rays having a common focus.

homogeneous (ho"mo-je'ne-us). 1. Consisting of elements of like nature; of the same kind; of a uniform quality throughout. 2. Pertaining to radiant energy consisting of only one wavelength, or radiant energy from so small a region of the spectrum as to include no perceptible differences of hue.

homokeratoplasty (ho-mo-ker'ah-to-plas"te). Keratoplasty in which the transplanted tissue is obtained from another individual. Cf. *autokeratoplasty.*

homonymous (ho-mon'ih-mus). 1. Pertaining to or designating uncrossed images of an object seen double, e.g., homonymous diplopia. 2. Pertaining to or designating symmetric halves of the visual fields, e.g., the nasal half of one field associated with the temporal half of the other.

homotransplant, corneal (ho"mo-trans'plant). Transplantation of corneal tissue obtained from the cornea of another human. See also *allotransplant; autotransplant; heterotransplant.*

Honi phenomenon (ho'ne). See under *phenomenon.*

Hooft syndrome. See under *syndrome.*

hook-over. Clip on.

hordeolum (hor-de'o-lum). A purulent infection of a sebaceous gland along the eyelid margin (external) or of a Meibomian gland on the conjunctival side of the eyelid (internal). It has the characteristic appearance of a markedly hyperemic, elevated area which increases in size and swelling and comes to a head with yellowish pus which breaks through and discharges.

external h. A purulent infection of a sebaceous gland along the eyelid margin. Syn., *sty.*

internal h. An acute purulent infection of a Meibomian gland on the conjunctival side of the eyelid. Syn., *Meibomian sty.*

horizon, retinal. The meridian of the retina which lies in a plane containing the x and the y axes and the horizontal meridian of the eye. It is the retinal meridian which coincides with the plane of fixation when the head is held erect and the two eyes look out in directions parallel to the median plane toward the far-off horizon.

von Hornbostel cube (fon hōrn′bos-tel). See under *cube.*

Horner's (hōr′nerz) **law; muscle; ptosis; syndrome; test.** See under the nouns.

Horner-Trantas points (hōr′ner-tran′tas). See under *point.*

Hornstein contact lens (hōrn′stīn). See under *lens, contact.*

◆

HOROPTER

horopter (ho-rop′ter). 1. The locus of object points in space simultaneously stimulating corresponding retinal points under given conditions of binocular fixation. 2. Any of several schematic representations of loci of object points in binocular space perception fulfilling specific criteria of singleness, position, alignment, direction, or distance, under given conditions of binocular fixation and presumed to represent manifestations of retinal correspondence.

h. circle. Vieth-Mueller horopter.

concave h. A horopter concave toward the observer.

convex h. A horopter convex toward the observer.

depth h. 1. The locus of points in the horizontal plane of regard which appears to be located at a distance from the observer equal to that of the fixation point, thus the empirical longitudinal horopter determined by the criterion of equidistance. See *equidistant horopter.* 2. An empirical longitudinal horopter, of doubted reliability, determined according to the criterion of maximal differential stereoscopic sensitivity, i.e., greatest awareness of small displacements of points toward or away from the observer. 3. An empirical horopter represented as having thickness corresponding to Panum's areas expressed in anteroposterior ranges of displacement of the test object.

empirical h. A horopter determined experimentally as opposed to a geometrical horopter or a theoretical horopter.

h. of equal convergence. Vieth-Mueller horopter.

equidistant h. An empirical longitudinal horopter based on the criterion that all points appear at the same distance from the observer as the fixation point. Except in the extreme periphery, it differs little from the apparent frontoparallel plane horopter.

frontal plane h. Apparent frontoparallel plane horopter.

frontoparallel plane h., apparent. An empirical longitudinal horopter based on the criterion that all points appear to lie in the frontoparallel plane containing the fixation point. Syn., *frontal plane horopter; frontoparallel plane horopter.*

fusion h. The locus of longitudinal horopter points at which test objects do not induce fusional movements, i.e., points of zero retinal disparity, a theoretical criterion not yet demonstrated experimentally.

general h. The location of all object points in three-dimensional space simultaneously stimulating corresponding retinal points under given conditions of binocular fixation, especially the complex theoretical horopter form derived by Helmholtz from assumptions of the location of corresponding retinal points.

geometrical h. A horopter based on theoretical or geometrical concepts as opposed to an empirical horopter. See *Vieth-Mueller horopter.*

haplopic h. An empirical horopter represented as having thickness corresponding to Panum's areas, expressed by the anteroposterior limits through which a nonfixated test object may be displaced and still be seen as single.

Hering-Hillebrand h. Hering-Hillebrand deviation.

identical visual direction h. An empirical horopter determined using the criterion of identical visual direction whence a single point in object space lying on the identical visual direction horopter gives rise to a percept in the same direction (from the self) for each eye. See also *nonius horopter.*

longitudinal h. The horopter for corresponding horizontal meridians of the two eyes, or the horopter represented as contained in the plane of regard of the two eyes, the possible presence of small degrees of cyclophoria in the latter representation being disregarded during experimental determination by the use of vertically oriented linear test objects or bars which eliminate vertical disparity effects.

Mueller's h. Vieth-Mueller horopter.

nonius h. An empirical longitudinal horopter utilizing the criterion of identical primary subjective visual direction for the two eyes. In practice, a central vertical rod or line is bifixated while other, peripherally located, vertical rods or lines, whose upper halves are visible to one eye only while the lower halves are visible to the other eye only, are individually moved until the two halves appear aligned. Syn., *similo-directional horopter; vernier horopter.*

similo-directional h. Nonius horopter.

theoretical h. A horopter based on theoretical concepts as opposed to an empirical horopter.

vernier h. Nonius horopter.

Vieth-Mueller h. The circle defined by the fixation point and the anterior nodal points of the two eyes, hence having the property that any two points lying on the circle will subtend equal angles at the two nodal points. Syn., *Vieth-Mueller circle; horopter of equal convergence; Mueller's horopter.*

◆

horopter-curve (ho-rop'ter-kurv). In the mathematical derivation by Helmholtz of a theoretical horopter, the complete spatial locus of all points whose projection will be simultaneously imaged on corresponding retinal points in the two eyes during a given condition of fixation. In the most general case, the horopter-curve is a curve of the third degree (one which pierces a plane in three points) formed by the intersection of two surfaces of the second degree (an hyperboloid and the surface of a cone or a cylinder), which passes through the point of fixation and the centers of the two eyes. In special cases of fixation (e.g., fixation in the median plane, or in the horizontal visual plane), the horopter-curve becomes a straight line joined to a conic section (circle or ellipse); or, in the case of fixation at infinity in the midline of the horizontal plane, it becomes a plane surface coinciding approximately with the floor plane upon which the observer stands. Thus, in general, the horopter-curve contains the entirety of the theoretical horopter (which may be defined as the visible portion of the horopter-curve, i.e., that portion which lies outside of the observer's head and body) plus the small portion which passes through and between the two eyes.

horror fusionalis (hor'ror fu-se-o-nal'is). Horror fusionis.

horror fusionis (hor'ror fu-se-ōn'is). The inability to obtain binocular fusion or superimposition of haploscopically presented targets, or the condition or phenomenon itself, occurring frequently as a characteristic in strabismus, in which case the targets approaching superimposition may seem to slide or jump past each other without apparent superimposition, fusion, or suppression. Syn., *fusion aversion.*

Horton syndrome (hōr'tun). Migraine.

Horton-Magath-Brown syndrome. See under *syndrome.*

Houstoun's (hu'stonz) **tests; theory.** See under the nouns.

Hovius' (ho've-us) **circle; plexus.** Circle of Hovius.

Howard's stereomicrometer (how'-ardz). See under *stereomicrometer.*

Howard-Dolman test (how'ard-dōl'man). See under *test.*

Hruby lens (hru'be). See under *lens.*

Ht. Abbreviation for *total hypermetropia.*

Hubbard-Kropf theory. See under *theory.*

Hubble effect. Red shift.

Hudson's brown line (hud'sonz). Superficial senile line.

Hudson-Stähli line (hud'son-sta'le). Superficial senile line.

hue. The attribute of color sensation ordinarily correlated with wavelength or combinations of wavelengths of the visual stimulus and distinguished from the attributes *brightness* and *saturation.*

extraspectral h. A hue sensation that cannot be matched by monochromatic light, but which can be matched by an additive mixture of wavelengths, e.g., the mixture of extreme ends of the visible spectrum to produce purple.

invariable h. 1. A hue that remains constant for all luminances. There are considered to be four, one each in the red, yellow, green, and blue regions of the spectrum. 2. A hue that remains constant wherever it is seen in the visual field, i.e., regardless of the area of the retina stimulated.

Munsell's h. Any one of the hue classifications in the system of Munsell color notations.

Ostwald h. Any one of the 24 hue classifications in the Ostwald system.

primary h's. 1. Any three hues, normally a red, a green, and a blue, so selected from the spectral scale as to enable one with normal color vision to match any other hue by their additive mixture in varying proportions; often called physical primary hues or colors, or the physical color primaries. 2. Four hues, red, green, blue, and yellow, which seem qualitatively individualistic or fundamental rather than mixed or composite; often called the psychological primary hues or colors, or the psychological color primaries. Syn., *unitary hues*.

unitary h's. Primary hues.

Hueck's ligament (heks). Uveal meshwork.

Hüfner rhomb. See under *rhomb*.

Hughes test. Three-disk test.

Hughlings-Jackson sign. See under *sign*.

humor (hu'mor, u'mor). Any normal fluid or semifluid of the body.

aqueous h. The clear, watery fluid which fills the anterior and the posterior chambers of the eye. It has a refractive index lower than the crystalline lens, which it surrounds, and is involved in the metabolism of the cornea and the crystalline lens. Syn., *aqueous fluid*. **plasmoid a.h.** The fluid that is rapidly formed after the normal aqueous humor is drained, or the modified aqueous that is formed following trauma or inflammation of the anterior segment of the eye. It contains a greater amount of protein than normal aqueous, approaching blood plasma in composition, and forms a diffuse cloud or aggregates into clumps. Syn., *secondary aqueous humor*. **secondary a.h.** Plasmoid aqueous humor.

crystalline h. Crystalline lens of the eye. *Obs.*

Morgagni's h. Morgagnian fluid.

ocular h. Either the aqueous or the vitreous humor of the eye, or both.

vitreous h. 1. The gelatinous, colorless, transparent substance filling the vitreous chamber of the eye, i.e., the space between the crystalline lens, the ciliary body, and the retina. It is considered to be derived from the surrounding ectoderm, especially the retina, and has a chemical composition similar to that of the aqueous humor, with the exception of two proteins, peculiar to the vitreous, the mucoid and the vitrein. Syn., *vitreous body*. 2. The vitreous body minus the vitrein and the mucoid thus a sol instead of a gel. **plasmoid v.h.** A modified vitreous humor formed following trauma or inflammation of the ciliary body, choroid, and/or retina. It contains a greater amount of protein than normal vitreous and forms a diffuse cloud or aggregates into clumps.

Humorsol. A trade name for *demecarium*.

Humphrey (hum'fre) **lenses; Vision Analyzer.** See under the nouns.

Humphriss method (hum'fris). See under *method*.

Hunt separator (hunt). See under *separator*.

Hunt-Giles test (hunt-jīls). See under *test*.

Hunter syndrome. See under *syndrome*.

Huntington's (hunt'ing-tunz) **chorea; disease.** See under *disease*.

Hurler's (hoor'lerz) **disease; syndrome.** See under *disease*.

Hurvich-Jameson theory (hur'vik-ja'meh-son). See under *theory*.

Huschke's valve (hoosh'kēz). See under *valve*.

Husted tonometer (hu'sted). See under *tonometer*.

Hutchinson's (huch'in-sunz) **chart; disease; patch; pupil; sign; syndrome; triad.** See under the nouns.

Hutchison's syndrome (huch'ih-sunz). See under *syndrome*.

Huygens' (hi'genz) **eyepiece; principle; theory.** See under the nouns.

Hx. History.

hyaline (hi'ah-lin). Vitreous humor. *Obs.*

hyalinosis cutis et mucosae (hi"ah-lin-o'sis). Lipid proteinosis.

hyalitis (hi-ah-li'tis). Inflammatory involvement of the vitreous humor or the hyaloid membrane. Since the vitreous body is a clear homogeneous gel, is physiologically inert, and has no demonstrable metabolism, the term "hyalitis" for pathological reactions of the vitreous is currently avoided. The term has been employed to cover secondary disturbances of the vitreous as a result of diseases of adjacent structures which produce infiltration into the vitreous.

asteroid h. Asteroid hyalosis.

punctate h. A degeneration of the vitreous humor characterized by the formation of small opacities.

suppurative h. A purulent inflammation in the vitreous humor due to exudation of cells from surrounding pathologically involved structures, as occurs in panophthalmitis.

hyalocytes (hi-al'o-sīts). Cells in the vitreous body of mammals and birds, adjacent to the ciliary body and retina, which are considered to be connective tissue cells of the macrophage type.

hyalogen (hi-al'o-jen). An albuminous substance occurring in the vitreous humor and in other parts of the body.

hyaloid (hi'ah-loid) **artery; body; canal; cataract; cyst; fossa; membrane.** See under the nouns.

hyaloiditis (hi"ah-loid-i'tis). Hyalitis.

hyalomucoid (hi"ah-lo-mu'koid). A mucoid substance present in the vitreous humor.

hyalonyxis (hi"ah-lo-nik'sis). Surgical puncture of the vitreous body.

hyalosis (hi"ah-lo'sis). Degeneration of the vitreous humor.

asteroid h. The presence of numerous, small, discrete, spherical or oval-shaped bodies in the vitreous humor, occurring essentially as a senile phenomenon, more common in males than in females, and more frequently unilateral than bilateral. The asteroid bodies usually show no orderly arrangement, and, when viewed ophthalmoscopically, appear white and shiny. The vitreous humor retains its solidity, and vision is but little affected. Syn., *Benson's disease*.

hydatoid (hi'dah-toid). 1. Aqueous humor. 2. Hyaloid membrane. 3. Pertaining or relating to the aqueous humor.

hydranencephaly (hi"dran-en-sef'ah-le). A developmental anomaly of the cerebral hemispheres which are reduced, in whole or in part, to membranous sacs composed of meninges fused with glial cortical remnants and filled with cerebrospinal fluid. The head is of normal size or slightly enlarged, and the cranium, being filled with fluid, readily transilluminates. Frequent ocular signs include cortical blindness with retention of the pupillary light reflex, strabismus, and ocular motility disturbances.

hydrargyrophthalmia (hi-drar"ji-rof-thal'me-ah). Inflammation of the eye or the conjunctiva from mercury or a mercuric compound.

hydroblepharon (hi-dro-blef'ah-ron). Edema of the eyelid.

hydrodiascope (hi-dro-di'ah-skōp). A device consisting of a fluid-filled chamber, tightly taped over the eye, with an anterior glass window before which correcting lenses are placed. Its purpose is to neutralize the anterior refracting surface of the cornea and eliminate the aberrations of keratoconus, irregular astigmatism, etc.

hydrogel (hi'dro-jel). A gel in which the liquid is water, commonly used in the manufacture of soft contact lenses.

hydrophthalmia (hi-drof-thal"me-ah). Hydrophthalmos.

hydrophthalmos (hi-drof-thal'mos). A condition in which congenital, structural abnormalities in the region of the angle of the anterior chamber offer an obstruction to the drainage mechanism of the intraocular fluids, so that the pressure of the eye is raised and a condition of congenital glaucoma results. The plasticity of the coats of the eye causes them to stretch under the increased pressure, and the whole eye enlarges. The most striking changes are in the cornea, which is enlarged and becomes globular in shape, and thinned, especially at the periphery. The iris may appear atrophic and may be tremulous, owing to the lack of support from the crystalline lens, which is smaller than normal and usually displaced backward. There is generally a marked cupping of the optic disk, and vision is subnormal. Syn., *buphthalmos*.

hydrophthalmoscope (hi-drof-thal'-mo-skōp). An instrument, used in ophthalmoscopy, which neutralizes the refractive power of the anterior surface of the cornea by means of a layer of water. It consists essentially of an eyecup with a flat glass bottom that serves as a viewing window.

hydrophthalmus (hi-drof-thal'mus). Hydrophthalmos.

hydrops, corneal (hi'drops). An accumulation of watery fluid, presumably aqueous humor, in the stroma of the cornea as a result of rupture of the posterior surface of the cornea involving the endothelium and Descemet's membrane.

hydroxyamphetamine hydrobromide (hi-drok"se-am-fet'ah-min). An adrenergic drug closely related to Benzedrine which in its hydrobromide form is said to act as a mydriatic without producing cycloplegia. It is sometimes used in combination with atropine or homatropine to exert a synergistic action and heighten the cycloplegic effect. The generic name for *Paredrine*.

hydroxyethylmethacrylate (hidrox"se-meth"il-meth-ak'ril-āt). A hydrophilic polymer, also known as ethylene glycol monomethacrylate, a common component of hydrogel materials used in the manufacture of soft contact lenses. Abbreviated HEMA.

hygroblepharon (hi-gro-blef'ar-on). An abnormally moist condition of an eyelid.

hyoscine (hi'o-sin). An alkaloid which, in its hydrobromide form, paralyzes the peripheral endings of the parasympathetic nerves, acting as a mydriatic, like atropine, but less powerfully. Syn., *scopolamine*.

hyperchromatopsia (hi"per-kro"mahtop'se-ah). A defect of vision in which colorless objects appear colored.

hypercyclophoria (hi"per-si"klo-fo're-ah). Combined hyperphoria and cyclophoria.

hyperdacryosis (hi"per-dak"re-o'sis). Abnormally profuse lacrimation.

hyperemia, retinal (hi"per-e'me-ah). Congestion of the retinal blood vessels, with some tortuosity, and increased redness and edema of the fundus, in whole or in part.

   active retinal h. Congestion of the retinal arteries characterized by their fullness and tortuosity and by a pinkish color of the optic disk, due to capillary engorgement. It may occur from a systemic cause that raises the blood pressure, or from local inflammation.

   passive retinal h. Congestion of the retinal veins due to some obstruction in the venous outflow.

hyperesophoria (hi"per-es"o-fo're-ah, -ēs"o-fo're-ah). Combined hyperphoria and esophoria.

hyperesthesia, optic (hi"per-esthe'ze-ah). Abnormal sensitivity of the eye to light.

hypereuryopia (hi"per-u-re-o'pe-ah). Abnormally large palpebral fissures.

hyperexophoria (hi"per-ek"so-fo're-ah). Combined hyperphoria and exophoria.

hyperkeratosis (hi"per-ker-ah-to'sis). Hypertrophy of the cornea.

hyperkinesia (hi"per-kih-ne'ze-ah). Hyperkinesis.

hyperkinesis (hi"per-kih-ne'sis.). Excessive muscular movement, as may be associated with spasm.

hyperlipemia, essential familial (hi"per-li-pe'me-ah). A familial disease, usually occurring in children, characterized by a milky blood serum (due to a rise in neutral fats), hepatosplenomegaly, and cutaneous xanthomatosis. Retinal lipemia and lipid keratopathy may also be present. Syn., *Bürger-Grütz disease; idiopathic hyperlipemia; essential hyperlipemic xanthomatosis*.

hyperlipemia, idiopathic. Essential familial hyperlipemia.

hypermetrope (hi"per-met'rōp). One who has hypermetropia.

◆

HYPERMETROPIA

hypermetropia (hi"per-me-tro'pe-ah). The refractive condition of the eye represented by the location of the conjugate focus of the retina behind the eye when accommodation is said to be relaxed, or the extent of that condition represented in the number of diopters of convex lens power required to compensate to the optical equivalent of emmetropia. The condition may also be represented as one in which parallel rays of light entering the eye, with accommodation relaxed, focus behind the retina. Syn., *farsightedness; hyperopia*.

   absolute h. The portion of hypermetropia which cannot be compensated for by accommodation, hence present in those having a total hypermetropia greater than the amplitude of accommodation. Cf. *facultative hypermetropia*.

   acquired h. Postnatal increase in hypermetropia, usually exclusive of the increase normally occurring in early infancy, and, more particularly, increases related to senility, surgery, and pathology.

   atypical h. Hypermetropia resulting from congenital abnormalities, degenerative changes, trauma, or disease. Syn., *complicated hypermetropia*.

axial h. Hypermetropia attributed to shortness or decreases in the axial length of the eye.

benign h. Simple hypermetropia.

complicated h. Atypical hypermetropia.

component h. Hypermetropia attributable to the abnormal refractive role of a single component of the eye, especially reduced axial length, observed by Sorsby to prevail among hyperopes greater than 6.00 D. Cf. *correlation hypermetropia.*

congenital h. Hypermetropia existing since or at the time of birth.

correlation h. Hypermetropia in which the individual refractive components are within the ranges of magnitude found in emmetropic eyes, observed by Sorsby to prevail among hyperopes of 6.00 D or less. Cf. *component hypermetropia.*

curvature h. Hypermetropia attributed to excessive increases in the radius of curvature of one or more of the refractive surfaces of the eye, and especially of the radius of the corneal surface.

deformational h. Hypermetropia of high degree, attributable to extreme pathological or developmental anomalies, as in microphthalmos or an extremely flat cornea.

facultative h. The portion of hypermetropia which can be compensated for by accommodation. Cf. *absolute hypermetropia.*

high h. Hypermetropia of high degree, usually of 5.00 D or more.

index h. Hypermetropia attributed to variations in the index of refraction of one or more of the ocular media.

latent h. The portion of the total hypermetropia compensated for by the tonicity of the ciliary muscle. It may be wholly or partially revealed by the use of a cycloplegic.

lenticular h. Hypermetropia attributed to a below average refractive power of the crystalline lens.

low h. Hypermetropia of a low degree, usually of 2.00 D or less.

manifest h. The portion of the total hypermetropia which may be demonstrated or measured by the relaxation of accommodation occurring with the simple reduction in stimulus

to accommodation, as in the increase of convex lenses in a routine refractive examination.

medium h. Hypermetropia of a medium degree, usually between 2.00 and 5.00 D.

pathological h. Hypermetropia resulting from pathological deformation of the eye; a type of atypical hypermetropia.

position h. Hypermetropia attributed to an excessive, or increase in, distance of the crystalline lens from the cornea.

refractive h. 1. Hypermetropia attributed to the condition of the refractive elements of the eye, including axial length, in distinction from deformational or pathological hypermetropia. 2. Hypermetropia attributed to the condition of the refracting elements of the eye in distinction from axial hypermetropia.

relative h. Facultative hypermetropia which permits clear vision but induces overconvergence or convergent strabismus for the point of fixation.

simple h. 1. Hypermetropia uncomplicated by any associated condition, disease, trauma, or abnormality. Syn., *benign hypermetropia; typical hypermetropia.* 2. Hypermetropia occurring without an associated astigmatism.

total h. The sum of the manifest and the latent hypermetropia.

typical h. Simple hypermetropia.

◆

hypermetropic (hi″per-me-trōp′ik, -trah′pik). Pertaining to or having hypermetropia. Syn., *hyperopic.*

hyperope (hi′per-ōp). Hypermetrope.

hyperopia (hi″per-o′pe-ah). Hypermetropia.

hyperopic (hi″per-op′ik). Hypermetropic.

hyperostosis, infantile cortical. A familial condition, occurring in infants up to age six months, characterized by soft tissue swelling and tenderness around the eyes which may be either unilateral or bilateral and which may have an associated conjunctivitis, proptosis, or soft tissue swelling and tenderness over the mandible, skull, clavicles and ribs. Its course is benign and self-limiting. Syn., *Caffey's disease; Caffey-Silverman syndrome; Silverman-Caffey disease.*

◆

HYPERPHORIA

hyperphoria (hi"per-fo're-ah). The upward deviation, or the amount of upward deviation, of the line of sight of one eye with reference to that of the other eye, as manifested in the absence of an adequate fusion stimulus or when fusion is made impossible. The condition of hyperphoria may be designated as one of hypophoria when the opposite eye is used as a reference.

alternating h. Double hyperphoria.

alterocular h. Double hyperphoria.

anatomic h. The manifestation of hyperphoria or that portion of the total hyperphoria attributable to structural (anatomical) anomalies or variation.

concomitant h. Hyperphoria which does not vary in amount with direction of gaze. Syn., *static hyperphoria.*

dissociated h. Double hyperphoria.

double h. The condition in which, under dissociation, the line of sight of the right eye deviates upward when the left eye is fixating and the line of sight of the left eye deviates upward when the right eye is fixating. Syn., *dissociated vertical deviation; alternating hyperphoria; alterocular hyperphoria; dissociated vertical divergence; alternating supraduction.*

innervational h. The manifestation of hyperphoria, or that part of the total hyperphoria, not attributable to structural (anatomical) anomalies or variation.

intrinsic h. Hyperphoria attributable to primary structural, myological, or neurological anomalies, distinguished from pseudohyperphoria attributable to spurious manifestations of neurological origin or to temporarily induced effects of lenses or prisms.

left h. Hyperphoria in which the line of sight of the left eye deviates upward with respect to that of the right eye.

nonconcomitant h. Hyperphoria varying in amount with changes in direction of gaze.

paretic h. Hyperphoria attributable to paresis of one or more of the extraocular muscles.

physiological h. Double hyperphoria which is considered to occur as a result of the nonfixating eye reverting toward the so-called position of rest assumed when both eyes are closed.

right h. Hyperphoria in which the line of sight of the right eye deviates upward with respect to that of the left eye.

spastic h. Hyperphoria attributable to overaction of one or both inferior oblique muscles, manifested pronouncedly with lateral fixation movements and presumed to be due to congenital check ligament deficiencies.

static h. Concomitant hyperphoria.

◆

hyperphoric (hi"per-fōr'ik). Pertaining to or affected with hyperphoria.

hyperplasia (hi"per-pla'ze-ah). An abnormal increase in the number of normal cells in normal arrangement in a tissue. It is usually the response to continued irritation and may occur in pathology of the epithelium of the conjunctiva and the cornea.

hyperpresbyopia (hi"per-pres-be-o'pe-ah). 1. Absolute presbyopia. 2. Hypermetropia. *Obs.*

hyperrhinoplaty, interocular (hi"-per-ri'no-plat-e). Ocular hypertelorism.

hyperstasis (hi"per-sta'sis). A term used by Lancaster to designate the static position of the covered eye during a cover test when its line of sight deviates upward.

hyperstereoscopy (hi"per-ster-e-os'ko-pe). Exaggeration of apparent depth relationships by increasing the lateral separation of the stereocamera lens system.

hypertelorism, Greig's (hi"per-tel'ōr-izm). Ocular hypertelorism.

hypertelorism, ocular (hi"per-tel'ōr-izm). A congenital malformation of the skull characterized by an enlarged sphenoid bone, extremely wide bridge of the nose with great width between the eyes, exophthalmos, divergent strabismus, and optic atrophy. Syn., *Greig's hypertelorism.*

hypertension, arterial (hi"per-ten'shun). See *retinopathy, hypertensive.*

hypertonia bulbi (hi"per-to'ne-ah bul'bi). The condition of consistently elevated intraocular pressure without associated destruction of the intraocular structures or the optic nerve.

hypertrichophrydia (hi"per-trik-of-rid'e-ah). Excessively long eyebrows.

hypertrichosis (hi"per-trih-ko'sis). The condition in which the length and/or the number of the eyelashes is increased.

hypertrophy (hi-per'tro-fe). An increase in the size of individual cells or fibers, without an increase in the number, resulting in enlargement of a tissue or an organ.

hypertropia (hi"per-tro'pe-ah). Strabismus characterized by the upward deviation of the line of sight of the nonfixating eye with reference to that of the fixating eye, hence similar to hyperphoria, except that the condition is continuous and unrelated to the presence or the absence of fusion stimuli.

   alternating h. Double hypertropia.

   double h. Strabismus characterized by the upward deviation of the line of sight of either eye while the other fixates. Syn., *alternating hypertropia.*

hyphema (hi-fe'mah). A sanguineous exudate in the anterior chamber of the eye; bloody hypopyon.

hyphemia (hi-fe'me-ah). Hemorrhage into the anterior chamber of the eye.

hypoblepharon (hi"po-blef'ah-ron). 1. A swelling beneath the eyelid. 2. An artificial eye.

hypocyclosis (hi"po-si-klo'sis). Deficient accommodation.

   ciliary h. Deficient accommodation due to weakness of the ciliary muscle.

   lenticular h. Deficient accommodation due to extreme rigidity of the crystalline lens.

hypoesophoria (hi"po-es"o-fo're-ah, -ēs"o-fo're-ah). Combined hypophoria and esophoria.

hypoexophoria (hi"po-ek"so-fo're-ah). Combined hypophoria and exophoria.

hypokinesia (hi"po-kih-ne'ze-ah). Hypokinesis.

hypokinesis (hi"po-kih-ne'sis). Decreased muscular movement, as of an extraocular muscle.

hypometropia (hi"po-me-tro'pe-ah). Myopia.

hypophasis (hi"po-fa'sis). Incomplete closure of the eyelids, leaving the sclera visible.

hypophoria (hi"po-fo're-ah). The downward deviation, or the amount of downward deviation, of the line of sight of one eye with reference to that of the other eye, as manifested in the absence of an adequate fusion stimulus or when fusion is made impossible. The condition of hypophoria may be designated as one of hyperphoria when the opposite eye is used as a reference.

   alternating h. Double hypophoria.

   double h. The condition in which, under dissociation, the line of sight of the right eye deviates downward when the left eye is fixating, and the line of sight of the left eye deviates downward when the right eye is fixating. Syn., *alternating hypophoria.*

hypoplasia (hi"po-pla'ze-ah). Defective or incomplete development of a tissue.

hypopyon (hi-po'pe-on). An accumulation of pus in the anterior chamber of the eye associated with infectious diseases of the cornea, the iris, and the ciliary body. The pus characteristically sinks to the bottom, filling the lower angle of the chamber, where it may be visible through the cornea.

   h. recidivans. Behçet's disease.

hyposcleral (hi"po-skler'al). Beneath the sclerotic coat of the eye.

hypostasis (hi"po-sta'sis). A term used by Lancaster to designate the static position of the covered eye during a cover test when its line of sight deviates downward.

hypostereoscopy (hi"po-ster-e-os'ko-pe). Diminution of apparent depth relationships by decreasing the lateral separation of the stereocamera lens systems.

hypotelorism (hi"po-tel'or-izm). A congenital malformation of the skull characterized by abnormal narrowness of the interorbital distance. Syn., *stenopia.*

hypothalamus (hi"po-thal'ah-mus). The portion of the diencephalon of the forebrain located in the floor of the third ventricle, consisting mainly of the posterior lobe and infundibulum of the pituitary gland, the optic chiasm, the tuber cinereum, and the paired mammillary bodies.

hypothesis (hi-poth′e-sis). An assumption, a supposition, or a conjecture; a tentative theory used provisionally to explain certain facts or to guide in the investigation of others.

albedo h. The perceived lightness (albedo) of a reflecting surface is judged only after the intensity of illumination of the surface is mentally evaluated.

cluster h. The hypothesis that color perception is due to specific retinal elements, grouped in clusters throughout the retina, which act as selective receptors to certain wavelengths of light. That is, one type of retinal cell acts in the perception of red, another in green, etc.

constancy h. The hypothesis that sensation is correlated directly with stimulation. That is, a given stimulus, if repeated, will produce the same sensation, providing the sense organ remains unchanged.

Cord's h. The hypothesis that a deep parietal lobe lesion in the area of the internal and external sagittal strata will cause an asymmetric horizontal optokinetic response associated with hemianopsia, whereas a lesion involving the optic tract, lateral geniculate body, temporal lobe, or occipital lobe may cause hemianopsia, but optokinetic responses remain normal.

Ogata-Weymouth h. Night myopia is due in part to the greater axial length of the eye outside the outer fovea when parafoveal fixation occurs in dim light. Subsequent investigation indicates that it must be a minor factor.

Ségal's h. The retina contains lightsensitive structures other than the rods and cones, such as the synaptic terminals of rods and cones and the cells of the pigment epithelium layer.

three-channel h. Normal trichomatic color vision is mediated by three pathways, channels, or mechanisms which selectively transmit color information. They may be three photosensitive pigments in the retina, three types of retinal receptors, or three selective "filters" in the visual pathways.

two-quantum h. The absorption of two quanta, within a given time interval, by a single sensitive unit under optimum conditions is sufficient for sensory detection.

Weymouth-Andersen h. The subconal angular values of the thresholds of binocular stereopsis and vernier visual acuity, which decrease with an increase in the length of the lines, the result of a comparison of the percepts of average oculocentric position of the lines derived from the pattern of stimulation of many cones.

Whittle's h. The perception of depth resulting from viewing a Helmholtz stereogram is caused by a disparity of similar gradients of brightness, and is not due to disparity of similar spatial contours, as stated by Helmholtz.

hypotonia oculi (hi-po-to′ne-ah ok′u-li). Ocular hypotony.

hypotony, ocular (hi-pot′o-ne). Abnormally low ocular tension. Syn., *hypotonia oculi.*

hypotrichosis (hi″po-trih-ko′sis). A condition in which the eyelashes are underdeveloped or absent.

hypotropia (hi″po-tro′pe-ah). Strabismus characterized by the downward deviation of the line of sight of the nonfixating eye with reference to that of the fixating eye, hence similar to hypophoria, except that the condition is continuous and unrelated to the presence or absence of fusion stimuli.

alternating h. Double hypotropia.

double h. Strabismus characterized by the downward deviation of the line of sight of either eye while the other fixates. Syn., *alternating hypotropia.*

Hyrtl's valve (hēr′tlz). See under *valve.*

hysterope (his′ter-ōp). One suffering from hysteropia.

hysteropia (his-ter-o′pe-ah). Disordered vision resulting from hysteria.

Hz. Abbreviation for *hertz.*

I

I. Symbol for *luminous intensity.*

IAB. See *International Association of Boards of Examiners in Optometry.*

IAOE. See *International Association of Optometric Executives.*

ianthinopsia (i-an″thin-op′se-ah). Ianthopsia.

ianthopsia (i-an-thop′se-ah). A very rarely reported perversion of color vision identified by the sensory attribution of the color violet to perceived objects.

ICI. See *International Commission on Illumination,* the English translation for *Commission Internationale de l'Eclairage* (abbreviated CIE).

ichthyosis (ik″the-o′sis). Hypertrophy of the corneous layer of the skin, usually congenital, in which the skin becomes dry, hard, and scaly, with an absence of secretion from the sweat and sebaceous glands. When affecting the eyelids, it may result in the loss of the eyelashes and in ectropion; when affecting the eye, it may result in chronic catarrhal conjunctivitis or keratosis of the cornea.

ichthyosis follicularis (ik″the-o′sis fol-lik″u-la′ris). A rare sex-linked hereditary condition characterized by keratosis and follicular formation in hairy regions resulting in sparseness of the eyelashes and loss of the outer halves of the eyebrows and manifesting corneal changes associated with photophobia. Syn., *keratosis follicularis spinulosa decalvans; keratosis pilaris decalvans.*

ICO. Institut et Centre d'Optometrie.

iconometer (i-kon-om′eh-ter). An instrument or a scale within an instrument, for measuring the size of a viewed image to determine the size or distance of the corresponding object. Cf. *eikonometer.*

iconoscope (i-kon′o-skōp). An instrument devised by Javal for testing binocular perception of depth, designed to vary the binocular relative parallactic angle and thereby determine the threshold of stereopsis.

icterus, scleral (ik′ter-us). A jaundiced pigmentation of the sclera associated with biliary or liver disease.

identification. *Optometric Extension Program:* The total process of cortically receiving impulses derived from the retinal image and integrating this input with other sensory information and past experience, with a resultant recognition and interpretation of the stimulus.

idiocy. The lowest of the three grades of mental deficiency, which describes those whose defectiveness is of such degree as to render them unable to guard themselves against common physical dangers. On the basis of intelligence tests, it includes those who have IQ scores of less than 25. Cf. *imbecility; moronity.*

  amaurotic family i. See under *amaurotic.*

  Mongolian i. Down's syndrome.

idiopathic (id″e-o-path′ik). Pertaining to a primary disease of unknown cause or origin.

idioretinal (id″e-o-ret′ih-nal). Pertaining to the retina alone, as in *idioretinal light.*

IERI. See *Illuminating Engineering Research Institute.*

IES. See *Illuminating Engineering Society of North America.*

ILAMO. See *International Library, Archives, and Museum of Optometry, Inc.*

illaqueation (il"ak-we-a'shun). A surgical operation in which a displaced or an ingrown eyelash is drawn into a correct position by use of a loop or a snare.

illuminance (ih-lu'mih-nans). Illumination.

illuminant (ih-lu'mih-nant). Any source of light or visible radiant energy, such as candle flame or fluorescent lamp.

 A, B, C, D i's. Light sources having specified spectral distributions adopted by the CIE in 1931 as international standards in colorimetry. A is the color temperature of a blackbody, approximately that of a tungsten lamp, at 2855.6°K. B is illuminant A in combination with a specified filter and approximates noon sunlight, having a color temperature of 4874°K or a blackbody operating at that color temperature. C is illuminant A in combination with a specified filter and approximates daylight provided by a combination of direct sunlight and clear sky, having a color temperature of 6774°K. D_{65} is an approximation of daylight at a correlated color temperature of 6504°K.

illuminate (ih-lu'mih-nāt). To supply with light.

Illuminating Engineering Research Institute. A self-governing trust affiliate of the Illuminating Engineering Society created in 1944 to raise funds and to underwrite university-based research in lighting as it relates to human function.

Illuminating Engineering Society of North America. An association, founded in 1906, of persons and firms concerned with all aspects of lighting.

◆

ILLUMINATION

illumination (ih-lu"mih-na'shun). 1. The photometric term for the intensive property of the luminous flux passing through a cross section of a beam or falling on a surface; the density of luminous flux incident on a surface. It is the quotient of the luminous flux divided by the area of the surface when the flux is uniformly distributed. Symbol: E. Common units are lumen per sq. ft (foot-candle) or per sq. m (lux, meter-candle). Syn., *illuminance.* 2. The act or process by which light is made to be incident on a surface.

 axial i. Illumination from light transmitted along the optical axis of a lens or a mirror.

 bright field i. See *microscopy, bright field.*

 contact i. Illumination of the interior of the eye by placing a light source directly on the conjunctiva or the cornea.

 critical i. 1. The minimum amount of light which will provide optimal performance in terms of any one criterion. For example, the footcandle level which will permit the practical maximum rate of reading of a specific sample of printed matter. 2. In microscopy, illumination of the specimen by focusing the image of a diffuse light source directly on it by means of a condenser whose aperture size is equal to that of the microscope objective.

 dark field i. See *microscopy, dark field.*

 diffuse i. 1. Illumination by light sources having dimensions relatively large with respect to the distance from the point being illuminated and emitting or scattering light in all directions, or illumination by light incident from all directions. It is characterized by a relative lack of shadow if an object is interposed between the light source and the illuminated area. 2. In slit lamp biomicroscopy, illumination obtained with a wide slit and out of focus beam, to provide an over-all view of the surface being studied.

 direct i. Illumination from a light source without being reflected from any surface. Cf. *indirect illumination.*

 i. of empty space, perceived. Perception of the intensity and chromaticity of light prevailing in the space between objects or in a neighboring room.

 equivalent sphere i. The level of sphere illumination which produces task visibility equivalent to that produced by a given lighting environment.

 focal i. 1. Illumination by focusing the image of a light source on an object, by means of an optical system. 2. Illumination at the focal plane of an optical system. 3. In slit lamp biomicroscopy, illumination with beam and microscope both sharply focused on the structure being studied.

 indirect i. 1. Illumination by means of reflected light. Cf. *direct illumination.* 2. Proximal illumination.

Kohler i. In microscopy, illumination of the specimen by collimated light obtained by imaging the light source at a diaphragm located at the primary principal focus of the condenser.

lateral i. Proximal illumination.

multidirectional i. Illumination produced by several separated light sources, characterized by the formation of multiple shadows when an object is interposed between the light sources and the illuminated area. Cf. *diffused illumination.*

i. of an object, perceived. Perception of the intensity and chromaticity of illumination of an object derived from surface cells such as shadows and light spots.

oblique i. Illumination used with certain instruments, such as the slit lamp, in which the beam of light is incident from such an angle that it is not reflected into the objective lens of the viewing system.

oscillatory i. In slit lamp biomicroscopy, illumination in which the light beam is oscillated to provide alternate direct and indirect illumination.

parafocal i. Proximal illumination.

proximal i. In biomicroscopy, illumination of a structure by focusing a small beam of light on nontransparent, translucent tissue adjacent to the structure under observation. Syn., *indirect illumination; lateral illumination; parafocal illumination.*

retinal i. The luminous flux incident per unit area on the retina.

retro i. See *retro-illumination.*

sclerotic scatter i. In biomicroscopy, a method of illumination in which the beam of light is focused on the corneoscleral limbus to create internal reflection through the cornea. The light will pass through normal tissue unimpeded and unobserved, but will be scattered by any disturbance of transparency (nebula, keratocele, etc.), rendering it visible.

sphere i. The illumination on a task from a source providing equal luminous intensity from all directions, such as in an illuminated sphere with the task located at its center.

sunset i. In biomicroscopy, illumination of a structure with an oblique tangential or surface grazing beam.

surround i. Illumination with respect to the area surrounding an object of reference.

through i. Transillumination.

unidirectional i. Illumination produced by a single light source of relatively small dimensions and characterized by the formation of a sharply defined shadow when a small object is interposed between the light source and the illuminated area.

◆

illuminator (ih-lu′mih-na″ter). Any device which is used to illuminate a surface; that which illuminates.

Barkan Focal I. A hand-held lamp which provides a focused beam of light; used to examine the eye, as in gonioscopy.

Luckiesh-Moss i. An appliance for uniformly illuminating visual acuity test charts.

microscope i. A light source designed to illuminate the specimen being viewed in a microscope.

illuminometer (ih-lu″mih-nom′eh-ter). Photometer.

illusion, Cornsweet edge. Similar to the O'Brien edge illusion except that the complex transition strip consists of a central sharp luminance edge with a gradual increase of luminance to that of the adjacent broad area on one side and a gradual decrease of luminance to that of the adjacent broad area on the other side, the two broad areas being of equal luminance but the former broad area appearing darker and the latter appearing brighter. Syn., *Cornsweet effect.*

illusion, O'Brien edge. The darkened appearance of the broad area adjacent to the more abrupt luminous intensity drop-off edge of a narrow, luminous transition strip combined with the lighter appearance of the broad area adjacent to the more gradual luminous intensity drop-off edge of the same strip separating the two adjacent areas. Syn., *O'Brien effect.*

illusion, optical (ih-lu′zhun). 1. Visual illusion. 2. An apparent visual illusion induced by optical design or optical circumstances unknown to the observer, as obtained with curved mirrors, trick projectors, or mirages.

McLean's o.i. Phenakistoscope.

◆

ILLUSION, VISUAL

illusion, visual (ih-lu′zhun). The visual perception of a pattern, a view, or a performance, which does not reflect, represent, or convey the actual physical characteristics of the stimulus conditions; or the pattern, the view, or the performance itself. Syn., *optical illusion.*

assimilative v.i. A visual illusion induced by nearby objects, suggestion, attitude, or past experience.

associative v.i. A type of contrast visual illusion in which the length of lines, or areas, is either overestimated or underestimated.

autokinetic v.i. The apparent motion of a small, single, stationary object when continuously observed in a surrounding dark environment. Syn., *visual autokinesis; autokinetic effect; Charpentier's visual illusion; autokinetic phenomenon.*

Baldwin's v.i. A visual illusion in which a dot, placed midway between a small circle and a large one, appears to be nearer the large one.

Bourdon's v.i. A geometrical visual illusion arising when viewing two wedge-shaped areas, joined at their apices, and whose upper borders form a common, continuous, straight line. The pattern appears curved, although the one line is straight.

cameo-intaglio v.i. The apparent reversal of normal depth relationships in a scene or an object, due to shadows which result from an unusual and unnoticed direction of illumination.

Charpentier's v.i. Autokinetic visual illusion.

chessboard visual v.i. The perception of straight, vertical, and horizontal rows of squares of equal width when viewing a figure, the chessboard of Helmholtz, at its center, from a specific distance. The figure actually does not consist of squares, as the rows are hyperbolic instead of straight. When the figure is viewed at its periphery, from the same distance, it has the appearance of a shallow bowl.

contrast v.i. A visual illusion due to the effects of the relationship of various components of a geometrical figure or pattern. Cf. *assimilative visual illusion.*

Delboeuf v.i. A small circle concentrically contained within a slightly larger circle appears larger than another of the same size concentrically contained within a much larger circle.

double interpretation v.i. Reversible visual illusion.

Ebbinghaus' v.i. The apparent increase in a linear dimension when it is "filled" rather than "empty," as illustrated when viewing two equal lines or spaces, one "filled" with a series of intersecting lines or narrow bands, and the other left "empty."

false reference v.i. A visual illusion leading to false aircraft orientation in which slanting clouds or aircraft are mistaken as horizontal, or in which stars are mistaken for ground lights, or vice versa, creating a false horizon.

following gaze v.i. The appearance that the eyes of a full-faced photograph or picture seem to follow the observer no matter at what angle the picture is viewed.

Frazer v.i. A pattern of concentric rings each consisting of a series of overlapping short arcs with successively narrower spaces between medially successive rings giving the illusion of a centrally receding conic spiral.

geometrical v.i. A visual illusion dependent on the arrangement of lines, angles, and spaces, rather than on color, light, and shade.

Hering's v.i. A geometrical visual illusion in which a pair of parallel lines appear bowed, or abruptly bent, by the placement of diagonals on or adjacent to them, as when a number of radiating lines are crossed by two parallel lines on opposite sides of the point of radiation.

Hermann's v.i. See *Hermann's grid.*

Höfler's v.i. A geometrical visual illusion arising when two curved bands or lines, each of equal length and radius, are placed one above the other, the band nearer the centers of curvature appearing longer.

horizontal-vertical v.i. A geometrical visual illusion arising when a horizontal line is near or touching a vertical line. When the bottom of the vertical line is placed at or near the midpoint of the horizontal, and the two lines are of equal length, the vertical appears to be longer. If the figure is rotated to any other position, the same line will still appear longer.

Jastrow v.i. A geometrical visual illusion arising when two curved bands of equal length and radii of curvature are placed one above the other, the band nearer the centers of curvature appearing longer.

Kundt's v.i. A geometrical visual illusion occurring when attempting to bisect a horizontal line viewed by only one eye, the middle point being placed too far toward the nasal side.

linear surround v.i. The apparent motion of stationary vertical stripes adjacent to a rotating stimulus drum which is inducing horizontal optokinetic nystagmus.

Mach's v.i. A geometrical visual illusion in which a drawing, resembling a partially open book, first appears to open toward and then away from the observer, or vice versa, on continuous fixation.

moon v.i. A visual illusion in which the moon appears to be larger when viewed near the horizon than when viewed high in the sky.

Mueller-Lyer v.i. A geometrical visual illusion in which two lines of equal length do not appear equal when different appendages are placed at their ends, as when viewing two equal lines, one of which has arrowheads on both ends and the other has quills on both ends. (See Fig. 22.)

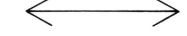

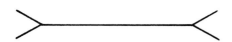

Fig. 22 Mueller-Lyer visual illusion.

oculoagravic v.i. Apparent movements or displacement of an object in space associated with reduced gravity or weightlessness, as in aircraft maneuvers.

oculogravic v.i. The apparent rising of an observed object coincident with a sensation of tilting backward created by high acceleration, attributed to stimulation of the vestibular apparatus.

oculogyral v.i. The apparent movements of viewed objects subsequent to rotatory acceleration of the observer's head in one direction. The initially observed movement is opposite to the direction of rotation and is followed by movement in the same direction. Syn., *optogyral visual illusion.*

Oppel-Kundt v.i. A geometrical visual illusion in which a divided, interrupted, or filled area is estimated to be larger than an empty or blank area of equal size.

optogyral v.i. Oculogyral visual illusion.

Poggendorff's v.i. A geometrical visual illusion arising from viewing a bandlike rectangular area overlaying a diagonal line. The two visible portions of the line, one on each side of the band, do not appear to be parts of a continuous line. (See Fig. 23.)

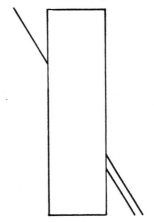

Fig. 23 Poggendorff's visual illusion.

Ponzo v.i. A geometrical visual illusion in which two parallel lines of equal length do not appear equal when viewed on a background of radiating straight lines emanating from a common point, the parallel line nearest the point of radiation appearing to be longer.

railroad v.i. The illusion of motion of one's own stationary vehicle when viewing another nearby parallel moving vehicle.

reverse optokinetic v.i. The apparent movement of a small stationary light, in a dark surround, in a direction opposite to the continuous movement of a previously viewed series of stripes oriented perpendicular to their movement, usually provided by means of a rotating striped drum.

reverse rotation v.i. The apparent movement of a stationary pattern of stripes in a direction opposite to that just previously observed when the stripes were in actual motion in a direction perpendicular to their orientation.

reversible v.i. The moment to moment variation in the interpretation of an ambiguous or a reversible figure. Syn., *double interpretation visual illusion.*

Schroeder's staircase v.i. A geometrical visual illusion arising from viewing a figure formed by parallel, steplike lines drawn from the upper corner of a parallelogram to the lower opposite corner. When observed continuously, the impression is, at one time, that one is viewing a staircase from underneath, and at another, that he is viewing the staircase from above.

stroboscopic v.i. The altered apparent speed of motion of a rotating, segmented pattern induced by rapid intermittent exposures, frequently observed when a revolving fan is illuminated by fluorescent light or when the spokes of a turning wheel are viewed in a motion picture. The segmented pattern may appear to move slowly, stand still, or to move in the opposite direction, depending on the relation of the amount of radial motion during each cycle of intermittency and the distance between the segments of the pattern.

Thiéry's v.i. A geometrical visual illusion in which a reversible perspective drawing first appears to be a solid rectangular box to which is attached the base and the side of another such box. Following fixation, the figure appears to change so that either two solid rectangular boxes are seen or the base and the side become a solid box and the solid box becomes the base and the side.

Tschermak-Seysenegg v.i. A geometrical visual illusion occurring in the attempt to bisect a vertical line, the inferior field being underestimated, resulting in subjectively locating the midpoint too far upward.

waterfall v.i. A visual illusion of motion induced as a temporary aftereffect of viewing an endlessly moving pattern, such as a waterfall or an endless belt. A subsequently viewed stationary object appears to move slowly in the opposite direction. Syn., *waterfall phenomenon.*

Wertheimer-Benary v.i. A simultaneous contrast effect; a gray on a black background appears lighter than the same gray on a white background.

Wundt's v.i. A geometrical visual illusion in which a pair of parallel straight lines appear bowed when crossed by lines radiating toward, and meeting, each other from two points, one on each side of the parallel lines.

Zöllner's v.i. A geometrical visual illusion in which a series of parallel lines appear to converge toward or diverge from each other when crossed by short diagonal lines. The diagonals on each line are parallel to each other, but are angled opposite to those of the adjacent line.

◆

IMAGE

image. 1. In general, a likeness, a copy, a replica, a symbol, or a mental representation of an object. 2. The optical counterpart of an object produced by a lens, a mirror, or other optical system. 3. The perceived counterpart of a viewed object subjectively projected in visual space.

accidental i. An afterimage.

aerial i. 1. An image, especially a real image, formed by an optical system but perceived by alignment of the viewing eye with the path of light emerging from the optical system, instead of being focused first as an image on a receiving screen. Cf. *direct image.* 2. An image perceived in the air by reflection or refraction by strata of different atmospheric densities, as in a mirage.

after i. See *afterimage.*

apparent i. Virtual image.

body i. The picture or mental representation of one's own body, at rest or in motion at any moment, as derived from internal sensation, postural change, contact with others, emotional experience, or fantasy.

catoptric i. An image formed by regular reflection, as from a mirror, or by reflection at refracting surfaces, as the Purkinje-Sanson images.

chemical i. The retinal image as represented by photochemical changes in the visual cells from light stimulation, as distinguished from *energy image.*

chiasmal i. A figurative image representing the pattern of impulses from a retinal image at a cross section of the optic chiasm.

cone-halo stellar i. A star's appearance of having a bright core and a relatively bright surrounding halo, especially when viewed with a large aperture telescope, probably attributable to the light distribution characteristic of the retinal image.

congruous i's. 1. Ocular images having the same area representation in the visual cortex, as opposed to incongruous images present in aniseikonia. 2. Diplopic images seen under conditions of normal retinal correspondence.

corneal i. Either of the two catoptric images of an object or a light source, produced by reflection at one or the other surface of the cornea. See also *Purkinje-Sanson images.*

cortical i. The topographical representation of the image of external objects at the terminal region of the neurological visual pathway in the visual cortex. It is the representation in the brain of the nervous impulses originating with the retinal image and conditioned by the anatomy of the retina, the physiological processes involved in transmission, and the anatomy of the visual cortex. Syn., *ocular image.*

curvature of i. See *curvature of the field.*

cyclopic i. The single, fused image of one's eyes obtained when each eye fixates its own image in a mirror.

diffusion i. A blurred image of an object point, formed on a surface not located in the focal plane of a lens or an optical system; an out-of-focus image.

dioptric i. 1. An image formed by a refracting optical system, distinguished from a *catoptric image.* 2. The retinal image.

direct i. 1. A virtual image, such as the erect image seen in direct ophthalmoscopy. Cf. *indirect image.* 2. An image, especially a virtual image, formed by an optical system, but perceived by alignment of the viewing eye with the path of light emerging from the optical system, instead of being focused first as an image on a receiving screen. Cf. *aerial image.*

double i. A pair of images of a single object, obtained either perceptually, as in diplopia, or optically by a doubling system.

eidetic i. An extraordinarily experienced, mental picture based on the recall of a previous visual experience and characterized by its clearness, apparent realness, and accuracy of detail.

energy i. The retinal image as represented by the light energy received at the retina, as distinguished from *chemical image.*

erect i. An image that is not inverted with respect to the object, such as a virtual image produced by a concave lens or a convex mirror.

extraordinary i. The image formed by the extraordinary rays in double refraction.

false i. 1. The anomalously projected image in monocular diplopia or associated with the deviating eye in strabismus. 2. In physiological diplopia, the image which seems to be incorrectly localized in space when attempts are made to reach for it.

following i. of von Kries. Second positive afterimage.

foot-piece i. A figurative image representing the pattern of impulses from a retinal image at the foot pieces of the visual cells.

functional i. The image on the retina considered or analyzed in terms of the number of retinal elements (rods and cones) within it or stimulated by it.

ghost i. An unwanted secondary image, as may be formed by internal reflection in a lens or an optical system, irregularity of spacing in a diffraction grating, or incomplete polarization by a Polaroid filter. Syn., *ghost.*

half i. One of the two images present in diplopia. (Helmholtz)

heteronymous i's. The images of an object, seen in physiological diplopia, when fixation is for a point farther than the object.

heterotopic i's. A pair of diplopic images separated in space. Cf. *homotopic images.*

homonymous i's. The images of an object, seen in physiological diplopia, when fixation is for a point nearer than the object.

homotopic i's. A pair of diplopic images, each arising from a different object, which are perceived at the same point in space, i.e., they are superimposed. Cf. *heterotopic images.*

incidental i. The bleached impression of an image remaining on the retina subsequent to the removal of the object. See also *optogram.*

incongruous i's. 1. Diplopic images seen under conditions of anomalous retinal correspondence. 2. Images which are not of the same size and/or shape, due either to aniseikonia or to the difference in direction of view created by the separation of the eyes in the head. **asymmetric i.i.** In aniseikonia, images which result from asymmetric magnification or minification in specific meridians. Syn., *irregular incongruous images.* **irregular i.i.** Asymmetric incongrous images. **regular i.i.** Symmetric incongruous images. **symmetric i.i.** In aniseikonia, images which result from symmetrical magnification or minification in specific meridians. Syn., *regular incongruous images.*

indirect i. A real image, such as the inverted image seen in indirect ophthalmoscopy. Cf. *direct image.*

inverted i. An optically formed image reversed in meridional orientation in relation to the object, i.e., upside down or right for left, usually implying reversal in all meridians unless otherwise qualified. Syn., *reversed image.*

leading i. The image seen by one eye in a direction farther from the primary position than the image seen by the other eye, in testing for paralysis or paresis of extraocular muscles.

i. line. See under *line.*

mental i. 1. A mental picture based on the recall of a previous visual experience. 2. A perceptual image. 3. A visual hallucination.

mirror i. 1. An image of an object formed by a mirror. 2. An object, or a part of an object, having the symmetrical attribute of replicating another object, or the other part of itself, as though it were its reflected image in a plane mirror.

negative i. 1. An image with features complementary to those of its correlated object in respect to luminance, color, or relief, as obtained, for example, in photographic negatives, negative afterimages, and contact lens molding processes, respectively. 2. A virtual image.

neural i. A pattern of neural activity represented at any specific point in the visual pathway as the correlate of a retinal image.

ocular i. 1. The cortical image. 2. The retinal image. 3. The image formed by the refracting system of the eye, the presence or the position of the retina being disregarded.

optical i. An image formed by the refraction or the reflection of light.

ordinary i. The image formed by the ordinary rays in double refraction.

orthoscopic i. An image exactly similar to its object in its entire extent, hence formed by an optical system corrected for distortions.

palinoptic i's. Images perceived in palinopsia.

perceptual i. That which is perceived and interpreted as an object in the visual field; hence, an object in terms of its perceived attributes and localization rather than in terms of its physical attributes or location. Syn., *psychological image.*

pinhole i. An image formed by rays that have passed through a pinhole aperture.

pipper i. A spot of light seen coincident with the pipper of an optical sight when the aim is correct.

pressure i. See *phosphene.*

primary i. The initial sensory effect of photic stimulation of the retina, distinguished from afterimage.

psychological i. Perceptual image.

Purkinje i's. Purkinje-Sanson images.

Purkinje-Sanson i's. The catoptric images of a light source, produced by reflection from the anterior and the posterior surfaces of the cornea and the crystalline lens.

pursuant i. of von Kries. Second positive afterimage.

real i. An optical image that can be received on a screen; one formed by the meeting of converging rays of light.

recurrent i's. A succession of afterimages following the primary image.

retinal i. The image formed on the retina by the refracting system of the eye.

reversed i. Inverted image.

satellite i. of Hamaker. Second positive afterimage.

schlieren i. The image formed by a schlieren optical system, consisting essentially of two components, one represented in the illumination of the field and the silhouette of opaque objects, and the other represented by intensity gradations resulting from refractive index gradients in the schlieren field.

shell i. See under *shell*

space i. The image of an object perceived through a binocular instrument. **homeomorphous s.i.** A space image which duplicates the object in shape but may differ in size. **hyper-**

plastic s.i. A space image in which the depth dimensions are greater in proportion to the frontal dimensions than those of the object. **hypoplastic s.i.** A space image in which the depth dimensions are less in proportion to the frontal dimensions than those of the object. **orthoplastic s.i.** A space image in which the ratio between depth and frontal dimensions exactly duplicates that of the object. **porrhallactic s.i.** A space image which does not duplicate the shape of the object. **tautomorphous s.i.** A space image which exactly duplicates the real object in all dimensions when a pair of stereophotographs of the object are viewed in a stereoscope.

specular i. An image produced by regular reflection.

stereoscopic i. A single perceptual image resulting from sensory fusion of the two ocular images, so as to induce the attribute of depth, solidity, or the third dimension.

total i. The single image perceived in simultaneous binocular vision.

true i. The image associated with the normally fixating eye in strabismus.

virtual i. An optical image that cannot be received on a screen; one formed by the backward prolongation of diverging rays to the point of apparent origin. Syn., *apparent image.*

visual i. 1. A mental picture based on the recall of a previous visual experience. 2. A perceptual image. 3. A visual hallucination.

window i. The image of a window or other object formed by reflection from the surface of the cornea.

◆

image plane. See under *plane.*
image point. See under *point.*
image ray. See under *ray.*
imagery (im'ij-re, -er-e). 1. The process of recalling actual past visual experiences. 2. Images taken collectively.

eidetic i. The process of recalling actual past visual experiences with marked clearness, apparent realness, and accuracy of detail, often demonstrated or experienced by children.

imbalance. Lack of balance.

binocular i. An inequality in some aspect of binocular vision, such as *anisometropia, aniseikonia, heterophoria,* or *strabismus.*

muscular i. The condition of either heterophoria or strabismus. **compound m.i.** A combination of lateral and vertical muscular imbalance. **lateral m.i.** Esophoria, exophoria, or convergent or divergent strabismus. **vertical m.i.** Hyperphoria, hypophoria, hypertropia, or hypotropia.

ocular i. Binocular imbalance.

imbecile (im'be-sil). A person who has imbecility.

imbecility (im″be-sil'ih-te). One of the three major grades of mental deficiency which describes those persons incapable of managing themselves or their affairs with ordinary prudence. On the basis of intelligence tests, it includes those persons who have IQ scores between 25 and 50. Cf. *idiocy; moronity.*

Imbert-Fick (im'bert-fik) **formula; law.** See under the nouns.

imperception (im-per-sep'shun). Defective perception.

impingement. The energy reaching a sense organ, regardless of whether effective or not. A stimulus is an effective impingement.

implant. A material inserted or grafted into intact tissue, such as an inert filler placed in the eye socket in surgical enucleation, or in the scleral shell in evisceration, to replace the interior volume of the eyeball.

Allen's i. A hollow, half-sphere, buried orbital implant with holes in each quadrant near its flat face to receive the four rectus muscles.

anterior chamber i. A lens placed in the anterior chamber, at the pupillary aperture adjacent to the iris, to replace the crystalline lens following cataract surgery. Syn., *anterior chamber lens; lenticulus.*

Arruga's i. An integrated orbital implant completely buried at the time of surgery with its one or two pegs at its summit covered by conjunctiva. Each peg erodes through the conjunctiva soon after surgery, at a site other than that of the original wound, and serves as an attachment for an artificial eye.

attached i. An implant attached directly to the extraocular muscles, but not directly to the artificial eye.

Binkhorst i. Iris clip lens.

Boberg-Ans i. A form of the Strampelli lens in which the plate to which the lens is secured is modified in shape and fenestrated.

buried i. An orbital implant which is completely covered with Tenon's capsule and conjunctiva.

Choyce i. Any of several anterior chamber implants designed by Choyce.

Cogan i. A modified form of the Strampelli lens in which the plate to which the lens is secured is fenestrated.

corneal i. A lens made of transparent inert material which is placed in the cornea in lieu of tissue transplantation. Syn., *keratoprosthesis*. **mushroom c.i.** A small, mushroom-shaped plastic lens used in combination with a lamellar corneal graft. The pedicle is placed through a central perforation of the cornea, its base extending into the anterior chamber, and the lamellar graft is sutured over its head.

Cutler's i. A semiburied implant consisting of a half-sphere of plastic surmounted with tantalum mesh, with a rectangular plastic peg protruding from its summit. The rectus muscles are attached to the mesh and covered with Tenon's capsule and conjunctiva, with the peg serving as attachment to the artificial eye.

Dannheim i. Dannheim lens.

Epstein i. Epstein lens.

external fixation i. An anterior chamber implant consisting of a convex lens held in position by loops of nylon filament which are passed through superior and inferior limbal incisions whereby it is fixed to the external surface of the sclera.

eyelid i. An acrylic or silicone implant placed in the upper eyelid to fill an area which is hollow due to surgery.

integrated i. An implant attached directly to both the artificial eye and the extraocular muscles.

intrascleral i. An implant inserted into the scleral cavity after evisceration of the eye.

Iowa i. A buried orbital implant having four mounds on its anterior face. The rectus muscles are sutured to the front of the implant with each muscle lying in a hollow between two mounds.

magnetic i. An orbital implant containing a magnet for holding the artificial eye.

mesh i. An orbital implant containing metal mesh to which the rectus muscles are sutured.

Mules's sphere i. A spherical implant with no direct attachment to either the artificial eye or the extraocular muscles.

orbital i. An inert filler placed in the eye socket in surgical enucleation, or in the scleral shell in evisceration, to replace the interior volume of the eyeball. Tenon's capsule and the conjunctiva are usually sutured over it.

posterior chamber i. A lens placed in the posterior chamber, between the iris and posterior lens capsule, in the approximate position of the removed crystalline lens, following cataract surgery. Syn., *posterior chamber lens*.

Roper-Hall i. A buried orbital implant in the shape of a hollow hemisphere with a magnet in its summit and a hole in each quadrant to receive the rectus muscles.

scleral i. A substance embedded into the sclera, usually for the purpose of impressing the choroid toward the retina for the repair of a retinal detachment.

semiburied i. An orbital implant, a portion of which is not covered with conjunctiva, thus affording a means of attachment to an artificial eye.

sponge i. A buried orbital implant consisting of polyvinyl sponge, on the front of which are sutured the rectus muscles.

Strampelli i. Strampelli lens.

subconjunctival i. An orbital implant completely covered by the conjunctiva; a buried orbital implant.

Torres-Ruiz i. Torres-Ruiz lens.

tunnel i. An orbital implant containing apertures through which the rectus muscles are placed.

vitreous i. A substance injected into the vitreous chamber to replace or supplement the vitreous humor.

impletion (im-ple'shun). A filling out, such as the normal lack of awareness of the physiological blind spot or of a sensory gap in a pattern that traverses it.

impression. 1. A perceptor effect produced on the mind by sensory stimuli. 2. A mold.

absolute i. The perceived magnitude of one of the psychological dimensions (such as intensity) of a singly presented stimulus.

visual i. An impression activated by visual stimuli. **homeomorphous v.i.** Orthoplastic visual impression.

hyperplastic v.i. An exaggerated or enhanced impression or percept of relief or relative distance. **hypoplastic v.i.** A diminished or reduced impression or percept of relief or relative distances. **orthoplastic v.i.** A quantitatively correct impression or percept of relief or relative distances. Syn., *homeomorphous visual impression.*

incandescence (in″kan-des′ens). The glowing or radiation of visible energy by a body, produced by heat.

inch. A unit of length.

    Austrian i. A unit of length equal to 26.34 mm, used in the specification of focal length of early lenses.

    English i. A unit of length equal to 25.4 mm; used in the USA.

    Parisian i. A unit of length equal to 27.07 mm, used by Donders in specifying focal power.

    Prussian i. A unit of length equal to 26.15 mm, used in the specification of focal length of early lenses.

incidence, grazing. The limiting direction of the incidence of a ray traveling from a less dense to a more dense optical medium along the interface between the two media, representing the largest angle of incidence from which a refracted ray will result.

inclinometer (in″klih-nom′eh-ter). An instrument for measuring or determining angles or inclinations, e.g., the axes of astigmatism.

incomitance (in-kom′ih-tans). Noncomcomitance.

incomitancy (in-kom-ih-tan′se). Nonconcomitance.

incomitant (in-kom′ih-tant). Nonconcomitant.

incongruity, retinal (in″kong-gru′ih-te). 1. The lack of correspondence, in the two retinae, of the anatomical positions of sensory receptors which do correspond in visual direction. 2. A normal condition in which the nasal and temporal halves of the retina do not contain the same number or distribution of receptor elements.

incontinentia pigmenti (in-kon″tih-nen′she-ah pig-men′ti). Infantile pigmentary dermatosis occurring in either of two forms, one characterized by slate-gray cutaneous pigmentation in reticular formation which occurs at about two years of age without ocular involvement, the other characterized by patches of wavy streaks of slate-gray cutaneous pigmentation and ocular anomalies in about one fourth of cases (*Bloch-Sulzberger syndrome,* q.v.).

incyclofusion (in-si″klo-fu′zhun). Relative rotation of the two eyes around their respective anteroposterior axes or response to a cyclofusional stimulus, so that the upward extensions of the vertical meridians rotate nasalward.

incyclophoria (in-si″klo-fo′re-ah). The turning, or the amount of turning, of the two eyes relative to each other around their respective anteroposterior axes or lines of sight, as manifested in the absence of an adequate fusion stimulus, so that elongations of their respective vertical meridians of reference cross superiorly, i.e., above the horizontal plane of the eyes. Syn., *minus cyclophoria; encyclophoria.*

incyclotropia (in-si″klo-tro′pe-ah). The turning, or the amount of turning, of the two eyes relative to each other around their respective anteroposterior axes or lines of sight, as manifested in the presence or the absence of a fusion stimulus, so that elongations of their respective vertical meridians of reference cross superiorly, i.e., above the horizontal plane of the eyes. Syn., *encyclotropia.*

incyclovergence (in-si″klo-ver′jens). The turning, or the amount of turning, of the two eyes with respect to each other around their respective anteroposterior axes, so as to converge the upward extensions of the vertical meridians of reference. Syn., *encyclovergence.*

index. The ratio, or the formula expressing the ratio, of one measurement to another.

    i. of absorption. The constant κ (kappa) in the expression for the exponential reduction in intensity of light passing through an absorbing medium:

$$I = I_0 e^{-\frac{4\pi n\kappa}{\lambda} x}$$

where n is the refractive index of the medium, and x is the distance traversed. The expression is more usually stated as

$$I = I_0 e^{-ax}$$

where a, the *coefficient of absorption*, is defined as

$$a = \frac{4\pi n\kappa}{\lambda}$$

alpha i. The percentage of time the alpha rhythm shows on an electroencephalographic record.

Arden i. The highest potential attained in an electro-oculogram when the subject is in the light divided by the lowest potential achieved in the dark, multiplied by 100 to express in percentage. Syn., *Arden ratio.*

blackout i. The time the brain is deprived of visual stimuli during a blink, divided by the frequency of occurrence of the blink. Normally, visual stimuli are absent 0.3 sec. each 2.8 sec. or 10.7% of the time. **modified b.i.** A blackout index which considers the periods of unreliable vision immediately before and after the blink, as well as the time the brain is deprived of visual stimuli during the blink. Normally this period lasts 0.55 sec. each 2.8 sec. or 19.6% of the time.

i. of blur. A measure of blur which can be applied to a line, point, or contrast border. As applied to the spread function for a border, it represents the ratio of the difference in luminance on the two sides of the border to the slope of the line connecting the points representing 25% and 75% of the difference between the two levels.

i. of blurredness. The visual angle of the bar width of a test character for which increase of the bar width does not reduce the threshold visibility of the character.

Broca's orbital i. The ratio of the height to the breadth of the orbital entrance, multiplied by 100.

cephalic i. The ratio of the breadth to the length of the skull, multiplied by 100.

discrimination i. Discrimination factor.

extraordinary i. In a double refracting medium, the index of refraction for the extraordinary ray.

optical i. The index of refraction.

orbital i. Broca's orbital index.

orbitonasal i. The ratio of the sum of two lines each extending from the front point of the outer edge of one of the orbits to the lowest point on the root of the nose, to the direct distance between the two orbital points, multiplied by 100; hence, a ratio denoting the relative projection of the root of the nose anterior to the plane of the eye orbits.

position i. A mathematical value, P, representing the angular separation of the light source from the subject's line of sight in the Luckiesh-Guth empirical equation describing the relationship of the angular separation to functions of the solid angle of subtense, the BCD brightness of the source, and functions of the field brightness.

reading efficiency i. The rate of words read per minute, multiplied by the percentage of comprehension.

i. of refraction. The ratio of the speed of light in vacuum, air, or other medium of reference, to the speed of light in a given medium, obtained by Snell's law as the ratio of the sine of the angle of incidence to the sine of the angle of refraction, and usually designated by the letter n. Syn., *optical index.* **absolute i. of r.** The ratio of the speed of light in vacuum to the speed of light in a given medium. **mean i. of r.** The index of refraction determined for a line of the spectrum which lies midway between two spectral lines of reference. **relative i. of r.** The ratio of the speed of light in a medium of reference other than vacuum to the speed of light in a given medium.

indicator. 1. An apparatus or a device which indicates or points out, such as a gauge or a dial. 2. A chemical substance which indicates, usually by color change, the condition, such as acid or alkaline, of a solution, or the end points of reactions.

Berens-Tolman Ocular Hypertension I. A tonometer designed for glaucoma screening which indicates ocular tension as being above or below 20 mm Hg.

Helmholtz' i. An instrument for the detection and differentiation of palsies of the cyclomotor muscles, consisting of a vertical card marked with a horizontal line with a spot at its center and supported on a horizontal rod, the proximal end of which is held in the patient's teeth so that tilting movements of the head are communicated to the card. The relative tilt and displacement of the two images of the line seen in diplopia indicate the character of the palsy.

muscle i. An instrument designed by Savage to show the interrelationship of muscle action to monocular and binocular eye movements, consisting of a metal ring on which are mounted a pair of mechanical schematic eyes with telescoping rods for visual axes which meet at a variable fixation point on the metal ring. The centers of rotation of the mechanical eyes are on the ring, and the ring can be tilted around a cord connecting the centers of rotation of the eyes.

Prentice's phoria i. A phoria measuring instrument consisting of a vertical row and a horizontal row of transilluminated green disks seen by one eye, and a single transilluminated red disk seen by the other eye through a red filter or a Maddox rod.

indigo (in'dih-go). 1. The hue attribute of visual sensation typically evoked by stimulation of the normal human eye with radiation of wavelengths approximately 436 mμ. 2. A color of the visible spectrum between the blue and the violet wavelengths.

induction (in-duk'shun). 1. The act or process of bringing in, initiating, or introducing. 2. Arousal by indirect stimulation.

color i. The modification of response to a color stimulus, due either to simultaneous perception of another color in a neighboring area or to a previous retinal excitation.

mutual i. The mutual modification of response to adjacent fields simultaneously stimulating the eye through the process of spatial induction.

spatial i. The modification of response to a part of the visual field, occasioned by simultaneous stimulation from another part of the visual field. Syn., *surface induction*.

successive i. Temporal induction.

surface i. Spatial induction.

temporal i. The modification of response to a stimulus, occasioned by a preceding stimulus. Syn., *successive induction*.

infiltration, peripheral annular (in-fil-tra'shun). A ring abscess.

infinity, optical (in-fin'ih-te). 1. The location of an optical image at infinity, so that rays emerging from a given point on the image are parallel. 2. Clinically, a test object distance great enough to be considered equivalent to infinity for certain test purposes, usually 20 ft or 6 m.

informative sequence. *Optometric Extension Program*: A group of clinical visual test findings systematically tabulated in reference to norms or to each other, for purposes of diagnosing the visual condition.

infradextroversion (in"frah-deks-tro-ver'zhun). Conjugate rotation of the eyes, downward and to the right.

infraduction (in"frah-duk'shun). 1. The downward rotation of an eye. 2. In vertical divergence testing, the downward rotation of one eye with respect to the other in response to increases in baseup prism, or the equivalent. Syn., *deorsumduction; subduction*.

infralevoversion (in"frah-leh-vo-ver'zhun). Conjugate rotation of the eyes, downward and to the left.

infraorbital (in"frah-ōr'bih-tal). Situated beneath or on the floor of the orbit.

infrared (in-frah-red'). Radiant energy of wavelengths longer than light or visible radiant energy, generally including 770 mμ to more than 50 μ.

infravergence (in-frah-ver'jens). The downward rotation of an eye, the other eye remaining stationary. Syn., *deorsumvergence*.

infraversion (in-frah-ver'shun). Conjugate rotation of the eyes downward. Syn., *deorsumversion; subversion*.

infula (in'fu-lah). A horizontal band of specialized retina extending through the fovea of certain birds, such as winchats, geese, or swans, which provides acute vision.

inheritance. The acquisition or the reception of characteristics or qualities by transmission from parent to offspring.

autosomal i. The hereditary mechanism in which the genes are located in any pair of chromosomes other than the sex (X and Y) chromosomes.

polygenic i. The hereditary mechanism in which more than a single locus on a pair of chromosomes determines the trait. Two or more loci and two or more sets of genes are involved. Refractive errors and eye color are now believed to be so inherited.

sex-linked i. The hereditary mechanism in which the genes involved are located in the sex (X or Y) chromosomes.

inhibition. 1. The act of holding back, restraining, or hindering. 2. A stopping, restraining, or arrest of the action of an organ, a nerve reflex, a cell, or a chemical. 3. A restraining of one physical activity by another.

i. of accommodation. The reduction or prevention, or the effecting of reduction or prevention, of accommodation or of the stimulus to accommodation.

i. of convergence. The reduction or prevention, or the effecting of reduction or prevention, of convergence or of the stimulus to convergence.

Hering-type i. Hering phenomenon.

lateral i. Neural pathway inhibition between spatially separated regions on the eye. **nonrecurrent l.i.** Lateral inhibition with its site of action neurally subsequent to its site of origin. **reciprocal l.i.** Lateral inhibition in which each stimulated receptive facet of the eye influences the other. **recurrent l.i.** Lateral inhibition with its site of action neurally preceding its site of origin, as in negative feedback.

reciprocal i. The phase or portion of the reciprocal innervation pattern producing inhibition of the antagonist muscle.

retinal i. Inhibition of response (to visual stimuli) occurring as a function of, or in, the retina, as distinguished from inhibition at higher or more central levels.

Wedensky i. Failure of the lateral geniculate body to conduct more than six impulses when the optic nerve is subjected to a long train of electric shocks in the frequency range from 150 to 600 per second.

injection. Increased redness of an area due to dilatation and engorgement of the small blood vessels of the region, e.g., in conjunctivitis.

ciliary i. A pinkish area around the limbus of the eye caused by dilatation of small, deeply seated blood vessels which appear to radiate from the cornea, seen in diseases of the cornea, the iris, and the ciliary body. Syn., *circumcorneal injection.*

circumcorneal i. Ciliary injection.

conjunctival i. A diffuse, brick-red discoloration of the conjunctiva fading toward the limbus, due to congestion of the superficial conjunctival vessels.

scleral i. A diffuse, purplish redness of the sclera, sometimes localized, due to a congestion of the deep vessels.

innervation, reciprocal (in-er-va'-shun). Innervation which simultaneously stimulates an agonist and inhibits its antagonist.

Inouye's (in'oo-yēz) **cubes; disk.** See under the nouns.

insectorubin (in-sek-to'ru-bin). Pig-

ments of unknown composition and function found in the eyes of insects.

insertion, foot-plate. An abnormal tendon insertion of an extraocular muscle extending posteriorly a greater distance than normal, although correctly positioned from the limbus both in distance and direction.

insertion, secondary. An abnormal tendon insertion of an extraocular muscle in which fibers leave the main tendon and attach farther back.

inset. The nasalward displacement of the segment of a multifocal lens with respect to the mechanical center or other reference point or line in the lens.

insistence. The power of a bright or highly saturated colored region of the visual field to gain attention and fixation. Cf. *target valve.*

instability, binocular. Difficulty in the maintenance of clear, single, binocular vision, attributed to deficiencies in motor or sensory fusion.

instinct, binocular. A presumed inborn tendency to use the two eyes as a single unit for the attainment of single, binocular vision.

Institut et Centre d'Optometrie. A nonprofit foundation at Bures-sur-Yvette, France, which provides preparatory, correspondence, and continuing education programs and facilities for optometrists.

Institut d'Optique Raymond Tibaut. A school for the training of opticians-optometrists founded in 1925 in Brussels by l'Association Professionnelle des Opticiens de Belgique and registered as a national institute in 1938, offering courses in Flemish and French. Syn., Flemish: *Instituut voor Optica Raymond Tibaut.*

instrument, optical. A single mirror, prism, or lens, or a combination of such elements, together with the mountings, stops, and diaphragms, which refracts, reflects, or in some way alters the incident light or its path.

insufficiency. The state or quality of being incompetent, unfit, deficient, or inadequate.

i. of accommodation. See under *accommodation.*

i. of convergence. See under *convergence.*

i. of divergence. See under *divergence.*

i. of the externi. 1. Paralysis or paresis of the external rectus muscles.

2. Presumed relative insufficiency of the external rectus muscles in relation to the internal rectus muscles, in cases of esophoria or low divergence ability.

i. of the eyelids. A condition in which a conscious effort is required to close the eyelids.

i. of the interni. 1. Paralysis or paresis of the internal rectus muscles. 2. Presumed relative insufficiency of the internal rectus muscles in relation to the external rectus muscles, in cases of exophoria or low convergence ability.

integral, Fourier's. A mathematical expression for any arbitrary, non-periodic, waveform in terms of the frequency distribution of the amplitude of component waves differing only by infinitesimal increments of wavelength.

integrals, Fresnel. Integrals, derived by Fresnel, which represent the x and y co-ordinates of Cornu's spiral.

integration, binocular. 1. Sensory fusion. 2. The organization of a binocular percept as a function of two monocular stimuli or percepts.

intensity. 1. The state, quality, or condition of being intense. 2. A specific measure of the effect of a physical agent such as light.

luminous i. In a given direction, the ratio of the luminous flux emitted by a source, or by an element of a source, in an infinitesimal cone containing this direction, to the solid angle of this cone; luminous flux per unit solid angle in a given direction. Symbol: I. Unit: *candela*.

radiant i. Radiant energy emitted per unit time, per unit solid angle about the direction considered, expressed in watts per steradian. Symbol: J.

specific i. Radiant intensity expressed for a specific source or element of a source.

interaction, contour (in"ter-ak'shun). The phenomenon of decrease or enhancement in vision performance (such as visual acuity, brightness, or color) induced by the proximity or juxtaposition of one or more contours in the visual field.

intercept, focal (in'ter-sept). The focal length or the focal distance of a lens or lens system.

intercilium (in"ter-sil'e-um). The space between the eyebrows. Syn., *glabella*.

interface. A plane or surface forming a common boundary between two optical media.

interference. 1. The act or process of interposing or intervening. 2. The phenomenon of modification of light intensity due to the combined effect, or mutual action, of two or more coherent trains of light waves superposed at the same instant at the same point in space.

constructive i. Interference in which trains of light waves are superposed in such phase relationship that they mutually aid or enhance each other.

contour i. 1. The perceptual covering or overlapping of the contour or border of an object in space by a nearer object, or the simulation of this effect in a drawing or photograph; one of the clues to depth perception. 2. Border suppression.

destructive i. Interference in which the trains of light waves are superposed in such phase relationship that they partially or completely neutralize or destroy each other.

multiple-beam i. Interference resulting from parts of a beam of light being reflected several times back and forth between a pair of reflecting surfaces prior to being reflected or transmitted from the pair.

selective i. Interference in which specific wavelengths of light are enhanced or neutralized, producing a considerable variation in light intensity throughout the spectrum.

interferogram (in"ter-fēr'o-gram). A reproducible recording of an interference pattern.

interferometer (in"ter-fēr-om'eh-ter). An instrument providing for the adjustable superposition of two coherent beams of light for constructive and destructive interference, and thus useful in measuring wavelength of light, small distances and thicknesses, and optical surface quality.

Burch i. An interferometer used to test large aperture optical systems in which interference is produced by a pair of identical scattering plates of random surface structure, one of which is optically superimposed on the other at the center of curvature of the reflecting surface under test, or at one of the conjugate foci of a system. The image path of one plate suffers wave distortions by reflection or refraction at the test surfaces and recombines to form interference patterns with the undisturbed image path of the other plate.

Dyson i. An instrument used for testing optical systems in which birefringent crystals are used to produce two interfering beams polarized at right angles to each other and subsequently brought into coincidence with a quarter wave plate.

Fabry-Pérot i. An interferometer in which interference fringes are produced in the transmitted light after multiple reflection in the air film between two plane plates thinly silvered on the inner surfaces.

Fizeau i. An interferometer with two parallel slits immediately behind an object lens so that the maximum and minimum of two equally bright fringe systems of a double star of a given diameter coincide to form a uniform band, thus measuring the star's angular diameter.

Jamin i. An interferometer for the measurement of the index of refraction of gases which utilizes interference fringes produced by reflection from two plane-parallel plates inclined at a slight angle to each other. (See Fig. 24.)

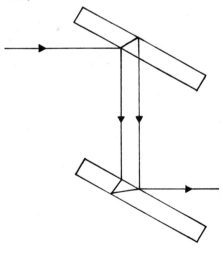

Fig. 24 Jamin interferometer.

Lummer-Gehrcke i. An instrument used to study spectrum lines in which interference is produced by multiple reflections from a pair of parallel reflecting surfaces at a fixed separation, and where the angles of incidence are large enough to produce total internal reflection, thereby eliminating the need for reflection coatings.

Michelson's i. An interferometer in which light from an extended source is divided into two beams by partial reflection. The two beams travel in different directions and are recombined after reflection from plane mirrors, to form interference fringes.

multiple-beam i. An interferometer such as the Fizeau or Fabry-Pérot in which a beam of light is reflected back and forth several times between a pair of parallel plane surfaces.

Rayleigh i. An instrument for the measurement of index of refraction of gases, which uses two interference beams formed by a double slit placed in front of a collimating lens. A reference diffraction pattern from one beam is compared to the lateral shift in the other beam which passes through the gas medium.

stellar i. An optical interferometer attached to a telescope for measuring interference rings at the telescope focus and used for determining the angular diameter of stars.

Twyman and Green i. A modification of the Michelson interferometer in which the illumination is parallel monochromatic light produced by a point light source at the principal focus of a corrected lens. It is used for testing the perfection of prisms and lenses.

interferometry (in"ter-fĕr-om'eh-tre). The study, measurement, utilization, and production of wave interference and interaction phenomena.

internal rectus (in-ter'nal rek'tus). See under *muscle.*

International Association of Boards of Examiners in Optometry. An association of boards of optometric examiners of the United States and Canada, founded in 1913 as the International Board of Boards and reorganized under the present title in 1919.

International Association of Optometric Executives. An association of persons holding administrative, executive and managerial positions in organizations, associations, and agencies serving or representing optometrists or optometric functions, founded in 1950 to provide continuing education in managerial skills for its members.

International Commission on Illumination. See *Commission Internationale de l'Eclairage* (CIE).

International Library, Archives, and Museum of Optometry, Inc. A corporate affiliate of the American Optometric Association formed in 1973, the successor to the Library of the Physiological Section of the Association established in 1902, to provide staff, facilities, and support for the development, maintenance, and cataloging of the archival, library, and museum collections for professional and public use.

International Optical League. See *International Optometric and Optical League.*

International Optometric and Optical League. An organization for many years called the International Optical League, founded in 1927 and cooperatively sustained by member organizations of various nationally and regionally recognized groups of optometrists and optometric institutions in many countries.

internus (in-ter'nus). Internal rectus muscle.

interocular (in"ter-ok'u-lar). Between the eyes.

interorbital (in"ter-ōr'bih-tal). Between the orbits.

interpalpebral (in"ter-pal'pe-bral). Between the eyelids.

interposition (in"ter-po-zish'un). The position of an object between another object and an observer, or the simulation of this effect in a drawing or a photograph so that contour interference results. Syn., *overlay.*

interpretation, visual. The involvement of meaning in a visually sensed situation.

interpupillary (in"ter-pu'pih-lār-e). Between the pupils.

interpupillary distance (in"ter-pu'pih-lār-e dis'tans). See *distance, pupillary.*

intersect, sighting. The point of intersection of the lines of sight for various directions of gaze of an eye.

Inter-Society Color Council. A federation founded in 1931 of 30 national societies and various individuals concerned with all aspects of color.

interval. 1. A period of time between two events or between the recurrence of similar states or conditions. 2. A space between objects or things. 3. A range or a gap between different states or qualities.

    achromatic i. A range of low degrees of light intensity which produces visual sensation but not color sensation; the range between the absolute threshold for light perception and the threshold for hue. Syn., *colorless interval; photochromatic interval.*

    astigmatic i. Interval of Sturm.

    class i. In statistics, a range of continuous values considered as being in a single numerical class, e.g., ages 5 to 9 may be in one group, ages 10 to 14 in another, etc.

    colorless i. Achromatic interval.

    corneal i. The site of the cornea considered as an interruption of the most anterior portion of the scleral tissue. Syn., *anterior scleral foramen; corneal foramen; rima cornealis.*

    focal i. 1. Interval of Sturm. 2. The distance from the anterior to the posterior principal focus of a lens or an optical system.

    hyperfocal i. The linear distance between the focus of the paraxial rays and the focus of the peripheral rays of a lens or an optical system.

    lucid i. of Vogt. The peripheral, clear zone of the cornea, located between the limbus and the circular opacity in arcus senilis.

    photochromatic i. Achromatic interval.

    i. of Sturm. The linear distance between the two focal lines of an astigmatic eye or optical system. Syn., *astigmatic interval; focal interval.*

intorsion (in-tōr'shun). 1. The real or apparent turning of the two eyes relative to each other and around their respective anteroposterior axes, so that the upward extensions of their respective vertical meridians of reference converge toward each other. 2. The real or apparent turning of an eye around an anteroposterior axis, so that the upward extension of its vertical meridian of reference rotates nasally from the true vertical.

intort (in-tōrt'). To turn toward a position of intorsion or away from a position of extorsion.

intorter (in'tōr-ter). An extraocular muscle which acts to intort the eye.

intraciliary (in"trah-sil'e-er-e). Within the region of the ciliary body.

intraocular (in"trah-ok'u-lar). Within the eye.

intraocular (in"trah-ok'-u-lar) **modification; pressure; tension.** See under the nouns.

intraorbital (in"tra-ōr'bih-tal). Within the orbit.

intraretinal (in"trah-ret'ih-nal). Within the retina.

intrascleral (in"trah-skler'al). Within the sclera.

intravitreous (in"trah-vit're-us). Within the vitreous humor.

invariant, optical (in-va'rih-ant). The product of the index of refraction and the sine of the angle between a ray and the normal before or after refraction at a surface.

inversion. 1. In an optical image, the reversal of orientation with respect to the conjugate object, i.e., upside down and left to right. 2. In space perception, the reversal of the perceived object with respect to its normal orientation, i.e., upside down and left to right, as when viewed through an inverting optical system. 3. The reversal of written characters, as in mirror writing. 4. The nasalward rotation of the eye.

inversion of the disk. A congenital anomaly in which the retinal vessels emerge from the temporal side of the optic disk and then course nasally.

invisible. 1. Incapable of being seen. 2. Visually indistinguishable from the surrounding field.

iodopsin (i-o-dop'sin). A photosensitive substance considered to be in the retinal cones which subserves photopic vision, as does rhodopsin in the retinal rods for scotopic vision. It has not been isolated from the human retina, but has been extracted from the retina of the chicken.

ionophose (i'o-no-fōz"). A subjective sensation of violet light.

iontophoresis (i-on"to-fo-re'sis). The introduction of drugs in ionic form into superficial intact tissues by means of a low tension direct electric current. It may be accomplished on the eye by means of a nonconductive spectacle-type frame designed by Erlanger with a two-compartment eyecup, one compartment containing a dry cell and two electrodes and the other the dilute drug solution which contacts the cornea through an absorbent pad. One electrode leads to the drug solution and the other to the side of the head through the earpiece of the frame.

IOL. See *International Optometric and Optical League.*

IOOL. See *International Optometric and Optical League.*

IOP. Intraocular pressure.

IORT. See *Institut d'Optique Raymond Tibaut.* Flemish: Instituut voor Optica Raymond Tibaut.

IOT. Intraocular tension (measured clinically as with a tonometer).

ipsilateral (ip"se-lat'er-al). Situated on the same side.

iralgia (i-ral'je-ah). Iridalgia.

iridal (i'rid-al, ir'id-). Pertaining to the iris.

iridalgia (ir"id-al'je-ah, i"rid-). Pain in the iris.

iridallochrosis (ir"ih-dal-o-kro'sis). A pathological change in the color of the iris. *Obs.*

iridauxesis (ir"id-awk-se'sis). A thickening or a swelling of the iris.

iridavulsion (ir"id-ah-vul'shun). Iridoavulsion.

iridectomesodialysis (ir"id-ek"to-me-so-di-al'is-is). A surgical procedure for the formation of an artificial pupil by detaching and excising a portion of the iris at its periphery.

iridectomize (ir"id-ek'to-mīz). To remove a part of the iris by surgery.

iridectomy (ir"ih-dek'to-me). Surgical removal of part of the iris.

   antiphlogistic i. Surgical removal of a part of the iris to reduce intraocular pressure in inflammatory conditions of the eye.

   basal i. An iridectomy which includes the root of the iris.

   complete i. Sector iridectomy.

   optical i. Surgical removal of part of the iris to enlarge the existing pupil, or to form an artificial pupil, when the natural pupil is ineffectual.

   peripheral i. Surgical removal of a portion of the iris in the region of its root, leaving the pupillary margin and sphincter pupillae muscle intact.

   preliminary (preparatory) i. Surgical removal of part of the iris preceding cataract extraction.

   sector i. Surgical removal of a complete radial section of the iris extending from the pupillary margin to the root of the iris. Syn., *complete iridectomy; total iridectomy.*

   stenopeic i. Surgical removal of a narrow slit or a minute portion of the iris, leaving the sphincter pupillae muscle intact.

   therapeutic i. Surgical removal of a portion of the iris for the cure or prevention of an ocular disease.

   total i. Sector iridectomy.

iridectropium (ir″id-ek-tro′pe-um). Eversion of a portion of the iris.

iridelcosis (ir″ih-del′ko-sis). Ulceration of the iris. *Obs.*

iridemia (ir″id-e′me-ah, i″rid-). Hemorrhage from the iris.

iridencleisis (ir″ih-den-kli′sis). A surgical procedure for glaucoma, in which a portion of the iris is incised and incarcerated in a limbal incision.

iridentropium (ir″id-en-tro′pe-um). Inversion of a portion of the iris.

irideremia (ir″id-e-re′me-ah). Congenital absence of all or part of the iris.

irides (ir′id-ēz, i′rid-). The plural of iris.

iridescence (ir″ih-des′ens). The rainbowlike play of colors as in mother-of-pearl or soap bubbles. Syn., *schiller*.

iridescent (ir″ih-des′ent). Having or demonstrating iridescence.

iridesis (ir-id′e-sis, ir″ih-de′sis). A surgical procedure in which a portion of the iris is brought through and incarcerated in a corneal incision.

iridiagnosis. Iridodiagnosis.

iridic (i-rid′ik, ir-id′-). Pertaining to the iris.

iriditis (ir″ih-di′tis). Iritis.

iridization (ir″id-ih-za′shun). The perception of a rainbow-colored halo around bright lights, in glaucoma.

irido- (ir′id-o, i′rid-do). A combining form denoting the iris.

iridoallochrosis (ir″id-o-al-o-kro′sis). Iridallochrosis.

iridoavulsion (ir″id-o-ah-vul′shun). Complete tearing away of the iris from its peripheral attachments.

iridocapsulitis (ir″id-o-kap″su-li′tis). Inflammation of the iris and the capsule of the crystalline lens.

iridocele (ih-rid′o-sēl, ir′id-o-). Hernial protrusion of a portion of the iris through a wound or ulcer in the cornea.

iridochisma (ir″id-o-kis′mah). Iridoschisis.

iridochoroiditis (ir″id-o-ko″roid-i′tis). Inflammation of both the iris and the choroid.

iridocinesia (ir″id-o-sin-e′ze-ah). Iridokinesia.

iridocinesis (ir″id-o-sih-ne′sis). Iridokinesia.

iridocoloboma (ir″id-o-kol″o-bo′mah). Coloboma of the iris.

iridoconstrictor (ir″id-o-con-strik′tor). 1. Any of the elements of the short ciliary nerve fibers to the sphincter pupillae muscle. 2. Any chemical which causes constriction of the sphincter pupillae muscle. 3. The sphincter pupillae muscle.

iridocorneosclerectomy (ir″id-o-kōr″ne-o-skler-ek′to-me). The surgical removal of a portion of the iris, the cornea, and the sclera.

iridocyclectomy (ir″id-o-si-klek′tome). Surgical removal of the iris and the ciliary body.

iridocyclitis (ir″id-o-si-kli′tis, i-rid-o-). Inflammation of the iris and the ciliary body, usually characterized by ciliary flush, exudates into the anterior chamber, deposits on the posterior surface of the cornea and the anterior surface of the crystalline lens capsule, aqueous flare, constricted and sluggish pupil, discoloration of the iris, and the subjective symptoms of radiating pain, photophobia, lacrimation, and interference with vision.

> **exudative i.** A severe iridocyclitis characteristic of gonorrhea usually without corneal precipitates and characterized by profuse fibrinous exudation into the anterior chamber which forms a translucent gray gelatinous mass.

> **heterochromic i. of Fuchs.** Complicated heterochromia.

> **plastic i.** The most common and severe type of iridocyclitis characterized by plastic exudates into the anterior chamber which consist essentially of fibrinous matter especially prone to the formation of synechiae and by a virtual absence of keratic precipitates.

> **i. recidivans purulenta.** Behçet's disease.

> **sarcoidal i.** See *sarcoidosis*.

> **i. septica.** Behçet's disease.

> **syphilitic i.** Iridocyclitis occurring in syphilis, especially that characterized by yellowish or pinkish nodules on the iris (roseola of the iris) or by fulminating exudates or hemorrhage.

> **tubercular i.** Iridocyclitis occurring in tuberculosis in either of two forms: (1) the miliary form characterized by the absence of marked vascular engorgement, and the presence of mutton fat keratic precipitates and small nodules (Koeppe's nodules) on the iris; or (2) the conglomerate form characterized by a single, yellowish-gray mass on the ciliary zone of the iris with keratic precipitates.

iridocyclochoroiditis (ir″id-o-si″klo-ko-roid-i′tis). Inflammation of the iris, the ciliary body, and the choroid; uveitis.

iridocystectomy (ir″id-o-sis-tek′to-me). Surgical removal of a portion of the iris to form an artificial pupil.

iridodesis (ir″id-od′e-sis). Iridesis.

iridodiagnosis (ir″id-o-di″ag-no′sis). 1. Diagnosis of systemic disease by the appearance of the iris. 2. Determination of personality traits by examining the structure of the iris.

iridodialysis (ir″id-o-di-al′is-is). A localized separation or tearing away of the iris from its attachment to the ciliary body.

iridodiastasis (ir″id-o-di-as′tah-sis). A colobomatous defect of the iris at its ciliary border.

iridodilator (ir″id-o-di-la′tor). 1. Any of the elements of the sympathetic ciliary nerve fibers innervating the dilator pupillae muscle. 2. Any chemical which causes constriction of the dilator pupillae muscle. 3. The dilator pupillae muscle.

iridodonesis (ir″id-o-do-ne′sis). Tremulousness of the iris, as may occur when the crystalline lens is absent or subluxated.

iridokeratitis (ir″id-o-ker-ah-ti′tis). Inflammation of both the iris and the cornea.

iridokinesia (ir″id-o-kih-ne′ze-ah). The expansion and contraction of the iris, normal or otherwise.

iridokinesis (ir″id-o-kih-ne′sis). Iridokinesia.

iridokinetic (ir″id-o-kih-net′ik). Pertaining to the expansion and contraction of the iris.

iridoleptynsis (ir″id-o-lep-tin′sis). Attenuation or atrophy of the iris.

iridology (ir″ih-dol′o-je). The study of the structure, markings, and color of the iris for the purpose of iridodiagnosis.

iridomalacia (ir″id-o-mah-la′she-ah). Degeneration or softening of the iris as a result of disease.

iridomedialysis (ir″id-o-me-di-al′is-is). Iridomesodialysis.

iridomesodialysis (ir″id-o-me″so-di-al′is-is). The loosening of adhesions of the inner border of the iris.

iridomotor (ir″id-o-mo′tor). Pertaining to movements of the iris.

iridoncosis (ir″ih-don-ko′sis). Swelling of the iris.

iridoncus (ir″ih-don′kus). Tumefaction of the iris.

iridonesis (ir″ih-don-e′sis). Iridodonesis.

iridoparalysis (ir″id-o-pah-ral′is-is). Paralysis of the iris; iridoplegia.

iridoparelkysis (ir″id-o-par-el′kis-is). An induced prolapse of the iris to displace the pupil artificially.

iridoparesis (ir″id-o-pah-re′sis, -par′es-is). Partial paralysis of the iris.

iridoperiphakitis (ir″id-o-per″e-fah-ki′tis). Inflammation of the iris and the capsule of the crystalline lens.

iridoplania (ir″id-o-pla′ne-ah). Iridodonesis.

iridoplegia (ir″id-o-ple′je-ah). Partial or total immobility or rigidity of the iris.

   accommodative i. Failure of the sphincter pupillae muscle of the iris to contract in association with accommodation.

   complete i. Total paralysis of the iris; failure of the iris to respond to any stimulation.

   reflex i. Absence of the pupillary light reflex.

   sympathetic i. Failure of the pupil to dilate on irritation of the skin.

   i. traumatica. Paralysis of the iris as a result of trauma.

iridoptosis (ir″id-op-to′sis). Prolapse of the iris.

iridopupillary (ir″id-o-pu′pih-ler″e). Pertaining to the iris and the pupil.

iridorhexis (ir″id-o-rek′sis). 1. Rupture of the iris. 2. The tearing away of the iris from its attachment or from an adhesion.

iridoschisis (ir″id-os′ke-sis). Separation of the anterior layers of the iris from the posterior layers and multiple rupture of the iris fibers. Fibers, which remain attached only at the ciliary body and at the sphincter, bulge forward, and the ends of those torn in two float forward into the aqueous. The posterior layer is usually intact and the sphincter and dilator fibers function normally. It usually occurs in the lower half of the iris in those over 65 years of age, with senile atrophy considered a major cause.

iridoschisma (ir″id-o-skiz′mah). A simple coloboma occurring in the iris in the presence of a normally closed fetal fissure.

iridosclerectomy (ir″id-o-skle-rek′to-me). The surgical removal of a portion of the sclera and of a portion of the iris in the region of the limbus, for the treatment of glaucoma.

iridosclerotomy (ir″id-o-skle-rot′o-me). The surgical puncture of the sclera and the margin of the iris, in glaucoma.

iridoscope (ir″id′o-skōp). A type of ophthalmoscope.

iridosis (ir″ih-do′sis). Iridesis.

iridosteresis (ir″id-o-ste-re′sis). Loss or absence of all or part of the iris.

iridotasis (ir″ih-dot′ah-sis). A surgical procedure for glaucoma in which the iris is stretched and drawn into a limbal incision, where it is incarcerated.

iridotomy (ir″ih-dot′o-me). An incision into the iris.

  peripheral i. An incision into the ciliary zone of the iris.

  radial i. A meridional incision into the iris.

iridotromos (ir″ih-dot′ro-mos). Iridodonesis.

iridovalosis (ir″id-o-val-o′sis). A condition in which the pupil is oval-shaped.

irin (i′rin). A chemical extracted from iris tissue which, when instilled into the eye, causes marked constriction of the iris which cannot be blocked by atropine or any other similarly acting drug. It is thought to be released by sensory nerve fiber endings in the iris through an axon reflex upon traumatizing the iris or the cornea, or stroking the trigeminal nerve.

irinic (i-rin′ik). Pertaining to or of the iris.

iris (i′ris). The most anterior portion of the uveal tract, consisting of a circular pigmented membrane, perforated to form the pupil, situated between the cornea and the crystalline lens and separating the anterior and posterior chambers. Its anterior surface is divided into two portions, a peripheral ciliary zone extending from its root at the anterior surface of the ciliary body to the collarette, and a pupillary zone extending from the collarette to the pupillary margin. The iris contains the sphincter pupillae muscle in the pupillary zone, which encircles the pupil, and the dilator pupillae muscle, whose fibers extend radially from the region of the sphincter pupillae muscle to the ciliary body. Its layers, anterior to posterior, are endothelium, the anterior border layer (both are absent at the crypts of Fuchs), the stroma, the region of the dilator pupillae muscle, and pigmented epithelium. The blood supply is from the anterior and long posterior ciliary arteries, which anastomose to form the greater arterial circle, from which branches anastomose to form the lesser arterial circle. The nerve supply consists of parasympathetic fibers via the third cranial nerve to the sphincter pupillae muscle, sympathetic fibers to the dilator pupillae muscle, and sensory fibers from the nasociliary branch of the ophthalmic nerve.

  i. bombé. A condition in which the iris is bulged forward by the pressure of aqueous humor contained in the posterior chamber by a total posterior synechia.

  i. dehiscence. Accessory holes or slits in the iris in addition to the normal pupil.

  detached i. An iris which is separated at its root from its junction with the ciliary body. See also *iridodialysis*.

  i. diastasis. Small holes in the iris at its ciliary border, similar to that occurring in iridodialysis.

  i. frill. The line of junction of the ciliary zone and the pupillary zone of the iris. Syn., *collarette*.

  piebald i. An irregularly pigmented iris of spotted appearance. Syn., *variegated iris*.

  plateau i. An abnormality of the iris in which its root inserts anteriorly into the ciliary body, lying in close apposition to the trabecular meshwork, with the iris having a less convex bulge than usual, tending to lie in a flat plane as it extends toward the crystalline lens.

  prolapse of i. Protrusion of a portion of the iris into a perforating corneal wound. It may form an anterior synechia if the iris remains fixed in the wound by scar tissue.

  tremulous i. A condition in which the iris shakes or quivers, usually caused by the absence of the crystalline lens from its normal position. Syn., *iridodonesis*.

  umbrella i. Iris bombé.

  variegated i. Piebald iris.

irisdiagnosis. Iridodiagnosis.

irisopsia (i-ris-op′se-ah). A defect of vision in which objects appear to be surrounded by rings of colored light.

iritic (i-rit′ik). Pertaining to or of the iris.

iritis (i-ri′tis). Inflammation of the iris usually characterized by circumcorneal injection (ciliary flush), aqueous flare, keratic precipitates, constricted and sluggish pupil, discoloration of the iris, and the subjective symptoms of radiating pain, photophobia, lacrimation, and interference with vision.

acne rosacea i. Neovascularization and swelling of the iris, especially in its ciliary zone, associated with acne rosacea of the face.

i. blennorrhagique à rechutes. Iritis with recurrent hypopyon.

catamenialis i. Iritis occurring before or during menstruation.

diabetic i. A mild plastic iritis occasionally occurring with diabetes, and sometimes accompanied by hypopyon or hemorrhage into the anterior chamber.

i. glaucomatosa. Increased intraocular pressure occurring in association with iritis or iridocyclitis, usually due to acute hyperemia and obstruction of the drainage channels by the inflammatory products.

gouty i. Iritis occurring with gout, characterized by sudden onset, intense injection of the conjunctiva, aqueous flare, steaminess of the cornea, keratic precipitates, and extreme pain. It is usually preceded by, or associated with, scleritis or episcleritis. Syn., *uratic iritis.*

guttate i. of Doyne. Nodular iritis.

hemorrhagic i. Iritis characterized by numerous petechial hemorrhages.

herpetic i. Iritis occurring with herpes zoster in either of two forms: (1) plastic iritis; (2) iritis characterized by swollen areas of acute vascular dilatation and hyphema, resulting in white atrophic scars (vitiligo iridis).

nodular i. Iritis due to a focal lesion and characterized by the presence of a nodule or nodules formed by aggregations of cells producing edema and tissue distortion. Syn., *guttate iritis of Doyne.*

i. obturans of Schieck. A low grade, chronic iritis, occurring with tuberculosis, persisting over a period of years without serious symptoms other than a slight loss of vision.

plastic i. The most common and severe type of iritis characterized by plastic exudates into the anterior chamber which consist essentially of fibrinous matter especially prone to the formation of synechiae and by a virtual absence of keratic precipitates.

purulent i. Iritis characterized by the presence of a pus discharge into the anterior chamber.

rheumatic i. A recurrent iritis associated with rheumatoid arthritis or muscular rheumatism. It is usually acute, with plastic exudates, keratic precipitates, synechiae, and pronounced subjective symptoms.

serous i. Iritis characterized by the presence of a serous discharge into the anterior chamber.

spongy i. Iritis characterized by the presence of a spongy mass of fibrinous exudates in the anterior chamber.

sympathetic i. See *sympathetic ophthalmitis.*

syphilitic i. See *syphilitic iridocyclitis.*

tubercular i. See *tubercular iridocyclitis.*

uratic i. Gouty iritis.

i. urica. Gouty iritis.

iritoectomy (ir″ih-to-ek′to-me, i-rih-to-). Surgical removal of the iritic deposits of aftercataract, together with a part of the iris, to form an artificial pupil.

iritomy (ir-it′o-me, i-rit′o-). Iridotomy.

irotomy (i-rot′o-me). Iridotomy.

irradiance (ir-ra′de-ans). Radiant flux incident per unit area, measured in watts per sq. cm or per sq. m.

irradiation (ir-ra″de-a′shun). 1. The impact of radiant energy on a receiver. 2. A phenomenon in which bright areas or objects appear enlarged against a dark background, as demonstrated in the overestimation of the size of stars, incandescent cinders, narrow illuminated slits, and white objects on a black background, or the apparent displacement of a straight edge held in front of a bright light. 3. Exposure to or application of x-rays, radium rays, or other radiation, as for therapeutic purposes. 4. The dispersion of a nervous impulse beyond the immediate or normal path of conduction. 5. The spreading of light by reflections from particle to particle in a photographic emulsion, causing the developed image to be larger and more diffuse at the edges than the optical image. 6. Emission of supposed influence or an immaterial fluid from the eyes. *Obs.*

irritation, sympathetic. Irritation of an organ secondary to irritation of its fellow, as in sympathetic ophthalmitis.

Irvine's method; syndrome; prism displacement test. See under the nouns.

ISCC. See *Inter-Society Color Council.*

ischemia of retina (is-ke'me-ah). A very pronounced anemia of the retina which may occur after profuse hemorrhage from any part of the body. A fixed, dilated pupil accompanies the condition, although the ophthalmoscopic picture varies.

iseiconia (īs"ih-ko'ne-ah). Iseikonia.

iseiconic (ī-ih-kon'ik). Iseikonic.

iseikonia (īs"ih-ko'ne-ah). A condition in which the size and the shape of the ocular images of the two eyes are equal.

iseikonic (īs-ih-kon'ik). Pertaining to or of the condition of iseikonia.

Ishihara (ish-e-hah'rah) **charts; plates; test.** See under the nouns.

isoametropia (i"so-am-e-tro'pe-ah). Ametropia in which the refractive error is similar in the two eyes. Cf. *anisometropia.*

isochromatic (i"so-kro-mat'ik). Possessing the same color throughout. Syn., *isochroous.*

isochroous (i-sok'ro-us). Isochromatic.

isochromes (i'so-krōmz). In the Ostwald color system, a series of surface color samples of approximately equal dominant wavelength and nearly constant purity, varying in luminous reflectance only, and arranged vertically in the Ostwald triangle parallel to the gray series. Syn., *shadow series.*

isoclinal (i"so-kli'nal). Isoclinic.

isoclinics (i"so-klin'iks). 1. Lines of equal inclination. Cf. *isotorsional lines.* Syn., *isoclinals.* 2. The lines of zero intensity, representing zero transmitted light, as may be observed in the examining of a material with a polariscope.

isocoria (i"so-ko're-ah). Equality in size of the two pupils.

iso-**cyanopsin** (i"so-si-an-op'sin). A photosensitive pigment with λ max at 575 mμ, formed from the reaction of cis_2 retinene$_2$ with chicken cone opsin.

isodynamic (i"so-di-nam'ik). Pertaining to dynamic retinoscopy in which the subject fixates a target in the plane of the peephole.

isofluorophate (i"so-floo'ro-fāt). Diisopropyl fluorophosphate. See *DFP.*

isogyre (i'so-jīr). A dark band in an interference pattern that corresponds to directions of transmission in which polarization of the incident light is not affected by passing through the crystal plate.

iso-iconia (i"so-i-ko'ne-ah). Iseikonia.

iso-ikonia (i"so-i-ko'ne-ah). Iseikonia.

iso-indicial (i"so-in-dish'al). Having the same index of refraction.

iso-**iodopsin** (i"so-i-o-dop'sin). A photosensitive pigment with λ max at 515 mμ, formed from the reaction of *iso-a* retinene$_1$ with chicken cone opsin.

isometropia (i"so-me-tro'pe-ah). Equal refractive states of kind and degree in the two eyes.

isomorphism (i"so-mōr'fizm). In gestalt psychology, the presumed or implied similarity of organization or pattern of conscious content, such as visual perception, and the simultaneously present cerebral cortex activity.

iso-oxyopia (i-so-ok"se-o'pe-ah). Equality of acuity of the two eyes fully corrected for ametropia. Cf. *anisooxyopia.*

isophoria (i"so-fo're-ah). 1. Lack of variation in phoria or muscular imbalance, with changes in the direction of gaze. Cf. *anisophoria.* 2. Vertical orthophoria.

isopia (i-so'pe-ah). Equality of visual acuity in the two eyes.

isoplanasie (i"so-plān'ah-se). Isoplanatism.

isoplanatism (i"so-plan'ah-tizm). The condition of an optical system free of spherical aberration and coma. Syn., *isoplanasie condition.*

iso-**porphyropsin** (i"so-por"fih-rop'sin). An iso-pigment with maximum absorption at 507 mμ, obtained, by incubation with opsin, from the cis_2 fraction of a mixture of retinene$_2$ isomers.

isopter (i-sop'ter). In visual fields, a contour line representing the limits of retinal sensitivity to a specific test target, usually designated by a fraction, the denominator of which represents the testing distance and the numerator the diameter of the test target.

iso-**retinene**$_1$ (i"so-ret'ih-nēn). Either of two of the isomers of retinene$_1$ known as *iso-a* and *iso-b.*

iso-**rhodopsin** (i"so-ro-dop'sin). 1. An isomeric photosensitive pigment resulting from a combination of *iso-a* retinene$_1$ with scotopsin having λ max at 487 mμ. 2. Regenerated rhodopsin derived from *neo-b*-retinene$_1$ and scotopsin.

isoscope (i'so-skōp). An apparatus for observing the effects of ocular torsional movements and cyclophoria subjectively, by comparison of the orientation of two parallel wires seen by one eye to a single wire seen by the other.

isotints (i'so-tints). In the Ostwald color system, the series of semichromes of constant white content.

isotones (i'so-tōnz). In the Ostwald color system, the series of semichromes of constant black content.

isotonography (i″so-to-nog'rah-fe). Constant pressure tonography.

isotropic (i″so-trop'ik). Having uniform properties of refraction, or of radiation of light, in all directions.

Ivanoff's theory (i-van'ofs). See under *theory*.

Ives' colorimeter; gratings; test; theory. See under the nouns.

Iwanoff's edema (e-wan'ofs). Cystic degeneration of the retina.

J

J. 1. Symbol for *radiant intensity*. 2. Abbreviation for *Jaeger*.

Jackson's (jak'sunz) **crossed cylinder lens; test.** See under the nouns.

Jacob's (ja'kubz) **membrane; syndrome; ulcer.** See under the nouns.

Jacobson's retinitis (ja'kub-sunz). Diffuse syphilitic neuroretinitis.

Jacod's (ja'kodz) **syndrome; triad.** See under the nouns.

Jadassohn-Lewandowsky syndrome (yah'das-ōn-lev-an-dow'ske). See under *syndrome*.

Jaeger (ya'ger) **chart; ocular micrometer; test type.** See under the nouns.

Jahnke's syndrome (yahn'kēz). See under *syndrome*.

James's waterfall (jāmz'ez). See under *waterfall*.

Jamieson's occluder (ja'mih-sunz). See under *occluder*.

Jamin (zhah-min') **interferometer; refractometer.** See under the nouns.

Jansky-Bielschowsky disease (yan'-ske-be-el-show'ske). See under *disease*.

Jarisch-Herxheimer reaction (yah'rish-herks'hīm-er). See under *reaction*.

Jastrow visual illusion (jas'tro). See under *illusion, visual*.

Javal's (zhah-valz') **N chart; grid; method; rule; stereoscope; theory.** See under the nouns.

jaw-winking. An abnormal associated movement of the eyelid and the jaw in which a ptosed eyelid raises when the jaw is opened or is moved laterally. Syn., *Gunn's jaw-winking phenomenon; Marcus Gunn phenomenon; Gunn's jaw-winking sign; pterygoid-levator synkinesis; Gunn's jaw-winking syndrome*.

reverse j. An abnormal associated movement of the eyelid and the jaw in which a partially ptosed eyelid droops farther when the jaw is opened or moved laterally. Syn., *inverse jaw-winking phenomenon; reversed Marcus Gunn phenomenon; Marin Amat syndrome*.

Jayle-Ourgaud syndrome. Ataxic nystagmus. See under *nystagmus*.

Jefferson syndrome (jef'er-sun). Cavernous sinus syndrome. See under *syndrome*.

Jellinek's sign (yel'in-eks). See under *sign*.

Jendrassik's sign (yen-drah'siks). See under *sign*.

Jenning's test (jen'ingz). See under *test*.

Jensen's (yen'senz) **choroiditis; disease; retinitis.** See under the nouns.

Jessen's chart (jes'enz). See under *chart*.

jnd. Just noticeable difference.

Joffroy's sign (zhof-rwahz'). See under *sign*.

Johnson syndrome (jon'sun). Adherence syndrome. See under *syndrome*.

Johnson-Stevens disease (jon'sun-ste'vens). Stevens-Johnson syndrome. See under *syndrome*.

joint, butt. A hinged juncture of the temple butt and endpiece of a spectacle frame for which the mating surfaces are not mitered, hence the squared-off end of one and the flat side of the other directly abut each other when the temple is swung open for wearing.

joint, mitered. The hinged juncture of

the temple butt and endpiece of a spectacle frame for which the mating surfaces of both the front and the temple are mitered.

Jones's test. See under *test*.

Judd's criterion. See under *criterion*.

Judd's formulas. See under *formula*.

judgment, absolute. Judgment of the magnitude or quality of a stimulus without reference to a comparison standard.

jugum sphenoidale (ju'gum sfe"noidal'e). The junction of the great and small wings of the sphenoid bone.

Juler scotometer (yu'ler). See under *scotometer*.

Julesz random-dot stereogram. See under *stereogram*.

jump, prismatic. The apparent displacement of an object occurring in the transition of view across the borderline between the two lens powers of a bifocal or when the object is viewed alternately with and without a prism.

jump duction. See under *duction*.

junction, sclerocorneal. The union of the cornea and the sclera in the region of the limbus.

Jungschaffer contact lens (yung'shafer). See under *lens, contact*.

just noticeable difference. The smallest difference between two stimuli that for a given individual gives rise to a perceived difference in sensation. Abbreviation *jnd*. Syn., *differential limen; differential threshold*.

K

K. 1. Symbol for karat gold. E.g., 14 K means alloy of 14/24 gold. 2. Symbol for the central corneal curvature of longest radius, as measured by a keratometer.

Kagenaar prism (kag'en-ahr). See under *prism.*

kaleidorama (kah-li"do-rah'mah). Phenakistoscope.

kaleidoscope (kah-li'do-skōp). 1. A viewing instrument consisting of a pair of long plane mirrors, usually mounted inside a long tube at an angle of about 60° to each other, so that small colored beads or fragments loosely confined between two transparent plates at one end of the tube can be viewed through an opening at the other end as a striking, complex, symmetric pattern produced by multiple reflection in the mirrors and endlessly variegated in design by the rotation of the tube rearranging the beads or fragments. 2. A visual training instrument employing the kaleidoscopic principle or presenting kaleidoscopically produced views.

Kalischer's (kah'lish-erz) **disease; syndrome.** See under the nouns.

kalopsia (kal-op'se-ah). The perceptional attribution of beauty to anything seen.

Kalt's contact lens (kaltz). See under *lens, contact.*

Kant's theory (kahnts, kants). See *nativism.*

Kaposi's disease (ka-po'sēz). Xeroderma pigmentosum.

kappa (κ). The Greek letter used as the symbol for (1) *angle kappa;* (2) *angle of meridional direction.*

kataphoria (kat"ah-fo're-ah). Cataphoria.

katatropia (kat"ah-tro'pe-ah). Catatropia.

katophoria (kat"o-fo're-ah). Cataphoria.

katotropia (kat"o-tro'pe-ah). Catatropia.

Katz's laws of field size. See under *law.*

Kayser's disease (ki'zerz). See under *disease.*

Kayser-Fleischer (ki'zer-flīsh'er) **ring; sign.** See under the nouns.

Kearns syndrome. See under *syndrome.*

Keeler Headband Trial Frame; Magnifying Spectacles. See under the nouns.

Kehrer's reflex (ker'erz). The aural blinking reflex.

Keiner's theory (ki'nerz). See under *theory.*

Keith's theory (kēthz). See under *theory.*

Kellner eyepiece (kel'ner). See under *eyepiece.*

Kelvin scale (kel'vin). See under *scale.*

Kennedy's syndrome (ken'eh-dēz). See under *syndrome.*

Kepler telescope (kep'ler). See under *telescope.*

keratalgia (ker"ah-tal'je-ah). Pain in the cornea.

keratectasia (ker"ah-tek-ta'ze-ah). A protrusion or forward bulging of the cornea due to pathological thinning or weakening of the corneal tissue. It differs from a corneal staphyloma in that it does not contain adherent uveal tissue. Syn., *kerectasis.*

keratectomy (ker"ah-tek'to-me). Surgical removal of a portion of the cornea. Syn., *kerectomy.*

keratic (ker-at'ik). 1. Pertaining to horny tissue. 2. Pertaining to or of the cornea.

keratic precipitates (ker-at'ik pre-sip'ih-tāts). See under *precipitates*.

◆

KERATITIS

keratitis (ker"ah-ti'tis). Inflammation of the cornea usually characterized by loss of transparency and dullness, due to cellular infiltration and vascularization from enlargement of limbal and anterior ciliary vessels. Keratitis is accompanied by circumcorneal injection, conjunctivitis, and the subjective symptoms of pain, lacrimation, photophobia, blepharospasm, and reduction of vision. If severe, ulceration and suppuration may result, and the iris and the ciliary body may become involved.

k. a frigore. Keratitis from exposure to cold.

acne rosacea k. Rosacea keratitis.

actinic k. Keratitis due to exposure to ultraviolet light.

alphabet k. Striate keratitis.

anaphylactic k. Keratitis appearing as an anaphylactic response as in *Morawiecki's, von Szily's,* or *Wessely's phenomena.*

annular k. Keratitis in which plastic exudates are deposited on the posterior corneal surface in the form of a hazy ring, with the center and the periphery of the cornea relatively free, as may occur in syphilitic interstitial keratitis. Syn., *keratitis parenchymatosa annularis.*

k. arborescens. Dendritic keratitis.

artificial silk k. Keratitis occurring among workers in the artificial silk industry.

aspergillus k. Keratitis due to infection with the *Aspergillus* fungus and characterized by a corneal ulcer with a dull, dry surface, surrounded by a yellow line of demarcation. It may be accompanied by hypopyon and the ulcer may perforate.

band k. Band keratopathy.

bullous k. Bullous keratopathy.

catarrhal ulcerative k. A relatively benign ulceration of the cornea, usually near the limbus, which may occur secondarily to conjunctivitis, or in elderly or debilitated persons.

deep k. Interstitial keratitis.

deep pustular k. A dense suppurative infiltration of the deeper corneal layers due to tuberculosis or syphilis, with an associated hypopyon, iritis, and periorbital pain, presumed to be due to an actual lodgment in the eye of the tubercle bacilli or of the treponema. Syn., *keratitis pustuliformis profunda.*

dendritic k. A form of herpetic keratitis characterized by the formation of small vesicles, which break down and coalesce to form recurring dendritic ulcers, characteristically irregular, linear, branching, and ending in knoblike extremities. Syn., *keratitis arborescens; furrow keratitis.*

desiccation k. Keratitis e lagophthalmo.

Dimmer's k. Nummular keratitis.

disciform k. A deep, localized, subacute, nonsuppurative keratitis, generally chronic and benign, characterized by a central discoid opacity and due to a virus infection or occurring as a sequel to trauma.

k. e lagophthalmo. Keratitis due to exposure and drying of the cornea from incomplete closure of the eyelids, characterized by a haziness and desiccation of the corneal epithelium which may result in fissures, exfoliation, and keratinization. Syn., *desiccation keratitis; exposure keratitis; lagophthalmic keratitis.*

k. electrica. A superficial punctate keratitis caused by exposure to an intense electric spark.

epithelial diffuse k. A rare, bilateral, superficial, punctate keratitis, usually associated with uveitis, and possibly vitamin B_2 deficiency, characterized by multiple, minute, epithelial flecks without vesiculation. Syn., *diffuse superficial keratitis.*

epithelial punctate k. Superficial punctate keratitis of Fuchs. See under *punctate keratitis.*

k. epithelialis marmorata. A rare, bilateral, mosaiclike, chronic, superficial, punctate keratitis involving the lower half of the corneal epithelium in the deep layers above Bowman's membrane. Vacuoles are present in the epithelium, and the surface layers are broken.

k. epithelialis vernalis. A corneal dystrophy, presumably due to disturbances of corneal nutrition, secondary to vernal conjunctivitis, in which dustlike, discrete, epithelial opacities develop, accompanied by edema and cystic subepithelial spaces. An extensive epithelial necrosis is found microscopically, and a peripheral degeneration in the interstitial tissue may also be present, causing an opaque white band resembling an arcus senilis.

k. epithelialis vesiculosa disseminata. A chronic, usually recurrent, form of punctate keratitis characterized by a relatively small number of opacities primarily in the area of the palpebral fissure, without vascularization. The superficial stroma is often infiltrated, although the condition is essentially epithelial.

exfoliative k. A corneal, epithelial denudation accompanied by corneal ulcers and degenerative interstitial keratitis, as may occur in a toxic, hypersensitive reaction to arsenic.

exposure k. Keratitis e lagophthalmo.

fascicular k. An inflammatory process secondary to phlyctenular keratitis, in which a limbal phlycten ulcerates and wanders toward the corneal apex, the periphery of the ulcer healing while the central margin remains active. A narrow band of neovascularization, extending from the limbus, follows in the furrow of the centrally advancing ulcer. The condition remains superficial, without perforation, and terminates in a linear opacity.

filamentary k. Filamentary keratopathy.

k. filiformis. Filamentary keratopathy.

furrow k. Dendritic keratitis.

herpetic k. 1. In herpes simplex: a superficial, epithelial, virus infection of the cornea characterized by the presence of groups of small vesicles which may break down and coalesce to form dendritic ulcers (dendritic keratitis). 2. In herpes zoster ophthalmicus: lesions in the subepithelial layers of the cornea, composed of minute dot opacities, which group together into large, well-defined, round areas. Usually epithelial vesicles appear over them, which may result in ulcers and secondary infection. **filamentary (superficial) h.k.** A rare form of filamentary keratitis due to the herpes virus. **geographic h.k.** The late stage of superficial herpetic keratitis characterized by loss of epithelium between the branches of a dendritic ulcer, resulting in an irregularly shaped, sharply demarcated geographic ulcer. **punctate (superficial) h.k.** Superficial punctate keratitis due to the herpes virus. See also *herpetic keratitis.* **striate (superficial) h.k.** A rare form of herpetic keratitis characterized by numerous, minute, punctate opacities in linear formation. **vesicular (superficial) h.k.** Vesicular keratitis due to the herpes virus.

hypopyon k. A purulent keratitis with accompanying hypopyon, as may result from a virulent corneal ulcer accompanied by quantities of leukocytes and fibrin which gravitate to the bottom of the anterior chamber to form the hypopyon.

infectious k. An acute, subacute, or chronic infectious keratoconjunctivitis of livestock. Syn., *pink eye; infectious ophthalmia.*

interstitial k. Any deep corneal inflammation primarily involving the substantia propria. See also *syphilitic keratitis.* Syn., *deep keratitis; parenchymatous keratitis.*

lagophthalmic k. Keratitis e lagophthalmo.

lattice k. Latticelike corneal dystrophy.

leprotic k. Keratitis associated with leprosy and occurring in three forms: keratitis punctata leprosa, leprotic pannus, and interstitial keratitis.

k. linearis migrans. A condition of obscure etiology in which a line of granular opacity slowly migrates from one portion of the cornea to another, as from limbus to limbus, from one layer to another, or both.

lipid k. Lipid keratopathy.

macular k. Superficial punctate keratitis of Fuchs. See under *punctate keratitis.*

k. marginalis miliaris. Keratitis characterized by a sudden onset of minute, subepithelial infiltrations which tend to occur in groups and seldom ulcerate.

k. marginalis profunda. An interstitial keratitis occurring rarely in elderly persons as a yellowish or gray infiltration, 1 to 2 mm wide, continuous with the sclera, and usually in the superior cornea, although it may form a complete ring.

Mauthner's k. Deep punctate keratitis.

k. metaherpetica. A corneal

ulceration which may follow the primary healing of a dendritic ulcer, consisting of single or confluent round ulcers of the epithelium and accompanied by slight congestion and pain.

k. molluscum. A rare superficial punctate keratitis, phlyctenular keratitis, peripheral infiltration, or corneal ulcer due to molluscum contagiosum.

mustard gas k. Keratitis due to exposure to mustard gas vapor, commencing after a 6 to 8 hour latent period, with edema, swelling, and cellular infiltration of the cornea. The edema and other clinical symptoms diminish in about one week followed by recurrence of the symptoms and vascularization for several weeks and subsequent recurrence and ulceration after a latent period of many years.

mycotic k. Inflammation of the cornea caused by a fungus infection.

neuroparalytic k. A stippled and edematous corneal inflammation accompanied by conjunctival hyperemia and iritis and followed by vesiculation. It is marked by epithelial exfoliation, due to abnormal epithelial metabolism and inability to resist trauma, desiccation, and infection following loss of sensory nerve control in Vth nerve lesions. Syn., *neuroparalytic ophthalmia.*

neurotrophic k. Keratitis due to loss of sensory nerve supply to the cornea and the consequent loss of trophic influence.

nummular k. A slowly developing, benign keratitis characterized by disk-shaped infiltrates in the superficial substantia propria. It occurs mainly among young land workers, is usually unilateral, and the surface epithelium over the opacities eventually sinks, forming a pathognomonic, faceted depression. Ulceration is rare, but vascularization is common. Syn., *Dimmer's keratitis.*

oyster-shuckers' k. A suppurative keratitis produced by pieces of oyster shell embedded in the cornea.

k. parenchymatosa annularis. Annular keratitis.

parenchymatous k. Interstitial keratitis.

k. periodica fugax. A bilateral condition consisting of migrating opacities in the deeper layer of the corneal stroma and associated with corneal swelling and keratic precipitates.

peripheral furrow k. Peripheral corneal ectasia.

k. petrificans. Band keratopathy.

phlyctenular k. A primary corneal inflammation, or one secondary to phlyctenular conjunctivitis, in which gray nodules (phlyctens) occur on the corneal surface near the limbus. The epithelium may break down to form shallow ulcers, which may heal without opacification, or the ulcers may migrate centrally to form a fascicular keratitis. Syn., *scrofulous keratitis.*

k. profunda. An interstitial keratitis, usually unilateral, affecting adults, and associated with anterior uveitis. In the early stages, the cornea is edematous and stippled, and a deep interstitial haze develops. Keratic precipitates occur frequently, and deep vascularization is usually minimal. Etiology may be varied, but it is probably an allergic reaction to some mild, chronic infection.

k. punctata leprosa. The most common form of leprotic keratitis, consisting of scattered, irregular, minute, white spots in the substantia propria, extending downward from the superior margin of the cornea gradually to cover its upper half, the area involved being wedge-shaped in section with the base upward.

k. punctata profunda. Deep punctate keratitis.

k. punctata superficialis. Superficial punctate keratitis.

k. punctata tropica. A nummular keratitis occurring in epidemics among rice field farmers in Java. Syn., *sahwah keratitis.*

punctate k., deep. Keratitis which may occur with acquired or hereditary syphilitic iritis, characterized by small, sharply defined, punctate opacities in an otherwise clear cornea. There is no accompanying irritation or vascularization, and the opacities may quickly appear and disappear. Syn., *keratitis punctata profunda; Mauthner's keratitis.*

punctate k., superficial. A group of corneal, inflammatory diseases characterized by discrete opacities in the superficial corneal layers.

s.p.k. of Fuchs. An acute keratitis characterized by the appearance of small, sharply defined, punctiform infiltrates on either side of Bowman's membrane. No vesicles are present. It usually commences as a catarrhal conjunctivitis, is frequently associated with a respiratory infection, and may be of viral, bacterial, neurotrophic, or parasitic etiology. A similar condition may develop after ultraviolet light exposure. Syn., *epithelial punctate keratitis; macular keratitis; keratitis subepithelialis.* **s.p.k. of Thygeson.** A bilateral coarse punctate epithelial keratitis chronically remittent without conjunctivitis, with gray and usually centrally located opacities, typically round or oval, though sometimes stellate or irregular, and visible only under magnification.

k. pustuliformis profunda. Deep pustular keratitis.

reapers' k. A suppurative, corneal inflammation following wound of the cornea by a particle of grain.

reticular k. Latticelike corneal dystrophy.

ring k. One or two concentric rings of interstitial keratitis encircling a previously established lesion in the corneal stroma and separated from it by clear cornea.

rosacea k. The corneal involvement in ocular acne rosacea characterized initially by a superficial, marginal, loop-type vascularization in a zone of gray infiltration and followed by subepithelial infiltrates which at first are small, round or oval, delimited areas near the limbus and later become larger, less defined, and progress toward the center of the cornea. Ulceration may occur.

sahwah k. Keratitis punctata tropica.

sclerosing k. Keratitis secondary to scleritis, characterized by hyperplasia and opacification of the substantia propria of the cornea.

scrofulous k. Phlyctenular keratitis.

serpiginous k. A diffuse keratitis characterized by a disk-shaped ulcer with a tendency to travel in one direction in a serpentlike manner, associated with iridocyclitis, hypopyon, and posterior corneal abscess, and due to infection by the pneumococcus.

k. sicca. A chronic keratitis resulting from insufficient lacrimal secretion, characterized by punctate or linear opacities in the deeper layers of the cornea, mainly in its inferior portion, and usually associated with epithelial filaments and a slight viscid secretion. See also *keratoconjunctivitis sicca.*

stellate k. A form of dendritic keratitis characterized by a rosette or a star-shaped ulcer.

striate k. Any keratitis in which localized radial or intersecting linear formations are found in or on the cornea. Syn., *alphabet keratitis.*

k. subepithelialis. Superficial punctate keratitis of Fuchs. See under *punctate keratitis.*

superficial k. Keratitis primarily involving the superficial layers of the cornea. **diffuse s.k.** Epithelial diffuse keratitis. **disseminated s.k.** A type of superficial punctate keratitis in which there are numerous widely scattered opacities. **linear s.k.** A keratitis associated with low intraocular pressure and characterized by folds in Bowman's membrane, the concavities of which are filled with fibrous tissue without vascularization. The lesion forms a linear pattern of gray ridges on the corneal surface, and nodes are found along the course of the ridges. **marginal s.k. of Fuchs.** A rare bilateral keratitis commencing with a band of superficial infiltrates around the periphery of the cornea with the central area remaining clear. It may stop at this stage or ulceration may develop to form a ring ulcer. It mainly affects the middle aged or older, and photophobia and severe pain are accompanying symptoms. **sequestrating s.k.** A condition in which pieces of corneal scar tissue undergo spontaneous necrosis and are thrown off by an inflammatory process to form an ulcer.

syphilitic k. 1. Interstitial keratitis due to inherited syphilis characterized by an early, localized, grayish infiltrate in the deep layers and by bedewing of the corneal epithelium. The infiltrate spreads to fill the entire stroma, deep brushlike vascularization appears, giving rise to yellowish-red discolorations (salmon patches), following which the cornea clears and vision improves, with the remnants of the vascularization remaining in the deep layers. It is usually bilateral, occurs between the ages of 5 and 15, and is part of a syndrome consisting of impaired hearing, notched teeth, saddle bridge nose, and rhagades at the corners of the mouth. 2. Interstitial keratitis, usually unilateral and affecting adults, due to acquired syphilis similar to the inherited form but milder and much rarer.

trachomatous k. Keratitis appearing in trachoma, characterized by an early, avascular, superficial inflammation and later by vascular changes at the limbus, which result in the formation of a trachomatous pannus.

trophic k. Keratitis due to disturbance of the sensory nerve supply to the cornea, as may occur in neuroparalytic keratitis.

k. urica. An extremely rare, corneal dystrophy in which the corneal stroma becomes infiltrated with crystalline deposits of urea and sodium urate. A yellow opacity forms near the limbus and progresses centrally. Isolated punctate opacities may also be present. Syn., *dystrophia uratica corneae; dystrophia urica.*

varicellar k. A vesicular corneal inflammation frequently resulting in ulceration and interstitial inflammation, due to ocular involvement in chicken pox.

vasculonebulous k. Pannus.

verrucose k. Keratitis resulting from prolonged infection by a wart on the margin of an eyelid, initially involving the epithelial layer producing a superficial punctate keratitis which tends to recur repeatedly with pain and photophobia and which may terminate with ulceration.

vesicular k. Keratitis characterized by the development of small epithelial vesicles. It is generally neurotrophic in origin, but may occur in blind degenerated eyes or may result from inflammation or trauma. **diffuse v.k.** A neurotrophic disturbance of the cornea resulting in epithelial vesiculation in the absence of concurrent inflammation or high intraocular pressure.

k. vesicularis neuralgica. A recurring, corneal vesiculation with exfoliation of the epithelium, frequently of traumatic origin.

volcano-like k. A benign condition of unknown etiology and with no subjective symptoms, consisting of 5 to 30 punctate lesions beneath the corneal epithelium, resembling tiny volcanos covered with snow with the bases in the superficial stromal layers and the apices at the level of Bowman's membrane. It occurs in the tropical areas of South America.

xerotic k. A corneal degeneration characterized by a dry, lusterless appearance of the cornea, due to deficient or disturbed metabolism. It may follow a debilitating disease or result from malnutrition with vitamin A deficiency, and usually develops into keratomalacia.

zonular k. Band keratopathy.

◆

kerato- (ker′ah-to-). A combining form denoting the cornea.

keratocele (ker′ah-to-sēl). Hernia of Descemet's membrane of the cornea. Syn., *descemetocele; keratodermatocele.*

keratocentesis (ker″ah-to-sen-te′sis). Puncture of the cornea.

keratochromatosis (ker″ah-to-kro″-mah-to′sis). Discoloration of the cornea.

◆

KERATOCONJUNCTIVITIS

keratoconjunctivitis (ker″ah-to-kon-junk″tih-vi′tis). Inflammation involving both the cornea and the conjunctiva. See also *conjunctivitis; keratitis.*

atopic k. Keratoconjunctivitis caused by hypersensitivity of the tissues to an allergen, not by a local organismal infection.

eczematous k. Phlyctenular keratoconjunctivitis.

epidemic k. An acute keratoconjunctivitis, highly contagious, characterized by edema of the eyelids and the conjunctiva, subepithelial corneal infiltration, petechial hemorrhages, hyperemia, and involvement of the regional lymph nodes, considered to be due to a virus. Syn., *shipyard conjunctivitis; Sanders' disease; shipyard keratoconjunctivitis; Sanders' syndrome; Sanders-Hogan syndrome.*

garlandiform k. Keratitis characterized by wreathlike intraepithelial infiltrates within the palpebral fissure. It is considered to be of virus origin, is usually bilateral, and clears without leaving corneal scars.

lymphatic k. Phlyctenular keratoconjunctivitis.

k. medicamentosa. Keratoconjunctivitis caused by ingestion of a drug such as arsenic or gold.

phlyctenular k. Keratoconjunctivitis characterized by the appearance of small gray nodules (phlyctens) on the conjunctiva, the limbus, and the cornea. See also *phlyctenular conjunctivitis; phlyctenular keratitis.* Syn., *eczematous keratoconjunctivitis; lymphatic keratoconjunctivitis; scrofulous keratoconjunctivitis.*

rosacea k. Acne rosacea involving both conjunctiva and cornea. See *acne rosacea conjunctivitis* and *rosacea keratitis.*

scrofulous k. Phlyctenular keratoconjunctivitis.

shipyard k. Epidemic keratoconjunctivitis.

k. sicca. Keratoconjunctivitis characterized by insufficient lacrimal secretion, keratinization of the superficial epithelial cells, signs of chronic catarrhal conjunctivitis with dry mucoid secretion, and punctate or linear opacities of the cornea. Associated with the eye symptoms may be generalized dryness of the skin and of various mucous and synovial membranes, particularly the mucous membranes of the mouth. See also *keratitis sicca; Sjögren's syndrome.*

superior limbic k. Inflammation of the tarsal conjunctiva of the upper eyelid and of the upper bulbar conjunctiva, showing fine punctate fluorescein staining of the cornea at the upper limbus and the adjacent conjunctiva, superior limbic proliferation, and in about one third of cases filaments at the upper limbus. It affects both sexes of all ages, usually bilateral, with etiology unknown. Abbreviation *SLK.*

tric virus k. A follicular conjunctivitis with all the features of inclusion conjunctivitis associated with the epithelial and subepithelial punctate keratitis typical of trachoma.

◆

keratoconometer (ker″ah-to-ko-nom′-eh-ter). An instrument for determining the degree or condition of keratoconus.

keratoconus (ker″ah-to-ko′nus): A developmental or dystrophic deformity of the cornea in which it becomes cone-shaped, due to a thinning and stretching of the tissue in its central area. It usually manifests itself during puberty, is usually bilateral, and is more common in women than men. Syn., *conical cornea.*

k. posticus. A rare deformity of the cornea in which the curvature of its posterior surface increases while the curvature of its anterior surface remains normal. The central area thus becomes abnormally thinner than the peripheral area. **k. posticus circumscriptus.** A localized keratoconus posticus. **k. posticus totalis.** Keratoconus posticus involving the entire posterior surface of the cornea.

keratocyte (ker′ah-to-sīt″). Corneal corpuscle.

keratodermatocele (ker″ah-to-dermat′o-sēl). Keratocele.

keratoectasia (ker″ah-to-ek-ta′se-ah). Kerectasis.

keratoglobus (ker″ah-to-glo′bus). A bilateral developmental anomaly in which the cornea is greatly enlarged and protruded, intraocular pressure being normal. Syn., *cornea globosa; keratomegalia; megalocornea; anterior megalophthalmus.*

keratohelcosis (ker″ah-to-hel-ko′sis). Ulceration of the cornea.

keratohemia (ker″ah-to-he′me-ah). Blood deposits in the cornea.

keratoiditis (ker″ah-toid-i′tis). Inflammation of the cornea; keratitis.

kerato-iridocyclitis (ker″ah-to-ir″id-o-si-kli′tis). Inflammation involving the cornea, the iris, and the ciliary body.

kerato-iridoscope (ker″ah-to-ih-rid′o-skōp, ker″ah-toir′id-). A microscope for examining the cornea and the iris.

kerato-iritis (ker″ah-to-i-ri′tis, ker″ah-to-ih-ri′-). Inflammation involving both the cornea and the iris.

keratokeras (ker′ah-to-ker″as). A rare tumor of the cornea due to extreme epidermalization of the epithelium.

keratoleptynsis (ker″ah-to-lep-tin′sis). A surgical procedure in which the anterior surface of the cornea is removed and replaced by bulbar conjunctiva for cosmetic reasons.

keratoleukoma (ker″ah-to-lu-ko′mah). A dense white opacity of the cornea.

keratomalacia (ker″ah-to-mah-la′she-ah). A corneal degeneration characterized by early loss of luster, dryness, and reduced sensitivity, and later by infiltration, opacification, pannus, exfoliation of the epithelium, necrosis, ulceration, and often perforation, with an absence of inflammatory reaction. There is an accompanying xerosis epithelialis of the conjunctiva and usually degenerative changes in medullated nerves. It is part of a general systemic condition of deficient or disturbed metabolism following debilitating disease or resulting from malnutrition with vitamin A deficiency.

keratomegalia (ker"ah-to-meg-al′e-ah). Keratoglobus.

keratomeninx (ker"ah-to-me′ninks). The cornea. *Obs.*

keratometer (ker"ah-tom′eh-ter). An instrument for measuring the anterior curvatures of the cornea, consisting of a luminous pattern of mires whose images, produced by reflection on the cornea, are viewed through a telescope with which is combined a doubling and image-size measuring system. Syn., *ophthalmometer.*

keratometry (ker"ah-tom′eh-tre). Measurement of the anterior curvatures of the cornea with a keratometer. Syn., *ophthalmometry.*

keratomileusis (ker"ah-to-mih-lu′sis). A surgical procedure for the reduction or elimination of myopia in which a thin segment of the cornea, sliced off with a microkeratome, is frozen, tooled with a lathe to alter its curvature, replaced on the cornea, and held in place by a contact lens temporarily sutured to the cornea.

keratomycosis (ker"ah-to-mi-ko′sis). A fungus infection of the cornea.

keratonosus (ker-ah-ton′o-sus). Any degenerative disease of the cornea.

keratonyxis (ker"ah-to-nik′sis). Surgical puncture of the cornea, especially in needling for soft cataract.

◆

KERATOPATHY

keratopathy (ker"ah-top′ah-the). 1. A morbid condition or disease of the cornea. 2. A noninflammatory disease of the cornea, as distinguished from *keratitis.* For types of, see *corneal dystrophy* and *keratitis.*

   band k. A degenerative disorder of the cornea characterized by the slow development of a horizontal, gray, band-shaped opacity in the intrapalpebral part of the cornea, first appearing as a slight turbidity at the level of Bowman's membrane in which are small, dark, round, pathognomonic holes. The most common form is secondary to iridocyclitis, a less common form is primary and occurs in the apparently normal eyes of the elderly, and the rarest form occurs in children, most of whom have rheumatism associated with chronic iritis. It may also follow trauma due to exposure to irritants. Syn., *band-shaped corneal dystrophy; keratitis petrificans; zonular keratopathy.*

   bullous k. A degenerative condition of the cornea characterized by the formation of recurring epithelial blebs or bullae, usually in the central area, which burst after a few days. It represents the advanced stage of a severe and prolonged epithelial edema consequent to ocular disease, such as glaucoma, iridocyclitis, or Fuchs' epithelial dystrophy.

   chloroquine k. Keratopathy associated with the prolonged ingestion of chloroquine, an antimalarial drug used also in the treatment of lupus erythematosus and rheumatoid arthritis. It is characterized by corneal changes which may vary from edema only, to slight punctate or flocculent opacities of the corneal epithelium, which tend to form lines similar to the superficial senile line. See also *chloroquine retinopathy.*

   diffuse epithelial k. Idiopathic corneal edema in which the cornea loses its luster and appears as though sprinkled with sand. It is accompanied by a foreign body sensation and the appearance of halos.

   filamentary k. A corneal condition characterized by the occurrence of fine epithelial filaments, attached at one end to the cornea and having a bulbous extremity. It may occur idiopathically, following abrasions, in glaucoma, keratitis sicca, herpes, edema of the cornea, etc. Syn., *keratitis filiformis; filamentary keratitis.*

   Labrador k. A non-familial bilateral corneal degeneration observed in Labrador and attributed to exposure to climatic extremes characteristic of this region.

   lipid k. Any of several corneal diseases in which lipoid deposits are found in the cornea.

   nodular hyaline band-shaped k. A condition occurring in tropical countries which consists of an elevated brownish opacity located symmetrically in each cornea in a band-shaped distribution confined to the palpebral fissures and separated from the limbus by clear cornea. Of unknown etiology, the nodules are of hyalin accumulation between the epithelium and Bowman's membrane.

striate k. Wrinkling of Descemet's membrane, a common and temporary condition occurring after cataract surgery. Also see *striate keratitis*.

superficial polymorphic k. A degenerative change of the corneal epithelium occurring in advanced stages of starvation, characterized by hypesthesia of the cornea, variously shaped areas of granulation which may project above the corneal surface, and ulceration.

vesicular k. See *keratitis, vesicular*.

zonular k. Band keratopathy.

◆

keratophakia (ker″ah-to-fa′ke-ah). A surgical procedure for the reduction or elimination of hypermetropia in which a suitably curved lens is made from the tissue of a donor's cornea and implanted interlamellarly into the recipient's cornea.

keratoplasty (ker′ah-to-plas″te). Corneal grafting or plastic surgery of the cornea.

acrylic k. Keratoplasty in which a plastic lens is implanted in lieu of a tissue graft.

autogenous k. Autokeratoplasty.

circumscribed k. Partial keratoplasty.

lamellar k. A surgical procedure in which a section of superficial layer of an opaque cornea is removed and replaced by healthy corneal tissue.

optic k. Corneal transplantation for the purpose of improving vision.

partial k. A surgical procedure in which only a portion of the cornea is removed and replaced by healthy corneal tissue, forming a window. Cf. *total keratoplasty*. Syn., *circumscribed keratoplasty*.

penetrating k. A surgical procedure in which a section of the entire thickness of an opaque cornea is removed and replaced by transparent cornea.

refractive k. A surgical procedure for the reduction or elimination of ametropia in which a superficial layer of the central cornea is removed, mechanically reshaped to a desired curvature, and replaced.

rotating k. A surgical procedure in which a section of corneal tissue is removed, rotated so that transparent tissue is in the pupillary area with the opaque portion peripheral, and reinserted.

step k. A surgical procedure involving both lamellar and penetrating keratoplasty in which the central section of the graft involves the entire corneal thickness and is smaller in diameter than the superficial lamellar portion.

tectonic k. Corneal transplantation solely to replace lost tissue.

total k. A surgical procedure consisting of transplantation of the entire cornea, including some of the surrounding conjunctiva.

two-level k. Keratoplasty in which the graft has a different diameter for the anterior layer from that for the posterior layer.

keratopographometry (ker″ah-to-po″grah-fom′eh-tre). Measurement of corneal curvatures for the determination of corneal topography as may be performed by keratometry, photokeratoscopy, or profile photography.

keratopography (ker″ah-to-pog′rah-fe). Topography of the cornea.

keratoprosthesis (ker″ah-to-pros′thesis). Corneal implant.

keratorhexis (ker″ah″to″rek′sis). Rupture of the cornea due to a perforating ulcer or to trauma.

keratoscleritis (ker″ah-to-skle-ri′tis). Inflammation involving both the cornea and the sclera.

keratoscope (ker′ah-to-skōp). An instrument for examining the curvature of the cornea, consisting of a pattern of alternately black and white concentric rings seen reflected on the cornea through a convex lens mounted in an aperture at the center of the pattern. Syn., *Placido's disk*.

Photo-Electronic K. See under *Photo-Electronic*.

keratoscopy (ker-ah-tos′ko-pe). 1. Examination of the anterior surface of the cornea with a keratoscope. 2. Originally used by Cuignet to mean *retinoscopy*.

photoelectric k. A method of investigating the corneal surface by scanning the cornea with a light beam and determining the changes in direction of the reflected beam by photoelectric detectors.

keratosis conjunctivae (ker"ah-to'sis kon-junk-ti've). Cornification of the conjunctival epithelium, occurring in various forms.

keratosis follicularis spinulosa decalvans. Ichthyosis follicularis.

keratosis nigricans (ker"ah-to'sis nig're-kanz, -ni'gre-). Acanthosis nigricans.

keratosis palmaris et plantaris. A marked, symmetrical thickening of the skin of the palms and soles, usually hereditary and sometimes congenital, which is frequently accompanied by ectropion, trachomalike lesions of the conjunctiva, and superficial and deep corneal vascularization.

keratosis pilaris atrophicans faciei. A rare disease beginning in infancy and characterized by the appearance of erythema at, and loss of, the outer halves of the eyebrows, due to keratosis of the hair follicles.

keratosis pilaris decalvans. A rare hereditary disease beginning on the face in infancy and characterized by keratosis of follicles in hairy regions, resulting in sparseness of the eyelashes and loss of the outer halves of the eyebrows. Ectropion, corneal opacities, and pannus are accompanying symptoms.

keratotomy (ker-ah-tot'o-me). Surgical incision of the cornea.

   delimiting k. Surgical incision into the cornea near the advancing border of a serpiginous corneal ulcer.

keratotorus (ker"ah-to-tōr'us). A rare corneal ectasia in which the bulging is eccentric and has a toric surface which creates against the rule astigmatism, with Descemet's membrane remaining intact.

keratouveitis (ker"ah-to-u"ve-i'tis). Simultaneous keratitis and uveitis.

kerectasis (ker-ek'tah-sis). A pathological protrusion or bulging of the cornea. Syn., *keratoectasia*.

kerectomy (ke-rek'to-me). Surgical removal of a portion of the cornea. Syn., *keratectomy*.

keroid (ker'oid). Resembling the cornea.

Kerr cell; constant; effect; method; shutter. See under the nouns.

Kestenbaum's (kes'ten-baumz) **formula; sign; test.** See under the nouns.

KGF. Karat gold filled. E.g., 10 KGF means that the surface layer of gold alloy is 10 karat gold and, under the U.S. National Stamping Act, it must be equal in weight to at least 1/20 of all metal in the part or piece.

kilohertz. A unit of frequency equal to one thousand cycles per second. Cf. *hertz*.

Kiloh-Nevin syndrome. See under *syndrome*.

Kimmelstiel-Wilson syndrome (kim'el-stēl wil'sun). See under *syndrome*.

kinephantom (kin"e-fan'tom). Perception of a moving visual object, such as a silhouette or shadow, as other than its actual direction or pattern.

kinephantoscope (kin"e-fan'to-skōp). A device for projecting shadows or other forms lending themselves to the perception of various movement patterns.

kinescope (kin'e-skōp). 1. An instrument for determining the refraction of the eye, in which the subject observes the apparent "with" or "against" movement of a test object through a stenopaic slit moved across the front of the eye. 2. An instrument for recording television programs by contact exposure of movie film on a television picture tube.

kinescopy (kin-es'ko-pe). The measurement of ocular refraction by use of the kinescope. Syn., *Holth's method*.

Kinsey-Cogan theory (kin'se-ko'gan). See *theory, osmotic pump*.

Kirchhoff's (kirk'hofs) **law.** See under *law*.

Kirschmann's law (kursh'manz). See under *law*.

Kisch's reflex (kish'ez). The aural blinking reflex.

Kitahara's disease. See under *disease*.

Klauder syndrome (klow'der). See under *syndrome*.

Klein's syndrome. See under *syndrome*.

Klein-Waardenburg syndrome (klīn-vahr'den-burg). Waardenburg syndrome. See under *syndrome*.

klieg (klēg) **conjunctivitis; light.** See under the nouns.

klinokinesis (kli"no-kih-ne'sis). A change in direction of movement of a motile organism in response to changes in the intensity of light stimulation but not in response to the direction of the light stimulation.

klinotaxis (kli-no-tak'sis). An irregular or wavy movement of a motile organism toward or away from light, which may be mediated by only one receptor organ that responds by comparing differences in light intensity of successive stimuli as the organism turns. See also *tropotaxis; telotaxis; menotaxis; mnemotaxis.*

Kloepfer syndrome (klep'fer). See under *syndrome.*

Klumpke syndrome (kloomp'keh). Lower radicular syndrome. See under *syndrome.*

Knapps' (naps) **law; streaks; striae.** See under the nouns.

knee, temporal, of Flechsig. Meyer's loop.

Knies's sign (k-nēz'ez). See under *sign.*

knob, end. End bulb.

Koby's (ko'bēz) **cataract; corneal dystrophy.** See under the nouns.

Koch-Weeks conjunctivitis (kōk-wēks). Acute contagious conjunctivitis.

Kocher's sign (kōk'erz). See under *sign.*

Koenig's (ke'nigz) **bars; theory; color triangle.** See under the nouns.

Koeppe's (kep'ēz) **gonioscopic lens; nodules.** See under the nouns.

Kohler illumination. See under *illumination.*

Kohlrausch's bend (kōl'rowsh-es). See under *bend.*

Kohlrausch (kōl'rowsh) **effect; phenomenon.** Helmholtz-Kohlrausch effect.

Kölliker's (kel'e-kerz) **layer; theory.** See under the nouns.

Kollmorgen contact lens (kōl'mōr-gen). See under *lens, contact.*

Köllner's (kel'nerz) **effect; law; rule.** See under the nouns.

Konigsmark syndrome. See under *syndrome.*

kopiopsia (kop"e-op'se-ah). Copiopia.

Koplik's spots (kop'liks). See under *spots.*

korectomia (kōr"ek-to'me-ah). Surgical formation of an artificial pupil.

korectopia (kōr"ek-to'pe-ah). Corectopia.

Korector, Arneson (kōr-ek'tor). An instrument used in visual training consisting of a large rotating disk on which is mounted an adjustable and removable fixation target to be observed through prisms, lenses, or both.

Kornzweig-Bassen syndrome (kōrn'-zvīg-bas'en). Bassen-Kornzweig syndrome. See under *syndrome.*

koroscopy (ko-ros'ko-pe). Retinoscopy.

Korte's laws (kōr-tēz). See under *law.*

Köster's (kes'terz) **prism; sign; test.** See under the nouns.

KP. Abbreviation for *keratic precipitate.*

Kratoculator (kra-tok'u-la"tor). An instrument used in visual training, in conjunction with a Myoculator, which projects a fixation target onto a screen, the target being moved to various positions on the screen by a manual control.

Kratometer (kra-tom'eh-ter). An instrument used in visual training consisting essentially of batteries of prisms mounted in bars through which an observer fixates distant or near targets. The prism bars are moved through a holding slot, introducing increasing or decreasing prismatic power, in individual steps, before either eye. A Maddox rod and a red glass are included in each battery, and the instrument is provided with a chin rest and cells for trial case lenses.

Kraupa's dystrophy (krow'paz). See under *dystrophy, corneal, epithelial juvenile (of Kraupa).*

Krause's (krawz'ez) **bulbs; corpuscle; glands; syndrome; valve.** See under the nouns.

Kravkov's experiment (krahv'kovz). See under *experiment.*

KRGP. Karat Rolled Gold Plate. E.g., 1/40 10 KRGP means that the 10 karat rolled gold plate is 1/40 of the total weight of the metal part or piece.

von Kries (fon krēs) **law of coefficients; law of persistence; theory.** See under the nouns.

von Kries pursuant image (fon krēs). Second positive afterimage.

Krimsky's (krim'skēz) **method; Eyecup Perimeter.** See under the nouns.

Kronfeld's test (krōn'feldz). See under *test.*

Krukenberg's spindle (kroo'ken-bergz). See under *spindle.*

kryptok (krip'tok). See *lens, bifocal, kryptok.*

Kubelka-Munk method (ku-bel'-kah-munk). See under *method.*

Kuf syndrome. Early infantile amaurotic family idiocy. See under *amaurotic.*

Kühne's (ke'nēz) **optical box; cycle.** See under the nouns.

Kuhnt's (koontz) **meniscus; intermediate tissue; post-central vein.** See under the nouns.

Kuhnt-Junius disease (koont-yun'e-us). Senile disciform degeneration of the macula. See under *degeneration*.

Kundt's (koondtz) **monocular asymmetry; illusion; partition; rule.** See under the nouns.

Kupfer's method (kup'ferz). See under *method*.

Kurova (koor-o'vah). A trade name for a series of corrected curve ophthalmic lenses.

Kurova Shursite lenses. See under *lens*.

Kurz's syndrome (kurz'ez). See under *syndrome*.

kuttarosome (kut"ar'o-sōm). A series of parallel bars in the neck of a retinal cone cell, described by early microscopists.

kyanophane (ki'an-o-fān). A bluish pigment said to exist in oil globules of the retinal cones, probably absent in man.

kyanopsia (ki"ah-nop'se-ah). Cyanopsia.

L

L. Symbol for (1) *lambert;* (2) *luminance.*

lachry- (lak'rih-). For words beginning thus, see *lacri-.*

lacodacryostomy (lak"o-dak"re-os'to-me). An operation to restore the flow of tears into the lacrimal sac from the lacrimal lake when the canaliculi are obstructed or obliterated.

Lacrilens (lak'rih-lenz). A trade name for a scleral contact lens with an inverted V-shaped opening in the inferior scleral portion to facilitate the flow of lacrimal fluid.

lacrima (lak'rih-mah). A tear.

lacrimae cruentae (lak'rih-me kru-en'te). Bloody tears. Syn., *dacryohemorrhysis.*

lacrimal (lak'rih-mal). Pertaining to the tears, or to the structures conducting or secreting tears, or to the lacrimal bone.

lacrimal ampulla; apparatus; artery; bones; canal; canaliculus; caruncle; crest; diaphragm; duct; fluid; fossa; gland; lake; papilla; punctum; sac; tubercle. See under the nouns.

lacrimale (lak"rih-mal'e). The point of junction of the posterior lacrimal crest and the frontolacrimal suture.

lacrimalin (lak-rim'ah-lin). A chemical which causes tear production.

lacrimase (lak'rih-mās). An enzyme found in tears.

lacrimation (lak"rih-ma'shun). The secretion of tears, the common connotation being excessive secretion.

> **basic l.** Secretion of tears mainly derived from tarsal and conjunctival glands, the accessory glands of Krause and Wolfring, and the glands of Zeis and Moll which normally maintain the hydration of the outer surface of the eye. It is the only lacrimation in infants during their first weeks of life, occurs during sleep, and remains relatively constant until approximately age 60 after which it gradually decreases. Also see *reflex lacrimation.*

> **central l.** Psychic lacrimation.

> **paradoxical l.** Crocodile tears.

> **paroxysmal l.** Excessive lacrimation occurring suddenly and periodically.

> **primary l.** Lacrimation due to direct stimulation or to irritation of the lacrimal gland.

> **psychic l.** Lacrimation associated with emotional states or physical pain.

> **reflex l.** Lacrimation in response to neurogenic stimulation, such as irritation of the cornea or the conjunctiva, vomiting, or glare.

lacrimator (lak'rih-ma"tor). Any substance which stimulates the secretion of tears, usually through irritation of the conjunctiva.

lacrimonasal (lak"rih-mo-na'zal). Pertaining to, or in the region of, the lacrimal sac or duct and the nose.

lacrimotomy (lak"rih-mot'o-me). Surgical incision of the lacrimal sac, duct, or gland.

lacrymal. Lacrimal.

lacunae, corneal (lah-ku'ne). 1. Von Recklinghausen's canals. 2. Tiny spaces in the stroma of the cornea filled with tissue fluid.

lacus lacrimalus (la'kus lak"rih-mal'-is). Lacrimal lake.

Ladd-Franklin theory (lad-frangk'-lin). See under *theory.*

laevo- (le'vo-). For words beginning thus, see *levo-*.

Lafora's disease (lah-fō'rahz). See under *disease.*

lag. 1. Comparative or relative retardation or slowness in movement, function, or development. 2. The slippage or extent of slippage of a contact lens associated with gravity, blinking, or rotation of the eyes from the straightforward position.

    l. of accommodation. See under *accommodation.*

    blink l. A downward movement of a contact lens following a blink.

    l. of convergence. See under *convergence.*

    dynamic l. *Optometric Extension Program:* An empirical deduction from the gross dynamic retinoscopy finding to compensate for an estimated lag of accommodation.

    excursion l. A slippage of a contact lens occurring during eye movement. Syn., *movement lag.*

    globe l., Means's. Means's sign.

    gravity l. A downward movement of a contact lens attributed to its weight or weight distribution.

    movement l. Excursion lag.

Lagleyze-von Hippel disease (lah-glīz'fon hip'el). Von Hippel's disease.

lagophthalmia (lag″of-thal'me-ah). Lagophthalmos.

lagophthalmos (lag″of-thal'mos). Inability to close the eyelids completely. Syn., *hare's eye.*

    l. in sopore. Failure of complete eyelid closure in profound sleep.

lagophthalmus (lag″of-thal'mus). Lagophthalmos.

Lagrange's law (lah-grahnz'ez). See under *law.*

lake, lacrimal. The accumulation of tears in the triangular-shaped region between the eyelids at the inner canthus prior to draining into the lacrimal puncta. Syn., *rivus lacrimalis.*

lambda (λ) (lam'dah). The Greek letter used as the symbol for (1) *wavelength;* (2) *angle of elevation* in the field of regard (Fry); (3) *angle lambda.*

lambert (lam'burt). A unit of luminance equal to $1/\pi$ candelas per sq. cm, or to the uniform luminance of a perfectly diffusing surface emitting or reflecting light at the rate of 1 lumen per sq. cm. Symbol: L. See also *footlambert.*

Lambert's law (lam'burts). See under *law.*

lamella (lă-mel'ah). 1. A thin leaf, plate, or layer. 2. A medicated gelatin disk for insertion under the eyelid.

    l. iridis anterior. Anterior limiting layer of the iris.

    posterior border l. of Fuchs. A layer of the iris containing the fibrils of the dilator pupillae muscle, exclusive of their cell bodies, located between the anterior pigment layer of Fuchs and the stroma. Syn., *Bruch's layer; Bruch's membrane; Henle's membrane; posterior membrane of the iris.*

    posterior limiting l. Lamina vitrea of the choroid.

    vitreous l. Lamina vitrea of the choroid. *Obs.*

    zonular l. The superficial layer of the capsule of the crystalline lens.

lamina (lam'ih-nah). A layer; a thin plate.

    l. basalis. Lamina vitrea of the choroid.

    Bowman's l. Bowman's membrane.

    l. capsulopupillaris. The lateral portion of the tunica vasculosa lentis, consisting of embryological vascular mesoderm, which normally unites with the pars iridica retinae to form the iris. In embryotoxon it adheres to the periphery of the cornea.

    choriocapillary l. Choriocapillaris.

    l. ciliaris retinae. The zonule of Zinn, derived from the pars ciliaris retinae of the optic cup.

    l. cribrosa. A thin, sievelike membrane, composed of neuroglia and connective tissue, bridging the posterior scleral foramen and continuous with the choroid and the deepest third of the sclera. The fibers of the optic nerve and the central retinal vessels pass through its many openings. Syn., *cribriform plate.*

    l. cribrosa sclerae. Lamina cribrosa.

    cuticular l. 1. The portion of the lamina vitrea of the choroid secreted by the pigment epithelium of the retina, to which it is fused, and located internal to the lamina elastica. 2. The portion of the lamina vitrea of the ciliary body secreted by the pars ciliaris retinae and located internal to the avascular connective tissue which separates it from the lamina elastica.

    l. elastica. 1. The portion of the lamina vitrea formed by the choroid, located external to the cuticular layer of the lamina vitrea and internal to the choriocapillaris. 2. The portion of the lamina vitrea of the ciliary body located external to the avascular connective tissue, which separates it from the cuticular lamina, and internal to the vascular layer of the ciliary body. **anterior l.e.** Bowman's membrane. **posterior l.e.** Descemet's membrane.

l. fusca. 1. The thin, brown, inner layer of the sclera containing melanin in chromatophores and fibrous elastic tissue. 2. The suprachoroid. 3. The external layer of the ciliary body, containing fibroblasts, chromatophores, and reticuloendothelial cells in its posterior portion, while anteriorly it becomes more of a serous space (suprachoroidal space). Syn., *membrana fusca*.

l. iridopupillaris. Embryological, vascular mesoderm from the tunica vasculosa lentis, of which the central portion forms the fetal pupillary membrane and the peripheral portion unites with the pars iridica retinae to form the iris.

medullary optic l. The large, fanshaped group of projectional fibers in the optic radiations of the visual pathway, which leaves the lateral geniculate body and reaches the ipsilateral area striata or higher visual center.

l. papyracea. One of the thin, paired portions of the ethmoid bone which forms part of the medial wall of the orbit. Syn., *os planum*.

Sattler's l. Sattler's layer.

l. suprachoroidea. Suprachoroid.

l. vasculosa choroideae. The vessel layer of the choroid subdivided into Haller's layer of larger vessels and Sattler's layer of smaller vessels.

l. vitrea. The inner layer of the choroid consisting of an innermost layer related to the pigment epithelium of the retina (cuticular lamina), a middle layer composed of a zone of elastin surrounded and interspersed by a collagenous meshwork, and an outermost basement membrane related to the endothelium of the choriocapillaris of the choroid, the latter two layers constituting the lamina elastica. Syn., *posterior limiting lamella; vitreous lamella; lamina basalis; Bruch's layer of the choroid; basement membrane of the choroid; Bruch's membrane of the choroid; Henle's membrane of the choroid.* 2. The layer of the ciliary body between its vascular layer and its epithelium. It is

a forward continuation of the lamina vitrea of the choroid, but differs in that there is a layer of avascular connective tissue between the lamina elastica and the cuticular lamina. Syn., *Bruch's layer of the ciliary body; Bruch's membrane of the ciliary body.*

lamp. Any device for producing artificial light.

arc l. A lamp in which light is produced by an electrical discharge between two electrodes by raising the temperature of gaseous particles from the electrodes to incandescence.

Argand l. A lamp with a tubular wick which admits a flow of air inside as well as outside of the flame, recommended by Andrew Jay Cross for retinoscopy.

argon l. A glow lamp filled with an argon mixture radiating chiefly in the near ultraviolet region around 360 $m\mu$, used clinically in conjunction with fluorescein in the fitting of contact lenses and for the detection of corneal abrasions.

Burton l. A viewing instrument consisting essentially of a magnifying lens in a rectangular frame that half shields a pair of tubular lamps which provide ultraviolet light at 360 $m\mu$ toward the object to be viewed through the lens. It is used primarily in conjunction with certain dyes, such as fluorescein, to create fluorescence for diagnostic purposes, such as in the evaluation of the fit of contact lenses.

cadmium l. A mercury vapor electric discharge lamp with cadmium added to emit radiation in the red region to complement the mercury vapor's blue and green radiation.

carbon arc l. An arc lamp, consisting of carbon electrodes, which radiates light because of incandescence of the electrodes and luminescence of vaporized electrode material.

carcel l. A special type of oil lamp of standard size and construction which has been used as a photometric standard in France. See also *carcel*.

Duke-Elder l. A lamp which produces ultraviolet radiations for certain ophthalmologic therapy.

Edridge-Green l. A color perception test lamp containing color filters mounted in rotating disks for serial presentation.

electric discharge l. A lamp in which light is produced by the passing of electricity through a metallic vapor or gas contained in a bulb or a tube.

electric filament l. An electric incandescent lamp consisting of a glass bulb containing a filament which is heated to incandescence by an electric current.

electric incandescent l. Any lamp in which light is produced by electrically heating a material to incandescence, particularly an electric filament lamp.

fluorescent l. An electric discharge lamp in which the radiant energy from the electric discharge is absorbed by certain materials (phosphors) and re-emitted as light of longer wavelength. Typically, ultraviolet radiation is converted into visible radiation by a phosphor coating on the inside of a tube.

Hague cataract l. A portable luminaire providing ultraviolet light to fluoresce the crystalline lens for its inspection, and for use in examining the cornea and other ocular tissues stained with a fluorescent dye.

HID l. High intensity discharge lamp.

incandescent l. Any lamp in which light is produced by heating a material to incandescence. It includes combustion sources, such as gas mantles as well as electric incandescent lamps, but is commonly associated with the latter.

mercury vapor l. An electric discharge lamp that utilizes mercury vapor and produces a blue-green light relatively rich in ultraviolet and near infrared radiations.

PXA l. Pulsed xenon arc lamp.

slit l. An instrument producing a slender beam of intense light for illuminating any reasonably transparent structure or medium (such as the cornea, the aqueous humor, the crystalline lens, or the anterior vitreous) in a sectionlike manner for oblique viewing, usually through a microscope.

Lancaster (lan'kas-ter) **chart; test.** See under the nouns.

Lancaster-Regan chart. See under *chart*.

lance, perceptual. The tridimensional spearhead-shaped representation of the visual acuity of the various regions of the retina, in which the point of the spearhead corresponds to the point of fixation and the spearhead base corresponds to the degree of eccentricity of retinal stimulation. The height of a line from a point on the base to the surface of the spearhead corresponds to the visual acuity obtainable for that point.

Land's theory. See under *theory*.

Landolt's (lahn'dolts) **ball; chart; club; fibers; fringe; prism; projectionometer; ring; stereoscope; tests; theory; test type.** See under the nouns.

Landström's muscle (lahnd'stremz). See under *muscle*.

Lange's fold (lang'ez). See under *fold*.

Langerhans' cells (lahng'er-hahnz). See under *cell*.

Langrange (lahn-grahnj') **fusion band; method.** See under the nouns.

Langworthy's theory (lang'wor-thēz). See under *theory*.

lantern. A protective, usually framed, enclosure of a light source with one or more transparent or translucent openings.

magic l. Slide projector.

lap. A tool, or the face of a tool, used for grinding and polishing a refracting surface of a lens blank to the selected shape (curvature) of the face of the tool by means of sandlike abrasive and polishing compounds.

Lapicque's target (lah-pēks'). See under *target*.

lapping. Surfacing.

lapsus (lap'sus). The falling down or drooping of a part; ptosis.

l. palpebrae superioris. Ptosis or drooping of the upper eyelid.

lash. An eyelash.

laser (la'zer). An acronym for "light amplification by stimulated emission of radiation"; a device for producing an intense coherent beam of monochromatic light in a wavelength in or near the visible spectrum. Syn., *optical maser*.

excimer l. A near UV laser in which the lasing gas consists of excimers, most commonly the molecules of the rare gas monohalides such as argon fluoride, krypton fluoride, and xenon chloride.

Laser Refractor. An apparatus for the subjective determination of ametropia consisting of a slowly rotating drum on the surface of which is perceived a granular pattern resulting from illumination by a helium-neon gas laser beam. The grain of the pattern appears to move when the eye is not focused for the fixation distance; hence, the correcting lens which neutralizes the movement focuses the eye for the fixation distance.

laterality. The internal awareness of the two sides of the body; an important substrate skill in the development of directionality, q.v.

laterality, visual. Any difference exhibited between the two eyes, the two halves of the binocular visual field, or the temporal and the nasal halves of the monocular visual field. See also *visual dominance*.

lateroduction (lat"er-o-duk'shun). Rotation of an eye or vergence of the eyes in the horizontal plane.

laterotorsion (lat"er-o-tŏr'shun). Rotation of the eye about an anteroposterior axis.

lateroversion (lat"er-o-ver'zhun). Version of the eyes in the horizontal plane.

Lauber's disease. Fundus albipunctatus.

laurence (lahr'ens). A shimmering seen over a hot surface, such as a roadway, on a calm, cloudless day, caused by irregular refraction of light by numerous air columns of various temperatures and densities.

Laurence's (lah'ren-siz) **pupillometer; strabismometer.** See under the nouns.

Laurence-Moon-Biedl (lah'rens-moon-be'-dl) **dystrophy; syndrome.** See under the nouns.

Laurent half-shade plate (lah-rent'). See under *plate*.

◆

LAW

law. A statement of a sequence or an interrelation of phenomena which is invariable under the given conditions.

Abney's l. The luminosity of the combined spectrum is equal to the sum of the luminosities of its component parts.

l. of absorption. 1. As light passes through a homogeneous substance of a given thickness, the same percentage of light is absorbed regardless of the intensity of the incident light. 2. The intensity of transmitted light varies as an exponential function of the length of the light path in the absorbing medium. Syn., *Bouguer's law; Lambert's law of absorption*.

all or none l. The weakest stimulus capable of producing a response in cardiac muscle, fibers of striated muscle, or nerve fibers, produces a maximal response, i.e., if there is any response at all, it is maximum under the existing conditions.

Allard's l. The square of the visual range of a light source is equal to its intensity times the transmissivity of the medium (atmosphere) divided by the minimum perceptible illumination at the eye.

Angströms l. The wavelengths absorbed by a substance are the same as those emitted by the substance when it is luminous. Abbrev. A, Å.

Aubert-Förster l. An observation by Aubert and Förster that, peripheral to the foveal region, visual acuity is better for small letters and numbers at short distances than for large letters and numbers at greater distances, though they subtend the same visual angle. Syn., *Aubert-Förster phenomenon*.

Beer's l. The absorption of the intensity of radiant energy by a stable solution is an exponential function of the product of concentration and the length of path in the solution.

l. of binocular projection. Images of an object or objects stimulating corresponding retinal points are perceptually localized as coming from the same direction and distance in space.

l. of binocular rest and motion. The extrinsic muscles of normal eyes, under the control of brain centers, relate the two eyes so that their visual axes and horizontal retinal meridians always lie in the plane of the primary isogonal circle whether at rest or in motion, and so that the two visual axes will converge at some point on this circle, in the interest of both binocular single vision and correct orientation. (Savage)

Bloch's l. The intensity of light required to produce a threshold response is inversely proportional to the duration of the stimulus, expressed by the formula: $Lt = C$ in which L = luminance of the stimulus, t = stimulus duration, C = a constant; valid only for short exposures.

Blondel-Rey l. A modification of Bloch's law for stimuli of long exposure. The intensity of light required to produce a response at threshold is inversely proportional to a function of the duration of the light, expressed by the formula: $Lt = L_\infty (t + t_0)$, in which L = luminance of the stimulus, L_∞ = luminance for an indefinitely long exposure, t = stimulus duration, t_0 = a time constant varying with the subject and the experimental conditions. It does not apply after maximum time, t_2, beyond which summation does not occur.

Bonnet-Cochet l. The log of the angle between the normal to the cornea at any point and the line connecting that point to a fixed center of reference, such as the center of rotation of the eye, is directly proportional to the angle between the latter line and the centrally aligned ophthalmometer axis.

Bouguer's l. The intensity of transmitted light varies as an exponential function of the length of the light path in the absorbing medium. Syn., *law of absorption; Lambert's law of absorption.*

Brewster's l. In a dielectric, such as glass, the angle of polarization is equal to the angle of incidence for which the reflected light is at right angles to the refracted light. Under this condition, the angle of polarization is equal to that angle of incidence whose tangent equals the refractive index of the medium.

Bunsen-Roscoe l. In photochemistry, for a reaction to a light stimulus of moderate intensity and short duration, the product of intensity and duration is a constant. Syn., *law of reciprocity.*

Charpentier's l. Ricco's law.

l. of closedness. The tendency to see an incomplete form as complete, the process of completion being termed *closure.*

l. of coefficients. A law expressed by von Kries and sometimes attributed to Helmholtz, Fechner, and Hering, which states that when two regions of the retina under conditions involving either the photopic or scotopic, but not mixed (mesopic), mechanism are differently adapted, the brightness matching results are the same as if all stimuli acting on one region were multiplied by a certain coefficient (of adaptation), whence the shape of the luminosity curve for either the photopic or scotopic mechanism remains the same for a range of intensities of the test standard. Cf. *law of persistence.*

l. of conjugate planes. Conju-

gate planes are pairs of parallel planes perpendicular to the axis of an optical system, and any straight line drawn to one nodal point and continued as a parallel straight line from the other nodal point will pierce the conjugate planes in a pair of conjugate points.

l. of constant orientation. Donders' law.

l. of corresponding areas. When an object is seen singly under binocular conditions, the images of this object, one on each retina, fall on corresponding retinal areas.

cosine l. Lambert's cosine law.

cosine-cubed l. A mathematical extension of the law of illumination in which the illumination (E) of a surface is directly proportional to the luminous intensity (I) of a given point source and to the cosine cubed ($\cos^3$) of the angle (θ) of incidence and inversely proportional to the square of the perpendicular distance (h) of the source from the plane of the surface in which the point of reference is located, expressed by the formula: $E \propto I \cos^3 \theta / h^2$.

l. of decentration. Prentice's law.

Descartes' l. Law of refraction.

Desmarres' l. When a nonfixated object is beyond the crossing point of the visual axes, its diplopic images are uncrossed (homonymous diplopia); and when a nonfixated object is closer than the crossing point of the visual axes, its diplopic images are crossed (heteronymous diplopia).

l. of disuse. When a neural pathway is not used for a period of time, its reaction to a stimulus is retarded.

Donders' l. For any determinate position of the line of fixation with respect to the head, there corresponds a definite and invariable angle of torsion, independent of the volition of the observer and independent of the manner in which the line of fixation has been brought to the position in question. Syn., *law of constant orientation.*

Draper's l. Only that portion of the spectrum which is absorbed by the medium it traverses exerts any effect on that medium. The effects may be thermal, photochemical, or the production of fluorescence. Syn., *Grotthus' law.*

Ebbinghaus' l. When luminosity alone is contrasted, the increase of brightness of a patch on a dark ground depends only on the relative difference of the two intensities and not on their absolute values.

l. of effect. The linkage of a response to a stimulus is strengthened when the response is a success or satisfying and weakened when the response is a failure or unpleasant.

Emmert's l. A projected afterimage or an eidetic image is altered in size in proportion to the distance of the surface on which it is projected.

Ewald's l. When a semicircular canal, either horizontal or vertical, is maximally stimulated, it elicits a nystagmus with the quick phase toward its own side. Minimal stimulation causes a nystagmus with the quick phase toward the opposite side.

l. of exercise. The exercise of a response to a given stimulus makes this response more precise, efficient, and stabilized.

Fechner's l. The intensity of a sensation varies as the logarithm of the intensity of the stimulus. For example, according to this law, brightness varies with the logarithm of luminance. Syn., *psychophysical law; Weber-Fechner law.*

Fechner-Helmholtz l. Law of coefficients.

Fermat's l. The actual path pursued by light in going from one point to another is that route which, under the given conditions, requires the least time.

Ferry-Porter l. The critical flicker frequency is directly proportional to the logarithm of the stimulus intensity.

Flouren's l. Nystagmus initiated in a semicircular canal occurs in a plane parallel to the canal.

l. of frequency. Responses that are elicited frequently and repeatedly show more facile reaction to stimulation than those whose function is held in abeyance.

Fresnel's l. Fresnel's formula.

Fresnel-Arago l's. 1. Two rays of polarized light will interfere the same as ordinary light when polarized in the same plane but do not interfere when polarized perpendicularly to each other. 2. Two rays perpendicularly polarized from ordinary light do not interfere when brought into the same plane of polarization. 3. Two rays perpendicularly polarized from polarized light will interfere when brought into the same plane of polarization.

Giraud-Teulon l. A viewed object is seen projected onto the plane passing through the point of convergence, hence increased convergence produced by added prism power will make the object appear nearer.

Gladstone-Dale l. The index of refraction of the corneal stroma is equal to the sum of the indices of refraction of the collagen fibers and the surrounding watery ground substance times their respective volume fractions.

Granit-Harper l. In normal subjects, the critical fusion frequency increases logarithmically as the area of retinal stimulation increases.

Grassmann's l's. Laws of color mixture formulated by H. Grassman (1853), but now stated in various forms, which hold true only within a prescribed set of conditions with respect to brightness level, adaptation of the observer, size of the field, etc. Essentially the laws are: (1) Any color, no matter how it is composed, can be matched in appearance by a mixture of three suitably chosen primary colors. (2) Any mixed color, no matter how it is composed, must have the same appearance as a mixture of a saturated (spectral) color with white. (3) If two different spots of light give the same color sensation, they continue to do so when the brightness of each is increased or decreased by the same factor. (4) When one of two kinds of light that are to be mixed together changes continuously, the appearance of the mixture changes continuously also. (5) Colors that look alike produce a mixture that looks like them. (6) The total light intensity of a mixture is the sum of the intensities of the mixed lights.

Grotthus' l. Draper's law.

Gullstrand's l. If, when a strabismic is made to turn his head while fixating a distant object, the corneal reflex from either eye moves in the direction in which the head is turning, it moves toward the weaker or paralyzed muscle.

de Haan's l. The loss in visual acuity after the age of 30, expressed as a decimal, is equal to one tenth the increase in years of age. The law is now regarded as being fallacious.

Haig's l. The intensity of light required to produce a cone response at threshold is inversely proportional to the cross sectional area of cones stimulated, expressed by the formula: $L (s/a)$

$=C$, in which L = luminance of the stimulus, a = area of retina stimulated, s = total cross sectional area of the cones in area a, C = a constant.

Helmholtz' l. of magnification. Lagrange's law.

Helmholtz' l. of torsion. The torsion of each eye is a function only of the angles of altitude and azimuth when the lines of fixation are parallel. Accordingly, the cyclophoria is constant in all directions of gaze as long as convergence is zero, confirming the theory that convergence movements are not identical to the otherwise similar fixational movements of the eye.

Hering's l. of equal innervation. Innervation to the extrinsic muscles of one eye is equal to that to the other eye, resulting in movements of the two eyes that are equal and symmetrical or parallel.

Hering's l. of ocular movements. Hering's law of equal innervation.

Hering's l. of sensation. The distinctness or the purity of a sensation is dependent on the proportion of its intensity to the total intensities of all simultaneous sensations.

Heyman's l. The threshold value of a visual stimulus is increased in proportion to the strength of a simultaneous inhibitory stimulus.

Horner's l. Color blindness is transmitted from males to males through unaffected females. (Recent research indicates that the female must be a carrier.)

l. of identical visual directions. The stimulation of corresponding retinal points, either simultaneously or individually, will result in the same visual directionalization, i.e., objects will be localized in the same direction from the self.

l. of illumination. The illumination (E) of a surface is directly proportional to the luminous intensity (I) of a given point source and to the cosine of the angle (θ) of incidence and inversely proportional to the square of the distance (d) between the point of reference on the surface and the source, expressed by the formula: $E \propto I \cos\theta/d^2$.

Imbert-Fick l. The external pressure required to flatten a given area of an infinitely thin spherical membrane filled with fluid is equal to the product of the internal pressure and the flattened area on which it acts; a prin-ciple applied to applanation tonometry.

inverse square l. The effective intensity of a freely irradiating source (i.e., not focused or otherwise confined in its path) is inversely proportional to the square of the distance between the source and the receiving surface.

Katz's l. of field size. 1. An increase in area of a portion of a surface which is differently illuminated from the remainder produces an impression of changed illumination of the area, rather than of changed surface color of the area; the latter is the impression when the area is small. 2. Same as (1) but stated for an afterimage: An afterimage cast upon a surface will appear to change the illumination of the surface in the region of the afterimage. The area covered can be increased by increasing the observer's distance from the surface. The effect in (1) remains.

Kirchhoff's l. At a given temperature, the ratio of radiant emittance to radiant absorptance for a given wavelength is the same for all bodies.

Kirschmann's l. The greatest contrast in color is seen when the luminosity difference is small.

Knapp's l. When a correcting lens is so placed before the eye that its second principal plane coincides with the anterior focal point of an axially ametropic eye, the size of the retinal image will be the same as though the eye were emmetropic.

Köllner's l. Lesions of the outer layers of the retina cause a yellow-blue color vision defect, and lesions of the inner retinal layers and of the optic nerve cause a red-green defect. For example, pigmentary degeneration of the retina causes a yellow-blue defect while retrobulbar neuritis causes a red-green defect.

Korte's l's. A series of formulas which express the optimal conditions for phi movement in terms of spatial, temporal, and intensity factors. They are: (1) With time interval constant, optimal distance varies directly with intensity. (2) With distance between stimuli constant, the optimal intensity varies indirectly with the time between the stimuli. (3) With the intensity constant, the optimal time between the stimuli varies directly with the distance between the stimuli.

von Kries l. of coefficients. See *law of coefficients*.

von Kries l. of persistence. See *law of persistence*.

Lagrange's l. In paraxial optics, the product of the index of refraction of object space, object size, and slope angle for object space is equal to the product of the index of refraction of image space, image size, and slope angle for image space. See also *Abbe's sine condition*. Syn., *Helmholtz' law of magnification*.

Lambert's l. of absorption. Law of absorption.

Lambert's cosine l. The luminous flux emitted, reflected, or transmitted by a perfectly diffusing surface per unit solid angle is proportional to the cosine of the angle between the emitted, transmitted, or reflected ray and the normal to the surface. Syn., *cosine law*.

Listing's l. When the line of fixation is brought from its primary position to any other position, the torsional rotation of the eyeball in this second position will be the same as if the eye had been turned around a fixed axis perpendicular to the initial and final directions of the line of fixation.

Loeser's l. For foveal stimulation, the product of the square root of the threshold intensity of light stimulation and the angular diameter of the lighted retinal area is a constant.

Lorentz-Lorenz l. A relationship between the index of refraction, n, of a gaseous medium and its density, D, expressed by the formula:

$$\left(\frac{n^2-1}{n^2+2}\right)\frac{1}{D} = \text{constant}$$

Mach's l. A uniform movement has no effect in producing statokinetic reflexes, the only effective stimuli being the initiation of movement or the acceleration or retardation of movement.

Malus' l. The transmission of light through two consecutively placed polarizing media is proportional to the square of the cosine of the angle between their respective planes of polarization.

Malus-Dupin l. A bundle of rays normal to a surface, a so-called normal system, remains a normal system after refraction and reflection.

Maxwell's l. The dielectric constant for a transparent medium is equal to the square of its index of refraction as measured for very long waves only.

l. of monocular projection. The monocular visual projection of a retinal stimulus is outward in the direction of that path of light incident toward the nodal point which would, after refraction, reach the locus of the retinal stimulus.

Mueller's l. of specific nerve energy. Each nerve of special sense, however excited, gives rise to its own peculiar sensation.

Nasse's l. In X-linked recessive traits, the daughters of a male case are carriers and pass the trait to one-half of their sons, as in hemophilia.

Newton's l. of color mixture. Any one or a combination of the several rules of color mixing described by Newton. The following two are frequently cited: (1) If two color mixtures elicit the same sensation of light or color, the combination of the mixtures will arouse the same sensation. (2) The spectral nature of a color resulting from a mixture of two colors may be determined graphically in a schematic representation by dividing the line joining the two constituents inversely as to the quantities of each constituent in the mixture.

Newton-Mueller-Gudden l. In mammals, the relative number of uncrossed fibers in the optic chiasm is closely proportional to the degree of frontality of the eyes.

l. of persistence. A law expressed by von Kries which states that, for either the photopic or scotopic, but not mixed (mesopic), mechanism, a match of two lights of different spectral composition remains a match at other levels of adaptation. Cf. *law of coefficients*.

Pieron's l's. 1. For foveal images of moderate size, the luminance of the target at threshold is inversely related to the cube root of the retinal area stimulated, expressed by the formula: $L\sqrt[3]{A}=C$, in which $L=$ luminance of the stimulus, $A=$ area of the retinal image, and $C=$ a constant. 2. A modification of the Blondel-Rey law. The intensity of light required to produce a response at nonlinear function of the duration of the light, expressed by the formula: $Lt^n=C$, in which $L=$ luminance of the stimulus, $t=$ stimulus duration, $n=$ a value varying with retinal location, and $C=$ a constant. It does not apply after maximum time t_2, beyond which summation does not occur.

Piper's l. For small images in peripheral vision, the product of intensity and the square root of the area stimulated is a constant for threshold effect, expressed by the formula: $L\sqrt{A}=C$, in which L=luminance of the stimulus, A=retinal area, and C=a constant.

Pitt's l. Differential wavelength discrimination in the color defective is best where saturation is poorest.

Planck's l. Energy distribution in the spectrum of a blackbody is expressed by the formula:

$$W\lambda = C_1\lambda^{-5}\left(\epsilon^{\lambda T}-1\right)^{-1}$$

in which $W\lambda$=watts radiated by a blackbody per sq. cm of surface in each wavelength band, 1 μ wide, at wavelength λ; λ=wavelength in microns; T=absolute temperature; C_1=37,350 micron-degrees; C_2= 14,380 micron-degrees; $_\epsilon$=2.718+.

l. of Prägnanz. There is a tendency to interpret the form of an object, seen in perspective, as being one of certain favored simple familiar forms, such as a circle, a square, or a rectangle.

Prentice's l. The deviation, expressed in prism diopters, at a point on a lens is equal to the product of the dioptric power of the lens and the distance, in centimeters, of the point from the optical center of the lens. Syn., *law of decentration.*

l. of projection. Law of monocular projection.

l. of proximity. Objects or forms that are adjacent or close together tend to be grouped visually, thus often becoming parts of a singly perceived object or pattern.

psychophysical l. Fechner's law.

Rayleigh l. In a transmitting medium whose heterogeneities have average dimensions which are small in comparison to the wavelength of the incident energy, the fraction of the incident flux scattered is inversely proportional to the fourth power of the wavelength.

l. of reciprocity. Bunsen-Roscoe law.

l. of rectilinear propagation of light. Light travels in straight lines in a homogeneous medium.

l. of reflection. The angle of reflection is equal to the angle of incidence; the incident ray, the normal to the surface at the point of incidence, and the reflected ray lie in the same plane.

l. of refraction. The ratio of the sine of the angle of incidence to the sine of the angle of refraction is a constant equal to the relative index of refraction; the incident ray, the normal to the surface at the point of incidence, and the refracted ray lie in the same plane. Syn., *Descartes' law; law of sines; Snell's law.*

l. of reversibility. The directions of propagation in a path of reflected or refracted light are precisely reversible. Syn., *principle of reversibility.*

Ricco's l. For small images on the fovea, the product of image area and light intensity is constant for threshold effect, expressed by the formula: $LA = C$, in which L = luminance of the stimulus, A = retinal area, and C = a constant. Syn., *Charpentier's law.*

Schouten-Ornstein l. If any new brightness level is maintained indefinitely, the state of dark or light adaptation of the eye remains unchanged.

Sherrington's l. of reciprocal innervation. The contraction of each skeletal (including ocular) muscle is accompanied by a simultaneous and proportional relaxation of its antagonist.

l. of similarity. Objects or forms which are similar, as in content or pattern, tend to be grouped visually.

l. of sines. Law of refraction.

sine-squared l. The dioptric power in any meridian of a cylindrical lens is equal to the cylinder power multiplied by the square of the sine of the angle between that meridian and the axis of the cylinder.

l. of size constancy. The perception of the size of an object remains constant, or nearly constant, although the object be moved farther from or nearer to the observer, subtending varying visual angles.

Smith-Helmholtz l. Lagrange's law.

Snell's l. Law of refraction.

Stefan-Boltzmann l. The radiant emittance of a blackbody is proportional to the fourth power of its absolute temperature.

Stokes' l. In fluorescence, the wavelength of the emitted light is always greater than that of the exciting light; now known to have exceptions.

l. of symmetry. The perceptual grouping of objects or forms into larger wholes is dependent on various features of geometrical symmetry.

Talbot's l. Talbot-Plateau law.

Talbot-Plateau l. The brightness of rapidly intermittent light perceived as continuous and unvarying is equal to that which would be produced by a constant light of intensity equal to the mean value of the intermittent stimuli.

l. of use. The frequent use of a neural pathway facilitates its reaction to a stimulus.

Weber's l. The increase of stimulus which is necessary to produce a just noticeable difference in sensation bears a constant ratio to the stimulus from which the difference is noted.

Weber-Fechner l. Fechner's law or Weber's law, especially implying recognition of the identity of the two as can be shown by the mathematical derivation of one from the other when sensation is regarded as directly measurable in jnd units, q.v.

Wien's displacement l. The wavelength for which spectral emittance is a maximum for complete radiators is inversely proportional to its absolute temperature.

Wien's radiation l. An empirical formula derived by Wien to represent the relationship between energy emission, wavelength, and the temperature of a radiator, similar to a more generally applicable radiation formula derived by Planck from quantum considerations. See also *Planck's law.*

Wundt-Lamanski l. The oblique fixational movements of the eye, as inferred from afterimage studies by Wundt and Lamanski, do not follow the shortest route, i.e., the afterimage tracing the path of movement is curved rather than straight.

Zeune's l. A theory that climate has much to do with blindness, whence it is stated that the proportion of blindness is least in the Temperate Zone and increases in the direction of the Frigid Zone and in the direction of the equator.

◆

Lawford's syndrome. See under *syndrome.*

◆
LAYER

layer. A deposited substance of uniform, or nearly uniform, thickness; one thickness laid over or under another.

anterior border l. of the iris. Anterior limiting layer of the iris.

anterior limiting l. of the iris. The layer of the iris, between the anterior endothelium and the stroma, which is a condensation of the anterior stroma consisting of anastomosing and intertwining processes of connective tissue and pigment cells. Syn., *anterior border layer of the iris.*

anterior pigment l. of Fuchs. The anterior layer of the posterior pigmented epithelial layer of the iris containing myoepithelial, pigmented, spindle cell bodies. Their myofibrils constitute the dilator pupillae muscle. Syn., *layer of pigmented spindle cells.*

bacillary l. Layer of rods and cones.

Bowman's l. Bowman's membrane.

Bruch's l. 1. The lamina vitrea or innermost membrane of the choroid. 2. The lamina vitrea of the ciliary body. 3. The posterior border lamella of Fuchs.

cerebral l. of retina. One of two subdivisions of the retina which contains the inner nuclear, the inner molecular, the ganglion cell, and the nerve fiber layers and the internal limiting membrane, the other being the *neuroepithelial layer of the retina.*

Chievitz l. Transient fiber layer of Chievitz.

choriocapillary l. Choriocapillaris.

columnar l. Layer of rods and cones. *Obs.*

fiber l. of Henle. In the region of the macula lutea, the horizontally directed fibers of the rods and cones located in the outer molecular layer.

fiber l. of Mueller. Mueller's fibers.

ganglion cell l. The layer of the retina lying between the inner molecular and the nerve fiber layers and containing large cell bodies whose neurons send axons into the nerve fiber layer, into the ipsilateral optic nerve, and into both optic tracts to synapse in the lateral geniculate bodies, the pretectal areas, and the superior colliculi.

Haller's l. A layer of the choroid lying between the suprachoroid and

Sattler's layer, composed of connective tissue and large blood vessels whose capillaries are located in the choriocapillaris.

Henle's l. Fiber layer of Henle.

inner granular l. Layer IV of the cerebral cortex which thickens in the region of the visual cortex to comprise its most voluminous layer. It is composed of three sublayers, an inner and an outer cellular lamina and a middle lamina containing the outer line of Baillargèr.

Kölliker's fibrous l. The stroma of the iris.

lacrimal l. Precorneal film.

limiting l. of retina, external. The membrane of the retina lying between the layer of rods and cones and the outer nuclear layer, through which pass the processes of the rods and cones. It is thought to consist of the united ends of the fibers of Mueller or the remains of the original intercellular cement of the fetal retinal cells. Syn., *external limiting membrane of the retina*.

limiting l. of retina, internal. The membrane of the retina lying between the nerve fiber layer of the retina and the vitreous, forming the inner limit of the retina and the outer boundary of the vitreous, occasionally called the *hyaloid membrane of the vitreous*. It is continuous with the central meniscus of Kuhnt and is thought to be partially formed by the ends of the fibers of Mueller. Syn., *internal limiting membrane of the retina*.

lipid l. of the cornea. The fatty layer of the basement membrane located between its reticular layer and the basal cells of the corneal epithelium.

marginal l. of His. Marginal layer of the optic cup.

marginal l. of the optic cup. The outer, nonnucleated layer of cells of the optic cup in the early embryo bounding the primitive layer of the optic cup. Syn., *marginal layer of His*.

molecular l., inner. The layer of the retina between the inner nuclear and the ganglion cell layers in which the neurons of these two layers synapse and in which amacrine cells synapse. Syn., *inner plexiform layer*.

molecular l., outer. The layer of the retina between the outer and the inner nuclear layers in which the neurons of these two layers synapse and in which horizontal cells synapse. Syn., *outer plexiform layer*.

nerve fiber l. The layer of the retina lying between the ganglion cell layer and the internal limiting membrane, containing axons of the ganglion cells and arterioles and venules of the central retinal vessels.

neuroblastic l. of optic cup, inner. The inner of two collections of nuclei in the embryonic retina which forms amacrine and ganglion cells.

neuroblastic l. of optic cup, outer. The outer of two collections of nuclei in the embryonic retina which forms visual, horizontal, and bipolar cells.

neuroepithelial l. of retina. One of two subdivisions of the retina which contains the layer of rods and cones, the external limiting membrane, the outer nuclear layer, and the outer molecular layer, the other being the *cerebral layer of retina*.

nuclear l., inner. The layer of the retina lying between the inner and the outer molecular layers and containing amacrine, bipolar, and horizontal cell bodies, nuclei of the fibers of Mueller, and capillaries of the central retinal vessels. Syn., *membrana granulosa interna*.

nuclear l., outer. The layer of the retina lying between the external limiting membrane and the outer molecular layer containing the cell bodies of rods and cones. Syn., *membrana granulosa externa*.

pigment epithelium l. of retina. The layer of the retina lying between the lamina vitrea of the choroid and the layer of rods and cones of the retina, consisting of a single layer of hexagonal cells which contain the pigment fuscin and have processes that surround the outer segments of the rods and cones. One of its main functions is the transfer of oxygen and foods from the choriocapillaris to the rod and cone cells.

l. of pigmented spindle cells. Anterior pigment layer of Fuchs.

plexiform l., inner. Inner molecular layer.

plexiform l., outer. Outer molecular layer.

primitive l. of optic cup. The innermost, nucleated layer of cells of the optic cup in the early embryo whose periphery is bounded by the marginal layer of the optic cup. It is the embryonic layer which differentiates into the *inner* and the *outer neuroblastic layers.*

proliferating l. of optic cup. The outermost layer of cells of the optic cup where cell division occurs in the early embryo. It gives rise to the visual cells, the fibers of Mueller, all neurons of the retina, and the pars caeca retinae.

reticular l. of the cornea. The layer of the basement membrane located between its lipid layer and Bowman's membrane which may be subdivided into three layers of reticular fibers, the anterior being most dense and the middle being the least.

retinal l's. The 10 layers of the retina: the pigment epithelium layer, the layer of rods and cones, the external limiting membrane, the outer nuclear layer, the outer molecular layer, the inner nuclear layer, the inner molecular layer, the ganglion cell layer, the nerve fiber layer, and the internal limiting membrane.

l. of rods and cones. The layer of the retina containing the receptive portions of the rods and cones, excluding their nuclei. It is approximately 40 μ in thickness and is bounded posteriorly by the pigment epithelium layer and anteriorly by the external limiting membrane. Syn., *bacillary layer; Jacob's membrane.*

Sattler's l. The layer of the choroid, lying between Haller's layer and the choriocapillaris, containing the smaller arteries and veins. Syn., *Sattler's lamina.*

substantia propria l. The main connective tissue portion or stroma of a structure, as in the cornea, the sclera, the choroid, or the iris.

suprachoroid l. Suprachoroid.

tear l. Precorneal film.

transient fiber l. of Chievitz. The temporary layer which separates the primitive inner and the outer neuroblastic layers of the embryonic retina. It is a clear layer containing the inner processes of the fibers of Mueller.

◆

layout. In opticianry, the process of marking a blank or lens for positioning in the surfacing or edging machinery.

Lazich's test (lāz'iks). See under *test.*

LCO. See *London Course of Optometry.*

LE. Abbreviation for *left eye.*

leaf room. See under *room.*

Leavell (leh-vel') **Hand-Eye Co-ordinator; tests.** See under the nouns.

Lebensohn (la'ben-sōn) **astigmometer; chart.** See under the nouns.

Leber's (la-berz') **congenital amaurosis; miliary aneurysms; cells; venous circle; retinal degeneration; disease; plexus; retinitis; theory.** See under the nouns.

LED. Light emitting diode.

Lederer lenses (led'er-er). See under *lens.*

LEF. Lighting effectiveness factor.

LeGrand-Geblewics phenomenon (le-grahnd'geh-blev'iks). See under *phenomenon.*

Leigh syndrome. See under *syndrome.*

leiomyoma (li"o-mi-o'mah). A tumor derived from smooth muscle characterized histologically by elongated spindle-shaped cells and myoglia fibrils. It is usually benign and may involve the iris and less frequently the ciliary body or orbit. When involving the iris it has a predilection for the pupillary margin, is lightly pigmented, and may be well localized but is more often diffuse.

leiomyosarcoma (li"o-mi"o-sar-ko'-mah). A malignant tumor derived from smooth muscle which may involve the iris, ciliary body, or orbit.

Leiner's disease (li'nerz). See under *disease.*

leishmaniasis (lēsh-man-i'ah-sis). Ulceration of the face, eyelids, and cornea due to infection with the protozoan *Leishmania tropica.* The corneal lesions are deep and spread to involve the entire cornea.

LeJeune syndrome. Cat-cry syndrome. See under *syndrome.*

lema (le'mah). The dried and hardened Meibomian secretion collected at the inner canthus of the eye.

Leman prism (le'man). See under *prism.*

lemmocytes (lem'o-sīts). Cells intimately connected with unmyelinated nerve fibers, representing the equivalent of the elements of the sheath of Schwann which surround myelinated nerve fibers. They are found in the peripheral nervous system and in the nerve fiber layer of the retina. Syn., *Remak's cells.*

lemniscus, optic (lem-nis'kus). Optic tract.

length. The number of units expressing the result of measurement of a distance in one direction.

   focal l. The linear distance between a point of reference, usually a principal point, of an optical system and the corresponding primary or secondary focal point. **anterior f.l.** Primary focal length. **back f.l.** The linear distance between the back vertex of an optical system and the secondary focal point. Syn., *posterior vertex focal distance.* **equivalent f.l.** The linear distance between the secondary principal point of an optical system and the secondary focal point. **front f.l.** The linear distance between the front vertex of an optical system and the primary focal point. Syn., *anterior vertex focal distance.* **posterior f.l.** Secondary focal length. **primary f.l.** The linear distance from the primary principal point to the primary focal point of an optical system. Syn., *anterior focal length; anterior principal focal length; primary principal focal length.* **principal (anterior) f.l.** Primary focal length. **principal (posterior) f.l.** Secondary focal length. **principal (primary) f.l.** Primary focal length. **principal (secondary) f.l.** Secondary focal length. **reduced f.l.** The ratio of the primary focal length to the refractive index of the medium containing the incident light or to the ratio of the secondary focal length to the refractive index of the medium containing the emerging light. **secondary f.l.** The linear distance from the secondary principal point to the secondary focal point of an optical system. Syn., *posterior focal length; posterior principal focal length; secondary principal focal length.* **vertex f.l.** The focal length of an optical system as measured from the back or front vertex to the secondary or primary focal point, respectively.

   optical l. The product of the length of the path of a ray in a medium and the index of refraction of the medium.

Lenoble-Aubineau syndrome. Aubineau-Lenoble syndrome. See under *syndrome.*

◆

LENS

lens. A piece of glass or other transparent substance having two opposite regular surfaces, either plane or curved, and functioning as a part or all of an optical system. More generally, it may include opaque objects with regular reflecting surfaces (e.g., a mirror lens in a reflecting telescope) or an assembly of several individual lenses regarded as a single unit (e.g., a camera doublet or a multifocal spectacle lens).

   absorption l. A lens which absorbs a portion of the incident light. Syn., *lens plate filter.*

   absorptive l. Absorption lens.

   achromatic l. A compound lens designed to reduce or eliminate chromatic aberration. The most common form is a converging system consisting of a crown glass convex lens of low dispersive power combined with a flint glass concave lens of high dispersive power but of lower refractive power.

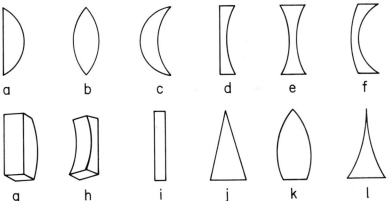

Fig. 25 Lenses: (a) planoconvex; (b) biconvex; (c) periscopic convex; (d) planoconcave; (e) biconcave; (f) periscopic concave; (g) convex cylindrical; (h) concave cylindrical; (i) plano; (j) plano prismatic; (k) convex prismatic; (1) concave prismatic.

actinic l. An absorption lens which primarily absorbs ultraviolet radiation.

adherent l. Contact lens.

afocal l. A lens of zero focal power in which rays entering parallel emerge parallel.

Allen-Braley fundus l. A planoconcave plastic scleral contact lens mounted by means of spring wire supports in a plastic speculum for use in slit lamp examination of the deep vitreous and fundus.

Alvarez l. A two-element variable-power spherical lens similar in principle to the *Humphrey lenses.*

Amici-Bertrand l. A polarizing microscope accessory lens which may be inserted between the eyepiece and the analyzer to focus on the rear focal plane of the objective where the diffraction patterns are formed. Syn., *Bertrand lens.*

anamorphote l. A lens which effects anamorphosis.

anastigmatic l. A lens with spherical surfaces and therefore said to have no cylindrical component. Anastigmatic lenses are one of two categories of ophthalmic lenses, the other being *astigmatic lenses.* Syn., *stigmatic lens.*

aniseikonic l. Iseikonic lens.

anterior chamber l. Anterior chamber implant.

Aolite l. A trade name for one of a series of plastic lenses made in both single vision and multifocal form.

aphakic l. A convex spectacle lens of high dioptric power, so named because its principal use is in the correction of vision in aphakia. Syn., *cataract lens.*

aplanatic l. A lens designed to correct for spherical aberration and coma.

apochromatic l. A compound lens designed to correct for spherical and chromatic aberrations.

Apollonio l. A small, plastic lens placed in the anterior chamber of the eyeball to replace the crystalline lens, following cataract surgery. It is held in position by a three-pronged plastic mount.

armor plate l. Case-hardened lens.

aspherical l. A lens in which one or both surfaces in the central sagittal section do not describe a circle, usually conforming instead to a parabola or some similar curve systematically deviant from a circle from the center to the periphery of the lens, so designed to correct for or reduce certain types of aberrations.

astigmatic l. A lens with one or both surfaces toric or toroidal, and therefore said to have a cylindrical component and to produce two perpendicularly oriented focal lines in the principal meridians instead of a single focal point. Astigmatic lenses are one of two categories of ophthalmic lenses, the other being *anastigmatic lenses.*

Astikorrect l. A variable power, cylindrical lens system designed for use with the Raubitschek test consisting of two counterrotating +1.00 D sph. −2.00 D cyl. lenses in a hand-held assembly. It provides powers ranging from plano to +2.00 D. sph. −4.00 D cyl. with the spherical power at any position being half the cylindrical power and of opposite sign.

Bagolini's l. See *glass, Bagolini's striated.*

balance l. A spectacle lens of undesignated power serving only to balance the weight and the appearance of its mate in front of the other eye.

Barkan goniotomy l. A thick, convex, contact lens used to provide a magnified view of the iris and filtration angle during goniotomy.

Barlow l. A concave achromatic lens placed between the objective and eyepiece of a telescope to provide greater magnification of the image with only a slight increase in focal length.

Baron l. A rectangular, plastic lens placed in the anterior chamber of the eyeball to replace the crystalline lens, following cataract surgery. Being larger than other such lenses, it has no mount and is held in position by its own edges.

baseball l. A double bifocal lens in which the two reading segments are rounded so that the lens resembles the seamline of a baseball.

Bertrand l. Amici-Bertrand lens.

best-form l. A corrected curve lens.

bicentric l. A lens with two optical centers.

biconcave l. 1. A lens with both surfaces concave. 2. A double concave lens in which both surfaces are equal in curvature. (See Fig. 25.)

biconvex l. 1. A lens with both surfaces convex. 2. A double convex lens in which both surfaces are equal in curvature. (See Fig. 25.)

bicylindrical l. A lens with both surfaces toroidal. Syn., *bitoric lens.*

Bietti l. A small plastic lens placed in the anterior chamber of the eyeball to replace the crystalline lens, following cataract surgery. The lens is held in position either by a four-pronged plastic mount or by a curved, rectangular, plastic plate into which the lens is secured.

bifocal l. A spectacle lens of two portions whose focal powers differ from each other. Usually the upper portion is larger and is for distant vision, and the lower portion is smaller and is for near vision. **baseball b.l.** See *lens, baseball.* **Bitex b.l.** An obsolete one-piece bifocal similar to the modern Ultex E bifocal lens. **blended b.l.** A one-piece bifocal lens in which there is a gradual transitional zone between the two curves of different radii instead of the line of demarcation contained in the conventional bifocal. **cement b.l.** A bifocal lens made by cementing a small wafer-thin lens to a larger lens. **CV (complete vision) b.l.** An obsolete monocentric multifocal lens designed by Andrew J. Cross. It consists of one piece of crown glass, ground on the inside surface into three different spherical curvatures, a large upper distance segment, a smaller lower reading segment, and two lateral areas of intermediate power. **depressed b.l.** An obsolete one-piece bifocal lens made by grinding the steeper curvature of the reading portion into the flatter surface required for the distance portion, causing the reading portion of the lens to be depressed and thinner. **double b.l.** A multifocal lens having two segments for near vision, one at the top and one at the bottom, with the portion for distance vision in between. **Executive b.l.** A monocentric, one-piece bifocal lens with a straight, horizontal line of junction, between the two portions, extending across the entire lens. **Franklin b.l.** The original bifocal invented by Benjamin Franklin in 1784. It consists of two half lenses mounted together in the same frame, the upper half for distant vision and the lower half for near vision. **Ful-Vue b.l.** A trade name for a fused bifocal lens with the optical cen-

ter of the reading segment 4 mm below its slightly curved top. **fused b.l.** A bifocal lens in which the added dioptric power required for near seeing is accomplished by countersinking into the surface of a crown glass lens a small lens, sometimes called a *button,* of barium crown, flint, or some other glass of higher index of refraction, and fusing the two types of glass in a high temperature oven for permanent adhesion. **Kryptok b.l.** A fused bifocal lens with a round flint glass reading segment, invented by John L. Borsch. **monaxial b.l.** An obsolete monocentric bifocal lens consisting of one piece of crown glass ground on the inside surface into three different spherical curvatures, similar in principle to the CV bifocal lens. **monocentric b.l.** A bifocal lens in which the optical centers of the two portions are coincident. **Nokrome b.l.** A trade name for a fused bifocal lens having a barium crown reading segment for the reduction of chromatic aberration. **one-piece b.l.** A bifocal lens consisting of a single piece of crown glass with two different curvatures ground on one surface. **Opifex b.l.** A cement bifocal lens having an extremely thin wafer reading segment. **Panoptik b.l.** A trade name for a fused bifocal lens with the optical center of the reading segment 3 mm below its slightly curved top. **Perfection b.l.** A bifocal lens invented by August Morck, similar in principle to the Franklin bifocal lens. It was made by removing an archshaped portion from the lower half of the distance lens and fitting in a lens of different power for near vision. **RedeRite b.l.** A trade name for a one-piece bifocal lens featuring a major portion of the lens for near vision and a small segment in the upper portion for distant vision. **solid b.l.** A one-piece bifocal lens. **solid upcurve b.l.** An obsolete one-piece bifocal lens invented by Isaac Schnaitmann. The process of manufacture consisted of grinding the top portion of a reading glass to the distance prescription. **split b.l.** Franklin bifocal lens. **Turay b.l.** A trade name for a series of one-piece bifocal lenses. **Twinsite b.l.** A trade name for a series of one-piece bifocal lenses. **Ultex b.l.** A trade name for a series of one-piece bifocal lenses. **Unisite b.l.** An obsolete monocentric one-piece bifocal similar to the modern Ultex B bifocal lens. **Univis b.l.** A trade name for a series of fused bifocal lenses, most of which are characterized by a straight top segment for near vision. **Widesite b.l.** A trade name for a series of fused bifocal lenses.

Billet's split l. Two halves of a convex lens divided along an axial plane and slightly separated to produce interference fringes in the overlapping images.

Binkhorst l. Iris clip lens.

Binkhorst-Weinstein-Troutman l. A lens placed in the pupillary opening following cataract surgery to render the eye emmetropic and to eliminate aniseikonia. It is a doublet consisting of an anterior concavoplano lens and a posterior convexoplano lens separated by an enclosed airspace, and is weightless in aqueous humor. Loops attached to the lens are fixed to the iris to hold it in position.

Bioptic telescopic l. A lens system used as a subnormal vision aid consisting of a small diameter Galilean telescope to magnify distant objects, mounted on the upper front surface of a plastic carrier lens having the patient's distance lens correction.

bispherical l. A lens that is spherical on both sides.

bitoric l. A lens having toroidal surfaces on both sides, used primarily in the correction of aniseikonia. **oblique b.l.** A bitoric lens in which the principal meridians of the two toroidal surfaces are not coincident, a type of lens used in the combined correction of a meridional aniseikonia and a cylindrical refractive error obliquely oriented with respect to each other.

l. blank. A molded piece of ophthalmic glass prior to grinding and polishing into a lens.

blended l. See *bifocal lens, blended.*

bloomed l. Coated lens.

Bonvue l. A trade name for a series of multibase curve lenses and for a series of fused bifocal and trifocal lenses.

Brücke's l. Brücke's loupe.

l. capsule. See under *capsule.*

Cartesian l. A lens proposed by Descartes to eliminate spherical aberration in which one surface is spherical and the other is ellipsoidal.

case-hardened l. A lens subjected to high temperature for superficial annealing of the glass to increase resistance to breakage by impact. Syn., *tempered lens.* Cf. *safety lens.*

cataract l. Aphakic lens.

Catmin l. A minifying spectacle lens consisting of a reversed Galilean telescope system of three glass lenses cemented together, designed to obtain equal binocular image size in the correction of monocular aphakia.

l. cement substance. The noncellular amorphous material secreted by the cells of the crystalline lens, found just within the lens capsule, posterior to the anterior epithelium, in the Y-sutures, in the more complicated lens stars, and between the individual lens fibers.

centered l. A lens whose optical center coincides with its geometrical center.

centering l. A plano lens having two etched lines, at right angles to each other, intersecting at its center, and used to align and center the cell of a trial frame with the center of the pupil.

Chavasse l. A spectacle lens with a rippled, multiple-facet back surface, designed by Chavasse to function as an occluder by its distortion of the retinal image, though still permitting the eye to be seen clearly through it.

Chevalier l. 1. A magnifier consisting of an achromatic negative lens separated by air from a positive front lens resulting in up to $10\times$ magnification and up to 7 cm object distance. 2. An achromatic doublet camera lens designed to make the focus of the photographically effective light coincident with that of visually effective light.

Choyce Mark VIII l. A transparent, polymethylmethacrylate, bilaterally symmetrical, quadrimerous, anterior-chamber implant with a centrally formed biconvex lens of about 6 mm diameter and an approximately 6 x 12 mm overall rectangular shape, V-notched at the two ends and somewhat rounded at the corners to provide four tonguelike shoulders which rest in the aqueous chamber angle of the eye.

Clear-Image L. A trade name for a magnifying telescopic spectacle lens designed and manufactured by Feinbloom.

l. clock. Lens measure.

coated l. A lens on whose surfaces is deposited a metallic salt, such as magnesium fluoride, about one-fourth as thick as a wavelength of light, to reduce, by interference, the amount of light reflected, and, if combined with a coloring ingredient, to reduce light transmission also.

cobalt l. A plano ophthalmic test lens made of cobalt glass, characterized by its relatively selective transmission of the red and blue spectral colors, hence useful in the bichrome testing of ametropia.

Coddington l. A magnifying lens consisting essentially of a cylindrical section through a solid sphere of glass, its two refracting surfaces being segments of the surface of the sphere.

collimating l. A lens placed in such a manner that the source or object is located at one of its focal points; hence, the refracted rays from an object point will leave the lens parallel to each other.

compound l. 1. A spectacle lens which functions as a combination of a simple spherical lens and a simple cylindrical lens. 2. A lens system composed of two or more coaxially placed lenses.

concave l. Diverging lens. (See Fig. 25.)

concavoconcave l. A lens which is concave on both surfaces.

concavoconvex l. A converging meniscus lens. Cf. *convexoconcave lens.*

concentric l. A meniscus lens whose two surfaces have a common center of curvature.

condensing l. A condenser.

congeneric l. In relation to another lens of reference, one which is of the same sign or dioptric character, whence a pair of converging lenses or a pair of diverging lenses are said to be congeneric. Cf. *contrageneric lens.*

conoid l. Volk conoid lens.

contact l. A small, shell-like, bowl-shaped glass or plastic lens that rests directly on the eye, in contact with the cornea or the sclera or both, serving as a new anterior surface of the eye and/or as a retainer for fluid between the cornea and the contact lens, ordinarily to correct for refractive errors of the eye. **A-B-C self-centering c.l.** A modification of the Feincone contact lens providing for minimum corneal clearance. **Accusoft c.l.** Trade name for a lathed, soft contact lens made of droxifilcon. **afocal c.l.** A contact lens whose optical section has no refractive power. **Akiyama c.l.** A narrow and approximately rectangular contact lens designed to rest on the lower portion of the cornea and to cover the pupil only when the eye rotates downward as in looking at a near object. **Allen-O'Brien c.l.** Allen's contact prism. **Amsof c.l.** Trade name for a lathe-cut, soft contact lens made of deltafilcon material. **Aosoft c.l.** A hydrophilic contact lens made from tetrafilcon material. **aperture c.l.** Palpebral contact lens. **Aquaflex c.l.** Trade name for a lathe-cut, semi-scleral, soft contact lens. **bandage c.l.** Any of several soft contact lenses used as a bandage on the cornea to protect it from air, foreign bodies, or bacteria, or as a conveyor of medication. **Bass c.l.** Trade name for a bifocal contact lens made of PMMA material. **Bayshore c.l.** A type of palpebral contact lens fitted with a base curve significantly steeper than the flatter principal meridian of the cornea to provide constant and definite apical clearance, a secondary curve approximating the cornea on which it rests, and a narrow peripheral curve of 17.0 mm radius to contain a reservoir of tear fluid at the rim. Syn., *B.T. contact lens.* **bicurve c.l.** A corneal contact lens having two curvatures on its posterior surface, one the central base curve forming the optic zone, and the other a flatter curve forming the annular peripheral zone. **Bier c.l.** Either the Contour contact lens or the Transcurve contact lens designed by Norman Bier. **bifocal c.l.** A contact lens having two portions of different focal powers, one for distant vision and one for near vision. **bifocal (alternating vision) c.l.** A bifocal contact lens so designed that the pupillary area of the eye is effectively covered by either the reading zone or the distance zone, but not by both. **bifocal (annular) c.l.** A bifocal contact lens having a central round zone for distance vision surrounded by an annular zone for near vision. **bifocal (Bicon) c.l.** A monocentric, shifting, alternating vision, bifocal contact lens having two curvatures on its front surface, providing a central round zone for distance vision surrounded by an annular zone for near vision. **bifocal (Bi-Profile) c.l.** An annular bifocal contact lens made from a single piece of plastic having four monocentric curvatures on its back surface, a central base curve, a slightly flatter secondary curve approximately 1.5 to 2.0 mm wide, which provides up to +1.00 D of additional power, and a flatter tertiary curve and bevel. A second peripheral curve commencing coincident with the margin of the central base curve is added to the front surface when more than a +1.00 D addition is required. **bifocal (bivisual) c.l.** A bifocal contact lens so designed that portions of the pupillary area of the eye are covered simultaneously by both the reading zone and the distance zone, e.g., *deCarle bifocal contact lens.* **bifocal (Black) c.l.** A shifting, alternating vision, bifocal contact lens made of a single piece of plastic with two different curvatures cut on the front surface to provide a reading portion below and a distance portion above, the junction line being a curve whose convexity is toward the bottom of the lens. **bifocal (Brucker) c.l.** A prism ballast, alternating vision, bifocal contact lens having an optical zone for distance vision decentered upward and surrounded by the reading addition, the power of which is determined essentially by the radius of the secondary curve. **bifocal (Camp) c.l.** A prism ballast bifocal contact lens, truncated at the base, having a round reading segment, of a plastic of higher index of refraction, fused into its posterior surface. **bifocal (Cinefro) c.l.** A shifting, alternating vision, bifocal contact lens made of a single piece of plastic with two different curvatures cut on the front surface to provide a reading portion below and a distance portion above, the junction line being a curve whose convexity is toward the top of the lens. **bifocal (Contour Comfort) c.l.** A truncated, prism ballast, alternating vision, fused, bifocal contact lens with a segment for near vision formed by pouring liquid plastic into a countersink cut on the back surface. The liquid plastic contains a dye which fluoresces under black light to facilitate its location. **bifocal (deCarle) c.l.** A bivisual, monocentric, bifocal contact lens having two curvatures on its posterior surface, providing a central, small, round distance portion surrounded by an annular reading portion. **bifocal (fused) c.l.** A bifocal contact lens constructed of two pieces of plastic, of different indices of refraction, fused together. **bifocal (Genevay) c.l.** An alternating vision, bifocal contact lens made of one piece of plastic and having two curvatures on its posterior surface, providing a central round zone for distance vision surrounded by an annular zone for near vision. **bifocal (No-Jump) c.l.** A prism ballast, alternating vision, bifocal contact lens, truncated at the base, made of a single piece of plastic having two curves on its front surface with a com-

mon center of curvature to eliminate prismatic jump. It provides a reading portion below and a distance portion above, the junction line being a curve whose convexity is toward the top of the lens. **bifocal (Paraseg K) c.l.** An oval-shaped, alternating vision, bifocal contact lens made of a single piece of plastic having two curvatures on its posterior surface to provide a reading portion below and a distance portion above, the junction line being a curve whose convexity is toward the bottom of the lens. **bifocal (piggyback) c.l.** A combination of a single vision contact lens and a half-moon-shaped lens which provides the additional power for near vision. The half-moon lens is placed by the patient on the lower half of the single vision lens with its straight edge upwards, after the single vision lens has been inserted. **bifocal (prism ballast) c.l.** A bifocal contact lens, usually of the alternating vision type, having a small amount of base-down prism to weight the lens and thus prevent rotation, to provide a low riding position, and to assist the propping effect of the lower eyelid. **bifocal (reverse centrad) c.l.** A hydrophobic bifocal contact lens with a fused, circular segment of higher index of refraction than the major portion of the lens, centrally located on the back surface for near vision, the major portion of the lens surrounding the segment being for distance vision. **bifocal (shifting) c.l.** A bifocal contact lens of the alternating vision type so designed that the lens will be displaced vertically, relative to the pupil, as the eye rotates upward or downward, so that the appropriate reading zone will effectively cover the pupil. **bifocal (target) c.l.** A bifocal contact lens having a central round zone for distance vision surrounded by an annular zone for near vision, hence resembling a target. **bifocal (U.V.) c.l.** An alternating vision, prism ballast, fused, bifocal contact lens having a circular reading segment in the lower portion of the lens impregnated with a dye which fluoresces under black light to facilitate its location. **bifocal (Wesley-Jessen) c.l.** A prism ballast, alternating vision, fused, bifocal contact lens having a circular reading segment in the lower portion of the lens which has been impregnated with a fluorescing substance to facilitate its location with black light. **bitoric c.l.** A contact lens, both surfaces of which are toric, usually fabricated so that the steepest radius of each surface lies in the same meridian. **blown c.l.** A contact lens formed by glass blowing. **B.T. c.l.** Bayshore contact lens. **channelled c.l.** A contact lens having one or more radial depressions on its posterior surface which serve as channels to facilitate tear circulation. **closed c.l.** A contact lens whose surface is continuous, that is, free of fenestrations. **Comberg c.l.** A contact lens containing radiopaque reference markings, used with x-ray photography for the localization of intraocular foreign bodies. **Comfortflex c.l.** Trade name for a lathed, soft contact lens made of delta-filcon A. **Concentra c.l.** Trade name for a type of bicurve corneal contact lens. **Con-O-Coid c.l.** The trade name for an aspheric PMMA contact lens specified in terms of the values *r*, the apical radius of curvature, and *c*, the degree of peripheral flattening. **Continuous Curve c.l.** A corneal contact lens having a spherical central base curve and an aspherical peripheral curve. **Contour c.l.** A corneal contact lens, approximately 9.5 mm in diameter, which has a molded ocular surface of three different curvatures: a central curve conforming to the central corneal curve, a flatter peripheral curve, and a transitional curve blending the two. **control c.l.** Trial contact lens. **corneal c.l.** A contact lens which rests primarily on the cornea rather than on the sclera and requires no auxiliary fluid. Syn., *corneal lens*. **cosmetic c.l.** A contact lens designed to alter or enhance the appearance of the eye, as to conceal a disfigurement or to change its color. It may range from a tinted lens to a completely opaque lens with a painted pupil, iris, and sclera. **Cycon c.l.** The trade name for a corneal contact lens having a toric base curve. The peripheral curves of the posterior surface and the anterior lens surface may be either toric or spherical. **Dallos c.l.** 1. A glass scleral contact lens molded from a casting of the patient's eye, with its anterior corneal surface ground to prescription, originally designed by Dallos in 1932. 2. A glass scleral contact lens, subsequently designed by Dallos, having a small perforating vent near the limbal area in the inferior temporal region. **diagnostic c.l.** 1. Trial contact lens. 2. A contact lens used in the diagnosis of ocular pathology, such as a goniolens. **Dura Soft c.l.** Trade name for a lathe-cut, soft contact lens made of phemicol. **facet (regular) c.l.** A

corneal contact lens with four slightly raised facets symmetrically distributed near the periphery of the otherwise spherical posterior surface. **facet (toric) c.l.** A corneal contact lens with two slightly raised facets symmetrically placed in the meridian of greatest curvature near the periphery of the posterior toroidal surface. **Feinbloom c.l.** Any one of several types of contact lenses made and supplied by Feinbloom, including: (1) a molded, scleral contact lens, designed by Feinbloom in 1936, consisting of a transparent glass corneal section and a translucent plastic scleral section, used in conjunction with a fluid; (2) a prefabricated, scleral contact lens, designed by Feinbloom in 1939, consisting of a transparent glass corneal section, 12 mm in diameter, and a translucent plastic scleral section 24 mm in diameter, used in conjunction with a fluid; (3) the Feincone contact lens; and (4) the A-B-C self-centering contact lens. **Feincone c.l.** A prefabricated, plastic, scleral contact lens, designed by Feinbloom in 1945, consisting of a spherical corneal section, not in contact with the cornea or the limbus, a conical section extending from the corneal section in contact with the sclera, and a temporal spherical flange to prevent the lids from striking the edge of the cone. It is used in conjunction with a fluid. Syn., *tangent cone contact lens*. **fenestrated c.l.** A contact lens containing one or more perforations for the more rapid transfer of air and/or tears between the lens and cornea. **fitting c.l.** Trial contact lens. **fluid c.l.** A scleral contact lens in which the distance between the posterior optical surface and the anterior surface of the cornea is such that the addition of artificial tear fluid is required to fill the space between the two surfaces. **fluidless c.l.** Minimum clearance contact lens. **focal c.l.** A contact lens whose optical section has a measurable degree of refractive power. **formed c.l.** A contact lens made by thermoforming sheet acrylic plastic to a die or eye model. **gas permeable c.l.** Any contact lens made of a material that transmits a useable amount of oxygen and carbon dioxide. **gel c.l.** A contact lens made of hydrophilic plastic which is hard and brittle when dry, but becomes soft and flexible when hydrated, in which state it is worn. **Gelflex c.l.** Trade name for a lathe-cut, soft contact lens made of dimefilcon. **glued on c.l.** A contact lens glued to the anterior surface of the cornea subsequent to surgical removal of the epithelium. **ground c.l.** Any contact lens whose corneal section has been ground and polished. **haptic c.l.** Any contact lens having a section designed to rest on the sclera. **hard c.l.** A contact lens made of a substance which absorbs little or no water, thus remaining in a hard state when worn. Syn., *hydrophobic contact lens; rigid contact lens.* **Heine afocal c.l.** A glass, scleral, afocal contact lens, designed by Heine in 1929, having a corneal section of a radius of curvature selected to provide a fluid lens of sufficient dioptric power to correct the ametropia. **Hersh palpebral traction c.l.** A hard contact lens having a groove on the front surface, near the edge, which aids the upper eyelid in lifting the lens during a blink. **Hornstein c.l.** A corneal contact lens designed to be fitted with a base curve steeper in curvature than the flattest central corneal curve, to provide definite central corneal clearance. **Hydrocurve II c.l.** Trade name for a lathed, soft contact lens made of bufilcon A. **hydrogel c.l.** Soft contact lens. **Hydromarc c.l.** Trade name for a lathed, soft contact lens made of etafilcon A. **Hydron c.l.** A lathe-cut, hydrophilic contact lens made from polymacon material. **hydrophilic c.l.** Soft contact lens. **hydrophobic c.l.** Hard contact lens. **Imcor c.l.** A trade name for a corneal contact lens formed to a model of the cornea which, in turn, is made from a corneal impression. It may be used either as formed or with a central base curve cut with a lathe. **impression c.l.** A contact lens prepared from the casting of the eye to which it is to be fitted. **intrapalpebral c.l.** Palpebral contact lens. **Jungschaffer c.l.** A diagnostic corneal contact lens of high concave dioptric power for examination of the vitreous and fundus in slit lamp biomicroscopy. **Kalt's c.l.** One of the early corneal contact lenses constructed of glass and designed by E. Kalt in 1888. **Keraform c.l.** A microlens with four slightly raised facets symmetrically distributed near the periphery of the otherwise spherical posterior surface. **Kollmorgen c.l.** Any one of several types of contact lenses made and supplied by Kollmorgen, including: (1) a ground and polished glass, scleral contact lens having spherical corneal and scleral sections, used in conjunction with an auxiliary fluid; (2)

a ground and polished glass, scleral contact lens having a spherical corneal and toroidal scleral section, used in conjunction with an auxiliary fluid; and (3) a molded glass, scleral contact lens used in conjunction with an auxiliary fluid. **lenticular c.l.** A corneal contact lens of high dioptric power with the prescription ground only in the central portion, permitting a reduced center thickness in convex lenses and a reduced edge thickness in concave lenses. **lenticular (tangential) c.l.** A corneal contact lens of high convex dioptric power in which, to reduce central thickness, only the central portion contains the prescription, with the second curve being flatter and cut on the anterior surface, tangent to the central curve, in order to present a smooth and continuous transition. **LoVac c.l.** A series of plastic diagnostic contact lenses which are fixed to the eye by a low vacuum created by a rubber bulb connected to the lens by a polyvinylchloride tube. The series includes lenses for gonioscopy, for inspection of the fundus, for electroretinography, and for foreign body location. **LoVac fundus c.l.** A LoVac corneal contact lens having a flat anterior surface, used with the slit lamp biomicroscope for viewing the deep vitreous body and the region of the fundus of the eye central to the equator. **LoVac peripheral fundus c.l.** A LoVac contact lens having a flat anterior surface set at a 30° angle with the visual axis, used with the slit lamp biomicroscope for viewing the peripheral fundus of the eye. **Meso c.l.** Trade name for a hydrophilic contact lens, either molded or lathe-cut, made of cellulose acetate butyrate. **Micro-V c.l.** A bicurve corneal contact lens having radial channels in the peripheral secondary curve portion to facilitate tear circulation. **minimum clearance c.l.** A scleral contact lens in which the posterior optical surface is in close approximation to the anterior surface of the cornea, the space between the two surfaces being filled with normal tear fluid, without requiring an auxiliary artificial tear fluid. Syn., *fluidless contact lens.* **molded c.l.** 1. A contact lens prepared from the casting of the eye to which it is to be fitted. Cf. *preformed contact lens.* 2. A contact lens prepared from dies, i.e., not cut by a machine. **monocurve c.l.** A corneal contact lens having a single curvature on each surface, exclusive of edge bevels. **monticule c.l.** A contact lens having one or more small elevations on its posterior surface. **Mueller c.l.** 1. A blown glass contact lens, designed by F. E. Mueller in 1887, to protect the cornea from exposure. It is considered to be the first of the modern contact lenses. 2. A blown glass contact lens, designed by F. E. Mueller in 1909, having a transparent corneal section and a white opaque scleral section, for the correction of ametropia. **Mueller-Welt c.l.** Any one of several types of contact lenses developed by Mueller-Welt, including: (1) a spherical, afocal, blown glass, scleral contact lens, developed in 1924, used in conjunction with an auxiliary fluid, for correcting ametropia; (2) a spherical, blown glass, scleral contact lens, developed in 1933, having refractive power and used in conjunction with an auxiliary fluid; (3) a blown glass, scleral contact lens, developed in 1935, having refractive power and a parabolic scleral section and used in conjunction with an auxiliary fluid; (4) a prefabricated, plastic, scleral contact lens, developed in 1945, having refractive power and a parabolic scleral section, used in conjunction with an auxiliary fluid; (5) a type of prefabricated, fluidless, plastic scleral contact lens; and (6) corneal contact lenses. **multicurve c.l.** A corneal contact lens having two or more curvatures on its posterior surface. **Naturalens c.l.** Trade name for a lathe-cut, semi-scleral, soft contact lens made of Bionite. **Natural Vision c.l.** The trade name for a PMMA, monocentric, bifocal contact lens having a crescent-shaped segment. **Naturvue c.l.** Trade name for a lathed, soft contact lens made of hefilcon A. **Neo-Phakic c.l.** The trade name for a PMMA contact lens tinted yellow to offset the high transmission of blue in aphakia. **offset c.l.** A preformed scleral contact lens in which the scleral section is aspherical and the centers of curvature of the radii do not coincide with the axis of symmetry of the corneal section. **open c.l.** A contact lens containing one or more fenestrations for the more rapid transfer of air and/or tears between the lens and cornea. **palpebral c.l.** A corneal contact lens usually of small diameter and designed to fit within the palpebral fissure, free of contact with the limbus and eyelid margins except during blinking. Syn., *aperture contact lens; intrapalpebral contact lens.* **Palsite c.l.** Trade name for a hy-

drophobic contact lens made of PMMA material, characterized by a constant increase of convexity from center to periphery as an aid for presbyopia. **Panofocal c.l.** The trade name for a PMMA contact lens having an aspheric front surface intended to neutralize the spherical aberration of the eye. **Para-Curve c.l.** A trade name for a type of corneal contact lens having an aspheric secondary curve. **pentacurve c.l.** A corneal contact lens in which the posterior optical zone is surrounded by four distinct and separate annuli, the surface of each being successively of less curvature. **peri ballast c.l.** A lenticular, minus carrier hard contact lens cut eccentrically so that a larger amount of carrier is on one side than is on the other side. **peripheral angle c.l.** A corneal contact lens in which the peripheral portion of the posterior surface is shaped to a solid angle by means of a cone-shaped cutting tool. **piggy-back c.l.** A half-moon-shaped lens placed, straight edge upwards, by the wearer on the lower half of a regular single vision contact lens which has been inserted, in order to provide additional power for near vision. **Polycon c.l.** A rigid, gas-permeable contact lens made from silafocon A, a copolymer containing silicon and methyl methacrylate. **prefabricated c.l.** Preformed contact lens. **preformed c.l.** A contact lens prepared from a stock model or die. Cf. *molded contact lens.* Syn., *prefabricated contact lens.* **prism ballast c.l.** A corneal contact lens having a small amount of prism to compensate for hyperphoria or to weight the lens in one meridional direction, either to effect a lower riding position or to aid in proper orientation of cylindrical corrections or bifocal segments. **rigid c.l.** Hard contact lens. **RX-56 c.l.** A semirigid, gas-permeable contact lens made from porofocon A, a polymer cellulose acetate butyrate. **Sauflon c.l.** Trade name for a gas-permeable, soft contact lens made of Sauflon material. **scleral c.l.** A contact lens which fits over both the cornea and the surrounding sclera, used with or without an auxiliary fluid to fill the space between the lens and the cornea. **Scleroform c.l.** A fenestrated scleral lens having a small scleral section and therefore a small overall diameter, designed primarily for use in sports. **Silcon c.l.** A trade name for a pliable, gas-permeable, hard contact lens made of silicone rubber. **silicone rubber c.l.** A pliable, gas-permeable, hard contact lens made of a silicone elastomer. **Soehnges Micro Pupil Multifocal c.l.** A multifocal corneal contact lens having a central zone for distance vision surrounded by a zone for near vision, in which the curvature on the anterior surface increases continuously toward the periphery to provide a continuously increasing addition. **Soflens c.l.** Trade name for a spincast, soft contact lens made of polymacon. **soft c.l.** A contact lens made of a water-absorbing substance which, when worn, is soft and flexible. Syn., *hydrophilic contact lens; hydrogel contact lens.* **Softcon c.l.** Trade name for a lathed, soft contact lens made of vifilcon A. **Sphercon c.l.** A corneal contact lens, of approximately 9 mm diameter and 0.2 mm thickness, which has a secondary flatter curve or bevel at its periphery. Its central portion is fitted to conform closely to the central curves of the cornea. **Spherex c.l.** A trade name for a type of bicurve corneal contact lens. **spherical c.l.** 1. A corneal contact lens whose inside surface is spherical. Cf. *toric contact lens.* 2. A scleral contact lens whose corneal and scleral portions are segments of spheres. **Sphertan c.l.** A trade name for a type of tangential lenticular contact lens. **Spiro Vent c.l.** A trade name for a corneal contact lens which has five curved, tongue-shaped channels equally spaced in a spiral pattern, extending from the lens edge toward the optic zone, to promote tear circulation. **sports c.l.** A corneal contact lens made larger in diameter than customary, or with an added narrow scleral flange, to minimize its dislodgement in active sports. **Stellar c.l.** The trade name for a PMMA contact lens molded with parabolic surfaces intended to aid centering and tear dispersion. **tangent cone c.l.** Feincone contact lens. **Tangential Periphery (TP) c.l.** A trade name for a type of tangential lenticular contact lens in which the peripheral portion of the anterior surface is conical and perpendicular to the radius of curvature of the central portion at their points of tangency. **Thorpe c.l.** 1. A contact lens containing radiopaque reference markings, used with x-ray photography for the localization of intraocular foreign bodies. 2. A diagnostic contact lens of high concave dioptric power, for examination of the fundus in slit lamp biomicroscopy. **Torbase c.l.** Trade name for a prism ballast, hard contact

lens having back toric and front spherical surfaces. **Torcon c.l.** A trade name for a corneal contact lens having a toric curvature on its front surface for the correction of residual astigmatism. **toric c.l.** A corneal contact lens with a toroidal inside surface. Cf. *spherical contact lens.* 2. A scleral contact lens having a toroidal inside surface on its scleral section. **Transcurve c.l.** A trade name for a preformed, minimum clearance, ventilated, scleral contact lens consisting essentially of a corneal section and a scleral section separated by a transition zone approximately 1.5 mm to 2.5 mm wide and of a curvature midway between the corneal and scleral curvatures. It is fitted with two trial sets, one to determine the corneal section dimensions and the other the scleral section dimensions. **Tresoft c.l.** Trade name for a lathed, soft contact lens made of ocufilcon. **trial c.l.** Any contact lens, usually one of a set of lenses having a range of specifications, used in preliminary fitting to determine the final specifications required to obtain a physical fit and the desired refractive power. Syn., *control contact lens; diagnostic contact lens; fitting contact lens.* **tricurve c.l.** A corneal contact lens in which the posterior optical zone is surrounded by two distinct and separate annuli, each of which is successively of less curvature. **Troncoso c.l.** Troncoso goniolens. **truncated c.l.** A corneal contact lens having one or more sections cut away so that it is no longer circular. **Tuohy c.l.** A monocurve corneal contact lens, with a narrow bevel of a curve flatter than the base curve, patented by Kevin M. Tuohy in 1948. In its original form it was approximately 11.5 mm in diameter and was fitted with a base curve flatter than the flattest central corneal curve. **Variable Focus c.l.** The trade name for a contact lens designed for presbyopes and aphakics having an ellipsoidal base curve and a spherical anterior surface such that plus power gradually increases from the apex to the periphery. **ventilated c.l.** Any contact lens containing an opening for the more rapid transfer of air and/or tears between the lens and the cornea. Examples are the Lacrilens and the Dallos contact lens. **wide angle c.l.** A preformed, minimum clearance, scleral contact lens having a flat, conical, transition zone between the corneal and scleral sections which is angled to be approximately tangent to the corneal section. The base of the transition zone is a constant of 16 mm diameter, and the base of the corneal section is a constant of 11.5 mm diameter. **X-Chrom c.l.** A contact lens of a specific red color designed to increase the range of colors seen by certain color deficients and worn only on the nondominant eye.

Contour l. See under *lens, contact.*

contrageneric l. In relation to another lens of reference, one which is opposite in sign or dioptric character, whence a converging lens and a diverging lens are said to be a pair of contrageneric lenses. Cf. *congeneric lens.*

contrameniscus l. A concave meniscus lens. *Obs.*

converging l. A lens which converges light. Syn., *convex lens; plus lens; positive lens.*

convex l. Converging lens. (See Fig. 25.)

convexoconcave l. A diverging meniscus lens.

Cooke l. A triplet consisting of a biconcave lens between two convex lenses designed to minimize longitudinal chromatic aberration.

Copeland l. A light-weight, plastic intraocular lens similar to the *Epstein Maltese Cross lens*, q.v.

coquille l. A deep curve lens cut from a blown glass sphere, formerly used in inexpensive sunglasses.

corneal l. 1. The cornea of the eye when considered as a lens. 2. A corneal contact lens.

corrected curve l. 1. A spectacle lens with surface curvatures chosen to eliminate or reduce aberrations resulting from the use of the peripheral portions of the lens. 2. An ophthalmic trial case lens with surface powers chosen to make the power designation precisely correct for the spectacle plane or other plane of reference when inserted correctly in a properly designed trial frame.

correcting l. An ophthalmic lens which corrects the error of refraction or other optically correctable deficiencies of the eye or eyes.

l. cortex. See under *cortex.*

crossed l. A form of lens with surface curvatures selected to provide for minimum spherical aberration for an infinitely distant object. In the case of a lens with an index of refraction of 1.5, the ratio of the two radii of curvature is -6, whence the lens must be biconcave or biconvex.

crossed cylinder l. A compound lens in which the dioptric powers in the principal meridians are equal but opposite in sign, usually mounted on a rotating axis or handle midway between the principal meridians, commonly used in the clinical measurement of the power and the axis of astigmatism, and designated in terms of the powers in the two principal meridians. **homokonic c.c.l.** A modified crossed cylinder lens, devised by P. R. Haynes, which has the same magnification in all meridians to eliminate the rotary deviation and differential magnification present in the Jackson crossed cylinder lens.

crystalline l. The biconvex, normally transparent and resilient, lenticular body directly behind the pupil of the eye and nested in the patellar fossa of the vitreous body, having a relatively high index of refraction and an anterior surface whose convexity responds to ciliary muscle action. It consists of capsule, anterior epithelium, cortex, and nucleus, the latter two containing the lens fibers. It is supported by the fibers of the zonule of Zinn and the hyaloideocapsular ligament which are attached to its capsule.

cylindrical l. 1. A lens on which one surface is plane and the other cylindrical, or on which one surface is spherical and the other toroidal, such that one meridian has zero power and a meridian 90° to it has maximum power. 2. An astigmatic lens.

Dannheim l. A small, biconvex, plastic lens suspended in the anterior chamber by means of a double loop of thin resilient plastic thread passing through the peripheral body of the lens. It is used to replace the crystalline lens following cataract surgery or to correct ametropia. Syn., *Dannheim implant.*

decentered l. A lens so constructed that its optical center does not coincide with its geometrical center.

depth l. A 2.50 D convex cylinder lens, axis 90°, used by artists to elicit perceptual depth in a realistic painting.

didymium l. A lens containing didymium to absorb yellow light and hence used for protection in glass-blowing and other occupations involving excessive exposure to sodium flare.

dispersing l. An inaccurate term for a diverging lens.

diverging l. A lens which diverges light. Syn., *concave lens; minus lens; negative lens.*

double concave l. A lens which is concave on both surfaces.

double convex l. A lens which is convex on both surfaces.

ectopic l. A crystalline lens which is displaced from its normal position.

eikonic l. Iseikonic lens.

Engel fundus l. A diagnostic contact lens of high concave dioptric power, with a flat or slightly convex anterior surface, for examination of the fundus and deep vitreous in slit lamp biomicroscopy.

Epstein collar-stud l. An intraocular lens in the shape of a double disk separated by a deep peripheral groove, resembling a collar button, which is positioned in the pupillary aperture, with the iris between its anterior and posterior disks, to replace the crystalline lens following cataract surgery. Syn., *Epstein collar-stud implant.*

Epstein Maltese Cross l. An intraocular lens which is positioned in the pupillary aperture following cataract surgery and is fixed in position by two solid limbs situated behind the iris and two fenestrated limbs, perpendicular to the solid limbs, situated in front of the iris. Syn., *Epstein Maltese Cross implant.*

equiconcave l. A double concave lens on which the two surfaces are equal in curvature.

equiconvex l. A double convex lens on which the two surfaces are equal in curvature.

equi-tint l. A lens with a uniform absorptive layer not affected by variations in lens thickness.

equivalent l. 1. A lens so located as to form on a screen the same size image as another lens or series of lenses. 2. A spherical lens equal in dioptric power to the mean spherical refracting power of an astigmatic lens. 3. Any one of two or more ophthalmic lenses having the same mean spherical refracting power.

Essel Atoral l. Trade name of a plastic lens on which the rear surface is both aspherical and toroidal and the front surface is spherical.

Eventone l. A type of uniform density lens fabricated from glass.

eye l. The lens nearest the eye in an eyepiece which renders light, from the objective or field lens, parallel prior to entrance into the observer's eye.

l. fiber. See under *fiber.*

field l. The lens in an eyepiece nearest the objective lens, serving to increase the usable field of view in a telescopic or microscopic system over that obtained in using a single lens.

fish-eye l. A camera lens having a total hemispheric, 180°, angular field, or nearly so.

flat l. A biconvex, biconcave, planoconvex, or planoconcave ophthalmic lens, differentiated from a *meniscus lens.* **plano-cylinder f.l.** A flat lens which is plane on one surface and cylindrical on the other. **spherocylinder f.l.** A flat lens which is spherical on one surface and cylindrical on the other.

fluid l. 1. A lens consisting of liquid held between two transparent solid media. 2. Lacrimal lens.

fogging l. The ophthalmic lens or combination of lenses which constitute a slight overcorrection of plus lens in hyperopia or a slight undercorrection of minus lens in myopia for the purpose of inducing or maintaining relaxation of accommodation during certain types of vision testing, as for astigmatism with a fan dial chart, or to blur the vision in one eye, when attempting to force the use of an amblyopic eye.

l. fossette. The depression in the secondary eye vesicle of the human embryo.

Four-Drop l. See *Welsh Four-Drop Aspheric Lens.*

Franklin l. Franklin bifocal lens.

Franklin gonioscopic l. A convex diagnostic contact lens fitted with a rubber scleral flange and handle for viewing the filtration angle of the anterior chamber, usually in conjunction with a hand-held biomicroscope and focal illumination.

Franklin 3 mirror l. A contact lens in combination with three inclined mirrors in a plastic cone assembly, used with a slit lamp biomicroscope for viewing the fundus, the vitreous body, and the filtration angle of the anterior chamber.

Fresnel's l. A lens with a surface consisting of a concentric series of simple lens sections or zones of the same power, thereby effecting the optics of a simple, large diameter, short focal length lens without the incumbent thickness.

Fresnel Press-On L. Trade name for a Fresnel lens of thin, transparent, flexible, plastic material which adheres to the surface of an ophthalmic lens when pressed in place.

frosted l. An otherwise transparent lens made translucent by grinding or etching.

Full Spectrum L. Trade name for an ophthalmic lens made from a plastic that transmits approximately 90% of the ultraviolet light, whereas a conventional plastic lens transmits only 10%.

Fyodorov l. An iris-supported, intraocular lens implant with three omega-shaped loops. The ends of the loops are attached to the posterior surface of the lens near its periphery and lie posterior to the iris with three radially extended knobbed posts or struts resting anteriorly, somewhat resembling the Sputnik satellite. Syn., *sputnik lens.*

Gauss objective l. An anastigmatic lens system consisting of two air separated doublets, one on each side of the stop. Syn., *Celor lens system.*

Goldmann fundus l. A diagnostic contact lens with a flat anterior surface, mounted in a plastic cone, for examination of the vitreous and fundus in slit lamp biomicroscopy.

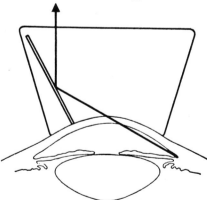

Fig. 26 Diagram of light rays emerging through a Goldmann lens. (From A. E. Kolker and J. Hetherington, *Becker-Shaffer's Diagnosis and Therapy of the Glaucomas*, 4th ed. St. Louis: C. V. Mosby, 1976)

Goldmann gonioscopy l. A diagnostic contact lens with a mirror attachment, mounted in a plastic cone, used in conjunction with a slit lamp biomicroscope for viewing the structures of the filtration angle of the anterior chamber. (See Fig. 26.)

Goldmann 3-mirror contact l. A contact lens in combination with three mirrors mounted in a plastic cone assembly and set at angles of 59°, 67°, and 73°, at 120° meridional intervals, used with a slit lamp biomicroscope for viewing the fundus, vitreous, and anterior chamber angle.

gonioscopic l. A thick convex or prismatic lens placed in contact with the eye for the purpose of viewing the structures of the filtration angle of the anterior chamber.

goniotomy l. A type of gonioscopic lens used in surgery of the filtration angle of the anterior chamber.

gradient density l. A lens having a continuously increasing change of light absorption from one edge to the other along a given meridian.

hardened l. Case-hardened lens.

Henkes electroretinography l. A diagnostic scleral-type contact lens used in electroretinography with or without a low vacuum retention attachment, and equipped with a limbal electrode and a protruding cone to hold the eyelids open, within which are mounted disks having various sized pupillary apertures.

Hersh Palpebral Traction l. A hydrophobic corneal contact lens having a concentric groove about .2 mm wide and .2 mm deep, located about 1 mm from the edge on the anterior surface to allow the palpebral conjunctiva of the upper eyelid to elevate and hold the lens in better position by traction.

High-Lite L. The trade name for a lens of high index glass (n = 1.70) which is thinner but heavier than crown, though lighter than flint, and can be chemically hardened. Trade names of other high index glass lenses include Hilite, Wide-Lite, One Dot Seven, and LHI (lightweight high index).

Hruby l. A spherical diverging lens of 55.0 D with a slightly convex anterior surface (+5.0 D) placed in front of the eye for the examination of its interior structures in conjunction with an ocular biomicroscope and slit lamp.

Humphrey l's. Paired lens slabs of square dimension, the slightly separated interfaces of which are of complementary, anamorphic, toric curvatures which provide zero power when flush. Continuously variable sphere and cylinder powers may be produced by the lateral and vertical translatory displacement of the slabs in relation to each other. They are an element in the Humphrey Vision Analyzer.

HyperAspheric L. Trade name for a plastic spectacle lens having a central spherical zone and an aspheric periphery, used for the correction of aphakia.

hyperchromatic l. A doublet lens having more chromatic aberration than a single lens of the same power.

Hyperocular L. A trade name for a plastic aspheric lens used in the correction of subnormal vision, available in 4×, 6×, and 8× magnifications.

immersion l. See *immersion microscope.*

intracorneal l. A small plastic lens placed between the layers of the cornea to substitute for the crystalline lens following cataract surgery.

iris clip l. An anterior chamber implant consisting of a biconvex lens positioned in front of the pupil and held to the iris by peripheral loops. Syn., *Binkhorst lens; Binkhorst implant; pupillary lens.*

iseikonic l. An ophthalmic lens designed to correct the image size difference between the two eyes in aniseikonia. Syn., *aniseikonic lens; eikonic lens.* **bitoric i.l.** An ophthalmic lens having a toroidal curvature on each surface, for the correction of aniseikonia. **doublet i.l.** A doublet consisting of two lenses separated by an air space, for the correction of aniseikonia.

isochromatic l. A tinted lens having the same absorption at all points, irrespective of variations in thickness.

isogonal l's. A pair of spectacle lenses which, though of different refractive powers, are designed to produce identical magnifications in corresponding meridians.

Isokrystar l's. A trade name for a series of corrected curve lenses.

Jackson crossed cylinder l. Crossed cylinder lens.

Johann Zahn's polyspheri- cal l. An early lens for testing sight, having six different powers ground in concentric annuli and held in a large lens ring with a handle.

Jungschaffer l. See under *lens, contact.*

Katral l's. A trade name for a series of lenses having an aspheric curvature on the inner surface with a spherical or spherocylindrical curvature on the other surface. It is made in convex powers from 7.0 D to 20.0 D and is said to correct marginal aberration for a 60° field of vision.

Koeppe gonioscopic l. A hemispheric diagnostic contact lens for direct viewing of the filtration angle of the anterior chamber, usually employed with a portable microscope and focal illumination.

Kurova l's. A trade name for a series of corrected curve lenses.

Kurova Shursite l. Trade name for a series of corrected curve lenses.

lacrimal l. The layer of tears between a contact lens and the cornea.

laminated l. A protective, relatively shatter-proof lens consisting of a layer of clear plastic between two layers of glass.

Lederer l's. A series of convex lenses of high dioptric power, corrected for oblique astigmatism and curvature of the field, designed by Lederer for use in subnormal vision.

lenticular l. An ophthalmic or spectacle lens of high dioptric power with the prescription ground only in the central portion, the peripheral (usually afocal) portion of the lens serving only to give dimensions suitable for mounting in a spectacle or trial frame, permitting a reduced center thickness in the case of convex lenses and a reduced edge thickness in the case of concave lenses.

Lieb l. A small plastic lens suspended in the anterior chamber by means of a double loop of thin, resilient plastic thread fitted into peripheral grooves on either side of the lens. It is used to replace the crystalline lens following cataract surgery or to correct ametropia.

Lookout L. Trade name for an afocal lens assembly designed for miniaturized wide-field viewing through the peephole of an apartment door and useful as a hand-held field expander and searching aid by persons with peripherally restricted visual fields.

LoVac direct gonioscopic l. A LoVac contact lens having a flat anterior surface set at a 45° angle with the visual axis, used with the slit lamp biomicroscope to provide a direct view of the filtration angle of the anterior chamber as well as of the iris and peripheral fundus.

LoVac six mirror gonioscopic l. A LoVac contact lens to which is attached a plastic cone containing six mirrors, all inclined at the same angle, to provide a composite view of the circumference of the filtration angle of the anterior chamber when directly viewed with a slit lamp biomicroscope.

Luboshez l. A lens designed so that the object point is at the center of curvature of the first surface and at the aplanatic point of the second surface.

luxated l. A crystalline lens that is completely displaced from the pupillary aperture, differentiated from a *subluxated lens*, which is displaced but remains in part within the pupillary aperture.

magnifying l. Any lens which will produce an apparent enlargement of an object viewed through it.

l. measure. See under *measure*.

medi-Flow L. The trade name of a PMMA scleral contact lens having a central hole into which a polyethylene tube is fastened, the other end being secured to a syringe or bottle, used for protection from movement of the eyelid over a damaged or infected eye and for continual delivery of medicinal fluids to the eye.

meniscus l. 1. A lens having a spherical concave curve on one surface and a spherical convex curve on the other surface. 2. A deep curve spectacle lens as distinguished from a *flat* or *periscopic lens*. 3. A spectacle lens having a 6.0 D base curve.

metallized l. A lens upon which a metallic film has been deposited to reduce the amount of light transmitted.

meter l. A converging lens of 1 m focal length.

mi-coquille l. A lens cut from a blown-glass sphere but of shallower curvature than a coquille lens.

microphakic l. See *microphakia*.

microscopic l. A magnifying spectacle lens, or a lens system, of short focal length for near viewing, designed to provide a flat field of view comparatively free from aberrations.

Micro-V l. See under *lens, contact*.

minifying l. Any lens which will produce reduction in the apparent size of an object viewed through it. Syn., *reducing lens*.

minus l. Diverging lens.

Motex L. A trade name for a laminated lens.

multifocal l. A composite spectacle lens with different dioptric powers in different segments, e.g., a bifocal or a trifocal lens.

Myo-disc L. A trade name for a lenticular lens used in the correction of high myopia, having a concave, central corrective area 20 to 30 mm in diameter on the back surface, both the front surface and the peripheral area of the back surface usually being flat.

negative l. Diverging lens.

nonshatterable l. A term sometimes applied to laminated lenses.

Normalsite l. Trade name for a series of corrected curve lenses.

objective l. The lens in a telescopic or microscopic system nearest the object, serving to converge light from points in the field of view. Syn., *objective glass; objective*.

occluding l. A spectacle lens for obscuring or preventing vision. It may be opaque, translucent, of irregular curvature, or of a dioptric power incompatible with the refractive state.

Omnifocal L. The trade name for a lens in which the dioptric power changes progressively from above to below to provide correction for variations from distance to near vision, usually used in the correction of presbyopia.

ophthalmic l. A lens used for correcting or measuring refractive errors of the eye and/or compensating for ocular muscle imbalances.

Orthogon l. A trade name for a series of corrected curve lenses.

orthoscopic l's. 1. A series of spectacle lenses designed by Tscherning to correct peripheral aberrations. 2. A symmetrical magnifying doublet, with a central aperture stop, which eliminates distortion, i.e., straight lines are reproduced as straight lines. Syn., *orthoscopic doublet; rectilinear lens.*

Ostwalt l. One of a series of corrected curve lenses based on the Ostwalt branch of the Tscherning ellipse, giving minimum marginal astigmatism and characteristically flatter than other corrected curve series.

panoramic l. A lens system which produces an image of a laterally extended field approximating a total of 360°.

pantoscopic l. A spectacle lens, for near vision only, approximating in shape only the lower half of a conventional spectacle lens, thus enabling the wearer to look over the top for distant seeing.

parabolic l. A lens having one or both surfaces of parabolic curvature.

pebble l. A spectacle lens made from quartz crystal; no longer in common use.

Percival l. Any of a series of lenses corrected for mean oblique astigmatic error, according to formulas by Percival.

periscopic l. 1. A lens with a 1.25 D base curve. 2. One of a series of deep corrected curve lenses designed by Wollaston in 1804. Syn., *Wollaston lens.*

l. pit. See under *pit.*

plano l. A lens of zero focal power, in which light entering parallel will emerge parallel. (See Fig. 25.)

planoconcave l. A lens which is plane on one surface and concave on the other. (See Fig. 25.)

planoconvex l. A lens which is plane on one surface and convex on the other. (See Fig. 25.)

planocylindrical l. A lens on which one surface is plane and the other cylindrical, or on which one surface is spherical and the other toroidal, such that one meridian has zero power and the meridian perpendicular to it has maximum power.

plastic l. A lens made of transparent plastic.

l. plate. See under *plate.*

plus l. A converging lens.

point-focal l. A corrected curve lens.

Polaroid l. 1. A laminated lens containing a layer of Polaroid sheeting. 2. A lens made of Polaroid material.

positive l. Converging lens.

posterior chamber l. Posterior chamber implant.

prismatic l. A lens with prism power. In a spectacle lens, one with prism power at the major reference point.

Punktal l. A trade name for a series of corrected curve lenses in which the curve for each power of lens is calculated independently to minimize aberrations.

pupillary l. 1. A lens placed in front of or in the pupillary opening to replace the crystalline lens following cataract surgery. 2. Iris clip lens.

rectilinear l. Orthoscopic lens.

red l. An ophthalmic filter primarily transmitting red light and used monocularly in binocular clinical tests and visual training procedures.

reducing l. 1. Minifying lens. 2. Diverging lens. *Rare.*

Richardson-Shaffer diagnostic l. A small version of the Koeppe gonioscopic lens for use on infant eyes.

Ridley l. A small plastic lens placed in the eyeball against the posterior wall of the capsule to replace the crystalline lens following extracapsular cataract surgery.

safety l. 1. A lens providing protection to the eyes, especially from injury due to impact. 2. A lens that meets standard specifications of construction and impact resistance, as determined by the *drop ball test.*

Sarwar l. A diagnostic contact lens of high divergent dioptric power for examination of the fundus and anterior chamber angle in slit lamp biomicroscopy.

Scharf l. A small plastic lens placed in the anterior chamber of the eyeball to replace the crystalline lens following cataract surgery. It is held in position by a four-pronged plastic mount.

Schreck l. A small plastic lens placed in the anterior chamber of the eyeball to replace the crystalline lens following cataract surgery. The lens is held in position by a curved plastic plate into which it is secured.

scleral l. Scleral contact lens.

simple l. A lens consisting of two spherical refracting surfaces.

single vision l. A spectacle lens having the same focal power (disregarding aberrations) throughout its useful area, thus distinguished from a *multifocal lens.*

size l. An iseikonic lens, usually

implying one with zero verging power. **meridional s.l.** A size lens having different magnification in the various meridians, the meridians of maximum and minimum magnification being at right angles. **over-all s.l.** A size lens giving equal magnification in all meridians.

slab-off l. A lens on which one surface is ground and polished in two segments having the same curvatures, but with separated centers of curvature. The expression "slab-off" refers to the method of grinding, in which, in effect, a prismatic slab of glass is removed from one portion of the lens.

Slidefocal l. Variable Focus Lens.

spectacle l. A lens used as a visual corrective aid and mounted a short distance in front of the eye, usually by means of a frame or attachment supported by the ears, the bridge of the nose, the cheeks, or the eyebrows. Specifically, a lens incorporated in a pair of spectacles, but, more generally, the term includes lenses used as monocles, pince-nez glasses, lorgnettes, etc.

Sphercon l. See under *lens, contact.*

spherical l. A lens in which all refracting surfaces are spherical.

spherocylindrical l. A lens which functions as a combination of a simple spherical lens and a simple cylindrical lens.

spherophakic l. The abnormally small and spherical crystalline lens characteristic of microphakia.

spheroprism l. A spherical lens eccentrically mounted or decentered to produce prismatic effect, or a combined spherical lens and prism.

sputnik l. Fyodorov lens.

l. stars. See under *star.*

Stigmagna l's. A series of convex lenses of high dioptric power, corrected to minimize oblique astigmatism and distortion, designed for use in subnormal vision.

stigmatic l. Anastigmatic lens.

Stokes's l. A combination of a planoconvex cylindrical lens and a planoconcave cylindrical lens of numerically equal power mounted with their flat surfaces almost in contact with each other in lens rings which are simultaneously but oppositely rotatable about their common axis, producing a maximum astigmatic resultant when the two lens power meridians are at right angles to each other, a minimum astigmatic resultant when the two lens power meridians are parallel, and intermediate astigmatic resultants for intermediate relative positions of the two lens power meridians.

Strampelli l. A small plastic lens placed in the anterior chamber of the eyeball to replace the crystalline lens following cataract surgery. The lens is held in position by a curved plastic plate into which it is secured. Syn., *Strampelli implant.*

subluxated l. A crystalline lens which is displaced from its normal position but remains in part within the pupillary aperture. Cf. *luxated lens.* **Vogt's s.l.** A spontaneous subluxation of the crystalline lens occurring in adults and considered to be due to a congenital abnormality of the zonule of Zinn.

symmetrical l's. A lens system consisting of two identical sets of thick lenses symmetrical about a stop placed between them.

tear l. Lacrimal lens.

telephoto l. A camera lens for obtaining large images of distant objects, consisting of a front positive lens combined with a back negative lens separated by about half the focal length of the positive lens, thereby effectively displacing the principal planes of the system substantially forward.

telescopic l. A short, lightweight, wide angle, fixed focus Galilean telescope mounted in front of the eye as a magnifying spectacle lens.

tempered l. Case-hardened lens.

Tessar L. Trade name of an anastigmatic, wide-field camera lens of triplet construction consisting of two single optical elements and a doublet.

Therminon L. Trade name for a light blue glass lens with low infrared and high visible transmission.

thick l. A lens or a system of lenses in which the two or more refracting surfaces are regarded in their separate positions rather than as if coincident.

thin l. A lens or a combination of lenses in which the two or more refracting surfaces are regarded as if coincident rather than in their separate positions. **equivalent t.l.** The value (refractive power, or focal length) of a thin lens placed at the principal plane of a thick lens or lens system which will give the identical optical effect of the thick lens or lens system.

thinflint l. An ophthalmic lens made of dense flint glass, containing lead oxide, of relatively high refractive index. The lens is appreciably thinner than a crown glass lens of equal power, but is heavier and has more chromatic aberration.

Thinlite L. A trade name for a thinflint lens.

Tillyer l. A trade name for a series of corrected curve lenses.

tinted l. A lens with color absorption properties designed to reduce light transmission and/or selectively absorb undesirable incident radiations. In contact lenses, the color may be also for facilitating location.

Topogon L. Trade name of a camera lens designed to correct moderate aperture and large-field aberrations, consisting of two thick positive meniscus lenses with mutually facing concavities and, usually, with two intermediately placed and similarly arranged plano-meniscus lenses.

toric l. Any one of a series of meniscus cylindrical and spherocylindrical spectacle lenses characterized by a toric convex surface with a minimum curvature (base curve) of 6.00 D refracting power. 2. A lens with a toric surface.

Torres-Ruiz l. A corneal implant consisting of a central glass cylinder, 3 mm in diameter, convex anteriorly and concave posteriorly, 1.5 to 3.0 mm long, surrounded by a metallic, annular, spherically curved flap 6 mm in diameter. The flap contains semicircular perforations through which the corneal tissue proliferates to hold the lens in position. Syn., *Torres-Ruiz implant*.

trial l. Any of a set of lenses used to test vision or to correct temporarily ocular muscle imbalances, or refractive or aniseikonic errors. 2. A trial contact lens.

trifocal l. A multifocal lens of three portions whose focal powers differ from each other. Usually the top portion is the largest and is for distant vision, the middle for intermediate distances, and the bottom for near vision. **Hawkins t.l.** One of the original trifocal lenses designed by Hawkins, consisting of three separate portions of lenses mounted in one frame after the manner of a Franklin bifocal.

Trioptic telescopic l. A subnormal vision aid with three components, a plastic carrier lens having the wearer's distance correction, a small diameter Galilean telescope, to magnify distant objects, mounted on the upper front surface of the carrier, and a small microscopic lens, to magnify near objects, mounted on the lower front surface of the carrier.

Triplex L. A trade name for a laminated nonshatterable lens.

Troncoso gonioscopic l. Troncoso goniolens.

Ultravue L. The trade name for a hard, resin, multifocal lens having a full-width spherical or spherocylindrical portion for distant vision, a spherical or spherocylindrical portion averaging 18-20 mm in width for near vision, and an intermediate aspheric corridor, 12 mm long, in which the power gradually and progressively changes from that of the upper portion to that of the lower portion.

uncut l. A lens that is completely surfaced but has not been cut or edged to its final size and shape.

Uni-Form l's. Trade name for a series of corrected curve lenses.

uniform density l. An absorptive lens whose color is distributed uniformly across the lens regardless of the power. This is achieved by making the body of the lens of clear glass or plastic, and applying the color in a thin layer to one or both surfaces. In glass lenses, this is done by fusing or cementing a thin plate of colored glass onto one surface or by depositing metallic oxides of the desired color onto the surfaces, and in plastic lenses by impregnating the lens surfaces with inorganic pigments.

variable focus l. 1. A lens system in which the focal length can be varied, usually by the differential moving of parts of the system along the axis. 2. A lens system mounted on a slide or rack, as in a projector, so as to permit variation of image distance by varying the distance of the lens unit from the object.

Variable Focus L. Trade name for a spectacle lens having one flexible wall and a hollow core filled with fluid which can be pumped in or out by means of a sliding cylinder on the temple of the frame to vary its refractive power. Syn., *Slidefocus lens*.

varifocal l. 1. A lens having a gradual and progressive change in dioptric power, either throughout its entire area or over a region intermediate between areas of uniform power, usually used in the correction of presbyopia. 2. Zoom lens.

Varilux L. Trade name for a multifocal lens consisting of an upper portion for distant vision, a lower portion for near vision, and a middle, aspheric portion in which the power gradually and progressively changes from that of the upper portion to that of the lower portion.

Varilux 2 l. A Varilux lens improved by diminution of distortion lateral to the optically usable portions.

Volk Catraconoid l. Trade name of any of a series of glass aspheric multifocal lenses for aphakia.

Volk conoid l. Any of a series of ten convex lenses of high dioptric power used as subnormal vision aids. Seven of the lenses each have one surface ellipsoidal and the other plano or spherical, while the other three, of highest power, have both surfaces hyperbolic.

Welsh 4-drop L. Trade name for a plastic aspheric spectacle lens with a 24 mm diameter central spherical zone and successive concentric peripheral power decreases of approximately one diopter per three mm totalling four diopters, used for the correction of aphakia.

wide-angle l. A corrected curve lens, so called because of the larger angle of field with reduced aberration.

Widesite l. A trade name for a series of corrected curve lenses and for a series of fused bifocal lenses.

Wollaston l. The original periscopic lens, a deep corrected curve lens, designed by Wollaston in 1804, based on the Wollaston branch of the Tscherning ellipse.

Worst's prismatic goniotomy l. A goniotomy lens having a flat anterior surface set at a 45° angle with the visual axis, a scleral rim containing four holes for suturing to the conjunctiva, a cannula through which saline solution is injected to eliminate air bubbles and obtain optical continuity between the lens and cornea, and an opening at the side of the lens for insertion of the goniotomy knife.

Worst's spherical goniotomy l. A hemispherical goniotomy lens of the Barkan type, modified by an added scleral rim containing four holes for suturing to the conjunctiva, a cannula through which saline solution is injected to eliminate air bubbles and obtain optical continuity between the lens and cornea, and an opening at the side of the lens for insertion of the goniotomy knife.

zero converging l. A lens for which the image position coincides with that of the object.

l. of zero curvature. A converging meniscus lens in which the axial thickness is equal to the distance between the centers of curvature of the two surfaces and in which the radii of curvature are equal.

zoom l. A lens or a lens system providing continuously variable magnification without a change in object and image positions.

Zoom B B L. The trade name for a multifocal lens consisting of an upper portion of uniform power for distant vision, a lower portion of almost uniform power for near vision, and an intermediate narrow portion of non-linearly increasing power, the separation of distance and near optical centers being 14 mm.

◆

Lenscorometer (lenz-ko-rom'eh-ter). The trade name for a micrometer-like device for measuring the distance between the posterior surface of a spectacle lens and the anterior surface of the closed eyelid.

Lensmark. The trade name for a relatively durable black dye used for marking contact lenses.

Lensometer (lenz-om'eh-ter). A trade name for an instrument which determines the vertex refractive power, the cylinder axis, the optical center, and the prismatic effect of ophthalmic lenses.

lenticele (len'tih-sēl). Phacocele.

lenticonus (len"tih-ko'nus). 1. A rare congenital anomaly in which either the anterior or the posterior surface of the crystalline lens has a conical or spherical bulging, as a consequence of which refraction may be excessive (myopic) through the central pupillary area. Syn., *lentiglobus.* 2. A rare congenital anomaly in which either the anterior or the posterior surface of the crystalline lens, usually in its axial region, has a conical bulging, as opposed to a spherical bulging *(lentiglobus).*

false l. A condition of abnormally high refractive index in the axial portion of the crystalline lens, hence simulating the optical effects of lenticonus, and usually attributed to sclerosing of the crystalline lens nucleus in the aged. Syn., *false cataract; pseudocataract.*

internal l. The condition of abnormally high convexity of the nucleus of the crystalline lens, hence simulating the optical effects of lenticonus.

lenticular (len-tik'u-lar). 1. Pertaining to, or resembling, a lens. 2. Pertaining to the crystalline lens of the eye. Syn., *lentiform.*

lenticulus (len-tik'u-lus). Anterior chamber implant.

lentiform (len'tih-form). Lenticular.

lentiglobus (len"tih-glo'bus). 1. A rare congenital anomaly in which either the anterior or the posterior surface of the crystalline lens, usually in its axial region, has a spherical bulging, as opposed to a conical bulging (*lenticonus*). 2. Lenticonus.

lentitis (len-ti'tis). Inflammatory involvement of the crystalline lens. Syn., *phacitis; phakitis.*

lentoids (len'toidz). White or yellowish, opaque, round or oval, lenslike structures, about 0.1 to 0.2 mm in diameter, consisting of newly formed lens tissue containing lens fibers and surrounded by a membrane resembling the lens capsule, appearing on the iris, posterior cornea, and in the vitreous following cataract surgery and in congenitally maldeveloped eyes.

lentoptosis (len"to-to'sis). Prolapse or hernia of the crystalline lens.

leprosy (lep'ro-se). A disease, common in tropical climates, caused by the *Mycobacterium leprae* and characterized by granulomatous lesions in the skin, the mucous membranes, and the peripheral nervous system. Two clinical types are recognized: (1) cutaneous or nodular; (2) neural or maculoanesthetic. The lesions may affect the structures of the eye or the eyelid and resultant interstitial keratitis and conjunctivitis are common. Syn., *Hansen's disease.*

leptomeningitis (lep"to-men"in-ji'tis). Inflammation of the pia mater and the arachnoid of the brain, the spinal cord, or the optic nerve. Cf. *pachymeningitis.*

leptospirosis (lep"to-spi-ro'sis). Weil's disease.

Lesser's method (les'erz). See under *method.*

Lester's sign. See under *sign.*

letters, confusion. 1. Letters on visual acuity test charts which may easily be mistaken for each other because of their similarity, e.g., *F* and *P*. 2. Letters included in a visual acuity test in excess of the minimum variety intended to measure acuity, to prevent or discourage memorization or pure chance guessing.

letters, Sloan. The letters C, D, H, K, N, O, R, S, V, and Z used in the *Sloan chart,* q.v.

letters, Snellen. Snellen test type.

Letter Separator. An instrument for the diagnosis and treatment of the crowding phenomenon in amblyopia ex anopsia, consisting of 25 randomly orientated letter E's mounted in radial slits on a flat vertical surface in a square formation, the distance between the E's being varied by a lever on the side of the instrument.

leucitis (lu-si'tis). Inflammation of the sclera. Syn., *scleritis.*

Leuckart's ratio (lūk'artz). See under *ratio.*

leukiridia (lu-kih-rid'e-ah). A condition in which the iris has whitish patches of depigmentation, as may occur in the secondary stage of syphilis.

leukokeratosis (lu"ko-ker"ah-to'sis). Leukoplakia.

leukokoria (lu"ko-kōr'e-ah). Any pathological condition, such as retrolental fibroplasia, which produces a white reflex from behind a clear crystalline lens.

leukoma (lu-ko'mah). A very dense, circumscribed, whitish opacity of the cornea. Cf. *macula; nebula.*

adherent l. A leukoma caused by scar tissue which encloses a prolapsed iris in a corneal wound.

leukophthalmos (lu"kof-thal'mos). A condition in which the sclera of the eye is unusually white.

leukoplakia (lu"ko-pla'ke-ah). A focal epithelial hyperplasia and keratinization affecting mucous membranes, especially of the mouth and occasionally of the conjunctiva. On the conjunctiva, it occurs most frequently in the limbal area, appears as a slightly elevated, white plaque and is considered to be the forerunner of an epithelioma. Syn., *leukokeratosis.*

leukopsin (lu-kop'sin). The colorless chemical end product resulting from the bleaching of rhodopsin by light and thought to be vitamin A plus a protein. Syn., *visual white*.

leukoscope (lu′ko-skōp). An instrument used by Hering to analyze the color mixture production of white, and later modified by Tschermak-Seysenegg for testing color vision by the mixture of colors to produce white.

leukotrichia (lu″ko-trik′e-ah). A condition in which the eyebrows and eyelashes are white, having a lack of pigment.

levator palpebrae superioris (le-va′tor pal′pe-bre su-pe″re-ōr′is). See under *muscle*.

level. Character, degree, quality, standard, or rank.

　　illumination l. The amount of illumination on a surface, expressed in footcandles, metercandles, phots, etc.

　　preadaptation l. The level of luminance for which the eye is adapted prior to submission to prolonged darkness.

　　reading capacity l. The highest level of difficulty at which a person can comprehend material read by, or to, him.

　　Talbot l. The level of brightness which results when intermittent stimuli are delivered at rates high enough to produce uniform sensation.

　　zero l. of accommodation. See *accommodation, zero level of*.

Levinsohn's theory (lev′in-sōnz). See under *theory*.

levoclination (le″vo-klih-na′shun). Levotorsion.

levocycloduction (le″vo-si″klo-duk′-shun). Intorsion of the right eye or extorsion of the left eye.

levocycloversion (le″vo-si″klo-ver′-zhun). Conjugate intorsion of the right eye and extorsion of the left eye. Syn., *negative cycloversion*.

levoduction (le″vo-duk′shun). Rotation of an eye to the left; abduction of the left eye or adduction of the right eye.

levophoria (le″vo-fo′re-ah). A tendency of the eyes to turn toward the left, manifested in the absence of a fixation stimulus.

levorotatory (le″vo-ro′tah-to″re). 1. Turning of the plane of polarization toward the left (as seen by an observer looking toward the source of light). 2. Pertaining to levoclination. Syn., *sinistrorotatory*.

levotorsion (le″vo-tōr′shun). Intorsion of

the right eye and/or extorsion of the left eye. Syn., *levoclination*.

levoversion (le″vo-ver′zhun). Conjugate rotation of the eyes to the left. Syn., *sinistroversion*.

Lex optometrica. Optometry law; the laws regulating or affecting the practice of optometry.

Lhermitte's (lār′mitz) **ophthalmoplegia; syndrome.** See under the nouns.

li test. See under *test*.

lichen planus (li′ken pla′nus). A disease of the skin and the mucous membranes, of unknown etiology, characterized by purplish papules and white opalescent spots and striae, and accompanied by intense itching. The conjunctiva is rarely involved.

lid. The eyelid.

Lie's experiment. See under *experiment*.

Lieb lens (lēb). See under *lens*.

Liebmann (lēb′man) **effect; phenomenon.** See under *effect*.

Liebreich's symptom (lēb′rīks). See under *symptom*.

ligament (lig′ah-ment). 1. A tough, flexible band of dense white, fibrous connective tissue which connects the articular ends of bones, or supports or retains an organ in its place. 2. Certain folds or processes of the pleura or peritoneum.

　　annular l. 1. Scleral spur. 2. A grouping of cells continuous with the corneal endothelium and extending to the anterior surface of the iris, filling the filtration angle of the anterior chamber, found in certain fishes, such as teleosteans, chondrosteans, cyclostomes, and holosteans.

　　l. of Campos. Extensions of the vitreous humor between the ciliary processes to the ciliary valleys. They pass between the zonular fibers and attach to the internal limiting membrane of the ciliary body.

　　check l. A band of fibrous connective tissue, with a small amount of smooth muscle, which leaves the surface of the sheath of an extraocular muscle and attaches to the periorbita, the orbital septum, the conjunctival fornix, the sheath of another muscle, or some neighboring ocular structure, serving to limit the action of the muscle. **extra c.l.** A check ligament arising parallel to the origin of the main check ligament of an extraocular muscle.

fused c.l. A series of several check ligaments forming a thick solid mass, especially observed to extend from the muscle sheath of the medial rectus to the orbital wall in congenital esotropes. **posterior c.l.** A check ligament having its muscle sheath origin farther back than normal and inserting into a greater portion of the orbital wall.

Hueck's l. Uveal meshwork.

hyaloideocapsular l. Noncellular attachments of the anterior limiting layer of the vitreous to the posterior capsule of the lens in the form of a ring about 9 mm in diameter. Syn., *ligament of Wieger.*

intermuscular l's. Connective tissue extensions between neighboring extraocular muscle sheaths which help bound the cone of muscles and separate the central adipose tissue from the peripheral adipose tissue of the orbit. Syn., *intermuscular membranes.*

intracapsular l's. Bands of fibers at the points of penetration of the extraocular muscles through Tenon's capsule, those of the superior rectus muscle being attached medially to the trochlea and laterally to the wall of the orbit, and those of the medial and lateral rectus muscles being attached inferiorly to the ligament of Lockwood; originally described by Lockwood but their presence has been denied by others.

l. of Lockwood. A hammocklike structure extending beneath and supporting the eyeball, formed by the fusion of the sheaths of the inferior rectus and the inferior oblique muscles, blending with the sheaths of the medial and the lateral rectus muscles (thus in effect thickening the inferior portion of Tenon's capsule), and inserting medially on the lacrimal bone and laterally on the orbital tubercle of the zygomatic bone.

palpebral l., inferior. The septum orbitale of the lower eyelid.

palpebral l., lateral. A band of fibrous connective tissue formed by the fusion of the lateral extremities of the tarsal plates of the upper and the lower eyelids and inserting on the orbital tubercle of the zygomatic bone. Syn., *external tarsal ligament.*

palpebral l., medial. A band of fibrous connective tissue formed by the fusion of the medial extremities of the tarsal plates of the upper and the lower eyelids and having two insertions, one superficially into the anterior lacrimal crest and the frontal process of the maxilla, and the other deep into the posterior lacrimal crest. Syn., *internal tarsal ligament.*

palpebral l., superior. The septum orbitale of the upper eyelid.

pectinate l. In lower mammals and birds, a group of large pigmented trabeculae stretching from the root of the iris to the cornea across the angle of the anterior chamber, forming the spaces of Fontana. In man, a vestigial structure after the sixth month of fetal life, the uveal meshwork. See also *meshwork of the angle of the anterior chamber.*

Soemmering's l. Trabeculae connecting the superior surface of the orbital portion of the lacrimal gland to the lacrimal fossa. Syn., *suspensory ligament of the lacrimal gland.*

suspensory l. Any ligament having as a principal function the support of another anatomical structure by suspension, e.g., the zonule of Zinn, the ligament of Lockwood, and Soemmering's ligament.

tarsal l., external. Lateral palpebral ligament.

tarsal l., internal. Medial palpebral ligament.

tarso-orbital l. Septum orbitale.

tenacular l. A ligament extending from the insertion of Brücke's muscle in the posterior region of the ciliary body to the sclera, found in the eyes of birds and reptiles.

transverse l. A condensation of the connective tissue running across the aponeurosis of the levator muscle of the upper eyelid and extending from the trochlea and the supraorbital notch to the lateral orbital margin. It probably checks excessive action of the levator muscle.

l. of Wieger. Hyaloideocapsular ligament.

Zinn's l. Annulus of Zinn.

ligamentum pectinatum iridis (lig″ah-men′tum pek″tin-a′tum ir′id-is). The pectinate ligament.

◆

LIGHT

light *(v.).* To illuminate.

light *(adj.).* 1. Bright, luminous; in reference to colors of high or very high brightness. 2. Having light; not dark or obscure, as, the room was *light.* 3.

Somewhat resembling white; pale in color, as a *light* complexion.

light (*n.*). 1. Radiant energy, approximately between 380 and 760 mμ, that gives rise to the sensation of vision on stimulating the retina. 2. The sensation of vision produced by stimulating the retina. 3. Radiant energy emitted at wavelengths in the ultraviolet, the visible, and the infrared bands of the electromagnetic grand spectrum. Syn., *physical light.* 4. A localized, usually named, source of illumination, e.g., a candlelight or windowlight.

accidental l. Stray light.

achromatic l. Light in which the quality of hue is absent. Syn., *neutral light.*

actinic l. Light capable of producing or serving to produce chemical changes.

l. adaptation. See under *adaptation.*

air l. Daylight scattered toward the observer along the path of sight, contributing to the apparent luminance of distant objects. Syn., *space light.*

ambient l. Light occurring in, and arising from, the surround of the object of regard.

l. area. See under *area.*

artificial l. Light produced by mechanical, electrical, thermal, and other man-made energy-transforming devices, in contrast to natural light received directly or by reflection from the sun and the sky.

axial l. Rays of light located on, or directly adjacent to, the axis of an optical system. Syn., *central light.*

l. beam. See under *beam.*

black l. Ultraviolet radiation near the visible spectrum, approximately between wavelengths of 320 mμ and 400 mμ, used in conjunction with certain dyes, such as fluorescein, to create fluorescence for diagnostic purposes, such as in the detection of corneal abrasions or the evaluation of the fit of contact lenses.

central l. Axial light.

l. chaos. The irregular, usually minute, fluctuations occurring in the idioretinal light. Syn., *light dust.*

chromatic l. Light having the quality of hue.

coagulation, l. Photocoagulation.

coherent l. See *coherence.*

cold l. 1. Light emitted by any body whose temperature is below that of incandescence. See also *luminescence.* 2. Any visible light essentially free of infrared radiation.

colored l. Chromatic light.

compound l. Light composed of more than one wavelength.

convergent l. Light directed toward a common point.

dark l. Idioretinal light.

diascleral l. Light entering the eyeball through the sclera.

l. difference. See under *difference.*

diffuse l. Light characterized as coming apparently from a source of extensive area and having no predominant directional component.

direct l. Light from a source falling directly on the eye or an object.

divergent l. Light directed away from a common point.

l. dust. Light chaos.

fluorescent l. Light emitted by a substance through the process of fluorescence.

l. flux. Luminous flux.

heterochromatic l. 1. Light composed of several noncontiguous wavelengths or of a spectral band broad enough so that it cannot be regarded as monochromatic light. 2. Light derived from a multiplicity of varicolored sources presented in mosaic pattern or in sequence.

heterogeneous l. Heterochromatic light.

homogeneous l. Monochromatic light.

idioretinal l. A sensation of light occurring in the absence of any photic or other external physical stimulus and attributed to physiological processes within the brain or the retina. Syn., *dark light; intrinsic light; self light.* Cf. *idioretinal gray; light chaos.*

incandescent l. Light emitted by a substance through the process of incandescence; especially light emitted by electric incandescent lamps.

incident l. Light falling on a surface.

infrared l. Infrared energy.

intensity l. Luminous intensity.

intrinsic l. Idioretinal light.

klieg l. A flood lamp employing an incandescent filament to produce an intense light, used in film studios.

metameric l's. Metameric colors.

l. minimum. See under *minimum*.

monochromatic l. 1. Light consisting of a single wavelength, as obtained in isolated lines of line spectra. 2. Light composed of a spectral band so narrow, or a series of spectral lines so close together, as to serve as the practical equivalent of a single wavelength.

neutral l. Achromatic light.

objective l. Light regarded as a physical entity, exclusive of its sensation-producing property. Cf. *physical light*.

oblique l. Light incident on an object from a direction oblique in relation to a given direction, as a line or an axis of observation, or in relation to a plane of reference, as the receiving surface itself.

parallel l. Light whose component rays are parallel.

parasitic l. Stray light.

l. pencils. See *rays, pencil of*.

photometric l. Radiant energy evaluated as to its capacity to evoke the brightness aspect of visual sensation. Syn., *luminous energy*.

physical l. Radiant energy in the ultraviolet, the visible, and the infrared bands of the electromagnetic grand spectrum. Cf. *objective light*.

polarized l. Light for which the presumed transverse wave motion is not uniform in amplitude in all directions in a plane perpendicular to the direction of propagation. **circularly p.l.** Light consisting of two plane-polarized components of equal frequency, perpendicular to each other, with a phase difference such that the resultant vibration in a transverse plane is a circle. **elliptically p.l.** Light consisting of two plane-polarized components of equal frequency, perpendicular to each other, with a phase difference such that the resultant vibration in a transverse plane is an ellipse. **linearly p.l.** Plane-polarized light. **plane p.l.** Polarized light in which the transverse wave vibrations are parallel to a plane through the axis of the beam. Syn., *linearly polarized light*.

primary l. The initial or first phase of the light stimulus in the sequence leading to the formation of afterimages. It alters the retinal sensitivity to the secondary light stimulus. Syn., *tuning light*.

psychological l. The sensation of light as given by any stimulus effective on the retina or on the central visual pathways. Thus, both the viewing of a lamp and the direct electrical irritation of the visual cortex arouse psychological light. Syn., *subjective light*.

quantity of l. Luminous flux per unit of time.

l. ray. See under *ray*.

reacting l. Secondary light.

reflected l. Light turned back, bent, or "rebounded" by the surface of a second medium so that it continues to travel in the first medium, but in an altered direction.

refracted l. Light whose pathway is altered from its original direction as a result of passing from one medium to another of different refractive index.

scattered l. Light deflected in various directions from its intended path, as by minute particles or irregularities in the transmitting medium, by irregularities at a reflecting surface, or by successive internal reflections at interfaces of a series of refracting layers.

secondary l. The second phase of the light stimulus in the sequence leading to the formation of a negative afterimage. The retinal response to this light is altered by the change in retinal sensitivity initiated by the primary light stimulus. Syn., *reacting light*.

self l. Idioretinal light.

solar l. Light from the sun, or light having the properties of light from the sun.

l. source. See under *source*.

space l. Air light.

stray l. Light reflected inside or passing through an optical system, but not involved in the formation of the image. Syn., *accidental light; parasitic light*.

subjective l. Psychological light.

transmitted l. Light which passes or has passed through a medium.

tuning l. Primary light.

Tyndall's l. Light from a transverse beam reflected or dispersed by small, otherwise invisible, particles in a transmitting medium, thus rendering these particles visible.

ultraviolet l. Ultraviolet energy.

l. wave. See under *wave*.

white l. 1. Achromatic light, or light perceived without the attribute of hue, such as may be obtained in proper mixtures of complementary hues, under conditions of scotopic vision, at the spectral neutral point of a dichromat, or under surround color conditions inducing the percept of white in a source. 2. Light produced by a source having an equal energy spectrum. 3. Light from any of several broadly heterochromatic sources adopted as standards for white light, such as sunlight and ICI illuminants A, B, and C.

Wood's l. A lamp which emits ultraviolet radiation in the region near the visible spectrum, used with certain dyes, such as fluorescein, to create fluorescence for diagnostic purposes, such as the detection of corneal abrasions or the evaluation of the fit of contact lenses.

◆

Lighthouse near acuity test (līt'hows). See under *test*.

lighting. An artificial supply of light, or the apparatus supplying it.

diffused l. Lighting from a source of extensive area and having no predominant directional components.

direct l. Lighting in which light reaches the area to be illuminated directly from the luminaire or the lighting equipment.

directional l. Lighting from a specific direction, generally from a light source of relatively small dimensions, such as a spotlight.

general l. Lighting providing a substantially uniform level of illumination throughout an area, exclusive of any provision for special local requirements.

indirect l. Lighting in which light reaches the area to be illuminated after reflection from a ceiling or other object external to the luminaire or the light equipment.

local l. Lighting arranged to provide illumination to a relatively small area.

lightness. An attribute of object colors whereby they can be rated on an achromatic scale from black to white for surface colors, or from black to colorless for transparent spatial colors. It implies a direction on the scale opposite to that implied by *darkness* and its physical correlate is *reflectance*.

limbal (lim'bal). Pertaining to, of, or situated near, the limbus corneae.

Lignac-Fanconi syndrome. See under *syndrome*.

limbosclerectomy (lim"bo-sklerek'to-me). Limboscleral trephining.

limbus (lim'bus). A border.

l. corneae. An annular transitional zone, approximately 1 mm wide, between the cornea and the bulbar conjunctiva and sclera. It is highly vascular and is involved in the metabolism of the cornea.

corneoscleral l. Limbus corneae.

l. luteus. Macula lutea.

l. palpebralis anterior. The anterior eyelid margin, in the region of the eyelashes, lined by skin.

l. palpebralis posterior. The posterior eyelid margin, lined by palpebral conjunctiva.

limen (li'men). Threshold.

liminal (lim'ih-nal). Pertaining to, or having the magnitude of, a limen or threshold.

limit, Dawes. An arithmetic modification of the formula for the Rayleigh limit to predict more precisely the actual resolution attained in optical systems.

limit of perception. Threshold of resolution.

limit of resolution. Resolving power.

limit, Rayleigh. A mathematical limit for the resolution of an optical system, without image deterioration from diffraction. The maximum difference in optical path distances for the rays meeting at the best focus is, as stated by Lord Rayleigh, a quarter of a wavelength of light.

limitation, eccentric. An irregular reduction in the limits of the visual field.

Lindau's disease (lin'dowz). See under *disease*.

Lindau-von Hippel (lin'dow-fonhip'el) **disease; syndrome.** Von Hippel-Lindau disease. See under *disease*.

Linder occluder. See under *occluder*.

Lindner's stenopaic spectacles; theory. See under the nouns.

◆

LINE

line. 1. A narrow, distinct furrow, ridge, seam, or band; a long mark or thread-like formation; a mark of division or demarcation; a boundary. 2. A succession of ancestors or descendants of a given person.

absorption l's. Dark lines in a spectrum resulting from absorption of specific wavelengths of light by the substance through which it passes. Syn., *Fraunhofer lines.*

l. of accommodation. The linear extent to which an object can be displaced toward and away from the eye in a given state of refraction without producing perceptible blurredness. Cf. *depth of focus.*

angular l. The collarette.

anti-Stokes's l's. New spectral lines occurring from a decrease in wavelength during scattering of monochromatic light. Cf. *Stokes's lines.*

arcuate l. A white crescentic line seen with the slit lamp in the posterior capsule of the crystalline lens, below the posterior pole in the region of the bifurcation of the posterior Y-suture. It encloses the area within which the vestiges of the hyaloid artery are found. Syn., *Vogt's line.*

Arlt's cicatricial l. A white line of scar tissue running horizontally across the tarsus in the region of the anastomosing of the terminal capillaries of the ascending and descending conjunctival vessels; the first indication of the cicatricial stage of trachoma.

Baillarger's outer l. The outer white band of myelinated nerve fibers in layer IV of the visual cortex which, in the area of the calcarine fissure, is known as the *line of Gennari.* Syn., *Baillarger's outer band.*

Barkan's white l. A white line observed in goniotomy following a circumferential incision of the root of the iris, representing the exposed scleral wall at the angle of the anterior chamber.

base l. The line joining the centers of rotation of the two eyes.

base-apex l. A line perpendicular to the intersection of two faces of a prism and bisecting the angle between the two faces.

cutting l. A horizontal line drawn on the 180° meridian of an uncut ophthalmic lens after the lens has been so placed that the cylinder axis and the optical center are in the desired position. It is the reference line for cutting and edging.

datum l. A line midway between the horizontal tangents of a spectacle lens shape at its highest and lowest points, used as a reference line in the cutting and edging of spectacle lenses.

Under certain conditions it may coincide with the cutting line. Syn., *mechanical axis; working axis.*

demand l. In the graphical representation of accommodation and convergence in a two coordinate system, the locus of points representing, for a given lens or prism correction, the accommodation and convergence stimulus values of a fixation object varying in position on the midline from an infinite distance to the nearest point of binocular vision. Syn., *orthophoria line.*

l. of direction. For a given point in space, the line connecting it with the anterior nodal point of the eye of reference. **principal l. of d.** The line joining the point of foveal fixation and the anterior nodal point of the eye; the visual axis. **secondary l. of d.** A line of direction other than the principal line of direction.

dividing l. The boundary line between two portions of a multifocal lens.

Donders' l. The demand line obtained with no lens or prism correction.

Egger's l. A line formed by the attachment of the hyaloideocapsular ligament to the posterior capsule of the crystalline lens, in a ring of about 9 mm diameter.

Ehrlich-Türk l. Line of Türk.

equidistant l. A type of horopter line characterized by the condition that all points on the line appear at the same distance as the fixation point. Syn., *iso-apostatic line.*

fixation l. Fixation axis.

Fleischer's l. Fleischer's ring.

focal l. A line image of a distant point source produced by an astigmatic optical system. Syn., *image line; Sturm's line.* **anterior f.l.** The more anterior of the two focal lines of the conoid of Sturm. **meridional f.l.** Tangential focal line. **posterior f.l.** The more posterior of the two focal lines of the conoid of Sturm. **radial f.l.** Sagittal focal line. **sagittal f.l.** The line image of a point source perpendicular to the sagittal section of a homocentric bundle of rays obliquely incident on an optical system containing spherical surfaces. The sagittal section is made up of two planes perpendicular to the tangential plane, one plane containing incident rays, the other plane containing emergent rays. Syn., *radial focal line.* **tangential f.l.** The line image of a point source, perpendicular to the tangential plane, formed by a homocentric bundle of rays obliquely incident on an optical system containing spherical surfaces. Syn., *meridional focal line.*

l. of force. Line of traction.

Fraunhofer's l's. A series of dark lines in the solar spectrum due to the absorption of specific wavelengths by elements in the atmosphere of the sun and the earth. The chief ones have been designated by the letters *A* through *K*, by Fraunhofer. Syn., *absorption lines.*

Fuchs' l's. of clearing. Clear lines occurring in various patterns in the midst of a corneal nebula or leukoma. They are associated with neovascularization of the cornea and follow the course of deep blood vessels.

l. of gaze. Any of variously defined lines of reference intended to represent the direction in which the eye is looking, e.g., line of sight, line of fixation, and visual axis.

l. of Gennari. A white line or stria formed in the middle of the fourth layer of the visual cortex or the area striata by the termination of the medullated fibers of the optic radiations. Syn., *outer band of Baillarger; band of Gennari; band of Vicq d'Azyr; stria of Gennari.*

Hudson's brown l. Superficial senile line.

Hudson-Stähli l. Superficial senile line.

image l. Focal line.

intermarginal l. A line of the margin of each eyelid corresponding to the anterior part of the tarsus and marking the union of the cutaneous and the tarsal portions of the eyelid.

iso-apostatic l. Equidistant line.

isocandela l. On any appropriate system of coordinates, the locus of points showing directions in space, with respect to an external light source, for which the candlepower is of a given and equal value.

isochromatic l's. Streaks or lines of the same color occurring when strains in photoelastic media are examined in polarized white light.

isofootcandle l. Isolux line.

isolux l. On a coordinate system representing a light-receiving surface, the locus of points for which the illumination is of a given and equal value. Syn., *isofootcandle line.*

isotorsional l's. In a fixation field plot, the contourlike lines representing the loci of points of equal degrees of ocular torsion.

keratoconus l's. Vertical lines in the corneal stroma which have the appearance of fibers of wood stretched apart, but still connected with each other at some points, seen with the slit lamp in keratoconus. Syn., *Vogt keratoconus stripes.*

least squares l. The line of best fit, for a series of values, determined by the *method of least squares.*

Lussi's l. A linear arrangement of leukocytes on the posterior corneal surface, found in normal eyes, usually of children, the pattern of distribution being attributed to thermal currents in the anterior chamber.

Marx l. A punctate line normally appearing with rose-bengal staining along the lid margin of the tarsal conjunctiva and sometimes absent or rudimentary in conditions of reduced tear secretion.

mounting l. of the face. A reference line for spectacle fitting, variously defined as one connecting the inner canthi, the outer canthi, or the centers of the pupils.

mounting l. of a frame. 1. In a metal rim or rimless type spectacle frame, the line which passes through the points on the eyewires or straps at which the guard arms are attached. 2. In a plastic spectacle frame: (*a*) the line which passes through the top points of attachment of the nose pads to the frame; (*b*) the line corresponding to the mounting line of the lens for which the frame is designed. 3. In a metal saddle bridge frame, the line which passes through the points at which the bridge is attached to the eyewires.

mounting l. of a lens. In an ophthalmic lens, a reference line parallel to the horizontal geometric axis at a vertical level defined more or less arbitrarily by the manufacturer of the "former" or pattern from which the lens is shaped and specified in terms of the distance above the geometrical center.

orthophoria l. Demand line.

Paton's l's. Fine folds in the retina resulting from lateral displacement of the retina adjacent to the optic disk in papilledema, seen ophthalmoscopically as arcuate stripes concentric with the optic disk.

primary sagittal l. A line in the primary position of the plane of regard which bisects the base line.

pupillary l. Pupillary axis.

l. of regard. A variously defined line intended to represent the direction of an object of either peripheral or central regard in relation to the eye or to a point of reference in the eye.

l. of regression. The line describing one variable (y) in terms of the other (x), when the relationship between the two variables is linear. The general equation is $y = a + bx$ where y is the dependent variable, x the independent variable, b the coefficient of regression or slope, and a the x-intercept.

rod l. The junction of the rodfree area in the fovea with the area of the retina containing rods.

Schwalbe's annular l. A gonioscopic landmark formed by the peripheral limit of Descemet's membrane of the cornea, indicating the anterior edge of the trabecular wall.

l. of sight. The line connecting the point of fixation and the center of the entrance pupil of the fixating eye.

sighting l. 1. Line of sight. 2. A line passing through two or more visually aligned object points, such as the sights of a gun.

spectral l. Any of a series of lines in the solar or other spectra which form distribution patterns characteristic of individual chemical elements in the gaseous state, each line representing light of a specific wavelength. These lines appear bright when due to emission or dark when due to absorption.

Stähli's l. Superficial senile line.

Stocker's l. 1. A yellowish-brown line of pigmentation in the clear superficial cornea near the head of a pterygium, attributed to ruptures in Bowman's membrane caused by a flattening of the cornea produced by the pterygium. 2. A fine line of melanotic pigmentation extending across the cornea and located in its epithelium, found by Stocker in a case exhibiting a tuberculosislike lesion of the uvea and sclera with accompanying corneal vascularization and infiltration.

Stokes's l's. New spectral lines occurring from an increase in wavelength during scattering of monochromatic light.

Sturm's l. Focal line.

superficial senile l. A brown, yellow, or green line, occurring in the apparently normal corneae of the elderly, which characteristically runs horizontally slightly below the center of the cornea. Syn., *Hudson's brown line; Hudson-Stähli line; Stähli's line; linea corneae senilis.*

temporary atropic l. The line normal to the secondary axis plane.

l. of traction. A line indicating the direction of force of an extraocular muscle on the eyeball on contraction. It extends from the origin to the point of tangential ocular contact of each of the extraocular muscles except the superior oblique, in which case it is from the trochlea to the point of tangential ocular contact. Syn., *line of force.*

l. of Türk. 1. A deposit of leukocytes on the posterior corneal surface, observed with the slit lamp as a vertical line, normally present in children of ages 7 to 16. 2. Any similar vertical line formed on the posterior corneal surface by the deposition of pigment or precipitates.

l. vergence. See under *vergence.*

vision, principal l. of. Line of sight.

visual l. Visual axis.

l. of visual direction. Line of direction.

Vogt's l. Arcuate line.

Zöllner's l's. Zöllner's figure.

◆

linea corneae senilis (lin′e-ah kōr′ne-e sen-il′is). Superficial senile line.

Linksz graticule; rule. See under the nouns.

Linnér's test. See under *test.*

Linnick microscope (lin′ik). See under *microscope.*

lipemia, retinal (lip-e′me-ah). A rare retinal condition due to abnormally high lipoid content of the blood. It occurs almost exclusively in association with diabetes mellitus and is characterized ophthalmoscopically by enlarged, flat, ribbonlike retinal arteries and veins which vary in color from salmon-pink to cream and are difficult to differentiate from each other.

lipoid granulomatosis (lip′oid gran″u-lo″mah-to′sis). Schüller-Christian-Hand disease.

lipoid histiocytosis, essential (lip′oid his″te-o-si-to′sis). Niemann-Pick disease.

lipoid spleno-hepatomegaly (lip'oid sple"no-hep"ah-to-meg'ah-le). Niemann-Pick disease.

lipoidosis, cerebroside (lip"oi-do'sis). Gaucher's disease.

lipoma (lip-o'mah). A tumor composed of fat cells.

liporrhagia retinalis, traumatic (lip"o-ra'je-ah ret"ih-nal'is). Purtscher's disease.

Lippich prism. See under *prism*.

lippitude (lip'ih-tūd). Marginal blepharitis.

lippitudo (lip"ih-tu'do). Marginal blepharitis.

liquor corneae (lik'er kōr'ne-e). The tissue fluid in the interstitial spaces of the cornea.

liquor Morgagni (lik'er mōr-gahn'ye). Morgagnian fluid.

Listing's (lis'tingz) **reduced eye; law; pearl specks; plane.** See under the nouns.

lithiasis conjunctivae (lith-i'ah-sis con"junk-ti've). A condition of the palpebral conjunctiva marked by the presence of minute, hard, yellow spots consisting of products of cellular degeneration contained in Henle's glands or glands of new formation. Only rarely are there calcareous deposits. Syn., *calcareous conjunctivitis; conjunctivitis lithiasis; conjunctivitis petrificans; uratic conjunctivitis.*

Little's disease (lit'elz). See under *disease*.

Littrow prism (lit'ro). See under *prism*.

Livingston's (liv'ing-stunz) **gauge; test.** See under the nouns.

Lloyd's (loidz) **experiment; method; mirror.** See under the nouns.

loa loa (lo'ah lo'ah). Filaria oculi.

lobe. A rounded or partly rounded projection of an organ; a division of an organ separated by a fissure or constriction, as those of the brain or the lungs.

occipital l's. The portion of the cerebral hemispheres posterior to the parietal lobes containing the area striata, the visual associational areas, the occipital eye fields, and higher convergence and accommodative centers.

optic l's. The superior colliculi in the midbrains of birds and lower vertebrates which lack cortical visual centers.

orbital l. That portion of the frontal lobe which rests above the bony orbit.

Lobeck ocular micrometer (lo'bek). See under *micrometer*.

Lobstein's disease (lōb'stīnz). Eddowes' disease.

Lobstein's syndrome (lōb'stīnz). Eddowes' syndrome.

localization, spatial. The reference of a visual sensation to a definite locality in space.

absolute spatial l. The localization of an object in visual space with the observer as the center of reference.

anomalous spatial l. The reference of a visual sensation to a locality in space significantly different from its physical correlate.

egocentric spatial l. The localization of an object in visual space with the self as the center of reference.

oculocentric spatial l. The localization of each direction in space with reference to the entrance pupil of the observing eye and its angular deviation from the line of sight.

partial spatial l. Localization of an object in visual space with reference only to direction and not to distance.

relative spatial l. The localization of an object in visual space with another object as the reference point.

similar spatial l. The localization of two or more objects to the same place in visual space.

Localizer. A visual training instrument designed by Bangerter to establish correct spatial localization, centric fixation, and normal visual acuity, in the treatment of amblyopia ex anopsia. Essentially it presents a series of various sized holes which are individually illuminated. With the nonamblyopic eye occluded, the amblyopic eye is made to fixate the illuminated hole such that the corneal reflex of the light source is properly positioned, that is, indicating centric fixation, and the patient is then instructed to touch the light source while maintaining his eye in this position.

Localizer-Corrector. A visual training instrument designed by Bangerter which incorporates the features of both the *Localizer* and the *Corrector*.

Lockwood's (lok'woodz) **ligament; tendon.** See under the nouns.

locus. 1. A place or locality in space. 2. The location of the plotted points on a coordinate chart or the path represented by a line joining these points.

blackbody l. The locus of points on a chromaticity diagram which represents the chromaticities of blackbodies having various color temperatures. Syn., *Planckian locus.*

egocentric l. The site or location of an object in visual space with reference to the self.

Planckian l. Blackbody locus.

spectrum l. The locus of points on a chromaticity diagram which represents the colors of the visible spectrum.

Loeser's law (lēs'erz). See under *law.*

Loewe's ring (leh'vēz). See under *ring.*

Loewi's sign (leh'vēz). See under *sign.*

logadectomy (log"ah-dek'to-me). Surgical removal of a portion of the conjunctiva.

logades (log-ah-dēz'). The "whites" of the eyes.

logaditis (log"ah-di'tis). Scleritis. *Obs.*

logadoblennorrhea (log"ah-do-blen"o-re'ah). Inclusion body blennorrhea.

logagnosia (log"ag-no'ze-ah). Alexia.

logagraphia (log"ah-graf'e-ah). Agraphia.

logamnesia (log"am-ne'ze-ah). The inability to comprehend either spoken or written words; sensory aphasia.

logaphasia (log"ah-fa'ze-ah). Motor aphasia.

Lomonosov's theory (lo-mon'o-sofs). See under *theory.*

London Course of Optometry. A six-week summer course started in 1956 and consisting of 180 hours of instruction designed especially for overseas opticians and optometrists eligible to practice in their home countries. Shortened versions have been provided in numerous other cities of the world.

London Refraction Hospital. A hospital opened in 1923 under sponsorship of the ophthalmic opticians as a center for the provision of a complete range of optometric services, especially for underprivileged patients, and as a clinical training center for optometry students and practitioners.

long-sightedness. A lay term for hypermetropia.

look. 1. To direct one's visual attention, as in "*look* toward the object." 2. To have resemblance, identity, or apparent quality, as in "to *look* new."

loop. A circular bend or fold in a cord or ribbonlike structure.

Archambault's l. Meyer's loop.

Axenfeld's intrascleral nerve l. A loop formed by a variation in the course of a long ciliary nerve. After traversing the perichoroidal space, the nerve pierces the sclera a few millimeters behind the limbus, turns back on itself, retraces the same path, and then enters the ciliary body.

Cushing's l. Meyer's loop.

Flechsig's l. Meyer's loop.

Meyer's l. A loop of inferior fibers of the optic radiations which extends forward in the temporal lobe at a level with and external to the optic tract, sharply bends downward and passes backward through the temporal and the occipital lobes to terminate in the lingual gyrus below the calcarine fissure. Syn., *Archambault's loop; Cushing's loop; Flechsig's loop.*

LP. Light perception.

LP & P. Light perception and projection.

Lorentz theory (lo'rents). See under *theory.*

Lorentz-Lorenz law (lo'rentz-lo'renz). See under *law.*

lorgnette (lōrn-yet'). Opera glasses, especially with a long vertical (sometimes folding) handle for holding the glasses poisedly with one hand; or spectacles held in place in the same manner.

lorgnon (lōrn-yon'). 1. Lorgnette. 2. A single spectacle lens mounted on a handle.

L.O.Sc. Licentiate of Optometric Science (granted by Victorian College of Optometry, Melbourne, Australia)

loss, Fresnel. Surface reflection.

Lotze's (lōt'zez) **sign; theory.** See under the nouns.

louchettes (loo-shets'). Goggles or similarly worn devices providing partial or total monocular occlusion as a treatment for strabismus.

Louis-Bar syndrome (loo-e'bahr). See under *syndrome.*

loupe (loop). Originally a simple convex lens for magnifying; now, any magnifying aid, monocular or binocular, held in the hand or mounted in front of the eye, for viewing very minute objects at very close range, but without image inversion as in a microscope.

Beebe l. A pair of spheroprisms with adjustable separation mounted on a several-centimeters-long anterior extension from a pair of "half-eye" trial lens holders with saddle bridge and

temples, giving approximately 2.3×
magnification.

Behr's l. A single or double lens
magnifier held in front of one of the
spectacle lenses by a clip attached to
the temple of the spectacle frame.

Berger's l. A binocular loupe
with the lenses mounted at the anterior
end of a light-excluding chamber fitting
over the eyes and held in place by an
elastic headband.

Boyle's l. A monocular loupe for
the inspection of soft contact lenses
having a 10× magnifying lens, red and
blue filters, and a clear lens used as a
holding device while examining edge
thickness, bevels, etc. The blue filter is
said to show lens damage, defects, and
protein buildup, the red filter containing a scale for diameter and bevel
width.

Brücke's l. A loupe formerly
used in dissecting, surgery, etc., essentially a Galilean telescope which magnifies from 4 to 6 diameters and permits
a working distance of from approximately 48 to 60 mm. Syn., *Brücke's
lens.*

Wollaston l. A highly magnifying laminated lens consisting of two
hemispherical lenses with a centrally
perforated aperture stop cemented between.

Zeiss l. A pair of adjustable
spheroprisms having 2× magnification
at a working distance of about 20 cm
which can be clamped to a pair of glasses or worn independently.

**LoVac contact lens; gonioscopic
lens; goniotomy lens.** See under
lens.

Lovibond Color Vision Analyzer.
See under *analyzer.*

Lowe's syndrome. See under *syndrome.*

**Lowe-Terry-MacLachlan syn-
drome.** Lowe's syndrome.

Lowenstein's (lo'en-stīnz) **climbing
pupil; descending pupil.** See
under the nouns.

**Lowenstein's low intensity reac-
tion** (lo'en-stīnz). Gunn's pupillary
phenomenon.

low-neutral. See under *neutral.*

Loxit (loks'it). A trade name for a rimless
spectacle mounting which is assembled
to the lenses with solder pins instead of
screws.

loxophthalmus (loks"of-thal'mus).
Strabismus.

LRH. See *London Refraction Hospital.*

Luboshez lens (lu'bo-shāz). See under
lens.

lucid interval of Vogt. See under *interval.*

luciferase (lu-sif'er-ās). A photoprotein
consisting of 19 amino acids which allows the oxidation of luciferin to produce bioluminescence.

luciferin (lu-sif'er-in). A chemical containing eleven carbon atoms arranged
into three rings found in certain organisms, such as the firefly, which,
when oxidized by the aid of luciferase,
emits light (bioluminescence). It also
has been produced synthetically.

lucifugal (lu-sif'u-gal). Avoiding bright
light.

Lucite (lu'sīt). The commercial name of
polymethyl methacrylate, produced by
E. I. du Pont de Nemours and Company. A chemically identical form,
marketed by Rohm & Haas Company,
is called Plexiglas. Both are lustrous,
water-white, lightweight, transparent
thermoplastics used in making contact
lenses, some spectacle frames, etc. They
were formerly used in the U.S.A. in the
manufacture of ophthalmic lenses, but
have been largely replaced in this application by more abrasion-resistant,
heat-hardened resins.

Luckiesh and Moss (lu'kēsh and maws)
illuminator; sensitometer. See
under the nouns.

Luckiesh-Taylor brightness meter
(lu'kēsh-ta'lor). See under *meter.*

Luer's clock (lu'erz). A cylindrosphe-
rometer.

Lumarith (lu'mah-rith). A trade name
for a cellulose acetate material used in
spectacle frames.

lumen (lu'men). The unit of luminous
flux; the flux emitted within a unit solid
angle (1 steradian) by a point source
having a luminous intensity of 1
candela (1 candlepower). Symbol: *lm.*

lumen-hour (lu'men-our'). A unit of
light; the quantity of light delivered in 1
hour by a flux of 1 lumen.

lumerg (lūm'erg). A unit of luminous energy representing that obtained from a
radiant energy source of 1 erg with a
luminous efficiency of 1 lumen per
watt.

lumeter, holophane (lu'me-ter). A portable photometer for measuring luminance.

Lumi-Cote. The trade name for a coating
applied to plastic contact lenses which
renders them opaque to ultraviolet

light without affecting the transmission of the visible spectrum.

Lumi-Mark. The trade name for a dye which is visible only when exposed to black light, used for reference markings on plastic contact lenses.

luminaire (lu'mih-nār). A complete lighting unit consisting of a light source, housing, supports, shields, etc; a complete lighting fixture.

luminance (lu'mih-nans). The photometric term for the intensive property of an emitting or reflecting surface; the luminous flux per unit of projected area per unit solid angle either leaving or arriving at a surface at a given point in a given direction; the luminous intensity in a given direction per unit of projected area of a surface as viewed from that direction. Previously termed *photometric brightness* and must be differentiated from *brightness*, the resulting visual effect. Symbol: *L*. Common units are *candela* per unit area, *stilb*, *footlambert*, *nit*, *lambert*, *apostilb*, and *millilambert*.

    absolute l. The luminance of a target in absolute units.

    apparent l. The luminance of an object or its background as viewed from a specific direction and through a given distance of atmosphere which attenuates and/or scatters light. Cf. *inherent luminance.*

    average l. of a luminaire. The luminous intensity (candlepower) of a luminaire in a given direction divided by the area of the directionally corresponding orthographic projection of the combined luminaire components which contribute to the candlepower, hence, its mean luminance from a given direction of view.

    average l. of a surface. Luminous exitance.

    inherent l. The actual luminance of an object or its background in a specified direction when it is unaltered by atmospheric attenuation or scatter, or by the presence of a glare source in the field of view. Cf. *apparent luminance.*

    relative l. The ratio of luminance of a target to luminance of the background.

lumination (lu"mih-na'shun). The emitting of light from a source.

luminator (lu'mih-na"tor). An emitter of light; a light source.

luminescence (lu"mih-nes'ens). Radiation which results primarily from the excitation of individual atoms, so scattered or arranged that each atom is free to act without much interference from its neighbors. As distinguished from radiation due to incandescence, it is not due to temperature; also, the radiation is apt to consist of discrete wavelengths, or colors, rather than forming a continuous spectrum. See also *bioluminescence; chemiluminescence; crystalloluminescence; electroluminescence; photoluminescence; thermoluminescence; triboluminescence.*

luminiferous (lu"mih-nif'er-us). Transmitting, producing, yielding, or conveying light.

luminophor (lu"min'o-fōr). A substance which has the property of absorbing energy and releasing it again in the form of luminescence, such as a fluorophor or phosphor.

luminosity (lu"mih-nos'ih-te). The luminous intensity or brightness sensation-producing attribute of radiant flux; brightness.

    absolute l. Spectral luminous efficacy of radiant flux. See under *efficacy.*

    l. contrast. See under *contrast.*

    l. curve. See under *curve.*

    l. factor. See under *factor.*

    minimum-field l. Luminosity determined by reducing the size of the test object (hence the area or "field" of the test object) until it matches the brightness of a fixed comparison standard or fulfills some other comparable criterion for determining luminous equivalence, e.g., the level of hue extinction.

    relative l. Spectral luminous efficiency of radiant flux. See under *efficiency.*

luminous (lu'mih-nus). 1. Emitting or reflecting light. 2. Having the property of exciting the visual receptors.

luminous dust. Light chaos.

luminous density; efficacy; efficiency; exitance; energy; flux; intensity. See under the nouns.

lumi-rhodopsin (lu'me-ro-dop'sin). An intermediate product in the chemical breakdown of rhodopsin by the action of light prior to the formation of meta-rhodopsin and then retinene.

Lumiwand. The trade name for a device used in visual field testing consisting essentially of a wand containing a 10.0 mm electroluminescent light source at one end, a battery and switch in the handle at the other end, and a control to regulate luminance. Auxiliary caps with apertures ranging from 1.0 mm to 5.0 mm in diameter may be fitted over the light source to vary the size of the test stimulus.

Lummer-Brodhun (lum'er-brod'hun) **cube; photometer.** See under the nouns.

Lummer-Gehrcke interferometer (lum'er-gärke). See under *interferometer*.

Luneburg's theory (lūn'eh-burgz). See under *theory*.

lupus erythematosus conjunctivae (lu'pus er"e-them-ah-to'sus kon"junkti've). A rare affection of the conjunctiva which almost invariably has spread from a neighboring lupus erythematosus of the eyelids. It commences with intense hyperemia and velvetlike edema and may be diffuse, limited to circumscribed patches, or scattered as dotted foci. The lesions later become bluish, then white and depressed as atrophy occurs. Symptoms include slight photophobia, itching, lacrimation, and mucoid discharge with little or no pain.

lupus pernio (lu'pus per'ne-o). Sarcoidosis.

Lüscher color test (loo'shur). See under *test*.

Luschka's nerve (lush'kahz). The posterior ethmoidal nerve.

Lussi's line (lus'ēz). See under *line*.

luster. 1. The appearance of two different surface colors viewed haploscopically and superimposed, the resulting percept being characteristically unstable and aptly described as one surface being seen through the other; also called *binocular luster*. 2. A glossiness or sheen associated with metallic surfaces, sometimes called *metallic luster*.

    achromatic l. Luster obtained from two different achromatic colors, e.g., black and white, viewed haploscopically and superimposed.

    polychromatic l. Luster obtained by the haploscopic superimposition of two different hues.

Lutes near point chart (lūtz). See under *chart*.

lux. A unit of illumination equal to 1 lumen per sq. m. Syn., *metercandle*.

luxation of the eyeball. See under *eyeball*.

luxation of the lens. Complete dislocation of the crystalline lens from the pupillary aperture. Cf. *subluxation of the lens*.

luxmeter. A photometer which measures illumination in luxes.

luxometer (luks-om'eh-ter). A portable photometer by which an illuminated surface is compared with an area illuminated by a standard lamp contained within the instrument.

Lyle and Jackson's method (līl and jak'sunz). See under *method*.

Lyman's ghosts (li'manz). See under *ghost*.

lymphangiectasis, hemorrhagic, conjunctival (lim"fan-je-ek'tah-sis). A rare condition in which a conjunctival blood vessel becomes connected with a lymphatic vessel, resulting in intermittent or permanent filling of the lymphatic with blood.

lymphangiectasis, ocular (lim"fan-je-ek'tah-sis). Dilatation of the lymphatic vessels of the eye, characterized in the bulbar conjunctiva by single or multiple, small, transparent, pearl-like blebs or cysts.

lymphangioma (lim"fan-ge-o'mah). A congenital, benign, slowly progressing tumor of the lymph-vascular system which may affect the eyelids, conjunctiva, or orbit, and rarely the eyeball.

lymphatic (lim-fat'ik) **nodes; rings; spaces; vessels.** See under the nouns.

lymphogranulomatosis, benign (lim"fo-gran"u-lo-mah-to'sis). Sarcoidosis.

lymphogranulomatosis of Schaumann (lim"fo-gran"u-lo-mah-to'sis). Sarcoidosis.

lymphoma (lim-fo'mah). Any tumor made up of lymphoid tissue.

lymphorrhagia retinalis traumatic (lim"fo-ra'je-ah ret-ih-nal'is). Purtscher's disease.

lymphosarcoma (lim"fo-sar-ko'mah). A form of malignant tumor of lymphatic tissue characterized by proliferation of masses of cells resembling lymphocytes and resulting in enlargement of lymph nodes and infiltration of other tissues. Of the malignant orbital tumors, it is one of the most common.

lysozyme (li'so-zīm). A bactericidal mucolytic enzyme present in tears (also in saliva, nasal secretions, egg white, and leukocytes).

Lythgoe (lith'go) **cycle; theory.** See under the nouns.

M

M. Abbreviation for *myopia* or *myopic;* symbol for *luminous exitance.*

m. Abbreviation for *meter.*

MA. Abbreviation for *meter angle.*

mμ. Symbol for *millimicron.*

Macbeth illuminometer; photometer. See under *photometer.*

McCarthy's reflex (mah-kahr'thēz). Supraorbital reflex. See under *reflex.*

McCollough effect (mah-kul'uh). See under *effect.*

McCulloch's rule (mă-kul'oks). See under *rule.*

McDougall's theory (mak-du'galz). See under *theory.*

Mach's (mahks) **band; figure; visual illusion; law; ring.** See under the nouns.

Mach-Dvŏrák effect; phenomenon. See under *phenomenon.*

MacKay-Marg Electronic Tonometer. See under *tonometer.*

Mackenzie's theory (mă-ken'zēz). See under *theory.*

macreikonic (mak″ri-kon'ic). Pertaining to the eye with the larger image in aniseikonia.

macroblepharia (mak″ro-bleh-far'-e-ah; -fa're-ah). An abnormally large eyelid.

macrocornea (mak″ro-kōr'ne-ah). An abnormally large cornea. Syn., *megalocornea.*

macrodacryocystography (mak″ro-dak″re-o-sis-tog'rah-fe). Radiography of the lacrimal canaliculus, lacrimal sac, and lacrimal duct performed at one to ten minute intervals after the instillation of a contrast material through a dilated punctum.

macroesthesia (mak″ro-es-the'ze-ah). Macropsia.

macroglia (mă-krog'le-ah). Astroglia.

macroglobulinemia (mak″ro-glob″u-lin-e'me-ah). Waldenström's syndrome.

macrophthalmous (mak″rof-thal'-mus). An abnormally large eye.

macropia (mă-kro'pe-ah). Macropsia.

macropsia (mă-krop'se-ah). An anomaly of visual perception in which objects appear larger than they actually are. Syn. *megalopsia.*

    accommodative m. Macropsia attributed to underaccommodation or reduced effort of accommodation in relation to the amount of accommodation normally required for the distance of the object in question.

    retinal m. Macropsia resulting from a disturbance of the retina in which the visual receptor cells are crowded together. It may be due to a detachment, a tumor, exudative or inflammatory process or cicatricial changes.

macropsy (mă-krop'se). Macropsia.

macroscopic (mak″ro-skop'ik). Large enough to be seen or distinguished by the human eye without magnification.

macula (mak'u-lah). 1. Any uniquely pigmented area such as the macula lutea of the retina. 2. A corneal macula.

    bull's eye m. A ring-like depigmentation surrounding the macula, seen ophthalmoscopically.

    corneal m. A moderately dense and circumscribed whitish opacity of the cornea. It is more dense than a *nebula* and less dense than a *leukoma.*

detached m. A detachment of the retina in the region of the macula lutea.

false m. In anomalous correspondence, the retinal area of the deviating eye corresponding in visual direction to the fovea of the fixating eye, hence, appearing to exhibit certain projective attributes of the normal fovea. Syn., *anomalous associated area; pseudomacula.*

m. flava. Macula lutea.

heterotopia of m. See under *heterotopia.*

hole in m. See under *hole.*

honeycombed m. Cystic degeneration of the macula.

m. lutea. An oval area in the retina, 3 to 5 mm in diameter, usually located temporal to the posterior pole of the eye and slightly below the level of the optic disk. It is characterized by the presence of a yellow pigment diffusely permeating the inner layers, contains the fovea centralis in its center, and provides the best photopic visual acuity. It is devoid of retinal blood vessels, except in its periphery, and receives nourishment from the choriocapillaris of the choroid. Rod and cone fibers from the visual cells in this area course obliquely to form the fiber layer of Henle. Syn., *limbus luteus; macula flava; punctum luteum; Soemmering's spot; yellow spot.*

sparing of m. The retaining of macular function in the presence of adjacent visual field losses, especially so identified in hemianopsia which circumvents the macula.

macular (mack'yoo-lur). Of, pertaining to, or identified with, a macula, especially the macula lutea.

Macular Integrity Tester-Trainer. An instrument primarily for diagnosis and treatment of eccentric fixation, consisting essentially of a rotating transilluminated Polaroid filter which, when viewed through a blue filter, produces rotating Haidinger's brushes localized in relation to a fixation point mounted on the instrument.

Macula-Scope, Rinaldi-Larson. A hand-held, battery-operated instrument which presents a transilluminated, rotating, polarizing filter subtending a field adjustable for size to induce the rotating Haidinger's brushes phenomenon for fixation-testing and orthoptic purposes.

maculopathy (mak"u-lop'ah-the). A morbid condition or disease of the macula lutea.

cystic m. Cystic degeneration of the macula lutea which may occur subsequent to cataract extraction or in senile macular dystrophy.

epinephrine m. Maculopathy occurring in the eyes of aphakics using adrenalin drops, characterized initially by intermittent blurring of vision with a subsequently constant loss of visual acuity accompanied by macular edema and petechial hemorrhages. Complete recovery of visual acuity is usual about six months after use of the drops has ceased.

nicotinic acid m. Maculopathy resulting from the daily ingestion of 3000 mg or more of nicotinic acid taken for the reduction of serum cholesterol. The condition is reversible with restoration of normal vision after discontinuation of the medication.

madarosis (mad"ah-ro'sis). Loss of the eyelashes. Syn., *milphae; milphosis.*

Maddox (mad'oks) **calculator; chart; cross; groove; prism; prism verger; rod; rule; oblique scale; strabismometer; tests; wing.** See under the nouns.

Maeder-Danis deep filiform corneal dystrophy. See under *dystrophy, corneal.*

Magder's test. Bailliart's test.

Magendie-Hertwig (mah-zhan'de-hert'vig) **sign; syndrome.** See under the nouns.

magenta (mă-jen'tah). 1. The hue attribute of visual sensation typically evoked by stimulation of the normal human eye by any combination of wavelengths which act as the complement of a wavelength of 515 mμ. 2. The hue attribute produced by the additive mixture of red and blue.

magneto-optics (mag-ne"to-op'tiks; mag"net-o-). That area of optics which treats of the interaction of light with magnetic fields.

magnification (mag"nih-fih-ka'-shun). An increase in the apparent size, the perceived size, or the actual size of an object, or of its image in relation to the object.

angular m. Magnification expressed as a ratio of the angle subtended by the image to that subtended by the object with respect to a viewing point of reference, such as the entrance pupil of the eye.

apparent m. In an optical viewing instrument, the ratio of the apparent size of the image to the apparent size of the object at a standard or assumed distance, conventionally 25 cm. Syn., *magnifying power*.

axial m. The ratio of the distance between two axially located points in image space to the distance between the corresponding two axially located points in object space. Syn., *longitudinal magnification*.

chromatic difference of m. In an optical system with chromatic aberration, the difference in magnification produced by different wavelengths or colors.

effective m. Traditionally, the ratio of the apparent size of the image as seen through a lens or optical system to the apparent size of the object as it would appear at a distance of 25 cm, the so-called "distance of distinct vision." For a simple lens in front of the eye, this magnification is expressed by the formula: $M = F/4$, where F = the dioptric power of the lens.

empty m. Magnification in excess of that necessary to afford comfortable discrimination of resolvable detail.

initial m. Objective magnification.

lateral m. The ratio of the distance between two points in the image plane to the corresponding two points in the object plane, distinguished from *axial* or *longitudinal magnification*. Syn., *transverse magnification*.

longitudinal m. Axial magnification.

meridional m. Magnification, as produced by a meridional iseikonic lens, in which the image is magnified maximally in one meridian and minimally in a meridian at right angles to it.

normal m. The maximum magnification under which a microscope can provide a retinal image having the same brightness or luminance as that obtained without the microscope, called *normal brightness*. The limiting factor is the area of the exit pupil of the microscope in relation to the area of the entrance pupil of the eye.

objective m. The magnification attributed to the objective of a microscope. Syn., *initial magnification*.

over-all m. Magnification, as produced by an over-all iseikonic lens, in which the image is magnified equally in all meridians.

peripheral m. The magnification obtained when the eye fixates through a peripheral portion of a spectacle lens, usually differing from the normally obtained magnification through the center because of the greater distance of the periphery of the lens from the eye.

power m. Magnification resulting from the power of an ophthalmic lens, represented by the fraction $\dfrac{1}{1-zF_v}$ in the formula

$$M = \left(\frac{1}{1-cF_1}\right)\left(\frac{1}{1-zF_v}\right)$$

where c = thickness divided by index of refraction, F_1 = refractive power of the front surface of the lens, z = distance from the back surface of the lens to the entrance pupil of the eye, and F_v = the effective power of the lens.

psychological m. The perceptual enlargement of an object not associated with an increase in size of the retinal image, e.g., the perceptual enlargement of the moon when seen at the horizon.

relative spectacle m. The ratio of the retinal image size in the corrected ametropic eye to that in the schematic emmetropic eye. Abbreviation *RSM*.

shape m. Magnification resulting from the shape of an ophthalmic lens, represented by the fraction $\dfrac{1}{1-cF_1}$ in the formula

$$M = \left(\frac{1}{1-cF_1}\right)\left(\frac{1}{1-zF_v}\right)$$

where c = thickness divided by index of refraction, F_1 = refractive power of the front surface of the lens, z = distance from the back surface of the lens to the entrance pupil of the eye, and F_v = the effective power of the lens.

spectacle m. See *power magnification*.

transverse m. Lateral magnification.

magnifier. 1. An optical device or visual aid, usually for close viewing, producing apparent magnification. 2. Any optical system producing magnification.

binocular m. A binocular magnifying instrument, usually consisting of simple convex lenses, and sometimes

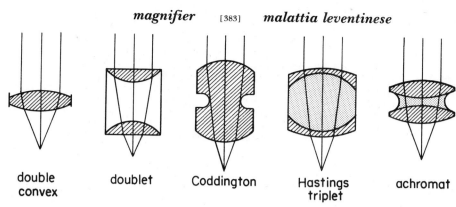

double convex   doublet   Coddington   Hastings triplet   achromat

Fig. 27 Common types of magnifiers. (From Jenkins and White, *Fundamentals of Optics*, 3d ed. New York: McGraw-Hill, 1957; copyright © 1957; used with permission of McGraw-Hill Co.)

prisms, supported before the eyes by an attachment to a spectacle frame or by a headband. Syn., *binocular loupe.*

Bishop Harman m. A binocular magnifying loupe consisting of two laterally adjustable, rectangular, convex, spheroprism lenses rigidly mounted anteriorly to a trial frame with single cells for auxiliary lenses.

Brungardt m. A 10× binocular lens assembly which can be attached to a focal illuminator for fitting and inspection of contact lenses and for locating foreign bodies.

hand m. A simple magnifier that typically is held close to the object, as distinguished from a spectacle magnifier that is held close to the eye.

Igard Hyperocular Spectacle M. A plastic, aspherical, biconvex, lenticular lens mounted in a spectacle frame having two anterior posts acting as stops against which reading material is held. It is available in 4×, 6×, and 8× magnifications, for use in subnormal vision.

measuring m. A small, hand-held, magnifying viewer used in the inspection of contact lenses, consisting essentially of a convex lens eyepiece with a transparent scale at its object focal plane.

projection m. An instrument which projects a magnified image of printed matter onto a screen by reflecting light from the surface of the matter through a system of mirrors and lenses. A type used for subnormal vision contains both the optical system and a translucent screen on the back of which the image is focused to be viewed from the front.

spectacle m. A magnifier mounted in a spectacle frame so that it is held close to the eye, as distinguished from a hand magnifier that is typically held close to the object.

Visolett m. A paperweight magnifier with a linear magnification of 1.8× that can be increased to 2.5× by lifting it 5 mm from the object surface. It is relatively distortion free, has a minimum of reflections, and is made in five diameters, ranging from 28 mm to 90 mm.

magnify. To produce magnification.

magnitude, apparent. 1. The perceived size of an object, or its image, when it is projected to, or identified with, a specific distance from the observer. 2. The size of an object, as measured by the plane angle which it subtends at the eye of the observer.

Magnocular (mag-nok'u-lar). A trade name for a binocular magnifying device consisting of two concave lenses mounted in a spectacle frame and two convex lenses anteriorly mounted on jointed arms.

Magnus (mag'nus) **formula; method.** See under the nouns.

Maier's sinus (mi'erz). See under *sinus.*

Maklakov's tonometer (mak'lah-kofs). See under *tonometer.*

Maksutov corrector. See under *corrector.*

malattia leventinese (mal-ah-te'ah leh-ven'tih-nēz). A slowly progressive, dominant, inherited degeneration of the retina found among inhabitants of the Leventine Valley in North Ticino, Switzerland. It is characterized in its later stages by numerous, closely grouped, round, yellowish spots of various sizes in the region of the macula and optic disk, and results in a gradual loss of central vision.

Malherbe's disease. See under *disease*.

malingering (mah-ling′er-ing). Feigning or deliberately giving false test responses, indicating illness or disability, to gain a desired award or compensation or to avoid doing a duty. Syn., *dissimulation*.

    negative m. Feigning or deliberately giving false test responses, indicating the total or partial absence of illness, disability, or damage.

    positive m. Malingering, distinguished from *negative malingering*.

Mallett Fixation Disparity Test. See under *test*.

Mallett Near Fixation Disparity Test Unit. See under *unit*.

malprojection (mal″pro-jek′shun). False projection.

Malus' law (mă-lūz). See under *law*.

Malus-Dupin law (mah-lu′-du-pen′). See under *law*.

mandrel (man′drel). A tapered hollow bar having a cross section shape of a spectacle lens and used to stretch and shape the rims of plastic spectacle frames.

Mangin mirror. See under *mirror*.

Mann's sign (manz). See under *sign*.

manometer (mă-nom′eh-ter). An instrument for determining the intraocular pressure, by direct contact with the aqueous humor. It consists essentially of a cannula introduced into the anterior chamber and a U-shaped tube filled with mercury, saline, or some other fluid to register the pressure.

    compensatory m. A manometer which has a compensating apparatus by which pressure may be applied or released to counter-balance any movement of fluid out of or into the eye during measurements.

manometry (mă-nom′eh-tre). Determination of intraocular pressure by means of a manometer.

manoptoscope (man-op′to-skōp). A hollow, truncated cone for testing ocular dominance on the principle of unilateral sighting. The subject holds the base of the cone against his face, covering both eyes, and views a distant object through the small end of the cone. Only one eye can fixate under these conditions, and that eye is considered to be the dominant eye. Syn., *manuscope*.

mantle, glial (peripheral). A layer of neuroglia located between the pia mater and the peripheral nerve fiber bundles of the optic nerve.

manuductor (man″u-duk′tor). An instrument used in visual training, based on the principle of the Brewster stereoscope, with large spheroprism lenses and a large target area especially adaptable for tracing, as in a cheiroscope, and for fusional convergence training.

manuscope (man′u-skōp). Manoptoscope.

Manz's (man′zez). **disease; gland; theory.** See under the nouns.

Marano's chart (mah-rah′nōz). See under *chart*.

March's disease (mar′chez). Exophthalmic goiter.

Marchesani's syndrome (mahr″ke-sahn′ēz). See under *syndrome*.

Marcus Gunn (mar′kus gun) **phenomenon; pupil.** See under the nouns.

Maréchal's box (mar″a-shalz′). See under *box*.

Marfan's syndrome (mar-fahnz′). See under *syndrome*.

margin. A boundary, border, or edge.

    ciliary m. The periphery of the root of the iris where it attaches to the ciliary body.

    orbital m. The anterior rim of the bony orbit formed by the frontal, the zygomatic, the maxillary, and, according to some, the lacrimal bone.

    pupillary m. The pigmented border of the iris that immediately surrounds the pupil.

    supraorbital m. Supraorbital arch.

marginoplasty (mar′jin-o-plas″te). Plastic surgery of the eyelid margin.

margo palpebrae (mar′go pal′pe-bre, pal-pe′-). The margin of the eyelid.

Marie's disease (mar-ēz′). See under *disease*.

Marie-Guillan syndrome (mahr-e′-ge-yăn). Rubrothalamic syndrome.

Marin-Amat syndrome (mah-rin′-ah-mat′). Reverse jaw-winking.

Marinesco-Sjögren syndrome (mar″ih-nes′ko-sye′gren). See under *syndrome*.

Mariotte's (mar-e-ots′). **experiment; blind spot.** See under the nouns.

Mark diplopia test. See under *test*.

marker, axis. A device used to locate and mark the cylindrical axis and the optical center of a spectacle lens preparatory to cutting.

Markus syndrome (mahr'kus). Adie's syndrome. See under *syndrome*.

Marlow's (mar'lōz) **prolonged occlusion; test.** See under the nouns.

Maroteaux-Lamy syndrome. See under *syndrome*.

Marsden ball (marz'den). See under *ball*.

Martegiani, area of (mar-tej-ah'ne). See under *area*.

Martens photometer (mar'tenz). See under *photometer*.

Martin-Albright syndrome (mahr'-tin-awl'brīt). Polyvisceral dystrophy. See under *dystrophy*.

Martius disk (mar'tih-us). See under *disk*.

Martorell's syndrome. Pulseless disease.

Marx effect; line. See under the nouns.

maser (ma'zer). An acronym for "microwave amplification by stimulated emission of radiation"; a device for producing coherent radiation at a frequency within the microwave band. Cf. *laser*.

    optical m. Laser.

Mason's disk (ma'sunz). See under *disk*.

mass, ciliary (of Whitnall). A thickening at the lateral margin of the eyelid formed by the uniting of the connective tissue of the tarsus with that around the follicles of the eyelashes.

Masselon's spectacles (mas-eh-lawnz'). See under *spectacles*.

Masson disk (mah-son'). See under *disk*.

Masuda's disease. See under *disease*.

match, Rayleigh. Rayleigh equation.

matching, color. 1. The selection of colors possessing the same hue, saturation, or brightness from a group of colors varying in hue, saturation, and brightness. 2. The mixing of two or more colors on a spinning color wheel to match the hue, saturation, and brightness of a uniform surface.

Matsuura Autocross (mah"tsu-oor'-ah). See under *Autocross*.

Matthiessen's ratio. See under *ratio*.

Mauriac syndrome (mo're-ak). See under *syndrome*.

Maurice's theory (mo're-sez). See under *theory*.

Mauthner's (mout'nerz) **keratitis; test.** See under the nouns.

maxima, principal (mak'sih-mah). The brightest bands produced in interference phenomena by reinforcement of two or more separate wave trains.

maxima, secondary (mak'sih-mah). The bright bands produced in interference phenomena adjacent to the principal maxima.

Max Pfister color pyramid test (max fiss'ter). See under *test*.

Maxwell's (maks'welz) **box; color curves; disk; law; ring; spot; table; test; theory; top; color triangle.** See under the nouns.

May's (māz) **ophthalmoscope; prism; sign.** See under the nouns.

Mazow pupilens (ma'zo). See under *pupilens*.

Means' sign (mēnz). See under *sign*.

measure, lens. An instrument designed to measure the sagitta of a curve and so calibrated as to give this measurement in terms of diopters of refractive power for a given index of refraction, usually that of crown glass ($n = 1.523$ or 1.53). It is shaped like a pocket watch, with three prongs attached to the edge, the outer two being fixed and the center one varying in length with the curve of the lens surface. Syn., *lens clock; lens gauge*.

measure, Maddox monocular phoria. A Maddox rod with a rotatable prism used to measure the subjective angle of deviation, either horizontal or vertical.

Mecholyl (mek'o-lil). A trade name for *methacholine*.

Meckel's (mek'elz) **cave; cavity; ganglion; space.** See under the nouns.

media (me'de-ah). Substances through which a force acts or an effect is transmitted.

    anisotropic m. Optical media in which the velocity of light is not constant for all directions.

    isotropic m. Optical media in which the velocity of light is constant for all directions.

    ocular m. The transparent substances of the eye through which light passes prior to stimulation of the retina. They include the tears, the cornea, the aqueous humor, the crystalline lens, and the vitreous humor.

    m. optica. See *medium, optical*.

    redirecting m. Media that change the direction of radiant energy without scattering.

mediaometer (me"de-ah-om'eh-ter). An instrument for determining the dioptric powers of the ocular media.

medi-Flow Lens. See under *lens.*

medium, optical. Any material, substance, space, or surface regarded in terms of its optical properties.

medulloepithelioma (me-dul″o-ep″-ih-the″le-o′mah). A tumor of the retina or of the central nervous system which is derived from the primitive retinal epithelium or from the medullary epithelium of the primitive neural tube of the brain.

Meekren-Ehlers-Danlos syndrome (mē′ren-a′lerz-dan′los). See under *syndrome.*

Meesmann's corneal dystrophy (mēz′mahnz). See under *dystrophy.*

megalocornea (meg″ah-lo-kōr′ne-ah). A bilateral developmental anomaly, in which the cornea is abnormally large in diameter in the presence of normal intraocular pressure. The cornea is otherwise normal, although there may be associated changes in the crystalline lens and the zonule of Zinn. Syn., *cornea globosa; keratoglobus; keratomegalia; anterior megalophthalmus.*

megalopapilla (meg″ah-lo-pah-pil′ah). A congenital condition in which the optic disk is abnormally large, but otherwise of normal appearance.

megalophthalmos (meg″ah-lof-thal′-mus). Megalophthalmus.

megalophthalmus (meg″ah-lof-thal′-mus). The condition of abnormally large eyes occurring as a developmental anomaly.

 anterior m. Megalocornea with associated changes in the crystalline lens and the zonule of Zinn.

megalopia (meg″ah-lo′pe-ah). Macropsia.

megalopsia (meg″ah-lop′se-ah). Macropsia.

Megascope (meg′ah-skōp). A projection magnifier for use in subnormal vision which provides either 12× or 25× magnification.

megaseme (meg′ah-sēm). Having an orbital index greater than 89; characteristic of the yellow races. See also *mesoseme; microseme.*

megophthalmus (meg″of-thal′mus). Megalophthalmus.

Meibomian (mi-bo′me-an) **cyst; glands.** See under the nouns.

meibomianitis (mi-bo″me-ah-ni′tis). Inflammation of the Meibomian glands.

meibomitis (mi-bo-mi′tis). Meibomianitis.

Meisling's colorimeter (mīs′lingz). See under *colorimeter.*

Meissner's test (mīs′nerz). See under *test.*

melange (meh-lahnzh′). A multi-component lubricant used in drilling lenses, commonly consisting of oil, turpentine, and camphor.

melanin (mel′ah-nin). A brown, black, or otherwise dark pigment derived from the metabolic activity of certain specialized cells and normally present in the skin, the hair, the choroid, the iris, the retina, the ciliary body, the cardiac tissue, the pia mater, and the substantia nigra of the brain. Melanin is found in melanoblasts, melanocytes, melanophages, and melanophores, is absent in true albinos, and its amount and distribution determine the color of the iris.

melanocataracta (mel″ah-no-kat-ah-rak′tah). Black cataract.

melanocytosis, ocular (mel″ah-no-si-to′sis). Melanosis bulbi.

melanocytosis, oculodermal (mel″-ah-no-si-to′sis). Oculocutaneous melanosis.

melano-hypostasis of Vogt (mel″-ah-no-hi-pos′tah-sis). Dust-like accumulation of pigment on the back surface of the cornea, iris, and chamber angle following iris atrophy, seen in angle closure glaucoma.

melanokeratosis, striate (mel″ah-no-ker″ah-to′sis). A condition occurring in Negroid eyes in which clear cornea is invaded by streaks of pigmented connective tissue growing from the limbus toward, and in response to, a corneal lesion.

melanoma (mel″ah-no′mah). A tumor arising from a pigmented nevus, as may occur in the conjunctiva, the choroid, the iris, the ciliary body, the optic nerve, etc.

melanosis (mel″ah-no′sis). A condition characterized by abnormal deposits of melanin.

 m. bulbi. Melanosis of the eyeball especially affecting the iris, the ciliary body, the choroid, and the sclera.

 m. corneae. A physiological or pathological deposition of melanin in the epithelial or endothelial layers of the cornea.

 m. iridis. Melanosis of the iris.

 m. lenticularis progressiva. Xeroderma pigmentosum.

 m. oculi. Melanosis bulbi.

oculocutaneous m. A syndrome of ocular and cutaneous melanosis, usually congenital, in which the skin lesions commonly follow the branches of the fifth cranial nerve, especially the ophthalmic. Syn., *oculodermal melanocytosis; nevus of Ota.*

m. of the optic nerve. A condition characterized by deposits of melanin in the optic nerve in the form of flecks, pigmented pits, uniform pigmentation, or melanomata.

m. of the retina. Pigmented paravenous retinochoroidal atrophy.

Riehl's m. A distinctive, brownish-gray, pigmentary affection of the skin of the face, forehead, and eyelids, marked by itchiness, reddening, and desquamation.

m. sclerae. A congenital condition characterized by flecks of melanin deposited in the sclera.

meliceris (mel″ih-se′ris). A chalazion.

Melkersson-Rosenthal syndrome. See under *syndrome.*

member, inner (of a rod or cone). The portion of a visual cell proper between the external limiting layer and the outer member of a visual cell in the retina. The thickness of an inner cone member is usually three to four times that of an inner rod member in the same region. Syn., *inner segment.*

member, outer (of a rod or cone). The portion of a visual cell proper between the inner member and the pigment epithelium layer of the retina. Rhodopsin is present in the outer member of a rod cell. Syn., *outer segment.*

membrana (mem-brah′nah). Latin for *membrane.*

m. capsularis. The hyaloid vascular network about the posterior pole of the embryonic crystalline lens or about a persistent hyaloid artery.

m. capsuli pupillaris. Capsulopupillary membrane.

m. coronae ciliaris. The suspensory ligament of the crystalline lens.

m. epipapillaris. Prepapillary membrane.

m. fusca. Lamina fusca.

m. granulosa externa. Outer nuclear layer of the retina.

m. granulosa interna. Inner nuclear layer of the retina.

m. hyaloidea plicata. Membrana plicata of Vogt.

m. limitans. Limiting membrane.

m. limitans perivascularis gliae. Perivascular limiting membrane.

m. nictitans. Nictitating membrane.

m. plicata of Vogt. A zone of vitreous condensation, appearing as a fine multifolded membrane, posterior to the capsule of the crystalline lens, which represents the anterior limit of the secondary vitreous, and bounds the anterior opening of the hyaloid canal. Syn., *tractus hyaloideus.*

m. ruyschiana. Ruyschian membrane.

m. vasculosa retinae. A dense network of blood vessels located in the vitreous, superficial to the retina, found in certain lower vertebrates.

◆

MEMBRANE

membrane. A thin layer of tissue which covers a surface, surrounds a part, lines a cavity, separates adjacent cavities, or connects adjacent structures.

amphiblestroid m. The retina. *Obs.*

anterior basal m. Bowman's membrane.

anterior elastic m. Bowman's membrane.

arachnoid m. The spiderweb-like tissue between the dura mater and the pia mater of the central nervous system and of the optic nerve. A subarachnoid space with cerebrospinal fluid is found between the arachnoid and the pia mater.

Barkan's m. A very thin membranous structure extending from Descemet's membrane to the iris and covering the filtration angle of the anterior chamber, said to be present in typical congenital glaucoma.

basal corneal m. Basement membrane of the corneal epithelium.

basement m. of choroid. Lamina vitrea.

basement m. of the corneal epithelium. The very thin noncellular layer of the corneal epithelium adjacent to Bowman's membrane, which is secreted by the basal cells and consists of two major layers, an anterior lipid and a posterior reticular layer. Syn., *basal corneal membrane.*

Bowman's m. The thin, non-cellular, second layer of the cornea, located between the anterior stratified epithelium and the substantia propria. Syn., *lamina elastica anterior; Bowman's lamina; Bowman's layer; anterior basal membrane; anterior elastic membrane.*

Bruch's m. 1. The lamina vitrea of the choroid. 2. The lamina vitrea of the ciliary body. 3. The posterior border lamella of Fuchs.

capsulopupillary m. The lateral portion of the tunica vasculosa lentis of the embryonic crystalline lens, formed by the anastomoses of the intraocular and extraocular blood vessels.

choroid m. Choroid.

cyclitic m. A layer of fibrous tissue formed in the anterior vitreous during certain acute purulent inflammations of the ciliary body. It is developed from macrophages from the region of the pars plana which emigrate through the ciliary epithelium and transform into fibroblasts.

Demour's m. Descemet's membrane. *Obs.*

Descemet's m. The strong, resistant, thin, noncellular fourth layer of the cornea, located between the endothelium (from which it is secreted) and the stroma. Syn., *lamina elastica posterior; posterior basal membrane.*

Döllinger's m. Ruyschian membrane.

Duddell's m. Descemet's membrane. *Obs.*

epipapillary m. Prepapillary membrane.

glass m. of the iris. A transparent membrane on the surface of the iris, similar to Descemet's membrane, formed by proliferation of the corneal endothelium and found in degenerated eyes having extensive pathological changes.

Henle's m. 1. Posterior border lamella of Fuchs. 2. Lamina vitrea of the choroid. *Obs.*

hyaloid m. The condensed gel at the surface of the vitreous, at the interface between the primary and secondary vitreous, and at the boundaries of the hyaloid canal. Posteriorly it is inseparable from the internal limiting layer of the retina. Syn., *vitreous membrane.*

intermuscular m's. Intermuscular ligaments.

Jacob's m. Layer of rods and cones.

limiting m., accessory. A delicate sheath surrounding retinal capillaries, external to the retinal perivascular glia and internal to the perivascular limiting membrane.

limiting m. of Elschnig. A thin, glial sheath, interspersed with large oval nuclei, that lines the physiological cup of the optic disk. If the central depression of the physiological cup is deep it may partly fill with a thicker layer of glial tissue known as the *meniscus of Kuhnt.*

limiting m., external (of the retina). External limiting layer of the retina.

limiting m., internal (of the ciliary body). A thin, homogeneous, structureless layer adjacent to the epithelium of the ciliary body. It is said to disappear both anteriorly and posteriorly.

limiting m., internal (of the iris). An extremely thin, homogeneous structure said to occur rarely on the posterior surface of the pigment epithelium of the iris.

limiting m., internal (of the retina). Internal limiting layer of the retina.

limiting m., intravitreal. The portion of the hyaloid membrane that separates the primary and secondary vitreous and forms the boundary of the hyaloid canal.

limiting m., perivascular. The external dense glial insulating sheath surrounding retinal capillaries. Syn., *membrana limitans perivascularis gliae.*

limiting m. of the vitreous. Hyaloid membrane. **anterior l. m. of the v.** Perilenticular capsule.

nictitating m. The third eyelid of lower vertebrates, supposedly represented in man by the vestigial plica semilunaris at the inner canthus.

periorbital m. The periosteum lining the bony orbit; the periorbita.

posterior basal m. Descemet's membrane.

posterior m. of the iris. The thin layer of the iris containing the dilator pupillae muscle fibers. Syn., *posterior border lamella of Fuchs.*

prepapillary m. A developmental anomaly consisting of remnants of embryonic tissue extending over or outward from the optic disk. Syn., *epipapillary membrane; prepapillary veil.*

preretinal m. Preretinal macular fibrosis.

pupillary m. The central thin portion of the lamina iridopupillaris of the fetus. Normally it degenerates during the seventh and eighth fetal month to form the pupil; at times strands of the membrane persist in the adult. Syn., *Wachendorf's membrane.* **persistent p.m.** Remnants of the fetal pupillary membrane which span the pupil or are adherent to the anterior lens capsule.

purpurogenous m. The pigment epithelium layer of the retina, so named because it was believed to form the visual purple.

Reichert's m. Bowman's membrane. *Obs.*

ruyschian m. The choriocapillary layer and lamina vitrea of the choroid combined with the layer of rods and cones and the pigment epithelium of the retina. Syn., *Döllinger's membrane.*

secondary m. Aftercataract.

superficial glial m. A delicate neuroglial sheath peripheral to the glial mantle of the optic nerve and over the surface of the central nervous system.

tarsal m. The tarsus or tarsal plate in the upper and lower eyelids.

Tenon's m. Tenon's capsule.

Verhoeff's m. The noncellular dense portion of the intercellular substance between cells of the pigment epithelium of the retina. In horizontal section it forms a net with hexagonal openings.

vitreous m. 1. Lamina vitrea of the choroid. 2. Descemet's membrane. 3. Hyaloid membrane.

Wachendorf's m. Pupillary membrane.

Zinn's m. The anterior surface of the iris. *Obs.*

◆

memory, plastic. The tendency of certain thermoplastic materials to resume their original shape after forced deformation under heat, either gradually if kept warm, or more rapidly when reheated.

memory, visual. The ability to recall previous visual experiences.

men. Abbreviation for *meniscus.*

Mende syndrome (men'de). Waardenburg syndrome. See under *syndrome.*

Mendel-Bechterew sign (men'del-bek-ter'yef). See under *sign.*

Ménière's (măn-e-ārz') **disease; syndrome.** See under the nouns.

meninges (me-nin'jēz). The three mesodermal coverings of the central nervous system and of the optic nerve: the dura mater, the arachnoid, and the pia mater.

meningioma (me-nin"je-o"mah). An essentially ectodermal nonmetastasizing neoplasm of the central nervous system thought to arise from the meningocytes of the arachnoid villi.

meningocele, orbital (me-nin'go-sēl). A congenital herniation of the meninges of the brain through the walls of the orbit, usually in the superior nasal region.

meniscus (me-nis'kus). A crescent shaped structure.

m. of Kuhnt. The thick deposit of neuroglia at the physiological cup of the optic disk, which is continuous at its periphery with the internal limiting membrane of the retina. Syn., *central connective tissue meniscus of Kuhnt.*

menotaxis. A phototactic movement of relatively high complexity of response in which the animal retains an impression of the distribution of the light stimulus over its retina and can orientate itself with respect to any selected part of its visual field. See also *klinotaxis; mnemotaxis; telotaxis; tropotaxis.*

mer. Abbreviation for *meridian.*

meramaurosis (mer"am-aw-ro'sis). Partial blindness.

meridian. The angular orientation of a great circle of the eye containing the line of sight or some other axis of reference and represented on an angular scale or protractor centered on and perpendicular to the axis of reference. In ophthalmic lens designations, the angular scale is considered parallel to the face plane with the 0°-180° meridian parallel to the base line or some other line of reference regarded as horizontal. See *axis scale.*

axis m. 1. The meridian of zero refractive power on a planocylindrical lens. 2. In a spherocylindrical lens, the meridian of zero power of the cylindrical component, whence it may be either principal meridian of the lens, depending on whether the designation is by minus or plus cylinder formula.

m. of the eye (horizontal). The meridian of the eye which coincides with the plane of regard when the foveal line of sight is straight forward and the head is held with the base line horizontal and the face plane vertical.

m. of the eye (vertical). The meridian of the eye which lies in a plane containing the foveal line of sight and which is perpendicular to the horizontal meridian of the eye.

iseikonic m's. The principal meridians of a meridional aniseikonic error or its correcting iseikonic lenses.

power m. 1. The meridian of greatest refractive power on a planocylindrical lens. 2. In a spherocylindrical lens, the meridian of greatest power of the cylindrical component, whence it may be either principal meridian of the lens, depending on whether the designation is by minus or plus cylinder formula.

principal m's. The meridians, normally located perpendicular to each other, of least and greatest curvature or refractive power of a toric surface or an optical system.

principal retinal m. The meridian of the retina which lies in a plane containing the y and z axes and the vertical meridian of the eye.

Merkel's (mer'kelz) **muscle; greater ring.** See under the nouns.

meropia (mer-o'pe-ah). Partial blindness or reduced vision.

Merseburg triad (mār-zeh-boorg). See under *triad*.

mesencephalon (mes"en-sef'ah-lon). The midbrain, consisting of a tectum dorsally, a cerebral aqueduct and paired cerebral peduncles ventrally. The tectum contains the superior colliculi, which are primary visual centers reflexly affecting skeletal muscle movements, and the cerebral peduncles contain oculomotor and trochlear motor nuclei.

meshwork. Any system of fibers, lines, or channels which cross or interlace like the fabric of a net.

m. of the angle of the anterior chamber. The meshwork of connective tissue located between the canal of Schlemm and the anterior chamber, containing spaces between intercrossing trabeculae which are involved in the drainage of aqueous humor. It is triangular on meridional section, the apex is attached to Descemet's membrane, and the base is continuous with the scleral spur, the anterior surface of the ciliary body, and the root of the iris. It is divided into three portions: uveal meshwork, corneoscleral meshwork, and endothelial meshwork.

corneoscleral m. The larger, anterior portion of the meshwork of the angle of the anterior chamber, consisting of a mass of trabecular tissue, each trabecula being a delicate flat band made of collagenous fibers, elastic fibers, hyaloid material, and endothelium. The corneoscleral meshwork lies between the canal of Schlemm and the uveal meshwork and extends from Descemet's membrane to the scleral spur. Syn., *corneal meshwork; scleral meshwork; corneoscleral trabeculum.*

endothelial m. of Speakman. A condensation of the trabecular meshwork of the angle of the anterior chamber which surrounds the canal of Schlemm. Syn., *pore tissue of Flocks.*

scleral m. Corneoscleral meshwork.

uveal m. The smaller, inner portion of the meshwork of the angle of the anterior chamber, consisting of a fine layer of loose connective tissue fibrils. It bounds the anterior chamber between Descemet's membrane and the root of the iris. Syn., *pectinate ligament; uveal trabeculum.*

mesiris (mes-i'ris). Substantia propria of the iris.

mesocornea (mes"o-kōr'ne-ah). Substantia propria of the cornea.

mesophryon (mes-of're-on). The glabella or its central point.

mesopia (mes'o-pe-ah). Mesopic vision.

mesopic (mes'op-ik). 1. Having the characteristics of mesopic vision or pertaining to levels of illumination between the photopic and scotopic ranges. 2. Having an orbitonasal index from 110 to 112.9 (or sometimes of 107.5 to 110). Cf. *platyopic; pro-opic.*

mesoramic (mes-ōr-am'ik). Weston's classification of a visual task at an intermediate distance of from 30 cm to 2 m. Cf. *ancoramic; teloramic.*

mesoropter (mes"o-rop'ter). 1. The normal position of the eyes when at rest. 2. The position of the line of sight of the eye when centered in its field of vision, as may be determined, e.g., by the orbital boundaries, spectacle rims, or an anterior field stop.

mesoseme (mes'o-sēm). Having an orbital index of 84 to 89; characteristic of the white race. See also *megaseme; microseme.*

mesothelium, corneal (mes″o-the′le-um). A single layer of flat hexagonal-shaped mesothelial cells lining the posterior surface of the cornea, more commonly termed *corneal endothelium*.

metacontrast (met″ah-kon′trast). The reduction in subjective brightness of a flash of light when it is followed closely by a second flash in a separate or an immediately adjacent portion of the visual field. Cf. *paracontrast*.

meta-iodopsin (met″ah-i-o-dop′sin). A form of cone pigment converted from iodopsin by irradiation with orange light and reconverted to iodopsin upon irradiation with blue light.

metamerism (me-tam′er-izm). The property of color perception which permits stimuli of different spectral composition to appear colorimetrically identical.

metamers (met′ah-merz). Metameric colors.

metamorphopsia (met″ah-mōr-fop′se-ah). An anomaly of visual perception in which objects appear distorted or larger or smaller than their actual size.

    retinal m. Metamorphopsia resulting from a displacement of the visual receptor cells of the retina. It may be due to detachment, tumor, exudative or inflammatory process, or cicatricial changes.

    m. varians. Metamorphopsia in which the shape and/or size of an object appear to change while fixated.

meta-rhodopsin (met″ah-ro-dop′sin). An intermediate product in the chemical breakdown of rhodopsin by the action of light, after the formation of lumi-rhodopsin and prior to the formation of retinene.

metastereoscopy (met″ah-ster-e-os′-ko-pe). The viewing of a stereopsis-inducing pattern in which objects in a given plane are reproduced in natural proportions, whereas objects in other planes are not. Cf., *orthostereoscopy*.

Méténier's sign. See under *sign*.

meter. 1. The basis for measuring length by the metric system. It is equivalent to 39.371 in. 2. An apparatus for registering and measuring quantity.

    absorption m. Absorptiometer.

    acuity m. An apparatus for measuring visual acuity. **Clason a.m.** An acuity-measuring instrument which projects test types of continuously variable size.

    m. angle. See under *angle*.

    Baylor visual acuity m. A portable semi-automated instrument with totally enclosed filmstrip, motor, light source, and optics into which the examinee peers through an aperture with eyecup, and, by button-pressing, reports the directions of the gaps of successively smaller or larger Landolt C's until his acuity threshold is reached.

    m. candle. See under *candle*.

    m. curve. See under *curve*.

    footcandle m. Light meter.

    illumination m. Light meter.

    m. lambert. See under *lambert*.

    light m. An instrument for measuring the illumination on a surface, by placing the meter in the plane of that surface, usually consisting of barrier layer cells connected to a scale calibrated in footcandles. Syn., *footcandle meter; illumination meter*.

    Luckiesh-Taylor brightness m. A small portable, self-contained visual photometer for measuring luminance or illumination.

    visibility m. An instrument for appraising the discernibleness of an object or a visual task in relation to that of a standard test object under a standard level of illumination.

metercandle. A unit of illumination equal to 1 lumen per m². Syn., *lux*.

methacholine (meth-ah-ko′lēn). A direct acting, parasympathomimetic agent used for the differential diagnosis of Adie's pupil, in which case a tonic pupil will contract upon topical application of a 2.5% solution.

◆

METHOD

method. A set form of procedure for examination, operation, treatment, or instruction. See also *test*.

    arc centune m. A method devised by Dennett for measuring the displacement or bending of light rays by a prism. The unit of measurement is the *centrad* (∇), representing the power of a prism which will deviate a ray of light 1 cm along an arc of 1 m radius at a distance of 1 m from the incidence of light on the prism. Syn., *Dennett's method*.

    average error m. A psychophysical method involving a series of repeated adjustments of a variable stimulus to subjective equality with a constant standard.

    Bachmaier's m. A refractive technique employing a Scheiner's disk with a red filter in front of one pinhole, a green filter in front of the other, and a test target consisting of a green line and a pair of mutually perpendicular red lines oriented 45° from, and intersecting each other at, the green line. The green line is seen to bisect the cross in emmetropia and is seen displaced from the center in ametropia, the distance on a scale indicating the degree. The lens power needed to center the line on the cross by rendering the eye emmetropic is also a measure of the ametropia.

Barlow's m. A method by which eye movements are followed by observing the position of a tiny droplet of mercury placed on the surface of the cornea or sclera. The mercury acts as a small convex mirror and reflects light directed on it.

boxing m. A system of measurement and specification of eye size of spectacle frames based on the vertical and horizontal dimensions of the smallest horizontally oriented rectangle that can enclose the lens oriented in the position in which it is to be mounted. It is the approved system for manufacturers and dispensers of eyewear. Syn., *boxing system.*

Bradley's m. An astronomical method for measuring the velocity of light based on the telescopic observation that a star located in a direction perpendicular to the earth's orbit appears displaced in the direction of the earth's velocity.

Brinker-Katz m. A method for the treatment of eccentric fixation and amblyopia ex anopsia in which a deep red filter, such as a Kodak Wratten #92, is worn before the amblyopic eye, the other eye being totally occluded.

Brock's luster m. A method for eliciting a sense of fusion in which a small spot on a neutral background is monocularly fixated while a flashing light is held against the lid of the other, closed, eye. An attempt is made to perceive the glow from the light as if it were emanating from the background surrounding the fixation spot.

cascade comparison m. A method for determining the luminosity curve by direct and systematic, step-by-step, matching of the brightness of adjacent spectral segments of nondiscriminable hue difference.

Charpentier's m. A method for determining the objective angle of strabismus with the perimeter. The subject is placed so that the deviating eye is aligned with a light source in the center of the arc while the nondeviating eye fixates a distant point straight ahead. The examiner moves his eye along the arc of the perimeter until the reflection of the light appears to lie in the center of the pupil of the deviating eye. One half of the angle at this position, plus angle kappa in convergent and minus angle kappa in divergent strabismus, is the objective angle.

color mixing m., additive. The mixing or fusing of colors by any technique which produces a resultant color whose spectral composition represents a direct summation of the spectral components of the separate colors, as by direct superimposing of projected light sources of different color, by rapidly alternating exposures of different colors on a color wheel, or by the viewing of a closely interwoven pattern of different colors at a distance at which the separate colors are nondiscriminable.

color mixing m., physical. Color mixing so as to produce a single color stimulus having the physical or spectral attributes of an additively or subtractively produced combination.

color mixing m., physiological. The perceptual mixing of colors, by presenting them in rapidly alternating sequence or by presenting simultaneously one color to one eye and another to the other eye.

color mixing m., subtractive. The production of a resultant color whose spectral composition represents the remainder of the spectral components of an original source of illumination after selective absorption by one or more media of different color, as obtained in pigment mixing or by the superimposition of filters.

Comberg's m. A method of localizing an intraocular foreign body, consisting of making anteroposterior and lateral x-ray photographs of the eye with a contact lens in place to permit alignment of the anteroposterior views on the major axis of the eye by centering with respect to four symmetrically located lead markers in the lens, and fore and aft positioning of the lateral view by reference to the plane of the four markers.

concentric m. An insertion method for making an eye impression in the fitting of molded contact lenses in which the molding shell does not have a handle, being placed on the eye in the same manner as a scleral contact lens.

Con-lish m. A method for contouring and polishing the edge of a contact lens, devised by Gilberto Cepero, in which the lens is placed with the concave surface first down, then up, for a specified number of seconds, on each of five angled polishing tools (40°, 60°, 90°, 140°, 180°) rotating at either 100 rpm or 500 rpm.

constant m. A psychophysical method in which each of a series of randomly varied stimuli is presented to be judged as "less than" or "more than" a fixed comparison stimulus. A third category response, "equal to" or "doubtful", also may be included. In the determination of an absolute threshold the two categories of response may be simply "observed" and "not observed," without reference to a fixed comparison stimulus.

corneal reflection m. Any method which utilizes the reflection of light from the cornea to determine the position or movement of the eye, as in measuring the objective angle of strabismus, photographing eye movements in reading, etc.

Crédé's m. The instillation of a few drops of dilute silver nitrate solution into the eyes of the newborn as a prophylactic measure against ophthalmia neonatorum.

critical frequency m. Any technique employing the critical flicker frequency of intermittent light as a criterion.

Cross's m. A method of retinoscopy, devised by Cross, in which the neutralizing lenses, obtained with the fixation target in the plane of the retinoscope at 1 m or nearer, is considered to represent the refractive error.

cross cylinder m. The determination of the axis and the amount of astigmatism by the use of a low power crossed cylinder lens mounted on a handle 45° from its principal meridians to facilitate quick changes of resultant cylindrical power, or resultant cylinder axis, of the test lens combination in front of the eye for direct comparison of relative blurredness.

Cuignet's m. Retinoscopy.

Cüpper's afterimage m. A method of treating amblyopia in which all of the nonmacular area of the retina is stimulated with intense light with a Euthyscope to create an afterimage in the peripheral retina and to render the macular area relatively more sensitive. After the positive afterimage in the macula becomes white, the macula is stimulated with various targets.

datum m. A system of measurement and specification of spectacle frame dimensions based on the use of the datum line. Syn., *datum system*.

Dennett's m. Arc centune method.

direct m. See *ophthalmoscopy, direct*.

direct comparison m. 1. A method for measuring aniseikonia in which a target containing polarized horizontal and vertical lines is projected onto a screen and viewed through Polaroid filters. The relative positions of the lines, as seen individually by each eye, indicate the magnitude and kind of aniseikonia. 2. A method for determining a spectral luminous efficiency curve by the direct matching of the brightness of each segment of the spectrum with a neutral standard.

displacement m. The dissociation of the two eyes by means of a prism of sufficient power to break or prevent fusion for the purpose of measuring phorias.

distance motivation m. A type of training in which subthreshold Koenig bars or Snellen letters are repetitively moved from a 20 ft distance toward the trainee until they become discriminable, with the objective of improving the visual acuity score by successively greater distances of discrimination or by the use of successively smaller test targets.

distortion m. The dissociation of the two eyes by the gross distortion of the imagery for one eye, as with a Maddox rod, for the purpose of measuring phorias.

Donders' m. The determination of false torsion by projecting afterimages, in different directions of gaze, onto a screen.

Drysdale m. A method for determining the radius of curvature of a short focal length mirror in which a light source in a modified microscope is placed in sharp focus at the mirror surface and at the center of curvature of the surface, the distance between the two being recorded on the instrument dial as the radius of curvature. This method is employed in design of instruments for measuring the curvature of contact lenses. Syn., *Drysdale principle.*

duochrome m. The determination of the refractive correction of the eye by comparison of the sharpness of imagery formed by two different spectral wavelengths, as in comparing black letters on red and green backgrounds, or the image pattern of a small light source through a cobalt glass. Syn., *bichrome refraction; duochrome refraction; bichrome test; duochrome test.*

Erb m. The deposition, by evaporation, of a thin transparent layer of titanium dioxide on the surface of a plastic contact lens to increase its wettability.

Fabry-Pérot m. The determination of the index of refraction of a prism by placing its emergent face perpendicular to the incident light beam and calculating the index from the angle of deviation.

fan dial m. The determination of the axis and the amount of astigmatism with the aid of a fan dial chart.

fixation disparity m. for AC/A ratio. Ogle's fixation disparity method for AC/A ratio.

Fizeau's m. A method for determining the velocity of light, devised by Fizeau in 1849, based on the interval of interruption of light by a rotating toothed wheel before and after traversing a long optical path reflected on itself.

flicker photometer m. In the photometric determination of the luminosity curve, the alternate presentation of the reference and test colors at a speed which just eliminates chromatic flicker, and the adjustment of the intensity of the test color until luminous flicker is abolished.

fogging m. The placement of more plus lens or less minus lens in front of the eye than is necessary to correct the refractive error, for the purpose of minimizing accommodative effects during tests for astigmatism, or as a means of forcing the use of an amblyopic eye by reducing the acuity of the nonamblyopic eye.

form emergence m. A method of visual training in which targets are projected out of focus onto a screen and gradually brought into focus while the subject attempts to identify them.

Fry's m. A method for eliciting normal retinal correspondence in a case of anomalous retinal correspondence, in which a small spot of light on a black background is fixated by one eye while a flashing ring of light on a black background is viewed by the other eye. The targets are presented in a major amblyoscope at the objective angle of strabismus, and an attempt is made to see the spot as being in the center of the ring.

geometrical m. Ophthalmoscopy by means of an instrument whose observation system and illumination system are conducted through separate portions of the pupil to eliminate the interference of corneal reflections.

Gibson's m. A method for eliminating suppression by attempting to obtain superimposition of two dissimilar, but superimposable, haploscopically presented targets, such as a bird and a cage.

GOMAC m. A method for specifying the dimensions of plastic spectacle frames, devised by a committee representing the countries of the European Common Market. It consists of four specifications: the maximum horizontal length of the lens; the minimum distance between the lenses; the distance between the midpoint of the datum line of one lens and the midpoint of the datum line of the other lens to the nearest millimeter; the width of bridge opening measured along the datum line to the nearest millimeter. Syn., *GOMAC standard.*

gradient m. See *gradient.*

graphic m. Graphic analysis def. 2.

Halldén's m. A method for determining the objective angle, the subjective angle, and the angle of anomaly in strabismus, utilizing a semicircular filament for producing an afterimage, and a pair of projectors containing Polaroid filters such that each eye can see only one of the images projected onto the screen. The objective angle is measured by fixating a target on the screen with one eye and adjusting a projected target, seen only by the nonfixating eye, such that it appears to be centered in a semicircular afterimage previously provided to the nonfixating eye. The distance between the fixated target and the projected target indicates the objective angle. The subjective angle is measured by adjusting the two projected targets until they appear to be superimposed, the distance on the screen between the two projected targets indicating the subjective angle. The angle of anomaly is measured by fixating a target on the screen with one eye, and adjusting a projected target, seen only by the fixating eye, such that it appears to be centered in a semicircular afterimage previously provided to the other, the nonfixating, eye. The distance of the projected target from the fixated target indicates the angle of anomaly in the fixating eye.

Harms's m. A method of perimetry in which test objects of various sizes, located at fixed positions in the visual field, are gradually increased in luminance to the threshold of visibility.

heterodynamic m. A method of dynamic retinoscopy in which the fixation target is in a plane other than that of the retinoscope peephole.

Hetzel m. A technique for viewing the entoptic shadows of opacities within one's own eye.

Hirschberg's m. A method for approximating the objective angle of strabismus by noting the position of the reflex of a fixated light on the cornea of the deviating eye.

Holt's m. An empirical method for computing compensation for loss of vision, based on the assumption that the total loss of vision of one eye is an 18% loss of the total function of the body.

Holth's m. Kinescopy.

Humphriss m. 1. A binocular subjective refraction technique in which foveal vision of the eye not being tested is suppressed by the addition of a +0.75 D lens to the approximated correcting lens, allowing for peripheral fusion to maintain binocular alignment of the two eyes during refractive refinement of the correction of the other eye. Humphriss refers to the induced anisometropia causing foveal suppression as a *psychological septum*. Syn., *Humphriss immediate contrast test*, abbreviated *HIC*. 2. A method for treating amblyopia ex anopsia in which a red lens is placed in front of the nonamblyopic eye for periodic general wear.

hydrodiascopic m. A seldom used method of ophthalmoscopy in which the cornea is immersed in water to eliminate unwanted reflections from the cornea.

indirect m. See *ophthalmoscopy, indirect*.

injection m. A technique for making an eye impression for the fitting of molded contact lenses, in which the impression material is injected into the molding shell through a hollow handle after the shell has been placed upon the eye. Cf. *insertion method*.

insertion m. A technique for making an eye impression for the fitting of molded contact lenses in which the perforated molding shell is filled with impression material before being placed on the eye. Cf. *injection method*.

Irvine's m. Irvine's prism displacement test.

isodynamic m. A method of dynamic retinoscopy in which the fixation target is in the same plane as the retinoscope peep-hole.

Javal's m. A method for determining the objective angle of strabismus with the perimeter. The subject is so placed that the deviating eye is at the center of the arc while the nondeviating eye fixates a distant point straight ahead. The examiner moves a light source, with his eye directly above it, until the corneal reflex appears to lie in the center of the pupil of the deviating eye. The angle at this position, plus angle kappa in convergent and minus angle kappa in divergent strabismus, is the objective angle.

Kerr cell m. A method for determining the velocity of light, similar to Fizeau's method, except that the light is interrupted by a shutter instead of by a toothed wheel. The shutter is operated by an electrical and an optical system and can interrupt the beam at a rate of many millions of times per second.

Krimsky's m. A method for determining the objective angle of strabismus in which the examiner, with his eye directly above a light source fixated by the subject, observes the position of the corneal reflexes. Prisms are placed before the deviating eye until the reflex appears to occupy the same relative position as that in the fixating eye. A variation is to place prisms before the fixating eye, causing the eyes to turn, until the reflex is centered in the pupil of the deviating eye. Syn., *prism reflex test*.

Kubelka-Munk m. A method of analysis for the formulation of a colorant layer, such as in paper, textiles, and paint, which both reflects and transmits light, utilizing a general expression for the reflectance, R, of any colorant layer of known absorption and scattering coefficients, K and S, on a background of reflectance Rg, as a function of the thickness, X, of the layer.

Kupfer's m. A method for the treatment of eccentric fixation in which the patient is instructed in which direction to move his eye with respect to the light source of the ophthalmoscope until he learns the fixational position for which the light is observed to be centered on the fovea. He then observes, through a pinhole, the same light at several feet, and subsequently large letters, with the newly learned sense of fixation.

Langrange m. A method for determining the horizontal limits of the field of binocular fixation, employing the fusion band of Langrange. See under *band*.

Lesser's m. A method for determining a recommended near point prescription by deducting from the gross dynamic retinoscopic finding a dioptric value computed from the near phoria and the amplitude of accommodation.

m. of limits. One of the psychophysical methods in which the test stimulus is adjusted to "just greater than" and "just less than" the comparison standard; the average of the two is taken as a measure of subjective equality while the difference between the two is a function of the threshold or sensitivity. Variations may include similar techniques for determining maxima or minima in which the variable is adjusted to obtain just noticeable decrements or increments on either side, as when a blind man locates the top of a hill.

Lloyd's m. A method of demonstrating the interference and the phase change of light on reflection at grazing incidence. Syn., *Lloyd's experiment*.

longitudinal horopter m. A method of determining aniseikonia in the horizontal meridian in which the magnitude of the rotation of the apparent frontal plane horopter about a vertical axis is measured.

Lyle and Jackson m. A method for eliciting normal retinal correspondence in a case of anomalous retinal correspondence by the rapid alternate fixation of two dissimilar targets

haploscopically presented at an angle other than the subjective angle of strabismus and then gradually moved through the subjective angle to the objective angle.

Magnus m. A method for computing indemnification for loss of earning ability as a result of visual disability by the use of a formula which considers central visual acuity, the extent of the visual field, muscle function, and the ability to compete.

meridional balance m. Any technique for determining the axis and power of astigmatism by successive comparison of the relative sharpness of a test character before and after each time a crossed cylinder lens is flipped 90° and the thereby indicated cylindrical correcting lenses are rotated or combined with compensating spheres to maintain a constant spherical equivalent until equality of sharpness is attained.

middle third m. The application of the clinical rule of thumb that visual discomfort is not induced as long as the convergence demand is in the middle third of the range of fusional convergence.

minus lens m., binocular. The determination of the amplitude of positive relative accommodation by the placing of consecutively stronger minus lenses binocularly before the eyes until the test type can no longer be seen clearly or until diplopia occurs; usually tested at a 16 or 13 in. distance.

minus lens m., monocular. The determination of the amplitude of accommodation by placing consecutively stronger minus lenses before an eye until the test type can no longer be seen clearly; usually tested at a 16 in. distance.

monocular diplopia m. A method for eliciting normal retinal correspondence, in a case of anomalous retinal correspondence, in which targets are presented in a major amblyoscope at the objective angle of strabismus and an attempt is made to obtain monocular diplopia which would indicate the simultaneous use of normal and anomalous correspondence.

multiple pattern m. Harrington-Flocks test.

nonius m. Any method of utilizing vernier acuity as a criterion, as in measuring fixation disparity, plotting the nonius horopter, etc. (Nonius is the

Latinized form of the name of Pedro Nunes, a Portuguese mathematician of the seventeenth century, a rediscoverer of the method of measuring first published by Vernier in 1631.)

Nott's m. A method of dynamic retinoscopy in which the fixation target is placed at a distance requiring 0.50 D more accommodation than the distance of the retinoscope, e.g., the retinoscope at 40 cm and the fixation target at 33.3 cm. This relationship is thought to compensate for the normal lag of accommodation.

Ogle's fixation disparity m. for AC/A ratio. The amount of lateral prism that induces a given level of fixation disparity and the amount of spherical lens power that does the same are plotted as a point on a coordinate scale representing binocular prism and sphere power. The line formed by several such points represents the AC/A ratio.

Parks-Hardesty three-step m. A testing procedure for determining an isolated cyclovertical muscle paresis or paralysis consisting of three steps: (1) measurement of a hyper deviation in the primary gaze; (2) measuring an increase in the hyper deviation on lateral gaze; (3) noting a further increase of the hyper on the Bielschowsky head tilt test. Cf. *Schwarting three-point test.*

Pascal's m. A method of dynamic retinoscopy in which a gross target is casually fixated in the plane of the retinoscope at a distance of 33 cm. The strongest convex lens power not giving an against motion (high neutral) is determined, and from this gross finding + 0.50 D is deducted to arrive at a near point correction.

Peckham's m. Peckham's test.

Pfund's m. A method for producing or analyzing polarized infrared rays in which light is reflected, at Brewster's angle, from the surfaces of selenium-coated glass mirrors.

polarization m. for ophthalmoscopy. Ophthalmoscopy in which Polaroid filters are used to eliminate unwanted reflections from the cornea.

Prentice's m. Tangent centune method.

Priestly Smith's m. A method for determining the objective angle of strabismus in which a fixation target is moved along a centimeter scale or tape, perpendicular to the midline and 1 m from the subject, until the corneal reflex of a light source, at zero on the tape, is centered in the pupil of the deviating eye. The observer's eye remains directly above the light source.

psychophysical m's. The methods utilized in determining thresholds of relationship between stimulus and response. The methods include, among others, the *average error method*, the *method of limits*, and the *constant method*.

push-away m. 1. An orthoptic technique for improving vergence ability, as when treating either divergence insufficiency or divergence excess, consisting of moving a fixation object away from the eyes, in the median plane, as the attempt is made to maintain bifixation. 2. The determination of the far point of convergence by moving a fixation point away from the eyes, in the median plane, to the farthest point of binocular fixation. See also *recession phenomenon*.

push-up m. 1. The determination of the near point of accommodation by moving a test object toward the eye or eyes until it blurs. 2. The determination of the near point of convergence by moving a fixation point toward the eyes, in the median plane, to the nearest point of binocular fixation. 3. Repetition of either of the above as an orthoptic exercise.

Römer's m. The first successful method for determining the velocity of light, devised by Römer in 1676 and based on the time interval between eclipses of the satellites of the planet Jupiter.

rotating mirror m. A method for determining the velocity of light suggested by Arago and applied by Fizeau and Foucault independently in 1850. It consists essentially of measuring the deviation in the path of light reflected by a rotating plane mirror before and after traversing a long path to a fixed mirror and back.

Rushton's m. The locating of the posterior pole of the eye in situ by the visibility of a narrow transverse beam of x-rays when the eye is dark adapted, for the purpose of determining the axial length of the eyeball.

Ryer-Hotaling m. A method for determining the correcting cylindrical lens by finding a lens, placed at the wearing distance before the eye, through which the ophthalmometer indicates 0.50 D with-the-rule astigmatism. This lens rotated 90° represents the astigmatic correction.

Schapero's anomalous correspondence m. A visual training procedure for breaking down anomalous correspondence, in which superimposition or fusion targets in a major amblyoscope are simultaneously presented to the two eyes at the subjective angle. The patient is required to alternate fixation for the monocularly perceived target elements and is made aware of the necessary eye movements, even though both targets appear to lie in the same direction. Training is continued until superimposition is lost, and then carried on at the new subjective angle. The procedure is repeated until the subjective angle is the same as the objective angle.

Schapero's pupil measurement m. Determination of the diameter of the pupil in dim illumination by directing a black light source onto the eye while a distant target is fixated. The crystalline lens will fluoresce under these conditions and clearly define the pupillary limits, enabling easy measurement.

Scheiner's m. See *Scheiner's experiment.*

schlieren m. Photographic and/or observational use of a schlieren system.

screen parallax m. The determination and measurement of a phoria by the apparent movement of a fixated object when the eyes are alternately occluded and by the prism power necessary to eliminate the movement.

sensitometric m. of refraction. The determination of the ophthalmic lens correction producing the best scores on the Luckiesh-Moss Ophthalmic Sensitometer.

Sheard's m. A method of dynamic retinoscopy in which a target is fixated in the plane of the retinoscope at a 40 cm distance. The weakest convex lens power not giving a with motion (low neutral) is determined; from this gross finding a deduction, based on the patient's age, is made to arrive at a near point correction.

Sugar's m. One of the psychological septum systems of performing binocular subjective refraction in which the eye not under test views the chart through a crossed cylinder lens which assumedly blurs the test type. Cf. *Humphriss method.*

Sweet's m. A method of localizing an intraocular foreign body in which two objects of known position are used to create radiographic images to assist in plotting the location of the foreign body.

Swenson's m. A method for treating eccentric fixation and anomalous retinal correspondence associated with esotropia, in which the temporal portion of the spectacle lens before the deviating eye is occluded. The occluder is positioned with its edge bisecting the pupil as the dominant eye fixates a light source in the midplane at a 30 cm distance.

Tait's m. A method of dynamic retinoscopy in which a target is fixated in the plane of the retinoscope at a 33 cm distance through +3.00 D fogging lenses. The lens power is reduced until a neutral point is reached. An allowance, dependent on the amount of accommodative convergence at this testing distance, is deducted from the gross finding to arrive at the distance correction.

Tajiri contacts-impression m. A method for examining the edge profile characteristics of a corneal contact lens in which a mold, made of a portion of the edge, is sectioned and studied under high magnification.

Tajiri custom-adjust m. A method for custom fitting plastic spectacle frames in which a soft plastic substance is fixed to the bridge and/or bends of the temples and allowed to harden while the frame is held firmly in the wearing position.

tangent centune m. A method devised by Prentice for measuring the displacement or bending of light rays by a prism. The unit of measurement is the *prism diopter* (Δ), which represents the power of a prism that will deviate a ray of light 1 cm along a straight line perpendicular to the original path of the light at a distance of 1 m. Syn., *Prentice's method.*

telescopic ophthalmoscopy m. See under *ophthalmoscopy.*

timed resolution m. The distance motivation method employing an intermittently illuminated target.

Treleaven's m. A method of dynamic retinoscopy with the fixation target and retinoscope at 33 cm and neutralization to high neutral, the results of which are used to recommend the power of the reading addition for 13 or 16 in. in accordance with a table formulated by Treleaven.

Updegrave's m. A method of visual training for increasing lens or prism acceptance in which intermittently illuminated reading material is fixated through the specific lens and/or prism power and an attempt is made to keep the print clear as the fixation distance is increased.

Van Orden star m. A vision therapy technique for testing and training consisting of simultaneous drawing of two pencil lines at a time, one pencil in each hand, on a haploscopically viewed card from diagonally opposite, temporally peripheral points with the pencils moving centrally toward each other. The resulting star-like pattern is clinically interpreted in terms of various characteristics such as symmetry, separation, and regularity of the radial lines.

Welsh zero error m. A trial lens method for determining the spectacle prescription for an aphakic in which the refraction is performed while the patient wears a pair of +12.00 D sphere lenses that are centered to his interpupillary distance and in a frame similar to his permanent frame set at the final tilt and vertex distance. Syn., *zero error refraction.*

Westheimer m. The assessment of the influence of various sizes and brightnesses of background on visual sensitivity by their effects on the increment threshold of a brief test flash.

◆

methylcellulose (meth"il-sel'u-lōs). A highly viscous lacrimal substitute used in artificial tears for protection of the cornea during gonioscopy, to moisten hard contact lenses, and to lubricate artificial eyes.

methyl methacrylate (meth"il meth-ak'ril-āt). The chemical name of a liquid ester which, when polymerized, forms a light, strong, transparent, thermoplastic resin, widely used in contact lens manufacture, and known commercially as Plexiglas or Lucite.

methyl methacrylate vinylpyrrolidone. A copolymer of methyl methacrylate with vinylpyrrolidone, used for hard contact lenses. Abbreviation MMA-VP.

metrec (me'trek). A unit of curvature rep-

resenting the reciprocal of the radius in meters.

metronoscope (met-ron'o-skōp). An instrument used in visual training, consisting essentially of three rectangular shutters placed horizontally end to end, which expose phrases of reading material at a controlled rate, on a scroll moving beneath them at a controlled speed. The instrument also contains rotary prisms and cells for trial lenses.

Meyer's (mi'erz) **experiment; loop; phenomenon; sign.** See under the nouns.

Meyer-Schwickerath-Weyers syndrome. Oculodentodigital dysplasia. See under *dysplasia.*

Meynert's (mi'nerts) **pyramidal cells; commissure; fibers; radiations.** See under the nouns.

Meyrowitz' test (mi'ro-vitz). See under *test.*

Michel's (mi'kelz) **flecks; spots.** See under the nouns.

Michelson's interferometer (mi'kel-sunz). See under *interferometer.*

micreikonic (mi"kri-kon'ic). Pertaining to the eye with the smaller image, in aniseikonia.

microblepharia (mi"kro-bleh-fa're-ah). Eyelids of abnormally short vertical dimension, a rare developmental anomaly.

microblepharism (mi"kro-blef'ah-rizm). Microblepharia.

microblepharon (mi"kro-blef'ah-ron). Microblepharia.

microblephary (mi"kro-blef'ah-re). Microblepharia.

microcoria (mi"kro-ko're-ah). Abnormally small pupils, usually congenital, and occurring with the absence of the dilator pupillae muscle.

microcornea (mi"kro-kōr'ne-ah). An abnormally small cornea. Syn., *anterior microphthalmus.*

microdensitometer (mi"kro-den"sih-tom'eh-ter). An instrument for measuring the transmission of light through an extremely small area of a photographic film, as needed, for example, for the determination of photographically recorded spectral line intensities. Syn., *microphotometer.*

microglia (mi-krog'le-ah). The phagocytic neuroglia of the central nervous system, the retina, and the optic nerve.

microgonioscope (mi"kro-go'ne-o-skōp). A magnifying gonioscope.

microinterferometer (mi"kro-in"ter-fēr-om'eh-ter). An instrument for the examination of very small optical components, such as the surface structure and cylindricity of glass fibers.

microlens (mi'kro-lenz). A plastic corneal contact lens characterized by its thinness and by its small diameter.

micromanometer (mi"kro-mah-nom'-eh-ter). A manometer with a closed system and with dimensions so small as to minimize errors. Usually it consists of a capillary tube closed at the top, filled with air both above and below a saline solution, and connected directly with a needle cannula.

micromegalopsia (mi"kro-meg"ah-lop'se-ah). The perception of objects as being smaller or larger than their true size, or alternately too small and too large.

micrometer (mi-krom'eh-ter). An instrument or attachment for measuring small distances or angles.

   Jaeger's ocular m. A device designed for attachment to the Zeiss slit lamp biomicroscope for measurement of corneal thickness or anterior chamber depth. It produces two identical overlapping images, one of which is moved until the anterior limit of the distance being measured is aligned with the posterior limit on the other image, the micrometer giving a direct reading of the distance.

   Lobeck's ocular m. A device designed for attachment to the Zeiss slit lamp biomicroscope for measurement of corneal thickness or anterior chamber depth. It splits the image into upper and lower halves, and the lower half is moved until the anterior limit of the distance being measured is aligned with the posterior limit on the upper half, the micrometer giving a direct reading of the distance.

   tonometer m. A device for checking the accuracy of a Schiötz tonometer over the full scale range by controlling the plunger so that the scale reading associated with any degree of projection can be determined.

   vertex m. A device for measuring the distance between the eye and the posterior surface of the lens.

micron (mi'kron). A unit of length equal to one thousandth of a millimeter. Symbol: μ.

micronystagmus (mi"kro-nis-tag'-mus). Minute oscillatory movements of the eye normally present on fixation.

micropapilla (mi'kro-pah-pil'ah). A congenital condition in which the optic disk is abnormally small, as may occur in such developmental disorders as cyclopia, anophthalmia, or microphthalmia.

microphakia (mi"kro-fa'ke-ah). A condition in which the crystalline lens is abnormally small. Syn., *microlentia*. Cf. *spherophakia*.

microphotometer (mi"kro-fo-tom'eh-ter). Microdensitometer.

microphthalmia (mi"krof-thal'me-ah). Microphthalmus.

microphthalmos (mi"krof-thal'mos). Microphthalmus.

microphthalmoscope (mi"krof-thal'-mo-skōp). An ophthalmoscope with high magnification.

microphthalmus (mi"krof-thal'mus). A rare developmental anomaly in which the eyeballs are abnormally small. When no other defects are associated, the condition is known as *nanophthalmos.*

   anterior m. Microcornea.

micropia (mi-kro'pe-ah). Micropsia.

micropsia (mi-krop'se-ah). An anomaly of visual perception in which objects appear to be smaller than they actually are.

   accommodative m. Micropsia resulting from an anomalous accommodative response, particularly from increased effort to accommodate, as in overcoming the effect of a partial cycloplegic.

   paresis m. Micropsia resulting from the increased effort to converge, induced by paresis of the internal rectus muscles.

   retinal m. Micropsia resulting from a disturbance of the retina in which the visual receptor cells are spread apart. It may be due to a detachment, a tumor, exudative or inflammatory process, or cicatricial changes.

microptic (mi-krop'tik). Affected by or pertaining to micropsia.

microrefractometry (mi"kro-re"frak-tom'eh-tre). Determination of the index of refraction of a tiny object by immersing it in a graded series of media of known refractive indices until it is invisible in a phase contrast microscope.

microsaccades (mi"kro-sah-kādz'). Minute rotatory movements or tremors of the eye through an angle of 5 to 15 sec. of arc with a frequency of usually 30 to 70 cycles per second, recorded only when highly magnified by electric methods.

◆

MICROSCOPE

microscope (mi'kro-skōp). A magnifying optical instrument for viewing minute objects.

Becker m. A microscope attached to a surgeon's headband.

binocular m. 1. A microscope with a binocular body consisting of two eyepieces and a beamsplitting prism, making the objective image identically visible to both eyes. 2. A stereomicroscope, consisting of two complete microscope systems mounted in a single unit.

comparison m. 1. A type of projecting microscope the image of which can be compared with a known pattern or template. 2. A combination of two microscopes for which the viewed fields are seen contiguously in the same ocular.

compound m. A microscope containing two or more lenses or lens systems, one, serving as the objective, to form an enlarged, inverted, real image of the object; the other, as the eyepiece, to form an enlarged, virtual image.

corneal m. A magnifying instrument, usually a stereomicroscope, for examining the anterior structures of the eye.

dark-field m. Ultramicroscope.

electron m. A microscope utilizing a beam of electrons instead of a beam of light. The beam is focused by means of an electric or a magnetic field onto a photographic plate or fluorescent screen. The magnification is 50 to 100 times that obtained with an optical microscope.

fluorescence m. A microscope used with a special light source and filters to observe fluorescent objects which may be naturally fluorescent or stained with a fluorescent dye.

Greenough m. A low power stereomicroscope with erecting prisms, used in dissecting, and with the slit lamp.

immersion m. A microscope with an objective lens designed to make direct optical contact with a drop of transparent liquid (oil or water) resting on the cover plate of the microscope slide.

interference m. A microscope that reveals optical path detail within a transparent specimen, or on the surface of a reflective opaque specimen, by combining coherent light beams from the specimen and its surround.

Linnik m. An instrument consisting of a light source whose beam is divided by a semireflecting mirror into two beams, one of which is focused by an objective onto a specimen surface and the other focused by another objective onto a comparison surface, following which the reflected light from each surface is channeled back through its respective objective with the two beams being reunited into the eyepiece to provide an interference pattern.

phase-contrast m. A compound microscope having an annular diaphragm at the front focal plane of the substage condenser and an annular phase plate, corresponding in area to the image of the annular diaphragm, at the back focal plane of the objective. Variations of phase on the wavefront leaving the object are converted into variations of light intensity in the plane of the image. Syn., *phase-difference microscope.*

phase-difference m. Phase-contrast microscope.

polarizing m. A microscope equipped with a polarizer and an analyzer, used to enhance the view of objects by polarized light.

projection m. A microscope which projects an enlarged image onto a screen.

proton m. A microscope utilizing protons instead of electrons, otherwise similar to the electron microscope, and having a magnification of 600,000 diameters.

simple m. A converging lens placed between the object and the eye to provide a larger retinal image of the object. Syn., *magnifier.*

slit lamp m. See under *lamp.*

stereoscopic m. A stereomicroscope.

ultraviolet m. A microscope employing quartz lenses and prisms, used with ultraviolet light.

◆

microscopic (mi-kro-skop'ik). 1. Of, pertaining to, conducted with, or attainable with a microscope or with microscopy. 2. So small as to be invisible or not clearly distinguishable without the aid of a microscope.

microscopy (mi-kros'ko-pe). Viewing or examination with the microscope; the use of the microscope.

> **bright field m.** Microscopy in which the light from the transilluminating source is directed to go through the microscope unimpeded, except as prevented by the specimen.

> **dark field m.** Microscopy in which the light striking or transilluminating the specimen does not enter the microscope objective except when scattered or reflected by the specimen itself.

> **phase-contrast m.** Microscopy with the phase-contrast microscope.

microseme (mi'kro-sēm). Having an orbital index less than 84; characteristic of the black races. See also *megaseme; mesoseme.*

microspherometer (mi"kro-sfe-rom'-eh-ter). An instrument for measuring the curvature of a contact lens, having an optical system employing the Drysdale method.

microstimulation, retinal (mi"kro-stim"u-la'shun). 1. Photic stimulation of very small retinal areas by means of an optical reduction system providing the observer with direct control of such variable factors as position, size, distance, wavelength, and luminance of the test object, the fixation object, and the surround. 2. Stimulation of small portions of the retina by microelectrodes.

microstrabismus (mi"kro-strah-biz'-mus). Strabismus in which the deviation is so minute that it is either not detectable by customarily used tests or is concealed by a small angle eccentric fixation in the deviating eye which is equal in direction and magnitude to the deviation. Syn., *microtropia.*

microtropia (mi"kro-tro'pe-ah). Microstrabismus.

microwave (mi'kro-wāv). A very short electromagnetic wave, usually one less than 10 m, and especially one less than 1 m.

microzonuloscopy (mi"kro-zōn-ūl-os'ko-pe). Examination of the zonule of Zinn and adjacent structures with the slit lamp biomicroscope.

midbrain (mid'brān). The mesencephalon.

MIDO. See *Mostra Internazionale di Ottica-optometria-e-oftalmologia.*

migraine (mi'grān, mih-grān', me'-grān). A headache characteristically confined to one side of the head, usually intense and recurrent, and often associated with nausea, vomiting, and visual disturbances, such as scintillating scotomata.

> **ophthalmic (ocular) m.** Migraine preceded or accompanied by characteristic visual sensory disturbances, especially peripheral scintillations and hemianopsia.

> **ophthalmoplegic m.** Migraine accompanied by paralysis of the extraocular and possibly the intraocular muscles, characteristically temporary, though the ophthalmoplegia may become permanent with repeated recurrence.

> **retinal m.** Ophthalmic migraine due to vasoconstriction of one or more retinal arteries, especially in instances where obscuration of vision alone is the chief manifestation and/or the disturbance is uniocular.

mikro-. For words beginning thus, see *micro-.*

Mikulicz' (mik'u-lich) **disease; syndrome.** See under the nouns.

Miles test (mīlz). See under *test.*

Millard-Gubler syndrome (me-har'-goob'ler). See under *syndrome.*

Miller's (mil'erz) **rule; syndrome.** See under the nouns.

Milles's syndrome. See under *syndrome.*

millilambert (mil"ih-lam'bert). A unit of luminance equal to $^1/_{1000}$ lambert, where 1 lambert is equal to $1/\pi$ candela per cm². See also *footlambert.*

millimeter (mil'ih-me-ter). A unit of length in the metric system equivalent to 0.03937 inches, approximately 25.4 millimeters equalling one inch.

millimicron (mil"ih-mi'kron). A unit of length equal to one millionth of a millimeter. Symbol, mμ. Syn., *nanometer.*

milliphot (mil'ih-fōt). A unit of illuminance equal to $^1/_{1000}$ lumen per cm².

Mills's tests (milz'ez). See under *test.*

milphae (mil'fe). Milphosis.

milphosis (mil-fo'sis). 1. Loss of the eyelashes or eyebrows. Syn., *madarosis.* 2. Permanent reddening of the eyelids.

minification (min"ih-fih-ka'shun). A decrease in the apparent size, perceived size, or actual size of an object, or of its image in relation to the object.

minima (min'ih-mah). The darkest bands, or areas of minimum intensity, appearing in interference of two or more wave trains. The minima usually occur between the principal maxima and are due to a nullification of intensity by wavelets whose algebraic sum approximates zero.

minimum. The least or lowest intensity or level; the threshold.

    m. cognoscible. The threshold for the identification of form.

    m. distinguishable change of contour. The threshold of vernier visual acuity.

    m. legible. The threshold for the identification of letters.

    light m. The threshold for light perception. It varies with the state of dark adaptation, the location of the retinal area stimulated, the size of the stimulus, the spectral nature of the stimulus, etc., and is a measure of the light sense.

    m. separable. The threshold of ability to resolve or perceive separately two small, nearly adjacent objects observed simultaneously; a measure of the sense of discrimination.

    m. visible. The smallest perceivable areal extension of light. See *minimum visible angle.*

Minsky's circles (min'skēz). See under *circle.*

Mintacol (min'tah-kol). An anticholinesterase used in the eye, in concentrations of 1:5,000 to 1:10,000, as a miotic.

minus. The opposite of *plus* or *positive* in the designation of data, systems, or observations, the values of which may be represented on a continuous numerical scale from minus, through zero, to plus values, whence it may represent *divergence* as applied to lenses, *convergence* as applied to wavefronts. Syn., *negative.*

minuthesis, visual (min-u-the'sis). A reduction in any specific visual sensibility while under the influence of the original stimulus, often spoken of as *visual fatigue*; the opposite of *visual auxesis.*

miosis (mi-o'sis). 1. Reduction in pupil size. 2. The condition of having a very small pupil, i.e., approximately 2 mm or less in diameter.

    accommodative m. Miosis associated with accommodation.

    irritative m. Spastic miosis.

    paralytic m. Miosis resulting from paralysis of the dilator pupillae muscle, due to a paretic lesion of the sympathetic nervous system. See also *Horner's syndrome.*

    spastic m. Miosis due to excessive contraction of the sphincter pupillae muscle. It may occur on sudden lowering of intraocular pressure, from irritative cerebral lesions, hysteria, pain, or action of drugs.

    spinal m. Paralytic miosis resulting from lesions of the cervical sympathetic chain.

miotic (mi-ot'ik). 1. Pertaining to, affected with, characterized by, or producing miosis. 2. A drug which produces miosis.

mirage (mih-razh'). 1. An optical phenomenon produced by atmospheric strata of varying density through which the observer sees inverted or remarkably displaced images of distant objects. 2. Something illusory, like a mirage.

mire (mēr). One of the luminous objects on the ophthalmometer. Images of these objects formed by reflection at the cornea are used for determining curvature of the cornea in any meridian.

MIRED. Acronym of *mi*cro-*re*ciprocal-*d*egree. The reciprocal of the color temperature times 10^6, used as a unit of visual sensitivity to change of color temperature.

mirror (mir'or). 1. A specular, smooth, or polished surface, or a substance having such a surface, forming optical images by reflection. 2. To reflect, as in a mirror.

    back surface m. A mirror which reflects from the back surface of a refracting layer, usually of glass. Ordinary household mirrors are common examples.

    cold m. A reflecting surface consisting of multiple thin coatings of different index which, because of interference, reflects visible light and transmits infrared. Usually used at an angle of incidence of 45°.

    concave m. A mirror with a spherical concave surface forming erect, magnified, virtual images when the object distance is less than the focal distance and inverted real images when the object distance is greater than the focal distance.

    convex m. A mirror with a spherical convex surface forming erect, virtual, and minified images.

dichroic m. A mirror having a special coating which reflects only certain colors of light and transmits all others.

Fresnel's m's. Two plane mirrors inclined at an angle of almost 180° so as to produce interference fringes from two reflected beams from a single slit light source.

front surface m. A mirror which reflects directly from its front surface, so that the reflected light does not penetrate the supporting medium. Examples are polished metal surfaces and glass with a reflecting coating on the front surface.

hot m. A reflecting surface consisting of multiple coatings of different index which, because of interference, reflects infrared light and transmits visible light. Usually placed perpendicular to the light path.

Lloyd's m. A front surface plane mirror used in conjunction with a slit light source in Lloyd's method for producing interference fringes.

Mangin m. A reflector consisting of a negative meniscus lens silvered on its convex surface and so designed that the reflected rays are corrected for spherical aberration by their incident and emergent refraction through the lens.

plane m. A mirror whose reflecting surface is plane.

spherical m. A mirror whose reflecting surface has a spherical curvature.

thick m. A reflecting optical system considered in terms of its equivalence to a simple mirror but consisting of a series of a mirror and one or more refracting surfaces as a unit, as obtains, e.g., in a back surface mirror or in a lens in which the front surface refracts and the back surface reflects.

thin m. 1. A front surface mirror. 2. A back surface mirror whose supporting refracting medium is so thin as to be considered negligible.

Wadsworth m. A plane mirror used in combination with a 60° prism to produce constant deviation of all wavelengths of incident light, used in spectroscopes and spectrometers.

Mirrorscope. A trade name for a magnifying telescopic spectacle lens containing a mirror system for gathering additional light, designed and manufactured by Feinbloom.

von Mises' marginal nerve plexus. See under *plexus.*

Mitchell's stability test. See under *test.*

Mittendorf's dot (mit'en-dorfs). See under *dot.*

mixer, color. Any device for combining two or more different color stimuli on the same area of the retina. The most common form is a rotating disk with colored sectors.

mixture, color. Two or more color stimuli combined by additive or subtractive methods to produce a single resultant color, as in superimposed colored lights, mixed pigments, colored surfaces presented in rapid succession, etc.

additive color m. Color mixture by the additive combination of lights of different color.

binocular color m. Color mixture by the perceptual fusion of a color stimulus seen by one eye with a different color stimulus seen by the other.

subtractive color m. Color mixture by the subtraction of wavelengths, usually by selective absorption, from the wavelength composition of the original source, as by placing a selectively absorbing filter before a color stimulus or by pigment mixing.

Mizukawa-Kamada test (me"zu-kah'wah-kah-mah'dah). See under *test.*

Mizuo's phenomenon (mih-zu'ōz). See under *phenomenon.*

mm. Abbreviation for *millimeter.*

MMA-VP. Methyl methacrylate vinylpyrrolidone.

Mnemoscope (ne'mo-skōp). An instrument designed by Bangerter which utilizes memory cues for the treatment of amblyopia ex anopsia. It projects individual targets of various sizes and complexities onto a stage where they are viewed by the amblyopic eye and copied, traced, or identified. The targets are presented in series, commencing with one large enough to be readily identified. Succeeding targets in the series are identical but successively smaller, the clue to identity being the memory of the previous larger target.

mnemotaxis. The movement or orientation of an animal, mediated in part by the memory of past experiences, as may be exemplified by navigational birds, and considered the most complex of five categories of motorial response to light. See also *klinotaxis; menotaxis; telotaxis; tropotaxis.*

modality. The property of a sensation which differentiates it from sensations of other sense organs; thus all visual sensations form a single modality.

mode. A perceptual attribute or generalized characteristic of a specific sensation.

Modern Arc. The trade name for an instrument for the inspection of ophthalmic lenses consisting essentially of an intense light source which is passed through a small aperture, transilluminating a lens held before it, and casting a shadow of the lens onto a screen so as to reveal defects in its structure.

modification, intraocular. Any modification of a visual stimulus caused by the structural characteristics of an eye, e.g., selective absorption, refractive aberrations, or scattering of light.

modulator (mod″u-la′tor). Granit's term for a retinal element which is sensitive to a narrow spectral band and considered by him to provide the basis for color determination. See also *dominator-modulator theory.*

module (mod′ūl). In illumination, one of a series of identical or nearly identical lighting units designed to be used in varied multiples for lighting extensive areas.

Moebius' (me′be-us) **disease; sign; syndrome.** See under the nouns.

Moeller-Barlow syndrome. See under *syndrome.*

moiré (mōr′a). See under *pattern.*

mold. 1. A negative form or replica of the anterior segment of the eye made by the introduction of a modeling material, usually a hydrocolloid, onto the eye. It is used for the preparation of positive models of the anterior segment of the eye, which, in turn, are used in the forming of contact lenses. Syn., *impression.* 2. A form for shaping a thermoplastic lens.

Moldent. The trade name for a solid material used on buffing wheels for rough polishing or small reductions in diameter of contact lenses.

Moldite. A trade name for an alginate hydrocolloid used in taking eye impressions for the fitting of impression contact lenses.

Moll's gland (molz). See under *gland.*

Moller test mark projector. See under *projector.*

Möller-Barlow syndrome (muh′ler bahr′lo). See under *syndrome.*

molluscum contagiosum (mol-lus′-kum kon-ta-je-o′sum). A mildly contagious disease of the skin, thought to be due to virus infection, chiefly affecting the eyelids, characterized by one or more pearly nodules which vary in size from a pinhead to a small pea and usually have a central depression. The lesions contain ovoid, sharply defined bodies (molluscum bodies) which are considered to be forms of epithelial degeneration.

Molyneux experiment (mol′ih-nōōks). See under *experiment.*

Monakow's (mon-ah′kovz) **fibers; syndrome.** See under the nouns.

mongolism (mon′gōl-izm). Down's syndrome.

monilethrix (mo-nil′eh-thriks). A sometimes hereditary and usually congenital condition in which hairs of the scalp, eyelashes, and eyebrows show alternate swelling and constrictions, giving them a beaded appearance. They are fragile, frequently break at the constrictions, and may be accompanied by abnormalities of the nails and teeth, cataract, and mental retardation.

monoblepsia (mon″o-blep′se-ah). A condition in which the visual acuity of one of the eyes is better than the binocular visual acuity. Syn., *monoblepsis.*

monoblepsis (mon″o-blep′sis). Monoblepsia.

monocentric (mon″o-sen′trik). 1. Pertaining to a bundle of light rays which meet or come to a focus at one point. 2. Pertaining to a lens with only one optical center or to a bifocal lens in which the optical centers of the two portions are coincident.

monochroic (mon″o-kro′ik). Monochromatic.

monochromasia (mon″o-kro-ma′se-ah). Monochromatism.

monochromasy (mon″o-kro′mah-se). Monochromatism.

monochromat (mon″o-kro′mat). One having the condition of monochromatism. Syn., *monochromate.*

　　cone m. A monochromat demonstrating a luminosity curve similar to the normal photopic luminosity curve, with normal visual acuity and dark adaptation and with no photophobia or nystagmus. Syn., *photopic monochromat.*

photopic m. Cone monochromat.

rod m. A monochromat demonstrating a luminosity curve similar to the normal scotopic luminosity curve under all intensities of light. He is usually affected with poor vision and photophobia and sometimes with nystagmus. Syn., *scotopic monochromat.*

scotopic m. Rod monochromat.

monochromate (mon"o-kro'māt). Monochromat.

monochromatic (mon"o-kro-mat'ik). 1. Pertaining to or having a hue produced by a very narrow band of the spectrum, or a single hue of the spectrum which may be produced by a wide band. Syn., *monochroic; monochromic.* 2. Pertaining to or affected with monochromatism.

monochromatism (mon"o-kro'mah-tizm). The condition of being unable to differentiate between the hues of the visible spectrum and in which all parts of the visible spectrum supposedly produce varying shades of gray. Syn., *achromatopsia; total color blindness; monochromasy; monochromatopia.*

cone m. A very rare atypical form of monochromatism in which the luminosity curve is similar to the normal photopic luminosity curve, and in which visual acuity and dark adaptation are normal with no photophobia or nystagmus. Syn., *cone achromatopsia.*

rod m. The typical form of monochromatism in which the luminosity curve is similar to the normal scotopic curve under all intensities of light, and with which reduced visual acuity, photophobia, and frequently nystagmus are associated. Syn., *rod achromatopsia.* **incomplete r.m.** Photanopia.

monochromatopia (mon"o-kro-mah-to'pe-ah). Monochromatism.

monochromator (mon"o-kro'mah-tor). A spectroscope provided with an exit slit for obtaining nearly monochromatic light.

monochromic (mon"o-kro'mik). Monochromatic.

monocle (mon'o-kl). A single ophthalmic lens which is worn by bracing it between the cheek and superciliary ridge.

monocular (mo-nok'u-lar). 1. Pertaining to or affecting one eye. 2. Pertaining to any optical instrument which is used with only one eye.

Barrett subnormal vision m. A Galilean-type telescope for use at near, having a + 20.00 D objective lens at one end of a tube and an eyepiece at the other end whose power is determined by trial and error. Accessory rectangular and round masks may be used to limit the aperture and assist in improving vision.

Sturman m. A simple telescopic magnifier for near vision designed to clip on to a spectacle frame.

monoculus (mo-nok'u-lus). 1. A monster with only one eye. 2. A bandage covering only one eye. Syn., *oculus simplex.*

monodiplopia (mon"o-dih-plo'pe-ah). Double vision with only one eye; monocular diplopia.

monofixation (mon"o-fiks-a'shun). 1. Monocular fixation. 2. A condition opposite to bifixation in which the center of the fovea of only one eye is fixating and participating in the act of seeing so that central foveal fusion is not occurring under binocular seeing conditions, e.g., foveal suppression of an eye. Also referred to as *monofixation pattern of Parks or monofixational syndrome of Parks.*

monophthalmia (mon"of-thal'me-ah). A rare developmental anomaly in which one eye is absent. The eye which is present is usually abnormal and microphthalmic. Syn., *unilateral anophthalmia.*

monophthalmos (mon"of-thal'mos). Monophthalmia.

monophthalmus (mon"of-thal'mus). Monophthalmia.

monops (mon'ops). Cyclops.

monopsia (mo-nop'se-ah). Cyclopia.

monoscopter (mon"o-skop'ter). Horopter.

Monrad-Krohn syndrome (mon'-rad-krōn). Raeder's syndrome. See under *syndrome.*

Monroe Visual Three test (mon'ro). See under *test.*

Montes-Lasala syndrome. Maculo-labyrinthine syndrome.

Moon-Bardet-Biedl syndrome. Laurence-Moon-Biedl syndrome.

Moore's lightning streaks. See under *streak.*

Mooren's ulcer (mōor'enz). Rodent corneal ulcer.

mope-eyed. Colloquial for *myopic.*

Morawiecki phenomenon. See under *phenomenon.*

Morax-Axenfeld conjunctivitis

(mōr'aks-ak'sen-felt). See under *conjunctivitis.*

Morgagni's (mōr-gahn'yēz) **humor; liquor.** See under the nouns.

Morgagnian (mōr-gahn'ye-an) **cataract; fluid; globules; spherules.** See under the nouns.

Morgan's (mōr'ganz) **test; theory.** See under the nouns.

moronity. The highest of the three grades of mental deficiency which include those who may need care, supervision, or control for either their own or others' protection. On the basis of intelligence tests, this group includes those with IQ scores of between 50 and 70 or 75. Cf. *idiocy; imbecility.*

Morquio's disease (mōr-ke'ōz). See under *disease.*

Morquio-Ullrich syndrome (mōr-ke'-o-ul'rik). See under *syndrome.*

Morton's pupillometer (mōr'tonz). See under *pupillometer.*

mosaic, retinal (mo-za'ik). The pattern formed by the distribution of the retinal rods and cones and their interspaces.

Moskowskij's sign (mos-kof'skēz). See under *sign.*

Mostra Internazionale di Ottica-optometria-e-oftalmologia. An annual ophthalmic optical products and equipment exhibition of international industrial scope started in 1970 in Milan, Italy.

motility, ocular. Capability or manifestation of spontaneous or induced movement of the eye or of its parts.

motion, apparent. See *movement, apparent.*

motor oculi (mo'tor ok'u-li). The third cranial or oculomotor nerve.

mouches volantes (moosh-vo-lahnt'). Muscae volitantes.

mounting. 1. Any device which holds spectacle lenses before the eyes, particularly a rimless mounting. 2. The attaching of a pair of ophthalmic lenses to a rimless mounting.

finger-piece m. A mounting without temples and held by small spring clips to the bridge of the nose. The spring clips are applied or released by small levers grasped between the thumb and finger.

Ful-Vue m. A mounting on which the endpieces are several millimeters higher than the datum line, so as not to obstruct the lateral view of the eyes.

Numont m. A rimless mounting supported by metal arms following the contour of the upper posterior edges of the lenses to the temples and attached nasally to the bridge to which the lenses are attached at their nasal edges only.

rimless m. A device for holding spectacle lenses before the eyes, usually consisting of a pair of temples with endpieces and a bridge which are fastened to the lenses by cement, screws, or clamps but without supporting eyewires.

rimway m. A Numont-like mounting containing additional straps to secure the lenses to the metal arms at the temporal edges.

Wils-Edge m. A rimless mounting, similar to the Numont, in which the lenses are gripped across their entire tops by the arms of the mounting, the lenses being grooved and cemented into slots in the arms.

◆

MOVEMENT

movement. Change or apparent change in position; the act of moving.

absolute m. The observed movement of an object when it is the sole object visible in a surrounding homogenous field, i.e., its movement is not relative to any other object.

afterimage of m. The apparent movement of a fixated object in a direction opposite to that of the actual movement of an object just previously fixated. Ex.: *waterfall illusion.*

against m. 1. In retinoscopy, the movement of the light reflex in a direction opposite to the movement of the retinoscopic beam of light. 2. In parallactic movement, the apparent direction of movement of the nearer stationary object when the observer moves.

alpha m. The apparent movement produced by serial presentation of the parts of an optical illusion, the parts being physically the same dimension but perceptually unequal. There is growth or contraction according to which part is presented first. The alternate presentation of the two "halves" of the Mueller-Lyer figures form a good example. Syn., *S movement.*

anorthoscopic m. 1. Illusory movements produced by an anorthoscope. 2. The movement corresponding to the illusory distortion of straight lines and other designs viewed in relation to or superimposed on conflicting, interrupting, delimiting, or contrasting patterns, e.g., the perceived displacement of the parallel lines in the Zöllner illusion.

antidiplopic m. A responsive turning of one eye opposite to that of the other eye so as to eliminate the diplopia effected by the deviation of their lines of sight from each other.

apparent m. The perception of movement of a physically stationary object, hence illusory in nature. Syn., *illusory movement.*

associated m's. 1. Muscular movements which, though not necessarily dependent on each other, are somewhat instinctively performed simultaneously, e.g., the swinging of the arms when walking. 2. Ocular movements resulting from a combination of actions of more than one extrinsic muscle.

autokinetic m. The apparent movement of a stationary object of fixation, as occurs in steadily fixating a single, stationary spot of light in a dark surround, considered to be due to spontaneous and involuntary eye movements.

ballistic (ballistiform) m. A type of movement having the acceleration characteristics of a projectile, used to describe certain fixational and pursuit movements (rotations) of the eye.

beta m. The apparent movement perceived when two or more slightly separated objects are seen in rapid sequence. Thus, when two slightly separated lights are alternately flashed, they appear as a single light jumping back and forth.

binocular m's. Movements of the two eyes, either conjugate or disjunctive, regarded as single or unitary responses.

bow m. An apparent movement in which the displacement does not occur in a single plane or straight line but "bows" out into space, e.g., the end portions of the Mueller-Lyer figure appear to hinge fore and aft·when the two halves are viewed alternately.

cardinal m. Movement of an eye from the primary position to a secondary position by rotation about the z axis or the x axis, i.e., either to the right, left, up, or down.

compensatory m. Any movement which functions to compensate

for a change in stimulus or posture, e.g., the involuntary, rolling movement of the eyes in the opposite direction of a head movement; the involuntary, fixational movement of an eye when a prism is placed in its line of sight; the involuntary, oscillatory, corrective, fixational movement of an eye when the previous fixation is inexact; the turning or tilting movement of the head to compensate for an imbalance of the extraocular muscles.

conjugate m. Movement of the two eyes in the same direction. Syn., *version movement.*

convergent m. A disjugate movement in which the eyes turn toward each other, as in changing binocular fixation from a distant to a near object.

cyclofusional m. A torsional movement of one or both eyes in response to disparate cyclofusional stimuli. **negative c.m.** A cyclofusional movement in which the top of the vertical meridian of one or both eyes rotates outward. **positive c.m.** A cyclofusional movement in which the top of the vertical meridian of one or both eyes rotates inward.

cyclovergence m. Disjunctive torsional movement.

cycloversion m. Conjugate torsional movement.

delta m. That one of the several types or phases of apparent movement, induced in stationary lights presented alternately or serially, which appears in a direction opposite the stimulus sequence when the later stimulus is brighter.

depression m. Movement of one or both eyes downward from the primary position.

disjugate m. Disjunctive movement.

disjunctive m. Movement of the two eyes in opposite directions, as in convergence or divergence. Syn., *disjugate movement; vergence movement.*

divergent m. A disjunctive movement in which the eyes turn away from each other, as in changing binocular fixation from a near to a distant object.

eidotropic m. An apparent displacement of a portion of a pattern to an expected position on momentary exposure, such as may be observed in viewing a number of points arranged in a circle with one slightly out of place.

elevation m. Movement of one or both eyes upward from the primary position.

fixation m. The movement of an eye which functions to position the retina to receive the image of an object of regard on the fovea.

following m. Pursuit movement.

fusional m. A binocular movement, made in response to disparate retinal stimuli, for obtaining or maintaining single binocular vision. **peripheral f.m.** 1. A fusional movement made in the interest of obtaining or maintaining single vision of objects in the peripheral portion of the visual field. 2. A fusional movement made in response to disparate stimuli in the peripheral retinae.

gamma m. The apparent contraction or expansion, or alternately both, of an object when its luminance is suddenly lowered or raised, e.g., the apparent swelling and subsequent shrinking of a light source when it is turned on.

illusory m. Apparent movement.

interfixation m. The movement of the eye or eyes in changing fixation from one point to another.

lateral m. Movement of an eye in a horizontal direction by rotation about its z axis.

monocular m. 1. The movement of one eye without regard to the movement of the other, as when one eye is occluded. 2. Ocular movement manifested in only one eye.

nystagmoid m's. Involuntary, oscillatory movements of the eye or eyes, such as occurs in nystagmus.

oblique m. Movement of an eye in a direction diagonal to a cardinal movement.

optokinetic m. 1. The nystagmoid movement occurring in optokinetic nystagmus. 2. An autokinetic movement.

parallactic m. The apparent movement of a distant stationary object in relation to a near stationary object, or vice versa, when the observer is moving.

parallel m. Movement (rotation) of the two eyes equally in the same direction.

phi m. The apparent movement created by two or more stationary stimuli, separated in space by a rela-

tively small distance, and presented to the eye alternately or successively in a specific temporal sequence. It is described as a perceptual "filling in" of the spaces between the stimuli and has been referred to as "pure" movement, in that it may be sensed even while the objects themselves are perceived to be stationary. Syn., *phi phenomenon.*

pursuit m. Movement of an eye fixating a moving object. Syn., *following movement.*

random m's. Wandering, ocular movements uninterrupted by fixations and apparently involuntary, as occur in the blind and the newborn.

real m. A perceived movement which correlates perceptually with the actual physical movement of the object of regard.

m. of redress. Movement of an eye to recover fixation and fusion after the removal of the occluder in a cover test.

reflex m. 1. Movement of an eye induced by reflex innervation. 2. Movement of the retinoscopic reflex.

relative m. Perceived movement of an object relative to other moving or stationary objects in the field of vision.

reversal m. In retinoscopy, the change from against motion to with motion, or vice versa.

rolling m. Torsional movement.

rotatory m. Any movement of the eye about an axis through its center of rotation.

S movement. Alpha movement.

saccadic m. A quick, abrupt movement of the eye, as obtained in changing fixation from one point to another.

scanning m. One of a series of movements of the eye, characteristically saccadic, obtained in an attempt to scan or view an extensive object in systematic detail. Cf. *tracing movement.*

scissors m. 1. Simultaneous movement of the retinoscopic reflex in opposite directions in different portions of the pupil, hence resembling scissors blades, present in irregular astigmatism and keratoconus. 2. The apparent movement of a crossed line target when viewed through a rotating cylindrical lens.

screw m. A combined translatory and rotatory movement of the eye.

searching m. Involuntary, aimless excursions of an eye, as sometimes occur in the blind or the newborn. Syn., *vagabond movement; vermiform movement.*

split m. A form of apparent movement when a vertical line followed by a line perpendicular to it at its base is seen to divide and rotate both to the right and to the left to form the long horizontal line.

stroboscopic m. An apparent movement created by the presentation of a series of related motionless stimuli, each representing successive phases of a movement, as typically occurs in motion pictures. This movement may also be created by viewing an intermittently illuminated rotating object, wherein the movement may be made to appear to slow down, stop, or reverse by changing its speed of rotation or the frequency of the illumination.

synergic m. The harmonious action of two or more extraocular muscles to produce a movement of an eye or correlated movements of the two eyes.

torsional m. A rotational movement of an eye about an anteroposterior axis, such as the line of sight or the y axis. Syn., *rolling movement; wheel movement; torsional rotation; wheel rotation.* **conjugate t.m.** Simultaneous torsional movement of both eyes in the same direction. Syn., *cycloversion movement.* **disjunctive t.m.** Simultaneous torsional movement of the two eyes in opposite directions. Syn., *cyclovergence movement.*

tracing m. The movement of an eye occurring when attempts are made to fixate along the path of a continuous pattern, such as a line, characterized by a rapid series of fixational jumps.

translatory m. The movement of an eye in which all points of the eye move in the same direction, such as forward, backward, to the side, etc., in contrast to or as distinct from *rotatory movement.*

vagabond m. Searching movement.

vergence m. Disjunctive movement.

vermiform m. Searching movement.

version m. Conjugate movement.

vertical m. Movement of an eye up or down by rotation about a transverse axis, such as the x axis.

wheel m. Torsional movement.

with m. 1. In retinoscopy, the movement of the light reflex in the same direction as the movement of the retinoscopic beam of light. 2. In parallactic movement, the apparent direction of movement of the more distant stationary object when the observer moves.

◆

MRP. Abbreviation for *major reference point.*

msec. Abbreviation for *millisecond.*

mu (μ). The Greek letter used as the symbol for (1) *micron;* (2) *angle of azimuth* in the field of regard. (Fry)

mucin (mu'sin). Glycoprotein, produced by goblet cells of the conjunctiva, the mucous membranes, the synovial membranes, and the salivary glands, which forms the basis of mucus.

mucocele (mu'ko-sēl). A pathological swelling of a cavity due to an accumulation of mucoid material, such as occurs in dacryocystitis or sinusitis.

mucoids (mu'koids). A group of glycoproteins found in cartilage, the sclera, the vitreous humor, the cornea, and the crystalline lens, similar to mucin, but differing in solubility and precipitation properties.

mucopolysaccharidosis (mu"ko-pol"-e-sak"ahr-ih-do'sis). A congenital aberration of metabolism of mucopolysaccharides, differentiated thus far into six types: MPS I, Hurler's disease; MPS II, Hunter's syndrome; MPS III, Sanfillipo syndrome; MPS IV, Morquio's disease; MPS V, Scheie syndrome; MPS VI, Maroteaux-Lamy syndrome.

mucoprotein (mu"ko-pro'te-in). A mucoid.

Mueller's (mūl'erz) **cells; center of rotation; fibers; ganglion; horopter; law; fiber layer; contact lens; muscles; reticulum; spots; theories; Electronic tonometer.** See under the nouns.

Mueller-Lyer (mūl'er-li'er) **figure; illusion.** See under the nouns.

Mueller-Welt contact lens (mūl'er-velt). See under *lens, contact.*

Mules's sphere implant (mūlz'ez). See under *implant.*

multifocal (mul-tih-fo'kal). See under *lens.*

multiple sclerosis. See under *sclerosis.*

Munsell's (mun-selz') **colors; circle; hue; notation; power; renota-**

tion; system; top; value. See under the nouns.

Munson's sign (mun'sunz). See under *sign.*

Münsterberg's monocular asymmetry; partition. See under *asymmetry.*

muscae volitantes (mus'se vol"ih-tan'-tēz, mus'ke). Small floating spots, "flitting flies," entoptically observed on viewing a bright uniform field, such as the sky, and seen to flit away with attempted fixation. Their presence is normal and attributed to minute remnants of embryonic structures in the vitreous humor. Syn., *mouches volantes.*

◆

MUSCLE

muscle. A contractile organ whose special function is to produce motion; also, the tissues of which such an organ is composed, consisting of individual muscle fibers or muscle cells. Classified by structure as nonstriated or striated; by control as voluntary or involuntary; by location as skeletal, cardiac, or visceral.

abducens m. External rectus muscle.

abducens oculi m. External rectus muscle.

accessory m's. of accommodation. The frontal, pyramidal, corrugator supercilii, and the orbicularis oculi muscles, supplied by the facial nerve, which contract vicariously when an extreme effort is made to see.

adducens m. Internal rectus muscle.

adducens oculi m. Internal rectus muscle.

agonistic m. A muscle yielding the desired movement; a prime mover or protagonist; one opposed by an antagonistic muscle.

antagonistic m. A muscle that has the opposite function of the muscle engaged in the movement of a part. The antagonist of an abductor is an adductor; of an elevator, a depressor; of a flexor, an extensor; etc.

anterior lacrimal m. The fibers of the pars tarsalis portion of the orbicularis oculi muscle, lying anterior to the fascia which covers the lacrimal sac. Syn., *muscle of Gerlach.*

Bowman's m. Ciliary muscle.

Brücke's m. The meridional or longitudinal fibers of the ciliary muscle

which attach in the scleral spur and uveal meshwork and extend to the choroid, where they usually end in branched stellate figures (muscle stars). Syn., *tensor choroideae muscle.*

bursalis m. In lizards, a muscle inserting into the posterior sclera near the optic nerve and encircled by the tendon of the nictitating membrane, which is drawn taut by its contraction.

capsulo-palpebralis m. Landström's muscle.

choanoid m. A retractor bulbi muscle found in land vertebrates but absent in the higher mammals. It pulls the eyeball into the orbit.

ciliary m. The intrinsic smooth muscle of the ciliary body. Its fibers course in three directions, meridionally (Brücke's muscle), radially, and circularly (Mueller's muscle). Innervation is from the ciliary nerves, and the blood supply from the anterior and posterior ciliary vessels. Its action, according to current theory, slackens the suspensory ligament of the crystalline lens, decreasing the tension of the capsule of the lens, permitting the lens to become more convex, as occurs in accommodation. Syn., *Bowman's muscle; musculus accommodatorius.*

contractor pupillae m. Sphincter pupillae muscle.

cornealis m. In lampreys, a large muscle arising outside of the orbit and inserting into the transparent dermal cornea, which acts to produce accommodation for distant objects by flattening the anterior eyeball on contraction and displacing the crystalline lens backwards to render the normally myopic eye emmetropic.

corrugator supercilii m. A small, striated muscle which arises at the medial end of the superciliary ridge, passes upward and outward, and inserts into the skin of the eyebrow at its middle. It draws the eyebrows toward the root of the nose, on contraction, as in frowning. Syn., *superciliary muscle.*

m. of Crampton. A muscle found in the eyes of birds and reptiles which arises from the inner peripheral surface of the cornea and inserts into the sclera in the ciliary region. It acts in accommodation by shortening the radius of curvature of the cornea.

cyclovertical m. Any of the vertical rectus or oblique extraocular muscles.

dilator pupillae m. An intrinsic, smooth, radial muscle of the iris, located posteriorly in both the pupillary and ciliary portions and extending into the ciliary body. Its myoepithelial fibers constitute the *posterior border lamella of Fuchs* and its spindle cells the *anterior pigment layer of Fuchs.* Innervation by the sympathetic fibers in the long ciliary nerves results in enlargement of the pupil.

external rectus m. A striated, extrinsic muscle of the eyeball that originates from the annulus of Zinn and from the spina recti lateralis and inserts laterally into the sclera about 6.9 mm from the limbus corneae. It is innervated by the abducens nerve and abducts the eyeball. Syn., *abducens oculi muscle; lateral rectus muscle.*

extraocular m's. The striated muscles, originating at the apex of the orbit or at the anterior medial portion of the orbit and inserting on the sclera, which rotate the eyeball. They are the extrinsic muscles of the eyeball and consist of the superior, inferior, internal, and external recti and the superior and inferior obliques. Syn., *oculorotary muscles.*

extrinsic m's. Muscles that have their origin outside of the structure under consideration but insert into that structure, such as the extraocular muscles.

frontalis m. A striated muscle which arises from the epicranial aponeurosis near the coronal suture and inserts vertically into the skin of the eyebrow. It is innervated by the facial nerve and causes horizontal wrinkling of the forehead as it lifts the eyebrows.

Horner's m. A thin layer of fibers that originates at the posterior lacrimal crest and passes outward and forward, dividing into two slips which surround the canaliculi, and becomes continuous with the pretarsal portion of the orbicularis oculi muscle and the muscle of Riolan. It affects tear drainage through action on the lacrimal sac and canaliculi. Syn., *pars lacrimalis muscle; tensor tarsi muscle.*

inferior oblique m. A striated, extrinsic muscle of the eyeball that originates from the anterior, medial portion of the orbital floor, passes beneath (external to) the inferior rectus and nasal to the external rectus to insert on the posterior, temporal portion of the eyeball, slightly below its horizontal meridian. It is innervated by the oculomotor nerve and elevates, abducts, and extorts the eyeball.

inferior rectus m. A striated, extrinsic muscle of the eyeball that originates from the annulus of Zinn and inserts inferiorly into the sclera about 6.5 mm from the limbus corneae. It is innervated by the oculomotor nerve and adducts, depresses, and extorts the eyeball.

internal rectus m. A striated, extrinsic muscle of the eyeball that originates from the annulus of Zinn and inserts medially into the sclera about 5.5 mm from the limbus corneae. It is innervated by the oculomotor nerve and adducts the eyeball. Syn., *adducens oculi muscle; medial rectus muscle.*

intraocular m's. The smooth muscles within the eyeball. They are the intrinsic muscles of the eyeball and consist of the *ciliary, dilator pupillae,* and *sphincter pupillae muscles.*

intrinsic m's. Muscles that have both origin and insertion within the structure under consideration, as the intraocular muscles.

Landström's m. Smooth muscle fibers which extend from the orbital septum over the anterior portion of the eyeball and blend with fascial expansions of the extraocular muscles just back of their insertions. When innervated by the sympathetic, they tend to move the eyeball forward. Syn., *capsulo-palpebralis muscle.*

lateral rectus m. External rectus muscle.

levator bulbi m. In amphibians, a skeletal muscle derived from the jaw mesoderm and innervated by the trigeminal nerve, which, on contraction, pulls the eyeball forward after it has been displaced backward by the retractor bulbi muscle.

levator palpebrae superioris m. A striated muscle that arises at the apex of the orbit from the small wing of the sphenoid bone and inserts via an aponeurosis into the skin and tarsus of the upper lid, the lateral orbital tubercle, the medial palpebral ligament, and the superior fornix conjunctivae. It courses forward under the roof of the orbit, from its origin, on the superior rectus muscle to which it is adherent by fascial sheaths. It is innervated by the oculomotor nerve and elevates the upper eyelid.

medial rectus m. Internal rectus muscle.

Merkel's m. The portion of the pars septalis muscle that arises superficially from the anterior portion of the medial palpebral ligament and extends laterally and inferiorly to insert fanlike into the skin of the medial half of the lower eyelid.

Mueller's annular m. The circular fibers of the ciliary muscle located in the anterior inner portion of the ciliary body and which run parallel to the limbus. Absent in the newborn, it develops after birth.

Mueller's orbital m. The smooth muscle fibers which arise in the periorbita and extend fanlike over the floor of the orbit, bridging the inferior orbital fissure, to the cavernous sinus. It is innervated by the sympathetic via a branch from the sphenopalatine ganglion. Its function in man is doubtful, although it acts as a protruder of the eye in some lower animals. Syn., *musculus orbitalis*.

Mueller's palpebral m., inferior. A small sheath of smooth muscle fibers which originates from the fascial sheath of the inferior rectus muscle and from its expansion to the inferior oblique muscle. It extends upward and divides into two layers, one of which attaches in the bulbar conjunctiva and the other inserts into the lower margin of the tarsal plate of the lower eyelid. It is innervated by the sympathetic, assists in retracting the lower eyelid, and may tend to protrude the eyeball.

Mueller's palpebral m., superior. A small sheath of smooth muscle fibers which originates from the levator palpebrae superioris muscle and extends downward and forward to insert into the upper margin of the tarsal plate of the upper eyelid. It is innervated by the sympathetic, assists in raising the upper eyelid, and may tend to protrude the eyeball.

occipito-frontalis m. A striated muscle located on the upper part of the cranium and consisting of two occipital and two frontal muscles united by an aponeurosis. The occipital portions originate from the occipital bone and insert into the aponeurosis. The frontal portions originate from the aponeurosis and insert into the skin of the eyebrows. It is innervated by the facial nerve. The frontal portions act to draw the scalp forward and raise the eyebrows, and the occipital portions act to draw the scalp backward.

oculorotary m's. The extraocular muscles.

orbicularis oculi m. An oval sheet of striated muscle in the eyelid running concentrically around the palpebral fissure and spreading out into regions of the forehead and face around the orbital margin. It consists of two portions, the *pars orbitalis muscle* and the *pars palpebralis muscle*, is innervated by the facial nerve, and functions as the sphincter of the eyelid. Syn., *orbicularis palpebrarum muscle; musculus dormitator; sphincter oculi; sphincter palpebrarum*.

orbicularis palpebrarum m. Orbicularis oculi muscle.

palpebral m's. 1. Mueller's inferior and superior palpebral muscles. 2. In aquatic mammals, striated muscular slips of the rectus muscles which insert into the eyelids.

pars ciliaris m. Muscle of Riolan.

pars lacrimalis m. Horner's muscle.

pars marginalis m. Muscle of Riolan.

pars orbitalis m. The peripheral portion of the orbicularis oculi muscle found in the eyebrow, the temple, and the cheek. The origin is from the inner orbital margin and the medial palpebral ligament. Its action is in forced or tight closure of the eyelids.

pars palpebralis m. That portion of the orbicularis oculi muscle present in the eyelids. It arises from the medial palpebral ligament and the adjacent bone and inserts in the lateral palpebral raphe, in the region of the external canthus. It consists of two parts, the *pars septalis muscle* and the *pars tarsalis muscle*, and acts in light or effortless closure or blinking of the eyelids.

pars septalis m. That portion of the pars palpebralis muscle which lies anterior to the septum orbitale. Syn., *preseptal muscle*.

pars subtarsalis m. Fibers of the muscle of Riolan which pass posteriorly to lie behind the openings of the ducts of the Meibomian glands.

pars tarsalis m. That portion of the pars palpebralis muscle which lies in the area of the tarsal plate. It consists of three parts, the *anterior lacrimal* muscle, *Horner's muscle* and *muscle of Riolan.* Syn., *pretarsal muscle.*

preseptal m. Pars septalis muscle.

pretarsal m. Pars tarsalis muscle.

protractor lentis m. A smooth muscle found in fishes, amphibians, and reptiles which acts to draw forward the crystalline lens in accommodation.

pupillary m's. The sphincter and the dilator pupillae muscles.

retractor bulbi m. A skeletal muscle found in amphibians to mammals, probably derived from the lateral rectus muscle and innervated by the abducens nerve, which, on contraction, pulls the eyeball backward into the orbit.

retractor bursalis m. In lizards, a muscle slip extending upwards from the bursalis muscle and inserting in the sclera, acting to keep the bursalis muscle and the tendon of the nictitating membrane free of the optic nerve upon contraction.

retractor lentis m. In fishes, an ectodermal muscle that arises from the fetal cleft and courses in the falciform process to insert into the lens.

m. of Riolan. The portion of the orbicularis oculi muscle originating from the posterior lacrimal crest and encircling the eyelid margins between the tarsal glands and the eyelash follicles, with some fibers passing posteriorly to lie behind the openings of the ducts of the tarsal glands. It brings the eyelid margins together as the eyes are closed. Syn., *pars ciliaris muscle; pars marginalis muscle.*

sphincter iridis m. Sphincter pupillae muscle.

sphincter pupillae m. An intrinsic, smooth, circular muscle of the iris, approximately 0.8 mm broad, located in the posterior stroma of the pupillary portion and forming a ring around the margin of the pupil. Innervation by parasympathetic fibers of the oculomotor nerve, which synapse in the ciliary or the episcleral ganglion, results in decreased diameter of the pupil. Syn., *sphincter iridis muscle.*

m. stars. Groups of smooth cell fibers arranged in star-shaped configurations, located in the suprachoroid in the region of the equator of the eyeball, where they are continuous with Brücke's muscle.

superciliary m. Corrugator supercilii muscle.

superior oblique m. A striated, extrinsic muscle of the eyeball that has its anatomical origin superior and medial to the optic foramen on the small wing of the sphenoid bone. It passes anteriorly and gives place to a rounded tendon about 1 cm behind the trochlea. The tendon passes through the trochlea, then bends downward, backward, and outward at an angle of about 54°, passes beneath the superior rectus muscle, and inserts on the superior posterotemporal portion of the eyeball. It is innervated by the trochlear nerve and depresses, abducts, and intorts the eyeball. Syn., *musculus amatorius; musculus patheticus.*

superior rectus m. A striated, extrinsic muscle of the eyeball that originates from the upper part of the annulus of Zinn and from the sheath of the optic nerve. It passes anteriorly and laterally beneath the levator palpebrae superioris muscle and inserts superiorly into the sclera about 7.7 mm from the limbus corneae. It is innervated by the oculomotor nerve, elevates, adducts, and intorts the eyeball and also assists in raising the upper eyelid. Syn., *musculus religiosus; musculus superbus.*

synergistic m's. Two or more muscles which act together to move a part, as the superior rectus and inferior oblique muscles in elevating the eyeball.

tensor choroideae m. Brücke's muscle.

tensor tarsi m. Horner's muscle.

tensor trochleae m. An abnormal slip of muscle extending from the levator palpebrae superioris muscle to the trochlea.

transverse m. In reptiles, a muscle derived from connective tissue between the ciliary body and sclera and inserting into the zonule of Zinn, thought to displace the crystalline lens nasally during accommodation.

yoke m's. Muscles of the two eyes which simultaneously contract to turn the eyes equally in the same direction, such as the right external rectus and the left internal rectus muscles in turning the eyes to the right.

◆

musculus (mus'ku-lus). Latin for muscle.

    m. accommodatorius. Ciliary muscle.

    m. amatorius. Superior oblique muscle.

    m. ciliaris. Ciliary muscle.

    m. dormitator. Orbicularis oculi muscle.

    m. orbitalis. Mueller's orbital muscle.

    m. patheticus. Superior oblique muscle.

    m. religiosus. Superior rectus muscle.

    m. superbus. Superior rectus muscle.

    m. tarsalis. The inferior or the superior palpebral muscle of Mueller.

mutton-fat deposits. See under *deposits*.

My. Abbreviation for *myopia*.

myasthenia gravis (mi"as-the'neah grav'is). A disease of obscure etiology characterized by abnormal fatigue and exhaustion of striated muscles, sometimes leading to muscular paralysis. It may affect any muscle of the body, especially those of the head and the neck. Ocular symptoms include external ophthalmoplegia, ptosis, and diplopia. Syn., *Erb-Goldflam disease; asthenic bulbar paralysis; myasthenic pseudoparalysis.*

myasthenia palpebralis (mi"as-the'ne-ah pal"pe-brah'lis). A deficiency in function of the orbicularis oculi muscles.

mycophthalmia (mi"kof-thal'me-ah). A conjunctivitis due to a fungus.

mydesis (mi-de'sis). Purulent discharge from the eyelids.

Mydriacyl (mih-dri'ah-sil). A trade name for a parasympatholytic drug used as a cycloplegic and mydriatic.

mydriasis (mih-dri'ah-sis, mi-). 1. Increase in pupil size. 2. The condition of having an abnormally large pupil, i.e., approximately 5 mm or greater in diameter.

    alternating m. Mydriasis alternately affecting each of the two eyes, due to a disorder of the central nervous system. Syn., *bounding mydriasis; leaping mydriasis; springing mydriasis.*

    amaurotic m. A condition in which the pupil of a blind eye is wider than that of its mate, the seeing eye.

    bounding m. Alternating mydriasis.

    leaping m. Alternating mydriasis.

    paralytic m. Mydriasis due to paralysis of the sphincter pupillae muscle, as may result from lesions in the pupillary center of the midbrain or its efferent pathways, after contusions to the eyeball, or increased intraocular pressure affecting the long ciliary nerves or muscle itself.

    psychic m. Mydriasis due to fright or violent emotion.

    spasmodic m. Spastic mydriasis.

    spastic m. Mydriasis due to irritation of the sympathetic pathway and spasm of the dilator pupillae muscle, accompanied by widening of the palpebral fissure and slight exophthalmos (Bernard's syndrome). The light and convergence pupillary reflexes are present, though limited, and the mydriasis is usually slight. Syn., *spasmodic mydriasis.*

    spinal m. Mydriasis due to irritation of the ciliospinal center of the spinal cord.

    springing m. Alternating mydriasis.

mydriatic (mid-rih-at'ik). 1. Pertaining to, affected with, characterized by, or producing mydriasis. 2. A drug or other agent which produces mydriasis.

myectomy (mi-ek'to-me). The excision of a portion of the belly of a muscle, sometimes done for the correction of strabismus.

myectopia (mi-ek-to'pe-ah). Abnormal placement of a muscle, either congenital or due to injury.

myectopy (mi-ek'to-pe). Myectopia.

myelinic dysgenesia (mi-el-in'ik dis-jen-e'ze-ah). A condition characterized by retardation or failure in the development of the myelin sheaths of nerve fibers of the central nervous system. Blindness, with little or no muscular coordination, is present at birth. Light perception and ocular fixations usually appear with postnatal development of the sheaths, but strabismus persists.

myelitis, neuro-optic (mi"eh-li'tis). Neuromyelitis optica.

Myerson's sign (mi'er-sonz). See under *sign*.

myiasis, ocular (mi'yah-sis). An infection of the conjunctival sac by maggots.

myiocephalon (mi"yo-sef'ah-lon). The protrusion of a minute portion of the iris through a perforation of the cornea; an iridocele.

myiodeopsia (mi"yo-de-op'se-ah). The perception of muscae volitantes.

myiodesopsia (mi"yo-des-op'se-ah). Myiodeopsia.

Myoculator (mi-ok'u-la-tor). An instrument used in visual training, consisting essentially of a motor-driven projector automatically controlled to move the projected fixation image meridionally or circularly under conditions of constant or intermittent illumination and often used in conjunction with a second manually controlled projector (Kratoculator).

myodeopsia (mi"o-de-op'se-ah). Myiodeopsia.

myodesopsia (mi"o-des-op'se-ah). Myiodeopsia.

myodiopter (mi"o-di-op'ter). The contractile force of the ciliary muscle necessary to increase the accommodation from zero to one diopter, said to be the unit of physiological accommodation.

myoid, visual cell (mi'oid). The nonrefractile inner portion of the inner member of a rod or cone cell located between the ellipsoid and the external limiting layer of the retina.

myokymia (mi"o-ki'me-ah, -kim'e-ah). Twitching or vibratory movements of individual muscle bundles, usually occurring in neurasthenics or following fatigue. In the eyelid, it is termed *clonic blepharospasm.*

superior oblique m. A condition of brief recurrent torsional diplopia associated with unilateral tremulous sensations and oscillopsia due to vertical and rotatory muscle microtremor.

myope (mi'ōp). One having myopia.

◆

MYOPIA

myopia (mi-o'pe-ah). The refractive condition of the eye represented by the location of the conjugate focus of the retina at some finite point in front of the eye, when accommodation is said to be relaxed, or the extent of that condition represented in the number of diopters of concave lens power required to compensate to the optical equivalent of emmetropia. The condition may also be represented as one in which parallel rays of light entering the eye, with accommodation relaxed, focus in front of the retina. Syn., *nearsightedness.*

acquired m. 1. Myopia which appears after infancy. 2. Myopia due to abnormal circumstances, such as a rise in blood sugar or a traumatic injury, wherein one suddenly becomes markedly more myopic than formerly. **a.m. of maturity.** Nonpathological myopia, typically of low or moderate amount, with onset after the attainment of physical maturity.

adventitious m. *Optometric Extension Program:* Myopia caused by near work.

apparent m. Hypertonic myopia.

associated m. A type of hypertonic myopia said to result from exophoria compensated for by accommodative convergence.

astigmatic m. 1. Myopia combined with astigmatism. 2. A type of hypertonic myopia said to result from accommodative efforts to compensate for uncorrected astigmatism.

atypical m. Malignant myopia.

axial m. Myopia attributed to excessive, or increase in, axial length of the eye.

benign m. Simple myopia.

complicated m. Malignant myopia.

correlative m. Simple myopia.

curvature m. Myopia attributed to excessive, or increase in, curvature of one or more of the refractive surfaces of the eye, especially of the cornea.

degenerative m. Myopia due to degenerative changes in the eyeball. One of three major groups of myopia, according to the Harding classification, the others being *hypertonic* and *fibrillar myopia.* See also *pathological, progressive,* and *malignant myopia.*

diabetic m. Myopia due to change in refraction associated with variation in blood sugar.

dietetic m. Nutritional myopia.

empty field m. Sky myopia.

false m. Pseudomyopia.

fibrillar m. Myopia attributed to faulty development of the fibroblasts of the sclera and the consequent reaction of the sclera to the intraocular pressure during the period of growth. One of three major groups of myopia, according to the Harding classification, the others being *hypertonic* and *degenerative myopia.*

functional m. Myopia attributed to a spasm of the ciliary muscle. Syn., *hypertonic myopia.*

m. gravis. High myopia.

healthy m. Simple myopia.

high m. Myopia of high degree, usually of 6.00 D or more.

hypertonic m. The refractive condition of myopia attributable to spasm of the ciliary muscle or incomplete relaxation of accommodation. One of three major groups of myopia, according to the Harding classification, the others being *degenerative* and *fibrillar myopia.* Syn., *apparent myopia; functional myopia; pseudomyopia.*

hysterical m. Psychogenic myopia occurring in hysteria.

index m. Myopia attributed to variation in the index of refraction of one or more of the ocular media.

infantile pyretic m. Myopia which appears or increases following a childhood disease accompanied by high fever, such as measles or scarlet fever.

innervational m. Myopia attributable to innervational anomalies, as distinct from myopia attributable to structural or index anomalies, hence a hypertonic myopia.

instrument m. The manifestation of more accommodation when looking at an image seen through an optical instrument than when looking at a real object placed at the optically equivalent true distance.

m. inversa. A conus or atrophic choroidal area located on the nasal side of the optic disk; considered to be due to a coexisting high myopia. Syn., *inverse crescent.*

lenticular m. Myopia attributed to excessive refractive power of the crystalline lens.

low m. Myopia of a low degree, usually of 3.00 D or less.

malignant m. Myopia characterized by marked fundus changes, such as posterior staphylomata, and associated with a high refractive error and subnormal visual acuity after correction. See also *degenerative, pathological,* and *progressive myopia.* Syn., *atypical myopia; complicated myopia; pernicious myopia.*

medium m. Myopia of medium degree, usually between 3.00 and 6.00 D. Syn., *moderate myopia.*

moderate m. Medium myopia.

night m. Myopia or an increase in ocular refraction occurring in low levels of illumination, as in twilight or at night. Syn., *twilight myopia.*

nutritional m. Myopia attributed to nutritional deficiencies, as a lack of certain minerals or vitamins. Syn., *dietetic myopia.*

occupational m. Myopia occurring, or regarded as, an occupational disorder or attributed to the excessive visual demands of an occupation. Cf. *adventitious* and *school myopia.*

pathological m. Myopia attributable to pathological causes, or in which visual acuity is subnormal after correction. See also *degenerative, malignant,* and *progressive myopia.*

pernicious m. Malignant myopia.

position m. Myopia attributed to an excessively forward position of the crystalline lens, i.e., near the cornea.

m. of prematurity. Myopia associated with premature birth.

primary m. Simple myopia.

prodromal m. The myopia which sometimes occurs in the early stage of lenticular cataract.

progressive m. Myopia which increases at an abnormally rapid rate or increases after maturity. See also *degenerative, malignant,* and *pathological myopia.*

pseudo m. Myopia due to spasm of the ciliary muscle. See *hypertonic myopia.*

psychogenic m. A hypertonic type of myopia of psychical origin, usually transitory, and ordinarily associated with other psychical phenomena or disorders.

refractive m. 1. Myopia attributed to the normal variation of the refractive elements of the eye, including axial length, as distinguished from *degenerative* or *pathological myopia.* 2. Myopia attributed to the condition of the refractive elements of the eye as distinguished from *axial myopia.* Cf. *curvature* and *index myopia.*

school m. Myopia attributed to the use of the eyes for close work during the school years.

secondary m. Myopia due to degenerative or pathological changes in the structure of the eye.

simple m. 1. Myopia due to normal growth of a healthy eyeball or to a chance combination of the optical elements. Characteristically, it ceases to increase after maturity and is associated with normal visual acuity after correction. It is differentiated from *degenerative, progressive, malignant,* or *pathological myopia.* Syn., *benign myopia; correlative myopia; stationary myopia; typical myopia.* 2. Myopia occurring without an associated astigmatism.

sky m. An increase in the refractive state of the eye noted in the absence of optical stimuli to accommodation, as occurs in viewing a clear, cloudless sky. Syn., *empty field myopia; space myopia.*

space m. Sky myopia.

stationary m. Simple myopia.

sulfanilamide m. A transitory myopia which follows administration of sulfanilamide. Typically, the myopia appears a day or two after taking sulfa drugs in patients who, on a previous occasion, have taken the drug with no ensuing visual disturbance. The degree of myopia is approximately 5.00 to 10.00 D, and lasts for a period of a few hours to a few weeks, most frequently about a week.

transitory m. Myopia which appears suddenly, lasts for a period of time, and then disappears. In this group are included myopia due to trauma, high blood sugar level (hyperglycemia), sulfanilamide therapy, etc.

traumatic m. Myopia resulting from a blow to the eye. The myopia develops shortly after the trauma (usually within 48 hours) and lasts from a few days to many years.

true m. Myopia, or that part of the total myopia, not attributable to spasm of the ciliary muscle or unrelaxed accommodation.

twilight m. Night myopia.

typical m. Simple myopia.

very high m. Myopia of extreme degree, over 10.00 D according to some authors, and over 15.00 D according to others.

◆

myopic (mi-op'ik). Pertaining to or having myopia.

myopic conus; crescent. See under the nouns.

myopiosis (mi"op-e-o'sis). Myopia.

myoporthosis (mi"o-por-tho'sis). The correction of myopia. *Obs.*

myopsis (mi-op'sis). Myiodeopsia.

Myoscope (mi'o-skōp). An instrument, similar to the Myoculator, used in visual training. It projects a circularly or meridionally moving target onto a screen.

myosis (mi-o'sis). Miosis.

myositis, orbital (mi-o-si'tis). 1. Inflammation of the extraocular muscles, either chronic or acute, which may be primary, but is usually secondary to other orbital inflammations, such as syphilis or tuberculosis. 2. A primary chronic inflammation of the extraocular muscles resulting in exophthalmos and external ophthalmoplegia, similar to that found in exophthalmic goiter. The condition is probably not a true inflammation.

myositis, myopic. Heavy eye phenomenon.

myotic (mi-ot'ik). Miotic.

myotomy (mi-ot'o-me). Surgical division of muscle fibers, particularly in the belly of the muscle.

myotonia congenita (mi"o-to'ne-ah kon-jen'ih-tah). Thomsen's disease.

N

N. Symbol for *radiance.*

n. Symbol for (1) *nasal;* (2) *index of refraction;* (3) *normal.*

nacreous (na'kre-us). Having iridescence resembling that of mother-of-pearl.

Naffziger syndrome. Scalenus anticus syndrome. See under *syndrome.*

Nagel's (nah'gelz) **adaptometer; test; empiristic theory.** See under the nouns.

nahastigmatismus. The additional cylindrical correction needed in the spectacle plane for correcting the astigmatism for a near object as compared to that needed to correct the same astigmatic error for a distant object, due to differential lens effectivity in the two principal meridians.

nanometer (nan-om'eh-ter, nan'o-me"-ter). A unit of length equal to one millionth of a millimeter. Symbol, *nm.* Syn., *millimicron.*

nanophthalmos (nan-of-thal'mos). A rare developmental anomaly in which the eyeballs are abnormally small but are without other deformities. See also *microphthalmos.*

naphazoline (naf-az'o-lēn). A sympathomimetic drug available in 0.12% to 0.05% concentration in over-the-counter products as an ophthalmic decongestant.

nasociliary (na"zo-sil'e-a-re). 1. Pertaining to or affecting the eyebrows and the bridge of the nose. 2. The nasociliary nerve.

nasolacrimal (na"zo-lak'rih-mal). Pertaining to the nasolacrimal duct.

Nasse's law (neh'sez). See under *law.*

National Board of Examiners in Optometry. An incorporated commission, created in 1951, consisting of five persons nominated by the International Association of Boards of Examiners in Optometry and three persons nominated by the Association of Schools and Colleges of Optometry to prepare and administer uniform examinations to students and graduates of accredited optometry schools and colleges, the passing of which is accepted by many state boards and agencies toward the fulfillment of licensure requirements.

National Eye Institute. One of the National Institutes of Health, specifically concerned with the eye and visual system.

National Eye Research Foundation. An organization of professionals and others, founded in 1956, to support eye and contact lens research and education.

National Institutes of Health. A part of the U.S. Public Health Service consisting of institutes, centers, and divisions which conduct and support biomedical research, training, and education related to the causes, prevention, and cure of diseases.

National Medical Foundation for Eye Care. See *American Association of Ophthalmology.*

National Optometric Association. An association of optometrists of minority ethnic groups originally founded by black optometrists in 1969 to represent special minority interests and needs and to promote better recruitment for the profession among minority populations.

National Society for the Prevention of Blindness. An incorporated, voluntary organization engaged in a program of eliminating preventable loss of sight through research, service, and education.

National Vision Research Institute. A Melbourne institute established in 1972 on the initiative of Australian optometrists in cooperation with the Victorian College of Optometry, supported by contracts, grants, and contributions from individuals, corporations, and agencies.

nativism. The theory, doctrine, or concept that certain aspects of behavior, knowledge, or perception are innate and independent of accumulated experience or learning. Cf. *empiricism.* Syn., *Kant's nativistic theory.*

Natural Environment Trainer. NET Orthoptor.

NBEO. See *National Board of Examiners in Optometry.*

near point of accommodation; convergence; fusion. Also, *nearpoint* or *nearpoint.* See under the nouns.

nearsight. Myopia.

nearsighted. Myopic.

nearsightedness. Myopia.

nebula (neb'u-lah). A faint or slightly misty corneal opacity. Cf. *leukoma; macula.*

Necker cube (nek'er). See under *cube.*

necroscleritis nodosa (nek"ro-skleri'tis no-dōs'ah). Nodular necrotizing scleritis.

necrosis (neh-kro'sis). The death of tissue or tissue cells, especially in a circumscribed portion of the body, as in gangrene, and/or the changes which take place in these cells after they have died.

Nederlandse Unie van Opticiens. A federation of several Dutch associations formed in 1950 to serve the various protective and developmental interests of member ophthalmic opticians and optometrists.

needling. A surgical operation for aftercataract or soft cataract in which the lens capsule is punctured to allow absorption of the lens substance. Syn., *discission.*

Negocoll (neg'oh-kol). A compound, having agar as a base, and containing cotton fibers for binding and strength, used in making impressions of an eye for the fitting of molded contact lenses.

Negri-Jacod syndrome (na'gre-ja'kod). Jacod's triad. See under *triad.*

Negro's sign (na'grōz). See under *sign.*

NEI. See *National Eye Institute.*

Nela wools test (ne'lah). See under *test.*

neo-retinene$_1$ (ne"o-ret'ih-nēn). Either of two of the isomers of retinene$_1$ known as *neo-a* and *neo-b.*

neostigmine (ne"o-stig'min). Prostigmine.

Neosynephrine (ne"o-sin-ef'rin). A trade name for *phenylephrine hydrochloride.*

neosynoptophore (ne"o-sin-op'to-fōr). A type of major amblyoscope with accessory attachments for creating Haidinger's brushes and afterimages.

neotocophthalmia (ne"o-to-kof'thal-me-ah). Ophthalmia neonatorum.

nephelometer (nef'eh-lom'eh-ter). A device for comparing the light scattered from particles in an unknown suspension to that of a standard, for the purpose of determining the amount of material in suspension; used in chemical and bacterial analyses, and in measurements of atmospheric scatter.

nephelometry (nef'eh-lom'eh-tre). Determination of the amount of particles in suspension in a gas or liquid with a nephelometer.

nephelopia (nef-el-o'pe-ah). Reduced vision resulting from cloudiness of the cornea.

NERF. See *National Eye Research Foundation.*

◆

NERVE

nerve. A cordlike structure of nervous tissue that connects parts of the nervous system with other tissues of the body and conveys nervous impulses to, or away from, these tissues. It is composed of bundles of nerve fibers, each bundle (funiculus) being surrounded by a connective tissue sheath (perineurium), and the whole is enclosed in a common sheath (epineurium).

abducens n. Cranial nerve VI. It has its deep origin from the abducens nucleus in the pons and its superficial origin from the pons-medulla junction, entering the orbit via the superior orbital fissure. It is the motor nerve innervating the ipsilateral external rectus muscle.

cervical sympathetic n. 1. Any sympathetic group of nerve fibers leaving the superior, inferior, or middle cervical ganglion. 2. In ocular neurology, any group of postganglionic axons leaving the superior cervical ganglion, the destruction of which yields Horner's syndrome.

ciliary n., long. One of a pair of

nerves that leaves the nasociliary nerve, pierces a posterior aperture of the sclera, courses in the suprachoroidal space nasally or temporally, and carries sympathetic fibers for the dilator pupillae muscle and the sensory fibers to the iris, the cornea, and the ciliary body.

ciliary n., short. One of six to ten nerves which arise from the ciliary ganglion, double in number, pierce the posterior sclera in a ring around the optic nerve, travel in the suprachoroidal space, and innervate the sphincter pupillae muscle, the ciliary muscle, and the cornea.

ethmoidal n., anterior. A terminal branch of the nasociliary nerve that supplies the cartilaginous portions of the nose and leaves the orbit via the anterior ethmoidal foramen. Syn., *nasal nerve.*

ethmoidal n., posterior. A branch of the nasociliary nerve that supplies the sphenoidal and ethmoidal sinuses and leaves the orbit via the posterior ethmoidal foramen. Syn., *nerve of Luschka; spheno-ethmoid nerve.*

facial n. Cranial nerve VII, a mixed nerve arising from the pons-medulla junction. It is efferent to the muscles of facial expression, including the orbicularis oculi, and to the lacrimal, submaxillary, and sublingual glands. It carries taste fibers from the anterior two thirds of the tongue.

fifth cranial n. Trigeminal nerve.

fourth cranial n. Trochlear nerve.

frontal n. A sensory branch of the ophthalmic nerve which divides into the supraorbital and supratrochlear nerves. It enters the orbit via the superior orbital fissure.

glossopalatine n. Intermediate nerve of Wrisberg.

infraorbital n. The continuation of the maxillary nerve as it passes the inferior orbital fissure to enter the orbit. It leaves the orbit by the infraorbital canal and gives origin to the inferior palpebral nerve, the nasal nerve, and the labial nerve.

infratrochlear n. A terminal branch of the nasociliary nerve that is sensory for the caruncle, the lacrimal sac, the canaliculi, and the medial portions of the eyelid and the conjunctiva.

intermediate n. of Wrisberg. A root of the facial nerve arising from the sensory nucleus, lateral and posterior to the motor root, containing parasympathetic fibers coursing to the lacrimal gland via the great superficial petrosal nerve which synapses in the sphenopalatine ganglion. It also contains sensory (taste) fibers to the anterior two thirds of the tongue and parasympathetic fibers to the glands of the palate and the nose and to the submaxillary and the sublingual salivary glands. Syn., *glossopalatine nerve.*

lacrimal n. A sensory branch of the ophthalmic nerve that enters the orbit by way of the superior orbital fissure and courses laterally to reach the lacrimal gland. Its superior division is sensory to the lacrimal gland and gives origin to the lateral palpebral nerve of the upper eyelid. Its inferior division has an anastomosis with the zygomaticotemporal nerve to receive sympathetic and parasympathetic fibers for the lacrimal gland.

n. of Luschka. Posterior ethmoidal nerve.

malar n. Zygomaticofacial nerve. *Obs.*

mandibular n. The third division of the trigeminal nerve consisting of two roots, a sensory root which comes from the Gasserian ganglion, and the motor root of the trigeminal. The two pass through the foramen ovale and join into one trunk. It is motor to the muscles of mastication and is sensory to the lower jaw region and the anterior two thirds of the tongue.

maxillary n. The second division of the trigeminal nerve which leaves the Gasserian ganglion, receives branches from the sphenopalatine ganglion, and then gives origin to the zygomatic nerve. After passing through the inferior orbital fissure into the orbit, it is known as the infraorbital nerve. It is sensory to the upper jaw and lower eyelid and contains autonomic fibers for the lacrimal gland. **superior m.n.** Maxillary nerve.

nasal n. 1. Anterior ethmoidal nerve. 2. A branch of the infraorbital nerve or of the sphenopalatine ganglion. 3. Nasociliary nerve.

nasociliary n. A branch of the ophthalmic nerve which receives most of the fibers of general sensation from the eyeball. It enters the orbit through the superior orbital fissure and gives origin to the anterior and posterior ethmoidal, the long ciliary, and the infratrochlear nerves and a sensory root to the ciliary ganglion.

oculomotor n. Cranial nerve

III. It originates from the lower ventral surface of the midbrain and is classified as a motor nerve. Its superior and inferior divisions enter the orbit through the superior orbital fissure. The superior division supplies the levator palpebrae superioris muscle and the superior rectus muscle. The inferior division supplies the medial and inferior rectus muscles and the inferior oblique muscle and also has parasympathetic fibers for the ciliary muscle and the sphincter pupillae muscle via a branch to the ciliary ganglion.

ophthalmic n. The first division of the trigeminal nerve which leaves the Gasserian ganglion, receives twigs from the III, IV, and VI cranial nerves, and divides into the nasociliary, the frontal, and the lacrimal nerves. It is sensory for the upper eyelids, eyebrows, forehead, eyeball, nose, and the air sinuses above and medial to the orbit.

optic n. Anatomically, cranial nerve II of the peripheral nervous system, but embryologically and histologically a "tract" of the central nervous system since it is a derivative of the forebrain containing neuroglia. The optic nerve receives over 800,000 fibers from the ganglion cells of the retina and contains some efferent fibers that end in the retina. Classified as a nerve of special sense, it is divided into intraocular, intraorbital, intracanalicular, and prechiasmal or intracranial portions. It leaves the orbit through the optic canal to enter the cranial cavity where it forms the optic chiasma.

orbital n. 1. The branches of the sphenopalatine ganglion which enter the orbit through the inferior orbital fissure and supply the periorbita and the orbital muscle of Mueller. 2. The zygomatic nerve. *Obs.*

palpebral n., inferior. A branch of the infraorbital nerve which supplies the lower eyelid.

palpebral n's., superior. Branches of the lacrimal, the frontal, and the nasociliary nerves which supply the upper eyelid.

pathetic n. Trochlear nerve. *Obs.*

petrosal n., deep. Sympathetic fibers from the carotid plexus for the lacrimal gland. It unites with the great superficial petrosal nerve to form the vidian nerve of the pterygoid canal.

petrosal n., great superficial. A branch of the facial nerve that carries parasympathetic fibers for the lacrimal gland and fuses with the deep petrosal nerve to form the vidian nerve of the pterygoid canal.

pterygoid canal n. Vidian nerve.

second cranial n. Optic nerve.

seventh cranial n. Facial nerve.

sixth cranial n. Abducens nerve.

spheno-ethmoid n. Posterior ethmoidal nerve.

sphenopalatine n. Either of two branches that join the sphenopalatine ganglion to the maxillary nerve and contain autonomic fibers for the lacrimal gland.

supraorbital n. The branch of the frontal nerve that passes through the supraorbital notch or foramen and is sensory for the upper eyelid, the conjunctiva, the eyebrow, the forehead, and the scalp up to the occipital bone.

supratrochlear n. The branch of the frontal nerve which anastomoses with the infratrochlear nerve and supplies the medial portions of the upper eyelid, the conjunctiva, and the eyebrow.

temporomalar n. Zygomatic nerve. *Obs.*

tentorial n. A branch of the ophthalmic division of the trigeminal nerve which supplies the tentorium and the dura mater over the posterior cranial fossa, and which, when stimulated intracranially, is considered to refer pain to the eyes or forehead.

third cranial n. Oculomotor nerve.

Tiedemann's n. The sympathetic fibers from the carotid plexus which course on the surface of the central retinal artery on into the retina. *Obs.*

trifacial n. Trigeminal nerve. *Obs.*

trigeminal n. Cranial nerve V. It originates from the lateral surface of the pons by a motor and a larger sensory root. The latter leads to the Gasserian ganglion which connects with the three divisions of the nerve, viz., ophthalmic, maxillary, and mandibular. It is sensory for the eyeball, the conjunctiva, the eyebrow, the skin of face and scalp, the teeth, the mucous membranes in the mouth and nose, and is motor to the muscles of mastication. Syn., *trifacial nerve.*

trochlear n. Cranial nerve IV. It

originates from the dorsal surface of the junction between the midbrain and the cerebellum and passes through the superior orbital fissure and is motor to the superior oblique muscle. Syn., *pathetic nerve.*

vidian n. The nerve of the pterygoid canal formed by the union of the deep petrosal and the great superficial petrosal nerves. It ends at the sphenopalatine ganglion and supplies parasympathetic and sympathetic fibers to the lacrimal gland. Syn., *pterygoid canal nerve.*

Wrisberg's n. See *nerve, intermediate of Wrisberg.*

zygomatic n. A branch of the maxillary nerve in the pterygopalatine fossa that enters the orbit by way of the inferior orbital fissure. It divides into the zygomaticofacial and zygomaticotemporal nerves and has sensory fibers for the skin of the cheek and the temple. It contains autonomic fibers for the lacrimal gland which enter a twig that leads to the lacrimal nerve. It leaves the orbit through the zygomatic foramen.

zygomaticofacial n. A terminal branch of the zygomatic nerve that supplies the skin just lateral to the eyelid and the skin of the cheek after passing through the zygomaticofacial canal.

zygomaticotemporal n. A terminal branch of the zygomatic nerve that passes through the zygomaticotemporal canal to enter the temporal fossa and supply the skin of the anterior temple and the forehead just above. The nerve may have a twig which conveys the autonomic fibers to the lacrimal nerve and gland. Syn., *malar nerve.*

◆

nerve fiber. See under *fiber.*

nerve loop, intrascleral (of Axenfeld). A loop formed by a variation in the course of a long ciliary nerve. After traversing the perichoroidal space, the nerve pierces the sclera a few millimeters behind the limbus, turns back on itself, retraces the same path, and then enters the ciliary body.

NET Orthoptor. A device designed for visual training in the home for the improvement of fusion, accommodative facility, and visual acuity. It is clamped to a spectacle frame and consists essentially of two apertures, both containing Polaroid filters, a mirror system before the right eye, controlled by a lever at the top to alter the direction of incident light, and lens holders for auxiliary trial lenses or Polaroid filters. Syn., *Natural Environment Trainer.*

Neumueller's tables. See under *table.*

neuralgia, trigeminal. Tic douloureux.

neurasthenia, optic (nu″ras-the′ne-ah). Neurasthenia accompanied by contraction of the visual fields. See also *neurasthenic visual field.*

neuritis (nu-ri′tis). Inflammation of a nerve or nerves.

hypertrophic n. A dominant, hereditary polyneuritis with symptoms including paresis of the extremities, muscular atrophy, peripheral sensory disturbances, possible lightning pains and visceral crises, pupillary disturbances such as anisocoria, myosis or pupillotonia and, occasionally, optic atrophy. Syn., *Déjerine-Sottas disease.*

optic n. Inflammation of the optic nerve that occurs in two principal forms, intraocular optic neuritis (papillitis) and retrobulbar optic neuritis. **axial o.n.** Optic neuritis in which there is a selective involvement of the papillomacular bundle in the optic nerve. **intraocular o.n.** Papillitis. **lactation o.n.** Optic neuritis occurring during the lactation period following childbirth. **orbital o.n.** Retrobulbar optic neuritis. **periaxial o.n.** Optic neuritis involving the peripheral interstitial tissues of the optic nerve, exclusive of the papillomacular bundle. **postocular o.n.** Retrobulbar optic neuritis. **pseudo o.n.** 1. A congenital abnormal elevation of the optic disk in which the nerve fibers are heaped and there is a neuroglial overgrowth. There are no accompanying hemorrhages or exudates and the vessels appear normal, although the disk margin may be ill-defined. 2. A mild hyperemia of the optic disk with slight blurring of its margins and some tortuosity and dilatation of the retinal vessels. The condition has been attributed to uncorrected errors of refraction, anemia, exposure to glare, or to congenital causes. **retrobulbar o.n.** Inflammation of the orbital portion of the optic nerve, usually without visible changes in the eyegrounds, and primarily occurring as an axial retrobulbar optic neuritis, although it may be periaxial or transverse. Characteristically there is a unilateral sudden loss of central vision with headache on the affected side, pain in the orbit, sluggishness of the pupil, and tenderness of the eyeball. The symptoms persist from two weeks to two months with gradual recovery, which is usually complete. The most common cause is multiple sclerosis, although it may be due to exogenous toxins and inflammatory general or local diseases. Syn., *orbital optic neuritis; postocular optic neuritis.* **spurious o.n.** Pseudo-optic neuritis. **transverse o.n.** Optic neuritis involving the entire cross section of the optic nerve.

optico-ciliary n. A rare orbital disease of unknown etiology characterized by lesions affecting the optic nerve and the ciliary ganglion. Symptoms include retrobulbar neuritis, iridoplegia, and cycloplegia.

n. papulosa. A rare disease, either unilateral or bilateral, occurring within the first two years of a syphilitic infection, characterized by a massive, sharply demarcated, grayish or yellowish exudate on the optic disk which protrudes into the vitreous and may extend onto adjacent retina. Vitreous opacities, patches of chorioretinitis, and hemorrhages, especially around the exudate, are also present. In the later stages the exudate becomes organized into connective tissue strands which extend from the disk and anchor in an atrophic patch of chorioretinitis. Vision is greatly reduced and may or may not be recovered.

postocular n. Retrobulbar optic neuritis.

n. retinae. Circumscribed exudative choroiditis.

neuroblastoma, retinal (nu″ro-blas-to′mah). Retinoblastoma.

neurochorioretinitis (nu″ro-ko″re-o-ret″ih-ni′tis). Inflammation of the optic nerve, the choroid, and the retina.

neurochoroiditis (nu″ro-ko″roid-i′tis). Inflammation of the optic nerve and the choroid.

neurocytoma (nu″ro-si-to′mah). A tumor of the retina or the central nervous system composed primarily of neurocytes.

neurodeatrophia (nu″ro-de″ah-tro′fe-ah). Atrophy of the retina.

neuroencephalomyelopathy (nu″ro-en-sef″ah-lo-mi″eh-lop′ah-the). Neuromyelitis optica.

neuroepithelioma, retinal (nu″ro-ep″e-the″le-o′mah). A congenital, malignant, neuroectodermal tumor of the retina, characteristically containing retinoblasts and large columnar cells which tend to arrange radially around a central cavity to form rosettes; a type of retinoblastoma.

neuroepithelium (nu″ro-ep″e-the′le-um). The epithelial structures containing receptor cells for special sense, as the neuroepithelial layer of the retina.

neurofibroma (nu″ro-fi-bro′mah). A fibrous tumor, usually benign, arising from the nerve sheath or the endoneurium. It occurs in either discrete or diffuse form (von Recklinghausen's disease) and in the eye may affect the choroid, the ciliary body, or the iris.

neurofibromatosis (nu″ro-fi-bro″mah-to′sis). Von Recklinghausen's disease.

neuroglia (nu-rog′le-ah). The nonconducting supportive structures of the central nervous system, the retina, and the optic nerve, occurring in three types, *astroglia, microglia,* and *oligodendroglia.*

neuromatosis, myelin (nu″ro-mah-to′sis). A congenital condition seen in infancy characterized by skull deformations, non-painful neurocytoma or neurinoma of the mucous membranes of the lips, tongue, esophagus, and eyes, facial freckles, and occasionally hypertrophic corneal nevi. Syn., *Froboese syndrome.*

neuromyelitis optica of Devic (nu″ro-mi″eh-li′tis op′te-kah). A self-limiting, demyelinating disease of the optic nerves, the optic chiasm, and the spinal cord, characterized by bilateral retrobulbar neuritis, usually accompanied by papillitis and transverse myelitis. Onset is usually acute, with almost complete blindness. In favorable cases there is restoration of vision, although central scotomata and hemianopsia may persist. The disease differs from multiple sclerosis in that relapses do not occur, it is more extensive, and results in greater destruction of the axis cylinders. Syn., *Devic's disease; encephalomyelitis optica; neuro-optic myelitis; neuroencephalomyelopathy; ophthalmoneuromyelitis.*

neuromyotonia, ocular (nu″ro-mi″o-to′ne-ah). A sudden extraocular muscle spasm initiated by peripheral-neurogenic pathological activity.

neuronal ceroid lipofuscinosis. Batten-Mayou disease.

neuro-ophthalmology (nu″ro-of″thal-mol′o-je). The branch of ophthalmology which deals particularly with the nervous system associated with the eye.

neuropapillitis (nu"ro-pap"ih-li'tis). Papillitis.

neuropathy, anterior ischemic optic (nu"rop'ah-the). An acute ischemic disorder of the anterior part of the optic nerve characterized by a cavernous degeneration of the optic nerve head, similar to a glaucomatous excavation, and believed to be due to sclerotic vascular disease within the optic nerve. A comparatively sudden partial or total loss of vision occurs in the presence of normal ocular tension and a normal facility of aqueous outflow. Abbreviation *AION.*

neuropathy, ataxic (nu-rop'ah-the). A syndrome of bilateral optic atrophy, nerve deafness, and posterior column myelopathy with or without polyneuropathy, occurring in poor Nigerians who eat cassava, a tuber with high cyanogenic glycoside content.

neuroretinitis (nu"ro-ret"ih-ni'tis). Inflammation of the optic nerve head and adjacent retina.

    n. descendens. Retinitis secondary to retrobulbar optic neuritis.

    diffuse syphilitic n. Neuroretinitis appearing in the second stage of syphilis characterized by swelling of the retina around the optic nerve head and blurring of the margins of the disk. The entire retina becomes gray, cloudy, and opaque, and dense, dustlike, vitreous opacities are usually present. Hemorrhages are few and the veins are tortuous and engorged. As the condition subsides, the vessels, particularly arteries, reduce in size and show marked sheathing, the disk becomes atrophic, and a migration of pigment assumes a characteristic bone corpuscle appearance, particularly in the periphery. Syn., *Jacobson's retinitis.*

    n. duplex. Bilateral neuroretinitis.

neuroretinopathy (nu"ro-ret"ih-nop'-ah-the). A disease of the optic nerve head and the retina.

neurotomy, opticociliary (nu-rot'o-me). Surgical cutting of the optic and ciliary nerves of one eye in an attempt to prevent sympathetic ophthalmia.

neutral. 1. Pertaining to a color which has neither hue nor saturation, such as gray, black, or white. 2. The absence of, or the transition between, "with" and "against" movement in the retinoscopic reflex.

    high n. In dynamic retinoscopy, the end point corresponding to the strongest convex or weakest concave lens in a range of dioptric values for which the reflex is neutral.

    low n. In dynamic retinoscopy, the end point corresponding to the weakest convex or the strongest concave lens in a range of dioptric values for which the reflex is neutral.

neutralization. 1. Hand neutralization. 2. The process or result of suppressing the perception of one eye while the other is fixating.

    absolute n. Constant involuntary neutralization as may occur in the deviating eye in strabismus. Syn., *suppression.*

    hand n. The method of determining the power of a spectacle lens by combining it with test lenses of known power until the resultant power is zero, especially when done by observing the motion or displacement of the image of an object viewed through the combination as it is held in the hand and moved back and forth in a plane perpendicular to the line of view.

    partial n. 1. Periodic involuntary neutralization. 2. Voluntary neutralization as may occur during the use of a monocular microscope. Syn., *suspenopsia; suspension.*

nevoxanthoendothelioma, intraocular (ne"vo-zan"tho-en-do-the"-le-o'mah). Nevoxanthoendotheliomatous involvement of the anterior uvea, and less frequently the epibulbar tissue, usually occurring in early life in association with skin lesions and characterized by yellowish-brown elevated lesions of the iris and ciliary body, spontaneous anterior chamber hemorrhages, and secondary glaucoma. Syn., *ocular juvenile xanthogranuloma.*

nevus (ne'vus). A circumscribed area of pigmentation or vascularization, usually in the form of a congenital benign neoplasm occurring in the skin or in various ocular tissues, as the conjunctiva, the iris, the choroid, the ciliary body, or the optic nerve.

    n. of Ota. Oculocutaneous melanosis.

Newman's theory (nu'manz). See under *theory.*

Newton's (nu'tonz) **color circle; colors; disk; formula; law; rings; color scale; color table; ring test; theory.** See under the nouns.

Newton-Mueller-Gudden law. See under *law.*

niacin (ni'ah-sin). Pyridine-3-carboxylic acid, a water soluble vitamin found in yeasts, egg yolk, liver, cereals, fresh meats, and some leafy vegetables. Deficiency in the diet is a main cause of pellagra and such eye signs as edema, dermatitis, and alopecia of the eyelids, conjunctivitis, keratitis, dustlike crystalline lens opacities, and optic neuritis. Syn., *nicotinic acid.*

nicking, A-V. The depression of a retinal venule into the tissue of the retina, where it is crossed by an overlying arteriole, primarily as a result of the thickening of the wall of the arteriole and the adventitial coat. It is one of the signs of hypertensive and/or arteriosclerotic retinopathy.

Nicol (nik'ol) **polarizer; prism.** See under *prism.*

nictation (nik-ta'shun). Nictitation.

nictitatio (nik"tih-ta'she-o). A clonic spasm of the eyelid.

nictitation (nik"tih-ta'shun). Winking.

Nieden syndrome. See under *syndrome.*

Niemann's disease (ne'manz). See under *disease.*

Niemann-Pick disease (ne'man-pik). See under *disease.*

night blindness. See under *blindness.*

night vision tester. A device for determining the lowest of eight scotopic levels of illumination at which an observer can discriminate the break in a large Landolt ring at a given test distance.

portable n. v. t. An instrument for measuring the threshold of dark adaptation at a testing distance of 15 in. It consists essentially of a black Landolt ring, subtending a visual angle of 2° on a background of self-luminous paint, the luminance of which can be controlled by a series of neutral density filters.

NIH. See *National Institute of Health.*

niphablepsia (nif'ah-blep'se-ah). Snow blindness. *Obs.*

niphotyphlosis (nif'o-tif-lo'sis). Snow blindness. *Obs.*

nit. A unit of luminance equal to 1 candela per sq. m. See also *footlambert.*

nivea (ni've-ah). Asteroid bodies.

nm. Abbreviation for *nanometer.*

NMFEC. National Medical Foundation for Eye Care. See *American Association of Ophthalmology.*

NOA. See *National Optometric Association.*

node. 1. A knot, knob, protuberance, or swelling, or an organ or a structure of such appearance. 2. The point on a wave or in a vibrating body which is absolutely or relatively free from vibratory motion; the point which undergoes minimum displacement. See also *antinode.*

Cajal's n's. Cytoid bodies.

cervical lymph n's., deep. Numerous lymph glands of varying size, located along the internal jugular vein, which drain lymph from the parotid and submaxillary lymph nodes and empty into the jugular trunk.

cervical lymph n's., superficial. Small lymph glands located at the ramus of the mandible bone and along the external jugular vein. They receive some lymph directly from ocular structures, but more lymph indirectly from the parotid and preauricular group of lymph nodes.

parotid lymph n's., deep. Lymph glands, located anterior to the ear and deep to the parotid salivary gland, which receive lymph from the conjunctiva of the entire upper eyelid and the lateral one third of the lower eyelid and drain into the deep cervical lymph nodes.

parotid lymph n's., superficial. Lymph glands, located anterior to the ear and superficial to the parotid salivary gland, which receive lymph from the lacrimal gland and the superficial structures of the lateral three quarters of the upper eyelid and the lateral one half of the lower eyelid. The glands drain into the superficial and deep cervical lymph nodes.

preauricular lymph n's. Superficial parotid lymph glands located anterior to the ear which receive lymph from the lacrimal gland.

submaxillary lymph n's. Four to six lymph glands, located between the lower jaw and the submandibular salivary gland, which receive lymph from the medial portions of the eyebrow, the eyelid, the conjunctiva, the caruncle, and the lacrimal drainage apparatus and drain into the deep cervical lymph nodes. Syn., *submandibular lymph nodes.*

nodule (nod'ūl). 1. A small, circumscribed, solid elevation. 2. A small node.

Bizzozero n's. Globular bodies arranged in regular rows between adjacent cellular membranes, found in the human corneal epithelium at the level of the basal and middle layers and considered to be related to, or a part of, the intercellular bridges (desmosomes).

Busacca's n's. Nodules frequently found in the iris of an eye affected with a low grade uveitis. They appear in the stroma as small, translucent, gray elevations and are formed by accumulations of epithelioid cells and lymphocytes, with no tissue loss. When appearing on the pupillary border, they are known as *Koeppe's nodules*.

Dalén-Fuchs n. A nodule found in isolated areas of the iris in eyes with sympathetic ophthalmia and caused by a swelling and proliferation of the cells of the pigment epithelium.

Koeppe's n's. Nodules frequently found in the iris of an eye affected with a low grade uveitis. They appear on the pupillary border as small, translucent, gray elevations and are formed by accumulations of epithelioid cells and lymphocytes, with no tissue loss. When appearing in the stroma of the iris, they are known as *Busacca's nodules*.

noncomitance (non-kom'ih-tans). Nonconcomitance.

noncomitancy (non-kom'ih-tan-se). Nonconcomitancy.

noncomitant (non-kom'ih-tant). Nonconcomitant.

nonconcomitance (non"kon-kom'ih-tans). The condition in which the angular relationship between the lines of sight of the two eyes is not constant, but varies with the direction of gaze, usually indicating paresis or paralysis of one or more extraocular muscles. Syn., *incomitance; incomitancy; noncomitance; noncomitancy.*

nonconcomitancy (non"kon-kom'ih-tan-se). Nonconcomitance.

nonconcomitant (non"kon-kom'ih-tant). Pertaining to or having nonconcomitance. Syn., *incomitant; noncomitant.*

nonius. See *method, nonius.*

Nonne-Marie syndrome (non'e-mar-e'). Marie's disease.

Nonne-Milroy-Meige disease (non'e-mil'roy-mehzh). See under *disease.*

nonreader. A child who has failed to learn to read although instructed by normally successful methods.

von Noorden-Burian experiment. See under *experiment.*

normal. 1. Perpendicular to the tangent of a curve or surface at the point of tangency. 2. Having a statistical value that can best be regarded as within the range of natural or normal distribution about the mean. 3. Typical, average, or natural, or free from disorders, distortions, or disease.

Normalsite lenses. See under *lens.*

Norrie's disease. See under *disease.*

Norris' theory (nōr'is). See under *theory.*

northlight. Daylight received only from northern sky areas. It is generally less variable in spectral quality than daylight received from other regions of the sky and the sun and has a bluish-white color.

No-scru. A type of rimless spectacle lens mounting employing a rivet and solder in place of a screw for holding the lenses in place.

nose glasses. See *spectacles, nose.*

nose pad. A guard.

nose piece. The bridge and guards of a spectacle frame or mounting.

notation. 1. The act, method, or process of representing by a system or a set of signs or figures. 2. Any system of signs, figures, or symbols used to express technical facts, quantities, etc.

Munsell n. Designation of hue, value, and chroma, in the 1,000 sample Munsell system. The original notation applies to the color samples of the 1929 Munsell *Book of Colors.* The Munsell renotation applies to a later method of designating the samples.

Ostwald n. Designation of the variables of the Ostwald system in the specification of a surface color. An arbitrary letter-number notation is used, the hue being designated by a number from 1 to 24, while the black content and the white content are indicated by arbitrary letters which are found by reference to charts of the system.

Snellen's n. See *fraction, Snellen's.*

Snell-Sterling n. The representation of visual efficiency as a function of visual acuity, according to the formula: $E = 0.836^{(1/s-1)}$ where s = the Snellen fraction. Syn., *Snell-Sterling visual efficiency scale.*

standard axis n. The spectacle lens axis scale for which the 0° is to the subject's left, 90° up, 180° to his right, adopted by an optical society in England in 1904, by the Technischer Ausschuss für Brillenoptik (TABO) in Germany in 1917, and by the Council of British Ophthalmologists in 1921. Syn., *TABO notation*. Cf. *axis scale*.

TABO n. Standard axis notation.

notch. An indentation or depression on the edge of a bone or other organ.

    Arnold's n. Frontal notch.

    frontal n. An indentation sometimes present just medial to the supraorbital notch on the medial superior orbital margin of the frontal bone which transmits medial branches of the supraorbital nerve, vein, and artery. Rarely, it becomes surrounded by bone to become the frontal foramen. Syn., *Arnold's notch; Henle's notch*.

    Henle's n. Frontal notch.

    supraorbital n. An indentation on the medial, superior, orbital margin of the frontal bone which transmits the supraorbital nerve, vein, and artery. Occasionally, it becomes surrounded by bone to become the supraorbital foramen.

Nothnagel's syndrome (nōt'nah-gelz). See under *syndrome*.

Nott's method (nots). See under *method*.

nox (noks). One thousandth of a *lux*.

NPC. Near point of convergence.

NSPB. See *National Society for the Prevention of Blindness*.

nu (*ν*). The Greek letter used as a symbol for the reciprocal of the *dispersive power* of a light-transmitting medium.

nubecula (nu-bek'u-lah). A nebula.

Nuckolls' test (nuk'olz). See under *test*.

◆

NUCLEUS

nucleus (nu'kle-us). 1. A collection of nerve cells in the central nervous system concerned with a common function. 2. A central mass, portion, or core.

    abducens n. A collection of the cell bodies of lower motor neurons located in the floor of the fourth ventricle in the lower portions of the pons. The axons from the nucleus enter the ipsilateral abducens nerve and supply the external rectus muscle.

    adult n. The outer portion of the nucleus of the crystalline lens between the infantile nucleus and the cortex, formed after puberty.

    anteromedian n. A group of parasympathetic preganglionic cell bodies lying rostroventral to both Edinger-Westphal nuclei and consid-

ered by some to be a rostral continuation of these nuclei. It is part of the oculomotor nuclear complex.

    basal optic n. Posterior optic tract nucleus.

    bulbospinal n. A group name for the principal sensory and the spinal nuclei of the trigeminal nerve.

    Cajal's n. Interstitial nucleus.

    caudal central n. An unpaired nucleus, separate from the nucleus of Perlia, which is thought to supply both the levator palpebrae superioris muscles.

    n. of the crystalline lens. The central core of the crystalline lens, surrounded by the cortex, which contains the oldest, more sclerosed, and less translucent lens fibers. Its zones of optical discontinuity are subdivided into *embryonic, fetal, infantile,* and *adult nuclei*. Y-sutures occur in the fetal nucleus and more complex lens stars occur in the infantile and adult nuclei.

    Darkschewitsch's n. A group of cells in the tegmentum of the midbrain, dorsal to the red nucleus, in the central gray matter near the aqueduct of Sylvius. It sends fibers into the medial longitudinal fasciculus. Syn., *nucleus of the posterior commissure*.

    dorsal n. 1. The main part of the external geniculate body, well developed in man and absent in lower vertebrates, which serves as a relay station for visual fibers in the optic tract. 2. A division of the lateral nucleus of the oculomotor nuclear complex.

    Edinger-Westphal n. The portion of the oculomotor nucleus containing preganglionic parasympathetic cell bodies of neurons which, via the oculomotor nerve, reach the ciliary ganglion and the episcleral ganglion to synapse with ganglionic neurons supplying the sphincter pupillae and ciliary muscles. It is the lower center for accommodation and pupillary constriction.

    embryonic n. The most central portion of the core of the crystalline lens formed during the first three months of intrauterine life and surrounded by the fetal nucleus. It contains the oldest lens fibers derived from the embryonic posterior epithelium of the lens.

    facial n. A collection of lower motor neuron cell bodies, located in the floor of the fourth ventricle in the lower pons, which are motor to the muscles of facial expression, including the orbicularis oculi, frontal, and corrugator supercilii.

fetal n. The portion of the nucleus of the crystalline lens lying between the embryonic and infantile nuclei and formed from the third to the eighth month of intrauterine life. It contains the Y-sutures of the lens.

Fuse's n. A supranuclear center for the co-ordination of lateral eye movements, located at the pons-medulla junction.

infantile n. The portion of the nucleus of the crystalline lens lying between the fetal and adult nuclei and formed from the eighth fetal month until puberty.

interstitial n. of Cajal. A scattered group of cells in the cerebral peduncle of the mid-brain, near the rostral end of the red nucleus, which extends dorsolaterally to send descending fibers into the medial longitudinal bundle. Fibers emerging from the superior colliculi and from the cortex, and going to the interstitial nucleus of Cajal, are considered to constitute pathways for cortical control of ocular movements.

lateral n. The portion of the oculomotor nucleus supplying the superior rectus, the inferior rectus, the internal rectus, and the inferior oblique muscles, and possibly the levator palpebrae superioris muscle.

mesencephalic n. of the trigeminal nerve. A group of unipolar cell bodies located lateral to the cerebral aqueduct of the mid-brain, which gives origin to the fibers of the mesencephalic root of the trigeminal nerve. It is involved in relaying sensory impulses from the muscles of mastication and possibly from the extraocular muscles.

oculomotor n. The nucleus of the oculomotor nerve located ventral to the superior colliculus of the midbrain and subdivided into the *Edinger-Westphal nucleus*, the *nucleus of Perlia*, the *lateral nucleus*, and the *caudal central nucleus*.

Perlia's n. A single (unpaired) mass of cells lying between the ventral nucleus and the dorsal nucleus of the oculomotor nuclear complex, not always present in man and of undetermined function.

pontine n. 1. Any collection of cell bodies of neurons in the pons, as in the abducens or the facial nuclei. 2. A

theoretical center for lateral gaze located near the abducens nucleus.

posterior accessory optic tract n. In quadrupeds, a group of cell bodies located ventrolaterally to the red nucleus, medial to the substantia nigra; and posterior to the mammillary body. It receives fibers from the posterior accessory optic tract and sends fibers to the substantia nigra, the oculomotor nucleus, the lateral reticular gray, and the interpeduncular nucleus. Syn., *basal optic nucleus; transverse peduncular tract nucleus.*

n. of the posterior commissure. Darkschewitsch's nucleus.

pregeniculate n. A small elongated mass of cells located within the lateral division of the optic tract, anterior to the main (*dorsal*) nucleus of the external geniculate body but having no continuity with it. In lower vertebrates it represents the entire geniculate, but is vestigial in man, probably having only photostatic functions. Syn., *ventral nucleus of external geniculate body.*

pretectal n. An oval group of cells located at the dorsal surface of the tecto-thalamic junction and internal to the superior colliculus, serving as a relay station for pupillary fibers.

principal sensory n. of the trigeminal nerve. A mass of cells located in the floor of the fourth ventricle, especially in the pons, where synapses occur with touch fibers in the sensory root of the trigeminal nerve.

spinal n. of the trigeminal nerve. The column of cells, extending from the lower pons to the middle of the cervical segments of the spinal cord, medially adjacent to the entire length of the spinal tract of the trigeminal nerve, in which the axons of the tract synapse. It is continuous with the principal sensory nucleus of the trigeminal nerve, courses through the medulla oblongata to end in the cervical cord, and is involved in relaying impulses for pain and temperature from the head region.

transverse peduncular tract n. Posterior accessory optic tract nucleus.

trochlear n. The collection of motor neuron cell bodies located in front of the inferior colliculus of the midbrain which supplies the contralateral superior oblique muscle.

ventral n. 1. A division of the lateral nucleus of the oculomotor nuclear complex. 2. Pregeniculate nucleus.

vestibular nuclei. A group of nuclei found in the region of the pons-medulla junction, named after Deiter, Bechterew, and Schwalbe, plus a descending spinal vestibular nucleus. They receive fibers from the vestibular nerve and send fibers into the medial longitudinal fasciculus to control the position of the eyes in relation to head position. The supranuclear center for lateral gaze may be located in this group.

◆

number. A symbol or digit expressive of a specified quantity, of a certain value, or of a designated place in a series or sequence.

Abbe's n. The nu (*v*) value.

blank n. A code number given to fused bifocal blanks which indicates the power of the reading addition of the finished lens for a specified base curve.

f n. The ratio of the focal length of an optical system to the diameter of the entrance pupil; reciprocal of the *relative aperture.*

T n. The lens f number adjusted to allow for loss by absorption and reflection, equal to the f number divided by the square root of the actual transmittance.

wave n. In light waves, the reciprocal of wavelength in centimeters; the number of waves per centimeter.

Numont. See *mounting, Numont.*

NUO. See *Nederlanse Unie van Opticiens.*

Nutt Auto-disc. See under *Auto-disc.*

NVOOB. Flemish: National Verbond der Optometristen en Opticiens van Belgie. See *Union Nationale des Optometristes et Opticiens de Belgique.*

NVRI. See *National Vision Research Institute* (Australia).

NVVO. See *Stichting Nederlandse Vakopleiding Voor Opticiens.*

nycotometer (nik″o-tom′eh-ter). An instrument for determining the threshold illumination for identifying form in the dark-adapted eye. It may also be used as an adaptometer.

nyctalope (nik′tah-lōp). An individual affected with nyctalopia.

nyctalopia (nik″tah-lo′pe-ah). A term used inconsistently to mean either night blindness or day blindness. Synonymous or autonymous with *hemeralopia.*

nyctotyphlosis (nik″to-tif-lo′sis). Nyctalopia.

Nyktometer (nik-tom′eh-ter). An instrument for testing visual acuity in the dark-adapted eye and changes in visual acuity upon sudden exposure to glare.

nystagmic (nis-tag′mik). Pertaining to or having nystagmus.

nystagmograph (nis-tag′mo-graf). An instrument for recording nystagmic movements of the eye.

nystagmography (nis″tag-mog′rah-fe). The study and recording of nystagmic movements of the eyes.

nystagmoid (nis-tag′moid). Resembling nystagmus.

◆

NYSTAGMUS

nystagmus (nis-tag′mus). A regularly repetitive, usually rapid, and characteristically involuntary movement or rotation of the eye, either oscillatory or with slow and fast phases in alternate directions. Syn., *spasmus oculi; talantropia.*

after n. Secondary nystagmus.

albinotic n. A hereditarily transmitted, pendular, usually horizontal, sometimes rotatory, nystagmus associated with albinism. General albinism is autosomal recessive, affecting both males and females, whereas ocular albinism is sex-linked recessive, affecting males only.

amaurotic n. A jerky or pendular nystagmus sometimes occurring in those who have been blind for a considerable time.

amblyopic n. Nystagmus associated with, or attributed to, reduced central vision.

aspiration n. Nystagmus produced by the aspiration of air from the external auditory meatus.

asymmetric gaze n. A horizontal nystagmus without a rotatory component, occurring in lateral gaze and commencing nearer the straightforward position, and more intensely on one side than the other. It indicates a lesion within the pons varolii, affecting one medial longitudinal bundle.

ataxic n. A unilateral nystagmus associated with impaired lateral conjugate movements occurring in disseminated sclerosis. In lateral movements the inturning eye is restricted and the outturning eye shows a lateral, jerky nystagmus. Syn., *Jayle-Ourgaud syndrome.*

aural n. Labyrinthine nystagmus.

Baer's n. A high frequency, fine nystagmus secondary to erosions or other superficial lesions of the cornea.

Bárány's n. Caloric nystagmus.

Bartels' cortical n. Nystagmus, reported by Bartels, due to paresis of conjugate ocular movements resulting from frontal lobe injury.

Bechterew's n. See *compensation, Bechterew's.*

caloric n. A vestibular nystagmus induced by thermal stimulation of the labyrinth of the inner ear, usually by the introduction of either cold or hot water into the external auditory canal. When cold water is used, the slow phase of the movement is toward the stimulated side; when warm water is used, it is toward the opposite side. Syn., *Bárány's nystagmus; thermal nystagmus.*

central n. A jerky nystagmus resulting from a lesion in either the vestibular nerve in its intracranial course, the primary vestibular nuclei, or their secondary connections.

central labyrinthine n. Central nystagmus.

cerebral n. A pendular nystagmus resulting from a lesion or a tumor of the cerebrum or its meninges.

coarse n. Nystagmus in which the angular range of excursion is over 15° . See also *fine nystagmus; medium nystagmus.*

compression n. An induced, labyrinthine nystagmus resulting from unilateral changes of pressure in the semicircular canals.

congenital hereditary n. A hereditarily transmitted binocular and pendular nystagmus, usually sex-linked dominant with variable penetrance, occurring in both males and females. It may be reduced in darkness. Close fixation may reduce the amplitude but increase the frequency, with the pendular motion becoming jerky; the response to optokinetic stimuli may be absent or inverted.

conjugate n. Nystagmus in which there is symmetry of amplitude, type, and direction of movement in the two eyes.

convergence n. An intermittent, abrupt, spasmodic, convergence movement in which the eyes move rhythmically toward each other and then slowly return to the original position, usually due to a tumor of the anterior aqueduct of Sylvius, the third ventricle, or the midbrain.

deficiency of light n. An ocular nystagmus sometimes occurring in children raised in dark surroundings.

deviational n. End-position nystagmus.

disjunctive n. Nystagmus in which there is symmetry of amplitude and type of movement in the two eyes but in opposite directions.

dissociated n. Nystagmus in which the amplitude, type, and/or direction of movement in the two eyes are unrelated.

down-beat n. Eccentric nystagmus in which the fast phase is downward and which is accentuated on gaze into the direction of the fast phase.

eccentric n. Nystagmus in which there is a position of gaze, usually eccentric, where the oscillatory movement is at a minimum and may be absent.

electrical n. Vestibular nystagmus induced by electrical stimulation of the labyrinth.

end-position n. A jerky, physiological nystagmus occurring in normal individuals when attempts are made to fixate a point at the limits of the field of fixation. Syn., *deviational nystagmus.*

essential n. Nystagmus occurring as a result of abnormal use of the eyes in certain occupations, such as *miners' nystagmus.*

ex amblyopia n. Variously pendular, jerky, and irregular nystagmus associated with extremely poor vision since birth for any reason, e.g., albinism, and inhibited by closing of the eyes.

fatigue n. Nystagmus as a result of fatigue caused by prolonged fixation at or near the limit of the field of fixation. Syn., *neurasthenic nystagmus.*

fine n. Nystagmus in which the angular range of excursion is less than 5°. See also *medium nystagmus; coarse nystagmus.*

first degree n. Nystagmus manifest only when fixation is in the direction of the quick component. See also *second degree nystagmus; third degree nystagmus.*

fixation n. 1. Nystagmus associated with attempts to fixate. 2. End-position nystagmus. 3. Ocular nystagmus.

Frenzel's hopping n. Nystagmus composed of two rapid phases with a short pause between, each phase starting and stopping abruptly.

galvanic n. A vestibular nystagmus induced by electrical stimulation of the labyrinth of the inner ear. When the anode is applied to one labyrinth, the slow phase of the movement is toward the stimulated side; when the cathode is used, it is toward the opposite side.

gaze-paretic n. Paretic nystagmus.

horizontal n. Lateral nystagmus.

hysterical n. Nystagmus occurring in hysteria and other psychopathic conditions in which the movements are generally rapid, pendular, and lateral.

idiopathic n. Nystagmus of unknown etiology.

inverse optokinetic n. An optokinetic nystagmus in which the more rapid excursion of horizontal movement occurs in the direction of the moving object, as may be manifested in subjects with congenital nystagmus of ocular origin, or with amblyopic nystagmus, or in normal persons when the fixation reflex is influenced by an eccentric afterimage during optokinetic stimulation.

irregular n. Nystagmus in which the movements are persistently unequal in duration, direction, and amplitude.

jelly n. A fine tremor of the eyes detectable only ophthalmoscopically by the rapid oscillation of the fundus structures. Syn., *quivering nystagmus*.

jerky n. Nystagmus characterized by a slow movement in one direction, followed by a rapid movement in the opposite direction to the original position. It is typical of vestibular nystagmus. Syn., *resilient nystagmus; rhythmic nystagmus; ruck nystagmus; springing nystagmus*.

labyrinthine n. A vestibular nystagmus resulting from stimulation, injury, or disease of the labyrinth.

labyrinthine end-position n. A first degree nystagmus, mixed lateral and rotatory, occurring when looking to the side and associated with other symptoms of labyrinthine irritation, such as vertigo.

latent n. Nystagmus induced by covering either of the two eyes but otherwise absent.

lateral n. Nystagmus in which the movements are from side to side.

medium n. Nystagmus in which the angular range of excursion is between 5° and 15°. See also *fine nystagmus; coarse nystagmus*.

miners' n. A nystagmus, usually pendular, occurring in coal miners after many years of working in dark, cramped conditions. The more complicated cases may develop an accompanying blepharospasm, photophobia, vertigo, loss of vision, and psychoneurosis.

mixed n. 1. Nystagmus in which a vertical or lateral movement is combined with a cyclorotatory movement. 2. Nystagmus which is pendular in one position of gaze and jerky in another.

motor-defect n. Nystagmus resulting from a neurological or labyrinthine lesion and usually of the jerky type. Cf. *sensory-defect nystagmus*.

muscle-paretic n. Paretic nystagmus.

neck-torsion n. In the newborn, nystagmus associated with horizontal ocular movements induced by torsion of the neck; in adults occurring when the vestibular reactions to rotation have been abolished by disease.

neurasthenic n. Fatigue nystagmus.

occupational n. Nystagmus acquired with prolonged exposure to working conditions prevailing in certain occupations.

ocular n. Nystagmus manifest when conditions of fixation are difficult or impossible. It includes *visual, end-position, optokinetic, paretic, latent*, and *miners' nystagmus*.

optical rotatory n. Optokinetic nystagmus.

opticomotor n. Optokinetic nystagmus.

optokinetic n. A physiological ocular nystagmus induced by the attempt to fixate objects rapidly traversing the visual field. Syn., *optical rotatory nystagmus; opticomotor nystagmus*.

oscillating (oscillatory) n. Pendular nystagmus.

paretic n. A first degree nystagmus occurring only in particular directions of gaze due to extraocular muscle paresis.

pendular n. Nystagmus in which there is a smooth, undulatory movement of equal speed in each direction. Syn., *oscillating nystagmus; undulatory nystagmus; vibratory nystagmus.*

periodic alternating n. A rare form of central nystagmus which alternately occurs for a finite period, ceases, and recurs in the opposite direction. The duration of the periods is from 1 to 6 minutes with pauses of a few seconds between.

peripheral n. 1. Vestibular nystagmus. 2. End-position nystagmus.

physiological n. Nystagmus which may be induced in normal individuals, such as *end-position nystagmus* or *optokinetic nystagmus.*

positional n. Nystagmus manifest or more pronounced when the head is in specific positions.

n. protractorious. The protrusion and retraction of the eyeball accompanying the pulse beat and respiration due to a slight variation of the amount of blood in the orbital tissues. Physiologically the displacement is slight, a few hundredths of a millimeter; pathologically it is more pronounced.

pseudo n. Pseudonystagmus.

pupillary n. A dilatation and contraction of the pupils occurring synchronously with nystagmus.

quivering n. Jelly nystagmus.

radiary n. Symmetric gaze nystagmus occurring during oblique eye movements and in the same meridian as the eye movements. It is usually indicative of multiple sclerosis or other related diseases.

railroad n. Optokinetic nystagmus, so named because it is manifested during observation of the passing landscape while riding on a railroad car or other rapidly moving vehicle.

reflex acoustic n. Nystagmus induced by a loud noise.

reflex sensory n. Nystagmus induced by sensory stimulation of the skin in the region of the ear.

resilient n. Jerky nystagmus.

retraction n. Nystagmus retractorius.

n. retractorius. A central nystagmus accompanied by a saccadic jerk of the eyeball backward into the orbit with each oscillation. It characteristically occurs on certain ocular movements and is considered to be caused by tumors or inflammatory conditions in or near the oculomotor nuclei, or by aberrant nerve innervation, as in Duane's syndrome.

rhythmic n. Jerky nystagmus.

rotary n. Rotatory nystagmus.

rotation n. A vestibular nystagmus induced by rotation of the head around any axis, clinically demonstrated by rotating a subject in a revolving chair.

rotatory n. Nystagmus in which the movements are in more than one plane, being a partial rolling of the eyeball around the anterior-posterior axis.

ruck n. Jerky nystagmus.

second degree n. Nystagmus manifest when fixation is straight ahead as well as in the direction of the quick component. See also *first degree nystagmus; third degree nystagmus.*

secondary n. A vestibular nystagmus manifest after the abrupt cessation of a rotation of the head, due to the tendency of the labyrinthine fluid to persist in its movement. Syn., *after nystagmus.*

seesaw n. A rare form of vertical nystagmus in which the movements of the two eyes are in opposite directions.

sensory-defect n. Nystagmus resulting from disturbances of vision and usually of the pendular type. Cf. *motor-defect nystagmus.*

springing n. Jerky nystagmus.

symmetric gaze n. A horizontal nystagmus without a rotatory component, occurring in lateral gaze and commencing before the end position, with equal movement to the right or left from the straightforward position and with equal intensity. It may be associated with nystagmus in upward gaze and is usually indicative of multiple sclerosis.

thermal n. Caloric nystagmus.

third degree n. Nystagmus constantly manifest regardless of the direction of fixation. See also *first degree nystagmus; second degree nystagmus.*

toxic n. Positional nystagmus induced by the ingestion of alcohol or of certain drugs such as barbiturates.

train n. Railroad nystagmus.

undulatory n. Pendular nystagmus.

unilateral n. 1. Nystagmus affecting only one eye. 2. Nystagmus manifest only when one eye is covered. See also *latent nystagmus*.

up-beat n. Eccentric nystagmus in which the fast phase is upward.

vertical n. Nystagmus in which the movements are up and down.

vestibular n. Nystagmus resulting from stimulation, injury, or disease of the labyrinth or of the vestibular nerves. It is typically jerky, fine, rapid, and of the lateral-rotatory type. Syn., *peripheral nystagmus*.

vibratory n. Pendular nystagmus.

visual n. An ocular nystagmus attributed to reduced central visual acuity.

voluntary n. A rapid alternating train of saccades, up to 80 per second, voluntarily producible by about 5% of the normal population.

◆

nystagmus-myoclonus. Rare congenital nystagmus associated with abnormal involuntary body movements.

nystaxis (nis-tak′sis). Nystagmus.

O. Abbreviation for *oculus*.

obcecation (ob″se-ka′shun). Partial or incomplete blindness.

obfuscate (ob-fus′kāt). To darken, as by reducing illumination; to dim, as by reducing vision; to obscure, as by creating mental confusion.

object. 1. That which is experienced as having location, dimensions, and physical properties. 2. That which is regarded in terms of its visible or luminous attributes, as the origin of reference for an optically formed image.

    o. distance. See under *distance*.

    o. glass. See under *glass*.

    o. plane. See under *plane*.

    o. point. See under *point*.

    o. ray. Incident ray.

    o. of regard. That object which is selectively receiving visual attention.

    o. space. See under *space*.

    test o. An object, pattern, or design used for vision testing.

objective. A single lens or doublet in a telescopic or microscopic system nearest the object, serving to converge light from points in the field of view.

    Dollond's o. The first achromatic doublet, designed by Dollond in 1757, consisting of a double convex crown glass lens cemented to a double concave flint glass lens.

    immersion o. A microscope objective used with the space between it and the cover glass filled with an oil having an index of refraction approximately the same as that of the objective and the cover glass, for the purpose of reducing loss of light from reflection.

oblique (ob-lēk′, ob-līk′). **astigmatism; axis; illumination; muscles; ray.** See under the nouns.

obliquity of the lens (ob-lik′wih-te). A tilted position of a lens, especially of the crystalline lens, which produces astigmatism.

O'Brien edge illusion; effect. See under *illusion*.

O'Brien test. See under *test*.

Obrig (o′brig) **Radius Dial Gauge.** See under *gauge*.

observer, standard ICI. A hypothetical observer whose color responses conform to those of a statistically computed mean derived from observers having normal color vision, as specified by the International Commission on Illumination.

occipitogram, visually evoked. Visual evoked cortical potential, as recorded through electrodes at the back of the head. Abbreviation *VEOG*.

occluder (ŏ-klūd′er). An opaque or translucent device placed before an eye to obscure or block vision.

    aero o. A rubber, cuplike occluder which completely covers the eye from the nose to the temple, containing holes for ventilation.

    Bangerter's graded o's. Adhesive plastic lens occluders of graded transparencies designed to reduce visual acuity in eight steps from 1.0 (20/20) to complete occlusion.

    Bell's o. A cuplike occluder which clips onto the back of a spectacle frame and is shaped so that its edges rest against the brow, the cheek, and the temple to block vision completely.

Chavasse o. Chavasse lens.

clip-over o. A plastic disk with clips to attach it to the front of a spectacle frame.

Doyne o. A cuplike occluder which clips onto the back of a spectacle frame and to the temple. It is so shaped that its edges rest against the brow, the cheek, and the temple to block vision completely.

expansion shield o. An occluder for blocking peripheral vision or for protecting the eye against air, dust, or glare, consisting essentially of a side shield that fits onto the eyewires of a spectacle frame and does not occlude vision through the spectacle lens.

half o. A lens, one half of which is covered with an opaque or translucent material.

Jamieson's o. A cuplike occluder of pliable rubber attached to the posterior surface of a spectacle lens by means of a small suction cup and shaped so that its edges rest against the brow, the cheek, and the temple to block vision completely.

Linder o's. Either of two types of soft plastic occluders, flesh color on the outside and black inside, each having three adjustable metal tabs for attachment to a spectacle frame. One, a patch type, covers the front of the lens, and the other, the cup type, covers the back of the lens and has an added flange to block peripheral vision.

Pap o. A cuplike occluder with clips for attachment to the back of a spectacle frame and with a cushioned ventilated edge which conforms to the brow, cheek, and temple to block vision completely.

polarizing o. An occluder consisting of two Polaroid lenses, one behind the other, with one lens in a fixed position and the other rotatable so as to vary the amount of light entering the eye.

Pugh's o. One of a series of four neutral filters of various densities which clip on to the front of a spectacle frame. Syn., *Pugh's visual acuity reducer.*

scientype o. Chavasse lens.

Vaccluder o. A plastic occluder with edges shaped to fit closely to the brow and orbital bone structure and attachable to the back surface of a spectacle lens by means of a rubber suction cup.

occlusio pupillae (ŏ-klu′ze-o pu′-pil-e).

Occlusion or covering of the pupil of the eye, as by a pathologically formed membrane.

occlusio pupillae lymphatica (ŏ-klu′ze-o pu′pil-e lim-fat′ik-ah). Occlusion or covering of the pupil of the eye by a pathologically formed membrane.

◆

OCCLUSION

occlusion (ŏ-klu′zhun). 1. The act of obscuring or blocking vision with an occluder, or the resulting condition. 2. Closure or blockage of a blood vessel.

bimesial o. Binasal occlusion.

binasal o. Obstruction of the nasal half of the field of view of each eye, used in the treatment of amblyopia and/or esotropia. Syn., *bimesial occlusion.*

blurring o. A reduction of vision by using a drug such as a cycloplegic, or a spectacle lens to induce a blur of the retinal image.

calibrated o. Graded occlusion.

chromatic o. A reduction of vision by the use of an optical color filter, usually red.

constant o. Occlusion during all hours other than during sleep.

diffusing o. A reduction of vision by diffusing the light entering the eye as with the use of an unpolished lens or a polished lens covered with frosted cellophane tape.

dimming o. A reduction of vision by the limiting of the quantity of light entering the eye as with a neutral density filter. Syn., *obscuring occlusion.*

direct o. Occlusion of the normal eye for the treatment of amblyopia and/or strabismus.

distorting o. A reduction of vision by distorting the retinal image with a rippled or pebbled surface lens, such as a Chavasse lens.

graded o. Partial obscuring of vision with one of a series of occluders, such as Bangerter's graded occluders, designed to reduce vision an intended amount. Syn., *calibrated occlusion.*

indirect o. Inverse occlusion.

inverse o. Occlusion of the amblyopic eye, a technique used in pleoptics before and between treatments for eccentric fixation. Syn., *indirect occlusion.*

Marlow's prolonged o. Occlusion of one eye for several days or weeks to determine more accurately the degree of heterophoria (especially vertical heterophoria) or to determine if symptoms of visual discomfort are due to binocular vision.

obscuring o. Dimming occlusion.

occasional o. Occlusion during specified or prescribed periods of activity.

opaque o. Exclusion of light from all or part of the field of vision by means of opaque material.

partial o. 1. The occlusion of a portion of the field of vision by covering part of the spectacle lens. 2. The reduction of vision, as with a neutral density filter. 3. Periodic or intermittent occlusion.

sneak o. A method used in the treatment of amblyopia in which a series of filters of increasing densities are placed before the nonamblyopic eye until it is totally occluded.

total o. 1. Occlusion of an eye in which both light and form vision are completely eliminated. 2. Occlusion of the entire visual field of an eye with a translucent or attenuating filter.

translucent o. Exclusion or partial destruction of form vision by means of translucent material such as an unpolished lens, or a polished lens covered with cellophane tape.

◆

ocellus (o-sel'us). A single light-sensitive cell or a group of such cells which function independently of each other; a primitive form of eye. Syn., *simple eye.*

composite o. A simple eye formed by the fusion of two or more ocelli.

ochronosis, ocular (o"kro-no'sis). Brownish pigmentation, usually bilateral, of the sclera in the intrapalpebral fissure in persons having an inherited inability to metabolize phenylalanine and tyrosine, resulting in the excretion of homogentisic acid in the urine (alkaptonuria). The pigmentation usually commences in middle age with patches or flecks which tend to merge into oval or triangular plaques. Pigmentation of the conjunctiva and cornea is a rare accompaniment.

octave, visible light (ok'tāv, -tiv). The visible spectrum regarded as a series of hues analogous in number to the tones in the musical octave, or as a spectral range fulfilling the condition that the longest wavelength is twice the shortest wavelength.

Ocucept. The trade name for an instrument consisting essentially of a clip to hold the upper eyelid up and away from the eyeball, and a tilted front surface mirror to permit viewing under the eyelid.

ocufilcon. The nonproprietary name of a hydrophilic material of which contact lenses are made.

ocul- (ok'ūl). A combining form denoting the *eye* or *ocular.*

ocular (ok'u-lar). 1. An eyepiece. 2. Pertaining to or of the eye.

ocular ballottement; bobbing; dominance; echogram; motility; myiasis; rosacea; spectres; tension; torticollis. See under the nouns.

ocularist (ok-u-lar'ist). One who designs, fabricates, and fits artificial eyes.

oculentum (ok"u-len'tum). An ophthalmic ointment.

oculi (ok'u-li). The plural of oculus; the eyes.

o. marmarygodes. Metamorphopsia.

o. unitas. Oculi uniter.

o. uniter. The two eyes as a unit, i.e., considered together or simultaneously, not separately. Abbreviation OU. Cf. *oculus uterque.*

o. uterque. Oculus uterque.

oculist (ok'u-list). A medical practitioner who limits his field to diseases and disorders of the eye and its appendages.

oculistics (ok-u-lis'tiks). The treatment of ocular diseases.

oculo- (ok'u-lo). A combining form denoting the *eye* or *ocular.*

oculoagravic (ok"u-lo-a-grav'ik). See *illusion, visual, oculoagravic.*

oculocentric (ok"u-lo-sen'trik). Pertaining to the eye as a center of reference. See *direction, oculocentric; localization, oculocentric spatial.*

oculodiagnostician (ok"u-lo-di"ag-nos-tish'an). One who practices iridodiagnosis.

oculofacial (ok"u-lo-fa'shal). Pertaining to both the eyes and the face.

oculofrontal (ok"u-lo-fron'tal). Pertaining to both the eyes and the forehead.

oculography (ok"u-log'rah-fe). The recording of eye positions and movements. See *electro-oculogram.*

photosensor o. Oculography effected by the differential photocell reception of red light reflected by the nasal and temporal limbi of the cornea.

oculogravic (ok″u-lo-grav′ik). See *illusion, visual, oculogravic.*

oculogyration (ok″u-lo-ji-ra′shun). Movement of the eyes.

oculogyric (ok″u-lo-ji′rik). Pertaining to or causing movements of the eyes. Syn., *ophthalmogyric.*

oculometer (ok″u-lom′eh-ter). Stigmatometer.

oculometroscope (ok″u-lo-met′re-skōp). An instrument used in retinoscopy, consisting of a battery of trial lenses mounted on a wheel to permit successive placement in front of the eyes.

oculomotor (ok″u-lo-mo′tor). 1. Pertaining to movements of the eye. 2. Pertaining to the oculomotor nerve.

oculomotorius (ok″u-lo-mo-tōr′e-us). Oculomotor nerve.

oculomycosis (ok″u-lo-mi-ko′sis). Any disease of the eye caused by a fungus.

oculonasal (ok″u-lo-na′zal). Pertaining to both the eye and the nose.

oculophrenicorecurrent (ok″u-lo-fren″ih-ko-re-kur′ent). Pertaining to the recurrent laryngeal and phrenic nerves involved in Horner's syndrome.

oculopupillary (ok″u-lo-pu′pih-lār-e). Pertaining to the pupil of the eye.

oculoreaction (ok″u-lo-re-ak′shun). See *reaction, ophthalmic.*

oculozygomatic (ok″u-lo-zi″go-mat′ik). Pertaining to both the eye and the zygomatic arch.

oculus (ok′u-lus) (pl. *oculi*). An eye.

   o. bovinus. Hydrophthalmos.

   o. bovis. Hydrophthalmos.

   o. bubulus. Hydrophthalmos.

   o. caesius. Glaucoma.

   o. dexter. The right eye. Abbreviation *OD.*

   o. duplex. A figure eight bandage covering both eyes. Syn., *binoculus.*

   o. elephantinus. Hydrophthalmos.

   o. lacrimans. Epiphora.

   o. laevus. The left eye. Abbreviation *OL.*

   o. leporinus. Lagophthalmos.

   o. purulentus. Hypopyon.

   o. simplex. A bandage covering only one eye. Syn., *monoculus.*

   o. sinister. The left eye. Abbreviation *OS.*

   o. unitas. Oculi uniter.

   o. uterque. The two eyes, both the one and the other, i.e., each one considered individually and separately. Abbreviation *OU.* Cf. *oculi uniter.*

OD, O.D. Abbreviation for: (1) *oculus dexter;* (2) *Doctor of Optometry.*

ODE. See *Optometric Development Enterprises.*

OEA. See *Optometric Editors Association.*

OEP. See *Optometric Extension Program Foundation, Inc.*

off-effect. The positive wave in an electroretinogram which follows, after a short latent period, the shutting off of the stimulus light.

Ogle's fixation disparity method for AC/A ratio. See under *method.*

Oguchi's disease (o-gōo′chēz). See under *disease.*

Ohara's disease. (o-har′ahz). Oculoglandular tularemia. See under *tularemia.*

OHS. See *Optometric Historical Society.*

OIC. See *Optical Information Council.*

OL. Abbreviation for *oculus laevus.*

OLA. See *Optical Laboratories Association.*

oligodacrya (ol″ih-go-dak′re-ah). A deficiency of tears.

Oliver's test (ol′ih-verz). See under *test.*

OMA. See *Optical Manufacturers Association.*

ommateum (om″ah-te′um). A compound eye, as in insects or crustaceans.

ommatidium (om″ah-tid′e-um). One of the group of functionally and structurally associated elements of the compound eye of arthropods. It consists of a surface corneal facet and an underlying crystalline cone which collect light, and a retinule, the receptor cells arranged in tubular form.

ommatophore (ŏ-mat′o-fōr). A movable tentacle bearing a compound eye at the tip, as found in some mollusks, such as the snail.

ommochromes (om-o-krōmz′). Pigments of unknown composition and function found in the eyes and integument of arthropods.

Omnitrainer (om″nih-trān′er). A haploscopic orthoptic instrument patterned after the Brewster stereoscope, with rotatable lenses for variable separation of optical centers, using both opaque and transilluminated targets, and having a built-in mechanism for providing variably intermittent illumination.

onchocerciasis (ong"ko-ser-si'ah-sis, -ki'ah-sis). Parasitic infection with the *Onchocerca volvulus,* characterized by nodules on the skin when caused by the adult filaria and by such ocular complications as keratitis, iridocyclitis, or retrobulbar neuritis when caused by the immature filaria. Syn., *Robles' disease.*

onyx (on'iks, o'niks). A gathering of pus behind the cornea, giving the appearance of a fingernail; hypopyon.

opacimeter (o"pah-sim'eh-ter). An instrument which measures the opacity, opaqueness, turbidity, or cloudiness of an optical medium.

opacity (o-pas'ih-te). 1. A discrete or generalized portion of certain normally transparent tissues or structures of the eye which has lost its usual degree of transparency and hence has become relatively opaque. 2. In photographic film, the ratio of incident to transmitted light.

   Berlin's o. The milky white opacity resulting from edema, seen in the macular area in commotio retinae.

   Caspar's o. A ring or latticelike opacity of the cornea resulting from contusion.

   Haab's band o. A circular opacity of the cornea characterized by the presence of bandlike stripes, which appear as glassy threads, on the posterior surface of the cornea. It is associated with buphthalmos and is due to tears in Descemet's membrane.

   peripheral concentric o's. Dustlike opacities of the crystalline lens which form circular lines and cloudy patches in the deep layers of the periphery, a form of *perinuclear punctate cataract.*

   senile annular o. Senile ring.

   Schirmer's o. A threadlike opacity of the cornea resulting from contusion of the cornea.

   Vossius ring o. Vossius ring cataract.

   whorl-shaped o. Vortex corneal dystrophy.

opalescence (o"pal-es'ens). The milky iridescence seen in certain media, such as the opal.

opalescent (o"pal-es'ent). Pertaining to the property of opalescence.

opaque (o-pāk'). Impervious to light; not transparent or translucent.

operculum oculi (o-per'ku-lum ok'-u-li). The eyelid.

ophryitis (of're-i'tis). Inflammation in the region of the eyebrow.

ophryosis (of're-o'sis). Spasm in the region of the eyebrow.

ophryphtheiriasis (of'rif-thi-ri'ah-sis). Infestation of the eyebrows and the eyelashes with lice. Also spelled *ophryphthiriasis.*

ophrys (of'ris). The eyebrow.

Ophthaine (of'thān). A trade name for proparacaine hydrochloride.

ophthalmacrosis (of-thal"mah-kro'-sis). Enlargement of the eyeball.

ophthalmagra (of'thal-ma'grah, -mag'-rah). Sudden pain in the eyeball.

ophthalmalacia (of'thal-mah-la'she-ah). Ophthalmomalacia.

ophthalmalgia (of'thal-mal'je-ah). Pain in the eyeball.

ophthalmatrophia (of'thal-mah-tro'fe-ah). Atrophy of the eyeball; phthisis bulbi.

ophthalmecchymosis (of'thal-mek"-ih-mo'sis). An extravasation of blood into the tissue of the conjunctiva.

ophthalmectomy (of'thal-mek'to-me). Surgical removal of the eyeball; enucleation or excision of the eyeball.

ophthalmencephalon (of'thal-men-sef'ah-lon). The neural mechanism of vision: the retina, the optic nerves, the optic chiasm, the optic tracts, the optic radiations, the visual centers, etc.

ophthalmia (of-thal'me-ah). Inflammation of the eye, particularly one involving the conjunctiva; conjunctivitis.

   actinic o. Actinic conjunctivitis.

   ante-partum o. Inflammation of the fetal eye, prior to birth. Syn., *ophthalmia fetalis.*

   o. arida. Xerosis of the conjunctiva; xerophthalmia.

   Brazilian o. Xerosis of the conjunctiva resulting from malnutrition.

   catarrhal o. Catarrhal conjunctivitis.

   caterpillar hair o. Nodular conjunctivitis.

   eczematous o. Phlyctenular conjunctivitis.

   Egyptian o. Trachoma.

   electric o. Conjunctivitis resulting from excessive exposure to a high tension electric spark or arc.

   o. externa. Paralysis of the extraocular muscles.

   o. fetalis. Ante-partum ophthalmia.

   gonorrheal o. Gonococcal conjunctivitis.

   granular o. Trachoma.

o. hepatica. Degenerative changes in the uveal tract and the retina and xerosis of the conjunctiva, associated with disease of the liver.

infectious o. Infectious keratitis.

o. lenta. Behçet's disease.

o. migratoria. Sympathetic ophthalmia attributed to bacterial transmission via channels in the intervaginal spaces of the optic nerves and the chiasm.

military o. Trachoma.

o. neonatorum. Gonococcal conjunctivitis in the newborn.

neuroparalytic o. Neuroparalytic keratitis.

o. nivialis. Snow blindness.

o. nodosa. Nodular conjunctivitis.

phlyctenular o. Phlyctenular conjunctivitis.

purulent o. Purulent conjunctivitis.

pustular o. Phlyctenular conjunctivitis in which one or more phlyctenules have purulent contents.

scrofulous o. Phlyctenular conjunctivitis.

spring o. Vernal conjunctivitis.

strumous o. Phlyctenular conjunctivitis.

sympathetic o. Sympathetic ophthalmitis.

o. tarsi. Seborrheic meibomianitis.

varicose o. Conjunctivitis associated with varicosity of the conjunctival veins.

war o. Trachoma.

ophthalmiac (of-thal'me-ak). One affected with ophthalmia.

ophthalmiater (of-thal'me-a"ter, of-thal"me-a' ter). An ophthalmologist or an oculist. *Obs.*

ophthalmiatrics (of-thal"me-at'riks). Ophthalmology, especially with emphasis on medical treatment as distinct from the science itself. *Obs.*

ophthalmiatrist (of'thal-mi'ah-trist). One engaged in the medical treatment of the eye and its appendages. *Obs.* Syn., *ophthalmologist.*

ophthalmic (of-thal'mik). Pertaining to the eye or to related functions, services, or materials.

ophthalmic artery; ganglion; lens; nerve; optics; vein. See under the nouns.

ophthalmics (of-thal'miks). The science related to the testing, measurement, and treatment of the eye and its functions, especially in the nonmedical aspects.

ophthalmitic (of-thal-mit'ik). Pertaining to ophthalmitis.

ophthalmitis (of"thal-mi'tis). Inflammation of the eye.

sympathetic o. A bilateral inflammation of the uveal tracts following a uniocular perforating wound involving uveal tissue or the retention of a foreign body in an eyeball. The inflammation appears first in the injured eye (exciting eye) and follows in the other eye (sympathizing eye). It usually commences with an iridocyclitis and follows a progressive chronic course until all vision is lost, unless the exciting eye is enucleated. Syn., *sympathetic ophthalmia.*

ophthalmo- (of-thal'mo). A combining form denoting the *eye.*

ophthalmoblennorrhea (of-thal"mo-blen-o-re'ah). Purulent conjunctivitis.

ophthalmobrachytes (of-thal"mo-brah-kit'ēz). A myopic eye. *Obs.*

ophthalmocace (of"thal-mok'ah-se). Disease of the eye. *Obs.*

ophthalmocarcinoma (of-thal"mo-kar-sih-no'mah). Carcinoma of the eye.

ophthalmocele (of-thal'mo-sēl). Exophthalmos.

ophthalmocentesis (of-thal"mo-sen-te'sis). Surgical puncture of the eyeball.

ophthalmochromoscopy (of-thal"mo-kro-mos'ko-pe). Ophthalmoscopy utilizing colored light.

ophthalmocopia (of-thal"mo-ko'pe-ah). Asthenopia.

ophthalmodiagnosis (of-thal"mo-di"ag-no'sis). Diagnosis of an infectious disease, such as tuberculosis, by means of the sensitivity reaction of the conjunctiva to the instillation of a drop of a weak solution or suspension of the bacterial products, such as tuberculin.

ophthalmodiaphanoscope (of-thal"mo-di"ah-fan'o-skōp). An instrument for viewing the interior of the eye by means of transillumination.

ophthalmodiaphanoscopy (of-thal"mo-di"ah-fan-os'ko-pe). Examination of the interior of the eye by transillumination.

ophthalmodiastimeter (of-thal"mo-di"as-tim'eh-ter). An instrument for determining the separation of the lines of sight where they intersect the spectacle plane.

ophthalmodonesis (of-thal"mo-do-ne'sis). A trembling motion of the eye.

ophthalmodynamometer (of-thal"-mo-di"nah-mom'eh- ter). 1. An instrument for measuring blood pressure of the retinal vessels by determining the pressure necessary to collapse them. 2. An instrument devised by Landolt for determining the near point of convergence, consisting of a hollow cylinder containing a lamp and a tape marked in centimeters and in meter angles. A vertical, illuminated slit in the cylinder is moved toward the eyes until it appears double.

ophthalmodynamometry (of-thal"-mo-di"nah-mom'eh-tre). 1. Measurement of the blood pressure of the retinal vessels with the ophthalmodynamometer. 2. Determination of the near point of convergence with the ophthalmodynamometer.

ophthalmodynia (of-thal"mo-din'e-ah). Pain in the eye.

ophthalmo-eikonometer (of-thal"-mo-i-ko-nom'eh-ter). An instrument for measuring aniseikonia, the refractive error by stigmatoscopy, and the phoria.

ophthalmofluorescence (of-thal"mo-floo"o-res'ens). Fluorescence of tissues of the eye or its adnexa that have been stained with fluorescein or similarly acting solutions.

ophthalmofundoscope (of-thal"mo-fun'do-skōp). An apparatus for examining the fundus oculi under magnification; an ophthalmoscope.

Ophthalmograph (of-thal'mo-graf). An instrument which records eye movements during reading by photographing, on a moving strip of film, light reflected from the corneae.

ophthalmography (of'thal-mog'rah-fe). 1. Description of the anatomy of the eye. 2. Photography of eye movements with the Ophthalmograph.

ophthalmo-iconometer (of-thal"mo-i-ko-nom'eh-ter). Ophthalmo-eikonometer.

ophthalmokopia (of-thal"mo-ko'pe-ah). Asthenopia.

ophthalmoleukoscope (of-thal"mo-lu'ko-skōp). A color perception testing instrument in which the color intensities are controlled by polarizing filters to produce a white mixture.

ophthalmolith (of-thal'mo-lith"). A calculus of the lacrimal duct.

ophthalmologist (of'thal-mol'o-gist). A medical practitioner who is versed in and specializes in ophthalmology.

ophthalmology (of'thal-mol'o-je). 1. The profession or the professional services and applied science concerned with the medical and surgical care of the eye and its appendages. 2. The science which treats of the structure, the functions, and the disease of the eye and its appendages.

ophthalmoluminescence (of-thal"mo-lu"mih-nes'ens). Luminescence of the tissues of the eye or its adnexa.

    primary o. The luminescence of tissues of the eye or its adnexa resulting from illumination with ultraviolet light, without the use of fluorescein or similarly acting solutions.

    secondary o. The luminescence of tissues of the eye or its adnexa that have been stained with fluorescein or a similarly acting solution.

ophthalmolyma (of-thal"mo-li'mah). Destruction of the eye.

ophthalmomacrosis (of-thal"mo-mah-kro'sis). Enlargement of the eyeball; buphthalmos. *Obs.*

ophthalmomalacia (of-thal"mo-mah-la'she-ah, -se-ah). Abnormally low intraocular pressure of the eye; hypotension.

ophthalmomanometer (of-thal"mo-mah-nom'eh-ter). An instrument for determining intraocular pressure, consisting essentially of a glass tube partially filled with colored water having a rubber diaphragm at one end and a branched rubber tube at the other. One branch is attached to a mercurial manometer and the other to a rubber bulb. The instrument is placed with its diaphragm against a plane surface and the level of the colored water is noted. Then the diaphragm is placed against the eye, and the rubber bulb is employed to supply air pressure to return the colored water to its original level. The pressure in millimeters of mercury is then read directly from the manometer.

ophthalmomelanoma (of-thal"mo-mel"ah-no'mah). A melanoma of the eye.

ophthalmomelanosis (of-thal"mo-mel"ah-no'sis). 1. Abnormal pigmentation of the eye by melanin. 2. The formation of an ophthalmomelanoma.

ophthalmometer (of′thal-mom′eh-ter). An instrument for measuring the anterior curvatures of the cornea, consisting of a luminous pattern of mires whose images, produced by reflection on the cornea, are viewed through a telescope with which is combined a doubling and image size measuring system. Syn., *keratometer*.

ophthalmometrology (of-thal″mo-meh-trol′o-je). The science of measurement of visual functions.

Ophthalmetron, Safir. Trade name of an infra-red, electro-optical instrument which rapidly scans, tracks, and plots graphically the conjugate foci of the retina in all meridians to provide a printout of the eye's refractive status.

ophthalmometroscope (of-thal″mo-met′ro-skōp). An ophthalmoscope adapted or designed to determine the refraction of the eye.

ophthalmometry (of″thal-mom′eh-tre). The measurement of the curvature of the anterior surface of the cornea with the ophthalmometer. Syn., *keratometry*.

   reflection point o. A method used in peripheral ophthalmometry enabling the region of the cornea being measured to be located in reference to its distance from the corneal intersection of the line of sight. A precalculated table indicates this location for a given radius of curvature of the cornea and for a given rotation of the line of sight from the optical axis of the instrument.

ophthalmomycosis (of-thal″mo-mi-ko′sis). Any fungus disease of the eye or its appendages.

ophthalmomyiasis (of-thal″mo-mi′-yah-sis, -mi-i′ah-sis). Invasion of the eye by the larvae of flies.

   anterior o. Internal ophthalmomyiasis affecting the anterior chamber of the eye.

   external o. Ophthalmomyiasis affecting the conjunctiva.

   internal o. Ophthalmomyiasis affecting the interior of the eye.

   posterior o. Internal ophthalmomyiasis affecting the posterior chamber of the eye.

ophthalmomyitis (of-thal″mo-mi-i′-tis). Inflammation of the extraocular muscles. Syn., *ophthalmomyositis*.

ophthalmomyositis (of-thal″mo-mi″-o-si′tis). Ophthalmomyitis.

ophthalmomyotomy (of-thal″mo-mi-ot′o-me). Myotomy of the extraocular muscles.

ophthalmoncus (of″thal-mon′kus). A tumor involving the eye. *Obs.*

ophthalmoneuritis (of-thal″mo-nu-ri′tis). Inflammation of the ophthalmic nerve.

ophthalmoneuromyelitis (of-thal″-mo-nu″ro-mi-el-i′tis). Neuromyelitis optica.

ophthalmonosology (of-thal″mo-no-sol′o-je). The science which treats of, or classifies, diseases of the eye.

ophthalmopathy (of′thal-mop′ah-the). Any disease of the eye.

   external o. Any disease of the conjunctiva, the cornea, or the adnexa of the eye.

   internal o. Any disease of the retina, the crystalline lens, or other internal structure of the eye.

ophthalmophacometer (of-thal″mo-fa-kom′eh-ter). A modification of the ophthalmometer, using the principle of the Purkinje images, for determining the curvatures and positions of the surfaces of the crystalline lens and the cornea.

ophthalmophacometry (of-thal″mo-fa-kom′eh-tre). The determination of the curvatures and positions of the surfaces of the crystalline lens and cornea with the ophthalmophacometer.

ophthalmophantom (of-thal″mo-fan′-tom). A model of the eye used for demonstration or for practicing surgery.

ophthalmophasmatoscopy (of-thal″-mo-fas″mah-tos′ko-pe). Ophthalmospectroscopy.

ophthalmophlebotomy (of-thal″mo-fle-bot′o-me). Surgical opening of a conjunctival vein to relieve congestion.

ophthalmophore (of-thal″mo-fōr′). Ophthalmotrope.

ophthalmophthisis (of′thal-mof′thih-sis). 1. Phthisis bulbi. 2. Ophthalmomalacia.

ophthalmophyma (of-thal″mo-fi′mah). A tumor of the eyeball. *Obs.*

ophthalmoplasty (of-thal′mo-plas″te). Reparative or plastic surgery of the eye or of its appendages.

ophthalmoplegia (of-thal″mo-ple′je-ah). Paralysis of one or more ocular muscles.

   exophthalmic o. 1. Limitation of movement of the eyes occurring in exophthalmos. 2. Malignant exophthalmos.

   external o. Paralysis of the extraocular muscles. **hereditary e.o.** A hereditary and familial progressive external ophthalmoplegia, generally accompanied by ptosis, which usually develops in early life or is present at birth. Originally considered to be the result of degeneration of the nuclei of the nerves supplying the extraocular muscles, it is now thought to be a muscular dystrophy. Syn., *von Graefe's ophthalmoplegia; progressive nuclear ophthalmoplegia.*

Féréol-Graux o. Féréol-Graux ocular palsy.

von Graefe's o. External hereditary ophthalmoplegia.

internal o. Paralysis of the intrinsic muscles of the eye, i.e., the dilator pupillae, the sphincter pupillae, and the ciliary muscles.

internuclear o., anterior. Paralysis of an internal rectus muscle for lateral conjugate movements, considered to be due to a lesion in contralateral ascending fibers of the medial longitudinal fasciculus. The external rectus muscle on the side of the lesion functions normally, and both internal rectus muscles contract normally in convergence. Syn., *Lhermitte's ophthalmoplegia; anterior internuclear palsy; Bielschowsky-Lutz-Cogan syndrome.*

internuclear o., posterior. Paralysis of an external rectus muscle for lateral conjugate movements, considered to be due to a lesion in homolateral descending fibers of the medial longitudinal fasciculus. Both internal rectus muscles function normally in convergence and in lateral conjugate movements. Syn., *posterior internuclear palsy.*

Lhermitte's o. Anterior internuclear ophthalmoplegia.

nuclear o. Ophthalmoplegia due to lesions in the nuclei of the motor nerves of the eye. **progressive n.o.** External hereditary ophthalmoplegia.

partial o. Ophthalmoplegia in which only some of the muscles are affected.

progressive congenital o. Progressive nuclear ophthalmoplegia present at birth.

Sauvineau's o. Ophthalmoplegia in which there is paralysis of the internal rectus muscle of one eye and spasm of the external rectus muscle of the other.

supranuclear o. Ophthalmoplegia due to lesions in the upper brain stem above the nuclei of the motor nerves of the eye.

total o. Ophthalmoplegia affecting all the muscles of the eye and resulting in immobility of the eyes, ptosis, immobility of the pupil, and paralysis of accommodation.

ophthalmoplegic (of-thal″mo-ple′jik). Pertaining to paralysis of the ocular muscles (ophthalmoplegia).

ophthalmoplethysmography (of-thal″mo-pleth″iz-mog′rah-fe). Measurement of changes in the blood volume of the eye.

ophthalmoptosis (of-thal″mop-to′sis). Exophthalmos.

ophthalmo-reaction. See *reaction, ophthalmic.*

ophthalmorrhagia (of-thal″mo-ra′-je-ah). Hemorrhage of the eye.

ophthalmorrhea (of-thal″mo-re′ah). A discharge from the eye.

o. externa. A discharge from the eyelid.

o. interna. A discharge from the eyeball.

ophthalmorrhexis (of-thal″mo-rek′-sis). Rupture of the eyeball.

ophthalmos (of-thal′mos). The eye.

ophthalmoscope (of-thal′mo-skōp). An instrument for viewing the fundus and the interior of the eye, consisting essentially of: (1) a mirror, a prism, or other optical system used in conjunction with a light source for illuminating the interior; (2) a viewing aperture or optical system. More modern instruments have built-in illumination sources and auxiliary lens batteries for compensating for errors of refraction of the observer and patient, or for viewing anterior portions of the eye.

binocular o. A large, table model ophthalmoscope featuring a binocular viewing system permitting magnified, erect, stereoscopic observations of fundus structures. The optical paths of the two viewing systems and the optical path of the illuminating system penetrate the pupil in separate areas to prevent interference from corneal reflections. Syn., *stereo-ophthalmoscope.*

hand o. A simple ophthalmoscope which may be held in the observer's hand, usually consisting of a mirror or a reflecting prism to control the illumination and a peephole as the viewing system, though modern ones have attached sets of small lenses which may be revolved in front of the peephole, and built-in illumination systems in the handle and the body of the instrument.

luminous o. An ophthalmoscope with a built-in light source.

May o. A hand ophthalmoscope using a May prism.

nonluminous o. An ophthalmoscope which reflects light from a separate, external source.

photographic o. Fundus camera.

polarizing o. An ophthalmoscope in which the light in the illuminating system and the light in the viewing system are made to pass through oppositely oriented polarizing media, thus eliminating the reflexes from the specular surfaces of the ocular media.

reflecting o. An ophthalmoscope which does not contain its own light source, reflecting light from an external source into the eye.

ophthalmoscopic (of-thal″mo-skop′-ik). Pertaining to or with the ophthalmoscope.

ophthalmoscopist (of″thal-mos′ko-pist). One who does ophthalmoscopy.

ophthalmoscopy (of″thal-mos′ko-pe). The examination of the interior of the eye with the ophthalmoscope.

direct o. Direct ophthalmoscopic observation, at close range, of the virtual, upright, fundus image formed by the patient's eye in combination with whatever lenses are needed to correct for the refractive errors of the observer and patient; the technique normally employed with the hand ophthalmoscope.

fluorescein o. Ophthalmoscopic observation through a blue filter subsequent to intravenous injection of fluorescein.

indirect o. Ophthalmoscopic observation, usually at approximately arm's length, of the real, inverted, anteriorly located aerial image of the fundus as formed by the patient's eye itself in combination with whatever auxiliary lenses are needed to make the combination highly myopic, and ordinarily with the aid of a lens serving as a viewing eyepiece near the observer's eye. The conventional hand ophthalmoscope can be employed in this manner, and most table model ophthalmo-scopes are designed on the principle of indirect ophthalmoscopy.

metric o. Ophthalmoscopy done as a means of determining the refractive error.

red-free o. Ophthalmoscopic observation through a blue-green filter, rendering the nerve fiber structure more discernible, and blood vessels and hemorrhages more sharply outlined.

red light o. Ophthalmoscopic observation through a red filter, giving sharper contrast to the pigmentation and less contrast to blood vessels and hemorrhages.

telescopic o. Ophthalmoscopy employing a telescopic viewing system for virtual and erect magnification.

yellow-green light o. Ophthalmoscopic observation through a yellow-green filter rendering maximum definition and contrast to blood vessels and hemorrhages. Retinal nerve fibers are discernible, but not as clearly defined as in red-free ophthalmoscopy.

ophthalmospasm (of-thal′mo-spazm). A spasm of an ocular muscle.

ophthalmospectroscopy (of-thal″-mo-spek-tros′ko-pe). The ophthalmoscopic and spectroscopic examination of the interior of the eye. Syn., *ophthalmophasmatoscopy.*

ophthalmospintherism (of-thal″mo-spin′ther-izm). The visual sensation of luminous sparks without corresponding physical stimuli.

ophthalmostatometer (of-thal″mo-stah-tom′eh-ter). An exophthalmometer.

ophthalmostatometry (of-thal″mo-stah-tom′eh-tre). Exophthalmometry.

ophthalmosteresis (of-thal″mo-ste-re′sis). Absence or loss of one or both eyes. *Obs.*

ophthalmosynchysis (of-thal″mo-sin′kih-sis). 1. Effusion into the interior of the eye. *Obs.* 2. Mixing of the humors of the eye. *Obs.*

ophthalmothermometer (of-thal″-mo-ther-mom′eh-ter). An instrument for determining the local temperature of the eye.

ophthalmotomy (of″thal-mot′o-me). Incision, dissection, or enucleation of the eye. *Obs.*

ophthalmotonometer (of-thal″mo-to-nom′eh-ter). An instrument for determining ocular tension; a tonometer.

ophthalmotonometry (of-thal″mo-to-nom'eh-tre). Determination of ocular tension with the ophthalmotonometer.

ophthalmotrope (of-thal'mo-trōp). An apparatus for demonstrating the individual actions of the extraocular muscles, consisting essentially of a model eyeball to which are attached strings and pulleys to duplicate the lines of force of the muscles. Syn., *ophthalmophore.*

ophthalmotropia (of-thal"mo-tro'pe-ah). Strabismus.

ophthalmotropometer (of-thal"mo-tro-pom'eh-ter). Strabismometer.

ophthalmotropometry (of-thal"mo-tro-pom'eh-tre). Strabismometry.

ophthalmovascular (of-thal"mo-vas'-ku-lar). Pertaining to or of the blood vessels of the eye.

ophthalmoxerosis (of-thal"mo-ze-ro'-sis). Xerosis of the conjunctiva.

ophthalmula (of-thal'mu-lah). A scar of the eyeball.

ophthalmus (of-thal'mus). The eye.

ophthalmyalos (of"thal-mi'ah-los). Vitreous humor. *Obs.*

ophthalmyalus (of"thal-mi'ah-lus). Vitreous humor. *Obs.*

Ophthetic (of-thet'ik). A trade name for proparacaine hydrochloride.

ophthoscope (of'tho-skōp). A device for determining sighting ocular dominance. It consists essentially of a double-faced mirror covered on each side with cardboard, with tubes inserted into a hole in the cardboard on each side of the mirror. The subject is asked to look into one of the tubes and to look for an eye. The eye used is considered to be the sighting dominant eye.

-opia (o'pe-ah). A combining form denoting *eye*, especially in relation to a condition or defect.

-opy (o'pe). A combining form denoting *eye*, especially in relation to a condition or defect.

opifex circumductionis (o'pe-fex ser"kum-duk'she-on-is). Superior oblique muscle. *Obs.*

opisthosynechia (o-pis"tho-sih-nek'-e-ah, -sih-ne'ke-ah). Posterior synechia. *Obs.*

Oppel-Kundt visual illusion (op'el-koont). See under *illusion, visual.*

Oppenheim's (op'en-hīmz) **reflex; test.** See under the nouns.

-ops. A combining form denoting the *eye*.

-opsia (op'se-ah). A combining form denoting *vision.*

opsin (op'sin). A protein formed, together with retinene, by the chemical breakdown of *meta*-rhodopsin.

opsiometer (op"se-om'eh-ter). Optometer.

opsionosis (op"se-o-no'sis, -on'o-sis). Defective vision.

-opsis (op'sis). A combining form denoting *vision.*

opsoclonus (op-so-klo'nus). Irregular, nonrhythmic, rapid, noncontrollable conjugate movements of the eyes, in horizontal and vertical directions, as may occur as a sequel to nonepidemic encephalitis.

-opsy (op'se). A combining form denoting *vision.*

Opt. D. Abbreviation for *Doctor of Optometry. Obs.*

optepaphist (op-tep'ah-fist). One who is skilled in and practices optepaphy.

optepaphy (op-tep'ah-fe). The prescribing and adapting of corneal lenses to the human eye.

optesthesia (op"tes-the'ze-ah). Visual sensibility; the capacity to perceive visual stimuli.

optic (op'tik). Pertaining to or of vision, or the eye.

optic angle; atrophy; axis; bundle; canal; cap; capsule; center; chiasm; commissure; constants; cup; disk; foramen; ganglion; groove; lobes; nerve; neuritis; papilla; pedicle; peduncle; pits; plate; radiations; stalk; thalamus; tracts; ventricle; vesicle. See under the nouns.

optic pseudo-atrophy of the newborn. Papilla grisea.

optical (op'tih-kal). Pertaining to or of the science of optics, vision, the eye, or lenses.

optical activity; aphasia; axis; center; circle; constringence; contact; cross; density; diameter; glass; illusion; index; invariant; length; medium; path; rotation; surface; system; wedge; zone; zone of cornea. See under the nouns.

Optical Information Council. A public information disseminating agency sponsored by the optical industry of England.

Optical Laboratories Association. An American association of firms which fabricate and assemble prescription eyewear and related materials for delivery to dispensing ophthalmologists, optometrists, and opticians, formed in 1962 to serve the interests and needs of the industry. Formerly the Optical Wholesalers Association.

Optical Manufacturers Association. An American association of firms which manufacture eyewear, eyewear components, and related products, founded in 1916 to serve the interests and needs of the industry.

Optical Society of America. An organization formed in 1916 to increase and diffuse the knowledge of optics in all its branches, pure and applied, to promote the mutual interest of investigators of optical problems, of designers, manufacturers, and users of optical instruments and apparatus of all kinds, and to encourage cooperation among them.

Optical Wholesalers Association. See *Optical Laboratories Association.*

optically (op'tih-kal-le). With reference to optics; by optics or sight; by optical means.

optician (op-tish'an). 1. One whose vocation involves the design or manufacture of ophthalmic appliances or optical instruments or one who compounds and adapts ophthalmic prescriptions. 2. A dispensing optician. 3. An ophthalmic optician.

  dispensing o. One who fits and adapts eyewear to the wearer, especially on prescription of the ophthalmologist or optometrist. Syn., *ophthalmic dispenser.*

  laboratory o. Prescription optician.

  manufacturing o. One employed in the manufacture of optical instruments or eyewear.

  ophthalmic o. British designation, or equivalent, for *optometrist.*

  prescription o. One employed in the fabrication or assembly of spectacles to prescription.

  refracting o. Ophthalmic optician.

  wholesale o. One engaged in the sale of optical supplies and products in varying quantities to ophthalmic dispensers, ophthalmologists, optical retailers, and optometrists.

opticianry (op-tish'an-re). The work of the optician as a vocation.

opticist (op'tih-sist). A person skilled in the science of optics.

opticochiasmic (op"tih-ko-ki-as'mik). Pertaining to or of both the optic nerve and the optic chiasm.

opticociliary (op"tih-ko-sil'e-ar"e). Pertaining to or of both the optic nerve and the ciliary nerves.

opticocinerea (op"tih-ko-sin-e're-ah). The gray matter of the optic tract.

opticomalacia (op"tih-ko-mah-la'she-ah). A degeneration of tissue in the optic nerve usually due to lack of normal circulation.

opticopupillary (op"tih-ko-pu'pih-lār"e). Pertaining to or of both the optic nerve and the pupil.

◆

OPTICS

optics (op'tiks). 1. The science which treats of light, its nature, properties, origin, propagation, effects, and perception. 2. The elements and/or design of an optical system.

  acoustical o. The branch of optics concerned with the interaction of light and sound waves in a medium.

  adaptive o. The optics involved in a system which corrects or counteracts the undesired effect of atmospheric or other media turbulence on light propagation by sensing a wavefront distortion and adjusting quite instantly an optical element, such as an electronically deformable mirror, to neutralize or cancel the effect.

  atmospheric o. The branch of optics concerned with the optical and visual phenomena associated with atmospheric conditions.

  biological o. The branch of optics which deals with the effect of radiant energy on tissues, especially ocular tissues.

  coated o. The elements of an optical system that have been coated with a metallic salt to reduce, by interference, the amount of light reflected. See *lens, coated.*

  environmental o. The branch of optics concerned with environmental factors relating to vision and visually facilitated performance, especially as applied to groups and populations categorized by occupation or other behavioral identity. Syn., *environmental vision.*

  fiber o. 1. The branch of optics which deals with the conduction of light along a transparent dielectric cylinder such as a fiber of glass. 2. Very fine flexible glass rods which transmit light longitudinally by internal reflection.

Gaussian o. A simplified representation of the fundamental relations between object-space and image-space of an axially symmetrical optical system of small aperture and limited extent of field expressed in terms of the focal points or planes, a pair of conjugate points or planes, nodal or principal, and the ratio of the refractive indices of the first and last media of the system.

geometrical o. The branch of optics which deals with the geometric analysis of the paths of light in refraction and reflection.

matrix o. Optics expressed in terms of the algebra of matrices.

mechanical o. Ophthalmic optics.

mirror o. Catoptrics.

ophthalmic o. The branch of optics involving the design, manufacture, fabrication, assembly, and dispensing of spectacles.

physical o. The branch of optics which deals with the fundamental physical properties of light, especially in relation to its origin, propagation, spectrum, diffraction, interference, polarization, and velocity.

physiological o. The branch of optics concerned with visual perception; the science of vision.

psychological o. The branch of optics concerned with visual sensation and perception as psychological processes.

quantum o. The branch of optics which deals with the quantum theory of light emission.

schlieren o. See *system, optical, schlieren.*

wave o. The science of optics based on radiation as a wave function.

◆

opticus (op′tih-kus). Optic nerve.

optimeter (op-tim′eh-ter). Optometer.

optist (op′tist). Optometrist. *Obs.* A title proposed by Prentice before adoption of the title optometrist.

opto- (op′to). A combining form denoting *vision* or the *eye.*

optoblast (op′to-blast). A large ganglion cell in the ganglionic cell layer of the retina.

optogram (op′to-gram). The picture on the retina of a retinal image due to the bleaching of rhodopsin.

optokinetoscope (op″to-kih-net′o-skōp). An instrument to induce optokinetic nystagmus, consisting essentially of a revolving drum with alternate black and white vertical stripes parallel to the axis of rotation.

optomeninx (op″to-me′ninks). Retina.

optometer (op-tom′eh-ter). Any of several objective or subjective devices for measuring the refractive state of the eye. Syn., *opsiometer; optimeter; refractometer.*

Badal's o. A simple optometer mounted so that the focal point of the converging lens or lens system coincides with a variously specified point of reference of the eye, such as its anterior focal point, the entrance pupil, or the nodal point, for which a known fixed relationship between object and image size can be computed, and with reference to which point the dioptric stimulus to accommodation can be represented on a linear scale marking the distance from the test chart to the lens.

Cardell o. A subjective optometer containing miniature test types and astigmatic test charts scaled to correspond to standard test distances.

coincidence o. of Fincham. An objective optometer which forms the image of a fine line target on the subject's retina to be viewed by the examiner through a telescope with an optical doubling and displacing system so that the resulting two half lines are out of alignment, and blurred, in relation to the ametropia. The adjustment of the dioptric stimulus value of the fine line target necessary to obtain sharpness and alignment of the two half lines gives a measure of the ametropia.

Donders' wire o. A small rectangular frame across which are stretched several fine black vertical wires, to be viewed against a white background and brought toward the eye to determine the nearest point of distinct vision. A small handle and measuring tape are attached. Syn., *hair optometer.*

Guyton o. An examinee-operated subjective refractor which provides a line target for astigmatism measurement and Snellen letters for sphere and acuity determination and is combined with a semi-programmed examination sequence.

hair o. Donders' wire optometer.

infrared o. An optometer which utilizes infrared rather than visible energy to determine the refractive state of the eye without interference with vision.

laser o. Laser Refractor.

objective o. An optometer containing an optical system for determining the vergence of light reflected from the subject's retina.

prism o. Prisoptometer.

Schmidt-Rimpler o. An instrument consisting of a convex lens (+10.00 D) mounted on a sliding carrier near the distal end of a graduated rod, the proximal end of which rests on the inferior orbital rim of the subject, and with a spring-wound measuring tape mounted on the sliding carrier and attached to a concave mirror ophthalmoscope which reflects the light from an externally located luminous grid through the convex lens into the examinee's eye. When the examinee's retinal image of the luminous grid is seen distinctly by the examiner, the refraction may be computed from the positions of the convex lens and the mirror image of the luminous grid.

simple o. The combination of a simple plus lens and an independently movable test target for varying the dioptric stimulus and measuring the refractive state of the eye subjectively.

subjective o. An optometer employing the criterion of blurredness or sharpness of a test target.

Young's o. A simple optometer incorporating Scheiner's double pupillary aperture and a thread extended along the line of sight. The thread is seen double, crossing at the point for which the eye is focused.

Optometricana. A collection of facts, anecdotes, pictures, documents, relics, and other assorted archival materials pertaining to optometry as a cultural and historical entity.

Optometric Development Enterprises. An agency of the American Optometric Association operating as a business to print, publish, assemble, stock, and sell materials, books, and various other office and clinical supplies utilized primarily by optometrists.

Optometric Editors Association. An international association of editors of optometric journals and newsletters formed in 1957 in the United States as the Association of State Optometric Journal Editors and, for a period later, as the Association of Optometric Editors to work cooperatively toward the improvement of optometric publishing.

Optometric Extension Program Foundation, Inc. Originally the Optometric Extension Program, a non-profit organization founded in 1928 to provide support for research in vision and to offer continuing education programs and materials to optometrists and their assistants by subscriptions.

Optometric Historical Society. An international association, founded in 1969, consisting of persons interested in optometry's heritage and the preservation of optometricana.

optometrist. A person qualified and authorized to practice optometry in all of its aspects.

optometry. 1. The profession or the professional services and applied science concerned with vision, the practice of which may include any part or all of the services and care involved in the determination and evaluation of the refractive status of the eye and of other physiological attributes and functions directly subserving vision, and in the selection, design, provision, and adaptation of optical and optically related corrective measures, aids, and counsel for the preservation, maintenance, improvement, and enhancement of visual performance. 2. The use of an optometer.

differential o. (Archaic) Use of an optometer to measure the difference between the refractive errors of the eye in the principal meridians.

functional o. Tenets of optometric theory which as a group reflect the overriding view that most measurable ocular traits are potentially modifiable and that a structural anomaly should first be regarded as the result rather than the cause of visual stress. Cf. *structural optometry.*

public health o. The branch of optometry which deals with the epidemiology of clinical anomalies, the biostatistics of ocular conditions, the systems, regulations, and socio-economic factors affecting the delivery and quality of optometric services, and the role of the optometrist in community health maintenance.

structural o. Tenets of optometric theory which as a group reflect the overriding view that most measurable ocular traits are not readily modifiable by other than drastic measures and that a structural anomaly, from whatever cause, is usually irreversible and as such should be regarded as a potential cause of visual stress. Cf. *functional optometry.*

optomyometer (op"to-mi-om'eh-ter). An instrument for measuring phorias or fusional convergence consisting essentially of 2 tubes, 20 in. long, one of which can be moved horizontally and the other vertically, and through which targets at the distal ends are viewed.

optophone (op'to-fōn). An instrument which converts light waves into sound waves, enabling the blind to discern between light and dark.

optophore (op'to-fōr). An instrument for the stimulation of an amblyopic eye, consisting essentially of a horizontal viewing tube, pivoted on a vertical axis, fitted at its distal end with a slide carrier containing two highly colored, illuminated, transparent targets which may be rotated in opposite directions, producing a kaleidoscopic effect.

optostriate (op-to-stri'āt). Pertaining to the optic thalamus and the corpus striatum or, when these two structures are considered as one, the optostriate body.

optotype (op'to-tīp). Test type used for determining visual acuity. Snellen's original name for his test type.

ora serrata (o'rah seh-ra'tah). The serrated anterior border of the retina located approximately 8.5 mm from the limbus and adjacent to the pars plana of the ciliary body. It is one of the sites of attachment of the retina to the choroid, the other being around the optic disk.

orange. A hue simulating that of an orange, corresponding to the spectral wavelength of approximately 600 mμ, and having the qualitative aspect of a red and yellow additive mixture.

    transient o. An intermediate product of the decomposition of rhodopsin when exposed to light; an unstable carotenoid pigment which is transformed rapidly to xanthopsin and then to retinene.

orbicularis oculi (or"bik-u-la'ris ok'u-li). See under *muscle.*

orbiculus ciliaris (or-bik'u-lus sil"e-ar'is). Pars plana.

orbit (or'bit). One of the two cavities in the skull which contains an eyeball, orbital

fat, extraocular muscles, the optic nerve, etc. It is formed by parts of 7 bones: the maxillary, the palatine, the frontal, the sphenoid, the ethmoid, the lacrimal, and the zygomatic, and is shaped roughly like a quadrilateral pyramid.

orbita (or'bih-tah). The orbit.

orbital (or'bih-tal). Pertaining to or of the orbit.

orbital abscess; cellulitis; decompression; fascia; fat; fold; index; margin; periosteum; periostitis; phlegmon; septum; tubercle. See under the nouns.

orbitale (or"bih-tah'le, -ta'le). The lowest point on the inferior margin of the orbit.

orbitography (or-bih-tog'raf-e). The recording of the orbit and its contents, usually by means of x-ray photography subsequent to retrobulbar injection of a positive opaque or a negative gaseous material.

orbitonometer (or"bih-to-nom'eh-ter). An instrument for measurement of the compressibility of the orbital contents into the orbit.

orbitonometry (or"bih-to-nom'eh-tre). Measurement of the compressibility of the orbital contents into the orbit.

orbitopneumography (or"bih-to-nu-mog'rah-fe). X-ray photography of the orbit subsequent to the retrobulbar injection of air.

orbitopneumotomography (or"bih-to-nu"mo-to-mog'rah-fe). Sectional x-ray photography of the orbit subsequent to the retrobulbar injection of air.

orbitotomy (or"bih-tot'o-me). Surgical incision into the orbit.

organs, accessory of the eye. The appendages or adnexa of the eye, consisting of the *lacrimal apparatus,* the *conjunctiva,* the *cilia,* the *supercilia,* the *eyelids,* the *extraocular muscles,* and *Tenon's capsule.*

organs of Hesse. Large photosensitive ganglion cells in the ventral and lateral portions of the posterior end of the nerve cord in *Amphioxus,* giving it directional ability. Each cell has a ciliated margin capped by a crescentic pigment mantle and has an issuing nerve fiber.

organelle, optic (or"gan-el'). An ellipsoidal, transparent hyalinelike structure in the photosensitive cells of worms and molluscs which is surrounded by a dense neurofibrillar network (retinella). Light striking this structure from any direction is brought to a focus on the retinella and initiates impulses to its nerve fiber.

organization, perceptual. The sensory attribution of one or another pattern of organization to a complex field, possibly in the interest of meaningfulness or economy of comprehension or retention, as in perceiving the digits 3825 as 38 and 25.

organon visus (or'gan-on vi'sus). The organ of vision; the eye.

orthochromatic (or"tho-kro-mat'ik). Pertaining to or of the reproduction of natural color, as in color photography.

Orthofusor (or'tho-fu'sor). An orthoptic training device consisting of a series of vectographic stereo pictures representing varying degrees of stimulus to convergence and divergence when viewed binocularly through a pair of Polaroid filters oppositely oriented in front of the two eyes.

Orthogon (or'tho-gon). A trade name for a series of corrected curve spectacle lenses.

orthokeratology (or"tho-ker"ah-tol'o-je). The science or program of therapeutic application of contact lenses to alter the curvature of the cornea, especially to reduce myopia.

orthokinesis (or"tho-kih-ne'sis). Acceleratory or deceleratory random movements of a motile organism in response to changes in the intensity of light stimulation but not in response to the direction of the light stimulation.

Ortholite (or'tho-līt). A trade name for an incandescent lamp, with a dark purple filter attachment, used in conjunction with fluorescein dye in the fitting of contact lenses and for the detection of corneal abrasions, or ulcers.

orthometer (or-thom'eh-ter). Exophthalmometer.

Ortho-Nez Spring Clamp Spectacle Frame. See under *frame.*

orthophoria (or"tho-fo're-ah). The condition in which the lines of sight, in the absence of an adequate fusion stimulus, intersect at a given point of reference, this point of reference usually being the point of binocular fixation prior to the phoria test, or, more arbitrarily, at an infinite distance; the absence of heterophoria.

asthenic o. The condition of orthophoria in combination with low relative convergence reserves.

basic o. Orthophoria obtained with the test object at infinity and the eyes actually or artificially emmetropic, hence with accommodation relaxed.

relative o. Orthophoria with reference to a given fixation distance, said to be present when dissociation produces no deviation of convergence from that otherwise demanded for the fixation distance.

sthenic o. The condition of orthophoria in combination with normal relative convergence reserves.

orthophoric (or"tho-fōr'ik). Manifesting, or one who manifests, orthophoria.

orthophorization (or"tho-fo"rih-za'shun). A process presumed to be operative in producing a greater frequency of occurrence of orthophoria, or only small amounts of heterophoria, than would be expected in terms of chance distribution, as may be explained by postulating a control of binocular coordination by higher visual centers.

orthopic fusion (ōr-tho'pik). See under *fusion.*

orthopsia (or-thop'se-ah). The condition of having normal vision.

orthoptic (or-thop'tik). Pertaining to orthoptics, its procedures and instruments.

orthoptics (or-thop'tiks). 1. The teaching and training process for the improvement of visual perception and coordination of the two eyes for efficient and comfortable binocular vision. Syn., *visual training; vision training.* 2. The teaching and training process for the elimination of strabismus.

chrome o. Orthoptics based on the use and application of colored filters, usually with implications of therapeutic value in the colors themselves.

orthoptist (or-thop'tist). One who practices, directs, or supervises orthoptic services.

orthoptoscope (or-thop'to-skōp). A type of amblyoscope.

Ortho-Rater (or"tho-ra'ter). A Brewster-type stereoscopic instrument for visual screening, with targets for measuring visual acuity, phorias, stereopsis, and color perception.

orthoscope (or'tho-skōp). 1. A device which neutralizes the refracting power of the cornea by means of a layer of water in a small glass container held in contact with the eye. 2. A Brewster-type stereoscope having an adjustment for interpupillary distance and a lens system designed to reduce aberrations. It is used primarily for visual screening and for testing aniseikonia.

orthoscopic (or-tho-skop'ik). 1. Affording a correct and undistorted view. 2. Pertaining to an orthoscope, orthoscopy, or an orthoscopic lens or optical system. 3. Pertaining to an optical system which produces an image free of distortion or aberration. 4. Pertaining to the condition of normal vision.

orthoscopy (or-thos'ko-pe). 1. Examination of the eye with an orthoscope. 2. That condition of an optical system which produces an image free of distortion or aberration.

orthostatic (or"tho-stat'ik). Pertaining to the condition of orthostasis.

orthostasis (or"tho-sta'sis). A term used by Lancaster to designate the static position of the covered eye, during a cover test, when orthophoria is present.

orthostereogram (or"tho-ster'e-o-gram"). A stereogram which fulfills the condition of orthostereoscopy.

orthostereoscopy (or"tho-ster"e-os'-ko-pe). The viewing of a stereopsis-inducing pattern so as to perceive the original scene in true dimensional proportions, both as to size and distance, the retinal images being identical to those from viewing the actual scene. This relief is produced when the focal length of the stereocamera is the same as that of the stereoscope, and the separation of the stereocamera lenses is the same as the viewer's interpupillary distance. Cf. *heterostereoscopy*.

Orthotrainer (or"tho-trān'er). A Brewster-type, stereoscopic, visual training instrument with carriers for transilluminated split targets and a rotor for providing various flash patterns. The separation of the split targets may be held constant for various viewing distances or may be varied by means of a disparator attachment.

orthotropia (or"tho-tro'pe-ah). 1. The absence of strabismus. 2. With respect to a given meridian of reference, a strabismus of zero angle of deviation, e.g., lateral orthotropia with right hypertropia.

OS. Abbreviation for *oculus sinister;* the left eye.

OSA. See *Optical Society of America.*

os. A bone.

    o. ethmoidale. Ethmoid bone.

    o. frontale. Frontal bone.

    o. lacrimale. Lacrimal bone.

    o. opticus. A horseshoe-shaped formation of single or multiple pieces of bone in the cartilaginous cup surrounding the optic nerve head in some avian eyes. Syn., *ossicle of Gemminger.*

    o. planum. The lamina papyracea of the ethmoid bone.

    o. sphenoidale. Sphenoid bone.

    o. unguis. Lacrimal bone.

    o. zygomaticum. Zygomatic bone.

oscillopsia (os"ih-lop'se-ah). The condition in which viewed objects appear to oscillate; oscillating vision.

O'Shea's rule (o-shāz'). See under *rule.*

Osler's disease (ōs'lerz). Rendu-Osler disease. See under *disease.*

Osler-Vaquez disease. (ōs-ler'-vak'-āz). Vaquez' disease.

osmotherapy (oz"mo-ther'ah-pe). Intravenous injection of a hypertonic solution to produce dehydration, a procedure sometimes performed to reduce ocular tension.

ossicle of Gemminger (os'ih-kl). Os opticus.

ossicles, scleral (os'ih-klz). A ring of overlapping membranous bones which acts as a supporting structure at the centrally constricted area of the eyes of some birds and reptiles.

osteitis deformans (os"te-i'tis defōr'mans). Paget's disease.

osteitis fibrosa, disseminated (os"-te-i'tis fi-bro'sah). Polyostotic fibrous dysplasia.

osteodystrophy, fibrous (os"te-o-dis'-tro-fe). Polyostotic fibrous dysplasia.

osteogenesis imperfecta (os"te-o-jen'e-sis im-per-fek'tah). A familial disease characterized by brittle bones which fracture easily. It may be accompanied by blue sclerae and frequently by deafness. Syn., *periosteal dysplasia; fragilitas ossium; osteopsathyrosis.*

osteoma (os"te-o'mah). A slowly progressive benign neoplasm composed of osteoblastic connective tissue that forms new bone. It may occur in the choroid, sclera, or episclera, on the wall of the orbit, or it may invade the orbit from a neighboring sinus.

osteopetrosis (os"te-o-pe-tro'sis). A rare anomaly of osteogenesis, of hereditary tendency, in which the bones become dense, sclerosed, and marblelike. It frequently affects the orbit and maxillary bone, resulting in progressive proptosis of the eyeball and optic atrophy. Syn., *Albers-Schönberg disease.*

osteopsathyrosis (os"te-op-sath"ih-ro'sis, os"te-o-sath"-). Osteogenesis imperfecta.

Osterberg test; unit. See under the nouns.

ostium lacrimale (os'te-um lak-rih-mah'le). The inferior opening of the nasolacrimal duct, usually located on the lateral wall of the inferior meatus of the nose.

Ostwald (ost'valt) **colors; color circle; hue; notation; purity; semichrome; color solid; system; tints; tones; color triangle.** See under the nouns.

Ostwalt (ost'valt) **curve; lens.** See under the nouns.

Ota, nevus of. Oculocutaneous melanosis.

Otero theory (o-ter'o). See under *theory.*

otocephaly (o-to-sef'ah-le). Marked hypoplasia of the mandible, grossly deformed tongue, nose, and ears, and gross anomalies of the eyes such as bilateral anophthalmia.

OU. Abbreviation for *oculus uterque* or *oculi uniter.*

outlets of Ascher. Collector channels.

oval, Descartes'. See *Cartesian ovals.*

overcorrection. 1. Ophthalmic lens power in excess of that necessary to correct or neutralize a refractive error. 2. An aberration of a lens or an optical system in which the marginal rays intersect the optical axis at a point farther from the lens than the paraxial rays. It is sometimes employed to neutralize spherical aberration in other elements of an optical system.

overlap, scleral. A surgical procedure for shortening the eyeball in the treatment of retinal detachment in which the sclera is incised and sutured so that it overlaps. It is performed in conjunction with diathermy.

overlay. Interposition.

overshoot, dynamic. A secondary small saccade immediately following a primary saccade, giving, in oculography, the appearance of a tiny sharp peak.

OWA. See *Optical Laboratories Association.*

Owen's deviometer (o'enz). See under *deviometer.*

oxford. A type of eyeglass frame without temples in which a straight or slightly curved spring joins the two lenses at the top. The frame is held on the bridge of the wearer's nose by tension of the spring. Some styles are of a folding type.

oxyblepsia (ok"se-blep'se-ah). Acute vision.

oxycephaly (ok"se-sef'ah-le). A condition in which the skull is conical in shape (tower skull), due to abnormal union of the cranial and the facial bones. The ocular signs are shallow orbits, wide separation of the eyes, divergent strabismus, exophthalmos, loss of vision, and sometimes ptosis and/or nystagmus.

oxyopia (ok"se-o'pe-ah). Acute vision.

oxyopsia (ok"se-op'se-ah). Acute vision.

oxyopter (ok"se-op'ter). A unit for measurement of visual acuity proposed by Blascovics. It is the reciprocal of the visual angle expressed in degrees.

OZ. Optical zone.

P

P. Abbreviation for *pupil* or *papilla* (optic); symbol for *position index*.

P I. One of the three separate potentials whose algebraic summation is considered responsible for the generation of the electroretinogram; the slow cornea positive component which, in Granit's analysis, is largely responsible for the *c* wave. See also *P II; P III*.

P II. One of the three separate potentials whose algebraic summation is considered responsible for the generation of the electroretinogram; the fast cornea positive component which, in Granit's analysis, is largely responsible for the *b* wave. See also *P I; P III*.

P III. One of the three separate potentials whose algebraic summation is considered responsible for the generation of the electroretinogram; the fast cornea negative component which, in Granit's analysis, is responsible for the initial *a* wave and at least part of the *d* wave. See also *P I; P II*.

P_o. Symbol for the intraocular pressure prevailing just prior to tonometric measurement; the starting point of tonography.

P_t. Symbol for the intraocular pressure during tonometry.

P_v. Symbol for the average pressure in the small episcleral veins or in the aqueous veins, near the limbus.

pachometer, optical (pah-kom'eh-ter). A pachymeter used in connection with a slit-lamp biomicroscope to provide a split field which may be adjusted to effect alignment of the back surface of the cornea in one half of the field with the front surface in the other half, from which adjustment the thickness of the cornea may be computed.

pachyblepharon (pak"e-blef'ah-ron). An abnormally thick eyelid. Syn., *pachytes*.

pachyblepharosis (pak"e-blef"ah-ro'-sis). Abnormal thickening of an eyelid.

pachymeningitis (pak"e-men"in-ji'tis). Inflammation of the dura mater of the brain, the spinal cord, or the optic nerve. Cf. *leptomeningitis*.

pachymeter (pah-kim'eh-ter). An instrument for measuring thickness. See *pachometer, optical*.

pachytes (pak'ih-tēz). Pachyblepharon.

pad, annular. A broad radial outgrowth of the subcapsular epithelium in the equatorial region of the crystalline lens in some birds and reptiles; involved in the mechanism of accommodation through forces exerted by zonular fibers of the ciliary body attached to it.

pad arm. See under *arm*.

pad, nose. One of the pair of attachments or protuberances of a spectacle frame or mounting designed to rest against the side of the nose. Syn., *guard*.

Paget's disease (paj'ets). See under *disease*.

pair, isomeric. Isomeric colors.

pair, metameric (pār). Metameric colors.

palinopsia (pal-in-op'se-ah). The persistence or recurrence of mentally perceived visual images subsequent to removal of their corresponding object stimuli and at some variance with their normal visual space dimensions and projection; a condition occurring in association with acute visual and mental defects and with auditory and/or somatosensory hallucination. Syn., *visual perseveration*.

palinoptic (pal-in-op'tik). Pertaining to palinopsia.

palisades (pal-ih-sādz'). Grayish-white, thin lines, about 1 mm wide, that run radially from the sclera, at the limbus, to disappear in the clear cornea. Although not found in all eyes, they are frequently seen in slit lamp examination.

Palmer's theory. See under *theory*.

palpate (pal'pāt). To press the eyeball gently with the fingers to estimate ocular tension.

palpation (pal-pa'shun). The gentle pressing of the eyeball with the fingers to estimate ocular tension.

palpebra (pal'pe-brah, pal-pe'-). An eyelid.

    p. frontalis. An upper eyelid.

    inferior p. A lower eyelid.

    p. malaris. A lower eyelid.

    superior p. An upper eyelid.

    p. tertia. Nictitating membrane.

palpebrae (pal-pe'bre). The eyelids.

palpebral (pal'pe-bral). Pertaining to or of an eyelid.

palpebralis (pal"pe-brah'lis). The levator palpebrae superioris muscle.

palpebrate (pal'pe-brāt). 1. To wink. 2. Possessing eyelids.

palpebration (pal"pe-bra'shun). The act of winking.

palpebritis (pal"pe-bri'tis). Blepharitis.

palsy (pawl'ze). Paralysis, especially in reference to special types. See also under *paralysis*.

    abducens p. Palsy of the external rectus muscle resulting from involvement of the abducens nerve.

    Bell's p. Paralysis of the upper and lower muscles of the face on one side, due to inflammation of the facial nerve within the stylomastoid foramen. The palpebral fissure is wider on the affected side, and the eyelid on the affected side cannot be closed. Syn., *Bell's paralysis*.

    Collier's sphenoidal p. S-O syndrome.

    conjugate p. The inability to move the two eyes simultaneously in the same direction, either laterally or vertically, due to involvement of cortical or subcortical oculomotor centers.

    Féréol-Graux ocular p. An associated paralysis of the internal rectus muscle of one eye and the external rectus muscle of the other, affecting lateral conjugate movements. Syn., *Féréol-Graux ophthalmoplegia; Graux ocular palsy; Féréol-Graux paralysis*.

    Graux ocular p. Féréol-Graux ocular palsy.

    internuclear p., anterior. Anterior internuclear ophthalmoplegia.

    internuclear p., posterior. Posterior internuclear ophthalmoplegia.

    progressive supranuclear p. Steele-Richardson-Olszewski syndrome.

    pseudobulbar p. Pseudobulbar paralysis.

    trochlear p. Palsy of the superior oblique muscle resulting from involvement of the trochlear nerve.

panchromatization (pan"kro-mah-tih-za'shun). An evolutionary development making the original light-sensitive substance of the cones more sensitive to long waves, as postulated in the Schenck theory of color vision.

panencephalitis, subacute sclerosing (pan"en-sef"ah-li'tis). Diffuse inflammation of the brain due to slow infection with the measles virus, chiefly affecting children; characterized by chorioretinal lesions, personality changes, seizures, progressive dementia and, following a slow course of months or years, terminates in blindness and a febrile decerebrate state. Syn., *van Bogaert's disease; van Bogaert's subacute sclerosing leukoencephalitis*.

panmural fibrosis (pan-mu'ral fi-bro'sis). Hypopyon corneal ulcer.

pannus (pan'us). An abnormal, superficial vascularization of the cornea associated with a membranouslike infiltration of granulation tissue.

    p. carnosus. Pannus in which the vascularization and infiltration of granulation tissue is thick, producing a dense opacity. Syn., *pannus crassus; pannus sarcomatosus; pannus vasculosis*.

    p. crassus. Pannus carnosus.

    p. degenerativus. Pannus occurring in blind, degenerated eyes following diseases such as iridocyclitis, glaucoma, or detachment of the retina, as a part of a general degeneration of ocular tissue.

    eczematous p. Phlyctenular pannus.

    glaucomatous p. A thin fibrous membrane formed between the corneal epithelium and Bowman's membrane in advanced glaucoma.

leprotic p. Pannus associated with leprotic keratitis and resembling phlyctenular pannus.

phlyctenular p. A thin and lightly vascularized pannus, extending completely around the periphery of the limbus toward phlyctens located in the cornea, commonly associated with phlyctenular keratitis. Syn., *eczematous pannus; scrofulous pannus.*

retrocorneal p. Pannus growing from the anterior surface of the iris over the posterior surface of the cornea, a rare condition which may occur as a sequela to traumatic iritis.

p. sarcomatosus. Pannus carnosus.

scrofulous p. Phlyctenular pannus.

p. siccus. Pannus whose surface appears dry and glossy.

p. tenuis. Pannus of recent origin characterized by few blood vessels and slight corneal cloudiness.

p. trachomatosus. Pannus occurring in the inflammatory stage of trachoma and characteristically extending from the superior limbus toward the central cornea.

p. vasculosis. Pannus carnosus.

panophthalmia (pan″of-thal′me-ah). Panophthalmitis.

panophthalmitis (pan″of-thal′mi-tis). Inflammation of the eyeball throughout all of its structures. Syn., *panophthalmia.*

gas gangrene p. Panophthalmitis resulting from infection of the inner eye by a gas gangrene organism such as *Cl. welchii* and clinically characterized by the rapid development of a severely painful fulminating panophthalmitis, an early rise of ocular tension, a blood or thin coffee-colored discharge, gas bubbles in the anterior chamber, and rapid loss of vision.

Panoptik (pan-op′tik). See *lens, bifocal, Panoptik.*

panoramogram, parallax (pan″o-ram′o-gram). An autostereoscopic picture produced by photographing an object from continuously changing or discretely changed directions through a vertically gauged grid. It is viewed through a comparable grid, producing a parallactic movement with changes of position of the eye, or a stereoscopic effect when viewed binocularly. Prismatic furrows in the photographic emulsion may be substituted for the grid.

pantachromatic (pan″tah-kro-mat′-ik). Completely achromatic.

pantankyloblepharon (pan-tang″-kih-lo-blef′ah-ron). Complete ankyloblepharon.

Pantoscope (pan″to-skōp′). A trade name for an ophthalmoscope manufactured by Keeler Optical Products.

pantoscopic (pan″to-skop′ik). 1. Pertaining to or having a wide angle of view. 2. Pertaining to a lens which has foci for both distant and near objects; a bifocal lens. 3. Pertaining to the pantoscopic angle.

Panum's (pah′nōōmz) **area; phenomenon; fusional space.** See under the nouns.

pan-uveitis. Exudative inflammation affecting the entire uveal tract.

papilla (pah-pil′ah). A small, nipple-shaped elevation.

Bergmeister's p. A cone-shaped mass of glial cells, at the center of the embryonic optic disk, which becomes vascularized by the hyaloid artery, its cells forming the sheaths of this vessel and its branches. Syn., *primitive epithelial papilla.*

conjunctival p. One of the finger-like extrusions of the substantia propria of the conjunctiva, the interspaces being filled with epithelium to form a flat surface; found near the limbus and the lid margin.

p. grisea. A gray optic disk seen in retarded development of the myelin sheaths of the optic nerve fibers. See also *myelinic dysgenesis.*

lacrimal p. A slight elevation, one on each eyelid margin, at the inner canthus, containing a lacrimal punctum.

p. leporina. An optic disk in which medullated nerve fibers are present at its surface and extend to the surrounding retina.

optic p. Optic disk.

primitive epithelial p. Bergmeister's papilla.

vascular choroidal papillae. Conical vascularized papillae in the fundus of fruit-bats and flying foxes which nourish the visual cells of the avascular retina covering its surface.

papillary diameter (pap′ih-ler″e). Disk diameter.

papilledema (pap″ih-le-de′mah). Non-inflammatory edema of the optic nerve head, due to increased intracranial pressure, orbital tumor, blood dyscrasias, etc. As observed ophthalmoscopically, the optic disk appears raised above the level of the retina and its margins are blurred. Accompanying changes are dilatation, tortuosity, and engorgement of the retinal veins, with retinal edema most pronounced in the area of the disk. It is termed *choked disk* when due to increased intracranial pressure.

papillitis (pap″ih-li′tis). Inflammation of the optic nerve head characterized initially by partial or complete loss of vision, lowering of dark adaptation, failure to maintain pupillary contraction under bright illumination, pain in and behind the eye, headache, and nausea. Ophthalmoscopically, the optic nerve head is hyperemic, has blurred margins, and is slightly edematous. The blood vessels are dilated, hemorrhages and exudates may appear, and fine diffuse opacities are usually present in the posterior vitreous. The condition is transient in nature, usually of short duration, and recovery may be complete. Syn., *intraocular optic neuritis.*

papilloma (pap″ih-lo′mah). A benign epithelial neoplasm which may arise from the skin, mucous membranes, or glandular ducts. It may affect the canaliculus, the lacrimal sac, the eyelid, or the conjunctiva.

papillomacular (pap″ih-lo-mak′u-lar) **bundle; fibers.** See under the nouns.

papilloretinitis (pă-pil″o-ret″ih-ni′-tis). Inflammation of the optic disk and the retina. Syn., *neuroretinitis.*

Pappataci's disease (pap-pah-tah′siz). Sandfly fever. See under *fever.*

parablepsia (par″ah-blep′se-ah). False or perverted vision, such as visual hallucination or illusion. Syn., *parablepsis; paropsia: paropsis.*

parablepsis (par″ah-blep′sis). Parablepsia.

paracentesis bulbi (par″ah-sen-te′-sis). Surgical puncture of the eyeball, usually into the anterior chamber for the drainage of aqueous humor or the removal of foreign matter.

paracentesis oculi (par″ah-sen-te′-sis). Paracentesis bulbi.

parachromatism (par″ah-kro′mah-tizm). Partial color blindness. Syn., *parachromatoblepsia; parachromatopsia.*

parachromatoblepsia (par″ah-kro″-mah-to-blep′se-ah). Parachromatism.

parachromatopsia (par″ah-kro″mah-top′se-ah). Parachromatism.

paracontrast (par″ah-con′trast). The reduction in subjective brightness of a flash of light when it is preceded by another flash in an adjacent region of the visual field. Cf. *metacontrast.*

paradox, Fechner's. A decrease in the binocularly perceived brightness of a surface occurring with the increase in luminance presented to one of the eyes from a very low intensity (as obtained by occlusion) to an intermediate intensity (as through a dark filter), while the stimulus to the other eye remains constant at a relatively high level of luminance.

parafovea (par″ah-fo′ve-ah). A band, approximately 0.5 mm wide, immediately surrounding the fovea centralis and surrounded by the perifovea.

parafoveal (par″ah-fo′ve-al). Beside or near the fovea.

parakinesis (par″ah-kih-ne′sis, -ki-ne′sis). Irregular action of an individual extraocular muscle.

paralexia (par″ah-lek′se-ah). A partial alexia in which words or syllables are substituted or transposed.

parallax (par′ah-laks). The apparent change in direction or lateral displacement of a viewed object when the eye is moved from one position to another, or when the object is viewed first with one eye and then with the other.

absolute p. The apparent difference in direction of an object from two points of view, either simultaneously or successively and usually measured in angular units, e.g., the difference in direction of a star from two points on the earth.

binocular p. Parallax effected by viewing with the two eyes separately, or in succession, and in their respective positions, i.e., without head movements.

chromatic p. The differential, apparent, lateral displacement of two objects of different color when observed through a narrow vertical slit moved horizontally across the pupil of the eye.

crossed p. The perceived relative displacement of the two images of an object seen in crossed binocular diplopia, i.e., under dissociation, particularly when perceived as a sudden movement of the fixated object in alternate monocular occlusion, hence manifested for the condition of exophoria. Syn., *heteronymous parallax.*

entoptic p. Relative entoptic parallax.

heteronymous p. Crossed parallax.

homonymous p. Uncrossed parallax.

instantaneous p. The relative parallax value of one point with respect to another when the other point is fixated; hence the relative parallax of any point with respect to a given point of fixation. (Helmholtz)

monocular p. Parallax effected by the movement or displacement of one eye.

motion p. Relative parallax resulting from the continuous motion of the observer and perceived as differences in speeds or direction of movement of objects at different distances, e.g., as may be observed in viewing the landscape from the window of a moving train.

relative p. The apparent relative displacement of one object with respect to another when seen from two points or directions, either simultaneously or successively, and usually measured in angular units representing the difference in angle subtended at the two points of view by the two objects. **binocular r.p.** Relative parallax effected by viewing with each of the two eyes separately while they remain in their respective positions, i.e., without head movements. **entoptic r.p.** The motion of the projected image of the retinal shadow of an opacity in the ocular media, relative to the field of view, when the illumination source is moved transversely with respect to the optical system of the eye. **monocular r.p.** Relative parallax effected by the movement or displacement of the viewing eye.

stereoscopic p. The relative parallax effected or stimulated by a stereogram so as to induce stereopsis.

uncrossed p. The perceived relative displacement of the two images of an object seen in uncrossed binocular diplopia, i.e., under dissociation, in particular when perceived as a sudden movement of the fixated object in alternate monocular occlusion, hence manifested for the conditions of esophoria. Syn., *homonymous parallax.*

vertical p. The perceived, relative, vertical displacement of the two images of an object seen in binocular vertical diplopia, i.e., under dissociation, in particular when perceived as a sudden movement of the fixated object in alternate monocular occlusion of the two eyes, hence manifested for the condition of vertical heterophoria.

parallelepiped, corneal (par″ah-lel″e-pi′ped). The section of the cornea, transilluminated by the narrow beam of a slit lamp, having the geometrical shape of a curved parallelepiped when viewed obliquely.

paralysis (pă-ral′ih-sis). Loss or impairment of muscle function or sensation.

abducens p. Sixth nerve paralysis.

p. of accommodation. Absence of accommodation due to paralysis of the ciliary muscle.

asthenic bulbar p. Myasthenia gravis.

basilar p. Ocular paralysis due to a peripheral lesion of the nerve before it enters the orbit.

Bell's p. Bell's palsy.

congenital oculofacial p. Moebius' syndrome.

congenital spastic p. Little's disease.

conjugate p. Paralysis resulting in the loss of one or more of the conjugate movements of the eyes.

convergence p. A pronounced limitation or absence of binocular convergence ability with monocular fixational eye movements intact. This clinical classification of paralysis implies or presumes a lesion involving the convergence control centers.

divergence p. The inability to diverge the eyes, characterized by a fixed state of convergence with monocular fixational eye movements intact.

Féréol-Graux p. Féréol-Graux ocular palsy.

fifth nerve p. Lack of sensation in the cornea, the conjunctiva, and parts of the face and head, and absence of the blink reflex, due to involvement of the ophthalmic branch of the fifth cranial nerve.

fourth nerve p. Paralysis of the superior oblique muscle due to involvement of the fourth cranial nerve. Syn., *trochlear paralysis.*

Foville's p. Conjugate paralysis of gaze with or without facial paralysis on one side, and contralateral paralysis of the arm and the leg, due to lesions of the pons varolii.

p. of gaze. The inability to move the eyes conjugately, either laterally or vertically, due to involvement of cortical or subcortical oculomotor centers.

Gubler's p. Millard-Gubler syndrome.

irritative cervical sympathetic p. Horner's syndrome.

oculomotor p. Third nerve paralysis. **cyclic o.p.** Cyclic oculomotor spasm.

orbital p. Ocular paralysis due to a peripheral lesion of a nerve within the orbit.

pseudobulbar p. Progressive loss of voluntary eye movements, with reflex eye movements intact, due to bilateral involvement of the frontal cortex. Syn., *pseudobulbar palsy.*

pupillary p., absolute. Immobility of the pupil, regardless of stimulation, due to paralysis of both the sphincter and dilator pupillae muscles.

pupillary p., amaurotic. Loss of direct and consensual pupillary reactions to light on ipsilateral stimulation of an eye blind from a completely destructive lesion in the retina or the optic nerve, with retention of the consensual pupillary reaction by contralateral stimulation.

pupillary p., hemianopic. Pupillary hemiakinesia.

pupillary p., reflex. Absence of direct and indirect pupillary reflexes to light with retention of the near and orbicularis pupillary reflexes, due to a lesion in the efferent pupillomotor pathway between the point of departure of the pupillomotor fibers from the optic tract and the constrictor center. Miosis and anisocoria are frequent accompaniments.

sixth nerve p. Paralysis of the external rectus muscle due to involvement of the homolateral sixth cranial nerve. Syn., *abducens paralysis.*

tegmental mesencephalic p. Benedikt's syndrome.

third nerve p. Paralysis of the levator palpebrae superioris, the superior rectus, the internal rectus, the inferior oblique, the ciliary, and the sphincter pupillae muscles, due to involvement of the third cranial nerve and resulting in ptosis, cycloplegia, iridoplegia, and exotropia. Syn., *oculomotor paralysis.*

trochlear p. Fourth nerve paralysis.

Weber's p. Homolateral oculomotor paralysis and contralateral hemiplegia of the face and limbs, produced by a lesion in the region of the cerebral peduncle affecting the third cranial nerve. Syn., *Weber's syndrome.*

paramacular (par″ah-mak′u-lar). Beside or near the macula lutea.

paraphimosis oculi (par″ah-fi-mo′sis o′ku-li, -fih-mo′sis). Paraphimosis palpebrae.

paraphimosis orbicularis (par″ah-fi-mo′sis or-bik″u-lar′is, -fih-mo′sis). Paraphimosis palpebrae.

paraphimosis palpebrae (par″ah-fi-mo′sis pal-pe′bre, -fih-mo′sis). Ectropion resulting from spastic contraction of the palpebral portion of the orbicularis oculi muscle. Usually it is of short duration, affects the upper eyelid, and is due to birth trauma. Syn., *paraphimosis oculi; paraphimosis orbicularis.*

paraplegia, familial spasmodic (par″ah-ple′je-ah). Familial spasmodic hypotonic paresis of pyramidal origin, without ataxia, sensory disturbances, or muscular atrophy, usually appearing in the second decade. Ocular involvements may include extraocular muscle paralysis, strabismus, macular degeneration, pupillary defects, and optic atrophy. Syn., *Strümpell-Lorrain disease.*

parastereoscopy (par″ah-ster″e-os′kope). The viewing of a stereopsis-inducing pattern so as to perceive essentially the original scene but with diminished depth or distance, although the objects within the scene appear to have full natural relief. This relief is produced by increasing the focal length of the stereocamera lenses and by increasing the parallactic base in the same proportion.

paratrachoma (par″ah-trah-ko′mah). Inclusion blenorrhea.

paraxial (par-ak′sih-al). Pertaining to light rays or the space closely surrounding the axis of an optical system.

Paredrine (par-ah-drēn′). A trade name for *hydroxyamphetamine.*

paresis (pah-re′sis, par′e-sis). Incomplete or partial paralysis.

amblyopic p., pupillary. Diminished direct and consensual pupillary reactions to light on ipsilateral stimulation of an eye which is amblyopic due to an incomplete lesion in the retina or the optic nerve, with retention of the consensual pupillary reaction for contralateral stimulation.

parfocal (par-fo'kal). Pertaining to sets of eyepieces or objectives which may be interchanged on an optical instrument without varying the focus of the instrument.

parhelion. Any one of several patches of concentrated light, usually somewhat colored, occasionally appearing on the *parhelic circle.* Syn., *mock sun; sun dog.*

Parinaud's (pah-rih-nōz') **conjunctivitis; syndrome; theory.** See under the nouns.

Parks monofixational pattern; syndrome. See *monofixation.*

Parks-Hardesty three-step method. See under *method.*

parophthalmia (par″of-thal′me-ah). Inflammation of the tissues around the eye.

parophthalmoncus (par″of-thal-mong′-kus). A tumor near the eye.

paropsia (par-op′se-ah). Parablepsia.

paropsis (par-op′sis). Parablepsia.

    p. glaucosis. Glaucoma. *Obs.*

    p. longinqua. Presbyopia. *Obs.*

    p. lucifuga. Day blindness. *Obs.*

    p. noctifuga. Night blindness. *Obs.*

    p. propinqua. Myopia. *Obs.*

paroptic (par-op′tik). Extraretinal.

parorasis (par″o-rah′sis). Any perversion of vision, such as color blindness or a visual hallucination.

paroxysms, conjunctivo-ciliary (pahr′oks-izms). Paroxysmal conjunctival and episceral congestion, unilateral or alternate, lasting a few days and recurring at varying intervals of weeks to months and associated with sinusitis or a nasal disturbance.

Parrot's sign (par-ōz′). See under *sign.*

Parry's disease (par′ēz). Exophthalmic goiter.

Parry-Romberg syndrome. Romberg's disease. See under *disease.*

pars (pahrz). A part.

    p. caeca oculi. The optic nerve head.

    p. caeca retinae. The parts of the retina which are not sensitive to light, i.e., the pars ciliaris retinae and the pars iridica retinae.

    p. ciliaris retinae. The epithelium of the ciliary body which represents the forward continuation of the

retina and is subdivided into the *pars plana* and the *pars plicata.*

    p. iridica retinae. The posterior pigmented epithelium of the iris.

    p. lacrimalis. Horner's muscle.

    p. optica hypothalami. The portion of the optic chiasm and its surrounding area which lies in the optic recess of the hypothalamus.

    p. optica retinae. The retina proper; the light-sensitive retina extending from the optic disk to the ora serrata.

    p. plana. The heavily pigmented, innermost portion of the ciliary body, composed of epithelial tissue, extending anteriorly from the ora serrata to the ciliary processes. It is approximately 3.6 to 4 mm wide and appears smooth to the naked eye. However, under low magnification, slight dark ridges (striae ciliaris) are seen running parallel to each other from the ora serrata to the ciliary processes. Syn., *orbiculus ciliaris.*

    p. planitis. A form of granulomatous uveitis occurring in the region of the pars plana.

    p. plicata. Corona ciliaris.

Parson's test (par′sunz). Manoptoscope test.

partial. One who has suonormal but some usable vision.

partition of Kundt. Kundt's monocular asymmetry.

partition of Münsterberg. Münsterberg's monocular asymmetry.

Pascal's (pas-kalz′) **method; schema.** See under the nouns.

Pascal-Raubitschek test (pas-kal′-row′bih-shek). See under *test.*

Pascheff's conjunctivitis (pas′shefs). See under *conjunctivitis.*

passband. The wavelength band or narrow range of wavelengths transmitted with maximum efficiency by an optical interference filter, or within which the transmittance is high.

Passow syndrome. See under *syndrome.*

past pointing. See under *pointing.*

pastel (pas′tel). 1. Lightly tinted; of relatively high brightness and low hue saturation. A color with these characteristics. 2. A picture made with a crayon composed of paste and ground pigments. 3. A crayon composed of paste and ground pigments.

Patau syndrome. Trisomy 13 syndrome. See under *syndrome*.

patch. A circumscribed area differing from the tissue surrounding it.

cotton-wool p's. White, fluffy-appearing patches occurring in edematous areas of the retina, as may occur in renal or hypertensive retinopathy. They are coagulated exudates of plasma and fibrin from the retinal capillaries. Syn., *cotton-wool spots*.

Hutchinson's p. A salmon-colored, localized area of the cornea seen in syphilitic interstitial keratitis, due to neovascularization of the deep corneal tissues. Syn., *salmon patch*.

Roth's p's. Roth's spots.

salmon p. Hutchinson's patch.

path difference. See under *difference*.

path, optical. The product of the length of path of a ray of light in a medium and the refractive index of that medium. It is equivalent to the distance that would be traversed by that ray in a vacuum in the same time taken to traverse the medium.

patheticus (pah-thet'ih-kus). 1. Trochlear nerve. 2. Superior oblique muscle.

pathology, ophthalmic (pă-thol'o-je). The branch of biological science which is concerned with the nature of disease of the eye and its surrounding structures and of the structural and functional changes which cause or are caused by such disease.

pathway. The course of the nerve structures, or the structures themselves, along which impulses are conducted.

centrifugal p. The motor pathway of the visual reflex arc; that portion of the visual pathway conducting impulses from the visual cerebral centers to the intrinsic and extrinsic muscles of the eye and to the skeletal muscles of the body.

centripetal p. The sensory pathway of the visual reflex arc; that portion of the visual pathway conducting impulses to the visual cerebral centers.

geniculocalcarine p. Geniculocalcarine tract.

visual p. The neural path of visual impulses starting in the retinae and ending in the visual cortex. The structures most commonly included are: the *retinae*, the *optic nerves*, the *optic chiasm*, the *optic tracts*, the *external geniculate bodies*, the *optic radiations*, and the *visual cortical areas*. **higher v.p.** The neural path of visual impulses starting at the external geniculate bodies and ending in the visual cortical areas. The pathway includes the *external geniculate bodies*, *optic radiations*, and the *visual cortical areas*. **lower v.p.** The neural path of visual impulses commencing in the retinae and ending at the external geniculate bodies. The pathway includes the *retinae*, the *optic nerves*, the *optic chiasm*, the *optic tracts*, and the *external geniculate bodies*.

patient. A person on whom a study is being made, or to whom treatment is being given, for any aberration of normal organization, particularly in matters of health.

Paton's lines; sign; syndrome. See under the nouns.

pattern. A specific arrangement or interrelation of parts; a design; a model.

A p. Exotropia in which the deviation increases as the eyes rotate straight downward, or esotropia in which the deviation increases as the eyes rotate straight upward. Cf. *V, X, Y, λ, patterns*. Syn., *A phenomenon; A syndrome*.

binocular fixation p. The refixation response time of the usually fixating eye of a strabismic infant following removal of a briefly placed occluder to force fixation by the usually deviating eye, graded I, immediate; II, momentarily delayed; III, following first blink; and IV, following second blink; and successively interpreted as levels of decreasing probability of presence of monocular amblyopia. Abbreviation *BFP*.

diffraction p. The alternate dark and light bands representing the distribution of light intensity due to diffraction of light at an aperture or an edge. See also *diffraction fringes*.

Donders' pseudoisochromatic p's. Patterns of colored threads wound in stripes around a piece of wood for detecting color blindness. See also *Donders' test for color blindness*.

equilibrium p. *Optometric Extension Program:* The relationships between the positive relative convergence finding (#16 A) and the negative relative convergence finding (#17 A) and between the positive relative accommodation finding (#20) and the negative relative accommodation finding (#21), in estimating the maximum amount of convex lens power (or minimum amount of concave lens power) which can be prescribed for the patient's near-point use.

Foucault p. A resolution test pattern consisting of alternate black and white stripes of equal width. Syn., *square wave pattern; grating pattern.*

grating p. Foucault pattern.

interference p. The alternate light and dark bands representing the distribution of light as a result of interference phenomena. See also *interference fringes.*

inverted Y (λ) p. Exotropia which increases as the eyes rotate straight downward with orthotropia in the primary position and on upward gaze. Cf. *A, V, X,* and *Y patterns.* Syn., *λ or lambda phenomenon; λ or lambda syndrome.*

isochromatic fringe p. A uniform pattern of colored bands such as may be seen in glass under strain when viewed in a polariscope.

lens p. A jig, of metal or plastic, which is attached to a lens cutting or edging machine to produce the desired shape of a lens.

moiré p. A pattern of alternate dark and bright bands, especially if wavelike or watery in appearance, as may be seen in the misaligned superimposition of a transilluminated pair of identical gratings. Syn., *moiré effect.*

monofixation p. of Parks. See *monofixation.*

receptor-type distribution p. The pattern of distribution of the rod and cone cells in the foveal area of the retina. Abbreviated *RDP.*

square wave p. Foucault pattern.

V p. Exotropia in which the deviation increases as the eyes rotate straight upward, or esotropia in which the deviation increases as the eyes rotate straight downward. Cf. *A, X, Y, λ, patterns.* Syn., *V phenomenon; V syndrome.*

visual p. A characteristic or apparent interrelationship or consistency in a group of visual test data.

X p. Exotropia in which the deviation increases as the eyes rotate either straight upward or straight downward. Cf. *A, V, λ,* and *Y patterns.* Syn., *X phenomenon; X syndrome.*

Y p. Exotropia which increases as the eyes rotate straight upward with orthotropia in the primary position and on downward gaze. Cf. *A, V, X,* and *λ*

patterns. Syn., *Y phenomenon; Y syndrome.*

pause, fixation. See under *fixation.*

PCB. Abbreviation for *punctum convergens basalis;* the near point of convergence.

pcc. Abbreviation for *periscopic concave,* in reference to periscopic concave lenses.

pcx. Abbreviation for *periscopic convex,* in reference to periscopic convex lenses.

PD. Abbreviation for *prism diopter; pupillary distance* (or, more correctly, *interpupillary distance*).

PD, monocular. A misnomer, relating to interpupillary distance, used to identify the lateral distance from the midplane of the bridge of the nose to the center of the pupil.

P-D Scope. The trade name for an instrument for measuring interpupillary distance, the distance of each pupil from the center of the bridge of the nose, and the size of the pupil, cornea, or palpebral fissure.

pearls, Elschnig. Elschnig bodies.

pearls, leprotic. Minute whitish nodules on the iris, usually between the collarette and ciliary margin, which are pathognomonic of leprosy.

pearl specks of Listing. The bright spots seen entoptically as a result of vacuoles in the crystalline lens of the eye.

pebble. Transparent and colorless quartz; rock crystal; a lens made of quartz or rock crystal.

Pechan prism (pek'an). See under *prism.*

Peckham's (pek'amz) **method; test.** See under *test.*

pecten (pek'ten). A black, heavily pigmented, typically pleated or vaned structure in avian eyes, composed primarily of small blood vessels projecting into the vitreous from the optic disk and functioning primarily to nourish the retina and inner eye.

pecten sclerae (pek'ten skler'e). The edge of the sclera surrounding the optic nerve.

pedicle (ped'ih-kul). A narrow supporting part; a stem or stalk.

cone p. Cone foot.

optic p. 1. The embryonic link between the optic vesicle or optic cup and the forebrain or diencephalon, which becomes the optic nerve. Syn., *optic stalk.* 2. In cartilaginous fish such as sharks or skates, a cartilaginous stalk extending from the cranium into the orbit and terminating in an expanded concave head against which the eyeball rests and receives support.

peduncle (pe-dung'k'l). A narrow supporting part; a stem.

    cerebral p's. Portions of the midbrain, ventral to the aqueduct of Sylvius, crossed by the optic tracts and connecting the cerebrum with the pons. Each is subdivided into a dorsal tegmentum, a substantia nigra, and a basis pedunculi; the dorsal tegmentum contains the oculomotor and trochlear nuclei. Syn., *crus cerebri*.

    optic p. The fibers of the optic radiations as they leave the lateral geniculate bodies and enter the internal capsule prior to the formation of the fan-shaped medullary optic lamina.

peephole. The retinoscope aperture, or the entrance pupil of the retinoscopist's own eye, through which is observed the reflected light from the subject's eye and which is at the conjugate focus of the subject's retina when the motion of the light reflexed is neutralized.

PEK. Photo-Electronic Keratoscope.

pelopsia (peh-lop'se-ah). A perversion of vision in which objects appear to be abnormally near.

Pel's (pelz) **crisis; syndrome.** See under *crisis*.

pemphigus foliaceus (pem'fih-gus). A condition of unknown etiology characterized by erythematous or bullous lesions and general exfoliation of the skin and by loss of eyelashes and eyebrows, ectropion, conjunctivitis, iritis, pannus, and cataract in the late stages. Syn., *Cazenave's disease*.

pemphigus, ocular (pem'fih-gus). Bullous eruptions or ulcerations of the conjunctiva, usually associated with bullae on other mucous membranes and on the skin, with invasion of the conjunctiva by newly formed connective tissue, which subsequently contracts, resulting in shrinkage of the conjunctiva. Syn., *essential shrinkage of the conjunctiva*.

penalization. See *attenuation*.

pencil of rays. See under *rays*.

penetration. The depth of focus of a lens or an optical system.

Penfield syndrome. See under *syndrome*.

pentachromic (pen"tah-kro'mik). 1. Pertaining to partial color blindness in which only five colors can be distin-

guished. 2. Pertaining to, or of, five colors.

penumbra (pe-num'brah). The region of gradually diminishing darkness surrounding the region of complete darkness (umbra) in the shadow cast by an opaque object in the presence of an extensive light source.

percept (per'sept). 1. The meaningful impression of an object obtained in response to sensory stimuli. 2. Formerly, the object perceived.

perceptible (per-sep'tih-b'l). Discernible; perceivable; apprehendable through the senses.

perception (per-sep'shun). 1. The appreciation of a physical situation through the mediation of one or more senses. 2. The process of discriminating between two or more stimulus presentations.

    after p. 1. An afterimage. 2. An aftereffect.

    albedo p. Perception of surface attributes as a function of diffuse reflection values rather than in terms of luminance.

    ambiocular p. Perception as obtained in ambiocular strabismus.

    binocular p. 1. Perception from simultaneous use of the two eyes. 2. Perception resulting from fusion of the images of the two eyes.

    color p. Perception of hue.

    depth p. Perception of relative or absolute difference in distance of objects from the observer; perception of the third dimension.

    dermo-optical p. The perception or identification of reading material or colors through stimulation of the skin and exclusive of stimulation of the eyes, an unverified skill.

    form p. Perception of shape or contour.

    haptic p. 1. Sense of touch. 2. Mental visual imagery derived from tactile-kinesthetic clues.

    immediate p. Perception resulting only from direct sensation, i.e., not influenced by memory of previous experience.

    light p. Perception of the brightness attribute of light.

    selective p. Perception of some but not all of the exposed environment, presumably in relation to motivation and past experiences.

    simultaneous p. Perception of the images of the two eyes simultaneously, with or without sensory fusion.

visual p. Perception through the sense of vision.

perceptivity (per″sep-tiv′ih-te). The ability to apprehend or perceive.

perceptual lance; organization; visual skill. See under the nouns.

Percival's (per′sih-valz) **criterion; formula; lens; rule.** See under the nouns.

periarteritis, retinal (per″ih-ar″ter-i′tis). Inflammation of the perivascular sheaths and adventitia of the retinal arterioles.

peribrosis (per″ih-bro′sis). Ulceration of the eyelid in the area of the canthus.

peribulbar (per″ih-bul′bar). Surrounding the eyeball.

perichoroid (per″ih-ko′roid). Perichoroidal.

perichoroidal (per″ih-ko-roi′dal). Surrounding the choroid.

periconchitis (per″ih-kong-ki′tis). Inflammation of the periorbita.

pericorneal (per″ih-kōr′ne-al). Surrounding the cornea.

pericranium (per″ih-kra′ne-um). The periosteum on the outer surface of the cranial bones; it is considered as the deepest layer of the eyebrow.

peridacryocystitis (per″ih-dak″re-o-sis-ti′tis). Infection in the area of the lacrimal sac, but not involving its interior or the lacrimal canals.

peridectomy (per″ih-dek′to-me). Surgical removal of a strip of conjunctival tissue from around the cornea for the relief of pannus. Syn., *perimitry; periotomy; peritectomy; peritomy; syndectomy.*

perifovea (per″ih-fo′ve-ah). A band, approximately 1.5 mm wide, immediately surrounding the parafovea and representing the outer limit of the macular area.

perifoveal (per″ih-fo′ve-al). Around or encircling the fovea.

perikeratic (per″ih-ker-at′ik). Surrounding the cornea.

perilenticular (per″ih-len-tik′u-lar). Surrounding the crystalline lens.

perimeter (per-im′eh-ter). An instrument designed to determine the angular extent and characteristics of the visual field peripheral to the direction of fixation, or of the field of fixation peripheral to a forward direction of reference. Types of test targets, fixation controls, illumination, recording apparatus, head and chin rests, mechanical features, and auxiliary attachments vary.

arc p. A perimeter employing an arc scale for peripheral angular specifications and the test object path, pivoted on an axis coinciding with the straightforward position of the line of sight of the eye being tested, the eye being located at the center of curvature of the arc. The pivot permits orientation of the measuring arc to coincide with any desired meridian of exploration.

hand p. A simplified, lightweight perimeter held in position by the examiner instead of being mounted on a stand.

hemispherical p. A perimeter consisting essentially of a large segment of a hollow sphere instead of a pivoting arc.

Krimsky Eyecup p. A translucent plastic hemisphere of about 5 cm radius placed in front of the eye to be tested so that the patient can fixate the examiner's eye through a 12 mm aperture at the hemispheric pole and report on the visibility of the light of an exposed ophthalmoscope bulb placed in contact with the outer hemispherical surface in various field positions.

projection p. A perimeter that has a projection system for target presentation and is typically controlled from behind the instrument, the location of the target being simultaneously indicated on a recording chart.

perimetric (per″ih-met′rik). 1. Pertaining to perimetry. 2. A trade designation of a spectacle lens shape.

perimetry (per-im′eh-tre). The determination of the extent of the visual field for various types and intensities of stimuli, usually for the purpose of diagnosing and localizing disturbances in the visual pathway.

black light p. Perimetry performed under ultraviolet light and with luminescent test targets.

electroencephalographic p. Objective perimetry in which alterations of the recorded alpha rhythm are used to determine the visual field while a narrow beam of light from a perimeter arc is projected through the pupil to various positions on the retina.

flicker fusion p. Determination of the integrity of the visual field by plotting the critical fusion frequency (CFF) throughout its extent.

kinetic p. Exploration of the visual field with a moving test object of fixed luminance.

light sense p. Static perimetry.

projection p. Perimetry performed with an instrument that provides projected luminous targets which are typically controlled from behind the instrument with the location in the field being simultaneously indicated on a recording chart.

qualitative p. Perimetry performed with test targets of the same size but of different stimulus intensity.

quantitative p. Perimetry performed with test targets of various sizes but of the same content, to determine the smallest visual angle for which each retinal area is sensitive.

static p. Exploration of the visual field in which test objects of various sizes, located at fixed positions, are gradually increased in luminance to the threshold of visibility. Syn., *light sense perimetry*.

ultraviolet p. Black light perimetry.

perimitry (per-im'ih-tre). 1. Peritomy. 2. Peridectomy.

perineuritis, optic (per"ih-nu-ri'tis). Inflammation of the sheaths of the optic nerve, usually in association with involvement of the optic nerve itself. It is classified into two main types, *pachymeningitis*, affecting the dura mater, and *leptomeningitis*, affecting the pia mater and the arachnoid.

perineuritis, retrobulbar (per"ih-nu-ri'tis). Optic perineuritis affecting the sheaths of the orbital portion of the optic nerve.

periocular (per"ih-ok'u-lar). Surrounding the eyeball.

period. 1. The interval of time during which anything occurs. 2. The interval of time between regular occurrences in an ordered series.

action p. Action time.

latent p. The time interval between the application of a stimulus and the response to that stimulus. In vision, it varies with light intensity, wavelength, state of light adaptation of the eye, and with location and size of the retinal area stimulated.

p. of light wave. The time interval for one complete cycle of periodic motion of a light wave; the reciprocal of the wave frequency.

refractory p., absolute. A short interval of time following the excitation of a nerve or muscle fiber during which the application of a second stimulus is not effective in producing a response.

refractory p., relative. The interval of time, immediately following the absolute refractory period, during which a stimulus greater than threshold is necessary to produce a response.

periophthalmia (per"ih-of-thal'me-ah). Periophthalmitis.

periophthalmic (per"ih-of-thal'mik). Situated around the eyeball.

periophthalmitis (per"ih-of"thal-mi'-tis). Inflammation of the tissues around the eye. Syn., *periophthalmia*.

perioptic (per"ih-op'tik). Situated around the eyeball.

perioptometry (per"ih-op-tom'eh-tre). The measurement of the limits of the visual field or of peripheral visual acuity.

periorbita (per"ih-ōr'bih-tah). The periosteum within the orbit. It is loosely attached to the bone, except at sutures, fossae, foramina, and the orbital margin where it is firmly attached. At the optic canal it is continuous with the dura mater of the optic nerve; at the orbital margin, where it is continuous with the periosteum of the face, it is thickened to form a ridge, the arcus marginale, to which the orbital septum is attached.

periorbital (per"ih-ōr'bih-tal). Situated around the orbit or pertaining to the periorbita.

periorbititis (per"ih-ōr"bih-ti'tis). Inflammation of the periorbita.

periosteum, orbital (per"ih-os'te-um). Periorbita.

periostitis, orbital (per"ih-os-ti'tis). Periorbititis.

periotomy (per"ih-ot'o-me). Peridectomy.

peripapillary (per"ih-pap'ih-ler-e). Situated around the optic disk.

periphacitis (per"ih-fah-si'tis). Presumed inflammation of the capsule of the crystalline lens.

periphakitis (per"ih-fah-ki'tis). Periphacitis.

periphakus (per"ih-fak'us, -fa'kus). The capsule of the crystalline lens.

peripheraphose (peh-rif'er-ah-fōz"). A perceived dark spot, shadow, or interruption of light, originating in the optic nerve or the eyeball.

peripherophose (peh-rif'er-o-fōz). A subjective sensation of light or color originating in the optic nerve or the eyeball.

periphlebitis, retinal (per"ih-fle-bi'-tis). Inflammation of the external walls and the surrounding tissues of the retinal venules.

periphoria (per"ih-fo're-ah). Cyclophoria.

peripupillometer (per"ih-pu"pih-lom'eh-ter). An instrument for measuring the extent of the pupillomotor area of the retina by determining the extent of the visual field in which the pupillary reaction to light is elicited.

periscope (per'ih-skōp). An optical instrument enabling an observer to see around an obstruction in the line of view, or to obtain a view otherwise impossible for a given position of the observer's eye, used in submarines, tanks, trenches, and in other circumstances in which the observer may be recessed or hidden.

periscopic (per"ih-skop'ik). Pertaining to a periscopic lens or to a periscope.

peritectomy (per"ih-tek'to-me). Peridectomy.

peritomy (peh-rit'o-me). 1. The cutting of the conjunctiva at the limbus prior to enucleation or for the relief of pannus. Syn., *perimitry.* 2. Peridectomy.

perivasculitis, retinal (per"ih-vas"-ku-li'tis). Inflammation of the perivascular sheaths and adventitia of the retinal vessels.

    primary r.p. Eales's disease.

Perkins tonometer (pur'kins). See under *tonometer.*

Perlia's (per'le-ahz) **nucleus; test.** See under the nouns.

PERRLA. Acronym for *P*upils, *E*qual and round, *R*eact *R*egularly to *L*ight and *A*ccommodation.

perseveration, visual (per-sev"er-a'shun). Palinopsia.

perspective. The perceptual attribute of three-dimensional space, or its graphic representation on a plane or a curved surface.

    aerial p. 1. Perspective as influenced by the state of clarity of the atmosphere. In clear atmosphere contours remain sharp, colors are essentially unaltered, and objects appear nearer than in hazy atmosphere, in which contours are less distinct and colors altered. 2. Perspective in a painting effected by gradations of color and distinctness.

    ambiguous p. Perspective which changes or alternates, as that obtained in viewing an ambiguous figure.

    geometrical p. Perspective identified with the apparent converging of receding parallel lines. Syn., *linear perspective; mathematical perspective.*

    inverse p. Perspective as seen through a pseudoscope, in which near objects appear far, and far objects appear near.

    linear p. Geometrical perspective.

    mathematical p. Geometrical perspective.

    movement p. Apparent slowing of the motion of an object crossing the visual field, in proportion to its distance from the observer, i.e., the greater the distance the slower the apparent velocity.

    reversible p. Perspective which reverses or alternates, as that obtained in viewing a reversible figure.

Perspex. Trade name for an acrylic plastic consisting essentially of polymerized methyl methacrylate.

Peter's anomaly. See under *anomaly.*

Petit's canal (ptēz). See under *canal.*

Pettit's test. See under *test.*

Petzval's (pets'valz) **condition; curve; formula; surface; theory.** See under the nouns.

Peutz-Touraine syndrome. See under *syndrome.*

Pfund's (fundz) **absorption cell; gold-plated glass; method.** See under the nouns.

phacentocele (fah-sen'to-sēl). Dislocation of the crystalline lens into the anterior chamber.

phacitis (fah-si'tis). Presumed inflammation of the crystalline lens. Syn., *crystallitis; phacoiditis.*

phaco- (fak'o, fa'ko-). A combining form denoting a lens or the crystalline lens of the eye.

phaco-anaphylaxis (fak"o-an"ah-fih-lak'sis). Hypersensitivity to the protein of the crystalline lens, following extracapsular cataract surgery of one eye, so that breakage of the capsule of the other eye allows anaphylactic reaction.

phacocele (fak'o-sēl). Hernia of the crystalline lens, as when extruded out of the eyeball, through a rupture of the sclera near the limbus, to lodge beneath the conjunctiva. Syn., *lenticele.*

phacocyst (fak'o-sist). The capsule of the crystalline lens.

phacocystectomy (fak"o-sis-tek'to-me). Excision of a portion of the capsule of the crystalline lens.

phacocystitis (fak"o-sis-ti'tis). Presumed inflammation of the capsule of the crystalline lens.

phacodonesis (fak"o-do-ne'sis). Tremulousness of the crystalline lens.

phacoemulsification (fak"o-e-mul"sif-ih-ka'shun). A procedure for removal of the crystalline lens in cataract surgery in which an anterior capsulectomy is performed by means of a needle inserted through a small incision at the temporal limbus, allowing the lens contents to fall through the dilated pupil into the anterior chamber where they are broken up by the use of ultra-sound and aspirated out of the eye through the incision.

phacoerisis (fak"o-er'ih-sis). Surgical removal of the crystalline lens in cataract by means of pneumatic forceps which adhere to the anterior surface of the lens by suction.

phacoerysis (fak"o-er'ih-sis, -er-e'-sis). Phacoerisis.

phacoglaucoma (fak"o-glaw-ko'-mah). Changes produced in the crystalline lens secondary to glaucoma.

phacohymenitis (fak"o-hi"men-i'-tis). Presumed inflammation of the capsule of the crystalline lens.

phacoiditis (fak"oid-i'tis). Phacitis.

phacoidoscope (fah-koi'do-skōp). Phacoscope.

phacolysin (fah-kol'ih-sin). An albumin used in the treatment of cataract.

phacolysis (fah-kol'ih-sis). 1. Dissolution of the crystalline lens. 2. Surgical discission of the crystalline lens.

phacolytic (fak"o-lit'ik). Pertaining to or causing dissolution of the crystalline lens.

phacoma (fah-ko'mah). A tumorlike swelling of the crystalline lens, due to an overgrowth of lens fibers.

phacomalacia (fak"o-mah-la'she-ah). Softening of the crystalline lens as may occur in hypermature cataract.

phacomatoses (fak"o-mah-to'sēz). A group of congenital and familial diseases characterized by the appearance of multiple tumors and cysts in various parts of the body, particularly in the retina and the central nervous system. Included in this group are *Bourneville's disease, von Hippel-Lindau disease, von Recklinghausen's disease,* and *Sturge-Weber disease.*

phacometachoresis (fak"o-met"ah-ko-re'sis). Luxation or subluxation of the crystalline lens.

phacometecesis (fak"o-met"eh-se'-sis). Displacement of the crystalline lens into the anterior chamber.

phacometer (fah-kom'eh-ter). Lensometer.

phacoplanesis (fak"o-plah-ne'sis). A wandering or free-floating crystalline lens.

phacosclerosis (fak"o-skle-ro'sis). Hardening of the crystalline lens.

phacoscope (fak'o-skōp). An instrument for observing the crystalline lens, especially its accommodative changes. Syn., *phacoidoscope.*

phacoscopy (fah-kos'ko-pe). Examination of the crystalline lens with the phacoscope.

phacoscotasmus (fak"o-sko-taz'mus). Darkening or clouding of the crystalline lens.

phacoscotoma (fak"o-sko-to'mah). A lenticular opacity or cataract.

phak-. For words beginning thus, see *phac-.*

phakomatous choristoma (fah-ko'-mah-tus). An unusual benign congenital tumor bearing some tissue resemblance to cataractous lenses and occurring in the nasal part of the lower eyelid.

Phakometer, Entoptic (fa-kom'eh-ter). The trade name of an instrument for viewing shadows of lenticular and other opacities within one's own eye.

phalangosis (fal"an-go'sis). An abnormality in which the eyelashes grow in multiple rows.

phantasm (fan'tazm). A visual hallucination or illusion.

phantasmagoria (fan-taz"mah-go're-ah). 1. An optical effect whereby figures projected on a screen are made to appear to dwindle markedly into the distance, or to rush toward the observer with enormous increase of size. 2. A hallucination of a shifting succession of figures or objects.

phantasmascope (fan-taz'mah-skōp). Phenakistoscope.

phantasmoscopia (fan-taz" mah-skōp'-e-ah). Hallucinations of ghosts; the experiencing of phantasms with visual attributes.

phantom. A phantasm.

phase difference. See under *difference.*

phase of light wave. A point or stage in the periodic changes of a light wave considered in relation to a point of reference in the periodic change of the same wave or of an interacting wave.

phemicol. The nonproprietary name of a hydrophilic material of which contact lenses are made.

phenakistoscope (fe"nah-kis'to-skōp). A device consisting of a slotted disk containing a series of pictures representing the successive stages in the movement of objects or persons. It is held with the side containing the pictures facing a mirror and rotated while an observer on the other side of the disk sees the pictures, individually and instantaneously, in the mirror through the slots, obtaining the effect of animation. Syn., *magic disk; fantascope; McLean's optical illusion; kaleidorama; phantasmascope; stroboscope.*

phengophobia (fen"go-fo'be-ah). A morbid dread of light.

◆

PHENOMENON

phenomenon. 1. A remarkable or an unusual event or appearance, or one of unique significance. 2. A fact or an event which may be described or explained scientifically.

A p. A pattern.

Abney's p. A hue change resulting from a change in purity or saturation. The hues of colors having a dominant wavelength near 488 mμ (blue-green) become increasingly different from the hue of 488 mμ with increase of purity, whereas the hues of colors having a dominant wavelength near 577 mμ (yellow) become increasingly like the hue of 577 mμ. Syn., *Abney's effect.*

anorthoscopic p. Anorthoscopic movement.

aqueous influx p. The filling of the laminary vein, which normally carries blood and aqueous, with aqueous when the junction of the aqueous vein and the recipient vein is partially occluded by pressure of a glass rod, indicating higher pressure within the aqueous vein than within the recipient vein. Syn., *Ascher's positive glass rod phenomenon.*

ascension p. The persistence of elevated position of the walls of Cloquet's canal instead of the normal immediate gravitational settling, seen with the biomicroscope after abrupt vertical movements of the eye. It is attributed to pathologic conditions which change the specific gravity of the components of the vitreous humor. Syn., *Busacca's phenomenon.*

Ascher's negative glass rod p. Blood influx phenomenon.

Ascher's positive glass rod p. Aqueous influx phenomenon.

Aschner's p. Reduction of the pulse rate on exerting pressure on the eyeball, indicating cardiac vagus irritability. Syn., *oculocardiac reflex.*

Aubert's p. The apparent tilting in one direction of a bright vertical line, viewed in a dark room, when the head is slowly tilted in the opposite direction, due to the absence of compensatory postural changes.

Aubert-Förster p. Aubert-Förster law.

autokinetic p. Autokinetic visual illusion.

Bartley p. See *Brücke-Bartley effect.*

Becker's p. Pulsation of the retinal arteries, associated with exophthalmic goiter.

Behr's abduction p. In syphilitic sixth nerve palsy, attempted conjugate movement of the eyes toward the affected side produces an inequality of size of the pupils, the abducting eye having the smaller pupil.

Behr's pupillary p. Anisocoria associated with hemianopsia wherein the pupil on the hemianopic side is larger than its fellow and reacts less markedly to light, considered to be due to a lesion in the contralateral optic tract.

Bell's p. The normal upward and outward rotation of the eyes on bilateral closure, or attempted closure, of the eyelids.

Bell's inverse p. Downward rotation of the eyes on bilateral closure, or attempted closure, of the eyelids.

Bell's paradoxical p. Absent or abnormal (downward or lateral) rotation of the eyes on bilateral closure, or attempted closure, of the eyelids.

Bell's perverse p. Lateral rotation of the eyes on bilateral closure, or attempted closure, of the eyelids.

Bezold-Brücke p. A change in perceived hue of some, but not all, spectral colors with change in intensity. Syn., *Bezold-Brücke effect.*

Bielschowsky's p. The downward movement of the nonfixating hypertropic eye in some strabismics on placing a dark lens or a filter before the fixating eye.

blood influx p. The filling of the laminary vein, which normally carries blood and aqueous, with blood when the junction of the aqueous vein and the recipient vein is partially occluded by pressure of a glass rod, indicating higher pressure within the recipient vein than within the aqueous vein. Syn., *Ascher's negative glass rod phenomenon.*

blue-arc p. An entoptic sensation of two bands of blue light arching toward the blind spot from above and below a spot of light stimulating the temporal parafoveal area.

Broca-Sulzer p. Broca-Sulzer effect.

Busacca's p. Ascension phenomenon.

cattle-truck p. The appearance of the arterial or venous blood column in retinal vessels when segmentation occurs due to such abnormal processes as retinal ischemia, dysproteinemia, obstruction of circulation, or external pressure on the globe. The blood moves along in intermittent fashion, causing an appearance of linked sausages. Syn., *freight-car phenomenon.*

chromatic dimming p. Loss of saturation of a colored surface on steady fixation.

colored shadow p. The tendency of shadows cast on a gray surface to appear complementary in color to the intercepted illuminant, e.g., when shadows are cast on a neutral screen by an opaque body from two equidistant light sources of equal intensity, one white and the other colored, the shadow cast by the white light appears to be the color of the colored light and the shadow cast by the colored light appears to be its complement.

constancy p. The tendency of an object to retain its associated perceptual attribute, such as hue, size, and shape, under conditions altering its correlated physical stimulus value.

contrast p. A form of interinfluence between different perceptual processes whereby one perception induces a characteristic opposite to itself in another perception. The phenomenon occurs in *successive contrast* (time) and in *simultaneous contrast* (space).

co-variation p. A phenomenon observed in strabismics with anomalous correspondence in which the objective angle of deviation and the angle of anomaly change simultaneously such that the subjective angle remains constant.

crowding p. The increased difficulty in identifying targets which are closely adjacent to other targets, as clinically demonstrated by poorer visual acuity when using closely grouped multiple targets instead of an isolated single target. It is a normal phenomenon but is more pronounced in amblyopia ex anopsia. Syn., *crowding; dissociation difficulty; separation difficulty.*

depth contrast p. The perceived backward inclination of a vertical line when viewed binocularly between a bilaterally displaced pair of lines inclined slightly forward.

Dietzel-Roelofs p. The apparent movement of a fixated stationary light in a direction opposite to that of a second similar light, both being located in an otherwise empty, dark field.

doll's head p. Rotation of the eyes in a direction opposite to a sudden head movement, through an angle equal to the head movement, with a subsequent return toward the original position, in a case of a destructive lesion of the central mechanism for voluntary eye movements when the lesion is above the pontine centers. Syn., *head turning reflex; Cantelli's sign; doll's eye sign; Roth-Bielschowsky sign.*

Duane's p. Duane's syndrome.

entoptic p. A visual sensation, such as muscae volitantes or phosphene, arising from stimuli within the eye and perceived illusorily as in the external visual field.

epithelial touch p. A briefly sustained epithelial indentation on the cornea due to the just previous pressure of a foreign body and the temporary loss of the tear layer in that area usually lasting from 4 to 6 minutes.

exhaustion p. Rapid decrease of the *b* potential in the electroretinogram following stimulation with repeated flashes of light when the retina is in a condition of anoxemia.

extinction p. Imperceptibility of a stimulus in one portion of the visual field, or extinction of sensation, evoked by simultaneous stimulation elsewhere in the visual field.

Fick's p. Sattler's veil.

flicker p. Rapid variation or wavering of perceived luminance or hue associated with intermittent, interrupted, or suddenly varying stimulus intensity or quality; flicker.

fluttering heart p. Apparent fluttering of a colored figure drawn on a background of a very different hue when the drawing is moved back and forth laterally at a certain rate.

Fraunhofer's diffraction phenomena. Diffraction phenomena in which both the light source and the screen on which the diffraction is observed are effectively at infinite distances from the aperture or edge causing the diffraction.

freight-car p. Cattle-truck phenomenon.

Fresnel's diffraction phenomena. Diffraction phenomena in which either the source of light, or the screen on which the phenomena are observed, or both, are at a finite distance from the aperture or the edge causing the diffraction.

Fuchs' p. Paradoxical retraction of a formerly ptotic eyelid associated with eye movements and occurring during the healing stage of oculomotor paralysis or paresis; usually indicative of aberrant regeneration of fibers of the oculomotor nerve.

Galassi's pupillary p. Orbicularis pupillary reflex.

glass rod p., negative. Blood influx phenomenon.

glass rod p., positive. Aqueous influx phenomenon.

von Graefe's pupillary p. Pupillary constriction, after a forced abduction movement, in the presence of absolute and reflex paralysis of the iris to light.

green flash p. See *green flash*.

Gunn's arteriovenous p. Gunn's crossing sign.

Gunn's jaw-winking p. Jaw-winking.

Gunn's pupillary p. In unilateral disease of the retina or optic nerve, e.g., retrobulbar neuritis, minimal pupillary contraction of the affected eye followed by dilatation, on illumination of the affected eye with the sound eye simultaneously covered, due to an impaired direct reflex to light in the affected eye, with a dominant, consensual, darkness dilatation reflex from the covered sound eye. Syn., *Gunn's pupillary sign.*

heavy eye p. The manifestation of smaller excursions of the more myopic or less hyperopic eye than of the other eye in peripheral, especially upward, fixational movements in high anisometropia with strabismus. Syn., *myopic myositis.*

Helmholtz floating heart p. Red spots on blue paper appear to float above the surface upon oscillation of the paper.

Hering p. A pair of bands, one bright, the other dark, on either side of a contrast border, less intense and extending much farther from the border than the Mach ring. Syn., *Hering-type inhibition.*

Hering-Hillebrand p. A characteristic departure of the experimentally determined horopter from the Vieth-Mueller circle, explained by the asymmetry in the effective spatial positions of the corresponding elements in the two eyes. Syn., *Hering-Hillebrand deviation.*

Honi p. A failure of certain inductive, visual, environmental influences to produce an expected distortion of size or shape of a person with close emotional or sociological ties to the observer; named after the woman who first failed to report the usual perceived distortion of her husband seen in an Ames room.

inflection p. A perceived distortion of a straight contour toward the center of the physiological blind spot when the image of the contour falls on the edge of the blind spot.

interareal inhibitional p. Any of several demonstrations of the effect which stimulation of one retinal area may have on adjacent or remote retinal areas, including *border contrast*, *metacontrast*, and *paracontrast.*

inverted Y (⋏) p. Inverted Y (⋏) pattern.

jack-in-the-box p. Sudden appearance of an object when the eye shifts its fixation from the actual direction of the object through a peripheral portion of a strong convex spectacle lens, where the prismatic deviation renders it out of sight, to a more central direction, enabling the object rays to be received through the pupil. Syn., *jack-in-the-box effect.*

jaw-winking p. Jaw-winking.
inverse j.w.p. Reverse jaw-winking.

Kohlrausch p. Helmholtz-Kohlrausch effect.

LeGrand-Geblewics p. Perception of an indirectly observed colored flickering light (40-50 times per sec.) as a constant white light.

Liebmann p. Liebmann effect.

Mach-Dvořák p. The apparent displacement of a laterally moving object farther or nearer than its actual distance when viewed binocularly through the paired slits of an episcotister disk so that the rapidly successive exposures to one eye are slightly delayed, or advanced, with respect to the exposures to the other eye. Cf. *Pulfrich effect.* Syn., *Mach-Dvořák effect.*

Marcus Gunn p. Jaw-winking. **reversed M.G.p.** Reverse jaw-winking.

Meyer's iliac p. Transient, fixed, pupillary dilatation produced in psychotics or psychoneurotics by the exertion of pressure on the abdomen over McBurney's point.

Mizuo's p. In Oguchi's disease, characterized by a gray-colored fundus, the return of a normal red appearance to the fundus after several hours in the dark. Upon re-exposure of the eye to light, the fundus quickly returns to its former gray color.

Morawiecki's p. A response similar to *Wessely's phenomenon* wherein the infiltration is in the form of a ring concentric with the limbus.

on-off p. The alternate opening and closing of the filtration angle of the anterior chamber, during goniosopic examination, as the illumination is alternately turned on and off.

orbicularis p. Orbicularis pupillary reflex.

Panum's p. The appearance of one line nearer than another line when a single vertical line presented haploscopically to one eye is fused with one of two vertical lines close together, presented haploscopically to the other eye.

paradoxical pupil p. Paradoxical pupillary reflex.

phi p. Phi movement.

Piltz-Westphal p. Orbicularis pupillary reflex.

pseudo-Graefe's p. Pseudo-Graefe's sign.

Pulfrich stereo p. Pulfrich effect.

Purkinje's p. The relatively greater brightness of blue and green in comparison with red on adaptation to low, scotopic levels of illumination, corresponding to a shift of the relative luminosity curve toward the shorter wavelength during transition from light to dark adaptation. Syn., *Purkinje's effect; Purkinje's shift.*

Purkinje's pupillomotor p. Light from the green portion of the spectrum produces the maximal constriction of the pupil in the dark-adapted eye, instead of yellow, which produces the maximal constriction in the light-adapted eye.

recession p. Maintenance of bifixation over an extended distance, by an esotrope classified as having divergence insufficiency, while an object of fixation is moved slowly farther away from a fused near point. See also *push-away method.*

red spot p. Faintly visible, minute red spots occurring occasionally on the surface of hydrophilic contact lenses due to rusting of embedded ferrous particles.

Redlich's p. A transient, fixed, pupillary dilatation produced in psychotics or psychoneurotics by voluntary muscular effort, such as movement of the eyes in any direction or squeezing an object in the hand. Syn., *Redlich's symptom.*

Roenne's p. In viewing two isolated spots of light in the midsaggital plane, one nearer and one farther than the crossing point of the visual axes, also in the midsaggital plane, the resulting percept is two spots of light lying in a frontal plane, one to each side of the point of intersection of the visual axes.

Rosenbach's p. 1. Tremor of the upper eyelid on its gentle closure. 2. The inability to close the eyes on command in neurasthenia.

Scheerer's p. Entoptic appearance of red blood corpuscles circulating in the paramacular blood vessels on looking at a homogeneous blue field, such as the sky or a snowfield through a blue filter.

Schlesinger's p. Constriction of the pupil on forcible raising of the eyebrows, even in the absence of a normal reaction to light.

size constancy p. The relative apparent stability, or lack of perceived change, in the size of an object despite a change in viewing distance, actual size, or other related stimulus factors.

von Szily's p. An anaphylactic

keratitic response to a second injection of horse serum into the corneal stroma of a rabbit's eye, characterized by gray patches of leucocytic infiltrate from remnants of new vessels.

Troxler's p. The temporary and irregular fading or disappearance of a small object in the visual field during steady fixation of another object, e.g., during fixation of one of several spots drawn on a sheet of paper with disappearance and reappearance of the other spots. The phenomenon is also identified by some with the disappearance of a fixated spot with stabilized retinal imagery.

Tyndall p. Tyndall effect.

V p. V pattern.

wallpaper p. The change of perceived distance of a uniformly repeating pattern, such as wallpaper, when viewed binocularly with varying amounts of convergence so as to fuse different pairs of elements in the pattern.

waterfall p. Waterfall visual illusion.

Weber's p. The visibility of an incandescent body to the dark-adapted eye as a gray glow at about 400° C, at which temperature the glow is not yet visible to the light-adapted eye.

Wessely's p. An anaphylactic keratitic response of a rabbit's eye which has been injected with horse serum 10 to 14 days earlier to a similar but 10 to 14 days later injection into the other eye or subcutaneously, characterized by an interstitial clouding of the cornea of the first sensitized eye from the limbus and progressing centrally.

Westphal-Piltz p. Orbicularis pupillary reflex.

white with pressure p. A localized change of the normal orange-red choroidal color of the fundus into a translucent white or greenish-white color upon external scleral depression. It is attributed to pathology of the retina or overlying vitreous, such as retinal atrophy or vitreous traction. Syn., *white with pressure sign.*

Wilbrand's p. An abrupt refixation movement occurring in hemianopsia when prisms, to displace the images onto the blind sides of the retinae, are suddenly placed before the eyes while a small spot on a uniform background is fixated. According to Wilbrand, this movement indicates a cerebral lesion and its absence an optic tract lesion.

Wilson's p. Oculo-aural reflex.

winking-jaw p. Corneomandibular reflex.

X p. X pattern.

Y p. Y pattern.

◆

phenotype (fe'no-tīp). A type determined by the common visible characteristics of a group rather than by genetic characteristics.

phenylephrine hydrochloride (fen"il-ef'rin hi"dro-klo'rīd). A synthetic sympathomimetic amine chemically differing from epinephrine in having only one instead of two hydroxyl groups on the benzene ring, and used ophthalmically as a mydriatic and vasoconstrictor.

phi (ϕ) (fi, fe). The Greek letter used as the symbol for (1) *phi phenomenon;* (2) the *angle of longitude* in the field of regard. (Fry)

phimosis palpebrarum (fi-mo'sis pal"pe-brah'rum). Blepharophimosis.

phlebography, orbital (fle-bog'-rah-fe). A method of localizing and diagnosing an intraorbital hemangioma in which a series of x-ray photographs are made immediately after injecting a roentgen opaque material into the angular vein.

phlegmon, orbital (fleg'mon). Orbital cellulitis.

phlycten (flik'ten). A nodular pustule or minute subepithelial abscess on the conjunctiva or cornea in phlyctenular conjunctivitis or keratitis. Syn., *phlyctena; phlyctenula; phlyctenule.*

phlyctena (flik-te'nah). Phlycten.

phlyctenula (flik-ten'u-lah). Phlycten.

phlyctenule (flik'ten-ül). Phlycten.

phlyctenulosis (flik"ten-u-lo'sis). The presence of phlyctens, as in phlyctenular conjunctivitis or keratitis.

phobotaxis (fo-bo-tak'sis). Random trial and error light-avoiding movements of a motile organism.

phonism (fo'nizm). Synesthesia in which there is a sensation of sound created by the effect of sight, smell, taste, touch, or thought.

phonopsia (fo-nop'se-ah). Visual sensations, as of color, associated with, or induced by, the hearing of sounds.

phoria (fo're-ah). The direction or orientation of one eye, its line of sight, or some other reference axis or meridian, in relation to the other eye, manifested in the absence of an adequate fusion stimulus, and variously specified with reference to parallelism of the lines of sight or with reference to the relative directions assumed by the eyes during binocular fixation of a given object. Cf. *anisophoria; cyclophoria; esophoria; exophoria; heterophoria; hyperphoria; hypophoria; orthophoria.*

associated p. The amount of prism needed to neutralize a manifest fixation disparity.

habitual p. The phoria obtained through the patient's habitually worn lens prescription.

horizontal p. 1. Lateral phoria. 2. The phoria obtained with the fixation object in the horizontal visual plane.

induced p. 1. The phoria obtained through the subjectively determined lens correction. 2. A phoria obtained through any lens correction other than the one worn habitually.

lateral p. The phoria representing deviations in the plane of fixation.

monofixational p. A small angle strabismus, of about 1° to 4°, which persists after a greater deviation has been overcome to obtain peripheral fusion. It is of a greater magnitude than fixation disparity and is usually associated with central suppression of the deviating eye.

version p. 1. A tendency for both eyes to deviate in the same direction in the absence of a stimulus eliciting fixation attention, as in anaphoria or cataphoria. 2. Anisophoria.

vertical p. The phoria representing deviations perpendicular to the plane of fixation.

Phoriafractor, Smith (fo're-ah-frak"-tor). A trade name for a device, interposed between a refractor and a near-point chart, consisting essentially of a metal plate with two rectangular apertures through which each eye sees half of the target.

phoriagraph, Rosen (fo're-ah-graf'). A plastic rectangular chart of small numerals and letters with a centered transilluminated ruby-red aperture, to be viewed with a dark neutral or red filter in front of one eye and a light green filter in front of the other, making only the numerals and the letters visible to one eye and only the red spot to the other. The letter or the numeral on which the spot is seen superimposed gives a measure of the vertical and lateral phoria.

phoriascope (fo're-ah-skōp). An instrument containing prisms for use in visual training.

Phoro-Lenscorometer (fo"ro-lenz-ko-rom'eh-ter). A device for determining the distance of a phoropter lens from the cornea, consisting essentially of a rule, scaled to compensate for the thickness of the instrument, which is placed through the open aperture of the phoropter against the closed eyelid to provide a direct reading.

phorometer (fo-rom'eh-ter). 1. Any instrument or device for determining the kind and extent of phoria. 2. An instrument containing rotary prisms, Maddox grooves, and lens cells for determining phorias and vergences.

reflecting p. A phorometer containing mirrors to reflect separate targets into the two eyes.

Stevens' p. A phorometer consisting of two single, five prism diopter ophthalmic prisms, mounted one before each eye, so that the base-apex lines of the two prisms are parallel to each other but in opposite directions. The two prisms are so geared together that both rotate simultaneously in the same direction.

Wilson's p. A phorometer in which a revolving disk containing fixed prisms for dissociation is before the right eye and a rotary (variable) prism for measuring phorias and vergences is before the left eye.

phorometry (fo-rom"eh-tre). Measurement of the kind and extent of phoria with a phorometer.

phoro-optometer (fōr"o-op-tom'eh-ter). An instrument for determining phorias, vergences, and the refractive state of the eye, consisting essentially of rotary prisms, Maddox grooves, and lens cells.

phoropter (fōr-op'ter). An instrument for determining the refractive state of the eyes, phorias, vergences, amplitude of accommodation, etc., consisting essentially of a housing containing rotating disks with convex and concave spherical and cylindrical lenses, pinhole disks, occluders, and sometimes color filters and prisms. Attached to the front of the housing are crossed cylinder lenses, rotary prisms, and Maddox grooves.

phoroscope (fōr'o-skōp). 1. An instrument for reproducing an image, as of a photograph, conveyed by electric or other processes not necessarily optical, from a distance. 2. A variant of phorometer, sometimes applied to a trial frame with a bracket for attachment to a table.

phose (fōz). A subjective visual sensation, as of light or color.

phosgenic (fos-jen'ik). Light-producing.

phosis (fo'sis). Any condition of the eye, the optic nerve, or the brain, giving rise to a subjective visual sensation.

phosphene (fos'fēn). A subjective visual sensation of a luminous spot or an area in the external visual field, arising from mechanical or electrical stimulation of the eyeball.

  accommodation p. A luminous border appearing around the visual field following a conscious sudden relaxation of accommodation. Syn., *Czermak's phosphene.*

  Czermak's p. Accommodation phosphene.

  electrical p. A phosphene arising from electrical stimulation of the eyeball.

  flick p. A phosphene observed on sudden movement of a rested and dark-adapted eye, attributed by Nebel to instantaneous and transient deformation of the posterior surface of the vitreous.

  movement p. A phosphene appearing in the portion of the visual field corresponding to the physiological blind spot, arising from sudden movements of the eyes in the dark.

  pressure p. A phosphene which appears during local pressure on the eyeball in the sector of the visual field corresponding to the region of the retina receiving the pressure.

Phospholine Iodide. Trade name for *echothiophate iodide.*

phosphor. A substance which has the property of absorbing energy and releasing it again in the form of phosphorescence.

phosphorescence (fos"fo-res'ens). 1. The property of emitting light, without any apparent rise in temperature, or the light so produced, due to absorption of radiation from some other source, and lasting after exposure has ceased. The emitted light differs in composition and color from the absorbed radiation. Cf. *fluorescence.* 2. The glow, as of phosphorus, decaying wood, or certain living organisms, resulting from a slow process of oxidation.

phosphorescent (fos"fo-res'ent). 1. Pertaining to or exhibiting phosphorescence. 2. A substance which exhibits phosphorescence.

phot. A unit of illumination equal to 1 lumen per sq. cm.

photalgia (fo-tal'je-ah). Pain produced by excessive light. Syn., *photodynia.*

photanope (fo'tah-nōp). One having photanopia.

photanopia (fo"tah-no'pe-ah). A rare congenital condition resembling pure rod vision; characterized by deficient photopic vision, little, or no color vision, but may demonstrate cone spectral sensitivity. Syn., *incomplete typical achromatopsia; incomplete rod monochromatism; atypical achromasy.*

photanopic (fo"tah-nop'ik). Pertaining to or having photanopia.

photaugiaphobia (fo-taw"je-ah-fo'-be-ah). Abnormal intolerance of glare.

photerythron (fo"teh-rith'ron). A deuteranope

photerythrous (fo"teh-rith'rus). Deuteranopic.

photesthesia (fo"tes-the'ze-ah). Sensitiveness to light.

photic (fo'tik). Pertaining to light or the production of light.

photics (fo'tiks). The branch of physics dealing with light, including ultraviolet and infrared radiation.

photism (fo'tizm). Visual sensation, as of light or color, induced by another sense, body temperature, or by thought.

photo- (fo'to). A combining form denoting *light.*

photoactinic (fo"to-ak-tin'ik). 1. Pertaining to or emitting both visible and actinic light. 2. Capable of producing actinic effects.

photoallergy (fo"to-al'er-je). Marked hypersensitivity to light.

Photobrown. A trade name for an ophthalmic lens made of photochromic glass varying in light transmission from approximately 45% to 88%.

photocampsis (fo"to-kamp'sis). Refraction of light.

photocatalysis (fo"to-kah-tal'ih-sis). The acceleration of a reaction by radiant energy, particularly light, either directly, or indirectly, through excitation of an intermediate substance.

photocell (fo'to-cel). A cell which produces electric current when radiant energy is incident upon it.

photoceptor (fo"to-sep'tor). A photoreceptor.

photochemical (fo"to-kem'ih-kal). Pertaining to, capable of, or resulting in chemical change by the action of light.

photochromatic (fo"to-kro-mat'ik). 1. Pertaining to colored light. 2. Of or pertaining to color photography.

photochromic (fo-to-kro'mic). Pertaining to substances which change in color and in light transmission properties upon exposure to a change of light intensity or to ultraviolet radiation. The change may, or may not, be reversible.

photocoagulation (fo"to-ko-ag"u-la'-shun). Coagulation of tissue by the heat generated at the focus of an intense beam of light. In the eye, it is used in the treatment of retinal detachments, retinal holes, aneurysms, hemorrhages, and malignant and benign neoplasms.

photocoagulator, laser (fo"to-ko-ag'u-la-tŏr). A laser used for photocoagulation in the eye for the treatment of retinal detachment, retinal hole, aneurysm, neoplasm, or hemorrhage.

photocolorimeter (fo"to-kul"or-im'-eh-ter). A photoelectric colorimeter.

photoconductivity (fo"to-kon-duk-tiv'ih-te). Electrical conductivity of certain insulators and semiconductors, such as selenium, induced by radiation of suitable wavelength.

photodrome (fo'to-drōm). An apparatus consisting essentially of a rotating disk containing various patterns and a regulated flashing light. By varying the frequency of the flashes, the disk may be made to appear stationary, rotating at a different speed, or rotating in the opposite direction.

photodynamics (fo"to-di-nam'iks). The effect of light on organisms, especially the phototropic effect in plants.

photodynia (fo"to-din'ih-ah). Photalgia.

photodysphoria (fo"to-dis-fo're-ah). Photophobia.

photoelastic (fo"to-e-las'tik). Pertaining to the double refraction produced in a transparent material to which stress has been applied, patterns of which are observable with a polariscope.

photoelectric (fo"to-e-lek'trik). 1. Pertaining to the emission of electrons from liquid, solid, or gaseous bodies on exposure to radiations of certain wavelengths. 2. Pertaining to the decrease in electrical resistance of certain substances on exposure to radiations of certain wavelengths.

photoelectricity (fo"to-e-lek"tris'ih-te). 1. Electricity produced by the effect of radiation of suitable wavelengths on certain metals. 2. A change in electric resistance of certain metals on exposure to radiations of suitable wavelengths.

photoelectroluminescence (fo"to-e-lek"tro-lu"mih-nes'ens). Electroluminescence in which the electric current is created by light or other electromagnetic energy; a means of light amplification.

photoelectron (fo"to-e-lek'tron). One of a stream of electrons emitted from certain substances on exposure to radiations of suitable wavelengths.

Photo-Electronic Keratoscope (fo"-to-e-lek-tron'ik). An instrument for evaluating corneal topography and determining corneal curvatures consisting essentially of a target of black and white concentric rings of varying widths and a camera to photograph the reflected corneal image of the target. The photograph is analyzed with a densitometer.

photogene (fo'to-jēn). 1. A photograph. *Obs.* 2. An afterimage.

photogenesis (fo"to-jen'e-sis). The production or generation of light, as in certain bacteria or in the firefly; phosphorescence.

photogenic (fo"to-jen'ik). 1. Due to light; producing or generating light, as in certain bacteria or in the firefly; phosphorescent. 2. Pertaining to photography.

photogenous (fo-toj'e-nus). Photogenic.

photogrammetry (fo"to-gram'eh-tre). The use of aerial or other photography for measurement and cartographic purposes.

Photogray. A trade name for an ophthalmic lens made of photochromic glass varying in light transmission from approximately 45% to 85%.

photoisomerization (fo"to-i-som"er-i-za'shun). Isomerization from absorption of radiant energy, especially light.

photokeratograph (fo"to-ker'ah-to-graf). A photograph of the reflected corneal image of the target of a photokeratoscope, used to calculate corneal curvatures and evaluate corneal topography.

photokeratography (fo"to-ker"ah-tog'raf-e). Determination of corneal curvatures and topography by photographing and measuring the corneal image of the target of a photokeratoscope.

photokeratoscope (fo"to-ker'ah-to-skōp). An instrument consisting essentially of a Placido's disk with horizontal and vertical radial lines and attachments for viewing or photographing the image of the pattern on the cornea.

photokeratoscopy (fo"to-ker"ah-tos'-ko-pe). Determination of corneal curvatures and topography by observing or photographing the corneal image of the target of a photokeratoscope.

photokinesis (fo"to-kih-ne'sis). A movement or motion response of a motile organism to changes in intensity of light stimulation but not in response to the direction of the light stimulation.

photolabile (fo"to-la'bil). Affected by, or unstable in the presence of, radiant energy, especially visible radiant energy, as, for example, a photopigment which is converted by light to a different substance.

photology (fo-tol'o-je). The branch of physics which deals with light.

photoluminescence (fo"to-lu"mih-nes'ens). The emission of visible radiant energy by a substance on absorption of radiant energy of a different wavelength.

photolysis (fo-tol'ih-sis). Chemical decomposition by the action of light.

photoma (fo-to'mah). A visual hallucination consisting of sparks or flashes of light.

◆

PHOTOMETER

photometer (fo-tom'eh-ter). An instrument for measuring radiant energy in the ultraviolet, infrared, or visible regions of the electromagnetic spectrum. Syn., *illuminometer.*

  Abney's p. A direct, heterochromatic, comparison photometer for determining luminosity in which one portion of a beam of light passes through a wavelength-selecting spectroscopic system and the other portion through an episcotister-controlled system to form adjacent patches of light for comparison and luminance matching.

  acuity p. A photometer employing acuteness of vision as a measure of illuminance.

  bar p. Bench photometer.

  barrier-layer cell p. A photometer employing a barrier-layer cell which generates a current when exposed to light.

  bench p. A device consisting of a photometer head fixed to an optical bench between reference and test sources which are mounted on independently sliding carriers. It provides for an illumination match by varying the relative distances of the sources from the head and computing according to the inverse square law. Syn., *bar photometer.*

  Bunsen's p. A photometer employing a Bunsen disk, a translucent paraffined spot in the center of a substantially opaque white paper flanked by two mirrors forming an angle of 90° bisected by the paper, permitting a simultaneous view of both sides of the disk. When the spot disappears, the illumination on the two sides is equal. Syn., *grease spot photometer.*

  colorimetric p. A photometer utilizing color filters to measure the intensity of light in various regions of the spectrum.

  cosine p. 1. A photometer in which the illumination on the comparison surface is varied by tilting it relative to the direction of the incident light. 2. A light meter corrected for the cosine error introduced by the angle of incidence of the light.

  diaphragm p. A photometer employing a variable aperture for controlling the intensity of illumination from the reference or test source.

  distribution p. A photometer, used in conjunction with a goniometer, for determining the illumination of a light source in various directions. Syn., *goniophotometer.*

  extinction p. A photometer employing the criterion of just invisible, the intensity of the test light usually being controlled by a calibrated neutral wedge filter.

  flicker p. 1. A photometer employing the criterion of elimination of flicker when the test source and the reference standard are of equal luminance and alternately presented at a rate less than the critical flicker frequency for a given luminance difference, but greater than the critical flicker frequency for hue differences. 2. A photometer in which the critical flicker frequency for the alternate presentation of a test source and a reference standard is considered an index of the luminance of the test source.

Förster's p. A photometer with an adjustable diaphragm, used to determine the least amount of light that renders an object visible. Syn., *photoptometer.*

grease spot p. Bunsen photometer.

integrating p. A photometer with an integrating sphere or equivalent attachment for measuring the total output of light from a source, independent of the variation of intensity with direction.

integrating sphere p. A photometer employing a hollow sphere coated internally with a perfectly diffusing material such that the luminance at all points is equal and proportional to the total emitted by the source. Hence a measurement of the illumination on any segment of the sphere indicates the total flux of the source.

Lummer-Brodhun p. A photometer with a Lummer-Brodhun cube or head, in which two adjacent or concentric portions of a comparison viewing screen are separately illuminated by the test source and the reference or measuring standard.

Macbeth p. A portable bar photometer using a Lummer-Brodhun cube, an eyepiece, and a movable comparison lamp illuminating a diffusing surface seen as an annulus by reflection within the cube. The portion of the object to be measured is seen through the cube as a luminous area within the annulus. The brightness of the annulus is then adjusted to match the brightness of the central spot. Syn., *Macbeth illuminometer.*

Martens p. A photometer which, by means of a Wollaston prism, produces perpendicularly polarized images of the reference and test surfaces which are equated in brightness by rotating an analyzing prism.

meridian p. A photometer with telescopic and reflecting mirror arrangements for the simultaneous comparison of two stars.

photoelectric p. A photometer employing a calibrated photoelectric cell instead of the human eye.

physical p. A photometer consisting essentially of a radiant energy-sensitive element, such as a photoemissive cell, barrier layer cell, or thermopile, and an intensity indicator.

polarization p. A photometer employing light-polarizing elements to control intensity.

Pritchard p. A precision, portable photometer for measuring luminance in a selected portion of the visual environment, the size of the measured field being regulated by an aperture ranging from six minutes to two degrees of arc. Light from the selected area, focused directly onto the aperture plate by an objective lens, activates a photomultiplier. A built-in radium plaque serves as a standard. Syn., *Spectra-Pritchard photometer.*

Pulfrich p. A photometer which makes use of the Pulfrich effect to determine an illumination match. Syn., *stereo photometer.*

radiometric p. Any photometer employing a device, such as thermocouple or photoelectric tube, for converting incident radiant energy into another form of energy for purposes of measurement.

Ritchie p. A photometer consisting of a double diffuse reflecting viewing comparison screen, in the form of a wedge, arranged and housed to reflect separately from each surface the light from a reference source and a test source. Syn., *wedge photometer.*

Rumford p. A device for comparing two sources of light by placing a small opaque object or bar in front of a white screen and adjusting the distances of the two sources until the densities of the shadows cast by the object are equal. Syn., *shadow photometer.*

shadow p. Rumford photometer.

Simmance-Abady p. A pair of base-to-base, conical, diffuse reflecting surfaces rotated on an axis oblique to the apex-to-apex line and viewed through an aperture from a direction perpendicular to the axis of rotation so that the two conical surfaces, independently illuminated, one by a reference source and the other by a test source, are seen alternately, and hence flickering occurs if the separate illuminations are unequal.

Spectra-Pritchard p. Pritchard photometer.

stellar p. A photometer used in astronomy for measuring the luminance of a star, as by comparison with an artificial star of variable luminance.

stereo p. Pulfrich photometer.

thermopile p. A photometer employing a thermopile to measure intensity of illumination.

visual p. A photometer used to evaluate intensity in the visible spectrum and in which equality of brightness with a comparison standard is established through visual observation.

wedge p. Ritchie photometer.

◆

photometry (fo-tom'eh-tre). The measurement of light; the use of a photometer.

flicker p. Light measurement by means of a flicker photometer.

heterochromatic p. The measurement of light intensities of sources of different hue.

visual p. Photometry by means of intensity judgments with the human eye.

photomotor (fo"to-mo'tor). Pertaining to the response of a muscle to light stimuli, as in the contracting of the pupil.

photomultiplier (fo"to-mul"tih-pli'-er). A photoelectric device in which electrons from the cathode of a photoelectric cell or tube are caused to impinge on a second cathode, which in turn emits secondary electrons more numerous than the incident electrons, thus amplifying the current.

photomydriasis (fo"to-mih-dri'ah-sis). Enlargement of the pupil by destruction of the border tissue by means of an argon laser.

photon (fo'ton). 1. The basic unit of radiant energy, given by the equation: $E = h\nu$, where h = Planck's constant $(6.55 \times 10^{-27}$ erg sec.) and ν = frequency electromagnetic radiation concerned $(\nu = c/\lambda$, where c = velocity of light, approximately 3×10^{10} cm per sec., and λ = wavelength of radiation); the quantum. 2. Troland.

photone (fo'tōn). A visual hallucination or a visualization of light.

photonosus (fo-ton'o-sus). A disease due to exposure to excessive light. Syn., *photopathy*.

photo-ophthalmia (fo"to-of-thal'me-ah). Photophthalmia.

photopathologic (fo"to-path"o-loj'-ik). Pertaining to a disease due to exposure to excessive light.

photopathy (fo-top'ah-the). Photonosus.

photoped (fo'to-ped). A photometer head.

photoperceptive (fo"to-per-sep'tiv). Capable of perceiving light.

photophobia (fo"to-fo'be-ah). An abnormal intolerance or fear of light.

photophobic (fo"to-fo'bik). Pertaining to or affected with photophobia.

photophore (fo'to-fōr). A simple or complex organ that produces bioluminescence, such as may be found in certain worms, arthropods, insects, and deep sea fishes.

photophoresis (fo"to-fo-re'sis). Movement of very small suspended particles toward (negative) or away from (positive) a transilluminating source.

photophthalmia (fo"tof-thal'me-ah). Inflammation of the eyes from exposure to intense light, as in snow blindness or from a welder's arc.

photopia (fo-to'pe-ah). Photopic vision.

photopic (fo-top'ik). Having the characteristics of photopic vision or referring to the levels of illumination at which the eye is light adapted.

photopigment (fo"to-pig'ment). A pigment which is affected by, or unstable in the presence of, radiant energy, especially visible radiant energy, such that its chemical composition is altered. In the eye, the breakdown of photopigments by light is the first stage in the visual process.

photoprotein (fo"to-pro'te-in). A protein substance found in certain organisms which, when oxidized by a suitable substance, emits light (*bioluminescence*).

photopsia (fo-top'se-ah). An unformed hallucinatory perception of sparks, lights, or colors, frequently due to disease of the optic nerve, the retina, or the brain.

photopsins (fo-top'sinz). The photopigments in the retinal cones. Cf. *scotopsins*.

photopter (fo-top'ter). The unit of light transmission of Tscherning's filters designated by Tscherning to be $^1/_{10}$ of the incident light, hence 2 photopters represent a transmission of $(^1/_{10})^2$, or $^1/_{100}$, and x photopters represent a transmission of $(^1/_{10})^x$.

photoptic (fo-top'tik). Pertaining to photopsia.

photoptometer (fo"top-tom'eh-ter). An instrument for determining the light threshold which just permits objects to become visible or identifiable.

photoptometry (fo"top-tom'eh-tre). Determination of the light threshold which just permits objects to become visible or identifiable.

photoreceptive (fo"to-re-sep'tive). Capable of receiving and perceiving light; activated by light.

photoreceptor (fo"to-re-sep'tor). A receptor capable of being activated by light stimuli, as a rod or cone cell of the eye.

photoretinitis (fo"to-ret-ih-ni'tis). Inflammation of the retina due to exposure to intense light, as from viewing an eclipse or a welder's arc with insufficient protection. The condition results in a central scotoma, which may be temporary, and may be followed by pigmentary changes in the macular area.

photoscope (fo'to-skōp). 1. A statoscope. 2. A type of fluoroscope.

photoscopy (fo-tos'ko-pe). Retinoscopy. *Obs.*

photosensitive (fo"to-sen'sih-tiv). 1. Pertaining to the cells of an organ or organism that are capable of being stimulated to activity by light. 2. Pertaining to certain chemicals which have the property of reacting to light.

photosensitivity (fo"to-sen"sih-tiv'ih-te). 1. The capacity of the cells of an organ or an organism to be stimulated to activity by light. 2. The property of certain chemicals to react to light.

photosensitize (fo"to-sen'sih-tīz). To sensitize a substance or the cells of an organ or an organism to light stimulation.

photosensor (fo-to-sen'ser). A device designed to respond to light by transmitting an impulse or impulses for interpretation, measurement, or control operation.

photosensory (fo"to-sen'so-re). Pertaining to the act or process by which an organ or an organism responds to light stimuli.

photoskiascopy (fo"to-ski-as'ko-pe). An objective method of determination of the refractive error based on the pattern of light and dark areas appearing in the pupil when illuminated by the light of a stationary ophthalmoscope, and its modification by neutralization with ophthalmic lenses.

photostatic (fo'to-stat-ik). Of, constituting, or relating to postural, orientation, or equilibrium reflexes initiated by light stimulation.

photostimulator (fo"to-stim"u-la'-tor). An instrument which generates light pulses (flashes) of variable frequency, duration, and intensity.

Photosun. A trade name for an ophthalmic lens made of photochromic glass varying in light transmission from approximately 20% to 65%.

phototachometer (fo"to-tah-kom'eh-ter). A device for measuring the velocity of light by means of a rotating mirror.

phototaxis (fo"to-tak'sis). A purposive movement of a motile organism in response to the direction of light stimulation. It is positive when directed toward the light and negative when away from the light.

phototherapy (fo"to-ther'ah-pe). The treatment of a disease or condition by exposure to certain portions of the spectrum.

phototonus (fo-tot'o-nus). An irritable state of protoplasm to light stimulus; specifically applied to reciprocal coordination of muscle tone of certain symmetrical animals, when light is employed to induce motion.

phototopia (fo"to-to'pe-ah). A subjective light sensation.

phototrauma (fo"to-traw'mah). Injury from exposure to intense light, as in snow blindness.

phototropism (fo-tot'ro-pizm). The directional orientation of parts of sessile plants and animals toward (positive) or away from (negative) light stimulation.

phthiriasis ciliorum (thir-i'ah-sis sil-e-ōr'um). Infestation of the eyelashes or the eyelids with lice.

phthiriasis palpebrarum (thir-i'ah-sis pal-pe-brah'rum). Infestation of the lid margins by lice.

phthisis (thi'sis). A wasting away of tissue or of a part of the body.

p. bulbi. Shrinking, wasting, and atrophy of the eyeball; the sequela of panophthalmitis, absolute glaucoma, etc. Vision is completely lost, and intraocular pressure is abnormally low.

p. corneae. Shrinking, wasting, and atrophy of the cornea; the sequela of anterior staphyloma, etc.

essential p. Ophthalmomalacia.

physostigmine (fi"so-stig'mēn, -min). Eserine.

pi (π). The Greek letter used as the symbol for the *angle of eccentricity* in the field of regard. (Fry)

pia mater (pi"ah ma'ter). The innermost vascular member of the three meninges covering the brain, the spinal cord, and the optic nerve. It is closely attached to the central nervous system and all of its folds, and helps form the tela chorioidea or choroid plexus of each ventricle of the brain. From the optic nerve it becomes continuous for the most part with the sclera, but some fibers run into the choroid and some into the border tissue around the optic nerve.

Pick's (piks) **disease; sign; vision.** See under the nouns.

Pickford test. See under *test.*

picture, retinal. The retinal image.

Pierce's test (pĕr'sez). See under *test.*

Piéron's law; theory. See under the nouns.

piezometer (pi″e-zom'eh-ter). A type of orbitonometer in which the compressibility of the orbital contents is represented by the amount of depression produced by the addition of a 25 mg weight on a foot-plate resting on a vertically directed anesthetized cornea.

Pigeon-Cantonnet stereoscope (pe'je-ōn kan'ton-a). See under *stereoscope.*

pigment, photosensitive. Photopigment.

pigmentation, congenital, of the retina. Pigmented paravenous retinochoroidal atrophy.

pigmentum nigrum (pig-men'tum ni'grum). The pigment of the stroma of the choroid.

pili torti (pi'li tōr'te). A dominant inherited condition in which the eyelashes, and sometimes eyebrows and head hair, are short, scanty, twisted, and brittle. Affected children are usually born bald and remain so for one or two years.

Pillat's parenchymatous corneal dystrophy. See under *dystrophy, corneal.*

pilocarpine (pi″lo-kar'pēn, -pin). An alkaloid obtained from leaves of the South American shrubs *Pilocarpus jaborandi* and *P. microphyllus,* and used in salt form in a dilute solution as a miotic.

Piltz's reflex (piltz'ez). 1. Attention pupillary reflex. 2. Orbicularis pupillary reflex.

Piltz-Westphal (piltz-vest'fahl) **phenomenon; reaction; reflex.** Orbicularis pupillary reflex.

pimelopterygium (pim″eh-lo-teh-rij'e-um). Pinguecula.

pince-nez (pans'na″). Eyeglasses, without supporting temples, held on the nose by tension from springs attached to the nose pads.

pinguecula (ping-gwek'u-lah). A small, slightly raised, yellowish, nonfatty thickening of the bulbar conjunctiva on either side of the cornea, usually the nasal side, essentially formed by hyaline degeneration and proliferation of elastic fibers of the substantia propria.

pinhole. A pinhole pupil.

pink. Typically, a hue approximately complementary to a blue-green of 493 mμ; a desaturated or pastel red, orange-red, or bluish-red.

pink eye. See under *eye.*

Piper (pi'per) **law; syndrome.** See under the nouns.

piperocaine (pi'per-o-kān). A corneal anesthetic usually used in a 2% solution, having a relatively slow time of onset and long duration of action as compared with *benoxinate, proparacaine,* or *tetracaine.*

pipper. The bead at the center of a ring gunsight, or a small hole at the center of a sighting reticle.

pit. A surface depression, hollow, or indentation.

    foveal p. Fovea centralis.

    Gaule's p's. Gaule's spots.

    Herbert's p's. Facets in the cornea appearing in the chronic stage of trachoma, due to degeneration and sloughing of its superficial layer with subsequent filling by optically clear epithelium.

    lens p. A tiny depression formed by the invagination of the surface ectoderm or lens plate of the embryo, adjacent to the optic vesicle. It subsequently develops into the lens vesicle and the adult crystalline lens. Syn., *fovea lentis; lenticular sac.*

    optic p's. Paired pits formed by lateral depressions in the neural ectoderm of the forebrain during the stage of closure of the neural groove, the earliest embryonic stage in the development of the optic cups.

    p. of the optic disk. A rare, congenital, craterlike depression in the optic nerve head, typically located in its inferior temporal quadrant near the disk edge and generally between ⅓ to ⅙ disk diameter in size, between 2 and 8 diopters in depth, and round or oval in shape. The visual field may show an arcuate scotoma continuous with an enlarged blind spot and a central angiospastic retinopathy may be an accompaniment.

pitch. 1. Any one of several materials of various colors and sometimes transparent, characteristically sticky when warm, and hard or brittle at ordinary temperatures, used in ophthalmic laboratories for cementing a lens to a block, for impregnating polishing pads, and in molded form as a surfacing lap. 2. The distance between corresponding points in two adjacent threads of a screw, measured along the axis.

Pitt's law. See under *law.*

pityriasis rubra pilaris (pit″ih-ri′ah-sis). A chronic skin disease characterized by the formation of hard yellowish or reddish papules at the mouths of the hair follicles which may be accompanied by involvement of the conjunctiva and cornea. The conjunctiva may have a general thickening and may have typical mother-of-pearl papules on its bulbar portion, and the cornea may have a generalized epithelial thickening with pannus, ulceration, or interstitial keratitis.

placebo (plah-se′bo). A prescription or medicine given merely to satisfy a patient, irrespective of its corrective or therapeutic value.

Placido's disk (plah-si′dōz). See under *disk.*

placidoscope (plah-si′do-skōp). Placido's disk.

placode, lens (plak′ōd). Lens plate.

pladaroma (plad″ah-ro′mah). A soft tumor of the eyelid.

pladarosis (plad″ah-ro′sis). Pladaroma.

Planck's (planks) **constant; law; theory.** See under the nouns.

◆

PLANE

plane. A surface of zero curvature.

active p. The section of a cylindrical lens or prism in which the chief refraction occurs, as distinguished from the *passive plane,* perpendicular to this plane.

axial p. Muscle plane.

Broca's p. Visual plane.

cardinal p. Principal plane.

conjugate p's. The object plane and its corresponding image plane considered as a pair in the Gaussian representation of an optical system.

equatorial p. The plane, containing the transverse and vertical axes, which divides the eyeball into anterior and posterior halves.

face p. A plane taken to represent the geometric location and orientation of the face, such as one tangent to the two superciliary ridges and the point of the chin.

p. of fixation. The plane containing the axes of fixation of the two eyes.

focal p. 1. A plane, perpendicular to the optical axis, passing through one of the focal points of an optical system. 2. Occasionally, any image plane in an optical system. **anterior f.p.** Primary focal plane. **posterior f.p.** Secondary focal plane. **primary f.p.** A plane, perpendicular to the optical axis, passing through the primary focal point of an optical system. Syn., *anterior focal plane.* **secondary f.p.** A plane, perpendicular to the optical axis, passing through the secondary focal point of an optical system. Syn., *posterior focal plane.*

frontal p. A plane through two points of reference representing the two eyes, such as the entrance pupils, the centers of rotation, the nodal points, or the sighting intersects, and perpendicular to a plane connecting the same two points of reference with the point of fixation.

frontoparallel p. Any plane parallel to a frontal plane. **apparent f.p.** A surface containing the point of fixation and all other points judged by the observer to be equidistant from his frontal plane. **objective f.p.** A surface containing the point of fixation and all other points which are equidistant from the frontal plane.

horizontal p. of the eye. The plane, containing sagittal and transverse axes, which divides the eyeball into superior and inferior halves.

image p. A plane, perpendicular to the optical axis, through the axial image point of an optical system.

p. of incidence. The plane containing the incident light ray and the normal to the surface at the point of incidence.

Listing's p. A plane passing through the center of rotation perpendicular to the primary position of the line of sight. According to Listing, all fixational movements of the eye can be analyzed in terms of rotation of the line of sight about axes in this plane. Syn., *primary axis plane.*

median p. The plane, containing the sagittal and the vertical axes, which divides the eyeball into right and left halves.

meridional p. in oblique astigmatism. Tangential plane in oblique astigmatism.

muscle p. A plane containing the line of traction of an extraocular muscle and the center or rotation of the eyeball. Syn., *axial plane; plane of rotation; plane of traction.*

nodal p. A plane, perpendicular to the optical axis, passing through one of the nodal points of an optical system.

object p. A plane, perpendicular to the optical axis, through the axial object point of an optical system.

orbital p. 1. The plane approximating the surface of the maxillary bone which helps to form the floor of the orbit. 2. The visual plane.

passive p. The section of a cylindrical lens or prism in which no refraction occurs, as distinguished from the *active plane* perpendicular to this plane.

p. of polarization. The plane which is perpendicular to the plane of vibration of the electric vector of linearly polarized light.

primary axis p. Listing's plane.

primary p. in oblique astigmatism. Tangential plane in oblique astigmatism.

principal p. A plane in an optical system, perpendicular to the optical axis, at which refraction of the incident or emergent light may be considered to take place. Syn., *cardinal plane; unit plane.* **primary p.p.** The principal plane at which the total refraction with respect to the incident light may be considered to take place. It is located at the intersections of the incident rays from the primary focal point with the corresponding emergent parallel rays. **secondary p.p.** The principal plane at which the total refraction with respect to the emergent light may be considered to take place. It is located at the intersections of the emergent rays converging to the secondary focal point with the corresponding incident parallel rays.

principal p. of extraordinary ray. A plane in a crystal containing the optical axis and the extraordinary ray.

principal p. of ordinary ray. A plane in a crystal containing the optical axis and the ordinary ray.

principal section p. The plane containing the optical axis and normal to a surface of a doubly refracting crystal.

p. of refraction. The plane containing the refracted light ray and the normal to the surface at the point of refraction.

p. of reflection. The plane containing the reflected light ray and the normal to the surface at the point of reflection.

p. of regard. A plane passing through the point of regard and two points of reference for the two eyes, such as the centers of the entrance pupils, the centers of rotation, the sighting intersects, or the nodal points.

p. of rotation. Muscle plane.

sagittal p. in oblique astigmatism. A plane perpendicular to the tangential plane in oblique astigmatism. Syn., *secondary plane.*

secondary axis p. According to Listing's law, the plane containing the axes around which fixational rotations may occur when the eye is in a secondary position. It is described as a plane bisecting the angle made by the equatorial plane of the eye when it changes from the primary to the secondary direction of fixation.

secondary p. in oblique astigmatism. Sagittal plane in oblique astigmatism.

spectacle p. A plane taken to represent the geometric location and orientation of the spectacle lenses in relation to the eyes and usually considered to correspond with the posterior vertices of the two spectacle lenses and to lie from 12 to 15 mm anterior to the two corneal apices.

symmetrical p's. Planes perpendicular to the axis of an optical system and containing the symmetrical points.

tangent p. A modified Bjerrum's tangent screen having a black surface with a white fixation spot facing the patient with the reverse surface white and divided into squares or circles. The outlines of scotomata are shown on the white side by pins thrust through from the black surface.

tangential p. in oblique astigmatism. A plane containing the optical axis of the lens system and the off axis object point. Syn., *meridional plane; primary plane.*

tilting p. Tilting field.

p. of traction. Muscle plane.

transmission p. The plane of vibration of polarized light passing through a polarizer such as a Nicol prism.

unit p. Principal plane.

p. of vibration. The plane, perpendicular to the plane of polarization, indicating the direction of oscillation of the electric vector of linearly polarized radiation.

visual p. The plane containing the two visual axes. Syn., *Broca's plane; orbital plane.*

p. of visual projection. The plane in which a visually perceived object is subjectively localized.

xy p. The horizontal plane of the eye containing both the x axis and the y axis. When the eye is in the primary position, this plane cuts a circle on the eyeball called by Helmholtz the retinal horizon.

xz p. The vertical plane of the eye containing both the x axis and the z axis.

yz p. The vertical plane of the eye containing both the y axis and the z axis. When the eye is in the primary position, this plane cuts a circle on the eyeball called by Helmholtz the principal retinal meridian.

◆

plano (pla′no). Afocal; without dioptric power.

plano- (pla′no-). A combining form denoting that one surface is plane, e.g., planoconvex.

planoconcave (pla″no-kon′kāv). Pertaining to a lens that is flat on one surface and concave on the other. (See Fig. 25.)

planoconvex (pla″no-kon′veks). Pertaining to a lens that is flat on one surface and convex on the other. (See Fig. 25.)

plano-prism (pla′no-prizm). A prism with no dioptric power.

planum orbitale (pla′num ōr-bih-tal′-e). Orbital plane.

plaques, Hollenhorst's (plaks). Glittering, orange-yellow, atheromatous, cholesterin-containing emboli in the retinal arterioles, a sign of impending serious cardiovascular disease such as myocardial infarction, stroke, occlusion of the retinal arterioles, or aortic aneurysm.

plasmoma (plaz-mo′mah). A tumor consisting essentially of plasma cells, sometimes found on the conjunctiva in chronic inflammatory conditions such as trachoma.

plastic. 1. Pertaining to stereoscopic or third dimension effect, as in plastic relief. 2. Any of various materials showing plasticity, often used in lenses, spectacle frames, artificial eyes, etc.

◆

PLATE

plate. A flat, or nearly flat, structure or layer.

AO H-R-R p's. Pseudoisochromatic plates for testing color vision, each containing one or two variously located geometric figures (circle, cross, or triangle). Four plates are for demonstration; six are for screening into red-green deficient, blue-yellow deficient, and normal; ten are for further testing of the red-green deficient; and four are for further testing of the blue-yellow deficient.

Boström's p's. A series of 16 pseudoisochromatic plates for testing color vision, 12 containing digits, and 4 blank to detect malingering.

Boström-Kugelberg p's. A series of 20 pseudoisochromatic plates for testing color vision, 15 containing digits, 2 winding trails for illiterates, and 3 blank to detect malingering.

cribriform p. Lamina cribrosa.

Dvorine's p's. A series of pseudoisochromatic plates for testing color vision.

half-wave p. A thin sheet of crystalline material, such as mica or quartz, cut parallel to the optical axis and of such thickness as to produce a 180° phase difference between the ordinary and extraordinary ray vibrations. Its effect is to alter the direction of vibration of plane-polarized light.

Hardy-Rand-Rittler p's. AO H-R-R plates.

Hertel's p's. A series of 35 plates for testing color vision consisting of 2 for indoctrination and detection of malingering, 10 pseudoisochromatic plates (based on Stilling's plates) for the detection of red-green deficiencies, 6 pseudoisochromatic plates to differentiate protans from deutans, 4 plates incorporating marked brightness as well as color differences, 6 "selection" plates containing a random array of disks of similar hues, 3 plates to test the effect of adjacent stimuli on hue judgment, and 4 plates for the detection of yellow-blue deficiencies.

Ishihara p's. A series of pseudoisochromatic plates for testing color vision.

Laurent half-shade p. A semicircular half-wave plate of quartz or other crystal set between the polari-

plate   [483]   *plate*

zer and analyzer of an instrument to measure rotatory polarization.

lens p. The thickened surface ectoderm in the embryo, peripheral to the primary optic vesicle which forms, by its invagination, the lens pit and subsequently the lens vesicle and adult crystalline lens. Syn., *lens placode.*

optic p. That portion of the neural ectoderm in the embryonic forebrain, located at the anterior extremity of the neural fold, which gives rise to the retina and the pars caeca retinae.

orbital p. The portion of any facial or cranial bone that forms a part of the orbit, such as the lamina papyracea, the process of the frontal bone, or the process of the superior maxillary bone. **frontal o.p.** The portion of the frontal bone that forms most of the roof of the orbit. **maxillary o.p.** The portion of the maxillary bone that forms the floor of the orbit anterior to the palatine bone. **zygomatic o.p.** The portion of the malar or zygomatic bone that forms a portion of the lateral wall and floor of the orbit.

phase p. A layer of transparent material introduced into an optical system to advance or retard the direct light a fraction of a wavelength with respect to diffracted light originating from the same source. Syn., *phase disk.*

phase retardation p. A piece of doubly refracting material cut and polished so that it retards either the ordinary or extraordinary ray more than its companion ray, thereby chang-

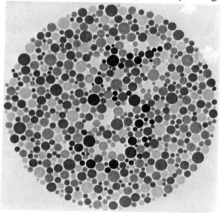

Fig. 28 A pseudoisochromatic plate.

ing the phase relationship between the two rays.

pseudoisochromatic p. A chart for testing color vision on which are printed numerous small disks, vary-

ing in color and brightness, some of which are oriented to form numbers, letters, or geometric figures so as to be perceived only by those with normal color vision and not by those with deficient color vision, or vice versa. (See Fig. 28.)

quarter-wave p. A thin sheet of crystalline material, such as mica or quartz, cut parallel to the optical axis and of such thickness as to produce a 90° phase difference between the ordinary and extraordinary ray vibrations. It is used to transform plane-polarized light into circularly or elliptically polarized light, or the reverse, or to analyze any form of polarized light.

Rabkin polychromatic p's. A set of 20 pseudoisochromatic charts designed by Rabkin to detect color vision abnormalities and to classify them according to type and severity of deficiency.

Savart p. A device consisting of two plane parallel plates of equal thickness, cut from a uniaxial crystal, such as quartz or calcite, such that the angle between the optic axis and the normal to the surface shall be the same for both. The two plates, shaped into squares, are mounted geometrically parallel but with one optical axis turned 90° with respect to the other. It is used to detect linearly polarized light in a pencil of natural light, to study elliptically polarized light, and to alter phase differences.

Schmidt p. A transparent aspheric refracting plate located at, or near, the center of curvature of a spherical telescope mirror for the purpose of "pre-correcting" the wavefronts of the otherwise parallel pencils entering the system so that they will be spherical after reflection by the mirror.

Stilling's p's. A series of pseudoisochromatic plates for testing color vision.

tarsal p. Tarsus.

Tokyo Medical College p's. See under *test.*

Velhagen's p's. A series of plates for testing color vision, of which some are pseudoisochromatic and others are based on color selection, color contrast, and brightness difference.

zone p. A screen consisting of a series of alternately opaque and transparent concentric rings whose common borders have radii successively proportional to the square roots of whole numbers. The rings will correspond to half-period zones for a given point of reference at which there will be a concentration of light from a source transmitting light through the screen.

◆

Plateau's spiral (plah-tōz). See under *spiral*.

plateau (plah-to'). 1. A leveling off or an interval of no increment in a curve otherwise showing continuous increase or growth, as, for example, in a learning curve. 2. A level elevated area.

  Stieda's p's. A series of low elevations, separated by Stieda's grooves, located in the palpebral conjunctiva between the tarsus and the fornix.

platoscope (plat'o-skōp). Stereoscope. *Obs.*

platycoria (plat″e-ko're-ah). A dilated or large pupil.

platycoriasis (plat″e-ko-ri'ah-sis). The condition of having a dilated or large pupil.

platymorphia (plate″e-mōr'fe-ah). A flatness in the shape of the eyeball, resulting in a short anteroposterior axis and hypermetropia.

platymorphic (plat″e-mōr'fik). Pertaining to the condition of platymorphia.

platyopic (plat″e-op'ik). Having an orbitonasal index below 110 (or 107.5). Cf. *mesopic; pro-opic.*

pleating, scleral. A surgical procedure for shortening the eyeball in the treatment of retinal detachment in which a fold is made in the sclera, at about the equator of the eyeball, and is fixed with a mattress suture. It is performed in conjunction with diathermy.

pleochroism (ple-ok'ro-izm). The property of certain crystals to exhibit different colors when the light transmitted through them is viewed from different directions, as in *dichroism* and *trichroism.* Syn., *polychroism.*

Pleopticon (ple'op-tih-kon). A device for the improvement of visual acuity and fixation in amblyopia, consisting essentially of a tube having a small circular aperture at one end and an opaque disk of 5° subtense with a central fixation point at the other end. The opaque disk is viewed through the aperture and fixated while a bright light source illuminates the area surrounding the disk. The opaque disk shields the central area of the retina from light stimulation, creating a positive afterimage having a dark center and a light sur-round. It is followed by a negative afterimage which is then centered on fixation targets.

pleoptics (ple-op'tiks). A method of treating amblyopia ex anopsia in which concentrated and intensive stimulation is provided to the fovea of the amblyopic eye. One procedure involves intense light stimulation of the nonfoveal area to render the foveal area more receptive to fixation stimuli; other procedures involve association of touch, hearing, and memory with visual perception.

Pleoptiscope (ple″op-tih-skōp'). An instrument which creates Haidinger's brushes for the diagnosis and treatment of eccentric fixation and the improvement of visual acuity in amblyopia.

Pleoptophor (ple-op'to-fōr). A visual training instrument designed by Bangerter for the treatment of amblyopia ex anopsia and eccentric fixation. It consists essentially of a telescope with a 40 degree field of view providing continuous observation of the fundus during treatment, with 18× magnification. The treatment consists of first stimulating the peripheral retina with bright light while shielding the central area with an opaque disk (dazzling phase), then stimulating the central and peripheral areas while shielding the pericentral area with a doughnut-shaped opaque disk (stimulating phase), and last, briefly repeating the initial phase. The treatment is designed to enhance foveal fixation and is immediately followed by fixation training on other instruments.

plesiopia (ple″se-o'pe-ah, ples″e-). Myopia.

Plexiglas (plek'sih-glas). A trade name for polymethyl methacrylate, marketed by Rohm & Haas Company.

◆

PLEXUS

plexus (plek'sus). A network of nerves, blood vessels, or lymphatics.

  annular p. Paramarginal plexus.

  anterior ciliary p. A plexus of veins in the longitudinal or outer portion of the ciliary muscle that empties into the intrascleral and episcleral plexuses.

  cavernous p. A network of nerve fibers derived from the internal carotid nerve and located on the medial side of the internal carotid artery in the cavernous sinus. It supplies sympathetic postganglionic axons to orbital effectors and the eyeball via the superior or orbital fissure.

ciliary p. 1. A network of thin vessels at the root of the ciliary processes, believed to serve in the absorption of aqueous humor. 2. Canal of Schlemm. *Obs.*

episcleral p. A plexus of veins in the anterior episclera which receives blood from the anterior ciliary, deep scleral, and superficial scleral plexuses and empties into the anterior ciliary veins.

episcleral limbal p. A network of branches of the episcleral arteries near the corneo-scleral junction which communicates with anterior conjunctival arteries.

Hovius' p. Circle of Hovius.

infraorbital p. The embryonic veins below the optic vesicle or optic cup, which later differentiate into the inferior ophthalmic vein.

intersphincteric p. A network of capillaries located between the fibers of the sphincter pupillae muscle in the iris.

intraepithelial p. The network of very fine fibers in the epithelial layer of the cornea.

intrascleral p. The deep scleral plexus and superficial scleral plexus in combination.

Leber's venous p. Circle of Hovius.

marginal nerve p. of von Mises. A plexus of nerve fibers surrounding the follicles of the eyelashes.

ophthalmic p. The network of sympathetic nerve fibers about the ophthalmic artery which are vasoconstrictor in function.

paramarginal p. A superficial network of sensory nerve fibers, about 1.5 mm wide, derived from subconjunctival and episcleral plexuses, located just beneath Bowman's membrane near the limbus, and terminating in receptors in the corneal epithelium. Syn., *annular plexus.*

pericorneal p. A network of vessels lying in a band around the limbus and formed by the anastomosing of conjunctival and anterior ciliary arteries. It lies superficially in the conjunctiva, where it is a branching network, and deeper in the episclera, where it follows a relatively straight course.

peripheral pericorneal p. Annular plexus.

posttarsal p. 1. A plexus of capillaries, running between the marginal and the peripheral arcades of the eyelid posterior to the tarsus, which supplies the conjunctiva. Syn., *retrotarsal plexus; subconjunctival plexus.* 2. The posttarsal lymphatic vessels.

pretarsal p. 1. A plexus of capillaries, running between the marginal and the peripheral arcades of the eyelid anterior to the tarsus, which supplies the tarsal glands and all structures anterior to the tarsus. 2. The pretarsal lymphatic vessels.

pterygoid p. The network of veins near the pterygopalatine fossa, which receives tributaries corresponding to the branches of the internal maxillary artery and the lower division of the inferior ophthalmic vein and communicates with the cavernous sinus and the anterior facial vein.

retrotarsal p. Posttarsal plexus.

scleral p., deep. A plexus of capillaries in the deep layers of the sclera, encircling the limbal area in close apposition to the canal of Schlemm, which receives aqueous humor from the canal of Schlemm via collectors and blood from the surrounding area. It drains into the superficial scleral plexus and anterior ciliary veins.

scleral p., superficial. A plexus of vessels, predominantly venous, in the anterior superficial sclera which receives blood from the deep scleral plexus and anterior ciliary plexus and communicates with the episcleral, Tenon's and anterior conjunctival plexuses.

stroma p. Superficial and deep networks of nerves in the substantia propria of the cornea.

subconjunctival p. Posttarsal plexus.

subepithelial p. The network of nerve fibers located immediately beneath Bowman's membrane of the cornea. It receives nerve fibers from the stratified epithelium and leads to the stroma plexus.

subsphincteric p. A network of capillaries located between the sphincter pupillae muscle and the pigment epithelium of the iris.

superficial marginal p. The network of small arteries and capillaries derived from the anterior ciliary arteries, located in the limbus of the cornea deep to the stratified epithelium.

supraorbital p. The embryonic veins above the optic vesicle or optic cup, which later differentiate into the superior ophthalmic vein.

◆

plica (pli′kah). A fold or a folded structure.

p. centralis. A fold in the retina coursing between the fovea centralis and the optic disk, observed only in postmortem examination.

p. ciliaris. Ciliary fold.

p. iridis. One of the many minute folds on the posterior surface of the iris.

p. lacrimalis. A fold of mucous membrane at the entrance of the naso-lacrimal duct into the inferior meatus of the nose. It represents the remains of the fetal septum. Syn., *Hasner's fold; lacrimal fold; Bianchi's valve; Cruveilhier's valve; Hasner's valve.*

p. lunata. Plica semilunaris.

p. semilunaris. The crescent-shaped conjunctival fold at the medial canthus lateral to the caruncle. It is a vestigial structure corresponding to the nictitating membrane of lower vertebrates. Syn., *plica lunata.*

pliers. A hand-held tool having two short handles and two grasping jaws working on a pivot, used for gripping, bending, or cutting.

angling p. 1. Pliers with jaws shaped to fit and hold the endpiece of a spectacle frame or mounting while the temples are angled. Syn., *endpiece pliers.* 2. Pliers with jaws shaped to fit and hold a saddle bridge while it is angled.

chipping p. Pliers with wide, flat-faced jaws used in chipping excess glass from the edge of a lens after it has been cut to approximate shape.

cutting p. Pliers with knife edge jaws used for removing the excess portions of screws of spectacle frames or mountings.

endpiece p. Angling pliers.

half-round p. Pliers with one round, tapered jaw and one flat-faced, tapered jaw, used in adjusting spectacle frames and mountings.

Numont arm p. Pliers with jaws that contain a small transverse groove for gripping the arm of a spectacle mounting, used for reshaping the arm or in angling the temple.

snipe nose p. Pliers with long, flat-faced jaws tapered to a point, used in adjusting spectacle frames and mountings.

strap p. Pliers with jaws designed for shaping the straps of spectacle mountings.

ploration (plo-ra′shun). Lacrimation. *Obs.*

plotter, ray. Any of a number of devices used to determine the path of a ray of light through optical media or an optical system.

plus. The opposite of *minus* or *negative* in the designation of data, systems, or observations, the values of which may be represented on a continuous numerical scale from plus, through zero, to minus values, whence it may represent *convergence* as applied to lenses, *divergence* as applied to wavefronts. Syn., *positive.*

plus acceptance. The acceptance, or the indication of acceptability, of convex sphere, or of an increased amount of convex sphere, as a dioptric correction either in a lens prescription or during a specific test or visual task, based on any one criterion or a combination of criteria related to blurredness, discomfort, and other clinical signs or symptoms.

PMMA. Polymethyl methacrylate.

pneumocele, orbital (nu′mo-sēl). An enclosed pocket of air in the orbit, usually caused either by forcible blowing of the nose or by trauma.

pneumatonograph. A pneumatic applanation tonometer which utilizes a probe consisting of a diaphragm pressed in contact with the eye which, according to the hardness of the eye, displaces a gimbaled sensing nozzle against the pressure of continuous flowing air so as to narrow the escape orifice and elevate the pressure in the air chamber of the sensor which, in turn, is recorded by means of a pneumatic-to-electric transducer.

pneumotography, orbital (nu-mo-tog′raf-e). Orbito-pneumotography.

Poggendorff's (po′gen-dorfs) **figure; illusion.** See under the nouns.

Poincaré sphere. See under *sphere.*

◆

POINT

point. 1. A place considered only as to its position, having definite location but no extent in space. 2. A condition or position attained; a step; a stage. 3. A unit of thickness of spectacle lenses equal to one fifth of a millimeter.

achromatic p. Any point in a chromaticity diagram which represents an achromatic color.

aplanatic p's. The object and image points as a pair in an optical system corrected for spherical aberration and satisfying the sine condition.

blur point. 1. Under a given set of test conditions, the point at which the fixation target appears blurred on the introduction of gradually increasing prism and/or lens power. 2. A point on a graph representing the limit of clear, single, binocular vision. **accommodative b.p.** A blur point induced by the addition of concave or convex lens power at a fixed test distance. **base-in b.p.** The point of blur obtained by gradually introducing base-in prism power or effect during binocular fixation at a fixed test distance. **base-out b.p.** The point of blur obtained by gradually introducing base-out prism power or effect during binocular fixation at a fixed test distance. **beginning b.p.** A just noticeable determination of a blur point. Cf. *blur-out point.* **convergence b.p.** 1. Base-out blur point. 2. Either base-in or base-out blur point. **minus lens b.p.** The point of blur obtained by gradually introducing minus lens power in front of one or both eyes at a fixed test distance. **plus lens b.p.** The point of blur obtained by gradually introducing plus lens power in front of one or both eyes at a fixed test distance.

blur-out p. The point at which a target becomes so blurred as to be illegible or unrecognizable. Cf. *beginning blur point.*

break p. The point at which diplopia occurs on gradually varying the prism or lens power during binocular fixation.

cardinal p's. Six points on the axis of an optical system, viz., the two principal foci, the two principal points, and the two nodal points. Cf. *Gaussian points.*

centration p. British equivalent to *major reference point.*

chief p. A point on the principal surface of an optical system corrected for coma where an incident ray intersects the surface.

conjugate p's. The object point and its corresponding image point considered as a pair in an optical system.

p. of convergence. 1. The point of intersection of the lines of sight. 2. The point to which a pencil of light converges.

corresponding p's. Corresponding retinal points.

demand p. The point in a graphical coordinate system representing the stimulus to accommodation and the stimulus to convergence in a given test situation. It may or may not represent a single target point in space.

disparate p's. Noncorresponding retinal points.

p. of divergence. 1. The point of intersection of diverging lines of sight. 2. The point from which a pencil of light diverges.

diving p's. Minute objects which approach the minimum visible threshold and appear to move or to disappear and reappear as stars do when constantly viewed.

entrance pupil p. The center of the entrance pupil.

equivalent p's. A pair of points on the axis of an optical system, corresponding simultaneously to the nodal and principal points, as when the object and image space have the same refractive index.

exit pupil p. The center of the exit pupil.

eye p. Eyepoint.

far p. of accommodation. See under *accommodation.*

far p. of convergence. See under *convergence.*

far p. of fusion. See under *fusion.*

p. of fixation. 1. The point in space to which one or both eyes are consciously directed. In normal vision its image is on the fovea. 2. Point of regard. **primary p. of f.** The point fixated when the eye is in the primary position.

focal p. The point of convergence or divergence of a pencil of light. **anterior f.p.** Primary focal point. **posterior f.p.** Secondary focal point. **primary f.p.** The point of convergence or divergence of a pencil of incident light rays which emerge parallel to the axis of an optical system. Syn., *anterior focal point; anterior principal focal point; primary principal focal point.* **principal f.p., anterior.** Primary focal point. **principal f.p., posterior.** Secondary focal point. **principal f.p., primary.** Primary focal point. **principal f.p., secondary.** Secondary focal point. **secondary f.p.** The point of convergence or divergence of a pencil of emergent light rays which are incident parallel to the axis of an optical system. Syn., *pos-*

terior focal point; posterior principal focal point; secondary principal focal point.

Gaussian p's. The two principal foci and the two principal points on the axis of an optical system. Cf. *cardinal points.*

homologous p's. Two points, one on each half of a stereogram, which are of identical target content.

homonymous p's. Corresponding retinal points.

Horner-Trantas p's. White pinpoint projections visible on the conjunctiva in vernal conjunctivitis which represent circumscribed areas of epithelial cells undergoing rapid and progressive degeneration. They are first situated in the deeper layers of the epithelium, extending later toward and breaking through the surface.

identical p's. Corresponding retinal points.

image p. The point at which an object point is imaged by an optical system.

p. of incidence. The point at which a ray of light is incident upon a refracting or reflecting surface.

infraorbital p. The lowest point on the margin of the orbit.

isosbestic p. A point on the spectral absorption curve of a photopigment that corresponds to the wavelength at which the optical density remains unchanged throughout the whole bleaching process, with increasing or decreasing densities at other points.

lacrimal p. Lacrimal punctum.

major reference p. The point of the front or back surface of a spectacle lens at which the prism power corresponds to that prescribed.

near p. of accommodation. See under *accommodation.*

near p. of convergence. See under *convergence.*

near p. of fusion. See under *fusion.*

neutral p. 1. In retinoscopy, the point at which the motion of the reflex cannot be detected, determined either by placing lenses before the eye or by moving the retinoscope to a point in space conjugate with the retina. 2. In certain types of color blindness, the point or points in the spectrum which appear colorless to an observer, or those spectral wavelengths which appear to match the chromaticity of a standard white.

nodal p's. A pair of points on the axis of an optical system which have the property that any incident ray directed toward the first, the anterior nodal point, leaves the system as though from the second, the posterior nodal point, and with its direction unchanged, i.e., parallel to the incident ray. **anterior n.p.** See *nodal points.* **negative n.p.** A pair of points on the axis of an optical system which have the property that the angle made by an incident ray directed toward the first, leaves the system as though from the second, at an angle of the same size but on the opposite side of the axis. **posterior n.p.** See *nodal points.*

noncorresponding p's. Noncorresponding retinal points.

object p. A point at which the object is represented in relation to an optical system.

p. of observation. *Illumination:* 1. The midpoint of the line connecting the centers of rotation of the eyes. 2. The center of the entrance pupil of the eye.

occipital p. 1. The pointed posterior extremity of the occipital lobe of the brain. 2. The most prominent point on the posterior protuberance of the occipital bone.

occipital p. of the field of fixation. A point behind the eye symmetrical to the point of fixation with respect to the center of rotation of the eye when the line of sight is in the primary position. (Helmholtz)

ophthalmometric axial p. The point of intersection of the axis of the ophthalmometer with the cornea.

orthoscopic p's. The centers of the entrance and the exit pupils of an optical system free from aberration.

principal p. In an optical system, the point of intersection of a principal plane with the optical axis. **anterior p.p.** Primary principal point. **negative p.p's.** Conjugate points on the axis of an optical system, lying at twice the focal length on opposite sides of the system, for which the lateral magnification is unity and negative. An object located at one such point will have an inverted image of the same size at the other point. Syn., *symmetrical points.*

posterior p.p. Secondary principal point. **primary p.p.** The point of intersection of the primary principal plane with the optical axis. Syn., *anterior principal point.* **secondary p.p.** The point of intersection of the secondary principal plane with the optical axis. Syn., *posterior principal point.*

quasi-corresponding p's. Quasi-corresponding retinal points.

recovery p. Under a given set of binocular test conditions, the point at which fusion is regained on gradual decrease of the prism or lens power which originally induced the diplopia.

reflection p. The point of incidence of a light ray on a surface from which it is reflected.

refraction p. The point of incidence of a light ray on a surface at which it is refracted.

p. of regard. 1. A point in space to which visual attention is directed. It may be independent of the point of fixation, as in giving attention to a peripherally located object. 2. Point of fixation.

retinal p's., abathic. A pair of retinal points, one in each eye, which binocularly give rise to a single impression of a distance equal to that of both the fixation point and the actual frontoparallel plane.

retinal p's., corresponding. A pair of points, one in each retina, which, when stimulated, give rise to a percept of common visual direction. Syn., *homonymous points; identical points.*

retinal p's., disparate. Noncorresponding retinal points.

retinal p's., noncorresponding. A pair of points, one in the retina of each eye, which, when stimulated, do not give rise to a percept of common visual direction. Syn., *disparate retinal points.*

retinal p's., quasi-corresponding. Noncorresponding retinal points lying within Panum's areas.

reversal p. 1. In retinoscopy, the point at which the motion of the reflex changes from with to against motion, or vice versa. 2. Neutral point.

symmetrical p's. Negative principal points.

tangential p. The point of ocular contact of an extraocular muscle nearest its origin, at which the muscle ac-

tion may be regarded as a tangential force on the eyeball.

visual p. The point of intersection of the line of sight with the back surface of a spectacle lens with the eyes either in the primary position (distance visual point) or in a given position for near vision (near visual point).

◆

pointing. To indicate the direction or position of a thing especially by extending a finger toward it.

fast p. A method for treating amblyopia ex anopsia in which, with the nonamblyopic eye occluded, rapid pointing movements are made toward small targets. With improved pointing ability target size is decreased toward print requiring normal acuity at 40 cm. Syn., *quick pointing.*

past p. Pointing too far in the direction of the displacement of an object of fixation presented monocularly in the field of action of a paretic extraocular muscle. A similar error may occur when an amblyopic eye with eccentric fixation is monocularly fixating.

quick p. Fast pointing.

short p. The kinesthetic directionalization of a gross object of fixation, presented monocularly in the field of action of an extraocular muscle affected with spasm, to a point nearer than it actually is.

Poisson diffraction; spot. See under the nouns.

Polack's stereoscope (pol'aks). See under *stereoscope.*

polarimeter (po"lar-im'eh-ter). An instrument for determining the amount of polarization of light or the amount of rotation of the plane of polarization.

polarimetry (po"lar-im'eh-tre). The measurement of the amount of polarization of light or the amount of rotation of the plane of polarization with a polarimeter.

polariscope (po-lar'ih-skōp). An instrument for examining substances in, or for studying the properties of, polarized light, consisting essentially of a polarizer and an analyzer with their planes of polarization at right angles to each other. One of its uses is to detect stress in glass.

Savart p. Savart plate.

polariscopic (po"lar-ih-skop'ik). Pertaining to the polariscope or to polariscopy.

polariscopy (po"lar-is'ko-pe). The science or process of using the polariscope.

polarization (po"lar-ih-za'shun). The act, process, or result of altering the presumed transverse wave motion of radiant energy, such that it is not uniform in amplitude in all directions in a plane perpendicular to the direction of propagation. See also *polarized light.*

polarize (po'lar-īz). To induce or effect polarization.

polarizer (po'lar-īz"er). 1. An agent or a medium which induces or effects polarization. 2. In a polarimeter or a polariscope, the first of two polarizing elements in sequence, the second being called the *analyzer.*

    Ahrens p. Ahrens prism.

    Glan-Foucault p. Glan-Foucault prism.

    Glazebrook p. Glazebrook prism.

    linear p. Polarizing material in sheet form, such as Polaroid, which maximally transmits perpendicularly incident light whose transverse wave motion is in one meridian and minimally transmits light whose wave motion is in the opposite meridian. Cf. *multilayer polarizer.*

    multilayer p. A laminated series of glass, plastic, of film sheets and air interstices, or of various combinations, through which obliquely transmitted light is polarized with wave motion parallel to the plane of lamination and perpendicular to the plane defined by the transmitted and reflected portions of the incident light. Cf. *linear polarizer.*

    Nicol p. Nichol prism.

    Rochon p. Rochon prism.

    Wollaston p. Wollaston prism.

Polaroid (po'lar-oid). A trade name for a manufactured polarizing medium available in sheet form, originally made of tiny iodoquinine sulfate crystals aligned and embedded in a cellulose film and now largely supplanted by a stretched sheet of polyvinyl alcohol containing polymeric iodine.

Polatest (po'lah-test). An instrument used in refraction and for investigating binocular functions which presents a series of vectograms to be viewed through Polaroid filters, for testing heterophoria, fixation disparity, aniseikonia, stereopsis, and visual acuity.

pole. 1. Either end of the axis of a body, farthest removed from its equator, as of the eyeball or the crystalline lens.

2. The point on a mirror or a lens at which the optical axis intercepts the surface.

    anterior p. 1. Of the eyeball, the point on the anterior surface of the cornea corresponding to the intersection of an anteroposterior axis of reference of the eye, or of the pupillary axis. 2. Of the crystalline lens, the geometric center of its anterior surface, or the intersection of the optical axis of the lens with its anterior surface.

    posterior p. 1. Of the eyeball, the point on the posterior surface of the sclera corresponding to the intersection of an anteroposterior axis of reference of the eye, located between the optic disk and the fovea centralis. 2. Of the crystalline lens, the geometric center of its posterior surface, or the intersection of the optical axis of the lens with its posterior surface.

polemophthalmia (pol"em-of-thal'me-ah). Trachoma.

polioencephalitis, superior hemorrhagic (pol"i-o-en-ceph"a-li'tis). Wernicke's disease.

poliosis of the cilia (pol"e-o'sis). A condition in which there is a loss of pigment in the cilia, resulting in gray eyelashes.

poliosis circumscripta (pol"e-o'sis ser"kum-skript'ah). A condition in which an isolated bundle of white eyelashes is set among normally pigmented eyelashes.

polishing. The final stage in the process of lens surfacing in which the lens is made smooth to provide regular light transmission or specular reflection.

polus (po'lus). A pole.

    p. anterior lentis. The anterior pole of the crystalline lens.

    p. posterior lentis. The posterior pole of the crystalline lens.

Polyak's theory (pōl'yaks). See under *theory.*

polyarthritis, juvenile (pol"e-ar-thri'tis). Rheumatoid arthritis in infants and children accompanied by lymphadenopathy, splenomegaly, and sometimes keratouveitis. Syn., *Still's disease.*

polyblepharia (pol"e-blef'ah-re-ah). Polyblepharon.

polyblepharon (pol"e-blef'ah-ron). A congenital anomaly in which there is an extra eyelid. Syn., *polyblepharia; polyblephary.*

polyblephary (pol"e-blef'ah-re). Polyblepharon.

polychroism (pol″e-kro′izm). Pleochroism.

polychromatic (pol″e-kro-mat′ik). Pertaining to or exhibiting many colors.

polycoria (pol″e-ko′re-ah). An anomaly consisting of more than one pupil in a single iris.

    p. spuria. Polycoria in which only one of the openings in the iris is a true pupil, having a sphincter pupillae muscle.

    p. vera. Polycoria in which each pupil has its own sphincter pupillae muscle.

polycythemia rubra vera (pol″e-si-the′me-ah). Vaquez′ disease.

polydacrya (pol″e-dak′re-ah). Excessive lacrimation.

polygon, rectangular frequency (pol′e-gon). Bar graph.

polymacon. The nonproprietary name of a co-polymer of which contact lenses are made.

polymethyl methacrylate (pol″e-meth′il meh-thak′ril-āt). Polymerized methyl methacrylate, a lightweight, transparent thermoplastic, used in the manufacture of contact lenses and spectacle frames. It was formerly used for ophthalmic lenses but has been replaced by more abrasion-resistant, heat-hardened resins. Abbreviation *PMMA*.

Polyophthalmoscope (pol″e-of-thal′-mo-skōp). An instrument with nine viewing tubes to allow simultaneous observation of the fundus and interior of the eye by nine observers.

polyopia (pol″e-o′pe-ah). A condition in which more than one image of a single object is perceived; multiple vision. Syn., *polyopsia; polyopy*.

    p. monophthalmica. Monocular polyopia.

polyopsia (pol″e-op′se-ah). Polyopia.

polyopy (pol′e-o″pe). Polyopia.

polystichia (pol″e-stik′e-ah). An anomalous condition in which there are two or more rows of eyelashes on a single eyelid.

polyvinyl alcohol (pol″e-vi′nil al′ko-hol). A viscous agent used as a lacrimal substitute and as a vehicle to increase the contact time of an ophthalmic medication.

pons varolii (pons va-ro′le-i). A white eminence consisting of fibers and nuclei located in the hindbrain between the cerebral peduncles of the midbrain and the medulla oblongata, and acting in the relaying of impulses. It contains the abducens and facial motor nuclei that supply the lateral recti and the facial muscles of expression, the supranuclear center for lateral gaze, the parasympathetic lacrimal nucleus, and ascending and descending tracts important in ocular neurology.

Pontocaine hydrochloride (pon′to-kān hi″dro-klo′rīd). A trade name for *tetracaine hydrochloride*.

Ponzo visual illusion. See under *illusion, visual*.

porofocon A. A polymer cellulose acetate butyrate used in the manufacture of RX-56 contact lenses.

porphyria (por-fi′re-ah). A disease due to abnormal metabolism of porphyrin and occurring in both a chronic and an acute form. The chronic form is inherited recessively, has an onset typically in infancy or early childhood, and affects twice as many males as females. It is characterized by a severe dermal sensitivity to sunlight resulting in bullous or vesicular lesions on exposed areas of the body which may mutilate the eyelids, conjunctiva, cornea, and sclera. The acute form appears in the third decade or later and is characterized by severe abdominal pain and nervous symptoms varying from peripheral neuropathy and mental disturbances to involvement of the autonomic nervous system. Ocular symptoms in the acute form include diplopia, ischemia of the retina, and exophthalmos.

porphyropsin (por″fih-rop′sin). A carotenoid protein, similar to rhodopsin, found in the retinal rods of some fresh water fish. Syn., *visual violet*.

Porro prism (pōr′o). See under *prism*.

port, entrance. In an optical system, the image of the field stop as formed in the object space. Syn., *entrance window*.

port, exit. In an optical system, the image of the field stop as formed in the image space. Syn., *exit window*.

porus opticus (po′rus op′tih-kus). The opening, in the lamina cribrosa of the sclera, through which the central retinal artery passes.

Posey's theory (po′sēz). See under *theory*.

◆

POSITION

position. A place; a posture; a condition.

    active p. The position of the eyes in binocular vision when attention is actively directed to an object and the oculomotor reflexes are operative. Syn., *functional binocular position.*

apparent p. The position at which a perceived object is mentally projected.

blind p. Physiological position of rest.

diagnostic p's. of gaze. The primary, the four secondary, and the four tertiary positions of ocular fixation attempted to demonstrate normal or defective eye movement. Cf. *diagnostic action field.*

dissociated p. The position assumed by the eyes in relation to each other in the absence of adequate fusion stimuli. Syn., *fusion frustrated position; phoria position.*

fixation p. The position of the eyes in relation to each other during binocular fixation of a single object.

fixation-free p. The position of the eyes in relation to each other when under the influence of normal muscle tonus and postural reflexes and free from fixational and fusional reflexes. Syn., *static position.*

functional binocular p. Active position.

fusion-free p. The position assumed by the eyes in relation to each other when fusion is suspended and the oculomotor system is free from control of fusional impulses, but is affected by postural and fixational reflexes and by normal muscle tonus. Syn., *functional position of rest; passive position.*

fusion-frustrated p. Dissociated position.

p. of gaze, primary. Primary position.

p. of gaze, secondary. Secondary position.

p. of gaze, tertiary. Tertiary position.

p. of meridional balance. The position for which the circle of least confusion of the interval of Sturm is on the retina.

orthophoric p. 1. The position or distance from the eyes at which a fixation target may be placed so as to elicit no lateral heterophoria, i.e., a zero prism scale reading in a phoria test. 2. In a haploscope, the position of the stimulus targets corresponding to orthophoria.

passive p. Fusion-free position.

phoria p. Dissociated position.

primary p. 1. The position of the eye, in relation to the head, from which vertical and lateral fixational movements may be made unassociated with torsional movements; not necessarily identical with the straightforward position. 2. The straightforward position.

primatial p. A downward, inward, and intorted position of the eyes in the binocular fixation of a near point.

p. of rest, absolute. Anatomical position of rest.

p. of rest, anatomical. The position of the eyes, in relation to each other, in the absence of neuromuscular control or innervation, as in death. Syn., *absolute position of rest.*

p. of rest, comparative. Physiological position of rest.

p. of rest, functional. Fusion-free position.

p. of rest, physiological. The position of the eyes in relation to each other under the influence of normal muscle tonus and free from accommodation, fixation, and fusion reflexes. Syn., *comparative position of rest; relative position of rest.*

p. of rest, relative. Physiological position of rest.

secondary p. Any position of the eye represented by a vertical or horizontal deviation of the line of sight from the primary position.

static p. Fixation-free position.

straightforward p. The position of the eye when the line of sight is perpendicular to the face plane. Cf. *primary position.*

tertiary p. Any position of the eye represented by an oblique, or a combination of vertical and horizontal, deviation of the line of sight from the primary position.

◆

Posner test (pōz'ner). See under *test.*

Posner-Schlossmann syndrome (pōs'ner-schlos'man). Glaucomatocyclitic crisis.

posterior. In man, dorsal; nearer to the back or toward the rear. The opposite of *anterior.*

posterior border lamella of Fuchs. See under *lamella.*

postocular (pōst-ok'u-lar). Situated or occurring posterior to the eye.

postopticus (pōst-op'tih-kus). Corpora quadrigemina.

postorbital (pōst-ōr'bih-tal). Situated or occurring posterior to the orbit.

Posture Board, Brock's. An instrument used for visual testing and training at a near fixation distance, consisting essentially of a transparent red plastic plate mounted parallel to a baseboard, such that a light source mounted on a wand can be placed between the two. It is used in conjunction with red-green complementary color filters so that any of a number of various targets clipped to the red plate are seen by one eye and the light source is seen by the other.

potential. The amount of work necessary to bring a unit positive charge from one point in an electrical field to another; strictly, a potential difference.

cone-receptor p. An electrical potential which is obtained in or at a region very close to the retinal cone receptors of the primate retina, and considered to account for the rapid cornea negative *a* wave and at least part of the *d* wave in the electroretinogram.

corneofundal p. Resting potential of the eye.

corneoretinal p. Resting potential of the eye.

dark p. of the eye. Resting potential of the eye.

early receptor p. A rapid electroretinogram response that can be detected when the retina is stimulated with an intense flash of light approximately 10^6 times brighter than that required to elicit the ERG, consisting of an initial corneal-positive peak (R_1) occurring at approximately 100 microseconds and a second (R_2) corneal negative peak occurring at approximately 900 microseconds. This potential appears to reflect molecular events within the photoreceptor outer segments and corresponds with the photochemical kinetics of these receptors. The human ERP is generated primarily by the cones.

focal p's. Intraretinal electrical potentials recorded in the frog retina and elicited only by illumination falling close to the recording electrode in the region of the bipolar cells; considered responsible for the generation of the internal electroretinogram.

oculorotary p. The electrical change in direct current potential resulting from rotation of the eye in the orbit, measured by electrodes placed on the skin at the eyelid margins or at the canthi.

oscillatory p's. The several wavelets superimposed on the ERG b-wave recorded under scotopic conditions with a light stimulus of high intensity, varying in number and appearance with different preadaptation and stimulus intensity conditions and probably originating from within the inner nuclear layer of the retina.

resting p. of the eye. The direct current potential difference which exists between the anterior and posterior poles of the eye, the cornea being positive relative to the retina. It is of the order of several millivolts in humans. Syn., *corneofundal potential; corneoretinal potential; dark potential of the eye; standing potential of the eye; static potential of the eye; steady potential of the eye.*

Schubert's p. An electrical potential recorded in the human ciliary muscle and considered to be related to the state of accommodation.

standing p. of the eye. Resting potential of the eye.

static p. of the eye. Resting potential of the eye.

steady p. of the eye. Resting potential of the eye.

visual evoked p. Visual evoked cortical potential.

visual evoked cortical p. The electrical discharge that occurs in the visual cortex in response to brief visual stimuli. Abbreviation *VECP.* Syn., *visual evoked potential; visual evoked response.*

Potts-Maurice theory. Metabolic pump theory.

power. The ability to act or to produce effect.

air equivalent p. The designated power of a lens in air which would have the same vergence effect on light traveling in air as a lens of reference has on light traveling in another medium of reference.

aligning p. 1. Vernier visual acuity. 2. The ability to place two or more objects on a straight line passing through the entrance pupil of the eye, as in aiming a gun, the center of the images of the aligned objects falling at the same point on the retina.

approximate p. The sum of the powers of the two surfaces of an ophthalmic or spectacle lens, as commonly determined with a lens measure, without regard to the form and thickness of the lens.

back p. Back vertex power.

defining p. Definition.

dioptric p. The vergence power of a dioptric system.

dispersive p. In a given medium, the ratio of the difference in the index of refraction for two extreme spectral lines (usually Fraunhofer F and C) to the difference in index for an intermediate line (usually Fraunhofer D) and unity. Syn., *relative dispersion.*

effective p. 1. The vergence power of an optical system designated with respect to a point of reference other than the principal point. 2. In a lens, the back vertex power.

emissive p. The time rate of emission of radiant energy, in all directions, per unit surface area of a radiating body at a given temperature.

equivalent p. 1. The vergence power of an optical system expressed with reference to the principal point. Syn., *true power.* 2. The mean spherical power of a cylindrical or spherocylindrical lens, determined by adding half the power of the cylindrical component to the spherical component.

focal p. Vergence power.

front p. Front vertex power.

magnifying p. 1. The ratio of image size to object size. Syn., *magnification.* 2. With reference to a magnifying optical viewing aid, the ratio of the angle subtended by the image at the nodal point of the eye to the angle subtended by the object when at the least distance of distinct vision from the eye, this distance conventionally being assumed to be 10 in. or 25 cm. Syn., *apparent magnification.*

mean oblique p. The arithmetic mean of the tangential and sagittal oblique vertex sphere dioptric powers.

Munsell p. The product of Munsell value and Munsell chroma.

neutralizing p. The power of a spectacle lens as indicated by the power of a trial case lens which neutralizes it when placed so that the back vertex of the trial case lens contacts the front vertex of the spectacle lens, and hence the front vertex power of the spectacle lens if the power of the neutralizing lens is designated by its back vertex power.

prismatic p. The angular deviation of the direction of light propaga-

tion, produced by a prism or other optical system.

reading p. A ratio representing visual acuity for reading, expressed as a fraction in which the numerator is the maximum distance at which the reading material can be read, and the denominator is the distance at which the letters subtend an angle of 5 minutes.

refractive p. The vergence power of a refracting optical system.

resolving p. 1. In an optical system, the ability to form a clearly defined image; the least separation of two optically imaged luminous points discernible as two, usually evaluated in terms of the separation of the maximum and first minimum of the intensity distribution curve of the diffraction pattern of the image of one of the luminous points. Syn., *limit of resolution.* 2. In the eye, the threshold of resolution. 3. In a grating or a prism, the ability to separate two wavelengths close together into two spectrum lines, usually specified in terms of the change in wavelength necessary to shift the central intensity maximum into the position of the first intensity minimum for the diffraction image of a given wavelength.

sagittal oblique vertex sphere p. The reciprocal of the distance, in meters, from the vertex sphere to the sagittal focus, as measured along the chief ray of the pencil.

stereo p. In a pair of prism binoculars or similar instrument, the ratio of the distance between the optical axes of the objectives to the distance between the optical axes of the eyepieces, multiplied by the magnifying power.

surface p. The vergence power of a single refracting or reflecting surface.

tangential oblique vertex sphere p. The reciprocal of the distance, in meters, from the vertex sphere to the tangential focus, as measured along the chief ray of the pencil.

thin lens p. The sum of the dioptric powers of the two surfaces of a lens of negligible thickness.

true p. Equivalent power.

vergence p. The ability of an optical system to change the vergence of a pencil of rays, usually designated quantitatively by the reciprocal of the focal length of the system. Syn., *focal power.*

vertex p., back. The vergence power expressed with reference to the posterior surface, at the optical axis, of a lens or an optical system instead of to the secondary principal point. Syn., *back power.*

vertex p., front. The vergence power expressed with reference to the anterior surface, at the optical axis, of a lens or an optical system instead of to the anterior principal point. Syn., *front power.*

PP. Abbreviation for *punctum proximum.*

PR. Abbreviation for *punctum remotum.*

Pr. Abbreviation for *presbyopia* or *prism.*

pragmatagnosia, visual (prag"-mat-ag-no'ze-ah). The inability to recognize by sight objects previously known, although the object is seen clearly. Syn., *object visual agnosia.*

pragmatamnesia, visual (prag"mat-am-ne'se-ah). The inability to recall the visual image of an object.

Prato's box (pra'tōz). See under *box.*

Pray's (prāz) **chart; test; test type.** See under the nouns.

precipitates, keratic (pre-sip'ih-tātz). Fibrinous and cellular deposits on the posterior surface of the cornea from exudates from the iris and the ciliary body into the anterior chamber, usually an accompaniment of iritis or iridocyclitis. Abbreviation *KP.*

glass k.p's. Keratic precipitates which persist after the causative inflammation has ceased and which appear as translucent rings with opaque centers.

mutton-fat k.p's. Keratic precipitates which have coalesced; found in long standing, severe cases of iritis or iridocyclitis, typically in the tubercular types.

plastic k.p's. Keratic precipitates in mass, usually appearing in severe iridocyclitis.

star-map k.p's. Keratic precipitates in the form of round deposits connected by fine line deposits, producing geometrical patterns.

preglaucoma (pre"glaw-ko'mah). A condition in which clinical and gonioscopic evidence indicates potential glaucoma.

prelacrimal (pre-lak'rih-mal). Situated or occurring anterior to the lacrimal sac.

Prentice's (pren'tis-ez) **phoria indicator; law; method; rule.** See under the nouns.

prepresbyope (pre-pres'be-ōp). One who has not yet manifested presbyopia.

prepresbyopia (pre-pres"be-o'pe-ah). The period or condition prior to the onset of presbyopia.

preretinal (pre-ret'ih-nal). Situated or occurring anterior to the retina.

presbyope (pres'be-ōp). One who has presbyopia.

presbyopia (pres"be-o'pe-ah). A reduction in accommodative ability occurring normally with age and necessitating a plus lens addition for satisfactory seeing at near, sometimes quantitatively identified by the recession of the near point of accommodation beyond 20 cm.

absolute p. 1. Presbyopia in which accommodative ability is completely absent. 2. Presbyopia in which some convex lens power is necessary for reading small print. Cf. *incipient presbyopia.*

incipient p. Beginning presbyopia, sometimes described as the stage in which small print may be read without the addition of convex lens power, but with effort. Cf. *absolute presbyopia.*

nocturnal p. A reduction in the apparent amplitude of accommodation induced by the reduction of the intensity of illumination.

premature p. Presbyopia manifested at an early age, as before the age of 40 years.

presbyopic (pres"be-op'ik). Pertaining to or having presbyopia.

presbytia (pres-bish'e-ah). Presbyopia. *Obs.*

presbytism (pres'bih-tizm). Presbyopia. *Obs.*

pressure, intraocular. The pressure of the intraocular fluid, measurable by means of a manometer. Cf. *ocular tension.*

normal intraocular p. Intraocular pressure within the range of values obtained in normal, healthy eyes, usually considered to represent an ocular tension of approximately 25 mm of mercury.

normative intraocular p. Intraocular pressure which is compatible with normal health and function of the eye. Cf. *normal intraocular pressure.*

Prevost's sign (pra-vōz). See under *sign.*

prezonular (pre-zōn'u-lar). Situated or occurring in the posterior chamber of the eye, anterior to the zonule of Zinn.

Priestley Smith's (prēst'le smiths) **pupillometer; tape; test.** See under the nouns.

primochrome (pri-mo-krōm'). Weale's term for *chlorolabe*.

Prince's (prinsz) **rule; rule test.** See under the nouns.

principle. 1. A fundamental law, doctrine, or assumption; a general or fundamental truth. 2. A rule or basis of action.

Babinet's p. The principle that complementary sets of obstacles, for which one set has openings where the other set is opaque, provide for superposition of diffraction pattern amplitudes without zero summation.

Drysdale p. Drysdale method.

Fermat's p. of least time. Fermat's law.

Huygens' p. Every point of any wavefront may be considered as the source of secondary spherical waves (wavelets) which, in combination with each other, constitute a new, further advanced, wavefront.

p. of reversibility. Law of reversibility.

◆

PRISM

prism (prizm). 1. A transparent body bounded in part by two plane faces which are not parallel. 2. An optical element or system, or the component of an optical system, which deviates the path of light as does a prism.

Abbe's p. Any of several prisms designed by Abbe. One is a constant deviation 30° –60° –90° prism with the internal reflecting face on the side opposite the 60° angle. Others include a modification of the Porro prism and a direct vision prism which invert and revert the image.

abducting p. An ophthalmic prism placed before a fixating eye with its base-apex line horizontal and its base nasal.

achromatic p. Two prisms of different refractive indices, combined so that the dispersion of one is offset by the dispersion of the other, thus producing deviation without dispersion.

adducting p. An ophthalmic prism placed before a fixating eye with its base-apex line horizontal and its base temporal.

adverse p. An ophthalmic prism placed before the eye so as to produce a displacement of the image seen through the prism in a direction opposite to that which would compensate for the deviation, or tendency to deviation, of the viewing eye. Cf. *relieving prism.*

Ahrens' p. A device, used in polarizing microscopes, consisting of three wedge-shaped prisms cemented together with Canada balsam to form a rectangular block which is coated black on its sides. Extraordinary rays pass straight through, while the ordinary rays undergo total internal reflection and are absorbed by the black coating. Syn., *Ahrens' polarizer.*

Allen's contact p. A totally reflecting plastic prism attached to a contact lens, used in conjunction with a biomicroscope to view the filtration angle of the anterior chamber. Syn., *Allen's gonioprism; Allen-O'Brien contact lens; contact prism.*

Amici p. Any one of several complex prisms designed by Amici. One, a roof prism, consists of a right-angled prism whose hypotenuse surface is replaced by an internally reflecting roof, so that a beam entering one of the other faces perpendicularly will be reflected successively at both surfaces of the roof and emerge from the last surface in a direction perpendicular to the incident path to form an inverted image. Another, a direct vision prism, consists of a prism of very dense flint glass cemented between two prisms of crown glass.

Barr and Stroud p. A very complex, ocular prism system used in fire control instruments, consisting of four single prisms and a cover, all cemented together.

base-in p. An ophthalmic prism placed before the eye with its base-apex line horizontal and its base nasalward.

base-out p. An ophthalmic prism placed before the eye with its base-apex line horizontal and its base templeward.

Brewster p's. Two identical prisms placed base to apex and hinged at the base of one and the apex of the other, so that the angle between the prisms may be changed. They are used to produce meridional magnification, without effective power for distance vision, the magnification occurring in the base-apex meridian and varying with the angle between the prisms.

Carl Zeiss p. Any of several very complex prism systems used in military fire control instruments.

combining p. Measuring prism.

compensating p. Relieving prism.

cone p. Quadrant prism.

constant deviation p. A prism unit with an internal or adjunct reflecting surface so constructed that, for each wavelength, the orientation of the unit which provides equal angles of entrance and emergence at the respective faces of the unit also provides for a constant total deviation of the emergent ray with respect to the entering ray.

contact p. Allen's contact prism.

Cornu p. A 60° prism consisting of one 30° right-handed quartz and one 30° left-handed quartz in contact, thus transmitting light at the minimum deviation position without double refraction because of the interchange in velocities at the interface.

Cornu-Jellet p. A Nicol prism modified by making a longitudinal cut, removing a small wedge, and cementing the cut surfaces together. It is used as an analyzer or polarizer in instruments for measuring rotatory polarization.

correcting p. Measuring prism.

Creté's p. A rotary prism, especially one designed with a sliding indicator on a long, radially protruding handle.

crossed Nicol p's. A pair of separate Nicol prisms placed in optical sequence with their optic axes perpendicular to each other so as to allow no light to pass through unless the plane of polarization of the light transmitted through the first of the pair is rotated by an interposed medium. The rotation of the plane of polarization is measured by the rotation of the second of the pair necessary for total extinction.

Delaborne p. Dove prism.

p. diopter. See under *diopter*.

direct vision p. 1. A combination of two (or more) prisms of different refractive indices, whose over-all effect is to produce spectral dispersion, but no deviation of the light corresponding to the D line, or other wavelength of reference. 2. Any prism for which the directions of propagation of the emerging and entering beams are the same.

dissociating p. A prism which, when placed before one of the eyes, so displaces the image of that eye that fusion is impossible and diplopia results.

double p. A pair of prisms, base to base, which serve to divide a beam of transmitted light into two separately deviated beams. When thin, it may be designed as a single, very obtuse prism with an apical angle of almost 180°, used with the incident light beam approaching normal to the base. See also *Fresnel biprism*. **Dove d.p.** A combination of two Harting-Dove prisms, their reflecting surfaces silvered and cemented together. **Maddox d.p.** Maddox prism. **Thorington d.p.** An ophthalmic test lens of ruby red, cobalt blue, or colorless glass, in the shape of an obtuse truncated prism, which consists of two lateral thin prism portions with bases toward each other, separated by a plano central portion or strip. A small light viewed through this lens is seen in triplicate with the three images connected by a streak produced by refraction at the borders of the plano central portion.

double image p. 1. A combination of two prisms composed of doubly refracting media with their optical axes so arranged in relation to each other that the ordinary and extraordinary beams are widely separated, producing separate images. 2. A double prism.

Dove p. An isosceles prism designed to refract light entering one side so as to reflect it internally on the base surface and refract it again on the opposite, emerging side, thus inverting the resulting image. The unused apical portion of the prism may be removed or absent, forming a frustum (Harting-Dove prism). Syn., *Delaborne prism*.

erecting p. A prism interposed in a refracting or reflecting optical system for the purpose of rendering an inverted image erect. Specifically applied to a prism attached to the eyepiece of a microscope to correct the inversion of the image. Syn., *erector*.

Fery p. A type of reflecting prism in which the surfaces of entrance and emergence are spherical curves.

Foucault p. A polarizing prism, similar in design to the Nicol prism, but employing an air film or space instead of balsam, thus to permit the transmission of ultraviolet light.

Frankford arsenal p. Any of several very complex prism systems used in military fire control instruments.

Fresnel's p. Fresnel's biprism.

Fresnel Press-On p. A *Press-On Fresnel lens* with prism instead of dioptric powers.

Glan-Foucault p. A polarizing prism made of two wedge-shaped pieces of calcite, so cut that the geometrical axis of the prism is parallel to the optic axis, and mounted with a thin air gap between their hypotenuses. It is used primarily for the polarization of ultraviolet light and transmits only the extraordinary ray. Syn., *Glan-Foucault polarizer.*

Glan-Thompson p. A polarizing prism designed to give a wider field and more perfect plane polarization than the Nicol prism. It must be cut with the optical axis parallel to the end faces, using more calcite than the Nicol prism.

Glazebrook p. A polarizing prism equivalent to half of an Ahrens prism cut in a plane perpendicular to the optic axis and transmitting only the extraordinary rays. Syn., *Glazebrook polarizer.*

Harting-Dove p. A Dove prism with the unused apical portion of the prism removed.

Herschel p. A type of rotary prism.

horizontal p. An ophthalmic prism placed base-in or base-out before the eye with its base-apex line horizontal. Syn., *lateral prism.*

Kagenaar p. A pair of thick slabs of plane glass mounted edge to edge at an angle of about 150° so as to separate, by displacement, the two halves of a beam of transmitted light, used in early ophthalmometers to double the mire images.

Kösters p. An interferometer element made from a pair of nearly identical prisms cut from a single 30° –60°–90° prism. A semireflecting film of aluminum or silver is applied to the face opposite the 60° angle of one prism, and this face is then cemented to the corresponding face of the other prism in various relationships, depending upon its intended use.

lacrimal p. The collection of lacrimal fluid at the margin of the lower eyelid.

Landolt p. Rotary prism.

lateral p. Horizontal prism.

Leman p. A complex, one-piece prism unit employing two flat internal reflecting surfaces and a reflecting roof. It inverts and reverts the transmitted beam without deviation, but with some displacement.

Lippich p. A Nicol prism so situated in the eyepiece of a polariscope or polarimeter as to cover half of the field of view.

Littrow p. One of the halves of a Cornu prism, with the interface side silvered to reflect the light back out through the face of incidence, the reversed orientation of the vibrations on reflection nullifying the double refraction, as does the second half of the Cornu prism.

Maddox p. A double prism with an apical angle of about 170°, sometimes made in ruby red or cobalt blue glass, used in ophthalmic clinical testing.

May p. A small, one-piece optical unit in the head of the May ophthalmoscope, consisting of a lower convex surface, at which light enters from a small source in the instrument handle, a pair of internal reflecting surfaces, and an oblique refracting surface which directs the light beam out of the unit, near its upper prism edge adjacent to the viewing aperture, so as to illuminate the eye under observation.

measuring p. A prism used for determining the amount of deviation in heterophoria and heterotropia, distinguished from the dissociating prism. Syn., *combining prism; correcting prism.*

Nicol p. A polarizing prism made from an Iceland spar or a calcite crystal, cut diagonally in half, with the two halves cemented together with Canada balsam; it transmits the extraordinary ray but totally reflects the ordinary ray. Syn., *Nicol polarizer.*

Pechan p. A direct vision, two-piece prism assembly which provides for five internal reflections of the transmitted beam, similar in function to the Dove prism, but usable with either convergent or divergent light.

Pellin-Broca p. A one-piece, quadrilateral, constant deviation, dispersing prism producing a deviation of 90°.

penta p. Any prism whose section is pentagonal. In particular, a prism with five faces, not including the end faces, in which light enters one face perpendicularly, reflects successively at two silvered faces, and emerges perpendicular from a fourth face at right angles to the first. The unused face results from the removal of a dihedral section between the two reflecting faces.

plano p. A prism of zero focal power.

polarizing p. A prism made of a doubly refracting material such as Iceland spar, calcite, or quartz, used for producing or analyzing polarized light.

Porro p. A triangular, totally reflecting prism with angles of 90°, 45°, and 45°, commonly used in pairs in telescopic systems such as prism binoculars. Light entering perpendicular to the hypotenuse surface is totally reflected in turn by the two opposite surfaces, to emerge from the hypotenuse surface parallel to the incident light.

Porro-Abbe p. A modification of the Porro prism, sometimes called a double right-angle prism, used successively in pairs to invert and revert an image.

quadrant p. An ophthalmic test lens in the shape of an obtuse pyramid with its apex at the center, through which an object is seen in quadruplicate. Syn., *cone prism; quadrilateral prism.*

quadrilateral p. Quadrant prism.

reflecting p. A prism in which the internally contained light is totally reflected at one or more of the plane surfaces before emerging. Syn., *total reflecting prism.* **double r.p.** A prism in which the internally contained light is totally reflected in turn at two of the plane surfaces before emerging. **single r.p.** A prism in which the internally contained light is totally reflected at one of the plane surfaces before emerging. **total r.p.** Reflecting prism.

relieving p. An ophthalmic prism placed before the eye so as to produce a displacement of the image seen through the prism in a direction which would compensate for the deviation, or tendency to deviate, of the viewing eye. Cf. *adverse prism.* Syn., *compensating prism.*

rhomboidal p. A long, narrow, rhomboid-shaped piece of glass used to displace a beam of light without deviation, reversion, or inversion of the image. The light enters near one end of a long rectangular side, reflects internally at the two inclined end surfaces, and emerges near the other end of the other long rectangular side.

Risley p. A type of rotary prism.

Rochon p. A rectangular polarizing unit consisting of two right-angled calcite or quartz prisms cemented together by their hypotenuse faces with the optic axis of the first prism perpendicular to its front surface, and with the optic axis of the second prism perpendicular to that of the first prism and parallel to the interface, producing an emergent ordinary beam undeviated, achromatic, and polarized, and a deviated, emergent, extraordinary beam which may be screened off easily at some distance from the prism. Syn., *Rochon polarizer.*

roof p. A complex prism unit which includes a pair of internally reflecting surfaces perpendicular to each other, thus resembling a roof externally. One type is an Amici prism, another has the plane of bisection of the reflecting surfaces parallel to and bisecting the incident beam, serving to reverse the resulting image by translating and inverting the two halves of the transmitted beam.

rotary p. A pair of equal power, thin prisms mounted one in front of the other, so that they can be rotated in opposite directions at equal rates to give a resultant power in a single meridian, varying from zero when the apex of one coincides with the base of the other to a maximum when the two apices coincide.

Schmidt p. A complex, one-piece prism unit which reverts and inverts the image and deviates the transmitted beam through an angle of 45° by a series of internal reflections.

slab-off p. The prism represented in a lens as a result of the bicentric grinding of one of its spherical surfaces, i.e., grinding the surface in two portions having separate centers of (equal) curvature, to compensate for the unequal prismatic effect produced when looking through the lower portions of an anisometropic prescription lens.

subducting p. An ophthalmic prism placed base up before a fixating eye, causing the eye to rotate downward.

superducting p. An ophthalmic prism placed base down before a fixating eye, causing the eye to rotate upward.

tank p. A long 90°–45°–45° prism used in military tank periscopes.

tear p. Lacrimal prism.

thick p. A prism in which the refracting angle is great enough to introduce a significant error in the mathematical assumption that the angle of deviation is arithmetically proportional to the refracting angle.

thin p. A prism in which the refracting angle is small enough to permit, without significant error, the mathematical assumption that the angle of deviation is arithmetically proportional to the refracting angle.

Thollon p. Young-Thollon prism.

Thorington p. Thorington double prism.

variable p. A rotary prism.

p. verger. See under *verger.*

vertical p. An ophthalmic prism placed before the eye with its base-apex line vertical.

Wadsworth p. A constant deviation, dispersing prism employing an auxiliary, externally located mirror instead of an internal reflecting surface.

Wernicke p. A composite of three glass prisms, two right-angle prisms of identical glass positioned on their hypotenuse faces to a triangular-shaped prism of nearly the same index for yellow light, but of different dispersion. It is used to obtain high dispersion with high transmission.

Wollaston p. 1. A double image prism consisting of two right-angled quartz or calcite prisms cemented together by their hypotenuse faces to form a rectangular unit, and with the optic axes of the two halves perpendicular to each other and to the direction of propagation of the incident light. The resulting two emerging beams are oppositely polarized and relatively free of dispersion. Syn., *Wollaston polarizer.* 2. A one-piece prism, with two internal reflecting surfaces, which will deviate a beam of light through an angle of 90° without inversion or reversion, and hence is useful in camera lucida systems.

Young-Thollon p's. A pair of 30° prisms, one of right-handed and one of left-handed quartz, arranged for additive dispersion in a spectrograph or monochromator, so that the incident light is normal to the first surface of the first prism and the emergent light is normal to the second surface of the second prism.

Zeiss p. Carl Zeiss prism.

Zenger p. A composite of two right-angle prisms, made of glass of nearly the same index for yellow light, but of different dispersion. The components are arranged hypotenuse to hypotenuse to form a right parallelepiped of glass. It is often used in direct vision spectroscopy.

◆

Prism Reader. An attachment of rotary prisms to the *Controlled Reader* for developing fusional convergence and divergence.

prismatic (priz-mat′ik). Produced by, pertaining to, or resembling, a prism or its action or effect.

prisme mobile. Creté's prism.

prismoptometer (priz″mop-tom′eh-ter). Prisoptometer.

prismosphere (priz′mo-sfēr). A spherical lens eccentrically mounted or decentered to produce prismatic effect; a combined spherical lens and prism. Syn., *spheroprism.*

prism-vergence (prizm-ver′gens). Vergence induced by prism effect.

prisoptometer (priz″op-tom′eh-ter). An instrument for determining ametropia, consisting essentially of a glass prism, the apical portion of which covers half of a central aperture in a revolving diaphragm. The subject views a circle at a distance of 20 ft, monocularly, through the aperture, with resulting monocular diplopia. The relative position of the doubled circle indicates the type of refractive error and the correction required. Syn., *prism optometer; prismoptometer.*

Pritchard photometer. See under *photometer.*

probability, visual comfort. Per cent of people who, if in the most undesirable location in a room, will be expected to find the lighting acceptable. Abbreviation *VCP.*

problem, alley. The problem of explaining the occurrence of the two types of Blumenfeld alleys.

problem, four-color. To determine whether any two-dimensional map can be constructed in four colors so that no two contiguous regions are of the same color.

procedure. See under *method, process,* or *test.*

process. 1. Any marked prominence or projecting part; an outgrowth or extension. 2. A course or method of procedure. 3. Any phenomenon which demonstrates a continuous change, such as an inflammatory process.

ciliary p's. Meridionally arranged projections, approximately 70 in number, extending from the ciliary body posterior to the iris, and forming collectively the corona ciliaris. Each process is a ridge about 2 mm long and 0.5 mm high, is almost white in color, and consists essentially of blood vessels, being the most vascular region of the eye. The ciliary processes serve as attachments for fibers of the zonule of Zinn and are considered to be involved in the formation of aqueous humor.

descending p. The inferior projection of the lacrimal bone which unites with the lacrimal process of the inferior nasal concha or turbinate to help bound the nasolacrimal canal.

filling-in p. Perceiving of areas in the visual field which correspond to the blind spot of Mariotte and to Arago's spot as of the same brightness, color, and pattern as their surrounds and not as dark or void spots.

frontal p. The upper medial projection of the maxillary bone which forms the anterior portion of the medial wall of the orbit and contains the anterior lacrimal crest and the anterior portion of the fossa for the lacrimal sac.

maxillary p. of the embryo. An embryological mass of visceral mesoderm, posterior and inferior to the optic vesicle, which gives rise to the connective tissue of the lower eyelid and to the orbital portions of the maxillary and zygomatic bones.

orbital p. of the palatine bone. The projection, at the upper end of the perpendicular portion of the palatine bone, which extends to the posterior portion of the floor of the orbit.

orbital p. of the zygomatic bone. The projection of the zygomatic bone that extends above the infraorbital process at the lateral wall of the orbit to form the anterior boundary of the temporal fossa.

photoreceptive p. The photochemical reaction which occurs when light energy strikes rhodopsin, iodopsin, or some other light-sensitive pigment in the outer segments of rods or cones and which initiates action currents.

pterygoid p. of the sphenoid bone. A projection, on either side of the junction of the body with the great wing of the sphenoid bone, which extends downward behind the lateral part of the hard palate and the last molar socket, forming the posterior boundary of the pterygopalatine fossa.

retinal p's. P I, P II, P III. Two excitational processes symbolized as PI and PII and one inhibitional process, PIII, the algebraic sum of which yields the resultant potential which registers in an electroretinogram. PI is related to the c wave, PII to the b wave, and PIII to the a wave.

visual p. The total sequence of events involved in the act of seeing from the incidence of light on the cornea to the cortical activity which results in a percept. **physiological v.p.** The portion of the total visual process involving the photochemical changes produced in the retina by light stimulation, the formation of an impulse, and its transmission to the brain. **physical v.p.** The portion of the total visual process involving the transmission of light through the transparent media of the eye and its incidence upon the retina. **psychological v.p.** The portion of the total visual process involving the cortical interpretation of visual impulses with the formation of a percept.

Professional Standards Review Organization. A peer review system created by U.S. Public Law 92-603 to develop and apply criteria, norms, and standards of health care, identify problem areas, and assess the effectiveness of federal and other third-party-financed health services.

projection. 1. The referring or localization of sensations from sense organs to the apparent source or place of origin of the stimulus. 2. A part that juts out or extends, or the act of jutting out or extending. 3. The act of causing a light, shadow, or optical image to fall into space or on a surface, or the light, shadow, or optical image itself.

anomalous p. The spatial localization of a visual sensation different from that which would have been predicted from the application of the laws of projection and the theory of local retinal sign for a given physical stimulus correlate in a normal eye, as occurs in anomalous retinal correspondence.

binocular p. The spatial localization of a binocularly perceived visual sensation. Cf. *cyclopean projection*.

center of p. See under *center*.

cyclopean p. Spatial localization of a binocularly perceived visual sensation with reference to a hypothetical single eye having certain attributes peculiar to the condition of binocular vision and presumed to resemble a cyclopean eye.

direction of p., absolute. The direction in which a perceived image is seen or projected in relation to a line of reference established by a given structural or functional characteristic of the eye or the subject.

direction of p., relative. The direction in which a perceived image is seen or projected in relation to a line of reference established by a given external point or object.

eccentric p. 1. Anomalous projection. 2. The spatial localization of an extrofoveally initiated visual sensation. 3. The aspect of the concept of projection that is concerned with localization external to the body or the sense organ itself.

erroneous p. False projection.

false p. 1. The reference of a visual sensation to a locality in space significantly different from its physical correlate, such as occurs in past pointing, and associated with extraocular muscle paresis. 2. Anomalous projection.

flash p. The optical projection of images onto a screen for brief exposures, i.e., tachistoscopically.

flicker p. The rapid and alternate projection of pictures viewed alternately by the two eyes through a device alternately occluding the eyes synchronously with the projector; used to create stereopsis.

minus p. *Optometric Extension Program:* A condition or syndrome represented by either the static retinoscopy finding being in minus lens power and the unaided distance visual acuity being 20/20 or better, or the net of near point crossed cylinder findings being in minus lens power and the unaided visual acuity at near being 20/20 or better.

monocular p. Spatial localization of a monocularly perceived visual sensation, especially in relation to the line of sight or other line of reference.

normal p. The spatial localization of a visual sensation in accordance with the laws of projection and the theory of local retinal sign.

optical p. Optical image formation on a surface or viewing screen, or the image so projected.

paradoxical p. Spatial localization represented in paradoxical diplopia, often manifested after corrective surgery on a strabismic in which

anomalous retinal correspondence previously existed.

postural p. The aspect of visual projection associated with proprioceptive impulses from the neck muscles and labyrinth and possibly from the extraocular muscles. Syn., *proprioceptive projection.*

proprioceptive p. Postural projection.

retinal p. 1. The aspect of visual projection associated with retinal local sign. 2. Visual projection in geometric reference to the retina. 3. Visual projection as influenced only by stimulation of the retina and exclusive of proprioceptive impulses.

visual p. Spatial localization identified with visual perception.

projectionometer, Alabaster's (pro-jek"shun-om'eh-ter). A device for the detection and measurement of false projection, consisting essentially of a platform extending out horizontally from the patient's face just below the eyes, supporting a peripheral metal railing on which a light is moved by the examiner. The patient with one eye occluded attempts to place a wooden ball, situated out of sight beneath the platform, underneath the light.

projectionometer, Landolt's (pro-jek"shun-om'eh-ter). A device for the detection and measurement of false projection, consisting essentially of a horizontal shelf above which a vertical fixation line is marked on a screen perpendicular to the shelf and below which is a continuation of the screen containing a tangent scale. The patient looks over the shelf, with one eye occluded, and places a finger on a point on the scale, out of sight beneath the shelf, which seems to be just below the fixation line.

Project-o-chart (pro-jek'to-chart). A trade name for an optical instrument that projects test types and other test targets onto a screen.

projector. An optical instrument for projecting an image on a screen.

acuity p. An optical instrument which projects targets used in the determination of visual acuity and in the refraction of the eyes.

Moller test mark p. A hand-held projector which produces colored or white spots of light, of various sizes, used as targets on a tangent screen.

opaque p. An instrument which projects by reflection an enlarged image of an opaque object, such as printed material, on a screen.

Polamatic acuity p. A 35 mm slide projector adapted for visual acuity testing and for refraction procedures which includes polarized slides for monocular testing while maintaining binocular fusion of peripheral contours.

slide p. An instrument which projects an enlarged image of a transilluminated transparency or slide on a screen. Syn., *magic lantern.*

spectrum p. An instrument which projects the spectrum on a viewing screen.

Projectoscope (pro-jek'to-skōp). A trade name for an ophthalmoscope having an assortment of graticules which are projected onto the fundus, including targets for the detection and treatment of eccentric fixation. (See Fig 29.)

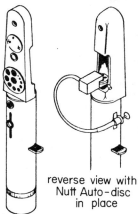

reverse view with
Nutt Auto-disc
in place

obverse view

Fig. 29 Projectoscope. (From J. R. Griffin, *Binocular Anomalies.* Chicago: Professional Press, 1976)

projicience (pro-jish'ens). The localization of a perceived sensation in the external environment.

prolapse of the iris (pro-laps'). Protrusion of the iris through a corneal wound.

prolapse of the lens (pro-laps'). A falling forward of the crystalline lens into a corneal wound.

prong, Snellen's. The letter U of various sizes and orientation, used as a test target for visual acuity.

pronouncedness. The perceptual, psychological, affective, or phenomenal attribute of quality or degree of "goodness" of a color perception, such as the whiteness of a white or the blueness of a blue.

pro-ophthalmus (pro-of-thal'mus). Exophthalmos.

pro-opic (pro-op'ik). Having an orbitonasal index above 113 (or 110). Cf. *mesopic; platyopic.*

prop, ptosis. Ptosis crutch.

proparacaine hydrochloride (propar'ah-kān hi"dro- klo'rīd). A synthetic topical anesthetic used on the cornea for procedures such as tonometry, gonioscopy, and removal of superficial foreign bodies. Chemically classed as a benzoic acid ester, it is commonly used in a 0.5% solution and has a rapid onset of action, usually within 20 seconds. It is the generic name for *Ophthaine, Alcaine,* and *Ophthetic.*

proprioception (pro"pre-o-sep'shun). Awareness of posture, balance, and muscular adjustment through sensory organs or receptors located within muscles, tendons, tendon sheaths, joints, and the vestibular apparatus of the inner ear.

proprioceptor (pro"pre-o-sep'tor). A receptor or sense organ located within muscles, tendons, tendon sheaths, joints, or the vestibular apparatus of the inner ear, which provides awareness of posture, balance, and muscular adjustment.

proptometer (prop-tom'eh-ter). Exophthalmometer.

proptosis ocular (prop-to'sis). Exophthalmos.

pro-sensation (pro-sen-sa'shun). A hypothetical, sensory response, presumed to be a fundamental hue, aroused by stimulation of a single retinal receptor or receptor-type, which cannot be experienced alone but only after combination with, or modification by, other pro-sensations or sensory processes.

prosopagnosia (pros"o-pag-no'se-ah). Inability to recognize a familiar face.

prosthesis, ocular (pros'the-sis). Specifically, an artificial eye or implant. More generally, all mechanical and/or optical devices worn as ocular or visual aids, e.g., ptosis crutches, spectacles, and occluders.

prosthokeratoplasty (pros"tho-ker'ah-to-plas"te). A surgical procedure in which diseased or opaque corneal tissue is replaced by a transparent prosthesis, usually of acrylic.

prostigmine (pro-stig'min). A trade name for a synthetic alkaloid (neostigmine) available only in its salts.

Prostigmine bromide instilled in the eye in diluted solution acts as a powerful miotic through its neutralizing effect on choline esterases, permitting the continued action of acetylcholine.

protan (pro'tan). Protanoid.

protanoid (pro'tah-noid). 1. Pertaining to, or having the properties of, protanopia or protanomalous trichromasy. 2. One whose color vision shows some or all of the characteristics of protanopia or protanomaly. Syn., *protan*.

protanomal (pro"tah-nom'al). One having protanomaly.

protanomalopia (pro"tah-nom"ah-lo'-pe-ah). Protanomaly. *Obs.*

protanomaly (pro"tah-nom'ah-le). A condition characterized by relatively lowered luminosity for long wavelength lights and, concomitantly, by abnormal color matching mixtures in which an excess of the red primary is necessary. Syn., *protanomalous trichromatism; protanomalous vision.*

protanope (pro'tah-nōp). One having protanopia.

protanopia (pro"tah-no'pe-ah). A form of dichromatism characterized by decreased luminosity for long wavelengths and an inability to differentiate the hues of red, orange, yellow, and green, or blue and violet, or blue-green and a neutral gray. A sex-linked, hereditary form of color blindness occurring in about 1% of the male population. Syn., *anerythropsia; red blindness.*

protanopic (pro"tah-nop'ik). Pertaining to or having protanopia.

proteinosis, lipid (pro"te-in-o'sis). A chronic recessive disease of unknown etiology occurring early in life characterized by extracellular deposits in the skin and mucous membranes which heavily involve the eyelid margins and sometimes the conjunctiva, uvea, or fundus. Syn., *Urbach-Wiethe disease; hyalinosis cutis et mucosae.*

prothesis (proth'e-sis). Prosthesis.

protometer (pro-tom'eh-ter). Exophthalmometer.

protractor. *Ophthalmic:* A chart containing a circle sectioned into degrees for positioning the axis of cylindrical spectacle lenses, and scales for positioning the optical center of lenses and multifocal segments.

protrusio bulbi (pro-trōō'ze-o bul'-bi). Exophthalmos.

protrusion, posterior, of von Ammon. Scleral ectasia in the region of the posterior pole of the eyeball, due to an incomplete closure of the fetal cleft and found in conjunction with a coloboma of the choroid.

prurigo estivalis (proo-rig'o es"tiv-ah'lis). Hydroa vacciniforme.

psammoma (sam-o'mah). A small, hard, fibrous tumor occurring in brain tissue and the optic nerve.

pseudagraphia (su"dah-graf'e-ah, -gra'-fe-ah). Pseudoagraphia.

pseudo-accommodation (su"do-ah-kom"o-da'shun). Apparent accommodation.

pseudoagraphia (su"do-ah-graf'e-ah, -gra'fe-ah). A condition in which written material can be correctly copied but in which meaningful original material cannot be written.

pseudoaphakia (su"do-ah-fa'ke-ah). Membranous cataract.

pseudoblepsia (su"do-blep'se-ah). Pseudoblepsis.

pseudoblepsis (su"do-blep'sis). A visual hallucination or illusion. Syn., *pseudopsia.*

pseudocataract (su"do-kat'ah-rakt). False lenticonus.

pseudochalazion (su"do-kal-la'ze-on). An eye lesion, such as a sarcomatous or syphilitic lesion, which resembles a chalazion.

pseudochromesthesia (su"do-kro"-mes-the'ze-ah). A type of synesthesia in which certain sounds induce characteristic color sensations. Syn., *color hearing; psychochromesthesia.*

pseudochromia (su"do-kro'me-ah). False perception of color.

pseudocoloboma (su"do-kol"o-bo'-mah). 1. A line or a scar on the iris resembling a coloboma. 2. Incomplete coloboma.

pseudocyclophoria (su"do-si"klo-fo'-re-ah). Optical cyclophoria.

pseudoepiphora (su"do-eh-pif'o-rah). Reflex hypersecretion of the orbital and accessory portions of the lacrimal gland, giving the appearance of a "wet eye," due to irritation resulting from hyposecretion of the accessory lacrimal glands of Wolfring and Krause, the mucin goblet cells, and the meibomian glands.

pseudoesophoria (su"do-es"o-fo're-ah, su"do-e"so-). An apparent esophoria attributable to spurious manifestations of accommodative convergence or positive relative convergence, or to temporarily or inadvertently induced effects of lenses or prisms.

pseudoexfoliation, capsular (su″do-eks-fo-le-a′shun). A disease in which small, gray, fluffy particles are deposited on the crystalline lens, zonule of Zinn, iris, cornea, and in the filtration angle. It is of undetermined etiology and pathogenesis and is often confused with a true exfoliation of the capsule of the crystalline lens.

pseudoexophoria (su″do-eks″o-fo′-re-ah). An apparent exophoria attributable to spurious manifestations, or failures of manifestation, of accommodative convergence, or to temporarily or inadvertently induced effects of lenses or prisms.

pseudogeusesthesia (su″do-gu″es-the′se-ah, su″do-ju″-). 1. A type of synesthesia in which certain tastes induce characteristic color sensations. 2. A false sensation of taste.

pseudoglaucoma (su″do-glaw-ko′-mah). Any anomaly of the optic disk which may appear to be of glaucomatous origin, as, for example, a congenitally large and pale physiological cup, a branching of the central retinal artery posterior to the lamina cribrosa, a congenital coloboma of the optic disk, or an excessively oblique connection of the optic nerve with the eyeball.

pseudoglioma (su″do-gli-o′mah). 1. An organized exudate in the vitreous body, caused by endophthalmitis, which simulates the reflex from the interior of the eye seen in retinoblastoma. 2. Any condition which simulates retinoblastoma, as retrolental fibroplasia or retinal detachment.

pseudohyperphoria (su″do-hi″per-fo′re-ah). An apparent hyperphoria attributable to spurious manifestations of neurological origin or to temporarily or inadvertently induced effects of lenses or prisms.

pseudoisochromatic (su″do-i″so-kro-mat′ik). Pertaining to the different hues which appear alike to the color blind.

pseudomacula (su″do-mak′u-lah). False macula.

pseudomonochromasy (su″do-mon-o-kro′mah-se). A term introduced by König for a type of total color blindness with luminosity functions corresponding to the known forms of congenital dichromasy but with normal visual acuity. Syn., *cone monochromatism*.

pseudomyopia (su″do-mi-o′pe-ah). Appearance of myopia due to spasm of the ciliary muscle or to failure of relaxation of accommodation. See also *hypertonic myopia*.

pseudoneuritis (su″do-nu-ri′tis). Pseudo optic neuritis.

pseudonystagmus (su″do-nis-tag′-mus). An accentuation of the normal oscillatory movements of the eyes occurring when fixation is changed from one point to another.

pseudo-ophthalmoplegia (su″do-of-thal″mo-ple′je-ah). Loss of voluntary eye movements, with reflex movements intact and possibly exaggerated, due to bilateral destructive lesions of the frontal cortex.

pseudopapilledema (su″do-pap″ih-le-de′mah). A condition of apparent papilledema, observed ophthalmoscopically, in the presence of normal visual acuity, normal size of the blind spot, and normal intracranial pressure.

pseudoparalysis, myasthenic (su″-do-pah-ral′ih-sis). Myasthenia gravis.

pseudophakia (su″do-fa′ke-ah). A congenital condition in which the crystalline lens has been invaded and replaced by mesodermal tissue.

　artificial p. An aphakic eye with an artificial lens implant. (Binkhorst)

　p. fibrosa. Pseudophakia in which the invading mesodermal tissue undergoes fibrous degeneration. Syn., *fibrous tissue cataract; cataracta fibrosa*.

　p. lipomatosa. Pseudophakia in which the invading mesodermal tissue undergoes fatty degeneration. Syn., *cataracta adiposa*.

　p. ossea. Pseudophakia in which the invading mesodermal tissue undergoes osseous degeneration. Syn., *cataracta ossea*.

pseudophotesthesia (su″do-fo″tes-the′ze-ah). Color or light sensation or attribution, induced by stimuli or irritants abnormal for vision, such as sound, taste, smell, pressure, thought, or anger.

pseudopolycoria (su″do-pol″ih-ko′-re-ah). Polycoria spuria.

pseudopsia (su-dop′se-ah). A visual hallucination or illusion. Syn., *pseudoblepsia*.

pseudopterygium (su″do-ter-ij′e-um). An adhesion of the conjunctiva to the cornea, as a result of an inflammatory process, which resembles a pterygium but which may occur at any part of the corneal margin and is attached only at its apex.

pseudoptosis (su″do-to′sis). A condition resembling ptosis, due to an abnormally small palpebral aperture (blepharophimosis), to lack of normal support to the upper eyelid by the eyeball, or to a fold of atrophic skin falling below the edge of the upper eyelid (blepharochalasis). Syn., *apparent ptosis; false ptosis; spurious ptosis.*

pseudoretinitis pigmentosa (su″do-ret′ih-ni′tis pig-men-to′sah). Any disease of the retina presenting the ophthalmoscopic picture of bone corpuscle pigmentation similar to that in retinitis pigmentosa, but without the other accompanying symptoms.

pseudoretinoblastoma (su″do-ret-ih-no-blas-to′mah). Any organized mass in the vitreous body which gives rise to a grayish-white pupillary reflex simulating that seen in retinoblastoma. Syn., *pseudoglioma.*

pseudosclerosis of Westphal (su″-do-skle-ro′sis). Wilson's disease.

pseudoscope (su″do-skōp). An instrument which transposes to the right eye the view normally seen by the left, and vice versa, usually by means of prisms and mirrors.

pseudoscopic (su″do-skop′ik). Seen in reversed stereoscopic relief, or pertaining to the effect obtained in, or tests done with, a pseudoscope.

pseudoscopy (su-dos′ko-pe). The viewing of targets in reverse stereoscopic relief, or in a pseudoscope.

pseudostereopsis (su″do-ster-e-op′sis). Binocular visual perception in reversed stereoscopic relief, as obtained in viewing a three-dimensional field in a stereoscope with the view for the two eyes transposed. Syn., *pseudoscopic vision.*

pseudostrabismus (su″do-strah-biz′-mus). Apparent strabismus.

pseudotrachoma (su″do-trah-ko′-mah). Nodular conjunctivitis.

    syphilitic p. Granular syphilitic conjunctivitis.

pseudotumor cerebri (su″do-tu′mor ser′e-bri). Increased intracranial pressure, without clinical evidence of tumor, which may be idiopathic or may occur following otitis media, upper respiratory infections, trauma, or thrombosis of the superior, sagittal, and lateral sinuses. The symptoms are primarily ocular and include blurring of vision, strabismus, diplopia, blindness, and papilledema.

pseudotumor, orbital (su″do-tu′-mor). Orbital myositis.

pseudotumor, retinal (su″do-tu′-mor). Retinal fibrosis.

pseudoxanthoma elasticum (su″do-zan-tho′mah e-las′tih-kum). A rare disease of the skin characterized by the appearance of elevated yellowish papules or plaques, particularly on the neck, chest, and abdomen, and infrequently on the eyelids. It is due to degeneration of dermal elastic tissue and is sometimes associated with angioid streaks (Grönblad-Strandberg syndrome).

psoriasis (so-ri′ah-sis). A disease of the skin of unknown etiology, characterized by sharply defined red patches covered with silvery scales which appear particularly in the regions of the elbows and knees, in the scalp, and rarely in the eyelids.

psorophthalmia (sōr″of-thal′me-ah). Blepharitis marginalis.

PSRO. See *Professional Standards Review Organization.*

psychalia (si-ka′le-ah). A depressed mental state associated with visual and auditory hallucinations. *Obs.*

psychanopsia (si-kah-nop′se-ah). Visual agnosia.

psychochromesthesia (si″ko-kro″-mes-the′ze-ah). Pseudochromesthesia.

psycho-optic (si″ko-op′tik). Pertaining to the relations between mental and optical processes or functions.

psychophysics (si″ko-fiz′iks). The branch of science that deals with the interrelationships of physical stimuli and their mental or perceptual correlates.

psychophysiology (si″ko-fiz″e-ol′o-je). Physiological psychology; the branch of science which deals with the interrelationships between psychological and physiological processes.

pterygium (teh-rij′e-um). A horizontal, triangular growth of the bulbar conjunctiva, occupying the intrapalpebral fissure, with the apex extending toward the cornea. The base is typically at the internal canthus, rarely at the external canthus, and the pterygium is fixed to the conjunctiva along its entire length, so that a probe cannot be passed entirely beneath it. It is highly vascularized during growth, is considered to be due to a degenerative process caused by long continued irritation, as from exposure to wind and dust, and, if not treated surgically, may encroach on the cornea and destroy Bowman's membrane.

p. carnosum. Pterygium crassum.

cicatricial p. Pseudopterygium.

congenital p. Epitarsus.

p. crassum. A thick, fleshy, vascular pterygium. Syn., *pterygium carnosum; pterygium sarcomatosum; pterygium vasculosum.*

false p. Pseudopterygium.

p. membranaceum. Pterygium tenue.

p. sarcomatosum. Pterygium crassum.

p. tenue. A thin, tendinous, stationary pterygium. Syn., *pterygium membranaceum.*

p. vasculosum. Pterygium crassum.

pterygoid (ter'ih-goid) **canal; plexus.** See under the nouns.

ptilosis (tih-lo'sis). Pathological loss of the eyelashes.

ptosed (tōst). Affected with ptosis.

◆

PTOSIS

ptosis (to'sis). 1. Prolapse or falling down of an organ or a part. 2. Drooping of the upper eyelid below its normal position. Syn., *blepharoptosis.*

p. adiposa. Folds of skin hanging from the upper eyelid over the free lid margin, once thought to result from an accumulation of fat, but it has been shown to result from relaxation of fascial bands which attach the levator to the skin of the eyelid. Syn., *Sichel's ptosis.*

apparent p. Pseudoptosis.

artificial p. Ptosis produced by surgical section of nerves to the levator palpebrae superioris muscle for the protection of the eyeball, as in lagophthalmos.

p. atonica. 1. Ptosis occurring in later stages of blepharochalasis in which atrophic, wrinkled, discolored, and venuled skin overhangs the upper eyelid margin and in which the power to raise the lid is diminished. 2. Pseudoparalytic ptosis.

p. atrophica. Blepharochalasis.

p. crutch. See under *crutch.*

false p. Pseudoptosis.

functional p. Partial closure of the eyelids to reduce the effective pupillary aperture.

Horner's p. Sympathetic ptosis present in Horner's syndrome.

hypertonic p. Ptosis associated with Parkinson's disease and due to increased tonicity of the opposing muscles, with a resulting rigidity and loss of voluntary movement.

p. iridis. Prolapse of the iris.

levator p. Ptosis attributable to inadequacy or paresis of the levator palpebrae superioris muscle.

p. lipomatosis. Mechanical ptosis due to lipoma of the eyelid.

mechanical p. Ptosis due to edema or inflammation of the conjunctiva or eyelid, to hypertrophy or atrophy of the eyelid tissue, to herniation of orbital fat into the eyelid, etc., without involvement of the levator palpebrae superioris muscle or its nerve supply.

morning p. Waking ptosis.

myogenic p. Ptosis due to disease of the levator palpebrae superioris muscle.

paralytic p. Ptosis due to lesion in the pathway of the oculomotor nerve.

periodic p. The intermittent ptosis associated with cyclic oculomotor paralysis.

pseudoparalytic p. Ptosis due to loss of normal tonicity of the levator palpebrae superioris muscle as may occur in senility, after prolonged bandaging, or after continued belpharospasm. Syn., *ptosis atonica.*

relative p. An apparent ptosis of a normally positioned eyelid in comparison with a contralateral upper eyelid retraction, presumed to be suggested by the asymmetry, but which may occur in part as a binocular compensatory effect of the unilateral retraction.

p. senilis. Pseudoparalytic ptosis occurring in the aged.

Sichel's p. Ptosis adiposa.

simple p. Congenital ptosis due to impaired development of the levator palpebrae superioris muscle or to absent or incomplete innervation to the muscle. It may be associated with paresis of the homolateral superior rectus muscle, but is unaccompanied by any other defect.

spurious p. Pseudoptosis.

sympathetic p. Ptosis due to paresis of Mueller's muscle; its association with other signs of sympathetic paresis constitutes Horner's syndrome.

synkinetic p. Ptosis associated with movements of the eye or jaw, as in jaw-winking.

voluntary p. 1. Voluntary closure of one eyelid to avoid diplopia. 2. Partial closure of the eyelids to reduce the effective pupillary aperture. Syn., *functional ptosis*.

waking p. Temporary paralysis of the upper eyelid on awakening from sleep. Syn., *morning ptosis*.

◆

ptotic (tot'ik). Pertaining to or affected with ptosis.

pucker, macular. Preretinal macular fibrosis.

Pugh's (pūz) **occluder; visual acuity reducer.** See under the nouns.

Pulfrich (pul'frik) **effect; phenomenon, photometer; refractometer; stereoscope.** See under the nouns.

pulse, corneal indentation. Pulse-pressure-induced variations of corneal indentation obtained with a continuously recording tonometer. Abbreviation *CIP*.

pulse, photic. A short duration of light, used in reference to a light stimulus and differentiated from a *flash*, the sensory correlate.

pulvinar (pul-vi'nar). The medial angular prominence of the posterior portion of the thalamus, thought to be associated with higher somatic functions, and with visual and auditory integration because of its connections with cortical areas adjacent to the primary cortical receptive areas for these types of impulses.

pump, lacrimal. The mechanism which acts to facilitate tear drainage in the lacrimal apparatus, primarily by action of the orbicularis oculi and Horner's muscles, initiated by blinking of the eyelids.

punctometer (punk-tom'eh-ter). 1. An instrument making use of the subjective appearance of a very small, in and out of focus, point of light for the determination of the conjugate focus of the retina and related refractive values. 2. A punctumeter.

punctometry (punk-tom'eh-tre). Measurement of the refractive state of the eye, or the status of accommodation, by use of an illuminated pinhole target subjectively adjusted in optical distance from the eye to appear maximally

bright, most sharply defined, and of minimum size.

punctum (punk'tum). A point.

p. caecum. The blind spot of Mariotte.

p. convergens basalis. The near point of convergence. Abbreviated PCB.

lacrimal p. The small, pointlike orifice in the lacrimal papilla which serves as the opening into the lacrimal canaliculus.

p. luteum. Macula lutea.

p. proximum of accommodation. Near point of accommodation.

p. proximum of convergence. Near point of convergence. Abbreviated PPC.

p. remotum of accommodation. Far point of accommodation.

p. remotum of convergence. The far point of convergence. Abbreviated PRC.

punctumeter (punk-tum'eh-ter). An instrument for determining the near and far points of accommodation.

Punktal (punk'tal). A trade name for a series of corrected curve ophthalmic lenses.

◆

PUPIL

pupil (pu'pil). 1. The aperture in the iris, normally circular and contractile, through which the image-forming light enters the eye. 2. *Zoology:* The dark central spot of an ocellus.

Adie's p. Tonic pupil.

apparent p. The entrance pupil of the eye, hence the pupil as normally seen, i.e., through the cornea. It is slightly larger than, and anterior to, the actual pupil.

Argyll Robertson's p. A pupil characterized by the loss of both direct and consensual reflexes to light, with normal contraction on accommodation and convergence and otherwise normal vision. Miosis may or may not be present. The condition usually indicates syphilis of the central nervous system. Syn., *Vincent's sign*. **inverse A. R's. p.** A pupil characterized by normal, direct, and consensual reflexes to light with loss of contraction on accommodation and convergence. It is due to a midbrain lesion of the connection of the convergence center with the constrictor center of the pupil.

artificial p. 1. A pupil made by iridectomy. 2. A perforation in a diaphragm or disk to be held or mounted in front of the eye to effect a small or constant pupil size.

bounding p. A pupil showing alternate dilations and contractions unassociated with illumination changes.

Bumke's p. A catatonic pupil found in neurotics.

cat's-eye p. A pupil with a narrow vertical aperture.

catatonic p. A pupil which transiently dilates and which may become inactive to light and convergence stimuli. The dilatation may persist for only a few seconds or for several days and is associated with catatonia and other psychotic states, hysteria, neuroses, syphilis, or alcoholism. Syn., *spasmus mobilis.*

climbing p. of Lowenstein. A pupil which contracts poorly to light and dilates in excess of the amount of original contraction and, upon repeated subsequent light stimulation, demonstrates a greater and greater dilatation.

cogwheel p. A pupil found in hysteria in which the contraction to light and the redilatation do not take place in a single continuous movement but in a series of steps, giving a cogged appearance to a continuous graphical recording of the pupillary diameter.

Cook's p. Hutchinson's pupil.

cornpicker's p. Mydriasis and cycloplegia induced by stramonium dust derived from jimson weed growing frequently in corn fields.

descending p. of Lowenstein. A pupil which contracts to light, does not demonstrate an equivalent redilatation on removal of the light stimulus, and, on repeated subsequent light stimulation, demonstrates a greater and greater contraction.

entrance p. The image of the aperture stop formed by the portion of an optical system on the object side of the stop.

exit p. The image of the aperture stop formed by the portion of an optical system on the image side of the stop.

fixed p. An immobile pupil, one which is inactive to all reflexes.

Hutchinson's p. An immobile, widely dilated pupil which is inactive to all reflexes, associated with intracranial hemorrhage, as may occur in fracture of the skull or with cranial neoplasm.

keyhole p. A pupil shaped like a keyhole, due to coloboma, surgery, or trauma of the iris.

Marcus Gunn p. The designation for the abnormal pupillary response in the *swinging flashlight test.*

miotic p. 1. A pupil which is reduced in size, as one constricted in response to the instillation of a miosis-producing drug. 2. A very small pupil, i.e., approximately 2 mm or less in diameter.

multiple p's. Polycoria.

mydriatic p. 1. A pupil which is increased in size, as one dilated in response to the instillation of a mydriasis-producing drug. 2. A very large pupil, i.e., approximately 5 mm or greater in diameter.

myotic p. Miotic pupil.

myotonic p. Tonic pupil.

neurotonic p. A pupil which contracts slowly on stimulation by light and, when contracted, remains immobile for some time.

nonluetic Argyll Robertson's p. Tonic pupil.

paradoxical p. A pupil which dilates on stimulation of the retina by light or has any other action opposite to that normally expected.

pinhole p. 1. An extremely small pupil. 2. A pupil or an aperture small enough to make the effects of refraction negligible; a pinhole.

pseudo-Argyll Robertson's p. Tonic pupil.

reverse Argyll Robertson's p. A pupil characterized by the loss of constriction on convergence and accommodation, with retention of the normal light reflexes.

Robertson's p. Argyll Robertson's pupil.

springing p. A sudden momentary dilation of one pupil, followed, after a short interval, by sudden momentary dilation of the other, seen in tabes, general paralysis, neurasthenia, veronal poisoning, and some times in apparently normal persons.

tonic p. A pupil in which the reaction to light, both direct and consensual, is almost abolished, being elicited only after prolonged exposure to dark or light, and in which there is a delayed reaction to changes in accommodation and convergence. It usually occurs unilaterally, with the affected pupil being the larger, and reacts normally to mydriatics and certain miotics. Syn., *Adie's pupil; myotonic pupil; nonluetic Argyll Robertson pupil; pseudo-Argyll Robertson pupil; pupillotonia.*

◆

pupilantoscope (pu″pih-lan′to-skōp). An instrument for examining one's own pupil, consisting essentially of a magnifying lens in front of a concave mirror, contained in a rim mounted on a handle.

pupilens, Mazow (pu′pih-lens). A corneal contact lens, opaque except for a small central aperture, giving the effect of a pinhole pupil, which increases the depth of focus of the eye and eliminates the necessity for a reading correction in presbyopia.

pupilla (pu-pil′ah). The pupil of the eye.

pupillary (pu′pih-lār-e). Pertaining to or of the pupil.

pupillary axis; block; distance; line; reaction; reflex; ruff. See under the nouns.

pupillography (pu″pih-log′rah-fe). 1. Photography of the pupil. 2. The recording of pupillary reactions.

pupillometer (pu″pih-lom′eh-ter). 1. An instrument for measuring the diameter of the pupil. Syn., *coreometer.* 2. Erroneously, an instrument for measuring the interpupillary distance.

    Broca's p. A pair of very small light sources or transilluminated pinholes placed in the anterior focal plane of the eye and varied in separation until the resulting circular out-of-focus images on the retina are seen in juxtaposition, whereupon the separation of the light sources or pinholes is a direct subjective measure of the diameter of the pupil.

    Haab's p. A series of graduated circles which are compared with the pupil for size.

    Laurence's p. A caliper-type pupillometer.

    Morton's p. A disk of graduated circles attached to Morton's ophthalmoscope for direct comparison with the pupil for size.

    Priestley Smith's p. A millimeter scale engraved on a convex lens through which an observer at the focal point views the pupil to be measured.

    projection p. A millimeter scale optically projected or mirrored in the plane of the pupil to be measured.

    Schlösser's p. A series of short parallel lines of graduated length engraved on a transparent scale for direct comparison with the pupil diameter.

pupillometry (pu″pih-lom′eh-tre). The measurement of the size of the pupil of the eye. Syn., *coreometry.*

pupillomotor (pu″pih-lo-mo′tor). Pertaining to motor activity affecting pupil size.

pupilloplegia (pu″pih-lo-ple′je-ah). Complete or partial paralysis of the pupillary reflexes.

pupilloscope (pu-pil′o-skōp). 1. An instrument for observing the pupil or its reactions. 2. A retinoscope.

pupilloscopy (pu″pih-los′ko-pe). 1. Retinoscopy. 2. Observation of the pupil or its reactions with a pupilloscope.

pupillostatometer (pu-pil″o-stah-tom′eh-ter). An instrument for measuring the interpupillary distance.

pupillotonia (pu″pih-lo-to′ne-ah). Tonic pupil.

pupillotonic pseudotabes (pu″pih-lo-ton′ik su″do-ta′bēz). Adie's syndrome.

purity. 1. A measure of the degree of freedom of a color from achromatic content; or, the degree to which a color approaches the condition required for maximum saturation. Various purity scales are used, all of which can be expressed as some mathematical function of the ratio of the spectral to the achromatic components of a color mixture. 2. Excitation purity.

    colorimetric p. The spectral purity of a color expressed as the ratio of the luminance of a monochromatic spectral component which, if mixed with an achromatic component, would match the color, to the luminance of the color itself. Syn., *luminance purity.*

    excitation p. The ratio of the distance, on the CIE standard chromaticity diagram, between the achromatic (white) point and the sample point to the distance in the same direction between the achromatic point and the point on the spectrum locus representing the dominant wavelength of the sample.

    luminance p. Colorimetric purity.

    Ostwald p. In the Ostwald system, the ratio of full color content to white content.

Purkinje's (poor-kēn′ēz) **afterimage;**

effect; figures; images; phenomenon; shadows; shift. See under the nouns.

Purkinje-Sanson images (poor-kĕn'e-san'son). See under *image*.

purple. 1. A mixture of blue and red, a nonspectral hue complementary to yellow-green of about 560 mμ. 2. One of a series of related hues ranging from blue to red on the nonspectral portion of the color scale.

 retinal p. Rhodopsin.

 visual p. Rhodopsin.

purpura (pur'pu-rah). A disease characterized by recurrent multiple hemorrhages in the skin, mucous membranes, serous membranes, and internal organs. The ocular manifestations may be hemorrhages into the eyelids, conjunctiva, iris, choroid, or retina, or palsies of the extraocular muscles due to hemorrhages in the brain.

 hyperglobulinemic p. Waldenström's syndrome.

pursuitmeter (pur-sūt'me-ter). A device for indicating degree of eye-hand coordination, utilizing an irregularly moving visual target that must be followed as accurately as possible by a handheld stylus.

Purtscher's (poor'cherz) **disease; retinopathy.** See under the nouns.

purulent (pu'roo-lent). Consisting of, containing, associated with, or identified by the formation of pus.

Px. Prognosis.

pyophthalmia (pi"of-thal'me-ah). Purulent inflammation of the eye, especially of the conjunctiva. Syn., *pyophthalmitis*.

pyophthalmitis (pi"of-thal-mi'tis). Pyophthalmia.

pyramid, color. A type of color solid.

pyridoxine (pir"ih-dok'sin). A watersoluble vitamin present in yeast, cereals, and liver and thought to be associated with the metabolism of unsaturated fatty acids. A deficiency in the diet may be a factor in nutritional amblyopia. Syn., *vitamin B$_6$*.

pyrometer, optical (pi-rom'eh-ter). An instrument to determine the temperature of a hot body by measuring the intensity of the emitted light of a given wavelength.

pyron (pi'ron). A unit of radiation intensity equal to a gram calorie per square centimeter of receiving surface per minute when the receiving surface is perpendicular to the direction of radiation.

quadra (kwod'rah). Having a predominantly square or rectangular shape; a British classification of spectacle lenses differentiated in outline from those predominantly round or oval.

quadrantanopia (kwod-ran"tah-no'pe-ah). Quadrantanopsia.

quadrantanopsia (kwod-ran"tah-nop'-se-ah). Blindness or loss of vision in a quarter sector of the visual field of one eye. Syn., *quadrantic anopsia; tetranopsia.*

    binasal q., crossed. Quadrantanopsia involving the lower nasal quadrant of the visual field of one eye and the upper nasal quadrant of the visual field of the other eye.

    bitemporal q., crossed. Quadrantanopsia involving the lower temporal quadrant of the visual field of one eye and the upper temporal quadrant of the visual field of the other eye.

    heteronymous q., lower. Quadrantanopsia involving either both lower temporal quadrants of the visual fields or both lower nasal quadrants of the visual fields.

    heteronymous q., upper. Quadrantanopsia involving either both upper temporal or both upper nasal quadrants of the visual fields.

    homonymous q., lower. Quadrantanopsia involving the lower nasal quadrant of the visual field of one eye and the lower temporal quadrant of the visual field of the other eye. Syn., *lower tetartanopsia.*

    homonymous q., upper. Quadrantanopsia involving the upper nasal quadrant of the visual field of one eye and the upper temporal quadrant of the visual field of the other eye. Syn., *upper tetartanopsia.*

quadrantic anopsia (kwod-ran'tik anop'se-ah). Quadrantanopsia.

quadrilopia (kwod"ril-o'pe-ah). The perception of a single object in quadruple, or double diplopia, as sometimes may occur with anomalous retinal correspondence.

quality, spectral. The color characteristic of a light source or a lighted area, as represented by the relative amounts of luminous energy of different wavelengths.

quantity of illumination. See *light exposure.*

quantity of light. The product of luminous flux and its duration, expressed in lumen-seconds. Cf. *light exposure.*

quantum of light (kwon'tum). A quantity of light energy equal to the product of the frequency of the light and Planck's constant (6.624×10^{-27} erg sec).

quartz. Silicon dioxide (SiO_2), a doubly refracting crystal, found in nature in a variety of forms, which is transparent to visible and ultraviolet radiation and is used in optics to produce polarized light.

    amorphous q. Silicon dioxide (SiO_2) not in crystal formation; fused quartz.

quasi-correspondence, retinal (kwa'-si-kōr"e-spon'dens). The faculty of vision which gives rise to the unitary percept of a binocularly seen object, or of a pair of objects viewed haploscopically, when the respective retinal images stimulate noncorresponding retinal receptors lying within Panum's areas.

Quincke's disease (kvink'ēz). Angioneurotic edema.

quizzing glass. Monocle.

quotient. A number obtained by dividing one number by another.

accomplishment q. The achievement age divided by the mental age.

achievement q. The achievement age divided by the chronological age.

intelligence q. The mental age multiplied by 100 and divided by the chronological age.

perversion q. The angle of anomaly divided by the objective angle of strabismus.

reading q. The reading age divided by the mental age.

r. Symbol for *radius of curvature.*

Rabkin charts; polychromatic plates; test. See under the nouns.

racemic (ra-se'mik). Pertaining to a compound or mixture having equal amounts of dextrorotatory and levorotatory components, which does not produce rotation of the plane of polarized light.

radiance (ra'de-ans). Radiant flux per unit solid angle per unit projected area of the source in a given direction. The usual unit is the watt per steradian per sq cm. It is the radiant analog of *luminance* (photometric brightness). Symbol: N.

radiant. Transmitted or emitted by radiation.

radiant energy; flux; intensity. See under the nouns.

radiation. 1. The process by which radiant energy is emitted and transmitted. Less appropriately, that which is radiated, thus synonymous with radiant energy. 2. A group of nerve fibers that diverge after leaving their place of origin.

  beta r. Radiation of negatively charged electrons which travel in a straight line at about the speed of light unless affected by a magnetic field. The electrons vary in penetrating power, travel about 9.0 to 10.0 cm in air and up to 1.0 cm in tissue. It may be derived from x-rays, radium, radon, radium D, or an isotope such as strontium 90, and, in the eye, is used for the treatment of rosacea keratitis, recurrent pterygia, and vernal conjunctivitis, and for the removal of corneal blood vessels prior to keratoplasty.

  blackbody r. The characteristic thermal radiation emitted by a heated blackbody; the radiation from a field in an enclosed cavity in thermal equilibrium with the matter surrounding it.

  coherent r. See *coherence.*

  infrared r. Infrared energy.

  luminous r. Luminous energy.

  r's. of Meynert. A large number of coarse, medullated fibers in the deep area striata that represent the continuation of the projection system of the optic radiations.

  optic r's. of Gratiolet. Geniculocalcarine tract.

  photochemical r. Radiation capable of producing chemical changes in materials.

  resonance r. Radiation emitted from a medium as the result of, and only during, the absorption of radiation from another source, the emitted radiation being of the same wavelength as that of the exciting radiation. Syn., *resonance fluorescence.*

  spectral r. Spectral energy.

  ultraviolet r. Ultraviolet energy.

radiator (ra'dih-a"tor). An emitter of radiant energy.

  complete r. Blackbody.

  ideal r. Blackbody.

  incomplete r. Graybody.

  isotropic r. An emitter of equal amounts of radiant energy in all directions.

  nonselective r. 1. A radiator for which spectral emissivity is constant throughout the spectrum. 2. A graybody.

perfectly diffusing r. Perfect diffusing surface.

Planckian r. Blackbody.

selective r. A radiator for which spectral emissivity varies for different wavelengths.

standard r. Blackbody.

total r. Blackbody.

radiolucent (ra-de-o-loo'sent). Permeable to x-ray and other forms of radiation. Cf. *radiopaque*.

radiometer (ra"dih-om'eh-ter). An instrument for detecting and measuring radiant energy.

Crookes' r. An exhausted glass globe in which is mounted a freely rotating shaft with several vanes, black on one side and silvered on the other, which rotate in reaction to radiant energy, with the blackened side of the vanes retreating, the velocity being roughly proportional to the energy received.

radiometry (ra"dih-om'eh-tre). The measurement of radiant energy; the use of a radiometer.

radiopaque (ra"de-o-pāk'). Opaque to x-ray and other forms of radiation. Cf. *radiolucent*.

radiotransparent (ra"de-o-trans-par'-ent). Completely permeable to radiation, especially x-ray.

radius. 1. The straight line extending from the center of a circle or a sphere to the curve or surface; the semidiameter of a circle or a sphere. 2. A circular limit defined by a fixed distance from an established point or center.

corneal r. The radius of curvature of the posterior surface of the corneal section of a contact lens.

scleral r. The radius of curvature of the posterior surface of the scleral section of a contact lens.

r. of stereoscopic vision. Range of stereopsis.

Radiuscope (ra'de-us-skōp). The trade name for an instrument for measuring the curvature of a contact lens; it has an optical system employing the Drysdale method.

radix nervi optici (ra'diks ner'vi op'tih-ki). Optic tract.

Raeder's syndrome (ra'derz). See under *syndrome*.

Ragona Scina experiment (rah-go'nah she'nah). See under *experiment*.

Raman effect (rah'man). See under *effect*.

Ramsay Hunt syndrome (ram'ze hunt). See under *syndrome*.

Ramsden (rams'den) **circle; disk; eyepiece.** See under the nouns.

ramus ophthalmicus (ra'mus of-thal'-mih-kus). Ophthalmic nerve.

range. The difference between the least and the greatest values in a series of measurements or values.

r. of accommodation. See under *accommodation*.

r. of convergence. See under *convergence*.

haplopic r. In the haplopic horopter, the anteroposterior distance through which a nonfixated test object may be displaced and still be seen as single.

r. of stereopsis. The linear distance from the eyes to the point just noticeably nearer than infinity as determined by the retinal disparity cue; the distance beyond which stereoscopic vision is not possible. Syn., *radius of stereoscopic vision*.

r. of vision. See under *vision*.

raphe (ra'fe). A line of union or demarcation, resembling a seam, between two more or less symmetrical halves of an organ or a structure.

r. palpebralis. A thin horizontal band of connective tissue which extends from the external canthus to the lateral margin of the orbit.

retinal r. A horizontal raphe on the temporal side of the macula in the nerve fiber layer of the retina above and below which the nerve fibers follow an arcuate course to the optic disk.

Rasin's sign. Jellinek's sign.

rate of aqueous outflow. The speed of drainage of aqueous humor, generally expressed in cubic millimeters per minute as $F = C(P_o - P_v)$, in which C = coefficient of facility of aqueous outflow, P_o = intraocular pressure just before tonometry, and P_v = episcleral venous pressure.

rate, reading. The rate at which an individual can read and comprehend, usually represented as the number of words read silently per unit time with a comprehension level of at least 80 percent.

Rateometer (rāt-om'eh-ter). The trade name for an instrument used in improving reading speed and comprehension, consisting essentially of a shutter which moves down over reading material at a preset speed, thus setting a pace for the reader.

rating, discomfort glare. A numerical assessment of the capacity of a combination of sources of brightness, such as luminaires, in a given visual environment for producing discomfort. Abbreviation *DGR*. Cf. *discomfort glare factor*.

◆

RATIO

ratio. A proportion; the quotient of one magnitude divided by another of the same kind.

ACA (AC/A) r. The ratio of accommodative convergence (AC) to accommodation (A), usually expressed as the quotient of accommodative convergence in prism diopters divided by the accommodative response in diopters. Syn., *gradient*.

aniseikonic r. A ratio representing the difference between the sizes of the two images in aniseikonia as determined by plotting the apparent frontoparallel plane horopter. It is the ratio of the angle subtended at the nodal point of one eye by the point of fixation and a peripheral point on the horopter to the angle subtended at the nodal point of the other eye by the same two points.

aperture r. The ratio of the diameter of the aperture of an optical system to its focal length. Syn., *relative aperture*.

Arden r. Arden index.

AV r. The apparent ratio of arterial to venous diameter in the retinal blood vessels, typically about 3:4, as observed ophthalmoscopically.

blank r. The ratio indicating the relationship of the index of refraction of the button of a multifocal lens to that of the carrier as expressed by the formula: $(n-1)/(N-n)$ in which n = index of refraction of the carrier and N = index of refraction of the button.

brightness r. The ratio, expressed as a fraction, indicating the luminance (photometric brightness) relationship between two areas.

Brunswik r. The expression, $S-S'/L-S'$, in which L = luminance of an unshadowed object, S' = luminance of the same object in shadow, and S = luminance of an experimental match to the shadowed object. It is used in experiments for determining the color constancy of an object when placed in shadow.

C/D r. Cup disk ratio.

ceiling cavity r. The computed effect of room dimensions above the luminaire plane on the coefficient of utilization. Abbreviation *CCR*. See also *FCR* and *RCR*.

contrast r. The ratio of the luminance of an object backed by black to that of the same object backed by white, and hence correlated with the transparency of the object.

cup disk r. The ratio of the horizontal diameter of the rims of the physiological cup to the horizontal diameter of the optic disk. Abbreviation C/D ratio.

floor cavity r. The computed effect of room dimensions below the working plane, usually table height, on the coefficient of utilization. Abbreviation *FCR*. See also *CCR* and *RCR*.

focal r. The ratio of the focal length of an optical system to the linear diameter of its entrance pupil, usually written as follows: f/5, f/4.5, etc. Syn., *f-value*.

Haller's r. A generalization that the size of animal eyes varies inversely with the size of the body.

Leuckart's r. A generalization that the size of animal eyes varies directly with swiftness of movement.

light-dark r. 1. In a repetitive, intermittent, light stimulus pattern, the ratio of light time to dark time in a cycle. 2. In a repetitive, intermittent, light stimulus pattern, the ratio of light time to the total time of the light-dark cycle.

light-dark, EOG r. The ratio of the potential of the light phase of the electro-oculogram to that of the dark phase, useful in differential diagnosis of disease affecting the functioning of the outer layers of the retina, especially of the retinal epithelium.

luminance r. The ratio of the luminance of one area to that of another area in the same field of view. Cf. *luminance contrast*.

Matthiessen's r. The radius of the crystalline lens × 2.55 is equal to the distance from the center of the lens to the retina, a constant in fishes, according to Matthiessen.

off/on r. The ratio between the stimulus thresholds for off and on responses of cells in the retina.

red-green r. Rayleigh equation.

room cavity r. The computed effect of room dimensions between the luminaire plane and the working plane on the coefficient of utilization. Abbreviation *RCR*. See also *CCR* and *FCR*.

Strehl intensity r. Strehl definition.

Thouless r. An alternate for the Brunswik ratio (q.v.), in which log luminances are substituted for luminances.

◆

Raubitschek chart; test. See under the nouns.

◆

RAY

ray. 1. A line representing the radiation or direction of the propagation of light, often regarded as an infinitesimally narrow pencil of light. 2. Light or radiant energy, especially in the sense of an element of light or radiant energy.

aberrant r. Stray light, or a ray of stray light.

actinic r. Radiant energy capable of producing or serving to produce chemical changes.

axial r. A ray coincident with the axis of an optical system.

bundle of r's. A cone or pencil of light. **direct b. of r's.** A homocentric bundle of rays emanating from or directed toward a point on the axis of an optical system. **homocentric b. of r's.** A bundle of rays which originate or meet at a common point. Syn., *monocentric bundle of rays*.

chief r. 1. An effective ray which passes through the center of the entrance pupil of an optical system. 2. A central or representative ray in a bundle of rays. **foveal c.r.** The ray or ray path represented in object space by the line connecting the point of fixation and the center of the entrance pupil, and, in image space, by the line connecting the center of the exit pupil and the fovea.

coherent r's. See *coherence*.

convergent r's. A pencil or a bundle of rays directed toward a common point.

Descartes' r. The path of a ray of light incident upon a transparent sphere reflected twice internally, and emerging in the approximate direction of its origin, as described by Descartes in explanation of the rainbow.

divergent r's. A pencil or a bundle of rays directed away from a common point.

effective r's. Rays which emanate from an object point and completely traverse an optical system.

emergent r. An effective ray in image space. Syn., *image ray*.

extraordinary r. In birefringence or double refraction, that ray which does not follow Snell's law; it is deviated even though the incident ray is normal to the surface.

grazing r. A ray which is presumed to travel along the interface between two media prior to incidence or after emergence. See also *grazing emergence; grazing incidence*.

Hertzian r's. Rays of radiant energy of wavelengths longer than infrared; used in radio and wireless transmission.

homocentric r's. Rays which originate or meet at a common point. Syn., *monocentric rays*.

image r. Emergent ray.

incident r. An effective ray in object space. Syn., *object ray*.

infrared r's. Rays of radiant energy in the region of the spectrum between the end of the visible red and the Hertzian rays, i.e., between 7,000 Å and 500,000 Å.

luminous r's. Rays from the visible region of the spectrum.

meridian r's. 1. Rays which lie in the plane containing the axis of the cylinder of a cylindrical refracting surface and the chief ray. 2. Tangential rays.

monocentric r's. Homocentric rays.

monochromatic r. A ray of monochromatic light.

normal r. A ray perpendicular to an optical surface.

object r. Incident ray.

oblique r. 1. A ray or one of a bundle of rays with a chief ray not parallel to the axis of the optical system. 2. A ray not perpendicular to a surface at the point of incidence.

ordinary r. In birefringence of double refraction, that ray which follows Snell's law; it is undeviated when the incident ray is normal to the surface.

parallel r's. 1. Rays parallel to each other. 2. Rays parallel to the axis of an optical system.

paraxial r. A ray which makes a very small angle with the axis of an optical system, lies close to the axis throughout the distance from object to image, and has a nearly normal incidence on the system.

pencil of r's. A narrow cone of rays coming from a point source or from one point of a broad source. **astigmatic p. of r's.** A nonhomocentric bundle of rays which has as a focus two mutually perpendicular lines, each centered along the chief ray and separated along this ray. **eccentric p. of r's.** A pencil of rays which is obliquely incident on a surface. **homocentric p. of r's.** A pencil of rays which have a common point of origin or which tend to meet at a common point.

reflected r. An image ray resulting from the impingement of an object ray on a reflecting surface.

refracted r. An effective ray after it has passed through an optical surface separating two transparent media of different indices of refraction.

residual r's. Rays of a narrow band of wavelengths which have been isolated by a series of reflections from selective reflection surfaces.

sagittal r's. 1. Rays which lie in the plane containing the chief ray and the perpendicular to the axis of the cylinder of a cylindrical refracting surface. 2. Rays of an oblique bundle which lie in the plane perpendicular to the plane of the tangential rays and containing the chief ray.

Schumann r's. Rays of radiant energy in the ultraviolet region of the spectrum between 1,850 Å and 1,200 Å.

secondary r. A nonaxial, effective ray which passes through the primary nodal point or the optical center of an optical system.

skew r's. Rays which are not in a plane containing the optical axis.

tangential r's. Rays which lie in the plane containing the axis of an optical system and the chief ray of the bundle. Cf. *meridian rays.*

r. tracing. See under *tracing.*

ultraviolet r's. Rays of radiant energy in the region of the spectrum between the end of the visible violet and the x-rays, i.e., between 4,000 Å and 136 Å.

◆

rayleigh (ra'la). A unit of luminous intensity equal to an emission rate of one megaphoton per square centimeter of a

column per second, used in photometry of the night sky and aurorae.

Rayleigh equation. See under *equation.*

Raymond Cestan syndrome (ramon'ses-tan'). See under *syndrome.*

Raynaud's disease (ra-nōz'). See under *disease.*

RCR. Abbreviation for *room cavity ratio.*

RDP. Abbreviation for *receptor-type distribution pattern.*

RE. Abbreviation for *right eye.*

reaction. A response to stimulation. For reactions not listed here, see under *reflex.*

Jarisch-Herxheimer r. An inflammatory reaction which may often include an acute iritis in a previously uninvolved eye 24 to 48 hours after the first therapeutic injection of arsenic or 10 to 16 hours after a treatment of penicillin for syphilis.

light-compass r. A type of menotaxis in which the animal travels at a fixed angle, the orientation angle, to a light source, in either a straight or a circular direction. See also *telomenotaxis; tropomenotaxis.*

Lowenstein's low intensity r. Gunn's pupillary phenomenon.

ophthalmic r. The reaction of the conjunctiva to toxins, as those of typhoid fever or tuberculosis, which have been instilled into the eye. The reaction is more severe in those affected with the disease.

ophthalmotonic r., consensual. Change in the intraocular pressure in one eye following or associated with change in intraocular pressure in the fellow eye.

r. time. See under *time.*

Reader, Craig. The trade name of an instrument for improving reading speed and comprehension, consisting essentially of a viewing screen on which reading material from film strips is projected and exposed sequentially at a controlled rate.

Reader, Franklin. The trade name of a projection magnifier for use in subnormal vision which provides either 3 × or 5 × magnification.

reader, retarded. An individual whose development of reading skills is below the normal performance for his age or grade placement.

readiness, reading. Capability of responding successfully to routine formal instruction in reading, especially in terms of maturational criteria.

Reading Accelerator. The trade name of an instrument for improving reading speed and comprehension, consisting essentially of an electrically controlled shutter which moves down over reading material at a preset speed, thus setting a pace for the reader.

reading, developmental. A program of instruction for improving reading rate and comprehension by training the component reading skills.

Reading Eye. A table model instrument which records eye movements during reading by photographing, on a moving film strip, light reflected from the corneae.

reading, mirror. Reading characterized by persistent left-right reversals and directional confusion of the printed symbols and word order.

Reading Pacer, Keystone. The trade name of an instrument for improving reading speed and comprehension, consisting essentially of an electrically controlled metal rod which moves down over reading material at a preset speed, thus setting a pace for the reader.

Reading Rate Controller. The trade name of an instrument for improving reading speed and comprehension, consisting essentially of a wide shutter which moves down over reading material at a preset speed, thus setting a pace for the reader.

reading, remedial. Systematic training for the development, improvement, or enhancement of reading ability.

Reading Trainer. The trade name of an instrument for improving reading speed and comprehension which rotates specially printed material past an opening at a controlled rate varying from 20 to 2,800 words per minute. The reverse side of the reading material has a comprehension test which is answered by pushing buttons on the instrument.

Reber's chart (ra'berz). See under *chart*.

receiver, photoelectric. A device in which electrical discharges are produced in response to incident radiant energy, as, for example, a photoelectric cell.

receptor, distance (re-sep'tor). A sense organ which responds to impressions from objects remote from the body. This would include such sense organs as the eyes, the ears, and the nose.

receptor, visual. A rod or a cone cell of the retina.

recess. A small groove, cleft, or cavity.

optic r. 1. In the young embryo, the portion of the cavity of the forebrain where the lumina of the optic stalks open. Syn., *preoptic recess*. 2. In the older fetus and the adult, the recess in the ventral and medial portion of the hypothalamus, in the floor of the III ventricle, occupied by the optic chiasm.

prelacrimal r. A groove on the medial wall of the maxillary sinus which forms a part of the bony passage for the nasolacrimal duct. Syn., *lacrimal groove*.

premarginal r. A small osteofibrous pocket containing adipose tissue in the region of the ascending portion of the zygomatic bone, between the orbital margin and the attachment of the septum orbitale to the periosteum a few millimeters below the margin.

recession (re-sesh'un). Surgical displacement of the insertion of an extraocular muscle posteriorly.

reciprocal (re-sip'ro-kal) **dispersion; inhibition; innervation; replacement.** See under the nouns.

von Recklinghausen's (fon rek'linghow"zenz) **canals; disease.** See under the nouns.

reclinatio palpebrarum (rek"lih-na'-she-o pal"pe-brah'rum). Ectropion.

reclusor palpebrarum (re-klu'sor pal"pe-brah'rum). Levator palpebrae superioris muscle.

recombiner. The second basic component of an interferometer which superposes the two coherent beams of light.

recovery. The binocular response to a fusion stimulus which eliminates diplopia and results in single binocular fixation of the test target, usually represented quantitatively in terms of the maximum amount of prism or other dissociating unit through which the response is made.

glare r. The ability to regain normal vision following exposure to a glare source such as an automobile headlight, usually specified in seconds of time.

involuntary r. A recovery response without voluntary effort on the part of the subject.

r. point. See under *point*.

voluntary r. A recovery response associated with or enhanced by voluntary effort on the part of the subject.

recruitment (re-kroot'ment). In neurophysiology, the gradual increase in response of a reflex when a given stimulus is repeatedly or consistently applied, believed to be due to the gradual increase in the number of motor units involved, additional ones being added during the stimulation.

rectangle, Tschermak's. A two dimensional arrangement of colors in which the four primals are located at the corners of a rectangle, with white at its center. The shorter sides of the rectangle represent colors between red and yellow and between blue and green, the longer sides colors between yellow and green and between red and blue.

rectus muscles (rek'tus). See under *muscle*.

red. The hue attribute typically evoked by stimulation of the normal retina with a combination of long and short wavelength radiation which is complementary to a blue-green of about 493 mμ and listed as one of the psychologically unique colors. Thus pure red does not occur in the spectrum, but long wavelength light, from about 650 mμ to the end of the spectrum, though slightly yellowish, normally is scarcely distinguishable from the pure or elementary extraspectral red.

red, visual. According to Kühne, the initial product of the decomposition of rhodopsin when exposed to light; an unstable carotenoid pigment which is transformed rapidly to visual yellow.

Redlich's (red'likhs) **phenomenon; symptom.** See under the nouns.

redout. Reddening of vision resulting from negative acceleration and due to blood being forced to the head. Cf. *grayout; blackout.*

reduced distance; eye; vergence. See under the nouns.

reducer, Pugh's visual acuity. Pugh's occluder.

reduction, color. Change in the perceived hue of an object when all environmental accessories are removed, as may be approximated by viewing the surface of an object through a tube.

Reed-Van Osdal test (rēd-van oz'-dal). See under *test*.

refixation (re-fiks-a'shun). Fixation movement from one object to another, or one of the series of saccadic movements in fixational pursuit of a moving object.

    active r. A volitional change of fixation from one object point to another.

    compensatory r. Refixation due to postural changes.

    passive r. Passive, nondeliberate reversion of fixation to an inconsequential object point on disappearance of, or discontinuation of attention to, a previously fixated object.

reflect. To turn, bend, send, or direct back within the same medium.

reflectance (re-flek'tans). The ratio of reflected flux to incident flux. Syn., *reflection factor.*

    adaptation r. For a given discrete area within the total visual field, the reflectance value of a contained, spectrally nonselective surface above which it would tend toward the hue of the illuminant and below which it would tend toward the hue of the complementary color.

    diffuse r. 1. The ratio of diffusely reflected flux to incident flux. 2. The reflectance of a sample relative to a perfectly diffusing, perfectly reflecting standard, with 45° incidence and perpendicular observation. Syn., *diffuse reflection factor.*

    directional r. Reflectance of a surface as determined for specific directions of incidence and viewing.

    hemispherical r. The total luminous flux reflected by a surface divided by the total incident flux. Cf. *hemispherical transmittance.*

    spectral r. Reflectance in reference to a specific wavelength or to a narrow band of wavelengths.

    specular r. The ratio of regularly reflected flux to corresponding incident flux. Syn., *specular reflection factor.*

    total r. The ratio of the total flux reflected, both diffusely and regularly, to incident flux. Syn., *total reflection factor.*

reflection. 1. A turning back, bending, or rebounding of light by the surface of a medium such that it continues to travel in the same medium but in an altered direction. 2. An image formed by a reflecting surface.

    coefficient of r. See under *coefficient.*

    dense-to-rare r. Internal reflection.

    diffuse r. Reflection in which the light is scattered in many or all directions, due to irregularities or roughness of the reflecting surface. Cf. *specular reflection.*

    direct r. Specular reflection.

external r. Reflection of light at the interface of two transparent media when the second medium is more dense (has a higher index of refraction) than the first. Syn., *rare-to-dense reflection.*

r. factor. See under *factor.*

internal r. Reflection of light at the interface of two transparent media when the second medium is less dense (has a lower index of refraction) than the first. Syn., *dense-to-rare reflection.*
total i.r. Internal reflection in which the angle of incidence is greater than the critical angle and in which no rays pass into the second (rarer) medium, but are all reflected at the interface.

irregular r. Diffuse reflection.

mixed r. A mixture of specular, diffuse, and preferential reflection; characteristic of glazed surfaces.

preferential r. Reflection characteristic of semipolished surfaces in which the light is not directly reflected but is distributed more in certain directions than in others. Syn., *spread reflection.*

rare-to-dense r. External reflection.

regular r. Specular reflection.

specular r. Reflection characteristic of smooth surfaces in which there is no scatter and in which the angle of incidence is equal to the angle of reflection. Syn., *direct reflection; regular reflection.*

spread r. Preferential reflection.

surface r. The perpendicularly incident light reflected at an optical surface or interface in accordance with *Fresnel's formula.* Syn., *Fresnel loss.*

veiling r. Reflection from an object which reduces its contrast with the surround and therefore reduces its visibility.

reflectivity (re"flek-tiv'ih-te). The property of a surface to return flux incident on it.

reflectometer (re"flek-tom'eh-ter). A device for measuring the percentage of light reflected by a surface.

Baumgartner r. A reflectometer consisting essentially of two spheres, one an integrating sphere photometer having two photovoltaic cells in its wall and an attached collimated light source which can be alternately directed toward the sphere wall and onto a reflecting test sample in a window for determining the reflectance of the sample, and the other sphere

housing a light source and having an opening to the window of the first, at which a transmitting sample may be alternately placed and removed for determining its transmittance to the first sphere.

Taylor r. A reflectometer consisting essentially of an integrating sphere photometer employing a Macbeth illuminometer as the measuring element.

reflectometry (re"flek-tom'eh-tre). The measurement of reflectance with a reflectometer.

retinal r. Reflectometry of an image on the retina.

reflector. That which reflects; in particular, the structure or the medium with which the reflection is identified.

perfectly diffusing r. Perfect diffusing surface.

reflectorize (re-flek'ter-īz). To provide with reflective properties, especially retroreflective properties.

reflet (reh-fla'). A quality of high metallic luster or brilliance on a surface, especially on ceramic ware.

◆

REFLEX

reflex. 1. A response to a stimulus without the necessary intervention of consciousness. 2. Pertaining to, or produced by, a stimulus without involving consciousness. 3. Reflected light or an image formed by reflection.

acceleratory r. Statokinetic reflex.

accommodation r. 1. Accommodative pupillary reflex. 2. The reflex initiated by an out-of-focus retinal image, as occurs when fixation is changed from far to near, resulting in increased convexity of the crystalline lenses. Syn., *ciliary reflex.*

accommodative r's. The reflexes initiated by an out-of-focus retinal image, as occurs when fixation is changed from far to near, resulting in constriction of the pupils, convergence of the eyes, and increased convexity of the crystalline lenses. **frontal a.r.** See *occipital accommodative reflex.* **harmonic a.r.** See *occipital accommodative reflex.* **occipital a.r.** One of the three reflexes postulated for accommodation by Chavasse, the other two of which are the *harmonic* and the *frontal accommodative,* differentiated on theoretical neurological presumptions.

accommodative-convergence
r. Convergence presumed to be induced reflexly by the lack of accommodation.

acoustic r. 1. Cochleopalpebral reflex. 2. Audito-oculogyric reflex.

acoustic nystagmus r. Nystagmus in response to stimulation by a sudden noise.

annular r. A ringlike light reflex around the macula lutea, sometimes seen in ophthalmoscopy.

Argyll Robertson's r. Argyll Robertson's pupillary reflex.

Aschner's r. Oculocardiac reflex.

associational r's. Psycho-optical reflexes.

attention r. Attention pupillary reflex.

audito-oculogyric r. Reflex movement of the eyes toward the source of an unexpected loud sound. Syn., *acoustic reflex; auditory reflex; cochlear reflex.*

auditory r. 1. Cochleopalpebral reflex. 2. Audito-oculogyric reflex.

auriculopalpebral r. Cochleopalpebral reflex.

auropalpebral r., acoustic. Cochleopalpebral reflex.

auropalpebral r., caloric. Momentary reflex closure of the eyelid on thermal stimulation of the outer ear near the tympanic membrane.

auropalpebral r., tactile. Momentary reflex closure of the eyelid on mechanical stimulation of the outer ear near the tympanic membrane.

Bechterew's r. 1. A quiver, followed by contraction, of the orbicularis oculi muscles of both lower lids after percussion of the bones of the forehead, the zygoma, and the root of the nose. It is marked in cases of trigeminal irritation and lost in complete facial or trigeminal paralysis. 2. Bechterew's pupillary reflex.

binocular attention r. Oriental fixation reflex.

blinking r., aural. Blinking on thermal or mechanical stimulation of the outer ear, near the tympanic membrane, usually accompanied by lacrimation on the ipsilateral side. Syn., *external auditory meatus reflex; Kehrer's reflex; Kisch's reflex.*

blinking r., optical. Blinking in response to stimulation of the eyes by light, as occurs in the *dazzle reflex* or the *menace reflex.* It is normally developed between the ninth month and second year of life and occurs only in the higher mammals. Syn., *opticofacial reflex; visual blink reflex.*

blinking r., protective. Blinking to protect the eyes from threatened injury, as occurs in the corneal, conjunctival, dazzle, and menace reflexes.

blinking r., sensory. Blinking in response to an irritative sensory stimulus of the eye, as occurs in the conjunctival and corneal reflexes.

caloric lacrimo-aural r. Bilateral lacrimation in response to thermal stimulation of the external auditory meatus, as by irrigating the ear with warm or cold water.

cat's eye r. A bright reflection observed at the pupil of the eye, as would appear from the tapetum lucidum of a cat, and due to such intraocular conditions as retinoblastoma or exudative choroiditis.

cerebral cortex r. Haab's pupillary reflex.

ciliary r. 1. Accommodative pupillary reflex. 2. Accommodation reflex.

ciliospinal r. Cutaneous pupillary reflex.

ciliovisceral r. Any vascular, respiratory, gastrointestinal, urinary or other visceral reflex that is initiated by pushing the eye into the orbit. See also *oculocardiac reflex; oculo-esophageal reflex; oculovisceral motor reflex.*

cochlear r. 1. Cochleopalpebral reflex. 2. Audito-oculogyric reflex.

cochleo-orbicular r. Cochleopalpebral reflex.

cochleopalpebral r. Momentary closure of the eyelid in response to an unexpected loud sound. Syn., *acoustic reflex; acoustic auropalpebral reflex; auditory reflex; auriculopalpebral reflex; cochlear reflex; cochleo-orbicular reflex; Gault's reflex.*

conjunctival r. 1. Blinking or winking in response to tactile stimulation of the conjunctiva. 2. Lacrimation in response to an irritation of the conjunctiva.

consensual light r. Consensual pupillary reflex.

convergence r. 1. Convergence pupillary reflex. 2. Convergence providing single, binocular vision in response to disparate retinal stimuli.

corneal r. 1. Blinking or winking in response to tactile stimulation of the cornea. 2. Lacrimation in response to irritation of the cornea. 3. Reflection of light from the cornea.

corneomandibular r. Contralateral deviation of the lower jaw simultaneous with closure of the eyelids, occurring when the mouth is open and the cornea of one eye is touched. Syn., *winking-jaw phenomenon; corneopterygoid reflex; mandibuloconjunctival reflex; pterygocorneal reflex.*

corneopterygoid r. Corneomandibular reflex.

crossed r. Response on one side of the body induced by stimulation of the other side, such as the *consensual pupillary reflex.*

Davidson's r. Light seen through the pupil when a light source is held in the mouth.

dazzle r. Blinking of the eyelids in response to sudden stimulation by bright light.

direct light r. Direct pupillary reflex.

external auditory meatus r. Aural blinking reflex.

eye closure r. Blinking or closure of the eyelids in response to any of a variety of stimuli, such as pressure on the supraorbital nerve, touching the cornea or the conjunctiva, or exposure to bright light.

eyeball compression r. Any reflex initiated by compression of the eyeball, such as the *oculocardiac,* the *oculoesophageal,* and the *oculovisceral motor reflexes.*

eyeball-heart r. Oculocardiac reflex.

fixation r. Fixation occurring in response to stimulation of an extrafoveal retinal area. Syn., *visual fixation reflex.* **compensatory f.r.** 1. Orientation of the eyes in response to proprioceptive impulses from the labyrinths and from muscles of the neck. Syn., *gravitational reflex.* 2. Movement of the eye to regain fixation when it is artifically disrupted, as by placing a prism before the eye. **conjugate f.r.** A fixation reflex in which both eyes move in the same direction to assume binocular fixation. Syn., *version fixation reflex.* **disjunctive f.r.** A fixation reflex in which the two eyes move in opposite directions, as in convergence or divergence, to assume binocular fixation. Syn., *vergence fixation reflex.* **oriental f.r.** Conjugate movement of the eyes and the head of primitive and lower animals to maintain the object of regard in the center of the field of binocular vision; this reflex is also said by some to be demonstrable in the newborn. Syn., *binocular attention reflex.* **vergence f.r.** Disjunctive fixation reflex. **version f.r.** Conjugate fixation reflex.

foveolar r. The small, dotlike reflex of light from the foveola observed during ophthalmoscopy.

fundus r. Light reflected from the fundus that appears as a red glow in the plane of the pupil, as observed in retinoscopy, due to the reflected light having passed through the choroid. Syn., *red reflex.*

fusion r. Movement of the eyes, providing single, binocular vision in response to disparate retinal stimulation. **corrective f.r.** Disjunctive movements, or myologic adaptations, of the eyes to compensate for a heterophoria or an artificial disorientation of binocular fixation, as by placing a prism in front of one eye, to provide fusion.

fusional convergence r. Convergence to provide single, binocular vision in response to disparate retinal stimulation.

Galassi's r. Orbicularis pupillary reflex.

Gault's r. Cochleopalpebral reflex.

Gifford's r. Orbicularis pupillary reflex.

von Graefe's r. Orbicularis pupillary reflex.

gravitational r. Compensatory fixation reflex.

gustolacrimal r. A profuse flow of tears from an eye on the affected side on tasting food, occurring during the stage of recovery from a facial palsy due to a lesion in the area of the geniculate ganglion.

Haab's r. Haab's pupillary reflex.

head turning r. Doll's head phenomenon.

indirect light r. Consensual pupillary reflex.

iris r. Pupillary reflex.

juvenile r. The glistening reflection of light from the fundus of young individuals, observed ophthalmoscopically.

Kehrer's r. Aural blinking reflex.

Kisch's r. Aural blinking reflex.

labyrinthine r. Any reflex originating from stimulation of the inner ear, such as the *tonic labyrinthine* or the *statokinetic reflexes*. **tonic l.r.** Orientation of the head and eyes from stimulation of the otolith apparatus, initiated by the position of the head in space. Syn., *otolith reflex*.

lacrimal r. Secretion of tears in response to irritation of the cornea or the conjunctiva and to other conditions or actions grossly identified with initiation of the reflex, such as eyestrain, glare, laughing, vomiting, etc. Syn., *weeping reflex*.

lid r. Orbicularis pupillary reflex.

light r. 1. Constriction of the pupil in response to light stimulation of the retina, as occurs in the consensual and direct pupillary reflexes. Syn., *photopupil reflex; Whytt's reflex*. 2. Reflected light.

McCarthy's r. Supraorbital reflex.

mandibuloconjunctival r. Corneomandibular reflex.

menace r. Blinking of the eyelids in response to a suddenly and rapidly approaching object. Syn., *threat reflex*.

miral r. The image of the mires of an ophthalmometer as mirrored by the cornea.

myopic r. Weiss's reflex.

nasolacrimal r. Profuse lacrimation in response to the touching of certain areas of the endonasal mucosa.

naso-ocular r. Hyperemia of the conjunctiva in response to irritation of the nasal mucosa.

nasopalpebral r. Blinking of the eyelids in response to stimulation of the nasal mucosa. It is absent in facial paralysis and is marked in Parkinsonism.

near r. 1. Near pupillary reflex. 2. Accommodation, convergence, and pupillary constriction on fixation of a near object. 3. Proximal accommodation and proximal convergence initiated by the awareness of a near object.

nose-bridge-eyelid r. See *orbicularis oculi reflex*.

nose-eye r. See *orbicularis oculi reflex*.

ocular frontalis r. In infants, lifting of the eyebrows, the producing of horizontal furrows on the forehead, and opening of the mouth upon looking upward and attentively fixating an object.

oculo-aural r. Pulling backward of the external ear by contraction of the transversus auriculae muscle on looking forcibly to the side. Syn., *Wilson's phenomenon*.

oculocardiac r. Slowing down of the rate of the heart beat following compression of the eyeballs. Syn., *Aschner's phenomenon; Aschner's reflex; eyeball compression reflex; eyeball-heart reflex*.

oculocephalogyric r. The synkinetic or associated movements of the eye, the head, and the body in fixating an object.

oculo-esophageal r. A diminution of esophageal contraction following compression of the eyeball, as by firmly pressing a finger on the lid of the closed eye.

oculofrontal r. Elevation of the ipsilateral eyebrow and depression of the contralateral upon concomitant lateral eye movement, occurring as a congenital anomaly.

oculolingual r. Homolateral deviation of the tongue upon concomitant lateral eye movement, occurring as a congenital anomaly.

oculomandibular r. Contralateral protrusion of the lower jaw upon rapid concomitant lateral eye movement, occurring as a congenital anomaly.

oculonasal r. Dilatation of the nostrils upon concomitant lateral eye movement, occurring as a congenital anomaly.

oculopharyngeal r. Rapid swallowing movements and closure of the eyelids in response to irritative stimulation of the bulbar conjunctiva.

oculopupillary r. Oculosensory pupillary reflex.

oculosensory r. Oculosensory pupillary reflex.

oculostapedial r. Unilateral blepharospasm and buzzing in the ears upon concomitant lateral eye movement, occurring as a congenital anomaly.

oculovisceral motor r. Contraction of the abdominal wall, the bladder, and the colon following compression of the eyeball, as by firmly pressing a finger on the lid of the closed eye.

Oppenheim's corneal r. Impairment of corneal sensation on the contralateral side in supratentorial lesions and on the ipsilateral side in infratentorial lesions.

optical righting r. Visual righting reflex.

opticofacial r. Optical blinking reflex.

orbicularis r. Orbicularis pupillary reflex.

orbicularis oculi r. Sudden, bilateral contraction of the orbicularis oculi muscle in response to any of a variety of stimuli, such as loud noises, bright lights, tapping of the bridge or tip of the nose, or tapping of the margin of the orbit.

orbiculomandibular r. Protrusion of the lower jaw upon forcible contraction of the orbicularis oculi muscle, occurring as a congenital anomaly.

otolith r. Tonic labyrinthine reflex.

palatopalpebral r. Closure of the eyelids when the palate is touched.

photoglycemic r. Alteration of sugar metabolism initiated by photic stimulation of the eye.

photo-pupil r. Light reflex.

Piltz's r. 1. Attention pupillary reflex. 2. Orbicularis pupillary reflex.

Piltz-Westphal r. Orbicularis pupillary reflex.

platysma r. Cutaneous pupillary reflex.

postural r. Righting reflex.

proprioceptive r. Orientation of the body and its parts in response to proprioceptive impulses from the labyrinth and from muscles of the limbs, the trunk, and the neck.

proprioceptive head turning r. Doll's head phenomenon.

protective r. Any defensive response to a noxious stimulus, as occurs in the *menace reflex*.

psycho-optical r's. Reflexes involving the eye or the eyelids which are involuntary and are mediated by the occipital cortex. They include the *accommodation*, the *protective blinking*, the *convergence*, the *fixation*, and the *fusion reflexes*. Syn., *associational reflexes*.

psychosensory r. Psychosensory pupillary reflex.

pterygocorneal r. Corneomandibular reflex.

pupillary r. 1. Constriction of the pupil in response to light stimula-

tion of the retina. 2. Any reflex involving the iris, with resultant alteration of the diameter of the pupil. **accommodative p.r.** Constriction of the pupils induced reflexly by the act of accommodation. Syn., *accommodation reflex; ciliary reflex*. **Argyll Robertson's p.r.** A pupillary reflex characterized by inactivity to light, both direct and consensual reflexes being absent, but with normal contraction on accommodation and convergence. See *Argyll Robertson's pupil*. **associated p.r.** Near pupillary reflex. **attention p.r.** Contraction of the pupil on sudden change of visual attention to an object. Syn., *Piltz's pupillary reflex*. **aurosensory p.r.** Pupillary dilation in response to stimulation of the middle ear by tactile or thermal means or by rapidly varying the air pressure. **Bechterew's p.r.** Dilatation of the pupils on exposure to light. Syn., *paradoxical pupillary reflex*. **cochlear p.r.** Bilateral, transitory, pupillary constriction followed by dilatation in response to intense sensory stimulation to the cochlea, as with a tuning fork. The effect is usually more pronounced on the pupil of the stimulated side. **cogwheel p.r.** Constriction of the pupil, in response to light, and subsequent redilatation, in a series of discrete steps instead of in the usual, single, continuous movement. Syn., *cogwheel pupillary reaction*. **consensual p.r.** Constriction of the pupil of one eye, in response to light stimulation of the retina of the other eye. Syn., *consensual light reflex; indirect light reflex; indirect pupillary reflex*. **convergence p.r.** Constriction of the pupils induced reflexly by convergence. **cutaneous p.r.** Dilatation of the pupils in response to scratching or pinching of the skin of the neck. Syn., *ciliospinal reflex; platysma reflex; skin pupillary reflex*. **direct p.r.** Constriction of the pupil of an eye in response to light stimulation of its retina. Syn., *direct light reflex*. **Galassi's p.r.** Orbicularis pupillary reflex. **Gifford's p.r.** Orbicularis pupillary reflex. **von Graefe's p.r.** Orbicularis pupillary reflex. **Haab's p.r.** Contraction of the pupils in a darkened room when attention is directed to a light source stimulating the peripheral retina without an ensuing eye movement. Syn., *cerebral cortex reflex; visuocortical reflex; Haab's sign*. **hemianopic p.r.** In hemianopsia, constriction of the pupil in response to light stimulation of the unaffected side of the retina and no pupillary response when light falls on the affected side. Syn., *hemianopic pupillary reaction; Wernicke's pupillary reflex; Wernicke's sign.* **indirect p.r.** Consensual pupillary reflex. **lid p.r.** Orbicularis pupillary reflex. **myotonic p.r.** A pupillary reflex in which the reaction to light, both direct and consensual, is almost abolished, being elicited only after prolonged exposure to dark or light and in which there is a delayed reaction to changes in accommodation and convergence. The condition usually occurs unilaterally, with the affected pupil being the larger, and the reaction to mydriatics and certain myotics is normal. It is usually associated with diminution or absence of tendon reflexes. **near p.r.** Constriction of the pupils induced by accommodation and/or convergence for a near object. Syn., *associated pupillary reflex.* **neurotonic p.r.** Delayed and slow constriction of the pupil in response to light, followed by delayed and slow dilatation. Syn., *neurotonic pupillary reaction.* **oculosensory p.r.** Bilateral, initial, slight dilatation of the pupils followed by sustained constriction in response to irritative sensory stimulation of the cornea, the ocular conjunctiva, or the eyelid. It is absent in the Argyll Robertson's pupil. Syn., *oculopupillary reflex; oculosensory reflex; trigeminal pupillary reflex.* **orbicularis p.r.** Unilateral constriction of the pupil when an effort is made to close eyelids which are forcibly held apart. Syn., *Galassi's pupillary phenomenon; orbicularis phenomenon; von Graefe's lid reaction; orbicularis pupillary reaction; Piltz-Westphal pupillary reaction; Gifford's pupillary reflex; Galassi's pupillary reflex; von Graefe's pupillary reflex; lid reflex; orbicularis reflex; Piltz's pupillary reflex; Piltz-Westphal pupillary reflex; Westphal's pupillary reflex; Westphal-Piltz pupillary reflex.* **pain p.r.** Dilatation of the pupil induced by pain. **paradoxical p.r.** 1. Reversed pupillary reflex. 2. Dilatation of the pupil on stimulation of the retina by light. Syn., *Bechterew's reflex.* **perverse p.r.** Dilatation of the pupil on converging the eyes to a near object. **Piltz's p.r.** 1. Attention pupillary reflex. 2. Orbicularis pupillary reflex. **Piltz-Westphal p.r.** Orbicularis pupillary reflex. **psychosensory p.r.** Dilatation of the pupil in response to stimulation of any sensory nerve other than those of the eye or its adnexa or in response to psychic stimuli, as emotion or fear. **reversed p.r.** An anomalous pupillary reflex in which the action is opposite to that normally expected, e.g., dilatation of the pupil on light stimulation of the retina or on converging the eyes to a near subject. Syn., *paradoxical pupillary reflex.* **Schlesinger's p.r.** Constriction of the pupil in response to forcible raising of the eyebrows. Syn., *Schlesinger's reaction.* **skin p.r.** Cutaneous pupillary reflex. **tonohaptic p.r.** An anomalous pupillary reaction to the onset and removal of a light stimulus, characterized by a long latent period preceding a short rapid constriction and a long latent period preceding a short rapid redilatation. Syn., *tonohaptic reaction.* **Tournay's p.r.** Inequality of the size of the pupils produced by extreme lateral conjugate movement of the eyes, the abducted eye having the larger pupil. Syn., *Tournay's reaction; Gianelli's sign; Tournay's sign.* **trigeminal p.r.** Oculosensory pupillary reflex. **vagotonic p.r.** Dilatation of the pupil in response to deep inspiration, and constriction in response to deep expiration. **vestibular p.r.** 1. Bilateral pupillary constriction followed by wide dilatation which passes into hippus, in response to thermal, rotation, or air compression stimulation of the labyrinth. Syn., *vestibulopupillary reaction.* 2. A pupillary constriction associated with the removal of the middle ear in rabbits. **visuocortical p.r.** Haab's pupillary reflex. **Wernicke's p.r.** Hemianopic pupillary reflex. **Westphal's p.r.** Orbicularis pupillary reflex. **Westphal-Piltz p.r.** Orbicularis pupillary reflex.

red r. Fundus reflex.

refixation r. See *refixation.*

retinal r. Light reflected from the fundus as observed with the retinoscope or the ophthalmoscope.

retinal accommodation r. Accommodation in response to an out-of-focus retinal image.

righting r. Any reflex which aids in maintaining the normal orientation of the body and its parts in space. Syn., *postural reflex.* **labyrinthine r.r.** Orientation of the head and the eyes from labyrinthine stimulation, as occurs in the *tonic labyrinthine* and the *statokinetic reflexes.* **neck r.r.** Tonic neck reflex. **visual r.r.** Orientation of the head in response to the perception of objects in the field of vision. Syn., *optical righting reflex.*

Robertson's r. Argyll Robertson's pupillary reflex.

Ruggeri's r. Quickening of the pulse induced by extreme convergence of the eyes.

Schlesinger's r. Schlesinger's pupillary reflex.

scissors r. A bipartite, retinoscopic (skiascopic) reflex showing opposite movements in the two sectors of the pupil, resembling the relative movements of scissors blades.

secondary light r. Increased constriction on consensual light stimulation of a pupil already constricted by direct light stimulation, or increased constriction on direct light stimulation of a pupil already constricted by consensual light stimulation.

senile r. A gray reflex seen in the pupil of the aged, due to light reflected from the crystalline lens.

shot silk r. Watered silk reflex.

skin r. Cutaneous pupillary reflex.

specular r. An image formed by a regularly reflecting surface, especially one so produced by a glossy surface coincidentally superimposed or interspersed on an otherwise rough or diffusing surface, as obtained by reflection of a bright source in a smooth wood table top.

static r. A righting reflex initiated by the position or change of position of the head, as occurs in the *tonic labyrinthine* and the *tonic neck reflexes*.

statokinetic r. Orientation of the eyes from stimulation of the semicircular canals, caused by changes in head movement (initiation, acceleration, or deceleration). When the head movement persists, a labyrinthine nystagmus results. Syn., *acceleratory reflex*.

supraorbital r. A quiver, followed by contraction, of the orbicularis oculi muscles of both lower eyelids after a tap on the supraorbital nerve. It is marked in cases of trigeminal irritation and lost in complete facial or trigeminal paralysis. Syn., *McCarthy's reflex*.

threat r. Menace reflex.

tonic neck r. Orientation of the head and the eyes in response to proprioceptive impulses from muscles of the neck, initiated by the position of the head in relation to the trunk. Syn., *neck righting reflex*.

Tournay's r. Tournay's pupillary reflex.

trigeminal r. Oculosensory pupillary reflex.

trigemino-facial r. Twitching of the jaw muscles following compression of the eyeball, as by firmly pressing a finger on the lid of the closed eye.

vagotonic r. Vagotonic pupillary reflex.

vergence r. Disjunctive fixation reflex.

version r. Conjugate fixation reflex.

vestibulo-palpebral r. Involuntary closure of the eyelids following rapid rotation of the body, as with Bárány's chair.

vestibulo-pupillary r. Vestibular pupillary reflex.

vestibulo-retinal r. Papillary stasis and hypertension of the retinal arteries associated with labyrinthine hyperexcitability.

visual r. Any reflex commencing with a pattern of stimulation on the retina and involving the use of the visual reflex arc, the intrinsic and the extrinsic muscles of the eye, and the skeletal muscles of the body, with the projection of the resultant sensation into space.

visual blink r. Optical blinking reflex.

visual fixation r. Fixation reflex.

visual righting r. See *righting reflex, visual*.

visuocortical r. Haab's pupillary reflex.

watered silk r. Glistening, shimmering reflections of light from the fundus, observed ophthalmoscopically, especially in the young. Syn., *shot silk reflex*.

weeping r. Lacrimal reflex.

Weiss's r. A crescent-shaped reflection of light on the nasal side of the optic disk, described by Weiss and considered by him to be an ophthalmoscopic sign of early myopia. It is attributed to a reflection of light from the surface of a posteriorly detached vitreous and may also be observed on the temporal side of the optic disk or around the posterior pole by changing the position of the viewing instrument. It also appears in nonmyopic eyes. Syn., *myopic reflex; Weiss's sign*.

Wernicke's r. Hemianopic pupilary reflex.

Westphal's r. Orbicularis pupillary reflex.

Westphal-Piltz r. Orbicularis pupillary reflex.

Whytt's r. Constriction of the pupil in response to light stimulation of the retina, first deduced by Robert Whytt to be of reflex nature.

winking r. Closure of the eyelids in response to any of a variety of stimuli, such as pressure on the supraorbital nerve, touching the cornea or the conjunctiva, or exposure to bright light.

◆

reflexio palpebrarum (re-fleks'ih-o pal"pe-brah'rum). Ectropion.

refract (re-frakt'). 1. To change the direction of light by refraction. 2. To determine the refractive and muscular state of the eyes.

◆

REFRACTION

refraction (re-frak'shun). 1. The altering of the pathway of light from its original direction as a result of passing obliquely from one medium to another of different index of refraction. 2. The refractive and muscular state of the eyes, or the act or process of determining and/or correcting it.

analytical r. 1. The specific routines and procedures for determination of the refractive correction as promulgated in the techniques and the papers of the Optometric Extension Program. 2. Any system or procedure for determination of the refractive correction not solely based on the subjective or retinoscopic examination but on supplementary testing of the visual functions.

angle of r. See under *angle*.

aplanatic r. Refraction in a system which meets the sine condition.

atmospheric r. Refraction due to varying density of the earth's atmosphere, which is greatest at the earth and decreases with increasing elevation, causing mirages and apparent displacement of heavenly bodies.

bichrome r. Duochrome refraction.

bicylindric r. A method of determining the error of refraction of the eye in which a cylindrical lens to correct the corneal astigmatism, as measured with the ophthalmometer, is first placed before the eye. The residual astigmatism is then determined by

means of a fan dial and the spherocylindrical equivalent of the combination is considered to be the correcting lens.

coefficient of r. Index of refraction. *Obs.*

conical r. 1. External and internal conical refraction. 2. Refraction by means of axicons. **external c.r.** An effect observed with biaxial crystals in which an external hollow cone of light is refracted into a narrow pencil of light inside the crystal. **internal c.r.** An effect observed with biaxial crystals in which an unpolarized ray entering such a crystal will form a cone of light within it.

cross cylinder r. See *method, cross cylinder.*

cycloplegic r. 1. The refractive state of the eye when accommodation is totally or partially paralyzed by a cycloplegic. 2. The process or act of determining the refractive state of the eye when accommodation is totally or partially paralyzed by a cycloplegic.

diffuse r. The scattering of light in many or all directions, due to irregularities or roughness of the refracting surface. Cf. *regular refraction.*

double r. The property of nonisotropic media, such as crystals, whereby a single incident beam of light traverses the medium as two beams, each plane-polarized, the planes being at right angles to each other. One beam, the ordinary, obeys Snell's law; the other, the extraordinary, does not. Along the optical axis the two beams travel at the same speed; in other directions the extraordinary beam travels at different speeds. Syn., *birefringence.* **electric d.r.** Double refraction which occurs when a strong transverse electric field is applied to a vapor through which light is passing. **magnetic d.r.** Double refraction which occurs when a strong magnetic field is applied to a vapor through which light is passing perpendicular to the field. Syn., *Voigt effect.*

duochrome r. A method of determining the error of refraction of the eye in which a test chart of two colors, usually one half red and one half green, is used. Correcting lenses are placed before the eye until the test letters on both halves of the test chart can be seen with equal clearness. It is based on the chromatic aberration of the eye. Syn., *bichrome refraction.*

dynamic r. 1. The refractive

state of the eye when accommodation is activated, as by fixating a near test target. 2. The act or process of determining the refractive state of the eye when accommodation is activated.

error of r. See under *error*.

r. of the eye. 1. The process or act of determining the refractive state of the eye. 2. The refraction of light effected by the media of the eye. 3. The error of refraction of the eye.

index of r. See under *index*.

laser r. The subjective determination of ametropia with the Laser Refractor in which corrective lenses are placed before the eye to eliminate the perceived motion of a granular pattern created by projecting a helium-neon gas laser beam onto a rotating drum.

manifest r. 1. The refractive state of the eye when accommodation is at rest, as by fixating a target at infinity, but not paralyzed. 2. The act or process of determining the refractive state of the eye when accommodation is at rest, but not paralyzed.

meridional r. Determination of the refractive state of the eye by refraction of selected isolated meridians of the eye.

oblique centric r. Astigmatism resulting from the passing of a pencil of light obliquely through a lens.

ocular r. Refraction of the eye.

over r. Determination of a residual error of refraction of the eye while the subject's eyeglasses or contact lenses are in place in front of the eyes.

principal point r. Refraction of the eye with respect to the anterior principal point of the eye.

regular r. Refraction at a regular, highly polished, smooth, nondiffusing surface. Cf. *diffuse refraction*.

sensitometric r. A method of determining the refractive error of the eye, in which the brightness and contrast of a test target of constant size are simultaneously varied by means of neutral filters and trial lenses until the smallest brightness difference between test target and background is recognized.

static r. 1. The refractive state of the eye when accommodation is at rest or paralyzed by a cycloplegic. 2. The process or act of determining the refractive state of the eye when accommodation is at rest.

stereo r. Refraction of the eyes performed while the patient is binocularly viewing a projected, colored stereo-inducing picture through Polaroid filters. The scene has a central blackened area on which polarized test targets are projected from a second instrument. The Polaroid filter on the acuity projector may be adjusted to provide central occlusion of one eye during monocular testing of the other eye.

subjective r. 1. The refractive state of the eye as determined by visual judgment of the patient. 2. The act or process of determining the refractive state of the eye utilizing the visual judgment of the patient.

terrestial r. Refraction phenomena observed in light originating from a source within the earth's atmosphere and caused by atmospheric inhomogeneities.

vertex r. Vertex power.

zero error r. Welsh zero error method.

◆

refractionist (re-frak'shun-ist). One skilled in determining the refractive state of the eyes, the state of binocularity, and the proper corrective lenses.

refractionometer (re-frak"shun-om'eh-ter). 1. Optometer. 2. An instrument which determines the vertex refractive power, the cylinder axis, the optical center, and the prismatic effect of ophthalmic lenses.

parallax r. An objective optometer, devised by Henker, consisting essentially of a Gullstrand ophthalmoscope modified by means of eccentric apertures in a test disk in the lens system to produce doubling of the test marks by parallactic displacement when the test disk is not focused precisely on the retina.

refractive (re-frak'tiv). Pertaining to refraction; capable of refracting.

refractivity (re"frak-tiv'ih-te). The ability to refract; the power of refraction; the quality of being refractive.

refractometer (re"frak-tom'eh-ter). 1. An instrument for determining the refractive index of a medium. 2. Optometer.

Abbe's r. An instrument designed to determine the index of refraction, based on measurement of the critical angle at the interface between the sample and a prism of known index of refraction. It contains two Amici compensating prisms which may be adjusted to neutralize chromatic dispersion of the unknown and thus permit the use of white light.

Jamin r. An instrument designed to determine the index of refraction of a gas, based on the production of interference fringes. A single beam of monochromatic light is broken into two parallel beams by reflection from the two parallel faces of a thick glass plate, one beam being passed through the sample and the other through a vacuum. The beams are recombined by a second thick glass plate to form the interference fringes.

Pulfrich r. An instrument designed to determine the index of refraction, based on measurement of the critical angle at the interface between the sample and a prism of known index of refraction. It is used in conjunction with a monochromatic light source.

Rayleigh r. An instrument designed to determine the index of refraction of a gas based on the production of interference fringes. A single beam of monochromatic light is made parallel by a lens and then split into two beams by a double slit, one beam being passed through the sample and the other through a vacuum. The beams are recombined by a lens to form the interference fringes.

Williams r. A modification of the Rayleigh refractometer which utilizes a prism instead of a double slit to split the collimated beam, thus enabling greater accuracy of measurement through increased intensity of the interference fringes.

refractometry (re"frak-tom'eh-tre). Determination of the refractive error of the eye or the index of refraction of a medium with a refractometer.

refractor (re-frak'tor). 1. An instrument containing spherical and cylindrical lenses, Maddox rods, rotary prisms, and other devices for measuring the refractive and muscular condition of the eyes. Syn., *phoroptor.* 2. A refracting telescope.

laser r. See *Laser Refractor.*

Leland r. An instrument utilizing polarized light to achieve monocular refraction while maintaining binocular fusion of peripheral contours.

refrangibility (re-fran"jih-bil'ih-te). The capability of being refracted.

refrangible (re-fran'jih-bl). Capable of being refracted.

refringent (re-frin'jent). Refractive; refracting.

Refsum's syndrome (ref'soomz). See under *syndrome.*

region. A part, a portion, an area, or a division.

r. of accommodation. See under *accommodation.*

ciliary r. The portion of the eyeball just anterior to the ora serrata which includes the ciliary body, the ciliary processes, and neighboring structures.

pretectal r. The nuclei or area between the superior colliculi or tectum and the diencephalon; a primary or lower visual center for the pupillary light reflex.

regression. 1. *Statistics: (a)* The systematic change in a dependent variable as a function of differences in the value of the independent variable. The quantitative relationship between the two variables is usually expressed as an equation, either linear or curvilinear, depending on the nature of the relationship. *(b)* The fact that in a group with a pair of imperfectly correlated attributes, x and y, the mean of the y values corresponding to a given value of x will be nearer the mean of the whole group than the y value for which the mean of the corresponding x values would have equaled the given value of x. Thus, the average weight of a group of 6'4" men will be 212 lb, but a group of men weighing 212 lb each will average less than 6'4" in height. 2. *Reading:* An eye movement to refixate words inadequately perceived at the first reading. 3. *Psychology:* A reversion to an earlier type of behavior no longer appropriate to the later situation.

phenomenal r. The approach of a mental percept of a stimulus toward a midpoint between the sensation which would be expected if the response were entirely a function of the receptoral stimulus and the sensation which would be expected on the basis of previous conditioning of the response function by factors extrinsic to the objective stimulus situation.

Reichert's membrane (ri'kerts). Bowman's membrane. *Obs.*

reinforcement. The influence of one neurological activity on another, such as to increase the intensity of the latter activity.

Reis-Bückler ring-like corneal dystrophy (rīs-bĕk'ler). Bückler's annular corneal dystrophy. See under *dystrophy, corneal.*

Reiter's (ri'terz) **disease; syndrome.** See under the nouns.

Rekoss' disk (re'kos). See under *disk.*

reliability. Repeatable results of a test or other measuring device. Cf. *validity.*

relief. 1. Projection of an object or parts of an object from the general plane or background in which it lies. 2. Alleviation or removal of pain or distress.

    plastic r. The effect of depth produced by stereopsis, as observed by viewing appropriate targets in a stereoscope.

    senile nuclear r. The patterned relief appearance of the anterior surface of the adult crystalline lens nucleus, especially in advanced years, with oblique illumination, due to shrinkage and optical irregularity of zones of the nucleus of the lens.

    stereoscopic r. The effect of depth produced by stereopsis.

religiosus (re-lij"e-o'sus). Superior rectus muscle. *Obs.*

relucency (re-loo'sen-se). The characteristic appearance of the cornea and crystalline lens in the beam of the slit lamp as created by the dispersion, irregular reflection, and scattering related to normal inhomogeneity of the tissue.

relucent (re-lu'sent). Radiant; reflecting light; shining.

Remak's cells (ra-maks'). Lemmocytes.

Rémy (ra'me) **diploscope; separator.** See under the nouns.

Rendu-Osler disease (ron-du'os'ler). See under *disease.*

Renier formula. See under *formula.*

renotation, Munsell (re-no-ta'shun). A revision of the Munsell notation based on further studies.

replacement. The act of replacing.

    complementary r. Reciprocal replacement.

    reciprocal r. A theory accounting for single image formation from binocular stimulation in which there is alternate, conscious acceptance of each of the pair of stimulated corresponding points, the other being mentally suppressed. See also *Verhoeff's theory.*

    total unitary r. Reciprocal replacement.

resection (re-sek'shun). Removal of a segment of tissue. In extraocular muscle surgery, it involves detachment of the muscle at its insertion, excision of a segment, and reattachment of the remaining muscle at the original site of insertion.

reserve, fusional. 1. That part of the range of fusional vergence measured from the fusional demand point, or from the vergence stimulus value, to the limit of clear, single, binocular vision in the direction opposite that represented by the phoria, accommodation being held constant. Hence, the amount of available fusional vergence in excess of that needed to overcome the phoria, clinically measured by the amount of vergence-inducing prism which can be overcome without blur or diplopia. 2. Relative vergence.

    negative f.r. Negative fusional reserve convergence.

    positive f.r. Positive fusional reserve convergence.

    vertical f.r. 1. Fusional reserve in terms of the vertical deviation of one line of sight with respect to the other, as measured by the vertical vergence in the direction opposite that represented by the vertical phoria. 2. Fusional reserve in terms of the vertical deviation of one line of sight with respect to the other in excess of that needed for normal binocular fixation, clinically measured by the amount of base-up or base-down prism which can be overcome without blur or diplopia.

resistance, glare. The ability to see objects in the presence of adverse ambient light, variously measured in terms of the intensity of an ambient source which obliterates the perception of a given test object or in terms of the threshold of luminance, contrast, or size of a test object in the presence of the ambient source.

resolution. See *resolving power.*

resolution, spurious. The return of visibility, usually with reversed contrast, of a grating target after it has ceased to be resolvable as the grating is progressively reduced.

resolution, visual. The ability to perceive two target elements as two. Syn., *resolution visual acuity.*

resolve. To distinguish between, or render visible, separate parts or elements.

response. The activity or reaction of an organism or its parts which results from stimulation.

abridgment of r. The shortening of the process of performing an act as a result of practice.

cortical r. The complex electrical potential recordable in or on the cerebral cortex as a result of brief peripheral (e.g., visual) stimulation.

excitatory r. On response.

fixation r. Fixation movement.

inhibitory r. The decrease of firing frequency or the cessation of the spike activity of a neuron due to an inhibitory effect resulting from stimulation of another functionally related neuron.

off r. The burst of spike activity from a neuron immediately after cessation of stimulation; probably a postinhibitory rebound phenomenon. Syn., *off discharge; Z-type discharge; off effect.*

on r. The commencement of spike activity from a neuron, or an increase in its firing frequency, in response to the onset of stimulation and continuing to cessation of stimulation. Syn., *maintained discharge; on discharge; X-type discharge; on effect; excitatory response.*

on-off r. The burst of spike activity from a neuron upon commencement and following termination of stimulation with no activity in between. Syn., *on-off discharge; Y-type discharge; on-off effect.*

pace r. The rate of accommodative response to a change of accommodative stimulus as manifested in convergence changes of the occluded eye measured by electro-oculography.

photo-oculoclonic r. The spikes and slow waves in an electro-encephalogram which are associated with photic stimulation.

pursuit r. Pursuit movement.

saccadic r. Saccadic movement.

SILO r. *Optometric Extension Program:* Smaller In Larger Out: The presumed change of perceived size of a test object for which an increase of base-out prism or minus lens power results in the object seeming to get smaller and nearer, whereas an increase of base-in or plus results in the object seeming to get larger and more remote.

visual evoked r. Visual evoked cortical potential.

rete mirabile in the vitreous (re'te). A profuse anastomoses of new blood vessels into the vitreous resulting from occlusion of a retinal artery.

reticle (ret'ih-k'l). Graticule.

reticule (ret'ih-kūl). Graticule.

reticulum of Mueller (re-tik'u-lum). A series of branched ridges on the surface of the cuticular lamina of the lamina vitrea of the ciliary body which fit into the depression of the pigment epithelium, helping to anchor it to withstand the traction of the zonule of Zinn.

◆

RETINA

retina (ret'ih-nah). The light receptive, innermost, nervous tunic of the eye which represents the terminal expansion of the optic nerve. It is a thin, transparent membrane lying between the vitreous body and the choroid and extending from the optic disk to the ciliary body, where it becomes continuous with the inner epithelium of the ciliary body. It is derived from the outer and the inner walls of the optic cup and consists essentially of nuclei and processes of three layers of nervous elements which synapse with each other, the visual cells (rods and cones), the bipolar cells, and the ganglion cells. The region providing best visual acuity is the macula lutea, near the posterior pole of the eye, containing in its center the fovea centralis. The inner layers receive blood from the central retinal artery and its branches and in some cases from the cilioretinal artery; the external layers and the fovea are nourished by the choriocapillaris. The retina is usually described as having 10 layers; from without to within they are: (1) the pigment epithelium layer; (2) the layer of rods and cones; (3) the external limiting membrane; (4) the outer nuclear layer; (5) the outer molecular layer; (6) the inner nuclear layer; (7) the inner molecular layer; (8) the ganglion cell layer; (9) the nerve fiber layer; (10) the internal limiting membrane.

anangiotic r. In the Leber classification of retinal vascularization in placentals, a retina which has no direct blood supply and is characteristic of primitive mammals including bats, sloths, armadillos, porcupines, chinchillas, beavers, and other rodents. Cf. *holangiotic retina; merangiotic retina; paurangiotic retina.*

anesthesia of r. Temporary reduction in vision and in the size of the visual field due to trauma of the eyeball.

r. caeca. The thin, double, pigmented epithelium extending from the ora serrata over the ciliary body as far as the pupillary margin of the iris.

central r. Macula lutea.

coarctate r. A funnel-shaped condition of the retina caused by effusion of fluid between the retina and the choroid.

converse r. Verted retina.

corrugated r. A retina, found in fruit-bats and flying foxes, having elevations and depressions due to underlying vascular choroidal papillae. Receptors at the tip of the papillae are considered to subserve distance vision, while those in the depressions to subserve near vision.

cortical r. 1. The representation of retinal points in the area striata. 2. The retina when considered to be a forward extension of the brain.

detached r. Separation of the retina from the pigment epithelium layer which generally stems from one of 4 main causes: (1) shrinkage of the vitreous; (2) effusion of fluid or a growth, such as a tumor, which pushes the retina forward; (3) degeneration of the retina in which holes or tears allow the vitreous to seep behind it; and (4) trauma. A detached retina is characterized ophthalmoscopically by being raised above the level of the surrounding retina, requiring more plus power to bring it into focus, and by appearing to be a grayish, uneven, tremulous surface on which the retinal vessels are seen as wavy black lines. Subjective symptoms include loss of vision in a portion of the visual field and prodromal sensations of flickering lights or color. **bullous serous d.r.** Retinal detachment secondary to central angioneurotic choriopathy. **exudative d.r.** A retina detached as a result of an accumulation of fluid beneath it. **flat d.r.** A detached retina in which the separated area is raised only slightly above the surrounding retina. **rhegmatogenous d.r.** A retina detached as a result of a retinal break or tear. **steep d.r.** A detached retina in which the separated area projects markedly from the surrounding area. **traction d.r.** A retina detached by the pull of organized tissue as a result of hemorrhagic or inflammatory lesions or by trauma.

duplicated r. A U-shaped retina, found in the tubular eyes of some deep sea fishes, in which the base, being further from the lens, subserves near vision and the sides, being nearer the lens, subserve distance vision.

E r. A retina dominated by rod function, especially with reference to the electroretinographic reaction to intermittent light, where onset of the stimulus evokes an increase in ERG potential followed by a decrease. This electrophysiological classification does not always correspond to the histological appearance of the retina, for E retinas (excitatory) are found in the rat, the mouse, the guinea pig, the rabbit, the dog, the cat, and in man.

holangiotic r. In the Leber classification of retinal vascularization in placentals, a retina which, except for the central fovea, receives direct blood supply from either a central retinal artery, cilioretinal arteries, or both. It is characteristic of primates and some insectivores, carnivores, and ungulates. Cf. *anangiotic retina; merangiotic retina; paurangiotic retina.*

I r. A retina dominated by cone function, especially with reference to the electroretinographic reaction to intermittent light, where onset of the stimulus evokes a decrease in ERG potential followed by an increase. I retinas (inhibitory) are found not only in diurnal snakes, pigeons, and turtles, which have nearly pure cone retinas, but also in frogs and owls, which have a plentiful number of retinal rods.

inverse r. Inverted retina.

inverted r. A retina typical of vertebrates and rare in invertebrates in which the visual cells are orientated so that their sensory ends are directed away from the incident light, whence light must traverse the cell bodies before reaching the end organs. See also *verted retina.* Syn., *inverse retina.*

ischemia of r. See under *ischemia.*

leopard r. Leopard fundus.

merangiotic r. In the Leber classification of retinal vascularization in placentals, a retina in which only the horizontal segment containing medullated nerve fibers receives a direct blood supply. It is characteristic of rabbits and hares. Cf. *anangiotic retina; holangiotic retina; paurangiotic retina.*

paurangiotic r. In the Leber classification of retinal vascularization in placentals, a retina in which the blood vessels are very small and extend only a short distance from the optic disk. It is characteristic of perissodactyla (horse, rhinoceros), elephants, hyracoidea, sirenia, and guinea pigs. Cf.

anangiotic retina; holangiotic retina; merangiotic retina.

peripheral r. The portion of the retina extending from the macula lutea to and including the ora serrata.

ramp r. A retina found in some selachians and ungulates for which portions differ in distance from the crystalline lens. The lower retina, nearer the lens, subserves distance vision, and the upper retina, farther from the lens, subserves near vision.

red fleck r. A condition similar to fundus flavimaculatus accompanied by a type of congenital night blindness characterized by a long adaptation period to attain the normal threshold, reportedly found in Japan.

shot silk r. Shot silk fundus.

tesselated r. Tesselated fundus.

tigroid r. Tesselated fundus.

verted r. A retina typical of invertebrates in which the visual cells are orientated so that their sensory ends are directed toward the incident light. See also *inverted retina.* Syn., *converse retina.*

◆

retinaculum, lateral (of Hesser) (ret"ih-nak'u-lum). The joined attachments of the check ligament of the lateral rectus muscle, the ligament of Lockwood, the lateral palpebral ligament, and the aponeurosis of the levator palpebrae superioris muscle at the lateral orbital tubercle of the zygomatic bone.

retinal. 1. Pertaining to or of the retina. 2. Retinaldehyde.

retinal, all-*trans*-. An isomer of 11-*cis*-retinal resulting from its exposure to light.

retinal, 11-*cis*-. A visual pigment chromophore which upon exposure to light isomerizes to *all-trans-retinal*, q.v.

retinal aplasia; correspondence; dehiscence; detachment; dysplasia; element; field; horizon; illuminance; image; incongruity; ischemia; principal meridian; picture; purple; reflex; rivalry; septum; slip; zones. See under the nouns.

retinaldehyde (ret-ih-nal'de-hīd). The chromophore of rhodopsin and product of its bleaching, first discovered by Wald and termed by him *retinene.* R.A. Morton later showed retinene to be vitamin A aldehyde, hence the name change to *retinal* or *retinaldehyde.* Vitamin A became *retinol.* It contains conjugated systems of alternate single and double bonds. One double bond is in a six-numbered ring and four more are in the side chain which can exist in either a *cis* or a *trans* configuration.

cis   *trans*

retinella (ret-ih-nel'ah). A dense light-sensitive neurofibrillar network surrounding the optic organelle in the photosensitive cells of worms and molluscs.

retinene (ret'ih-nēn). The original name given by Wald, its discoverer, to the chromophore of rhodopsin and product of its bleaching; later changed to *retinal* or *retinaldehyde.*

r. reductase. An enzyme which reduces retinene to vitamin A and the visual protein, opsin.

retineum (reh-tin'e-um). That part of an invertebrate eye which contains light receptor cells.

◆

RETINITIS

retinitis (ret"ih-ni'tis). Inflammation of the retina.

actinic r. Retinitis resulting from exposure to ultraviolet rays, as from acetylene torches or therapeutic lamps.

r. albi punctatus. Retinitis punctata albescens.

albuminuric r. Liebreich's (1859) term for lesions of the fundus characterized by hemorrhages and exudates occurring in association with albumen in the urine. It is now differentiated into *arteriosclerotic retinopathy, hypertensive retinopathy,* and *renal retinopathy.*

apoplectic r. Retinal apoplexy.

arteriosclerotic r. Arteriosclerotic retinopathy.

arteriospastic r. Arteriospastic retinopathy.

r. atrophicans. A hole in the macula through the entire thickness of the retina, a sequela of cystic macular degeneration.

azotemic r. Retinitis attributed to an accumulation of nitrogenous waste products occurring in association with renal disease.

Bright's r. Renal retinopathy.

r. cachecticorum. Pick's disease.

central r. Retinitis involving the macular area.

central angioneurotic r. Central angiospastic retinopathy.

central angiospastic r. Central angiospastic retinopathy.

central punctate r. A type of diabetic retinopathy characterized by soapy- or waxy-appearing, sharply defined, punctate exudates distributed irregularly in the macular area or forming a rough circle around the macula; sometimes associated with hemorrhages which are deep and round rather than flame-shaped.

central recurrent syphilitic r. A rare, recurring disease of the retina in which there is slight clouding of the macular area with small, whitish or yellowish dots and a characteristic, positive, central ring scotoma. Micropsia and metamorphopsia are often present, and the disease is often bilateral.

central serous r. Central angiospastic retinopathy.

central traumatic r. Traumatic macular degeneration of Haab.

r. centralis annularis. Central angiospastic retinopathy.

r. circinata. A degeneration of the retina characterized by a girdle of white exudates in the deeper retinal layers at a short distance from and around the macula, which are sharply defined, of various sizes, and may coalesce to form large irregular patches. The macular area may appear grayish or yellowish and may contain hemorrhages. The girdle contains no pigmentation, and the retinal vessels pass over it undisturbed. The disease occurs typically, but not invariably, in advanced age and is usually bilateral.

r. circumpapillaris. Retinitis occurring in the early stage of diffuse syphilitic neuroretinitis, characterized by intense localized swelling around the optic nerve head which completely blurs the margins of the disk.

Coats's r. Coats's disease.

congenital syphilitic r. Congenital syphilitic chorioretinitis.

diabetic r. Diabetic retinopathy.

diffuse syphilitic r. Diffuse syphilitic chorioretinitis.

disciform r. Senile disciform degeneration of the macula. See under *degeneration.*

eclamptic r. Toxemic retinopathy of pregnancy.

electric r. Retinitis due to exposure to intense electric light, as in electric welding or in the flash from a short circuit. It is characterized subjectively by a central, positive scotoma which may not completely disappear. Pigment changes may subsequently appear at the macula with permanent reduction in vision.

r. exudativa externa. Coats's disease.

exudative senile macular r. Senile disciform degeneration of the macula. See under *degeneration.*

foveo-macular r. A bilateral lesion of unknown etiology occurring in young males of average age 18 in the absence of retinal edema characterized by a yellow foveal exudate preceding formation of a retinal hole and permanent reduction of central vision.

r. gravidarum. Toxemic retinopathy of pregnancy.

gravidic r. Toxemic retinopathy of pregnancy.

gummatous r. A syphilitic gumma of the fundus.

guttate r. Choroiditis guttata senilis.

r. hemorrhagica externa. Coats's disease.

hypertensive r. Hypertensive retinopathy.

Jacobson's r. Diffuse syphilitic neuroretinitis.

Jensen's r. Jensen's disease.

juxtapapillary r. Jensen's disease.

Leber's r. Exudative retinitis giving the clinical appearance of pseudoglioma and detachment of the retina, occurring primarily in male children under age one in more than half of the cases.

leukemic r. Leukemic retinopathy.

lipemic r. Lipemia retinalis.

massive exudative r. Coats's disease.

metastatic r. Purulent retinitis due to lodgment of infective emboli in the retinal vessels as a result of septicemia or pyemia. In the very early stages, fluffy white exudates and numerous hemorrhages can be seen, the optic disk margins are blurred, and the retinal veins are dilated and tortuous. Within a few days the vitreous becomes opaque, obscuring the fundus from view, the iris, the ciliary body, and the choroid become involved, and panophthalmitis often follows.

nephritic r. Renal retinopathy.

photo r. Solar retinitis.

r. pigmentosa. A primary degeneration of the neuroepithelium of the retina with subsequent migration of the retinal pigment. The ophthalmoscopic appearance is of individual clumps of black pigment peripherally located and shaped like bone corpuscles, attenuated retinal vessels, and a pale waxy optic disk. The main symptoms are night blindness and progressive contraction of the visual field. It is familial, of unknown etiology, and usually bilateral. Syn., *primary pigmentary retinal dystrophy.* **inverse r.p.** Retinitis pigmentosa in which the pigmentation is either confined to, or commences in, the macular area. **pseudo r.p.** Pseudoretinitis pigmentosa. **r.p. sine pigmento.** A rare disease presenting all the symptoms and characteristics of retinitis pigmentosa except that the bone corpuscle-shaped pigment deposits are not present. A few scattered pigment dots and flecks may be seen in the periphery, or pigment deposits may be completely absent. Syn., *degeneratio sine pigmento.*

r. proliferans. Connective tissue proliferation and neovascularization extending into the vitreous and over the retinal surface as a result of the organization of hemorrhage into the vitreous, usually arising from the optic disk. Syn., *Manz's disease.*

pseudonephritic r. Stellate retinopathy.

r. punctata albescens. A bilateral, familial, degenerative disease of the retina, either congenital or beginning in early life, characterized by numerous discrete white dots scattered throughout a tesselated fundus except at the macula, by night blindness, and frequently by constricted visual fields. The dots always remain small, lie in a plane beneath the retinal vessels, and may contain pigment in their centers. It is differentiated from retinitis pigmentosa by the absence of optic atrophy and the lack of marked narrowing of the retinal vessels, and it occurs in two types, *progressive albipunctate dystrophy* and *stationary albipunctate dystrophy.* See

under *dystrophy.* Syn., *degeneratio punctata albescens; retinitis albi punctatus.*

purulent r. Infection of the retina by pus-forming organisms which may be exogenous, as from perforating wounds of the eye, or endogenous, as from metastasis.

renal r. Renal retinopathy.

Roth's r. Roth's disease.

rubella r. Pigmentary changes in the retina as a result of rubella. The pigment is typically deranged into small, irregularly round or filiform masses of a black or lead-gray color.

r. sclopetaria. Retinal disturbance of severe degree following trauma from the impact of a heavy foreign body, as a bullet.

r. septica of Roth. Roth's disease.

serous r. Retinitis characterized by serous infiltration, edema, and hyperemia, especially affecting the nerve fiber and the ganglion cell layers.

simple r. Serous retinitis.

solar r. Retinitis due to excessive exposure to sunlight, as from observing a solar eclipse without adequate protection or from sunlight reflected by snow. It is characterized subjectively by a central, positive scotoma which may not completely disappear. Pigment changes may subsequently appear at the macula with permanent reduction in vision. Syn., *photoretinitis.*

stellate r. Stellate retinopathy.

suppurative r. Purulent retinitis.

syphilitic r. Retinal inflammation as the result of syphilis, generally accompanied by choroidal and optic nerve involvement, which occurs in several clinical forms including: *congenital syphilitic chorioretinitis; diffuse syphilitic chorioretinitis; neuritis papulosa; diffuse syphilitic neuroretinitis;* and *central recurrent syphilitic retinitis.*

traumatic r. Inflammation of the retina due to injury; commotio retinae.

◆

retinoblastoma (ret"ih-no-blas-to'-mah). A congenital malignant tumor, usually observed before the age of 5, composed of embryonic retinal cells arising from the nuclear layers, and having a tendency to multiple origins in one or both eyes. It may invade the choroid and the optic nerve, may extend beyond the confines of the eyeball, and causes exophthalmos, cataract, and glaucoma. It is usually diagnosed initially by a yellowish or whitish reflex of light (cat's eye reflex) observed at the pupil, and the lesion characteristically appears in the vitreous as a pinkish-white mass with blood vessels extending over its surface or into its substance. Pathognomonic, pearly or chalky white, calcium deposits are usually present. Syn., *retinal glioma; retinal glioblastoma; retinal neuroblastoma; retinoma.*

diffuse infiltrating r. A retinoblastoma occurring flatly along the plane of the retina replacing all of the retinal layers with neoplastic cells. Syn., *glioma planum; retinoblastoma planum.*

r. endophytum. A retinoblastoma which extends into the vitreous chamber and does not cause retinal detachment.

r. exophytum. A retinoblastoma which grows in the subretinal space, detaches the retina, and in the early stages may not extend into the vitreous chamber. The ophthalmoscopic picture characteristically is of a funnel-shaped retinal detachment, some portions of which appear translucent and some opaque.

r. planum. Diffuse infiltrating retinoblastoma.

retinocele (ret"ih-no-sēl'). A congenital cyst of the retina typically located peripherally in the inferior temporal quadrant and giving a smooth bulbous appearance to the affected area. It may remain stationary or it may progress to cause retinoschisis or retinal detachment.

retinoception (ret"ih-no-sep'shun). The appreciation of the distance and direction of objects in space as a function of the stimulation of specific retinal receptors or of the rotation of the eye necessary to stimulate these receptors.

retinochoroidal (ret"ih-no-kó-roidal). Pertaining to both the retina and the choroid.

retinochoroiditis (ret"ih-no-ko"roidi'tis). Inflammation of both the retina and the choroid.

r. juxtapapillaris. Jensen's disease.

r. radiata. Pigmented paravenous retinochoroidal atrophy.

retinochoroidopathy (ret"ih-no-koroid-op'ah-the). Noninflammatory

disease involving both retina and choroid.

retinodialysis (ret"ih-no-di-al'ih-sis). A tearing of the retina from its attachment at the ora serrata. Syn., *retinal dehiscence; dialysis retinae; retinal disinsertion.*

retinograph (ret'ih-no-graf). A photograph of the retina or the fundus.

retinography (ret"ih-nog'rah-fe). Photography of the retina or the fundus.

retinol (ret'ih-nol). Vitamin A. Also see *retinaldehyde.*

retinoma (ret"ih-no'mah). Retinoblastoma.

retinomalacia (ret"ih-no-mah-la'she-ah). Retinosis.

retinomotor (ret"ih-no-mo'ter). Pertaining to the function of a retinal receptor in regulating the angular extent and direction of a fixational movement. See also *retinomotor value.*

retinopapillitis (ret"ih-no-pap"ih-li'tis). Inflammation of the optic nerve head and the retina; neuroretinitis.

◆

RETINOPATHY

retinopathy (ret"ih-nop'ah-the). 1. A morbid condition or disease of the retina. 2. Noninflammatory disease of the retina as distinguished from *retinitis.*

arteriosclerotic r. Sclerosis of the arterioles of the retina characterized ophthalmoscopically by widening of the light reflex resulting in a copper and silver wire appearance, increased tortuosity, arteriovenous crossing defects, perivascular sheathing, localized variations in caliber, and attenuation. Small, scattered hemorrhages and small, hard, sharply defined, white spots without surrounding edema may be seen. Syn., *arteriosclerotic retinitis.*

arteriospastic r. Retinopathy associated with persistent contraction of the retinal arterioles with reduction in size of the lumen, as in renal and hypertensive retinopathy. Syn., *arteriospastic retinitis.*

cellophane r. Preretinal macular fibrosis.

central angiospastic r. A disease of the retina characterized by a round or oval, restricted, macular edema which causes the macula to be swollen and indistinct. Small, yellowish or grayish white dots are frequently found in this area, and a light reflex usually encircles the edge of the swelling. The visual field shows a central relative scotoma for form and color, which in some cases may be absolute. The disease is usually unilateral, affects the young and the middle-aged, and has a tendency to recur. Subjective symptoms are metamorphopsia, micropsia, and misty vision or a central black spot. It is considered by some to be a disturbance in the circulation of the arterioles and the capillaries; prognosis is favorable. Syn., *preretinal edema of Guist; central angioneurotic retinitis; retinitis centralis annularis; central serous retinopathy.*

central disk-shaped r. Senile disciform degeneration of the macula. See under *degeneration.*

central serous r. Central angiospastic retinopathy.

chloroquine r. Retinopathy associated with the prolonged ingestion of chloroquine, an antimalarial drug used also in the treatment of lupus erythematosus and rheumatoid arthritis. It is characterized by retinal edeema, marked constriction of retinal arterioles, pigmentary degeneration resembling retinitis pigmentosa, paracentral scotomata, temporal field defects, and contraction of the peripheral fields.

circinate r. Retinitis circinata.

diabetic r. A disease of the retina associated with diabetes mellitus, characterized by small, punctate hemorrhages and numerous, smaller, round, red spots scattered around the posterior pole which are microaneurysms in the inner nuclear layer of the retina. In this same area are hard, sharply defined, white or yellowish, soapy or waxy exudates which may be isolated or coalesced into larger masses in a circinate manner around the macula. The disease is frequently found in association with arteriosclerotic and hypertensive retinal changes. Preretinal hemorrhages may occur, causing a retinitis proliferans. Syn., *diabetic retinitis.* **proliferative d.r.** An infrequent type of retinopathy associated with diabetes mellitus, characterized by proliferation of connective tissue and the formation of new blood vessels in the retina, and by hemorrhages into the vitreous. Typically, those affected have diabetes which began in childhood.

dysoric r. Retinopathy occurring in the debilitated and emaciated which is characterized by snow-white nodules, about one-fourth to one-half disk diameter in size, in the area of the optic disk. The nodules may remain without change for several weeks but eventually break down and disappear.

glomerulonephritic r. See *renal retinopathy.*

gravidic r. Toxemic retinopathy of pregnancy.

hemorrhagic r. Retinopathy characterized by profuse retinal hemorrhages as seen most commonly in diabetes, central vein occlusion, and hypertensive disease.

hypertensive r. A disease of the retina associated with essential or malignant hypertension. It may be classified into 4 grades of severity by the ophthalmoscopic picture. Grade I: The caliber of the arterioles is reduced to three-quarters to one-half the caliber of the corresponding vein, an occasional focal constriction of an arteriole may be present, and no hemorrhages, cotton-wool patches, or edema residues are seen. Grade II: Further reduction in the caliber of the arterioles to one-half to one-third of the corresponding vein, several focal constrictions of arterioles may be present and no hemorrhages, edema residues, or cotton-wool patches are seen. Grade III: Added to the changes in arteriole constriction are flame-shaped hemorrhages and/or cotton-wool patches and edema residues. Grade IV: Increased severity of the previous changes with the onset of papilledema which may range from mild blurring of the optic disk margins to pronounced edema and elevation with a star figure of edema residues at the macula. Arteriolosclerotic changes may accompany any of the four grades.

hypotensive r. Venous-stasis retinopathy.

leukemic r. A retinopathy found in all types of leukemia characterized by edema of the optic disk and the surrounding retina, marked engorgement, segmentation, and tortuosity of the veins, widely scattered superficial and deep hemorrhages of various sizes and shapes, some containing white centers, large, yellowish-white patches of exudate, and a yellowish-orange fundus. Syn., *leukemic retinitis.*

nephritic r. Renal retinopathy.

r. of prematurity. A bilateral retinal disease of premature infants, especially if placed in an abnormal oxygen environment, characterized by vascular proliferation and tortuosity, followed by intraocular hemorrhages, retinal edema and detachment, and finally by proliferation of fibrous tissue into the vitreous to form a dense retrolental mass. The cicatricial stage may terminate with only a small mass of opaque tissue in the peripheral retina, with useful vision, or it may progress to retrolental tissue covering the entire pupillary area, with no fundus reflex. Syn., *retrolental fibroplasia.*

proliferating r. Retinopathy resulting from absorption of intraretinal or vitreal hemmorhage and characterized by plaques of fine fibrous tissue associated with pigmentary migration and proliferation.

proliferative r. The growth of new blood vessels from the retina into the vitreous as a result of circulatory impairment in certain inflammatory conditions such as periphlebitis, diabetes, or degenerative vascular disease, resulting in a picture indistinguishable from retinitis proliferans.

Purtscher's traumatic angiopathic r. Purtscher's disease.

renal r. A disease of the retina associated with disease of the kidney (glomerulonephritis, nephrosclerosis, etc.) and hypertension, which presents the ophthalmoscopic picture of hypertensive retinopathy.

sickle-cell r. Retinopathy associated with sickle-cell disease or anemia, usually classified into four grades of severity. Grade I: Increased tortuosity and dilatation of the retinal venules and mild ischemia in the peripheral fundus. Grade II: Sheathing, neovascularization, microaneurysms, circumscribed narrowing, and telangiectasis of the peripheral venules. Grade III: The addition of retinal hemorrhages and exudates, and chorioretinal atrophy. Grade IV: Retinitis proliferans, vitreous hemorrhages, cholesterol deposits, central artery or vein occlusion, and occasionally papilledema.

solar r. Retinopathy due to excessive exposure to sunlight, as from observing a solar eclipse without adequate protection or from sunlight reflected by snow. It is characterized subjectively by a central, positive scotoma which may not completely disappear. Pigment changes may subsequently appear at the macula with permanent reduction in vision. Syn., *photoretinitis.*

stellate r. A retinal disease resembling hypertensive retinopathy, but not as a component of renal, arteriosclerotic, or hypertensive disease, characterized by pronounced retinal edema, exudates, hemorrhages, a macular star, and blurring of the optic disk. It may occur as a result of trauma, obstruction of a retinal artery or vein, papilledema, toxemia, etc. Syn., *pseudonephritic retinitis; stellate retinitis.*

thioridazine r. Retinopathy associated with the prolonged ingestion of large doses of thioridazine, a phenothiazine derivative used in psychotherapy. It is characterized by impairment of central vision, which may vary from slight and transient to severe and permanent, peripheral contraction of the visual fields with or without central scotomata, abnormal dark-adaptation curves, and pigmentary degeneration of the retina.

toxemic r. of pregnancy. A retinopathy associated with toxemia of pregnancy, characterized in the early stages by attenuation of the retinal arterioles, with a rise in diastolic blood pressure, occurring first in the nasal periphery, gradually spreading toward the optic disk, and becoming generalized. Local angiospasm may also appear. The later stages present the typical picture of advanced hypertensive retinopathy with exudates, hemorrhages, massive retinal edema, and possibly retinal detachment. The onset is acute and sudden, and restitution is equally rapid on the termination of pregnancy, with good prognosis for both vision and life. Syn.,*eclamptic retinitis; retinitis gravidarum; gravidic retinitis; gravidic retinopathy.*

venous-stasis r. Retinopathy resulting from the venous stasis occurring subsequent to total or partial occlusion of the internal carotid artery, characterized by irregular enlargement of the veins, sludging of the blood stream, petechial retinal hemorrhages, multiple micro-aneurysms, and sometimes the formation of new vessels. Syn., *hypotensive retinopathy.*

◆

retinopexy (ret"ih-no-peks'se). Surgical reattachment of a separated or detached retina, usually implying the use of high frequency electrical current.

retinophore (ret'ih-no-fōr). Vitrella.

retinophotoscopy (ret"ih-no-fo-tos'-ko-pe). Retinoscopy.

retinopiesis (ret"ih-no-pi-e'sis). The pressing of a detached retina back into its normal location, as by intravitreal silicone injection.

retinoschisis (ret"ih-no-skis'is). A splitting of the retina, usually at the outer plexiform layer, occurring as a slowly progressive hereditary disease, typically bilateral and affecting males. It appears ophthalmoscopically as a translucent, veil-like membrane emanating from the retina and carrying the retinal vessels in the inferior temporal quadrant, and spreads to involve the lower half of the fundus. It may also occur as a result of degenerative change at the retinal periphery, particularly in the elderly. Syn., *congenital vascular veils in the vitreous.*

retinoscope (ret'ih-no-skōp). An instrument for determining the conjugate focus of the retina, and hence the refractive state of the eye, consisting essentially of a transparent or perforated mirror which serves to reflect light on the retina from an external or contained light source and through which the observer views the light emerging through the subject's pupil from the retina and notes the apparent transverse motion of the emergent light in relation to the pupil and the motion of the source. Syn., *pupilloscope; skiascope.*

bi-vue r. An electric retinoscope having a plane mirror with two perforating apertures, 7 mm and 3 mm in diameter, either of which may be used.

concave mirror r. A retinoscope utilizing a concave mirror typically of short radius of curvature so that light entering the subject's eye diverges as though emanating from a point in front of the mirror and results in an "against" motion of the emerging light reflex in hypermetropia and a "with" motion in myopia, the opposite of that seen with a plane mirror retinoscope.

electric r. A retinoscope which contains an electric incandescent lamp as its light source, the current being supplied by batteries or through a transformer.

luminous r. Electric retinoscope.

nonluminous r. A retinoscope used with a separate source of light not contained in the instrument.

plane mirror r. A retinoscope utilizing a plane mirror so that light entering the subject's eye diverges as though emanating from a point behind the mirror and results in a "with" motion of the emerging light reflex in hypermetropia and an "against" motion in myopia.

spot r. A retinoscope which reflects a beam of light from a circular source into the patient's eye.

streak r. A retinoscope which reflects a beam of light from a transversely elongated or line source into the patient's eye. The beam is adjustable in width and is rotatable for meridional position.

V r. A streak retinoscope employing a light source with a right-angle-shaped filament, one leg of which provides the "streak" source for one principal meridian of measurement, and the other leg for the other principal meridian.

retinoscopy (ret"ih-nos'ko-pe). The determination of the conjugate focus of the retina, hence the objective measurement of the refractive state of the eye, with a retinoscope. The movement of the light reflex in the patient's pupil in relation to movement of the retinoscope and light source is noted and neutralized with suitable lenses. The power of the neutralizing lenses, less the dioptric equivalent of the working distance, is a measure of the refractive error of the eye. Syn., *koroscopy; pupilloscopy; retinoskiascopy; skiametry; skiascopy; shadow test; umbrascopy.*

book r. Retinoscopy performed while the subject is reading.

cylinder r. The secondary, confirmatory determination of the cylinder axis in retinoscopy by the rotation of the correcting cylinder axis away from its originally determined meridian, noting the reflex band, and redetermining the true axis by rotating the axis back until the band is eliminated.

dynamic r. Retinoscopy performed while the subject fixates a near object.

esoscopic r. Heteroscopic retinoscopy with the retinoscopist's peephole nearer to the subject's eye than the subject's point of fixation.

exoscopic r. Heteroscopic retinoscopy with the retinoscopist's peephole farther from the subject's eye than the subject's point of fixation.

heterodynamic r. Heteroscopic retinoscopy.

heteroscopic r. Retinoscopy in

which the subject's fixation target and the retinoscopist's peephole are at different distances from the subject's eye. Syn., *heterodynamic retinoscopy.*

isodynamic r. Isoscopic retinoscopy.

isoscopic r. Retinoscopy in which the subject's fixation target and the retinoscopist's peephole are at the same distance from the subject's eye. Syn., *isodynamic retinoscopy.*

near r. Retinoscopy performed on infants or very young children in a darkened room at 50 cm with the eye fixating the retinoscope light and the other eye occluded. Needed lens power is approximated by adding − 1.25 D to the dynamic spherical finding.

static r. Retinoscopy performed while the patient fixates a target at infinity or with accommodation otherwise relaxed.

retinosis (ret″ih-no′sis). Noninflammatory degeneration of the retina.

retinoskiascopy (ret″ih-no-ski-as′ko-pe). Retinoscopy.

retinula (reh-tin′u-lah). A group of light receptor cells located at the base of an ommatidium. Syn., *retinule.*

retinule (ret′ih-nūl). Retinula.

retractio bulbi (re-trak′she-o bul′bi). Duane's syndrome.

retraction of the eyelid. A condition said to exist for an otherwise normal eye when the margin of the upper eyelid rests at or above the limbus so that a band of white sclera is seen above the iris during relaxed straightforward fixation.

retraction, relative, of Heine. In high myopia, a bending of optic nerve fibers from their normal course in the region of the temporal margin of the optic disk, due to a temporal displacement of the margin of the lamina vitrea to which the fibers are attached.

retractor, Allen-Gulden plunger. An accessory pin on the handle of a Schiötz type tonometer which engages the edge of the weight and holds up the plunger until after the tonometer footplate is placed on the cornea.

retrobulbar (ret″ro-bul′bar). Situated, located, or occurring behind the eyeball.

retrography (re-trog′rah-fe). Mirror writing.

retro-illumination (ret″ro-ih-lu″mih-na′shun). Illumination of transparent or semitransparent media by reflecting light from tissues situated more posteriorly, as in slit lamp biomicroscopy.

direct r. Retro-illumination in which the tissue observed is in the direct path of the reflected light.

indirect r. Retro-illumination in which the tissue observed is not in the direct path of the reflected light.

retro-iridian (ret″ro-ih-rid′e-an). Situated, located, or occurring behind the iris.

retrolental (ret″ro-len′tal). Situated, located, or occurring behind the crystalline lens.

retrolental fibroplasia (ret″ro-len′tal fi″bro-pla′se-ah). See under *fibroplasia.*

retro-ocular (ret″ro-ok′u-lar). Situated, located, or occurring behind the eyeball.

retroreflection (ret″ro-re-flek′shun). Reflection of light back toward its origin regardless of its angle of incidence, as effected by three mirrors arranged to form the corner of a cube or by transparent beads of high refractive index, called retroreflectors or, more popularly, reflectorizers.

retroreflector (ret″ro-re-flek′tor). An optical element which reflects each incident light ray in a parallel path opposite in direction.

retroreflectorizer (ret″ro-re-flek′teh-rīz-or). See *retroreflection.*

retroscopic (ret″ro-skop′ik). Pertaining to the retroscopic angle.

retrotarsal (ret″ro-tar′sal). Situated or occurring behind the tarsus.

von Reuss's (von rois′ez) **chart; recuperative visual field.** See under the nouns.

Revilliod's sign (ra-ve-yōz′). Orbicularis sign.

revisualization (re-vizh″u-al-i-za′shun). The act or faculty of bringing an image again into view, especially a mental image.

rhabdom; rhabdome (rab′dom, -dōm). A rodlike refractile structure located along the central axis of an ommatidium and formed by the limiting membranes of the receptor cells.

rhabdomere (rab′dom-ēr). A subdivision of a rhabdome.

rhabdomyoma (rab″do-mi-o′mah). A benign tumor involving, and composed of, skeletal muscle tissue which appears rarely in the orbit.

rhabdomyosarcoma (rab″do-mi-o-sar-ko′mah). A malignant tumor of mesenchymal origin which in the orbit is one of the most common types and generally affects children in the first decade of life.

rhabdoscopy (rab-dos'ko-pe). Velonoskiascopy.

rhagades of eyelids (rag'ah-dēz). Cracks, fissures, or linear excoriations of the skin of the eyelids.

rhanter (ran'ter). Internal canthus.

rheobase (re'o-bās). The minimal electric current of indefinite duration which will produce an effect on tissue. Cf. *chronaxie.*

rheoophthalmography (re-o-of'thal-mog'rah-fe). Continuous recording of the changes of an electrical current passed through the eye.

rheum (room). A thin serous or catarrhal discharge from the eye. *Obs.*

rhinodacryolith (ri"no-dak're-o-lith). A concretion or stony formation in the nasolacrimal duct.

rhinommectomy (re"nom-mek'to-me). Surgical removal of a portion of the internal canthus.

rhinopsia (ri-nop'se-ah). Convergent strabismus. *Obs.*

rhitidosis (rit"ih-do'sis). Rhytidosis.

rho [ρ](rō). The Greek letter used as the symbol for (1) the *angle of torsion;* (2) the *coefficient of rank correlation.*

rhodogenesis (ro"do-jen'e-sis). The anabolism of rhodopsin.

rhodophane (ro'do-fān). A red pigment, or chromophane, in the retinal cones of birds and fishes.

rhodophylactic (ro"do-fi-lak'tik). Pertaining to rhodophylaxis.

rhodophylaxis (ro"do-fi-lak'sis). The property of the pigment epithelium of the retina to regenerate rhodopsin.

rhodopsin (ro-dop'sin). A purplish carotenoid protein in the outer segment of the rod cells of the retina which, on stimulation by light, bleaches and breaks down into transient orange, xanthopsin, and finally retinene and opsin. It is re-formed by the recombining of retinene and opsin. Syn., *visual purple.*

rhomb, Fresnel's. A crown glass block, rhomboidal in shape, which produces circularly or elliptically polarized light from plane-polarized light which is incident at a specific angle and then undergoes two internal reflections.

rhomb, Hüfner. A glass rhombohedron of such apical angles and index of refraction as to receive beams of light incident on two of its faces from separate illuminated surfaces to be compared after emerging in juxtaposition to each other from the two opposite faces, separated only by the fine line of demarcation of the apical edge.

rhythm, alpha. In electroencephalography, rhythmic oscillations in electrical potential in the cortex of the human brain, normally occurring at a rate of from 8 to 13 cycles per second and best recorded in the occipital region. Syn., *alpha wave.*

rhytidosis (rit"ih-do'sis). A wrinkling, especially of the cornea.

riboflavin (ri"bo-fla'vin). A water-soluble yellow crystalline powder present in milk, eggs, cheese, leafy vegetables, liver, kidney, and heart. It is necessary in cellular oxidation, and a deficiency in the diet results in lesions of the lips, cheilosis, glossitis, and seborrheic dermatitis. Eye signs include photophobia, blepharitis, peripheral vascularization of the cornea, and corneal opacities. Syn., *vitamin G.*

Ricco's law (re'kōz). See under *law.*

Richardson-Shaffer diagnostic lens. See under *lens.*

Riddoch's syndrome (rid'oks). See under *syndrome.*

riders, lenticular. V-shaped opacities which project from the surface of a zonular cataract like the spokes of a wheel, one limb of the V extending over the anterior surface of the main opacity and the other over the posterior surface.

ridge, superciliary. Arcus superciliaris.

ridge, supraorbital. Arcus superciliaris.

Ridgeway colors (rij'wa). See under *color.*

Ridley lens (rid'le). See under *lens.*

Rieger's (re'gerz) **anomaly; disease; syndrome.** See under the nouns.

Riehl's melanosis (rēlz). See under *melanosis.*

Riesman's sign (rēs'manz). See under *sign.*

rigidity, ocular. The resistance of the coats of the eye to distension; the summation of all factors in the eyeball and its adnexae, other than fluid pressure, which resists indentation. Its effect is considered in indentation tonometry. Syn., *scleral rigidity.*

rigidity, scleral. Ocular rigidity.

rima cornealis (ri'mah kor"ne-al'is). Corneal interval.

rima palpebrarum (ri′mah pal″pe-brah′rum). The palpebral fissure.

Rim-Cote. A trade name for a coating similar to Edge-Cote.

◆

RING

ring. Any circular or continuous round structure, line, or object; a circular or round arrangement of parts of a structure, a line, or an object.

anterior border r. of Schwalbe. A circularly arranged bundle of collagenous and elastic fibers located near the posterior surface of the cornea at the termination of Descemet's membrane. It gives rise to the scleral meshwork or corneoscleral trabeculae. A gonioscopic landmark. Syn., *Schwalbe's ring.*

benzene r. Benzene ring schema.

Brock's r's. Two complementary, colored rings viewed directly, or by projection onto a screen, through complementary colored filters, so that each ring is seen by only one eye. They are used in various visual training techniques, especially for the training of peripheral stereopsis.

Coats's r. A small, whitish-gray, ring opacity in the cornea, usually near the periphery, seen with the biomicroscope as a delicate, white, dotted circle, composed of lipoid deposits in Bowman's zone. It is variously considered to be hereditary, due to a disturbance in fat metabolism, or secondary to trauma or intraocular disease.

choroidal r. 1. A mottled, lightly pigmented ring around the optic papilla which is exposed choroid due to failure of the pigment epithelium of the retina to reach the disk. 2. An improperly used term for *pigmented ring.*

ciliary r. Annulus ciliaris.

conjunctival r. Annulus conjunctivae.

diffraction r. Airy's disk.

Döllinger's r. A thickening of Descemet's membrane in the region of the limbus.

Donders' r's. Rainbowlike halos seen around lights in glaucoma.

Fleischer's r. A thin, brownish or greenish, usually incomplete ring of pigment around the base of the cone in keratoconus, situated in the region of the basal epithelium and Bowman's membrane. It usually is visible only with the slit lamp. Syn., *Fleischer's line.*

Flieringa-Bonaccolto r. A thin stainless steel ring which is sutured to the sclera, between the limbus and the equator, to prevent vitreous loss in cataract extraction. It holds the sclera rigid and acts to prevent collapse of the anterior chamber and forward movement of the vitreous humor.

Flieringa-Legrand r. A device, consisting of two concentric rings with four equally spaced, interconnecting, radial arms, which is sutured to the anterior sclera as a supporting structure to prevent collapse of the anterior chamber during surgery, as in keratoplasty.

glaucomatous r. A light yellowish, circumpapillary ring of choroidal atrophy seen in the late stage of glaucoma.

greater r. of the iris. Ciliary zone.

greater r. of Merkel. Ciliary zone.

Kayser-Fleischer r. A pigmented ring in the periphery of the cornea, observed in Wilson's disease. It is about 1 to 3 mm wide, starts close to the limbus in a sharp border, and fades toward the center of the cornea. Characteristically it is brown or grayishgreen to the unaided eye and golden brown or reddish with the slit lamp and may be interspersed with any of the spectral colors. The pigment consists of fine, dense granules, believed to be deposits of copper, located in the deepest layers of the cornea.

Landolt r. An incomplete ring, similar to the letter *C* in appearance, used as a test object for visual acuity, especially in children and illiterates. The width of the ring and the break in its continuity are each one fifth of its over-all diameter. The break or gap is placed in different meridional positions with its location to be identified by the observer as evidence of its perception. The visual angle is represented by the subtense of the gap at the eye.

Lesser r's. Metal rings of various diameters with attached metal rod handles, used in visual training, especially for the elimination of suppression. The patient circles, with one of the rings, an area on one half of a haploscopically viewed stereogram corresponding to a target located on the other half.

lesser r. of the iris. Pupillary zone.

lesser r. of Merkel. Pupillary zone.

Loewe's r. A bright halo entoptically perceived surrounding Maxwell's spot when the eye is exposed to intermittent, uniformly diffused, blue or purplish light.

lymphatic r., pericorneal. An incomplete ring formed by two subconjunctival lymph collector channels located about 7 mm from the limbus and running circumferentially above and below it. It receives lymph from the limbal area and eventually drains into the preauricular nodes temporally and submaxillary nodes nasally.

Mach's r. A relatively bright or dark band perceived in a zone of brightness transition where the rate or gradient of change of brightness increases or decreases suddenly or rapidly, commonly referred to as Mach's ring because the phenomenon is usually demonstrated on rotating disks on which the brightness gradient is controlled by the proportions of black and white sectors at various distances from the center. Syn., *Mach's band.*

Maxwell's r. Maxwell's spot.

myopic r. A circular white area surrounding the optic papilla due to myopic degenerative changes of the choroid and the retina allowing the sclera to become visible.

Newton's r's. Concentric colored rings or interference fringes, produced when two glass lenses or plates are pressed together, due to interference of light in the thin film of air of varying thickness between the adjacent surfaces. See also *Newton ring test.*

pigmented r. A dark ring of pigment epithelium of the retina concentrated around the optic papilla.

postcorneal r. Embryotoxon.

posterior border r. of Schwalbe. The scleral spur, as observed gonioscopically.

Root red-green fusion r's. A target for testing and training sensory fusion consisting essentially of a pair of overlapping, complementary colored, red and green, oval rings encircling a smaller pair of similarly colored, overlapping, oval rings, which in turn encircle a white oval ring, all on a black background. When viewed through colored filters, and fused, the rings appear in stereoscopic relief.

Schwalbe's r. Anterior border ring of Schwalbe.

Schwalbe's posterior r. The scleral spur, as observed gonioscopically.

scleral r. A small, circular, white patch around the optic papilla which is the exposed sclera visible because both the pigment epithelium of the retina and the choroid stop short of the disk.

senile r. A circular opacity seen at a variable distance anterior to the optic disk, commonly present in senile myopic eyes and formed by torn portions of Cloquet's canal in posterior detachment of the vitreous. See also *Weiss's ring.* Syn., *senile annular opacity of Vogt.*

Soemmering's r. A doughnut-shaped ring of clear crystalline lens covered by a capsule, occurring as a result of physical destruction of the lens cortex and the nucleus, with the capsule and the subcapsular epithelium remaining intact. The central part, occupying the pupillary aperture, usually consists of a membrane composed of posterior capsule and fibrous tissue. Syn., *Soemmering's cushion.*

von Szily's r. Ring sinus of von Szily. See under *sinus.*

Verhoeff's r's. Verhoeff's circles.

Vossius lenticular r. Vossius ring cataract.

Wallach's r's. A two dimensional figure consisting of a series of four or five eccentric, but nonintersecting, rings placed one inside another, which, when rotated about an axis perpendicular to the plane of the figure, produces a three dimensional effect; used as a target in visual training.

Weiss's r. A gray circular opacity seen anterior to the optic disk, marking the posterior limit of the vitreous humor in an elongated myopic eyeball and considered to indicate a posterior detachment of the vitreous. See also *senile ring.*

white r. of the cornea. A small round or oval lesion of the cornea giving rise to no symptoms, appearing in the lower cornea at the level of Bowman's membrane, about 0.5 mm in diameter, made up of minute white dots of lipid material which coalesce and appear to form a continuous circular line, and presumed to be due to fatty infiltration secondary to trauma.

◆

Riolan's muscle (re"o-lanz'). See under *muscle.*

Ripault's sign (re-pōz′). See under *sign.*
Risley prism (riz′le). See under *prism.*
Ritchie photometer (rich′e). See under *photometer.*
Ritter's fibers (rit′erz). See under *fiber.*
rivalry. A competition or antagonism; a vying for supremacy.

> **binocular r.** Retinal rivalry.
> **border r.** Contour rivalry.
> **color r.** A form of retinal rivalry, or a sequence of alternate sensations, when the two eyes are separately but simultaneously exposed to different colors.
>> **contour r.** A form of retinal rivalry or alternation of sensations, when the two eyes are separately but simultaneously exposed to differently oriented contours which superimpose each other. Instead of an integrated pattern of contours, the borders of different orientation are alternately and intermittently suppressed. Syn., *border rivalry.*
>> **retinal r.** Alternation of perception of portions of the visual field when the two eyes are simultaneously and separately exposed to targets containing dissimilar colors or differently oriented borders. (See Fig. 30.) Syn., *figural alternation; binocular rivalry; strife rivalry.*

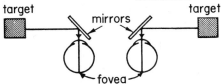

patchy rhythmical alterations of conflicting form sensations

target   target

mirrors

fovea

Fig. 30 Retinal rivalry resulting from simultaneous binocular stimulation with differently oriented borders. (From K. C. Swan, "The sensory physiology of binocular vision" in *Strabismic Ophthalmic Symposium* II, ed. by J. H. Allen. St. Louis: C. V. Mosby, 1958)

> **strife r.** Retinal rivalry.
> **r. of visual fields.** Retinal rivalry.
rivus lacrimalis (ri′vus lak″rih-mal′-is). Lacrimal lake.
Roaf's theory (rōfs). See under *theory.*

Robbins rock. See under *rock.*
Roberts Tachistoscreener. See under *Tachistoscreener.*
Robertson's (rob′ert-sunz) **pupil; reflex; sign.** See under the nouns.
Robin's syndrome. See under *syndrome.*
Robinson Cohen (rob′in-sun ko′en) **chart; slide; test.** See under the nouns.
Robles' disease. Onchocerciasis.
Robstein syndrome. Blegvad-Haxthausen syndrome. See under *syndrome.*
Rochester's sign (roch′es-terz). See under *sign.*
Rochon (ro-shon′) **polarizer; prism.** See under *prism.*
Rochon-Duvigneaud (ro-shon′-du-ve-nyo′) **bouquet of central cones; accessory fossa; scleral sinus; syndrome.** See under the nouns.
rock, accommodative. An accommodative exercise consisting of a series of accommodative responses to alternate monocular increases and decreases in dioptric stimulus to accommodation. It is usually performed clinically by having the right and the left eye alternately view a target through lenses which present different dioptric stimuli to each of the two eyes.
rock, Robbins. A training procedure for improving the facility of accommodative response in which a reduced Snellen chart is viewed at a 16″ distance through a phoropter and through a vertical dissociating prism. Fixation is alternated between the two images with lenses of different power placed before the two eyes, and the difference is increased in 0.25 D steps as the successive clearing of vision is demonstrated in each.
rod. A straight slender structure.
> **r. fiber.** See under *fiber.*
> **r. granule.** See under *granule.*
> **Maddox r.** A cylindrical glass rod used in measuring a phoria or heterotropia which, when placed in front of the eye, distorts the image of a light source into a long streak perpendicular to the axis of the rod.
> **r. proper.** The outer and the inner members of a rod cell; a rod cell in the restricted sense.
> **retinal r.** A rod cell.

Roenne's (ren'ēz) **effect; phenomenon; nasal step.** See under the nouns.

Roger's cone (roj'erz). See under *cone.*

Rolando's fissure (ro-lan'dōz). See under *fissure.*

Rollet syndrome. S–O syndrome. See under *syndrome.*

Romaña's sign (ro-mahn'yahz). See under *sign.*

Romberg's (rom'bergz) **disease; sign; syndrome.** See under the nouns.

Römer's method (re'merz). See under *method.*

Ronchi (ron'ke) **test; theory.** See under the nouns.

Rönne. See *Roenne.*

room, Ames. A room with trapeziform sides, or a miniature facsimile, designed so that all of the visible features on its walls, ceiling, and floor subtend, from a single point of reference, angles which are identical to those that would be subtended by a rectangular room with rectangular features with respect to the same point, whence it is perceived as a rectangular room when viewed monocularly with the eye at the predesigned point of observation, and normal-sized objects discretely placed in the room are simultaneously seen tilted and distorted in size and shape.

room, leaf. A room about 7 feet square, open at one end, set exactly level and with true right angles, the interior sides of which are covered with artificial leaves to reduce monocular depth clues so that depth judgment depends on the appreciation of binocular retinal disparity (stereopsis). It is used to demonstrate, detect, and measure spatial distortions resulting from aniseikonia.

root. 1. The portion of an organ by which it is attached. 2. The portion of a nerve adjacent to the center with which it is connected; in spinal and cranial nerves, the bundle of fibers connecting them with their respective nuclei and gray columns.

   ciliary ganglion r's. See *ganglion, ciliary.*

   r. of the iris. The portion of the iris attached to the ciliary body.

   mesencephalic r. of the trigeminal nerve. Dendrites of unipolar neurons originating in the mesencephalic nucleus of the trigeminus located in the lateral gray matter about the aqueduct of Sylvius. The root descends from the midbrain to the pons, and its fibers leave the brain to enter the motor root of the trigeminus. It carries proprioceptive impulses from the muscles of mastication and possibly from the extraocular muscles.

   sensory r. of the trigeminal nerve. The thickest portion of the fifth cranial nerve extending from the pons to the Gasserian ganglion. It contains the axons of general sensory neurons which course in the ophthalmic, the maxillary, and the mandibular divisions.

Root red-green fusion rings. See under *ring.*

Roper-Hall implant. See under *implant.*

Roque's sign (roks). See under *sign.*

rosacea, ocular (ro-za'se-ah). Acne rosacea involving the eye or its adnexa. See *rosacea blepharoconjunctivitis; rosacea episcleritis; rosacea keratitis.*

rose bengal. A stain clinically useful for the diagnosis of keratoconjunctivitis sicca and for locating the margins of corneal ulcers, especially in conjunction with a slit lamp.

Rosen phoriagraph (ro'zen). See under *phoriagraph.*

Rosenbach's (ro'zen-bahks) **phenomenon; sign; test.** See under the nouns.

Rosenmueller's (ro'zen-me"lerz) **gland; valve.** See under the nouns.

rosettes, Flexner-Wintersteiner (ro-zets'). A group of columnar cells with a peripheral basement membrane arranged in a radial manner around a central cavity, the spokes corresponding to the rods and cones, found in retinal embryonic tumors.

rosettes, Herbert's (ro-zets'). Slightly elevated, translucent nodules surrounded by a fine capillary network, appearing in the superior cornea or the limbus, in the early stages of trachoma.

rotation. The act or process of turning about an axis, as rotation of the eye.

   cardinal r. Rotation of the eye in the major field of action of any of the six extraocular muscles, i.e., to the right, the left, the left superiorly, the right superiorly, the left inferiorly, or the right inferiorly.

   center of r. See under *center.*

   excyclofusional r. Relative rotation of the two eyes around their respective anteroposterior axes in response to a cyclofusional stimulus, such that the upward extensions of their vertical meridians rotate templeward.

head r. A deviation in position of the head about a vertical axis of reference and away from a straightforward position, especially as a clinical symptom. Cf. *head tilt; shoulder tipping.* Syn., *head turn; face turn.*

incyclofusional r. Relative rotation of the two eyes around their respective anteroposterior axes in response to a cyclofusional stimulus, such that the upward extensions of their vertical meridians rotate nasalward.

optical r. 1. Optical activity. 2. The angular rotation of the plane of polarization by an optically active substance.

specific r. The angular rotation of a beam of plane-polarized light when passing through a solid medium of specified thickness or through a liquid medium of specified thickness and concentration.

torsional r. Wheel rotation.

wheel r. Rotation of an eye about an anteroposterior axis of reference, as the line of sight. Syn., *torsional movement; wheel movement; torsional rotation.*

Roth's (rōts) **disease; patches; retinitis; spots.** See under the nouns.

Roth-Bielschowsky (rōt'be-el-show'-ske) **sign; syndrome.** See under the nouns.

Rothmund's (rōt'mundz) **disease; syndrome.** See under the nouns.

Rothschild's sign (roths'chĭldz). See under *sign.*

Rotoscope (ro'to-skōp). A trade name for a visual training instrument which consists essentially of a modified Brewster stereoscope, a lighting system with rheostat controls, a flashing mechanism, and a motor for moving the target holders in a circular course. The target holders are separate for each eye, and the speed and the diameter of the excursion of the targets and the horizontal distance between them and their vertical alignment can be altered by manual controls.

Rototrainer (ro'to-trān"er). The trade name for an instrument consisting essentially of a manually or motor-activated rotating disk with interchangeable fixation targets mounted on it for viewing as a visual training exercise.

rouge. 1. A red powder consisting of ferric oxide, usually prepared by calcining ferrous sulphate, used in polishing glass, metal, and gems. 2. Any powdery substance used for polishing lenses.

roughing. The grinding of a lens to its approximate curvature and thickness with a coarse abrasive.

Rousseau (ru'so) **construction; diagram.** See under *construction.*

Rowland's (ro'landz) **circle; ghosts; diffraction grating.** See under the nouns.

Rubenstein-Taybi syndrome. See under *syndrome.*

rubeosis diabetica (ru"be-o'sis di"ah-bet'ih-kah). Rubeosis iridis.

rubeosis iridis (ru"be-o'sis i'rid-is). Noninflammatory neovascularization of the iris occurring in diabetes mellitus, characterized by numerous, small, intertwining blood vessels which anastomose near the sphincter region to give the appearance of a reddish ring near the border of the pupil. The vessels may extend from the root of the iris to the filtration angle to cause peripheral vascular synechiae and secondary glaucoma. Syn., *rubeosis diabetica.*

rubeosis retinae (ru"be-o'sis ret'ih-ne). The formation of new retinal blood vessels in front of the optic disk, a condition seen in retinitis proliferans.

Rubin's vase (roo'binz). See under *vase.*

Rubino-Corrazza syndrome. Uveomeningitic syndrome.

Rucker sign. See under *sign.*

Rud syndrome. See under *syndrome.*

ruff, pupillary. The fringe of black pigment at the pupillary margin of the iris representing the anterior termination of the pigmented layer lining the posterior surface of the iris. Syn., *pigment frill.*

Ruggeri's reflex (ru-ja'rēz). See under *reflex.*

◆

RULE

rule. 1. A prescribed guide for action or procedure. 2. The usual, expected, or normal case or condition. 3. A graduated measuring instrument.

Babinet's r. In uniaxial crystals the direction of greater refractive index is also the direction of greatest absorption.

Duane's accommodation r. A device for determining the near point and the amplitude of accommodation, consisting of a flat wooden ruler calibrated on the top and sides in centimeters and diopters, with the calibration commencing 14 mm in front of the cornea. It is grooved at one end to fit the bridge of the nose and a test chart is moved along the rule, toward the eyes, until a blur is noticed.

Foster near point r. An aluminum rule for measuring the near point of accommodation calibrated in centimeters, diopters, and the mean near points of accommodation for various ages. It is provided with a double-sided sliding test card.

Gulden accommodation r. An opaque white plastic rod calibrated in centimeters, inches, diopters, and the mean near points of accommodation for various ages, used to measure the near point of accommodation by utilizing a sliding carrier with small test objects.

Javal's r. The total astigmatic correction of the eye approximates the ophthalmometrically determined astigmatism multiplied by 1.25 and combined with -0.50 cyl axis 90°.

Köllner's r. Köllner's law.

Kundt's r. 1. Divided or graduated distances appear greater than physically equal nongraduated distances. 2. In attempting to bisect a horizontal line with monocular vision, there is a tendency to place the middle point too far toward the nasal side.

Linksz r. A rule that approximately 2× magnification can be achieved with a loupe or hand-held magnifier by placing the target one-half focal length of the loupe nearer than the preferred reading distance and the loupe another one-half focal length nearer than the target.

Maddox r. 1. A recommendation credited by Maddox to Noyes that the spectacle prism correction should approximate half of the lateral heterophoria and that little is to be gained by a correction exceeding two degrees or four prism diopters. 2. The vertical phoria usually should be fully corrected.

McCulloch's r. The total astigmatic correction of the eye approximates the ophthalmometrically determined astigmatism increased by one eighth of itself and combined with -0.75 cyl axis 90°.

Miller accommodation r. A device for determining the near point and the amplitude of accommodation,

consisting of a light metal tubular rod, ½ in. in diameter and 35 cm long, scaled in inches and millimeters. One end of the tube is curved to fit against the nose, and an attached occluder may be rotated in front of either eye. Test charts mounted on a holder are moved along the tube, toward the eye, until a blur is noticed.

O'Shea's r. The total astigmatic and spherical correction of the eye approximates the ophthalmometrically determined astigmatism combined with -0.50 cyl axis 90°, added to a spherical "corneal equivalent" ametropia, and further modified by a calculated table for effectivity at 15 mm from the cornea.

PD r. A ruler calibrated in millimeters, used for measuring interpupillary distance.

Percival's r. Lateral imbalance should not be considered a source of discomfort beyond 33 cm when the binocular demand point is in the middle third of the range of relative convergence.

Prentice's r. Prentice's law.

Prince's r. A device for determining the near point and the amplitude of accommodation, consisting of a steel tape scaled in diopters on one side and in millimeters on the other. One end of the tape is held against the lower orbital margin, and a test chart is moved along the tape, toward the eye, until a blur is noticed.

RAF near point r. A device for measuring the near points of accommodation and convergence consisting essentially of a sliding four-sided rotatable target holder mounted on a rod calibrated in centimeters, diopters, the mean near points of accommodation for various ages, and a convergence scale rated "normal," "reduced," and "defective."

Ryer-Hotaling r. The correcting cylindrical lens is the lens placed at the wearing distance before the eye, through which the ophthalmometer indicates 0.50 D with the rule astigmatism when rotated 90°.

Sinclair's r. A rule used to set the distance of the patient from a tangent screen and to determine the position and the extent of a plotted scotoma. It consists of a flat wooden ruler, 25 mm wide and 1 m long, scaled on one side in degrees for a one meter testing distance and on the other side with degrees for a 2 m testing distance.

Sutcliffe's r. An empirical rule for estimating the total astigmatic correction of the eye: for with the rule astigmatism, using minus cylinders, add one-half the amount of the corneal astigmatism to itself and deduct 1 D. For against the rule astigmatism, using minus cylinders, add one-third to the astigmatism indicated by the ophthalmometer.

◆

Rumford photometer (rum'ford). See under *photometer*.

Rushton's method (rush'tonz). See under *method*.

Russell angles. See under *angle*.

Rx. Prescription.

Rydberg's theory. See under *theory*.

Ryer-Hotaling (ri'er-ho'tah-ling) **method; rule; spectacles.** See under the nouns.

rytidosis (rit"ih-do'sis). Rhytidosis.

S

Sabouraud syndrome (sab'oo-ro). See under *syndrome*.

sac. A baglike structure.

 conjunctival s. A continuous mucous membrane which begins at the posterior lid margins, lines the inner surface of the eyelids, and is reflected at the fornix to cover the sclera.

 lacrimal s. The membranous, saclike structure which receives tears from the canaliculi, via the sinus of Maier, and conveys them into the nasolacrimal duct. It is situated in the lower, anterior, medial wall of the orbit, in the lacrimal fossa, and is surrounded by periosteum (the lacrimal fascia). The upper portion, above the entrance of the sinus of Maier, is closed superiorly, forming the fundus of the sac and the lower portion is continuous with the nasolacrimal duct.

 lenticular s. Lens pit.

 tear s. Lacrimal sac.

saccade (sah-kād'). An abrupt voluntary shift in fixation from one point to another, as occurs in reading.

saccadic (să-kad'ik) **fixation; movement; speed.** See under the nouns.

sacculus lacrimalis (sak'u-lus lak"-rih-mal'is). Lacrimal sac.

saccus lacrimalis (sak'us lak"rih-mal'is). Lacrimal sac.

Sachs's (saks'ez) **disease; experiment.** See under the nouns.

Saemisch's corneal ulcer (sa'mish-ez). Serpiginous corneal ulcer.

Saenger's (zeng'erz) **sign; syndrome.** See under the nouns.

sag. Abbreviation for *sagitta* or *sagittal depth*.

sagitta (să-jit'ah). Sagittal depth.

St. Clair's disease (sānt klārz'). See under *disease*.

Sainton's sign (san-tonz'). See under *sign*.

Salmon's sign (sam'onz). See under *sign*.

Salon International de la Lunetterie et du Materiel pour Opticiens. An annual French international ophthalmic optics industry trade fair initiated in 1967 under sponsorship of the Union Nationale des Syndicats de Fabricants de Lunetterie.

Salus' (sal'uz) **arch; sign.** See under the nouns.

Salzmann's (salz'manz) **vitreous base; corneal dystrophy.** See under the nouns.

sample. A limited number of cases taken from a larger population for statistical treatment or analysis.

 purposive s. A selected group of cases from a larger population chosen in deliberate fashion to yield a cross section representation of the larger population.

 random s. A number of cases taken from a larger population without preference or regard to any characteristic and so chosen that each case has an equal chance of being included.

Sanders' (san'derz) **disease; syndrome.** Epidemic keratoconjunctivitis.

Sanders-Hogan syndrome (san'derz-ho'gan). Epidemic keratoconjunctivitis.

Sanfilippo syndrome. See under *syndrome*.

Sanger-Brown ataxia. See under *ataxia*.

[550]

Sanyal conjunctivitis. See under *conjunctivitis*.

SAO. See *Scottish Association of Opticians*.

SAOA. See *South African Optometric Association*.

Sappey's fibers (sap'ēz). See under *fiber*.

sarcoid, Boeck's (sahr'koid). Sarcoidosis.

sarcoidosis (sahr-koi-do'sis). A disease of unknown etiology characterized by tuberclelike, granulomatous nodules which may affect the skin, the lungs, the lymph nodes, the bones of the distal extremities, the conjunctiva, the lacrimal gland, the retina, and the uveal tract. The nodules are differentiated from true tubercles in that caseation or necrosis rarely occurs. It is a chronic, recurring, and relatively benign disease except when affecting the uveal tract. Syn., *Besnier-Boeck disease; Besnier-Boeck-Schaumann disease; lupus pernio; benign lymphogranulomatosis; lymphogranulomatosis of Schaumann; Boeck's sarcoid; Schaumann's syndrome.*

sarcoma (sahr-ko'mah). A malignant tumor arising from any nonepithelial, mesodermal tissue, such as fibrous, mucoid, fatty, osseous, cartilaginous, synovial, lymphoid, hemopoietic, vascular, muscular, or meningeal. Each form is specified by an appropriate combining form: fibro-, lipo-, osteo-, etc. In the eye, it may occur in the eyelid, the conjunctiva, the lacrimal gland, the choroid, etc.

Sarver's criteria. See under *criteria*.

Sarwar lens. See under *lens*.

satellite of Hamaker (sat'eh-līt). Second positive afterimage.

satiation (sa"she-a'shun). An alteration of a medium, as the visual cortex, through which impulses have been passing, as from fixating a figure, evidenced by a perceived displacement effect on figures or patterns subsequently imaged on the same area of the retina, or by a change in percept of a constantly fixated figure. Syn., *satiety*.

satiety (să-ti'eh-te). Satiation.

Sattler's (sat'lerz) **lamina; layer; veil.** See under the nouns.

saturation (sat"u-ra'shun). The quality of visual perception which permits a judgment of different purities of any one dominant wavelength; the degree to which a chromatic color differs from a gray of the same brightness.

Sauflon. Trade name for a gas-permeable hydrophilic material used in the manufacture of contact lenses.

Sauvineau's ophthalmoplegia (so'-vin-ōz). See under *ophthalmoplegia*.

Savart plate; polariscope. See under the nouns.

Save Your Vision Week. The first full week in March of each year, dedicated to cognition and observance of public measures to preserve and safeguard good vision, initiated as Eye Conservation Week in 1924 and continued by its present designation in 1927 under auspices of the American Optometric Association, and mandated in 1963 by a joint Resolution of Congress calling on the President to proclaim it annually.

sc. Abbreviation for *sine correctione* (without correction). Cf. *cc.*

scale. 1. A graduated instrument used for measuring. 2. A system of graduations for measuring.

    axis s. A protractorlike representation of the meridians of the eye for designating cylinder axis orientation in spectacle lenses. In the United States the 0° is to the subject's left, 90° up, 180° to his right, etc. In Europe two systems prevail, one as above, the other having 0° nasalward and 180° temporalward. Cf. *standard axis notation*.

    Barraga visual efficiency s. A test designed to measure the ability to visually discriminate and recognize reading readiness items which have been appropriately adapted and enlarged for children with low vision. The test items include recognition and discrimination of geometric forms in solid black as well as outlines, pictures, and words and letters singly and in groups.

    gray s. A graduated series of achromatic tones providing a full range of grays between black and white.

    Kelvin s. An absolute scale of temperature in which zero is equal to −273°C or −459.4°F. This scale is used to designate the temperature at which a blackbody yields a hue matching that of a given sample of radiant energy.

    Maddox oblique s. A linear scale with a centered light source and numbered or lettered gradations that is oriented halfway between the vertical and horizontal in a frontoparallel plane and used in conjunction with a Maddox groove or rod in front of one eye which provides the appearance of a streak of light. The number or letter at which the vertically or horizontally oriented streak intersects the scale seen by the other eye indicates the magnitude of the respective binocular deviation.

Newton's color s. 1. The sequence of interference colors observed in thin films with increasing optical path difference. It often is used to judge the magnitude of optical path differences semi-quantitatively. 2. Newton's division of the visible spectrum into seven intervals of widths corresponding to the intervals in the musical scale, thus giving seven principal colors: red, orange, yellow, green, blue, indigo, and violet.

saturation s. A graduated series of colors of constant hue and brightness which appear to vary by uniform steps of saturation from a neutral gray to the maximum attainable saturation for that hue.

Snell-Sterling visual efficiency s. Snell-Sterling notation.

spectral chroma s. A color scale or a color series consisting of equally bright spectral colors arranged in uniform steps of just noticeable, or equally perceptible, differences in chromaticity; a scale of wavelength discrimination in a spectrum of uniform brightness.

tangent s., Maddox. Maddox cross.

tangent s., orthops. A calibrated horizontal scale for measuring lateral phorias or tropias.

Ziegler prism s. A combined horizontal and vertical scale used to measure the deviation in centimeters of a prism placed at a distance of 1 m.

scanner, cathode ray tube. In fiber optics, a bundle of short fibers, one end of which is placed against the face of a cathode ray tube and the other against a photographic plate.

Scarpa's staphyloma (skahr'pahz). Staphyloma posticum of Scarpa.

scatter, sclerotic. A method of illumination used in examination of the cornea with the slit lamp, in which the beam of light is focused on the corneoscleral limbus to create internal reflection through the cornea. The light will pass through normal tissue unimpeded and unobserved, but will be scattered by any disturbance of transparency (nebula, keratocele, etc.), rendering it visible.

scattering. Diffusion or deviation of light in all directions by irregular reflection, as may be produced by particles in the medium through which the light passes.

Brillouin s. The scattering of light in a medium by interaction with extremely high frequency sound waves passing through, e.g., at 10^{12} hertz or higher.

Mie s. As described by G. Mie, the characteristics of scattering of light by molecular and dust particles as a function of their size in relation to wavelength, explaining the deep blue color of the sky in a pure atmosphere compared to its whitish blue color in a turbid atmosphere.

Rayleigh s. The scattering of light by molecules and other particles small in comparison to the wavelength, the intensity occurring as a function of the fourth power of the frequency of the incident light, whence the resulting color of the scattered light is typically blue, as in the blue sky.

Thomson s. The scattering of light by free electrons in an ionized gas plasma upon penetration by a pulse of intense laser light.

Schacher's ganglion (shah'kerz). Ciliary ganglion.

Schäfer's (sha'ferz) **fovea externa; syndrome.** See under the nouns.

Schapero's method. See under *method*.

Scharf lens (sharf). See under *lens*.

Schaumann's (shaw'manz) **disease; lymphogranulomatosis; syndrome.** Sarcoidosis.

Scheie syndrome; system. See under the nouns.

Scheiner's (shi'nerz) **disk; experiment; method; test.** See under the nouns.

schema, body. The pattern of a person's awareness of his own body; the characteristic way in which one is aware of his body; an acquired pattern that determines body image in a given situation.

schema, Gát's (ske'mah). A full circle graduated schematic, serving as a reference guide for designating the angular location of the insertions of the four rectus muscles for the right eye between 80°–103°, 169°–190°, 257°–282°, and 351°–13°, and for the left eye at symmetrically corresponding positions, on a scale for which 0° is at 3 o'clock, 90° at 12 o'clock, etc.

schema, Pascal's benzene ring (ske'mah). Any one of several mnemonics, invented by Pascal, resembling the conventional benzene ring of chemistry, used to represent such functions as the interrelationships of the cardinal optical points, the extraocular muscle actions, etc. (See Fig. 31.)

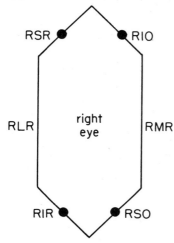

Fig. 31 Benzene ring schema from the examiner's view, illustrating action of the extraocular muscles by the position of the limb (principal action), the position of each dot in relation to the adjacent vertical limb, and the slant of the limb (secondary actions). (From H. W. Gibson, *Textbook of Orthoptics*. Kent, England: Hatton Press, 1955)

schemograph (ske'mo-graf). An instrument for tracing the limits of the visual field as determined with the perimeter.

Schenck's theory (shenks). See under *theory*.

Scherer cataract spectacles (shēr'er). See under *spectacles*.

scheroma (ske-ro'mah). Xerosis of the conjunctiva.

Schieck's iritis (shēks). Iritis obturans of Schieck.

Schilder's (shil'derz) **disease; test.** See under the nouns.

schiller (shil'er). Iridescence, especially the play of colors observed on some minerals and beetles, usually attributed to minute inclusions and cavities in the reflecting surface.

Schiötz tonometer (shuts). See under *tonometer*.

Schirmer's (shir'merz) **esthesiome-** ter; opacity; syndrome; test. See under the nouns.

schistoscope (skis'to-skōp). An early form of colorimeter employing a combination of Rochon prism, polarizing nicol, and cleavage plates of mica for producing variations in color.

schizoblepharia (skiz″o-bleh-fa're-ah). A cleft or fissure of the eyelid.

Schlemm's canal (shlemz). See under *canal*.

Schlesinger's (shla'zing-erz) **phenomenon; reaction; pupillary reflex.** See under the nouns.

schlieren (shle'ren). Streaks or optical inhomogeneities, especially in glass, negatives, and optical images. *German.*

schlieren (shle'ren) **field; head; optical system.** See under the nouns.

Schlösser's pupillometer (schles'-erz). See under *pupillometer*.

Schmidt's (shmitz) **corrector; plate; prism; sign; telescope.** See under the nouns.

Schmidt-Fracaro syndrome. Cat's eye syndrome.

Schmidt-Rimpler (shmit-rimp'ler) **optometer; test; theory.** See under the nouns.

Schnabel's (shnab'elz) **caverns; spaces.** See under the nouns.

Schneller test (shnel'er). See under *test*.

Schnyder's corneal dystrophy (shni'-derz). Crystalline corneal dystrophy.

Schober's theory (sho'berz). See under *theory*.

Schoen's theory (shānz). See under *theory*.

Schöler's theory (sha'lerz). See under *theory*.

Schönenberg syndrome (shān'enberg). See under *syndrome*.

Schouten-Ornstein law (shu'ten-orn'stīn). See under *law*.

Schreck lens (shrek). See under *lens*.

Schroeder's (shra'derz) **figure; visual illusion; staircase.** See under the nouns.

Schubert's potential. See under *potential*.

Schüller's disease (shil'erz). Schüller-Christian-Hand disease.

Schüller's syndrome (shil'erz). Schüller-Christian-Hand syndrome.

Schüller-Christian-Hand (shil'er-kris'chan-hand) **disease; syndrome.** See under the nouns.

Schultze's fiber basket (shoolt′sez). See under *fiber basket*.

Schwalbe's (shval′bēz) **contraction folds; structural folds; contraction furrows; structural furrows; annular line; ring; space.** See under the nouns.

Schwarting three-point test. See under *test*.

sciascopia (si″as-ko′pe-ah). Retinoscopy.

sciascopy (si-as′ko-pe). Retinoscopy.

sciascotometry (si″ah-sko-tom′eh-tre) Skiascotometry.

science, visual. The aggregate of knowledge considered to be particularly essential and pertinent to the understanding of the phenomena, processes, and functions of vision as a sense modality.

scieropia (si-er-o′pe-ah). An anomaly of vision in which objects appear shaded, darkened, or in a shadow.

scintillatio albescens (sin″tih-lah′-te-o al-beh′sens). Asteroid bodies.

scintillatio nivea (sin″tih-lah′te-o niv′e-ah). The shiny white bodies of calcium salts of fatty acids seen in asteroid hyalitis.

scintillation (sin″tih-la′shun). 1. A subjective visual sensation of sparks or quivering flashes of light. 2. An emission of sparks or a twinkling, as of stars.

  terrestial s. Scintillation phenomena observed in light from sources within the earth's atmosphere, variously identified as optical haze, atmospheric boil, twinkling, and shimmer.

scirrhencanthus (skir″en-kan′thus). A hard carcinoma of the lacrimal gland.

scirrhoblepharoncus (skir″o-blef′-ah-rong′kus). A hard carcinoma of the eyelid.

sclera (skle′rah). The white, opaque, fibrous, outer tunic of the eyeball, covering it entirely excepting the segment covered anteriorly by the cornea. It is surrounded by the capsule of Tenon and the conjunctiva, to which it is connected by the episclera; its inner, brown, pigmented surface (lamina fusca) forms the outer wall of the suprachoroidal space. It is essentially avascular and contains anterior apertures for the anterior ciliary vessels and the perivascular lymphatics, middle apertures for the venae vorticosae, posterior apertures for the long and the short posterior ciliary vessels and nerves, and a posterior foramen, which is traversed by the lamina cribrosa, for the optic nerve and the retinal vessels. It receives the tendons of insertion of the extraocular muscles and at the corneoscleral junction contains the canal of Schlemm.

  blue s. A sclera which appears bluish, due to the color of the blood and the pigment in the underlying ciliary body and the choroid, and which may occur normally, as in infants, or pathologically, as in Eddowe's disease.

scleral (skle′ral) **flange; radius; ring; spur; sulcus.** See under the nouns.

scleratitis (skle″rah-ti′tis). Scleritis.

sclerectasia (skle″rek-ta′ze-ah). A localized protrusion or outward bulging of the sclera.

sclerectasis (skle-rek′tah-sis). Sclerectasia.

sclerecto-iridectomy (skle-rek″to-ir″-ih-dek′to-me). Surgical removal of a portion of the sclera and of the iris, as for glaucoma.

sclerecto-iridodialysis (skle-rek″to-ir″id-o-di-al′ih-sis). Surgical removal of a portion of the sclera and a localized separation of the iris from its attachment to the ciliary body, as for glaucoma.

sclerectomy (skle-rek′to-me). Surgical removal of a portion of the sclera.

scleriasis (skle-ri′ah-sis). Sclerosis of an eyelid.

scleriritomy (skle″rih-rit′o-me). Incision of the sclera and the iris.

scleritis (skle-ri′tis). Inflammation of the sclera. It may occur in conjunction with an episcleritis, keratitis, uveitis, or tenonitis, or alone.

  annular s. Anterior scleritis which extends entirely around the cornea. The sclera is deeply injected with dark violet vessels and small whitish nodules may appear. Its course is protracted, it is extremely resistant to treatment, and there is an accompanying uveitis and keratitis.

  anterior s. Scleritis of the anterior portion of the eyeball which usually appears as a dark red or bluish swelling. More than one nodular area may appear, and they may fuse with each other.

  brawny s. A chronic, slowly progressive, virulent form of diffuse annular scleritis, occurring more commonly in the elderly, characterized by a gelatinous-appearing swelling of the episcleral tissue around the cornea. The affected area extends backward as the disease progresses, and keratitis and uveitis are an accompaniment. Syn., *gelatinous scleritis*.

gelatinous s. Brawny scleritis.

herpetic s. Herpes zoster involving the sclera, characterized by round nodules covered by glossy, smooth, hyperemic conjunctiva. The condition is painful, remains active for several months, and the lesions gradually heal, leaving permanent, slate-colored scars.

metastatic s. A pyogenic scleritis resulting from the lodgment of a bacterial embolus in a scleral vessel.

s. necroticans. Scleromalacia perforans.

nodular necrotizing s. A localized necrosis of the sclera characterized by the formation of nodules which break down and heal slowly to leave a thin sclera. Syn., *necroscleritis nodosa*.

posterior s. Inflammation of the posterior sclera and Tenon's capsule. It is diagnosed by the presence of ocular pain, edema of the eyelids, slight protrusion and immobility of the eyeball, and chemosis of the conjunctiva. Syn., *sclerotenonitis*.

pyogenic s. Scleritis resulting from the lodgment of a bacterial embolus in a scleral vessel, giving rise to the formation of an abscess.

suppurative s. Pyogenic scleritis.

sclero- (skle″ro-, skler′o-). 1. A combining form denoting *hardness*. 2. A combining form denoting the *sclera* or pertaining to the *sclera*.

sclerocataracta (skle″ro-kat″ah-rak′-tah). Hard cataract.

sclerochoroiditis (skle″ro-ko″roid-i′-tis). Inflammation of both the sclera and the choroid.

posterior s. Sclerochoroiditis occurring in malignant or pathological myopia together with posterior staphyloma.

sclerocleisis (skle″ro-kli′sis). A surgical procedure for glaucoma in which a flap of the sclera, approximately 3 mm wide and 6 mm long, based at the limbus, is inserted into the anterior chamber through an incision just anterior to the base.

scleroconjunctival (skle″ro-kon″junk-ti′val.) Pertaining to both the sclera and the conjunctiva.

scleroconjunctivitis (skle″ro-kon-junk″tih-vi′tis). Inflammation of both the sclera and the conjunctiva.

syphilitic s. A lesion of the secondary stage of syphilis, occurring in the conjunctival and the scleral tissues, characterized by a thickening of these tissues, which have a smooth, moist, waxy appearance like pink coral and are raised above to overlap the corneal margin and occasionally invade the cornea.

sclerocornea (skle″ro-kōr′ne-ah). The sclera and the cornea considered as a single structure.

sclerocorneal (skle″ro-kōr′ne-al). Pertaining to both the sclera and the cornea.

sclerocyclodialysis (skle″ro-si″klo-di-al′ih-sis). Cyclodialysis in which a scleral flap is inserted into the channel formed between the ciliary body and the sclera.

sclero-iridectomy (skle″ro-ir″ih-dek′-to-me). Sclerocleisis combined with a broad iridectomy.

sclero-iridencleisis (skle″ro-ir″ih-den-kli′sis). Sclerocleisis together with a radial incision of the iris and incarceration of the incised portion with the scleral flap.

sclero-iridotasis (skle″ro-ir″ih-dot′ah-sis). Sclerocleisis together with pulling the iris upward, out of the sclerocorneal incision, to be incarcerated with the scleral flap.

sclero-iritis (skle″ro-i-ri′tis). Inflammation of both the sclera and the iris.

sclerokeratitis (skle″ro-ker″ah-ti′tis). Inflammation of both the sclera and the cornea.

sclerokeratoiritis (skle″ro-ker″ah-to-i-ri′tis). Simultaneous inflammation of the sclera, the cornea, and the iris.

scleromalacia (skle″ro-mah-la′she-ah, -se-ah). Degenerative softening of the sclera.

s. perforans. A slowly progressing degeneration of the sclera occurring in the elderly, usually in females and in association with rheumatoid arthritis. It is characterized by localized atrophy and necrosis, without inflammation, resulting in perforation of the sclera. The lesions vary in number, may coalesce, and usually affect the anterior sclera. Syn., *scleritis necroticans*.

scleronyxis (skle″ro-nik′sis). Surgical perforation of the sclera.

sclero-optic (skle″ro-op′tik). Pertaining to both the sclera and the optic nerve.

scleroperikeratitis (skle″ro-per″ih-ker″ah-ti′tis). Inflammation of the sclera and the peripheral cornea.

sclerophthalmia (skle″rof-thal′me-ah). A rare condition in which scleral tissue has encroached on the cornea, leaving only the central area clear.

scleroplasty (skle′ro-plas″te). Plastic surgery of the sclera.

sclerosis, choroidal. Sheathing of choroidal vessels with secondary retinal pigment changes that allow these vessels to be seen with the ophthalmoscope; not related to any generalized vascular disease, and the vessels themselves show very little sclerotic changes.

sclerosis, disseminated (skle-ro′sis). Multiple sclerosis.

sclerosis, multiple (skle-ro′sis). An idiopathic disease in which there are disseminated areas of demyelinization and sclerosis of the spinal cord, the optic nerves, and white and gray matter of the brain. It is characterized by spastic paraplegia, nystagmus, speech defects, and frequently by retrobulbar neuritis, and diplopia due to involvements of the extraocular muscles. Syn., *Charcot's disease; disseminated sclerosis.*

sclerosis, tuberous (skle-ro′sis). Bourneville's disease.

sclerostomy (skle-ros′to-me). Surgical perforation of the sclera, as for the relief of glaucoma.

sclerotenonitis (skle″ro-ten″o-ni′tis). Posterior scleritis.

sclerotic (skle-rot′ik). 1. Pertaining to the outer coat of the eye; the sclera. 2. Hard, indurated, or sclerosed.

   blue s. One who is afflicted with a congenital, hereditary anomaly characterized by light blue sclerae. Fragility of the bones and deafness frequently are found concomitantly.

   s. scatter. See under *scatter.*

sclerotica (skle-rot′ih-kah). Sclera.

scleroticectomy (skle-rot″ih-sek′to-me). Surgical removal of a portion of the sclera.

sclerotico. (skle-rot′ih-ko-). For words beginning thus, see *sclero-.*

sclerotitis (skle″ro-ti′tis). Scleritis.

sclerotomy (skle-rot′o-me). Surgical incision of the sclera.

   anterior s. Surgical incision through the sclera into the anterior chamber of the eye, as for glaucoma.

   posterior s. Surgical incision through the sclera into the vitreous chamber of the eye.

sclerotonyxis (skle″ro-to-nik′sis). An obsolete operation for cataract in which the crystalline lens is depressed into the vitreous humor by a broad needle introduced through the sclera.

sclero-uveitis (skle″ro-u″ve-i′tis). Inflammation of both the sclera and uvea.

scopolamine (sko-pol′ah-min, sko″-po-lam′in). Hyoscine.

scoterythrous (sko″teh-rith′rus). Protanopic. *Obs.*

scotodinia (sko″to-din′e-ah). Vertigo and headache with a dimming of vision or black spots before the eyes.

◆

SCOTOMA

scotoma (sko-to′mah). An isolated area of absent vision or depressed sensitivity in the visual field, surrounded by an area of normal vision or of less depressed sensitivity.

   absolute s. A scotoma in which vision is entirely absent, i.e., light perception is not present.

   annular s. A circular scotoma, either a partial or complete ring, characteristically around the fixation area in the visual field.

   arcuate s. A scotoma which arches from the normal blind spot into the nasal field and follows the course of the retinal nerve fibers. A double arcuate scotoma extending both inferiorly and superiorly from the blind spot may form a ring scotoma. Syn., *comet scotoma; scimitar scotoma.*

   Bjerrum's s. A comet-shaped, arcuate scotoma, occurring in glaucoma, which extends from the superior or the inferior margin of the physiological blind spot into the nasal field, around the fixation area. It is usually located between the 10° and 20° circles and becomes wider as it leaves the blind spot.

   cecocentral s. A scotoma involving the physiological blind spot, the area corresponding to the macula lutea, and the area between. Syn., *centrocecal scotoma.*

   central s. A scotoma involving the area of the visual field corresponding to the macula lutea.

   centrocecal s. Cecocentral scotoma.

   color s. An area in the visual field for which color vision is absent or deficient.

   comet s. Arcuate scotoma.

congruous scotomata. Scotomata of equal size, shape, and intensity in both eyes and homonymous in position so that they superimpose in the binocular visual field.

cuneate s. A wedge-shaped scotoma which characteristically extends from the physiological blind spot into the temporal visual field with its apex toward the blind spot.

eclipse s. A small central scotoma resulting from observation of an eclipse of the sun without adequate protection.

facultative s. A scotoma considered to be due to suppression.

false s. A scotoma due to opacities obstructing the light from the retina, as in disease of, or hemorrhage into, the ocular media.

fleeting s. Wandering scotoma.

flimmer s. Scintillating scotoma.

flittering s. Scintillating scotoma.

Förster's ring s. A ring-shaped scotoma around the fixation area due to involvement of the nerve fiber layer of the retina in the acute stage of syphilitic chorioretinitis.

hemianopic s. A scotoma involving half of the central visual field. Cf. *hemianopsia.*

van der Hoeve's s. Enlargement of the physiological blind spot attributed to paranasal sinusitis. Syn., *van der Hoeve's sign.*

incongruous scotomata. Scotomata in both eyes of unequal size, shape, or intensity, but homonymous in position.

junction s. A defect in the visual field due to a lesion at the junction of the optic nerve with the chiasm, in the region where the nasal fibers of the contralateral optic nerve loop into the ipsilateral optic nerve before coursing into the body of the chiasm. Characteristically, it is manifested either as a superior temporal quadrantanopsia or as a temporal hemianopic scotoma in the field of the contralateral eye, usually in association with a defect in the peripheral field of the ipsilateral eye.

juxtacecal s. A scotoma adjacent to the physiological blind spot. Syn., *paracecal scotoma.*

motile s. A false scotoma of varying location due to a floating opacity of the vitreous humor.

negative s. A scotoma not perceived as such by the afflicted, i.e., one of which he is not aware except on demonstration of absence of vision in the involved area.

paracecal s. Juxtacecal scotoma.

paracentral s. A scotoma adjacent to the area corresponding to the macula lutea.

pericecal s. A scotoma surrounding the physiological blind spot. Syn., *peripapillary scotoma.*

pericentral s. A scotoma surrounding the area corresponding to the macula lutea. Syn., *perimacular scotoma.*

perimacular s. Pericentral scotoma.

peripapillary s. Pericecal scotoma.

peripheral s. A scotoma which does not involve the central or the fixation area.

physiological s. A negative scotoma corresponding to the site of the optic disk; the blind spot of Mariotte.

positive s. A scotoma directly perceivable by the afflicted, i.e., one of which he is continuously aware without proof of absence of vision in the involved area, usually seen entoptically as a black or a gray area.

quadrantic s. A scotoma involving the apex of one quadrant of the visual field.

relative s. 1. A scotoma of depressed sensitivity, or one blind to certain types and intensities of visual stimuli but not to others. 2. An area of depressed sensitivity in the visual field in which one or more colors cannot be recognized but in which achromatic stimuli are seen.

ring s. A circular scotoma around the fixation area in the visual field. It may be formed by two arcuate scotomata extending superiorly and inferiorly from the physiological blind spot.

roving ring s. A circular restriction in the peripheral field of view, due to the prismatic effect at the edge of a strong convex spectacle lens, which expands upon eye movement away from the center of the lens.

scimitar s. Arcuate scotoma.

scintillating s. A transient, shimmering, peripherally expanding scotoma with brightly colored, serrated edges which usually occurs as a prodromal symptom of migraine. Syn., *flimmer scotoma; flittering scotoma; spectrum scotoma.* See also *fortification spectrum.*

Seidel's s. A sickle-shaped scotoma appearing as an upward or downward prolongation of the physiological blind spot, found in glaucoma.

space s. In space physiology, the portion of visual space traversed by flight motion between the presentation and the perceptual awareness of a visual stimulus.

spectrum s. Scintillating scotoma.

suppression s. A unilateral scotoma found only when testing under binocular conditions, i.e., not present monocularly.

wandering s. A scotoma which changes its shape, position, size, or intensity in a relatively short period of time. Syn., *fleeting scotoma.*

zonular s. A curved scotoma which does not emerge from the blind spot and does not follow the lines of the nerve fibers. Its concavity is always toward the fixation area, it may occupy any part of the visual field, and is considered to be vascular in origin.

◆

scotomagraph (sko-to'mah-graf). An instrument for recording the size, the shape, and the position of a scotoma.

scotomameter (sko"to-mam'eh-ter). Scotometer.

scotomata (sko-to'mah-tah). Plural of *scotoma.*

scotomatous (sko-tom'ah-tus). Pertaining to or affected with a scotoma.

scotometer (sko-tom'eh-ter). An instrument such as a tangent screen, a perimeter, or a stereocampimeter, for detecting, measuring, and plotting scotomata.

Bjerrum's s. Tangent screen.

Elliot's s. A large black disk rotatable about a central fixation object with a movable, white, test bead on a black cord extending from center to periphery, used for plotting scotomata.

Fincham-Sutcliffe s. A visual field screening instrument consisting of a square tangent surface at one meter from the subject and extending 25° in each lateral and vertical direction on which assorted patterns of several small transilluminated spots may be flashed or displayed continuously. The

subject's failure to report the correct number of spots in each pattern is indicative of a scotoma.

Juler s. A device for projecting a circular patch of light of various diameters and colors onto a tangent screen to serve as a test target in plotting visual field defects.

scotometry (sko-tom'eh-tre). The detecting and plotting of scotomata with a scotometer.

scotopia (sko-to'pe-ah). Scotopic vision.

scotopic (sko-top'ik). Having the characteristics of scotopic vision or referring to the levels of illumination at which the eye is dark adapted.

scotopsins (sko-top'sinz). The photopigments in the retinal rods. Cf. *photopsins.*

scotoscopy (sko-tos'ko-pe). Retinoscopy.

scotosis (sko-to'sis). Scotoma.

scototaxis (sko-to-tak'sis). A purposive movement of a motile organism toward darkness and away from light; a negative phototaxis.

Scottish Association of Opticians. An association of Scottish ophthalmic opticians founded some 50 years ago to represent its members' professional interests, including the giving of qualifying examinations to candidates.

screen. A material, such as cloth, which affords a surface for receiving projected images or for plotting the visual fields.

apodizing s. An aperture of suitable shape and with non-uniform absorption which is placed in an optical system to reduce the intensity of, or eliminate, the peripheral portions of a diffraction pattern.

Bjerrum's s. Tangent screen.

Duane's s. A dull black tangent screen with small, light source, fixation targets placed in several positions on it, used to test the state of motility of the extraocular muscles in various directions of gaze. The test is performed in a darkened room with a red lens before one eye to create diplopia for the fixated light source. The patient locates with a pointer the positions of the diplopic images for each direction of gaze, first with one eye fixating, and then with the other eye fixating.

Hartmann s. A diaphragm consisting of a series of small holes, usually lying in a single meridian, which is used in the Hartmann test (q.v.) to confine the light striking the optical system to a series of narrow beams.

Hess s. A black cloth tangent screen for testing extraocular muscle function, calibrated both horizontally and vertically into 5° intervals by red lines, with red dots at the intersections of the 0°, 15°, and 30° lines. Two of three radially oriented, short, green threads of common origin are continuous with two black thread extensions leading to counterbalances attached to the upper corners of the screen. The patient, while wearing a red lens in front of one eye and a green lens in front of the other, attempts to superimpose the common origin of the green threads on each of the 25 red dots by means of a pointer attached to the third green thread.

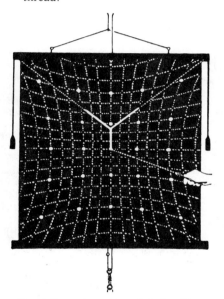

Fig. 32 Hess screen. (From S. Duke-Elder, *Textbook of Ophthalmology*, vol. 4. London: Henry Kimpton, 1949)

tangent s. A large plane surface of black cloth or other material mounted so as to be perpendicular to the straightforward direction of view of the subject and at a convenient distance, usually 1 m, and typically calibrated in degrees of subtense from the eye with reference to a central point of fixation. It is used for plotting the physiological blind spot, scotomata, and other visual and fixational field restrictions. Syn., *Bjerrum's scotometer; Bjerrum's screen.* **Auto-Plot t.s.** The trade name of a scotometer which projects a movable illuminated test spot on a gray tangent screen at one meter and instantly records the position on a paper chart.

screener, Harrington-Flocks visual field. A visual field screening instrument having a series of 20 large spiral-bound cards on which are printed patterns of dots and crosses visible only when illuminated under ultraviolet radiation. A chin rest, occluder, rack to support the targets, and an automatic timer for a one-quarter second flash exposure are provided. The serial presentation of the 20 card patterns systematically tests the integrity of all major sectors of the visual field.

screw tap. A device for rethreading the screw receptacles in ophthalmic frames or mountings.

S.D.O.N.Z. State Diploma in Optometry, New Zealand.

seam, pigment. The fringe of pigment epithelium at the pupillary margin of the iris. Syn., *pupillary ruff.*

seborrhea nigricans (seb"o-re'ah ni'-grih-kans). Seborrhea of the eyelids and adjacent skin in which they appear greasy and dark colored.

sebum palpebrale (se'bum pal"pe-brah'le). The secretion of the Meibomian glands of the eyelids.

seclusio pupillae (se-kloo'se-o pu'-pil-e). A complete blocking of the anterior chamber from the posterior chamber by a posterior annular synechia.

section, optic. In slit lamp biomicroscopy, the sagittal section of tissue illuminated by a very narrow focused beam of the slit lamp for the observation and localization of structural defects.

section, principal. A section lying in a plane perpendicular to the refracting edge of a prism.

sector defect. See under *defect.*

secundochrome (se-kun'do-krōm). Weale's term for *erythrolabe.*

see. 1. To perceive by the sense of sight. 2. To behold, as if with the eye, in imagination, dreams, hallucinations, or illusions. 3. To discern.

seeing. The using, or the act of using, the sense of sight; vision; sight; having the faculty of sight.

Seeligmueller's sign (za'lik-mil"erz). See under *sign.*

seg. Abbreviation for *segment,* as of a bifocal.

Ségal's hypothesis (sa-gahlz'). See under *hypothesis.*

segment. Any of the parts or portions into which an object is divided, naturally separated, or demarcated.

accessory outer s. of Engström. A ciliumlike structure lying beside the outer member of a visual receptor cell and originating from basal granules at the distal end of the inner member.

bifocal s. The smaller of the two dioptrically different portions of a bifocal lens.

inner s. (of a rod or cone). Inner member (of a rod or cone).

outer s. (of a rod or cone). Outer member (of a rod or cone).

Seidel's (si'delz) **formulas; scotoma; sign; test.** See under the nouns.

Seitz chart (sītz). See under *chart*.

Selectachart. The trade name for an attachment to an American Optical Co. acuity projector which permits remote control selection of target content.

selective cancellation. See under *cancellation*.

self-light. Idioretinal light.

sella turcica (sel'ah tur'sih-kah). The upper surface of the body of the sphenoid bone. On rare occasions the optic chiasm rests in its optic groove.

semichrome, Ostwald (sem'ih-krōm). An ideal Ostwald color having zero black content and zero white content, hence having a full color content of unity; thus a surface color with the maximum colorfulness which is theoretically possible. In terms of the theoretical ideal surface of the Ostwald system, this would be achieved by (1) complete absorption below a wavelength which has no spectral complement and complete reflectance for longer wavelengths, or vice versa, or (2) complete absorption in a band extending from one wavelength to its complementary wavelength and complete reflection of wavelengths outside this band, or vice versa. Syn., *full color*.

senopia (se-no'pe-ah). Unexpected, unaided improvement of vision, especially of near vision in the aged, regarded as a sign of incipient cataract. Syn., *gerontopia; second sight*.

sensation. 1. The apprehension of features of the external environment or bodily condition through the mediation of sense organs. 2. The afferent output of any sense organ. 3. Perception.

accommodative s. A sensation which indicates changes in ocular accommodation. A sensory attribute of the act of accommodating.

after s. 1. Afterimage. 2. A sensation lasting or occurring after the exciting stimulus has ceased to operate.

autokinetic s. The sensation of apparent motion of a fixated stationary object, as occurs in the autokinetic visual illusion.

color s. A visual sensation exhibiting hue, usually dependent on the selective use of portions of the spectrum as stimuli.

glass s. A visual sensation of a transparent solid which appears different from empty space, i.e., as if filled with substance.

light s. Any sensation whose proper stimulus is radiant energy between about 380 and 760 mμ, and mediated by the eye.

psychovisual s. A sensation having the perceived attributes of visual sensation but not mediated by the retinal cells.

visual s. A sensation produced by the sense of sight. **toned v.s.** A visual sensation evoked by stimulation with a chromatic color. **untoned v.s.** A visual sensation evoked by stimulation with an achromatic color.

sense. 1. Any of the faculties by which some aspect of the environment, or of body condition, may be apprehended, as that of sight, hearing, touch, smell, taste, hunger, or thirst. 2. The experiences or other end reactions from stimulation of sensory faculties. 3. To apprehend some aspect of the environment, or some bodily condition, through the use of a sense organ.

color s. The faculty by which hues are perceived and distinguished.

s. of direction. The faculty enabling the orienting of each of the various object points in external space to some direction in the visual field, either in reference to the self or to other object points.

discriminations s. 1. The faculty by which slightly separated objects in space are perceived as separate; the resolving power of the eye. 2. The faculty by which slightly differing stimuli are perceived as different, such as distinguishing between nearly equal spectral wavelengths.

distance s. The faculty of appreciating the spatial separation between the self and objects in the visual field or between two objects in the visual field. Cf. *stereopsis.*

form s. The faculty enabling one to distinguish the shapes of objects in the visual field.

fusion s. 1. The faculty of perceiving with the two eyes a single, integrated, fused image of a pair of haploscopically presented objects or an object viewed binocularly. 2. The faculty of perceiving continuously uniform light when the stimulus is intermittent.

light s. The faculty by which light (approximately 380 to 760 mμ) is perceived and by which gradations in its intensity are appreciated.

position s. The faculty enabling one to localize each of the various object points in external space either in reference to the self or to other object points. Syn., *space sense.*

space s. Position sense.

stereognostic s. The faculty by which objects in the visual field are perceived as solid, i.e., having three dimensions.

sensibilitometer, corneal. An instrument for determining the sensitivity thresholds of the cornea for touch, pain, or friction.

corneal s., Boberg-Ans. A device consisting of a nylon thread mounted in a handle such that its exposed length may be varied. Corneal sensitivity is measured by the greatest thread length which, when pressed against the cornea, causes a just noticeable sensation of pain.

sensitivity. 1. The capability of responding to stimulation or to receive sensations therefrom. 2. In psychophysical measurements, the reciprocal of the threshold.

contrast s. The ability to detect border contrast; the reciprocal of the minimum perceptible contrast. **relative c.s.** A percentage value of contrast sensitivity expressed relative to that obtained under a very high level of diffuse task illumination such as of 10,000 cd/m². Abbreviation RCS.

spectral s. The reciprocal of the radiant energy at each of various wavelengths, as represented by a curve or locus of points, which elicits a visual or photic response equal to that for a given reference standard, such as for illuminant C.

sensitometer (sen"sih-tom'eh-ter). An instrument for measuring sensitivity, as of the human eye.

Abney's s. Abney's colorimeter.

Luckiesh-Moss ophthalmic s. An instrument using brightness contrast threshold instead of acuity threshold for the subjective determination of the dioptric power producing maximum visibility. It consists essentially of a pair of neutral, graded density filters, one in front of each eye, a white target containing a vaguely defined vertical band of diffused light with a central gap in which a small, horizontal, black line is located. While the vertical band serves as a binocular fusion stimulus, a +2.50 D cylinder, axis horizontal, is placed before one eye to obliterate the horizontal black line, and the neutral filters are rotated before the eyes until the black horizontal line is just visible. Lenses of various power are placed before the other eye until the lens power is found which provides visibility of the test target through the greatest filter density.

sensitometry (sen"sih-tom'eh-tre). Determination of the ophthalmic lens correction producing the best scores on the Luckiesh-Moss ophthalmic sensitometer.

sensory-motor. Pertaining to the integration of both afferent and efferent pathway systems, as in binocular fusion.

separation difficulty. See under *difficulty.*

separation, reduced. Reduced distance.

separation, retinal. Separation of the retina from its pigment epithelium layer, commonly called *detachment of the retina.*

Separation Trainer. An instrument for the diagnosis and treatment of the crowding phenomenon in amblyopia ex anopsia, consisting of 25 randomly orientated letter Es mounted in radial tracks on a flat vertical surface in a square formation, the distance between the Es being varied by a lever on the side of the instrument.

separator (sep'ah-ra"tor). An instrument for separating the fields of vision of the eyes.

Hunt s. An instrument consisting of a drawing board divided by a perpendicularly mounted septum. The forehead is rested on the septum edge so that the field of vision of the two eyes is separated, a line drawing is placed on one side of the septum, and an attempt is made to copy it on the other side.

Rémy s. An instrument consisting of a vertical septum, with a handle below, which is attached to and bisects a target holder at one end. The other end of the septum is placed on the nose so that a target on either side of the septum is seen by only one eye and an attempt is made to fuse or superimpose them by voluntary effort.

septum (sep'tum). A dividing wall or partition, especially one which separates tissue, fluids, or two cavities.

s. orbitale. A thin membrane, containing collagenous and elastic fibers, which is attached to the arcus marginale at the orbital margin and extends to the tarsus of the upper and the lower eyelids. In the upper eyelid it fuses with the sheath of the levator palpebrae superioris muscle. Syn., *lid aponeurosis; palpebral fascia; tarso-orbital fascia; tarso-orbital ligament; orbital septum.*

psychological s. Foveal suppression of an eye by means of a filter or lens with maintenance of peripheral vision in order to keep the eyes in binocular alignment during the testing of the other eye. See also *Humphriss method.*

retinal s., congenital. A congenital condition characterized by gross folds or ridges of undifferentiated neural elements of the retina which arise from the optic disk and project into the vitreous. It is considered to arise from the inner layer of the embryonic optic cup and most often occupies the lower temporal quadrant of the retina. Syn., *ablatio falciformis congenita; congenital retinal fold.*

sequencing, visual motor. To remember a visual sequence, e.g., to string beads according to a specific pattern or to reproduce a pattern from memory.

serial reproduction. A visual training procedure in which a line drawing is flashed onto a screen and an attempt is made to reproduce the pattern. The procedure is repeated a number of times, and each time an attempt is made to improve without referring to the previous drawings.

series. A group of happenings or things in succeeding or progressing order.

Fourier's s. The components of a complex periodic wave form as resolved by Fourier's analysis.

light clear s. In the Ostwald system, a series of surface color samples of decreasing purity and increasing luminous reflectance which are arranged along the upper side of the Ostwald triangle.

shadow s. In the Ostwald system, a series of surface color samples of approximately equal dominant wavelength and nearly constant purity, varying in luminous reflectance only, and arranged vertically in the Ostwald triangle, parallel to the gray series. Syn., *isochromes.*

set, trial. An assortment of spherical, cylindrical, and prismatic lenses and variously perforated disks mounted in circular rims with tab handles on which are engraved the dioptric designations, systematically arranged in a slotted container, a trial case, for convenient ophthalmic use.

Sézary syndrome. See under *syndrome.*

Sforzini syndrome. See under *syndrome.*

shade. 1. A device used to diminish or intercept light from a lamp or other source to prevent full illumination in certain directions from the source. 2. The relative darkness of that side of an object which is turned away from a source of light, as distinguished from the shadow cast by the object. 3. Shadow, or the dimness or the relative darkness of, or within, a shadow. 4. A general term often used to designate a color not greatly different from another particular color. A gradation of color, or a slight variation of a color from a reference standard. 5. A mixture of black with a color. Thus, the antonym of *tint.* 6. Any color darker than median gray. 7. A term descriptive of a difference in hue only, as, "a redder shade than orange." 8. A variation in saturation or chroma only, when hue and lightness remain constant, as, "a paler shade of blue." Thus, synonymous with *tint.* 9. A variation in the lightness or brightness of a color. A darker shade of a color is one that has the same hue and saturation but a lower lightness. 10. A general term often used as a synonym for *color.* 11. To shield from light. To dim illumination by partially blocking light, as with a screen. 12. To create shadows. 13. To tone a drawing by increasing the thickness or the darkness of certain lines or portions of outlines. 14. To blend, as from one color to another.

Shado-Spector (shad'o-spek-tor). The trade name for an instrument that projects a 50× magnified image of a contact lens onto a calibrated viewing screen for the purpose of inspection.

Shado-Spectorette (shad'o-spek-to-ret"). The trade name for an instrument that projects a 25× magnified image of a contact lens onto a calibrated viewing screen for the purpose of inspection.

shadow. An obscure or darkened area from which rays from a source of light are cut off by an interposed opaque body.

> **Bowman's s.** The dark appearance, when viewed in profile, of the portion of the cornea which has become conical in advanced keratoconus.

> **color s's.** Shadows cast on a neutral screen by an opaque body from two equidistant light sources of equal intensity, one white and the other colored. The shadow cast by the white light appears to be the color of the colored light and the shadow cast by the colored light appears to be its complement.

> **iris s.** A shadow cast by the iris on the crystalline lens in oblique illumination, used as a guide to the depth of opacity in the lens. When the shadow on a cataractous lens can no longer be seen, the cataract is considered to be ripe.

> **Purkinje's s's.** Purkinje's figures.

> **scissors s.** Scissors movement of the retinoscopic reflex.

shadowgraph (shad'o-graf). The shadow of an object cast on a screen or photographically recorded, especially to display or measure profile features of the object, as, for example, the asphericity of a corneal mold.

shadowscope (shad'o-skōp). An instrument consisting essentially of an intense light source which is passed through a small aperture, transilluminating a lens positioned before it, and casting a shadow of the lens onto a screen for the purpose of inspection of the lens.

Shadowscope Reading Pacer. The trade name for an instrument used in improving reading speed and comprehension in which a rectangular band of light illuminates the material to be read, moving down over the reading material at a preset speed and thus setting a pace for the reader.

Shaffer system. See under *system*.

shagreen of the crystalline lens (shah-grēn'). The granular leatherlike

(shagreen leather) or pounded metal appearance of the anterior and posterior surface of the capsule of the crystalline lens when viewed with the biomicroscope under specularly reflected light.

shank. On a spectacle frame, that part of a metal saddle bridge connecting the strap or the eyewire to the crest of the bridge.

Shaxby's theory (shaks'bēz). See under *theory*.

Sheard's (shērdz) **chart; criterion; method.** See under the nouns.

sheath. A covering and/or supporting structure, usually one of connective tissue.

> **arachnoidean s.** The middle of the three meninges that cover the middle and the distal portions of the optic nerve. It consists of collagenous fibers and endothelium and connects through the subdural space with the dural sheath and by way of trabeculae through the larger subarachnoid space with the pial sheath.

> **dural s.** The outer of the three meninges that cover the optic nerve; blends with the sclera. It contains a thick collection of collagenous fibers, is lined with endothelium, and forms a tough protective layer around the nerve.

> **fascial s. of eyeball.** Capsule of Tenon.

> **glial s.** A sheath of neuroglial cells that protrudes from the optic disk of the fetus and encircles the proximal third of the hyaloid artery. It is an extension of Bergmeister's papilla and degenerates as the physiological cup is formed.

> **pial s.** The inner of the three meninges that cover the optic nerve. It is lined with the glial mantle, contains elastic and collagenous fibers, and carries capillaries into the nerve.

sheathing of retinal vessels. The appearance of white lines along the walls of the retinal blood vessels (*parallel sheathing*) or in extreme instances the appearance of the entire vessel as a white fibrous cord (*pipe-stem sheathing*). It may occur in normal and youthful eyes on or near the optic disk or, in conditions of sclerosis, first at arteriovenous crossings and may progress to pipe-stem sheathing.

shell. An outside covering, exterior, husk, or any similar hollow, usually frail, structure.

cosmetic s. A plastic shell placed over a disfigured eye and colored with opaque dyes to conceal the disfigurement and match the color of the fellow eye. It may have a clear or opaque scleral portion and does not possess any optical properties.

image s. The curved surface containing either all the sagittal, or all the tangential, foci of a homocentric bundle of rays obliquely incident upon an optical system containing spherical surfaces.

molding s. A shell of plastic, glass, or hard rubber, used to hold molding material while taking an impression or mold of the anterior segment of an eye in contact lens fitting. It consists of a small cup, curved to conform approximately to the anterior segment of the eye, is usually perforated, and often has a small handle affixed to the center of its convex side.

Walser s. A thin plastic shell, resembling the scleral portion of a scleral contact lens, which is placed on the bulbar conjunctiva to separate it from the palpebral conjunctiva to promote healing and to prevent adhesions of wounds, such as from burns.

shelves, lens. The intercellular cement substance in the Y-sutures of the crystalline lens or in the more complex lens stars which receive the ends of lens fibers.

Sheridan-Gardiner test type. See under *type, test.*

Sherrington's (sher'ing-tonz) **disk; experiment; law; theory.** See under the nouns.

shield, Buller's. A watch glass in a frame of adhesive tape secured over the nonaffected eye to protect it from infection from the other eye.

shield, eye. 1. A covering for the eye to protect it from light, infection, or injury. 2. An occluder.

shift, adaptive color. A change in perceived color due to chromatic adaptation.

shift, adjustment. A type of binocular vision present in some strabismics with harmonious, anomalous, retinal correspondence in which the perceived binocular field of vision is made up of portions of each uniocular field of vision. (Brock)

shift, Einstein. A slight shift of spectral lines of very dense stars toward red, explained by relativity theory in terms of a highly gravitational field.

shift, Purkinje's. Purkinje's phenomenon.

shift, red. A displacement toward longer wavelengths of spectral lines produced by an increasing distance between a light source and an observer. In astrophysics it is employed to determine rate of recession of celestial bodies. Syn., *Hubble effect.*

shimmer. See *laurence.*

shoe. The part of a rimless spectacle bridge or endpiece which rests against the edge of the lens.

short pointing. See under *pointing.*

shortsightedness. Myopia.

shoulder. The transitional zone between the corneal and the scleral sections on the inner surface of a scleral contact lens.

shoulder tipping. A tilting of the head toward one shoulder, especially as a clinical symptom.

shrinkage, essential, of the conjunctiva. Ocular pemphigus.

Shtremel's test (shtrem'elz). See under *test.*

shutter, electro-optic. A device which provides a nonmechanical method of interrupting or modulating a light beam. It consists of a Kerr cell placed between crossed polarizing filters and transmits light only when subjected to an electric field.

shutter, Kerr. See *electro-optic shutter.*

Shy-Drager syndrome. See under *syndrome.*

Sichel's ptosis. Ptosis adiposa.

siderophone (sid'er-o-fōn"). An instrument for detecting and locating iron particles in the eyeball by the electrical production of sound.

sideroscope (sid'er-o-skōp"). An instrument for detecting and locating iron particles in the eyeball.

sideroscopy (sid"er-os'ko-pe). The detection and location of iron particles in the eyeball.

siderosis (sid"er-o'sis). A deposit of iron in a tissue.

s. bulbi. Pigmentary and degenerative changes in the eyeball resulting from the prolonged presence of an iron foreign body in the ocular tissue. The changes may be localized to the immediate vicinity of the foreign particle, or they may be generalized and occur throughout the ocular structures. The typical clinical picture includes a rusty discoloration, together with the pigmentary and degenerative changes.

s. conjunctivae. Rusty discoloration in the conjunctiva and the sclera resulting from the prolonged presence of an iron foreign body.

siderostat. A mirror automatically rotated in synchrony with the earth's movements so that it reflects light from a star constantly in a chosen direction such as in the optical path of a stationary telescope. See also *coelostat.*

Siegrist's (se'grists) **spots; streaks.** See under the nouns.

Siemens' star (se'menz). See under *star.*

Siezel-Fusor. The trade name for a home training device utilizing the anaglyph principle to eliminate suppression, consisting of a special checkerboard with blue and black squares, reversible red and blue filters, and three sets of various-sized red and black checkers. The red and black checkers, but not the squares, can be seen through the red filter. The squares can be seen through the blue filter, with all the checkers appearing black.

sight. 1. The special sense by which objects, their form, color, position, etc., in the external environment are perceived, the exciting stimulus being light from the objects striking the retina of the eye; the act, function, process, or power of seeing; vision. 2. That which is seen. 3. A device to aid the eye in aiming. 4. To look at; to see. 5. To aim with the aid of a sight.

aging s. The lay term for presbyopia.

day s. Vision in higher levels of illumination, implying reduced vision in lower levels, or night blindness.

far s. Hypermetropia.

line of s. See under *line.*

long s. The lay term for hypermetropia.

near s. Myopia.

night s. Vision in lower levels of illumination, implying reduced or less than normal vision in higher levels, or day blindness.

old s. The lay term for presbyopia.

second s. Unexpected, unaided improvement of near vision in the elderly, resulting from senile sclerosis of the nucleus of the crystalline lens with a relative increase of its optical density. Syn., *gerontopia; senopia.*

short s. The lay term for myopia.

weak s. The lay term for reduced visual acuity or for asthenopia.

Sight Screener, American Optical. A Brewster-type stereoscopic instrument for visual screening, with targets for measuring visual acuity, phorias, stereopsis, and color perception.

◆

SIGN

sign. Objective evidence of a disease. See also *phenomenon; reflex; symptom; syndrome.*

Abadie's s. A spasm of the levator palpebrae superioris muscle in exophthalmic goiter.

Argyll Robertson's s. The Argyll Robertson pupil, indicating syphilis of the central nervous system.

Arlt's s. A triangular, base down, array of fine pigmented keratic precipitates on the endothelium of the inferior cornea, usually with a clear area between it and the limbus and indicative of low grade uveitis. Syn., *Arlt's triangle.*

Arroyo's s. Asthenocoria, as seen in hypoadrenia.

Aschner's s. The oculocardiac reflex, indicating cardiac vagus irritability.

Baillarger's s. Unequal size of the pupils in syphilitic meningoencephalitis.

Ballet's s. Partial or complete external ophthalmoplegia without internal ophthalmoplegia in exophthalmic goiter.

Bard's s. Increase of the oscillations of the eye in organic nystagmus in reflexly fixating a moving target and cessation of the oscillations under the same conditions in congenital nystagmus, as described by Bard.

Barré's s. Retarded contraction of the iris in mental deterioration.

Bechterew-Mendel s. Mendel-Bechterew sign.

Becker's s. Pulsation of the retinal arteries in exophthalmic goiter.

Behr's s. Paralysis of upward gaze associated with loss of the pupillary reflex to light, with slightly dilated pupils and with retention of convergence, considered to be due to a lesion of the midbrain. Syn., *hemianoptic tract sign.*

Bell's s. Outward and upward rotation of the eyeball on the affected side on attempt to close the eyelids in Bell's palsy. Syn., *Bordier-Fränkel sign.*

Berger's s. An elliptical or irregularly shaped pupil in the early stages of syphilis of the central nervous system.

Bielschowsky's s. Involuntary upward rotation of an eye when the head is forcibly tilted toward the shoulder on the same side as the eye, indicating a paretic superior oblique muscle of that eye.

Bjerrum's s. A comet-shaped, arcuate scotoma which extends from the superior or the inferior margin of the physiological blind spot into the nasal field, around the fixation area, indicating glaucoma. It is usually located between the 10° and 20° circles and becomes wider as it leaves the blind spot.

Bordier-Fränkel s. Bell's sign.

Boston's s. Spasmodic lowering of the upper eyelid on downward rotation of the eye, indicating exophthalmic goiter.

bowed head s. Gould's sign.

Cantelli's s. Doll's head phenomenon.

Cestan's s. Dutemps and Cestan sign.

Chvostek's s. A spasm of the facial muscles, including the orbicularis oculi, elicited by tapping the terminus of the seventh nerve in front of the ear, indicating tetany, hysteria, or chlorosis.

Cogan's lid twitch s. Twitching of a ptotic eyelid, a sign of myasthenia gravis.

Collet's s. The opening of the lid of one eye more quickly and more widely than the other on rapid, repeated, effortless opening and closing of the eyelids, indicating beginning paralysis of the orbicularis oculi muscle of that eye.

Collier's s. Mild retraction of the eyelids tending to give an appearance of cheerfulness and alertness, indicative of a diencephalic neoplasm.

conjunctival s. Multiple, isolated, saccular dilations of capillaries in the bulbar conjunctiva, seen with the slit lamp biomicroscope and attributed to vascular stasis, an indication of sickle-cell disease.

Cowen's s. A jerky, consensual, pupillary reflex to light in exophthalmic goiter.

Crichton-Browne s. Twitching of the outer corners of the eyes and the lips indicating syphilitic meningoencephalitis.

Crowe's s. Bilateral engorgement of the retinal veins on compression of the jugular vein on the healthy side, an indication of unilateral cavernous sinus thrombosis.

Dalrymple's s. Abnormal wideness of the palpebral fissures in exophthalmic goiter.

digito-ocular s. Pressing of the fingers or fist into the orbit by an infant, a sign of Leber's congenital amaurosis.

Dixon Mann's s. Mann's sign.

doll's eye s. Doll's head phenomenon.

Dutemps and Cestan s. A slight upward movement of the upper eyelid of one eye on attempted slow closure of the eyelids while looking straight ahead, indicating involvement of the orbicularis oculi muscle of that eye in peripheral facial paralysis.

Elliot's s. A jagged, irregular extension of the margin of the physiological blind spot, as plotted with an Elliot scotometer, consisting of several isolated scotomata, indicating glaucoma.

Enroth's s. Edematous swelling of the eyelids, especially the upper eyelids near the supraorbital margin, in exophthalmic goiter.

Flatau's s. Rapid mydriasis on gentle irritation of the skin, such as a scratch by the fingernail, in epidemic cerebrospinal meningitis.

Fodéré's s. Edema of the lower eyelids, indicating kidney malfunction.

Franceschetti's digital-ocular s. Franceschetti's digital-ocular symptom.

Froment's s. On closure of the eyelids while looking upward, one eye is closed imperfectly, indicating beginning paralysis of the orbicularis oculi muscle of that eye.

Gianelli's s. Tournay's pupillary reflex.

Gifford's s. Difficulty of eversion of the upper eyelid in exophthalmic goiter.

Goppert's s. Mydriasis produced on passive stretching of the neck muscles by bending the head backward, in epidemic cerebrospinal meningitis.

Gould's s. Turning of the head downward in walking to bring the image of the ground on the functioning portion of the retina, in destructive disease of the peripheral retina. Syn., *bowed head sign.*

von Graefe's s. Immobility or lagging of the upper eyelid on downward rotation of the eye, indicating exophthalmic goiter.

Griffith's s. Lag of the lower eyelid on upward gaze in exophthalmic goiter.

Guiat's s. Tortuousity of the retinal venules, an early indication of retinal arteriolar sclerosis.

Guist's s. Tortuosity of the retinal veins, especially of the smaller venules, an early sign of arteriosclerosis.

Gunn's crossing s. The compression of a retinal venule into the tissue of the retina, where it is crossed by an overlying arteriole so that it appears tapered and/or disconnected; one of the signs of hypertensive and/or arteriolosclerotic retinopathy. Syn., *Gunn's arteriovenous phenomenon.*

Gunn's jaw-winking s. Jaw-winking.

Gunn's pupillary s. Gunn's pupillary phenomenon.

Haab's s. Haab's pupillary reflex.

Haenel's s. Decrease in the sensation of pain on firm tactile pressure on the eyeball in tabes dorsalis.

hemianoptic tract s. Behr's sign.

Hensy's s. Orbicularis sign.

de Hertogh's s. Absence of the lateral portion of the eyebrows, occurring in certain hereditary anomalies of the skin.

Hertwig-Magendie s. Magendie-Hertwig sign.

van der Hoeve's s. Enlargement of the physiological blind spot in paranasal sinusitis.

Hughlings-Jackson s. The dilation of the pupil in response to cocaine, indicating that a drooping eyelid is levator rather than sympathetic ptosis.

Hutchinson's s. 1. Hutchinson's triad: interstitial keratitis, notched teeth, and deafness occurring together in congenital syphilis. 2. Hutchinson's triad, together with rhagades at the corners of the mouth and a saddle-shaped bridge of the nose.

Jellinek's s. Abnormal pigmentation of the skin of the eyelids, in exophthalmic goiter. Syn., *Rasin's sign; Tellais' sign.*

Jendrassik's s. Apparent paralysis of the extraocular muscles, in exophthalmic goiter.

Joffroy's s. Absence of the normal wrinkles in the forehead on looking upward with the head bent down, a sign of exophthalmic goiter.

Kayser-Fleischer s. The Kayser-Fleischer ring, indicating Wilson's disease.

Kestenbaum's s. In unilateral amblyopia, marked anisocoria with dilatation of the pupil of the affected eye, when it fixates a light source with the normal eye covered, and little or no anisocoria, when the normal eye fixates with the affected eye covered, indicating an organic lesion of the macula or the optic nerve in differentiation from a functional visual loss.

Knies's s. Unequal dilatation of the pupils in exophthalmic goiter.

Kocher's s. 1. Spasmodic retraction of the upper eyelid on attentive fixation in exophthalmic goiter. 2. Means's sign.

Koster's s. Failure of the upper eyelid to elevate, or ability to elevate only slightly, upon the administration of cocaine, indicating absence of the levator palpebrae superioris muscle in congenital ptosis.

Lester's s. Hyperpigmentation of the iris in a clover-leaf pattern.

Loewi's s. Ready dilatation of the pupil with instillation of adrenalin into the cul-de-sac, in exophthalmic goiter.

Lotze's local s. The subjective identification of a specific spatial direction from the self for each retinal element stimulated; a characteristic assumed to be inherent and present for any sensory receptor.

Magendie-Hertwig s. Spasmodic deviation of the eyes in opposite directions, in acute cerebellar lesions. It persists for all directions of gaze. Thus, if one eye looks down and in, the other eye will turn upward and outward. Syn., *skew deviation.*

Mann's s. The appearance of one eye being higher than its fellow, in exophthalmic goiter.

May's s. Ready dilatation of the pupil on instillation of adrenalin into the cul-de-sac, in glaucoma.

Means's s. Movement of the upper eyelids faster than the eyeballs on looking upward, thus exposing the sclera above the cornea, in exophthalmic goiter. Syn., *globe lag*.

Mendel-Bechterew s. Dilatation of the pupils on exposure to light (the paradoxical pupillary reflex) in cerebral syphilis, tabes dorsalis, or general paralysis.

Méténier's s. Extreme laxness of the eyelids resulting in easy eversion of the upper eyelid, sometimes even upon an upward pull of its loose skin, indicative of degeneration of elastic mesenchymal tissue.

Meyer's s. Swelling of the plica semilunaris after an initial "glassy eyes" appearance during the incubation period of measles and before the rash appears.

Moebius' s. Convergence weakness in exophthalmic goiter.

Moskowskij's s. Anisocoria, with dilatation of the pupil of the right eye, in acute abdominal disease, such as appendicitis, cholecystitis, or colitis.

Munson's s. A cone-shaped bulging of the margin of the lower lid when looking downward, such that the lower lid margin bisects the cornea, indicating keratoconus.

Myerson's s. A series of blinking movements in response to a tap on the forehead or to a sudden thrust toward the eyes, frequently seen in Parkinson's disease.

Negro's s. Overshooting of the eye on the more severely affected side on looking upward, in peripheral facial paralysis.

objective s. A sign apparent to the observer.

optokinetic nystagmus s., negative. Symmetric, horizontal, nystagmoid movements to both sides, as normally occur in optokinetic nystagmus. When present with homonymous hemianopsia, it is indicative of a lesion involving the optic tract, lateral geniculate body, the most anterior optic radiations in the temporal lobe, or the occipital cortex. Cf. *positive optokinetic nystagmus sign*.

optokinetic nystagmus s., positive. Horizontal optokinetic nystagmus less pronounced, or absent, to one side as compared to the other. When occurring with homonymous hemianopsia, it is indicative of a lesion involving the middle or posterior optic radiations. Cf. *negative optokinetic nystagmus sign*.

orbicularis s. Forced closure of the eyelids on the unaffected side on closure of the eyelids on the affected side, in hemiplegia. Syn., *Hensy's sign; Revilliod's sign*.

Parrot's s. Pupillary dilatation on pinching the skin of the neck, in meningitis.

Paton's s. Comma shaped dilations of the lower bulbar conjunctival vessels with sludging of the blood, pathognomonic of sickle-cell disease.

physical s. Objective sign.

Pick's s. Prominent injection limited to the exposed bulbar conjunctiva, associated with a burning sensation of pain and tenderness in the eyes, lacrimation, and photophobia, an indication of sandfly fever.

Piltz's s. 1. Attention pupillary reflex. 2. Orbicularis pupillary reflex. 3. Delayed and slow reaction of the pupils to light followed by slow dilation, in neurosis or psychosis.

Prevost's s. Turning the head and eyes toward the affected hemisphere and away from the palsied extremities, in hemiplegia.

pseudo-Graefe's s. Failure of the upper eyelid to follow the eyeball downward or the elevation of the upper eyelid when the eyeball turns downward, usually indicative of aberrant regeneration of fibers of the oculomotor nerve following paresis or paralysis. It is to be differentiated from *von Graefe's sign* in exophthalmic goiter. Syn., *pseudo-Graefe's phenomenon*.

Rasin's s. Jellinek's sign.

Revilliod's s. Orbicularis sign.

Riesman's s. 1. A decrease in ocular tension in diabetic coma. 2. A bruit heard stethoscopically over the closed eye, in exophthalmic goiter. Syn., *Snellen's sign*.

Ripault's s. A change in the shape of the pupil from external pressure on the eyeball, which is temporary during life and may be permanent after death.

Robertson's s. Failure to elicit pupillary dilatation on exerting pressure on an alleged painful area, an indication of malingering.

Rochester's s. The inability to maintain light closure of the eyelid on the affected side when the eyes are moved superiorly under lightly closed eyelids to a point beyond the limit of the field of fixation, an indication of beginning paresis of the seventh cranial nerve.

Romaña's s. Pronounced unilateral edema of the eyelids, with conjunctivitis and swelling of the regional lymph glands, an indication of Chaga's disease.

Romberg's s. Swaying of the body due to the inability to maintain equilibrium when standing with feet together and eyes closed, indicating tabes dorsalis.

Roque's s. Mydriasis of the left eye resulting from irritation of the cervical sympathetic chain, in exudative endocarditis.

Rosenbach's s. 1. Fine, rapid tremor of gently closed eyelids, an indication of exophthalmic goiter. 2. The inability to close the eyelids immediately on command, an indication of neurasthenia.

Roth-Bielschowsky s. Doll's head phenomenon.

Rothschild's s. Sparseness of the outer third of the eyebrows, in hypothyroidism.

Rucker s. Sheathing of retinal venules at the posterior pole, considered to be evidence of active retinal perivasculitis, and seen in about 15 percent of those with multiple sclerosis.

Saenger's s. The return of an absent pupillary light reflex after a short stay in the dark, indicating cerebral syphilis in differentiation from tabes dorsalis.

Sainton's s. Contraction of the frontalis muscle after the levator palpebrae superioris muscle has ceased to contract on looking upward, i.e., wrinkles in the forehead appear after the raising of the eyelids instead of during, an indication of exophthalmic goiter.

Salmon's s. Unilateral dilatation of the pupil in ruptured ectopic pregnancy.

Salus' s. An arch in a retinal venule, above or below a sclerosed arteriole, due to deflection from its normal course by the arteriole, an indication of hypertensive and/or arteriolosclerotic retinopathy. Syn.,*Salus' arch.*

Schmidt's s. A sign of manifest heterozygosity in carriers in X-linked diseases of protanomaly and protanopia, consisting of abnormal luminosity functions intermediate between those of normals and those of protanomals and protanopes without

any color-matching abnormalities. The sign is manifested in the relatively high brightness adjustment of a red light as compared to that of a blue light when she, the carrier, attempts to equate each of them to the brightness of green light.

Seeligmueller's s. Mydriasis on the affected side in facial neuralgia.

Seidel's s. 1. A sickle-shaped scotoma appearing as an upward or downward prolongation of the physiological blind spot, indicating glaucoma. 2. A green stain seen over the wound with a slit lamp through a cobalt glass filter after the instillation of fluorescein, subsequent to surgery for choroidal detachment, indicating a leak of aqueous humor.

Snellen's s. A bruit heard with a stethoscope placed over the closed eye, in exophthalmic goiter.

Stellwag's s. Infrequent and incomplete blinking, indicating exophthalmic goiter. Syn., *Stellwag's symptom.*

subjective s. A sign apparent only to the subject or the afflicted person.

Suker's s. The inability to maintain extreme lateral fixation of the eyes, indicating exophthalmic goiter.

Tay's s. The cherry-red spot in the region of the macula lutea of each eye in Tay-Sachs disease.

Tellais' s. Abnormal pigmentation of the skin of the eyelids in exophthalmic goiter. Syn., *Jellinek's sign; Rasin's sign.*

Terrien's s. Paralysis of downward gaze associated with loss of accommodation and convergence, considered to be due to a lesion of the midbrain.

Thies's s. Miosis occurring in lesions of the sigmoid flexure and the rectum.

Topalanski's s. Congestion of the pericorneal region of the eye in exophthalmic goiter.

Tournay's s. Tournay's pupillary reflex.

Uhthoff's s. The nystagmus associated with multiple sclerosis.

Vincent's s. Argyll Robertson pupil.

Vogt's s. Loss of the normal shagreen of the capsule of the crystalline lens in the affected area under slit lamp examination, indicating anterior capsular cataract.

Wartenberg's s. Reduced muscular control of the upper eyelid in facial paralysis.

Weber's s. Homolateral oculomotor paralysis and contralateral hemiplegia of the face and limbs, indicating a lesion in the region of the cerebral peduncle affecting the third cranial nerve. Syn., *Weber's paralysis; Weber's symptom; Weber's syndrome.*

Weiss's s. Weiss's reflex.

Wernicke's s. Hemianopic pupillary reflex.

Westphal's s. Dilated pupils which fail to contract to light in neurosis or psychosis.

white with pressure s. White with pressure phenomenon.

Wilder's s. A slight twitch of the eyeball on lateral movement, an indication of exophthalmic goiter.

Wood's s. Fixation of the eyeballs in a divergent position, and relaxation of the orbicularis oculi muscle in deep anesthesia.

◆

significance, statistical. The statistically evaluated extent to which a given quantitative relationship may be considered due to chance or to the operation of those factors whose influence the experimental procedure was designed to test.

silhouette (sil″oo-et′). 1. A representation of the contour or the outline of an object or a person filled with a uniform color differing from the surrounding field. 2. To represent by a silhouette.

SILMO. See *Salon International de la Lunetterie et du Material pour Opticiens.*

SILO response. See under *response.*

Silverman-Caffey disease. Infantile cortical hyperostosis. See under *hyperostosis.*

Simmance-Abady photometer (sim-mahnz′ah′bah-de). See under *photometer.*

simultanagnosia (si″mul-tan-ag-no′se-ah). Inability to perceive more than one object at a time.

Simultantest (si′mul-tan-test). Trade name for an attachment to be inserted in a lens aperture of a phoropter or trial frame to provide either (1) a pair of optically juxtaposed images of a distant test object each of which is seen through a +0.25 sphere −0.50 cylinder

lens system with their cylindrical axes perpendicular to each other, permitting simultaneous viewing for cross cylinder test comparison or, (2) alternatively by the turn of a knob, a pair of juxtaposed images of a distant test object, one of which is seen through a +0.25 sphere and the other through a −0.25 sphere, permitting simultaneous comparison of two spherically different lens corrections.

Sinclair's rule (sin-klārz). See under *rule.*

sine condition. See under *condition.*

sine correctione. Without correction. Abbreviation *sc.*

sinistral (sin′is-tral). 1. Showing preference for the left eye, hand, or foot. 2. Pertaining to, or on, the left side.

sinistrality (sin″is-tral′ih-te). Left-eyedness or left-handedness.

sinistroclination (sin″is-tro-klih-na′-shun). Rotation of the top of the vertical meridian of an eye toward the left; extorsion of the left eye or intorsion of the right eye. Syn., *levocycloduction; levotorsion; sinistrotorsion; sinistrocycloduction.*

sinistrocular (sin″is-trok′u-lar). Pertaining to the left eye or the condition of sinistrocularity.

sinistrocularity (sin″is-trok″u-lar′ih-te). A condition in which better vision exists in the left eye, or in which the left eye is dominant.

sinistrocycloduction (sin″is-tro-si″-klo-duk′shun). Sinistroclination.

sinistrocycloversion (sin″is-tro-si″-klo-ver′zhun). Rotation of the top of the vertical meridians of both eyes toward the left. Syn., *negative cycloversion; levocycloversion.*

sinistroduction (sin″is-tro-duk′shun). Rotation of an eye toward the left. Syn., *levoduction.*

sinistrogyration (sin″is-tro-ji-ra′shun). A turning to the left; motion, especially rotatory, to the left; said of eye movements and of the plane of polarization.

sinistrophoria (sin″is-tro-fo′re-ah). A phoria in which the nonfixating eye is turned toward the left. Syn., *levophoria.*

sinistrorotatory (sin″is-tro-ro′tah-to″re). 1. Turning of the plane of polarization toward the left. 2. Bending rays of light toward the left. 3. Pertaining to sinistroclination. Syn., *levorotatory.*

sinistrotorsion (sin"is-tro-tor'shun). Sinistroclination.

sinistroversion (sin"is-tro-ver'zhun). A conjugate rotation of both lines of sight to the left. Syn., *levoversion*.

sinus. A hollow space, cavity, or recess in the body.

s. of the anterior chamber. The space within the angle of the anterior chamber.

s. of Arlt. A small diverticulum sometimes found in the lower, lateral wall of the lacrimal sac.

cavernous s. One of the paired venous sinuses in the dura mater of the brain extending on each side of the pituitary body and the body of the sphenoid bone from the inner end of the superior orbital fissure to the petrous portion of the temporal bone. It receives blood from the superior and the inferior ophthalmic veins and the central retinal veins, empties into the superior and the inferior petrosal sinuses, and communicates with the pterygoid venous plexus. Its central spongy tissue contains the internal carotid artery with its sympathetic carotid plexus and the abducens nerve. Its lateral wall contains the oculomotor and the trochlear nerves and the first two divisions of the trigeminal nerve.

ciliary s. Ciliary cleft.

circular s. The venous ring around the pituitary gland formed by the two cavernous sinuses and the communicating anterior and posterior intercavernous sinuses.

s. circularis iridis. Canal of Schlemm.

intercavernous s's. Two sinuses in the dura mater of the brain which connect the two cavernous sinuses, one located anterior to and the other posterior to the pituitary body. Syn., *transverse sinuses.*

s. of Maier. A small diverticulum from the middle lateral wall of the lacrimal sac into which the canaliculi drain.

marginal s. Ring sinus of von Szily.

ring s. of von Szily. A circular space between the two layers of the optic cup, at the extreme tip of the growing edge in the developing iris, which appears at the end of the third month and disappears by the seventh month of fetal life. Syn., *von Szily's ring; marginal sinus.*

scleral s. Canal of Schlemm.

scleral s. of Rochon-Duvigneaud. Canal of Schlemm.

subscleral s. In the lamprey, a venous sinus composing the external portion of the choroid which drains blood from the choroid and empties, by way of four apertures, into extraocular venous sinuses surrounding the sclera.

transverse s's. Intercavernous sinuses.

s. venosus sclerae. Canal of Schlemm.

sinusotomy (si"nus-ot'o-me). Surgical cutting of a sinus, as, for example, the excision of a portion of the outer wall of Schlemm's canal and the overlying sclera to increase the facility of aqueous outflow.

situs inversus of the disk (si'tus inver'sus). A developmental abnormality in which the retinal vessels course nasally from the optic disk instead of temporally, giving the optic disk a reversed appearance.

size. Physical extent, bulk, or magnitude.

angular s. The size of an object expressed in terms of the angle subtended by it with respect to some point of reference, such as the nodal point of the eye or the center of the entrance pupil.

apparent s. 1. The size of an object represented by the angle or a trigonometric function of the angle it subtends at the eye. 2. The perceived size of an object, or the size attributed to the object, as distinguished from the actual size.

boxed lens s. Spectacle lens size specified in terms of the horizontal and vertical dimensions of the box which contains the lens.

s. constancy. The apparent relative stability or lack of perceived change in the size of an object despite a change in viewing distance, viewing angle, actual size, or other related stimulus factors.

datum lens s. Spectacle lens size specified in terms of the horizontal and vertical dimensions through the datum center.

s. diminution. The perceived relative decrease in size of elements in a stereopsis-inducing target which appear closer than other fused elements in the stereogram though they are the same actual size.

perceptual s. The perceived size of an object as distinguished from the actual size.

Sjögren's (syeh'grenz) **dystrophy; syndrome; test.** See under the nouns.

Sjögren-Larsson syndrome (syeh'-gren-lahr'son). See under *syndrome*.

skiakinescopy (ski"ah-kin-es'ko-pe). A method of determining the refractive state of the eye in which a pinhole is moved across the pupil while a distant light source is viewed through it. The light source appears stationary in emmetropia, appears to move in the same direction as the hole in myopia, and in the opposite direction in hypermetropia.

skiametry (ski-am'eh-tre). The determination of the refractive error by retinoscopy.

skiaporescopy (ski"ah-po-res'ko-pe). Retinoscopy.

skiascope (ski'ah-skōp). Retinoscope.

skiascopy (ski-as'ko-pe). Observation of the retinoscopic reflex.

skiascotometry (ski"ah-sko-tom'eh-tre). A method of measuring blind areas in the visual field in which test objects are moved automatically at a given rate of speed by means of an adaptation of the Goldmann perimeter.

skill, visual. The ability to perform a visual act, usually measured by psychophysical methods; the representation of a given aspect of a visual, ocular, or extraocular function as an attribute or a score.

motor visual s. A visual skill relating to the ability or function of the intrinsic and extrinsic muscles of the eye.

perceptual visual s. A visual skill relating to the perceptual aspect of vision, implying a more complex or higher level of interpretation than a sensory visual skill.

sensory visual s. A visual skill relating to the sensory aspect of vision, e.g., visual acuity or brightness discrimination.

skill, visual-motor. The ability to copy correctly that which is seen. It involves visual discrimination, perception and integration, motor planning, visualizing, and motor skill, as in the *Bender-Gestalt Visual Motor Test*. Syn., *visual-perceptual-motor skill*.

Ski-optometer (ski-op-tom'eh-ter). An instrument for determining the refractive state of the eye, phorias, vergences, etc., consisting essentially of a pair of rotating disks containing convex and concave spherical lenses, cells for trial cylindrical lenses, rotary prisms, and Maddox grooves.

skot (skot). One one-thousandth of an *apostilb*.

skylight. 1. Sunlight scattered by the atmosphere. 2. A window in a roof or a ceiling.

slab-off. A slab-off lens.

Slataper chart. See under *chart*.

slide. 1. A moving piece guided by the parts along which it slides. 2. A guiding surface or piece along which something slides. 3. A plate of transparent material on which is a picture to be projected.

Hamilton s. A slide containing letters, numerals, astigmatic dials, and other devices for vision testing, for use with the Clason acuity meter.

nodal s. An optical bench mount permitting adjustment of the perpendicular axis about which a lens or a lens system may be rotated to locate the nodal points.

Robinson Cohen s. A projector slide containing letters and other characters for vision testing and a rotatable astigmatic dial consisting of two broken black lines at right angles to each other on a red background, with an axis indicator on the control knob.

slip, retinal. Fixation disparity.

slip-on. Clip-on.

slip-over. Clip-on.

slit, stenopaic. Stenopaic disk.

slit lamp. See under *lamp*.

Slit-Lite. The trade name for a hand-held, portable slit lamp used in conjunction with a magnifier for examination of the anterior structures of the eye.

Sloan charts; letters; test. See under the nouns.

SMC. See *Worshipful Company of Spectacle Makers*.

Smith-Helmholtz law. See under *law*.

smoothing. Fining.

Smukler's deviometer. See under *deviometer*.

Sn. Abbreviation for *Snellen*.

SNADOC. See *Chambre Syndicate Nationale des Adaptateurs d'Optique de Contact*.

Snell's law (snelz). Law of refraction.

Snellen's (snel'enz) **visual acuity; chart; eye; formula; fraction;**

notation; prong; sign; test; test types. See under the nouns.

Snell-Sterling (snel-ster'ling) **notation; visual efficiency scale.** See under *notation*.

Societé d'Optometrie d'Europe. An association consisting mostly of western European ophthalmic opticians, founded in 1967 to encourage the distinction of those who would regard themselves as optometrists from those whose practices are more or less exclusively dispensing opticianry. Syn., *European Optometric Society (EOS).*

Society of Ocularists. An association of persons who design, fabricate, and fit ocular prosthetics.

socio-optometric. Pertaining to the interrelationships of optometry with social science and human welfare.

socket, eye. The bony orbit which contains the eye and adjacent structures.

SOE. See *Societé d'Optometrie d'Europe.*

Soehnges Micro Pupil Multifocal contact lens (sen'jēz). See under *lens, contact.*

Soemmering's (sem'er-ingz) **bone; cushion; foramen; ligaments; ring; spot.** See under the nouns.

Soleil compensator (so-leh'yeh). See under *compensator.*

solid, color. A representation in three dimensions of the quantitative or psychophysical relations of all possible colors with respect to their primary attributes of hue, brightness or lightness (value), and saturation (chroma). Brightness (lightness) is usually represented as the vertical axis of the solid, with hue and saturation represented as polar coordinates around this axis, the hues being arranged circumferentially and saturations radially. Although the boundaries of any such solid representation must necessarily be irregular because of the inequalities of maximal saturations of various hues, the solid is nevertheless represented variously as a cylinder, a sphere, a spindle, a double cone, or a double rectangular pyramid.

    Ostwald c.s. A three dimensional representation in the form of two cones placed base to base with white represented at the upper apex, black at the lower, and full color circumferentially at the center. Mixtures of full color with white and with black are represented, respectively, above or below the central circle. See also *Ostwald color system.*

somatagnosia (so"mah-tag'no-se-ah). The inability to recognize the existence, identity, or function of any part of one's body.

Sondermann, canals of (son'derman). See under *canal.*

sonohologram (so"no-ho'lo-gram). Acoustical hologram.

sonoholography (so"no-ho-log'rah-fe). Acoustical holography.

sonoptogram (so-nop'to-gram). Acoustical hologram.

sonoptography (so"nop-tog'rah-fe). Acoustical holography.

Sorsby's degeneration; dystrophy; syndrome. See under the nouns.

soule (sōō-la'). To cut from the lower nasal edge of a spectacle lens to give clearance for the nose.

source, light. Any source of visible radiant energy, such as a candle flame, incandescent lamp, or fluorescent lamp.

    A; B; C; D$_{65}$ l. s's. A; B; C; D$_{65}$ illuminants.

    anisophotic l.s. A light source that emits an uneven distribution of radiant energy throughout the visible range.

    coherent l. s's. Light sources which maintain a continual point-to-point phase relationship with each other.

    cool l. s. Luminescent light source.

    luminescent l. s. A light source which emits light without being heated, such as a fluorescent lamp. Syn., *cool light source.*

    standard l. s. A light source which has a specified spectral distribution and is used as a standard in colorimetry, such as illuminant A, B, or C (q.v.).

Souter's tonometer (sōō'terz). See under *tonometer.*

South African Optometric Association. A representative organization of South African optometrists founded in 1924 for general protective and professional development purposes.

Southall's double color circle. See under *circle, color.*

SOV-Stiftung. Acronym for Stiftung des Schweizerischen Optikerverbandes für die Förderung der Beruflichen Ausbildung, a Swiss foundation for the support of professional optometric education.

◆
SPACE

space. 1. A potential or an actual cavity within the body. 2. A delimited area, region, or interval, usually three dimensional.

central s. of the orbit. The retrobulbar space lying within the cone formed by the rectus muscles. Syn., *muscle cone space.*

circumlental s. Zonular space.

corneal s's. Tiny spaces between the lamellae of the corneal stroma containing tissue fluid. Syn., *interlamellar spaces.*

epichoroidal s. Perichoroidal space.

episcleral s. Tenon's space.

s's. of Fontana. In lower mammals and birds, large spaces formed by the trabeculae of the pectinate ligament. In man, smaller vestigial spaces, after the sixth month of fetal life, in the uveal meshwork of the angle of the anterior chamber, involved in the drainage of aqueous humor. Syn., *trabecular spaces; spatia anguli iridis; spatia iridis.*

free s. True space.

image s. The space containing rays emanating from an object after they have been refracted or reflected by an optical system.

interfascial s. Tenon's space.

interlamellar s's. Corneal spaces.

intermarginal s. The space on the surface of the eyelid margin.

intervaginal s's. The subarachnoid and the subdural spaces in the sheath of the optic nerve.

s's. of iridocorneal angle. Trabecular spaces.

Meckel's s. Meckel's cave.

muscle cone s. Central space of the orbit.

object s. The space containing rays emanating from an object prior to refraction or reflection by an optical system.

Panum's fusional s. The space enclosed between the anteroposterior limits of the haplopic horopter and within which fusion of a nonfixated target can occur, its images stimulating retinal points within Panum's areas.

perichoroidal s. The potential space between the choroid and the sclera across which fine lamellae stretch to blend the superficial layer of the choroid with the lamina fusca of the sclera. It is traversed by branches of the posterior ciliary arteries, the short and long ciliary nerves, and extends from the scleral spur to the opticoscleral foramen. Syn., *epichoroidal space; suprachoroidal space.*

perilenticular s. Zonular space.

peripheral s. of the orbit. The space between the cone formed by the rectus muscles and the periorbita.

perivascular s. Fluid-filled spaces around the orbital vessels, considered to act as lymph channels.

postlenticular s. of Berger. Retrolental space of Berger.

preseptal s. 1. A space in the upper eyelid, containing submuscular areolar tissue, bounded anteriorly by the orbicularis oculi muscle, posteriorly by the orbital septum and the fibers of the levator palpebrae superioris muscle, and superiorly by a preseptal cushion of fat. 2. A space in the lower eyelid, containing submuscular areolar tissue, bounded anteriorly by the orbicularis oculi muscle and posteriorly by the orbital septum.

pretarsal s. A space in the upper eyelid, containing submuscular areolar tissue, bounded anteriorly by the tendon of the levator palpebrae superioris muscle and posteriorly by the tarsus and the muscle of Mueller. It extends superiorly to the origin of the muscle of Mueller and inferiorly to the attachment of the fibers of the levator palpebrae superioris muscle to the tarsus.

prezonular s. The circular space between the iris and the anterior leaf of the zonule of Zinn, containing aqueous humor.

retrobulbar s. The area within the orbit outside Tenon's capsule, posterior to the conjunctiva, which contains orbital fat, extraocular muscles, vessels, and nerves.

retrolental s. of Berger. A potential space between the posterior surface of the crystalline lens and the hyaloid fossa of the vitreous body. Syn., *postlenticular space of Berger.*

retrolental s. of Erggelet. The optically empty space formed by anterior expansion of the hyaloid canal.

retrozonular s. A circular space filled with aqueous humor, peripheral to the retrolental space of Berger, and bounded by the posterior leaf of the zonule of Zinn, the ciliary body, and the anterior surface of the vitreous humor. Syn., *canal of Petit.*

Schnabel's s's. Small spaces in the optic nerve, posterior to the lamina cribrosa, resulting from degeneration or atrophy of nerve fibers, in glaucoma. According to Schnabel, their coalescence leads to glaucomatous cupping. Syn., *Schnabel's caverns.*

Schwalbe's s. Supravaginal space.

subarachnoid s. The space between the arachnoid and the pia mater which contains connective tissue trabeculae and is filled with cerebrospinal fluid. It is continuous from the cranium to the optic nerve and terminates in the region of the lamina cribrosa.

subdural s. A space between the dura mater and the arachnoid which is continuous from the cranium to the optic nerve where, unlike the corresponding space in the brain, it becomes very thin.

subperiosteal s. The potential space between the periosteum and the bony wall of the orbit.

suprachoroidal s. Perichoroidal space.

supraciliary s. The anterior portion of the perichoroidal space between the ciliary body and the sclera.

supravaginal s. A space, between the dura mater of the optic nerve and the orbital fat, described by Schwalbe and considered by him to contain lymph. Syn., *Schwalbe's space.*

Tenon's s. The space between Tenon's capsule and the sclera, containing interconnecting trabeculae. Syn., *episcleral space; interfascial space.*

trabecular s's. Small spaces between the intercrossing trabeculae of the meshwork of the angle of the anterior chamber, involved in the drainage of aqueous humor from the anterior chamber to the canal of Schlemm.

true s. A visual environment in which objects are seen directly and their positions or distances not altered by viewing through an optical device which has moved them to apparent positions not coincident with their actual positions. Syn., *free space.*

visual s. Space as perceived through the sense of vision, having dimensional and directional attributes similar to, but not necessarily commensurate with, physical space.

zonular s. The circumlental space between the equator of the crystalline lens and the ciliary processes, bounded by the anterior and posterior leaves of the zonule of Zinn, and containing aqueous humor. Syn., *Hannover's canal; circumlental space; perilenticular space.*

◆

Space Coordinator. An instrument primarily for the treatment of eccentric fixation designed by Cüppers and containing interchangeable fixation targets and a rotating transilluminated Polaroid filter which, when viewed through a blue filter, produces Haidinger's brushes localized in relation to the fixation target, both of which are projected to a more distant plane seen through the instrument.

Spache binocular reading test (spah'ke). See under *test.*

span. A limited interval of space or time, or the representation of that interval by its contents or circumstances.

attention s. The amount of material that is grasped or perceived and dealt with or mentally processed in a single, continuous, uninterrupted period of attention, or the duration of this period.

s. of recognition. The number of words, symbols, or digits, or the size of the field in which they are contained, that can be correctly identified or perceived during a time exposure sufficiently brief to exclude eye movement.

Spannlang-Tappeiner syndrome. See under *syndrome.*

sparganosis, ocular (spar"gah-no'-sis). Infestation of the eyelids, conjunctiva, episclera, or orbit with *Sparganum mansoni*, the larvae of tapeworms.

sparing of the macula. See under *macula.*

sparkle. To glitter, gleam, or shine with a brilliant and broken scintillating light.

spasm. An anomalous, involuntary muscular contraction.

s. of accommodation. A spasm of the ciliary muscle, producing excess accommodation. **clonic s. of a.** Alternate spasm and relaxation of the ciliary muscle. **tonic s. of a.** Prolonged uniform spasm of the ciliary muscle.

s. of convergence. A spasm of the extraocular muscles producing excess convergence.

cyclic oculomotor s. Alternating spasm and relaxation of the sphincter pupillae muscle with similar involvement of other muscles innervated by the third cranial nerve, and occasionally those innervated by the fourth and sixth cranial nerves. During the miotic phase the upper eyelid retracts, the eye converges, and accommodation undergoes a spasm, and during the mydriatic phase there is almost complete total ophthalmoplegia with ptosis. The onset is usually at birth or early in life, and it affects females more frequently than males. Syn., *cyclic oculomotor paralysis.*

nictitating s. Spasmus nictitans.

nodding s. Spasmus nutans.

oculogyral s. A spasm of the extraocular muscles occurring in oculogyric crisis.

winking s. Spasmus nictitans.

spasmus (spaz'mus). A spasm.

s. mobilis. Catatonic pupil.

s. nictitans. A clonic spasm of the orbicularis oculi muscle causing an increase in the rate of blinking and a prolongation of the phase of eyelid closure. Syn., *nictitating spasm; winking spasm.*

s. nutans. Head nodding associated with nystagmus and occasionally with torticollis, occurring usually in the first year of life. Head nodding is usually the first symptom, is frequently transient and inconstant, bears no relationship to the movements of the eyes, and does not occur when the head is supported. The nystagmus is constant, pendular, rapid, of small amplitude, may be horizontal, vertical, or rotary, is usually bilateral, with one eye affected more than the other, and disappears during sleep. The condition is of unknown etiology, but is thought to be related to a dimly illuminated environment with poor fixation control; the prognosis is favorable. Syn., *gyrospasm; nodding spasm.*

s. oculi. Nystagmus.

spatium (spa'she-um). A space.

spatia anguli iridis. Spaces of Fontana.

s. interfasciale. Tenon's space.

spatia intervaginalia nervi optici. Intervaginal spaces.

spatia iridis. Spaces of Fontana.

s. perichoroideale. Perichoroidal space.

s. zonularia. Zonular space.

Speakman's endothelial meshwork. See under *meshwork.*

spectacle, primary. A fixed transparent cutaneous structure constituting a dermal cornea underneath which the eye is free to rotate, found in cyclostomes, tadpoles, and adult aquatic amphibians.

spectacle, secondary. A transparent window in a moveable lower eyelid, or a fixed transparent structure formed by fusion of the two eyelids which have become transparent, found in reptiles and lizards.

◆

SPECTACLES

spectacles. A pair of ophthalmic lenses together with the frame or mounting.

anisometropic s. Spectacles in which one lens is of a significantly different refractive power from the other, for the correction of anisometropia.

Bartels' s. Spectacles with lenses of high refractive power (as +20.00 or −20.00 D) used to impair vision while inducing nystagmus by rotating a subject who is wearing them.

clerical s. Pantoscopic spectacles.

crutch s. Spectacles with a ptosis crutch attachment. Syn., *Masselon's spectacles.*

diver's s. Spectacles usually in some form of headgear and inserted in such a manner as to render them airtight and watertight, to enable the wearer to see under water.

folding s. Spectacles that are hinged or otherwise especially constructed so that the two lenses can be placed in apposition when not worn.

Franklin s. Spectacles containing Franklin bifocal lenses.

Frenzel s. Plano spectacles with a built-in light source for the purpose of dazzling the eyes and preventing fixation, used in a darkened room for the clinical detection of nystagmus.

Galilean s. Spectacles containing Galilean telescopic lenses, usually used as a subnormal vision aid.

half-eye s. Spectacles having semi-circular lenses for only the upper or only the lower part of the field of view, the other part of the field being seen by the unaided eye.

hemianopic s. Spectacles with a prism, of approximately 8$^\triangle$, affixed to one lens with its base toward the blind side of the visual field, used to increase the field of vision on the blind side in homonymous hemianopsia by reflecting light onto the seeing side of the retina.

industrial s. Spectacles made of frames and lenses designed with protective and other features (hardened or plastic lenses, side shields, etc.) especially suitable or necessary in certain types of hazardous industrial occupations.

Keeler Magnifying S. A binocular loupe consisting of a pair of telescopes mounted on a carrier spectacle frame and adjustable for interpupillary distance.

Lindner s. A spectacle frame with a single pinhole aperture for each eye.

Masselon's s. Crutch spectacles.

meshed s. Spectacles in which the lenses are etched with a number of fine lines at right angles to each other, used to obscure vision in experiments for determining effects of reduced vision on visual perception.

microscopic s. Spectacles containing lenses of relatively high convex power ($+10.00$ D or higher), used as a subnormal vision aid at near.

nose s. Spectacles held on the nose by spring pressure without the aid of temples, as in a pince-nez or an oxford.

orthopedic s. Spectacles with an attachment for the relief of an anatomical deformity, for example, spectacles with a ptosis crutch.

orthoscopic s. Spectacles in which the lenses are of strong convex power with base-in prism, used in fine, near tasks to magnify and to reduce convergence.

pantoscopic s. Half-eye spectacles used for reading, in which the top halves of the lenses are cut off so as not to affect distant vision. Syn., *clerical spectacles; pulpit spectacles.*

pinhole s. Spectacles having, in place of lenses, opaque disks with one or more small perforations, used as an aid in certain types of subnormal vision, or as protection from bright light or glare.

pulpit s. Pantoscopic spectacles.

recumbent s. Spectacles having right-angle prism lenses which enable the wearer to read or do other near work while recumbent.

reversible s. Spectacles that present either lens to either eye. It may

have either an X-shaped bridge with straight temples, or an arc-shaped bridge with doublejointed endpieces.

rimless s. Spectacles in which the lenses are fastened to the frame by cement, screws, or clamps but without supporting eyewires, the lens edges being exposed.

rising front s. A spectacle frame with an adjustable nosepiece which allows the entire frame to be lowered or raised so as to change the height of the bifocal segments.

Ryer-Hotaling cataract s. Spectacles having amber lenses with an untinted reading segment, for use with cataractous eyes.

safety s. Industrial spectacles.

Scherer cataract s. Spectacles in which the peripheral portion of the reading lens in front of the cataractous eye is covered with an opaque shield, leaving a 10 mm, central, circular aperture.

stenopaic s. Spectacles having, in place of lenses, opaque disks containing narrow slits or circular perforations, used as a subnormal vision aid or as protection against bright light or glare.

telescopic s. Spectacles containing telescopic lenses, usually used as a subnormal vision aid.

tubular s. Spectacles containing small tubes which shield the eyes from extraneous light, used as a subnormal vision aid in corneal or lenticular opacities.

variable focus s. See *lens, variable focus.*

◆

Spectograph (spek'to-graf). The trade name for an instrument that projects a magnified image of a contact lens onto a calibrated viewing screen for the purpose of inspection.

spectrocolorimeter (spek"tro-kul"or-im'eh-ter). A colorimeter employing a spectral source of light.

spectrogram (spek'tro-gram). The picture, or other record, of radiations taken by a spectrograph.

spectrograph (spek'tro-graf). An instrument for producing and photographing spectra of substances, consisting essentially of a diffraction grating, prism, or crystals, to disperse the radiations, and a camera to photograph them.

spectrometer (spek-trom'eh-ter). An instrument for producing and making measurements of a spectrum, for purposes of determining the index of refraction and other optical properties of a medium or source.

spectrometry (spek-trom'eh-tre). The measurement of wavelengths with the spectrometer.

spectrophotometer (spek"tro-fo-tom'-eh-ter). An instrument for measuring the photic intensities of the various lines or regions of a spectrum.

spectrophotometry (spek"tro-fo-tom'-eh-ter). Measurement of the intensity of various lines or regions of a spectrum with a spectrophotometer.

spectroprojector (spek"tro-pro-jek'-tor). An apparatus for projecting a spectrum onto a screen for group observation.

spectroradiometer (spek"tro-ra-dih-om'eh-ter). An instrument for measuring the radiant intensities of the various lines or regions of a spectrum.

spectroscope (spek'tro-skōp). An instrument for producing and observing spectra, consisting essentially of a diffraction grating, prism, or crystals to disperse the radiations and an eyepiece to view them.

> **direct vision s.** A spectroscope consisting of a direct vision prism and a collimator.

spectroscopy (spek-tros'ko-pe). Producing and observing spectra with the spectroscope; the study of spectra.

◆

SPECTRUM

spectrum (spek'trum). 1. The spatial arrangement or series of the dispersed components of radiant energy, in order of their wavelengths, emitted, absorbed, or reflected by a substance. 2. A series or a phenomenon, especially visual, having some of the attributes of a spectrum.

> **absorptance s.** A graphical representation of the radiant flux absorbed by a substance, plotted against wavelength.

> **absorption s.** A spectrum formed by passing light, which normally gives a continuous spectrum, through a selectively absorbing medium. The wavelengths which are absorbed give rise to dark lines or bands in specific positions in the spectrum, indicating the chemical structure of the medium. In the solar spectrum the dark lines are termed Fraunhofer lines. Cf. *emission spectrum.*

> **action s.** A graphical representation of the relative energy required to produce a constant biological effect, such as frequency of discharge in optic nerve fibers, plotted against wavelength.

> **atomic s.** Line spectrum.

> **band s.** A spectrum containing a series of bands, each with a sharply demarcated edge on one side called the *head.* Spectra of this type are produced by molecules and are distinguished from line spectra, which are produced by atoms. Syn., *molecular spectrum.*

> **bleaching s.** A graphical representation of the bleaching effectiveness of radiant flux on a photopigment, plotted against wavelength.

> **channeled s.** A bandlike spectrum formed by passing parallel white light through a plate or a thin film, producing alternate maxima and minima by selective interference.

> **chemical s.** The ultraviolet portion of the spectrum.

> **chromatic s.** That portion of the entire spectrum which includes visible radiations.

> **comparison s.** A line spectrum of known wavelengths which is used, by matching, to determine the wavelengths of another spectrum.

> **continuous s.** A spectrum ranging continuously, without lines or bands, from the long red wavelengths to the short blue wavelengths, characteristic of gases under high pressure or of hot solids.

> **difference s.** In densitometry or spectrophotometry, the change in spectral transmittance, absorbance, or reflectance of a substance which occurs as a result of exposure to radiant flux, or a graphical representation of such change as a function of wavelength.

> **diffraction s.** A spectrum formed by a diffraction grating. Syn., *grating spectrum; interference spectrum.*

> **discontinuous s.** A spectrum in which some wavelengths are not present, as in a line or band spectrum, characteristic of gases and vapors under low pressure.

> **electromagnetic s.** The spectrum including all known radiations, i.e., cosmic rays, gamma rays, x-rays, ultraviolet rays, visible rays, infrared rays, and radio waves. Syn., *energy spectrum; physical spectrum.*

emission s. A spectrum formed of radiations given off directly from excited bodies, as by heat or electric discharge. Cf. *absorption spectrum.*

energy s. Electromagnetic spectrum.

equal energy s. A spectrum characterized by equal flux per unit wavelength interval, i.e., the same amount of energy at each wavelength.

first-order s. A diffraction grating spectrum for which the path length difference from adjacent slits is one wavelength.

fortification s. The gradually expanding zigzag of colored light which forms the boundary of a scintillating scotoma, associated with migraine. Syn., *fortification figures.*

grating s. A spectrum formed by a diffraction grating. Syn., *diffraction spectrum.*

interference s. Diffraction spectrum.

invisible s. The portions of the entire spectrum which lie at wavelengths too long or too short to stimulate the retina, i.e., approximately outside of the range between 380 and 760 mμ.

irrational s. A spectrum whose dispersion is not uniformly proportional to the wavelength, as characteristically obtained by a prism.

line s. A spectrum consisting of a series of distinct lines which are monochromatic images of the slit of the spectroscope, each image being formed by light of a particular wavelength. Spectra of this type arise from single or uncombined atoms and are distinguished from band spectra, which arise from molecules. Syn., *atomic spectrum.*

molecular s. Band spectrum.

normal s. 1. A spectrum in which the dispersion is in direct proportion to the wavelengths, as in one produced by a diffraction grating. 2. Diffraction spectrum.

photopic s. The spectral range of wavelengths visible as colors, hence that included within the range of the photopic spectral luminous efficiency curve, and ordinarily represented as the array of spectral colors.

physical s. 1. Electromagnetic spectrum. 2. The visible spectrum, extending from red to violet and exclusive of the purples. Cf. *physiological spectrum.*

physiological s. A perceptual spectrum which contains all the hues perceived, i.e., the visible spectrum, extending from red to violet, with the addition of the purples. Cf. *physical spectrum.*

prismatic s. A spectrum formed by passing a beam of light through a prism.

rational s. A spectrum whose dispersion is uniformly proportional to the wavelength, as normally produced by a diffraction grating.

reversed s. A spectrum, or a portion of a spectrum, which has been reversed, as by reflection in a mirror, for superimposition on another spectrum, not reversed, for spectral color mixing.

scotopic s. The spectral range of wavelengths visible at scotopic levels of luminosity, hence that included within the range of the scotopic spectral luminous efficiency curve, and ordinarily represented as an array of grays of varying intensity.

secondary s. A small circular zone of color about each image point, due to chromatic aberration of the optical system.

solar s. The spectrum formed from sunlight, normally characterized by numerous Fraunhofer absorption lines.

thermal s. The infrared portion of the spectrum.

visible s. The portion of the electromagnetic spectrum which contains wavelengths capable of stimulating the retina, approximately between 380 and 760 mμ.

◆

specular (spek'u-lar). Pertaining to or having the properties of a mirror.

speculum, eye (spek'u-lum). An instrument for separating the eyelids. Cf. *blepharostat.*

speed of light. The speed of electromagnetic waves in vacuum; a constant equal to 299,792.4580 ±0.0012 kilometers per second.

speed of recognition. The time rate at which symbols, digits, or words of a specific angular subtense at the eye, can be correctly perceived or identified without eye movement. It is usually determined with the use of a tachistoscope.

speed, saccadic. The speed of movement of the eye in changing fixation from one point to another.

sph. Abbreviation for *sphere* or *spherical.*

sphere. 1. A body or a space bounded by a surface, all points of which are equidistant from a point within termed its center. 2. A spherical lens.

color s. A spherical color solid; an orderly arrangement of all colors according to hue, value (brightness or lightness), and chroma (saturation), represented by position coordinates within a sphere. Black and white are represented at opposite poles, hues are arranged longitudinally around the circumference at the equator, and chroma or saturation is represented by the distance from the polar axis. See also *color tree.*

far point s. of the eye. The locus of the far points of accommodation for all directions of gaze.

integrating s. A hollow enclosure with a highly reflective white diffusing internal surface which reflects light infinitely from an internally placed source so that the light flux measured at a small exit window is directly proportional to the total light emitted by the source irrespective of its original directional distribution. Syn., *Ulbricht sphere.*

Morgagnian s's. Morgagnian globules.

near point s. of the eye. The locus of the near points of accommodation for all directions of gaze.

Poincaré s. The graphic representation of the various types of polarization on a sperical surface on which the latitude represents the eccentricity and the longitude represents the major axis azimuth of the polarization ellipse.

Ulbricht s. A commonly used photometric integrating sphere.

vertex s. A surface, concentric with the center of rotation of the eye, on which the back vertex of the ophthalmic lens is situated.

spherocylinder (sfe″ro-sil′in-der). A spherocylindrical lens.

spherometer (sfe-rom′eh-ter). 1. An instrument for determining the curvature of a surface by measuring its sagittal depth, consisting essentially of three fixed legs in an equilateral triangle formation and a fourth adjustable central leg attached to a micrometer scale. 2. An instrument based on the Drysdale method for determining the curvature of a surface.

spherophakia (sfe″ro-fa′ke-ah). A congenital and bilateral condition in which the crystalline lens is abnormally small and spherical. Cf. *microphakia.*

spheroprism (sfe-ro-prizm′). A spherical lens eccentrically mounted or decentered to produce prismatic effect; a combined spherical lens and prism. Syn., *prismosphere.*

spherule (sfer′ūl). A small sphere.

Morgagnian s's. Morgagnian globules.

rod s. End bulb.

sphincter (sfingk′ter). A muscle which surrounds an orifice or opening and acts to close or reduce it.

s. iridis. Sphincter pupillae muscle.

s. oculi. Orbicularis oculi muscle.

s. palpebrarum. Orbicularis oculi muscle.

s. pupillae. Sphincter pupillae muscle.

sphincterectomy (sfingk″ter-ek′to-me). Excision of a sphincter muscle, such as the sphincter pupillae or orbicularis oculi.

sphincterolysis (sfingk″ter-ol′ih-sis). Surgical freeing of the iris from the cornea in anterior synechia.

sphincterotomy (sfingk″ter-ot′o-me). Surgical incision into the sphincter pupillae muscle of the iris.

Spielmeyer-Stock disease (spēl′ma-er-stok). Batten-Mayou disease.

Spielmeyer-Vogt disease (spēl′maer-fōgt). Batten-Mayou disease.

spike, blue. An entoptic phenomenon elicited by a spot of light stimulating the nasal parafoveal area. The subjective sensation is of a single strip of blue light running horizontally and downward to the blind spot.

spina (spi′nah). A spine.

s. recti lateralis. A small bony projection on the orbital plate of the great wing of the sphenoid bone, situated on the inferior margin of the superior orbital fissure at the junction of its wide and narrow portions. To it are attached the annulus of Zinn and a part of the lateral rectus muscle.

s. trochlearis. A small bony projection surmounting the trochlear fossa, in the anteromedial roof of the orbit, representing an ossification of the fibrocartilagenous attachment of the pulley for the superior oblique muscle.

spindle, color. A type of color solid.

spindle, Krukenberg's. A vertically oriented, spindle-shaped deposition of melanin pigment on the corneal endothelium in the region of the pupil, occurring bilaterally as a congenital or presenile pigmentation, or unilaterally as the result of uveitis.

spine, trochlear. The spina trochlearis.

spintherism (spin'ther-izm). Entoptic perception of sparks or flashes of light; photopsia. Syn., *spintheropia.*

spintheropia (spin"ther-o'pe-ah). Spintherism.

spiral, Cornu. A spiral of two oppositely coiled branches symmetrically located in opposite quadrants, each branch of which is the diagram of vector amplitudes corresponding to a half of a cylindrical wavefront.

spirals of Daniel. Simple or complex spirals of fibers of the oculomotor nerve encircling fibers of the extraocular muscles and considered to subserve proprioception.

spiral, Frazer. See under *illusion, visual.*

spiral, Plateau's. A circular white disk on which is painted a black spiral-like band with its origin at the center. When the disk is rotated and fixated at its center, the spiral band gives the illusion of moving forward or backward in a megaphonelike formation, with its small end toward or away from the observer, depending on the direction of rotation of the disk. Following exposure to the rotating disk, if another motionless object is fixated, it will appear to swell and come forward or shrink and move backward, the effect of this motion afterimage being opposite to the effect produced when fixating the rotating disk. (See Fig. 33.)

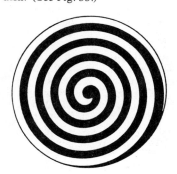

Fig. 33 Plateau's spiral. (From S. Duke-Elder, *Textbook of Ophthalmology,* vol. 4. London: Henry Kimpton, 1942)

spiral of Tillaux. A diagrammatic spiral line connecting the points of insertion of the four rectus muscles; used as a guide in approximating the distance of the insertions from the limbus.

Spitzka's bundle (spitz'kahz). See under *bundle.*

splitter. The first basic component of an interferometer which separates the incident light into two coherent beams.

Vicker's optical beam s. An optical apparatus comprised of a pair of separately rotatable rhomboidal prisms to which are respectively cemented a pair of right-angled prisms at a pair of partially reflecting, beam splitting interfaces, all arranged so that coincidence of the two images of two points on an object by the relative rotation of the rhomboidal prisms provides a measure of their separations.

spondylitis, ankylosing (spon"dih-li'tis). Rheumatoid arthritis of the spine occurring primarily in young males. Iridocyclitis is a frequent accompaniment. Syn., *Bechterew's disease; Strümpell-Marie disease; rhizomelic spondylosis.*

spondylosis, rhizomelic (spon"dih-lo'sis). Ankylosing spondylitis.

spongioneuroblastoma (spon"je-o-nu"ro-blas-to'mah). A malignant neoplasm composed of spongioblastic and neuronal components in different stages of maturity, occurring in the central nervous system, retina, and ciliary epithelium.

spongiosis choroideae (spon-je-o'sis ko-roi'de-e). Edema of the choroid, usually resulting from venous congestion.

◆

SPOT

spot. A small, circumscribed area differing, as in color or content, from its ground.

Arago's s. 1. A physiological negative scotoma present in low levels of illumination corresponding to the rod-free area at the center of the fovea. 2. Poisson spot.

Bitot's s's. Small, white or gray, sharply defined spots appearing on dried areas of the palpebral conjunctiva in xerosis of the conjunctiva from vitamin A deficiency. They have a soapy appearance, as of dried foam, and are at first oval in shape and then triangular, with the base toward the limbus.

blind s., baring of. The condition in which contraction of the temporal peripheral visual field is so marked that the temporal limit of the visual field lies on, or nasal to, the blind spot of Mariotte. Cf. *inverted uncinate visual field; uncinate visual field.*

blind s. of Mariotte. A physiological negative scotoma in the visual field corresponding to the head of the optic nerve which is insensitive to light stimulation. It is typically oval in shape, approximately 7.5° along its vertical axis and 5.5° along its horizontal axis, and its center is located 15.5° to the temporal side and 1.5° below the point of fixation. Syn., *punctum caecum; physiological blind spot; Mariotte's spot.*

blind s., physiological. Blind spot of Mariotte.

Brushfield's s's. Small, white or light yellow flecks on the iris of infant Mongolian idiots.

cherry-red s. A red spot in the center of a white, edematous, and/or atrophic macular area appearing in the fundus in Tay-Sachs disease and in occlusion of the central retinal artery. It has the coloring of the normal fovea, due to choroidal circulation, but appears redder by contrast to the surrounding whitened retina.

corneal s. An opacity of the cornea, as a leukoma, or a macula.

cotton-wool s's. White, fluffy-appearing patches, occurring in edematous areas of the retina, as may occur in hypertensive retinopathy. They are coagulated exudates of plasma and fibrin from the retinal capillaries distal to angiospastic arterioles. Syn., *cotton-wool patches.*

Dalén's s's. Small white spots, resembling drusen, which may occur in the fundus as an early sign of sympathetic ophthalmia, due to changes in the pigment epithelium layer of the retina.

Elschnig s's. Small bright red or yellow spots with isolated flecks of black pigment at their borders, appearing in the fundus in advanced hypertensive retinopathy.

eye s. Eyespot.

Fischer-Kuhnt s. Bluish transparency of the sclera anterior to the insertions of the horizontal rectus muscles, due to senile thinning and hyalinization of the sclera.

flame s's. Flame-shaped areas characteristic of hemorrhage into the nerve fiber layer of the retina.

Fuchs' s. A round and sharply defined black spot occasionally occupy-ing the macular area, due to degenerative changes in high myopia. Syn., *Förster-Fuchs fleck.*

Gaule's s's. Sharply circumscribed areas of degenerated corneal epithelium, sometimes appearing in neuroparalytic keratitis. Syn., *Gaule's pits.*

glaucoma s's. Multiple, circumscribed, white spots beneath the anterior lens capsule, occurring in association with glaucoma. See also *cataracta glaucomatosa acuta.*

von Graefe's s's. Areas over the vertebrae or near the supraorbital foramen which, when pressed, result in relaxation of the orbicularis oculi muscle in blepharofacial spasm.

green s. A spot occupying the macular area, similar to Fuchs' spot, but of a greenish coloration, due to degenerative changes in high myopia.

Koplik's s's. Pale whitish spots appearing in the mucous membrane of the mouth, and sometimes in the conjunctiva, in the prodromal stage of measles.

Mariotte's s. Blind spot of Mariotte.

Maxwell's s. An entoptically seen, darkened spot in the visual field corresponding to the fovea, observed on fixating a diffusely illuminated field, especially a field of dark blue or purplish-blue color, used clinically to detect anomalous fixation or the integrity of the foveal area.

Michel's s's. An atrophic patch of the iris, with the posterior pigment epithelium visible, as may result from a tuberculomatous nodule. Syn., *Michel's flecks.*

Mueller's s's. Small, white, depigmented areas on the iris resulting from local circumscribed atrophy, as may occur after an attack of smallpox.

Poisson s. A bright spot in the center of a shadow created by a circular or spherical obstruction in the path of a light source, due to diffraction. It is as bright as if no obstruction were present.

Roth's s's. Small white spots, frequently surrounded by hemorrhage so that the latter appears to have a white center, occurring in the fundus near the optic disk in Roth's disease. Syn., *Roth's patches.*

Siegrist's s's. Chains of pigmented spots which course along the paths of sclerosed choroidal vessels, occurring in the fundus in advanced hypertensive retinopathy.

snow bank s's. Cotton-wool spots.

Soemmering's s. Macula lutea.

Tay's s. The cherry-red spot seen in the macular area in Tay-Sachs disease.

yellow s. Macula lutea.

◆

S-potential. An intraretinal electrical potential assumed to be generated in the regions of the outer molecular or outer nuclear layers which has a square waveform whose amplitude remains nearly constant as long as the stimulus light is in effect. It is not considered to be a receptor potential nor to contribute directly to the ERG.

Spraing's test. See under *test*.

spread, illusory visual. A hallucinatory phenomenon in which an image seems to cover a greater area than would be expected, hence a brightly colored article of dress may appear to cover the face and hands of the wearer.

spread, line. See *line spread function*.

spur. A projecting structure or formation.

s. of Fuchs. A spur of indented, iridic, posterior pigment epithelium into the posterior surface of the sphincter pupillae muscle, about midway along its length, associated with the junction of a few fibers of the dilator pupillae muscle.

Grünert's s. A spur of indented, iridic, posterior pigment epithelium at the junction of the iris and the ciliary body, marking the peripheral termination of the dilator pupillae muscle.

Michel's s. A spur of indented, iridic, posterior pigment epithelium marking the peripheral border of the sphincter pupillae muscle and its juncture with fibers of the dilator pupillae muscle.

scleral s. A dense mass of circularly arranged scleral fibers at the level of the limbus, interposed between the posterior portion of Schlemm's canal and the anterior attachment of the ciliary muscle, terminating at the meshwork of the angle of the anterior chamber. Syn., *annular ligament; Schwalbe's posterior ring.*

Spurway's syndrome (spur'wāz). Eddowes' syndrome.

squint. Strabismus.

Squint Korector, Arneson. An orthoptic instrument consisting essentially of a large, circular, motor-rotated disk mounted vertically on a stand. On the surface of the disk are an E-shaped design in three colors and an eccentrically located, movable, small, ruby glass, fixation target.

SRx. Spectacle prescription.

Stähli's line (shta'lēz). Superficial senile line.

staining. The artificial coloration of tissue, usually in order to facilitate its study.

ocular s. Staining of ocular tissue (cornea and conjunctiva) by instilling a dye into the conjunctival sac. The tissue which retains the dye is either abraded, dead, or degenerated.

surface s. The usual form of ocular staining in which a 1 or 2% solution of fluorescein or rose bengal is instilled only once so as to stain only the superficial layers.

3 and 9 o'clock s. Corneal staining associated with contact lens wear due to inadequate blink frequency and/or amplitude and typically located at or below the 3 and 9 o'clock regions of the peripheral cornea and the sclera that are not covered by the contact lens.

vital s. A seldom used form of ocular staining in which a dye, such as a dilute solution of azure II, is instilled several times so as to stain debilitated living cells.

staircase, Schroeder's. Schroeder's figure.

stalk, lens. A pedicle of cells by which the newly formed lens vesicle in the embryo is still attached to the surface ectoderm. It atrophies, and the lens vesicle separates from the surface ectoderm at about the fourth or fifth week of embryonic life.

stalk, optic Optic pedicle.

standard, GOMAC. GOMAC method.

standard, Waidner-Burgess. The luminous intensity of a blackbody at the freezing point of platinum.

Stanford stereoscope (stan'ford). See under *stereoscope*.

Stanloscope (stan'lo-skōp). An instrument used in visual training which doubles the image from a motion picture projector. Each of the doubled images is passed through a Polaroid or color filter and is viewed through a Polaroid or color filter, so that each eye sees only one of the images.

Stanworth amblyoscope. See under *amblyoscope.*

staphyloma (staf″ih-lo′mah). A bulging or protrusion of the cornea or the sclera, usually containing adherent uveal tissue.

annular s. Ring staphyloma.

anterior s. 1. Corneal staphyloma. 2. Staphyloma anterior to the equator of the eyeball. **congenital a.s.** A corneal staphyloma existing since birth, characterized by a bulging opaque cornea lined on its posterior surface by an incarcerated iris.

ciliary s. Anterior scleral staphyloma occurring in the region of the ciliary body and lined with prolapsed tissue of the ciliary body.

s. corneae racemosum. Corneal staphyloma resulting from a number of corneal perforations in each of which is incarcerated iridic tissue.

corneal s. A bulging cicatrix of the cornea formed essentially by prolapsed iris partially converted into fibrous scar tissue. Syn., *anterior staphyloma.*

equatorial s. Scleral staphyloma occurring in the region of the equator of the eyeball, especially in the area of exit of the vortex veins.

intercalary s. Anterior scleral staphyloma occurring between the anterior extremity of the ciliary body and the iris and lined with tissue from the root of the iris.

posterior s. Scleral staphyloma occurring posterior to the equator of the eyeball, especially in the region of the posterior pole. **p.s. of von Ammon.** Posterior protrusion of von Ammon.

s. posticum of Scarpa. Posterior staphyloma occurring at the posterior pole of the eyeball, due to degenerative changes in high myopia. Syn., *Scarpa's staphyloma; staphyloma verum.*

ring s. An anterior scleral staphyloma around the cornea in the ciliary region formed by the confluence of smaller staphylomata. Syn., *annular staphyloma.*

Scarpa's s. Staphyloma posticum of Scarpa.

scleral s. A bulging or protrusion of a thin or weakened sclera, ordinarily lined with uveal tissue. **anterior s.s.** Staphyloma of the sclera anterior to the equator of the eyeball, occurring either as a *ciliary staphyloma* or as an *intercalary staphyloma.*

s. verum. Staphyloma posticum of Scarpa.

staphylomatous (staf″ih-lom′ah-tus). Pertaining to, resembling, or affected with staphyloma.

staphylotomy (staf″ih-lot′o-me). Surgical incision of a staphyloma.

star. A figure having five or more points representing a star, or anything which is like or suggests a star or such a figure.

lens s's. The starlike formations, one in the anterior and one in the posterior portion of the crystalline lens, formed by the sutures of the lens fibers.

macular s. Deposits of lipid material in Henle's fiber layer in a star formation radiating out from the macula in a previously edematous area. See also *macular fan.*

muscle s's. Groups of smooth cell fibers arranged in star-shaped configurations, located in the suprachoroid in the region of the equator of the eyeball, where they are continuous with Brücke's muscle.

Siemens' s. A target for testing the resolution of an optical system consisting of a circle containing alternate black and white wedgeshaped spokes of equal size whose apices all meet at a common point at the center of the circle. The resolution is determined by the diameter of the area of central blur resulting from lack of resolution of the spokes.

Van Orden s. The multiple-spoke radiating pattern traced, or perceived as being traced, by a subject undergoing the *Van Orden method,* q.v.

Winslow's s's. Whorls of capillaries in the choroid which drain into the vorticose veins. Syn., *stellulae vasculosae winslowii.*

stare. To gaze or look fixedly; a fixed gaze.

postbasic s. A stare characteristic of posterior basic meningitis in which the eyeballs are rotated downward and the upper eyelids are retracted.

Stargardt's (stahr′gahrtz) **disease; macular degeneration; foveal dystrophy.** See under *disease.*

Stark effect. See under *effect.*

stasis, papillary (sta′sis). Cessation of the flow of blood in the retinal vessels in the region of the optic disk, due to papilledema.

statometer (stah-tom′eh-ter). An instrument for determining the degree of proptosis in exophthalmos.

statoscope (stat'o-skōp). An instrument consisting essentially of a tube in which a light source, a blue filter, a diaphragm, and a lens are so arranged that parallel light is reflected into one eye by a plane mirror, to be fixated while the other eye is being examined with a retinoscope. Syn., *photoscope*.

status Bonnevie-Ullrich. Lymphatic edema of the hands and feet, pterygium colli, malformation of the ears, muscle defects (especially of the pectoralis), hypertelorism, epicanthus, syndactyly and other digital deformities, and paralyses of the third, sixth, seventh, and twelfth cranial nerves; occurring in girls as a hereditary congenital anomaly in two forms: a symmetrical form in which both internal and external malformations occur, and an asymmetrical form chiefly characterized by anomalies distributed asymmetrically near the body surface. Syn., *Bonnevie-Ullrich syndrome.*

status dysraphicus (sta'tus dis-ra'fihkus). A widespread condition caused by failure of normal closure of the neural tube which includes skeletal anomalies, changes in soft tissues, and vasomotor disturbances. The most common ocular sign is heterochromia iridum, either congenital or developed, and other ocular symptoms may include Fuchs' syndrome, Horner's syndrome, Duane's retraction syndrome, and Romberg's syndrome.

steatoma of the eyelid (ste"ah-to'mah). A sebaceous cyst or tumor, associated with the hairs of the eyelid, encapsulated by fibrous tissue and containing disintegrated epithelial cells, keratin, cholesterol crystals, and fatty granules. Syn., *atheroma of the eyelid.*

steatosis corneae (ste"ah-to'sis). Dystrophia adiposa corneae.

Steele-Richardson-Olszewski syndrome. See under *syndrome.*

Stefan-Boltzmann (shta'fahn-bōlts'-mahn) **constant; law.** See under the nouns.

Steiger's theory (sti'gerz). See under *theory.*

Steinert's disease (sti'nertz). Myotonic dystrophy.

Steinheil cone (stīn'hīl). See under *cone.*

stella (stel'ah). A star.

    s. lentis hyaloidea. The posterior pole of the crystalline lens of the eye.

    s. lentis iridica. The anterior pole of the crystalline lens of the eye.

stellulae vasculosae winslowii (stel'u-le vas"ku-lo'se wins-lo'ih-i). Winslow's stars.

Stellwag's (stel'vagz) **sign; symptom.** See under the nouns.

stenochoria (sten"o-ko're-ah). Stenosis, or narrowing, particularly of a lacrimal duct.

stenocoriasis (sten"o-ko-ri'ah-sis). Constriction of the pupil of the eye.

stenopaic (sten"o-pa'ik) **disk; slit.** See under the nouns.

stenopia (steh-no'pe-ah). Hypotelorism.

step, Roenne's nasal. A steplike defect in the nasal visual field, caused by asymmetrical involvement of the retinal nerve fibers on either side of the horizontal raphe, indicative of glaucoma.

stereo-acuity (ster"e-o-ah-ku'ih-te). The ability to perceive depth by the faculty of stereopsis, represented as a function of the threshold of stereopsis.

    dynamic s. Stereo-acuity obtained while the test targets are in motion, especially in motion in a frontoparallel plane.

stereocampimeter (ster"e-o-kampim'eh-ter). A haploscopic type of instrument used for examination of the visual fields, especially the central fields, in which the fields of view of the two eyes are separated and in which the eyes fixate similar targets to be fused, thus enabling the plotting of the visual field of one eye under conditions of binocular fixation. One type is similar to a Brewster stereoscope and another type has a movable mirror to reflect the test target into one eye while the target of the other is directly viewed.

stereocomparator (ster"e-o-kom-par'-ah-ter). A variable pair or a graduated series of disparately fused fiducial lines or reticles incorporated in the optics of a binocular viewing instrument to serve as a stereoscopic reference for judging the distances of viewed objects; a binocular instrument incorporating this feature.

stereocryptogram (ster"e-o-krip'togram). A typewritten stereogram in which the words or letters, constituting an otherwise unnoticed message or legend, are displaced horizontally so that they appear to stand out or recede from the plane of reference of the binocularly fused stereogram.

stereodisparator (ster"e-o-dis'pah-ra"ter). Disparator.

stereogram (ster'e-o-gram"). A target composed of a pair of drawings or similar photographs side by side such that, when viewed in a stereoscope, the right eye sees only the right side drawing or photograph and the left eye only the left side. If the corresponding parts of the drawings have been properly decentered, or the photographs are of a single scene taken from two directions, the stereogram, when properly fused, will give rise to the percept of relief or stereopsis. Syn., *stereograph.*

Dvorine animated fusion s's. A series of stereograms, each of which contains an aperture on the one side so that a rotatable disk mounted on this side may present a variety of pictures to the one eye. Thus, e.g., one side of the stereogram may present a cage and the other side may present either a tiger, a lion, or a bear.

Helmholtz s. An opposite contrast stereogram consisting of white lines on a black background in one half-field and black lines on a white background in the other half-field.

opposite contrast s. A stereogram in which the view presented to one eye is seen as a negative of that presented to the other, i.e., black lines and areas of one correspond to white lines and areas on the other. See also *Helmholtz stereogram.*

parallax s. A stereogram consisting of a composite photograph taken with a camera having two apertures and a grid interposed between the lens system and the film. The resultant photograph consists of alternate vertical parallel strips, each alternate strip being formed through one aperture. The stereogram is viewed through a screen of alternate opaque and transparent bands, so that the left eye is exposed to the portions of the photograph taken through the left aperture and the right eye through the right aperture.

Julesz random-dot s. A stereogram in which each eye sees an amorphously randomized but almost identical pattern of small printed characters or dots, differing only in the slight relative lateral displacement of nearly corresponding portions of each pattern, the shapes of which are recognized in stereoscopic relief by the observer as a result of the induced disparity during binocular fusion.

rotating s. A stereogram in which the two pictures may be rotated simultaneously, by a central cogwheel, to produce variations in the stereoscopic effect.

split s. A stereogram in two separate halves to permit variable vertical and lateral separations in the stereoscope.

stereograph (ster'e-o-graf"). Stereogram.

stereography (ster"e-og'rah-fe). The representing or delineating of three dimensional attributes in a single plane, as in a stereogram; making a stereogram.

stereomicrocamera (ster"e-o-mi'kro-kam"er-ah). A stereocamera which magnifies as it photographs.

stereomicrography (ster"e-o-mi-krog'-rah-fe). Photography with a stereomicrocamera.

stereomicrometer, Howard's (ster"-e-o-mi-krom'eh-ter). A binocular instrument with micrometer control of the lateral position of one of four vertical wires in the focal plane of the eyepieces, two seen by each eye, to be fused stereoscopically and adjusted for stereo judgments.

stereomicroscope (ster"e-o-mi'kro-skōp). Two complete microscope systems mounted in a single unit to permit binocular viewing of the object or specimen. Cf. *binocular microscope.*

stereomonoscope (ster"e-o-mon'o-skōp). An instrument which, by means of two separate and differently oriented lens systems, projects onto the same portion of a ground glass plate two images which appear in relief when viewed binocularly from the proper direction and distance.

Stereomotivator (ster"e-o-mo"tih-va'-tor). A visual training instrument consisting of a target holder for a laminar series of three projector slides or transparencies. The top two slides are of red and green color composition and synchronously and laterally displaceable in opposite directions to produce stereoscopic and prismatic effects when viewed by transillumination or by projection on a screen while wearing a red filter before one eye and a green filter before the other eye.

stereo-ophthalmoscope (ster"e-o-of-thal'mo-skōp). A binocular ophthalmoscope.

Stereo-orthopter (ster"e-o-ōr-thop'-ter). A visual training instrument, similar to a Wheatstone stereoscope, consisting essentially of two front surface mirrors joined at an angle at one end to reflect targets, one into each eye, and eyepieces of spherical convex lens power to reduce or eliminate accommodative demands. The angular separation of the mirrors may be varied to alter prismatic effect and a built-in motor provides for lateral rotation of the mirrors about a point where they meet and for introducing various flash patterns.

stereoperception (ster"e-o-per-sep'-shun). Stereopsis.

stereophantoscope (ster"e-o-fan'to-skōp). A stereoscope in which, instead of still pictures, rotating stroboscopic disks are used to impart apparent motion to the views.

stereophenomenon, Pulfrich (ster"-e-o-fe-nom'e-non). Pulfrich effect.

stereophorometer (ster"e-o-fo-rom'-eh-ter). A phorometer with an attachment for the use of stereograms.

stereophoroscope (ster"e-o-fōr'o-skōp). An early instrument for producing a series of images in apparent motion and in relief, consisting essentially of a series of stereograms attached to a many-sided prism rotating about a horizontal axis, to be viewed in rapid sequence in a Brewster stereoscope.

stereophotogram (ster"e-o-fo'to-gram). Paired photographs of the same scene taken from two stations which, when viewed through an appropriate haploscopic optical system, give rise to a three-dimensional percept.

stereophotogrammetry (ster"e-o-fo"to-gram'eh-tre). Photogrammetry utilizing stereopsis, as used, for example, for determining the contours of the cornea.

stereophotography (ster"e-o-fo-tog'-rah-fe). Photography to produce pictures which give rise to the percept of the third dimension when viewed through a device such as a stereoscope. Syn., *stereography.*

stereophotometry (ster"e-o-fo-tom'eh-tre). Subjective photometry based on the Pulfrich effect, in which the apparent path of a laterally moving spot or pendulum bob is changed from an ellipse, when the background luminosity differs for the two eyes, to its true on-plane motion when the background luminosity is the same.

stereopsis (ster"e-op'sis). 1. Binocular visual perception of three dimensional space based on retinal disparity. 2. Visual perception of depth or three dimensional space.

amplitude of s. See under *amplitude.*

anteroscopic s. Stereopsis in which objects appear closer than the plane of the stereogram.

axial s. Central stereopsis.

binocular s. Stereopsis based on depth clues present only when both eyes are in use, such as retinal disparity.

central s. Stereopsis based on retinal disparity within the foveal or the macular areas. Syn., *axial stereopsis.*

chrome s. Chromostereopsis.

global s. Stereopsis elicited by the disparity of portions and/or clusters within relatively large stereogram patterns, involving complex textured surfaces and repetitive elements for which many disparately paired details might provide ambiguous or even conflicting stereopsis clues without destroying the overlying percept of depth, believed by Julesz to represent a perceptual interpretation process differentiable from *local stereopsis.*

local s. Stereopsis elicited by a very simple disparity stimulus pattern such as, for example, a stereogram with two parallel vertical line segments seen by each eye with slightly differing lateral separations. Cf. *global stereopsis.*

monocular s. Perception of the third dimension based on depth clues not dependent on binocular vision, such as shadows, aerial perspective, or contour interference. Such clues are not exclusive to monocular vision, but are usually more effective in the absence of conflicting binocular clues, as may be noted by viewing a photograph monocularly. (Uncommon usage.)

peripheral s. Stereopsis based on retinal disparity stimuli peripheral to the maculae.

range of s. See under *range.*

retroscopic s. Stereopsis in which objects appear farther away than the plane of the stereogram.

reversible s. Stereopsis in which uncrossed disparate points appear to be nearer than the point of binocular fixation, as may occur when viewing bright targets in a dark field of view.

stereoplotting (ster"e-o-plot'ing). The cartographic plotting of contour lines by tracing loci of equal elevation as, for example, in stereoscopically viewed aerial photographs of the terrain.

stereopticon (ster″e-op′tih-kon). An instrument for projecting enlarged images of pictures on a screen, especially one with a double optical system to permit successive presentations so that one image appears to fade away as the other replaces it. A projector.

stereoptor, Verhoeff's (ster″e-op′-ter). A small, hand-size, transilluminated, black frame with three opaque, different-sized bars which can be presented in a variety of orders with one always being a fixed distance behind or in front of the other two; it is used to measure stereopsis by determining the maximum viewing distance at which the displaced bar can be identified.

stereoradiography (ster″e-o-ra″-de-og′rah-fe). Stereoroentgenography.

Stereo-Reader, Delacato (ster″e-o-re′der). A visual training instrument consisting essentially of a Brewster-type stereoscope with a flat platform on which target material is presented to either or both eyes. A reading guide attachment may be utilized before either eye.

stereorefraction (ster″e-o-re-frak′-shun). Refraction performed while the patient is binocularly viewing projected stereo-inducing targets through Polaroid filters. The usual procedure is to project a stereo picture or scene with a central clear area on which the polarized test targets are projected from a second instrument. Adjustments may be made for central occlusion of one eye during monocular testing of the other.

stereoroentgenography (ster″e-o-rent″gen-og′rah-fe). The making of a stereogram containing two roentgen ray photographs. Syn., *stereoradiography.*

◆

STEREOSCOPE

stereoscope (ster′e-o-skōp″). An instrument which separates the field of view of the two eyes, either by tubes, a septum, or an arrangement of mirrors, so that only certain portions of stereogram targets viewed through it are seen by one eye and other portions by the other eye to give rise to a combined binocular percept. Usually spheroprism eyepieces are used in conjunction with the septum or the tubes and spherical eyepieces with the mirrors.

Asher-Law s. A Brewster-type, hand stereoscope with a disparator attachment for use with split stereograms.

automatic s. A stereoscope with an attachment housing a number of stereograms, so that they may be successively viewed by manipulating a lever or turning a knob.

book s. A folding stereoscope.

Brewster's s. A pyramidal-shaped stereoscope consisting essentially of two tubes, acting to separate the fields of view of the two eyes, and containing double convex base-out spheroprism eyepieces of 6 in. focal length, which are adjustable for interpupillary distance and distance from the targets at the base of the instrument. Syn., *Brewster-Holmes stereoscope; lenticular stereoscope; prismatic stereoscope; refracting stereoscope.*

chain s. A Brewster-type stereoscope in which a series of stereograms are attached to a chain affixed to sprockets, so that the turning of a knob rotates successive stereograms into view.

Cross's s. A Brewster-type, hand stereoscope with a target holder consisting of a rotatable fourteen-sided drum, on each face of which is mounted a stereogram for individual viewing.

Cruise s. A Brewster-type, hand stereoscope in which the eyepieces may be rotated to provide variable prism power.

Derby's s. A Brewster-type stereoscope containing spheroprism eyepieces (+7.00 D lenses combined with 5△ base-out) which are attached to a screw mounting for adjustment of the interpupillary distance, and a target holder marked off in square centimeters on which are attached small, circular, split targets.

Dynamic s. Dynascope.

Ellis s. A Brewster-type, hand stereoscope containing +4.00 D spheroprism lenses, cells for use of auxiliary prisms or lenses, and a movable target carrier.

Engelmann s. Dynascope.

folding s. A simplified Brewster-type stereoscope in which the eyepieces are mounted in material which can be folded. It usually contains no target holder and is held manually before the eyes when viewing stereograms (usually those contained in books). Syn., *book stereoscope.*

Hartline's s. A Wheatstone-type stereoscope in which the angle between the two mirrors is adjustable.

Holmes's s. A Brewster-type, hand stereoscope with a movable target holder and eyepieces of +5.25 D spheres so decentered as to produce about 8^Δ base-out before each eye.

Javal's s. 1. A Brewster-type stereoscope in which narrow split targets may be moved laterally or vertically in the plane of the target holder. 2. A Wheatstone-type stereoscope in which two plane mirrors are hinged together, each of which in turn has attached at its opposite end a target holder at a 45° angle, providing a view of each target by one eye, while the angle between the two mirrors may be adjusted to the desired convergence stimulus.

kinetic s. A Brewster-type stereoscope having a variable separation split-target holder mounted on a rotatable grooved arc mechanism, providing for variations in direction of fixation in all meridians independent of the convergence demand.

Landolt's s. A box stereoscope, 166 mm long, in which the optical system consists of any pair of desired trial case lenses or prisms.

lens s. Lenticular stereoscope.

lenticular s. A stereoscope containing spheroprisms for eyepieces, together with a septum to separate the fields of view of the two eyes, as in the Brewster stereoscope. Syn., *lens stereoscope; prismatic stereoscope; refracting stereoscope.*

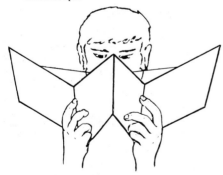

Fig. 34 Illustration of a mirror stereoscope. (From J. R. Griffin, *Binocular Anomalies*. Chicago: Professional Press, 1976)

mirror s. A stereoscope in which mirrors separate the fields of view of the two eyes, as in the Wheatstone ster-eoscope. (See Fig. 34.) Syn., *reflecting stereoscope.*

phoro-optometer s. A phoro-optometer with a target holder for stereograms.

Pigeon-Cantonnet s. A visual training instrument consisting of three black, stiff, cardboard leaves, 31.5 × 23 cm, hinged together at one end, as in a book, with a small plane mirror placed on one face of the middle leaf, and targets or patterns on the inner faces of the two outer leaves. When the middle leaf is held to the nose as a septum, one target may be seen directly by one eye and the other by reflection in the mirror, and the convergence demand may be controlled by the angle between the outer leaves and the position of the targets on their inner faces.

Polack's s. A Brewster-type, hand stereoscope containing two rotary prisms for eyepieces which may be synchronously rotated to provide prism effects varying from 0° to 18°.

prismatic s. 1. Lenticular stereoscope. 2. A Wheatstone-type stereoscope containing reflecting prisms in place of plane mirrors.

Pulfrich s. A Wheatstone-type stereoscope containing two 90° reflecting prisms for eyepieces.

reflecting s. Mirror stereoscope.

refracting s. Lenticular stereoscope.

Stanford s. A Wheatstone-type stereoscope for viewing roentgen ray stereograms.

Wheatstone s. A stereoscope consisting of two plane mirrors joined at one edge at a 90° angle and two target holders, one opposite one mirror and the other opposite the other, mounted on a screw base which, when turned, synchronously moves the targets toward or away from each other. Syn., *Wheatstone amblyoscope; reflecting stereoscope.*

Whittington s. A Brewster-type stereoscope designed primarily for cheiroscopic drawing.

◆

stereoscopic (ster″e-o-skop′ik). Pertaining to or producing stereopsis.

s. relief. See under *relief.*

stereoscoptometer (ster″e-o-skop-tom′-eh-ter). An instrument for determining the threshold of depth perception.

stereoscopy (ster″e-os′ko-pe). 1. The science treating of stereoscopic effects and the methods of producing them. 2. Seeing in the third dimension.

color s. 1. Chromostereopsis. 2. Stereoscopic viewing accomplished by means of a red filter in front of one eye and a green filter in front of the other and a composite picture or pattern whose red detail represents the view of one eye and the green detail the view of the other.

irradiation s. The perception of stereoscopic relief in a flat target resulting from retinal images of a different effective size, produced by reducing the irradiation of one eye by means of a neutral filter, the difference in effective image size causing an apparent rotation of the frontoparallel plane about a vertical axis. It may be observed by binocularly fixating a point on either side of which are white squares in the frontoparallel plane, with a neutral filter before one eye. Syn., *luminance aniseikonia.* See *Cibis test.*

stereostroboscope (ster"e-o-stro'bo-skōp). An apparatus for producing binocular relief effects by means of differential or asynchronous stroboscopic views presented separately but concurrently to the two eyes.

stereotest, Wirt (ster'e-o-test). Wirt test.

stereothreshold. Threshold of stereopsis.

Stevens' (ste'vens) **clinoscope; phorometer; test; tropometer.** See under the nouns.

Stevens-Johnson (ste'vens-jon'son) **disease; syndrome.** See under the nouns.

Stichtung Nederlandse Vakopleiding voor Opticiens. A Dutch educational foundation which provides and administers optometric correspondence courses and concerns itself with matters of educational policy.

Stieda's (ste'dahz) **grooves; plateaus.** See under the nouns.

Stifel's figure (sti'felz). See under *figure.*

stigma. Eyespot.

stigmas, hysterical (stig'mahz). The specific symptoms of hysteria including reversal of the color visual fields, contraction of the visual field, and transient amblyopia.

stigmatic (stig-mat'ik). Affected with or pertaining to stigmatism.

stigmatism (stig'mah-tizm). The condition in which light from a point source is brought to a point focus by a lens or an optical system.

stigmatometer (stig"mah-tom'eh-ter). An instrument for measuring refractive error by the criterion of sharpness of appearance or imagery of a very small pointlike source of light. Syn., *oculometer.*

stigmatoscope (stig-mat'o-skōp). 1. An instrument for observing the character or pattern of a very small pointlike source of light in relation to the refractive error. 2. A stigmatometer.

stigmatoscopy (stig"mah-tos'ko-pe). Observation or measurement of the refractive state of the eye by means of a stigmatoscope.

objective s. A modified method of retinoscopy in which the observer moves his head instead of the light source or the mirror.

stilb (stil'b). A unit of luminance equal to 1 candela per cm². See also *footlambert.*

Stiles theory. See under *theory.*

Stiles-Crawford effect (stīlz-kraw'-ford). See under *effect.*

Still's disease. Juvenile polyarthritis.

stillicidium lacrimarum (stil"ih-sid'-e-um lak-rih-mah'rum). Epiphora. *Obs.*

Stilling's (stil'ingz) **canal; charts; plates; test; theory.** See under the nouns.

Stilling-Türk-Duane syndrome. Duane's syndrome.

Stimson charts. See under *chart.*

stimulation. The act or the effect of applying a stimulus.

biretinal kinetic s. Stimulation of the peripheral retinae by viewing in an amblyoscope superimposition targets which are locked at the objective angle of strabismus and then moved laterally back and forth while the eyes remain motionless in the straightforward position; a method designed to reestablish normal retinal correspondence by attempting to obtain peripheral superimposition.

peripheral s. In visual training, the haploscopic presentation of peripherally located patterns to one eye, while the other eye fixates a centrally located object, to break down suppression.

stimulus. Any agent, condition, or environmental change having the capability or property of influencing the activity of living protoplasm or of initiating or controlling a response, a percept, or a sensation, especially through the medium of a sense organ or receptor.

achromatic s. Neutral stimulus.

adequate s. 1. A stimulus of sufficient magnitude and/or of appropriate character to elicit, control, or influence a response, a percept, or a sensation, with respect to a given type of receptor mechanism. 2. A stimulus of a type for which the receptor is especially sensitive, such as wavelengths within the visible spectrum for the rods and cones.

cardinal stimuli. Four standard visual stimuli by means of which three reference stimuli and the basic stimulus of any trichromatic system may be defined. Light of wavelengths 700, 546.1 and 435.8 mμ and Illuminant B have been adopted by the CIE.

color s. A photic stimulus capable of eliciting the sensation of color.

equal-energy s. Photic radiation whose irradiance per unit wavelength is equal throughout the spectrum.

inadequate s. 1. A stimulus of insufficient magnitude or of inappropriate character or type to elicit, control, or influence a response, a percept, or a sensation, with respect to a given type of receptor mechanism. 2. A stimulus of a type for which the receptor is not especially sensitive but to which it may respond, such as pressure on the eyeball producing phosphene.

liminal s. A stimulus of the least energy value capable of evoking an overt response. Syn., *minimal stimulus; threshold stimulus.*

maximal s. The stimulus which evokes the greatest response capable for that type of stimulation.

minimal s. Liminal stimulus.

neutral s. Photic radiation that does not produce a chromatic experience. Syn., *achromatic stimulus.*

subliminal s. A stimulus of insufficient magnitude to evoke an overt response. Syn., *subminimal stimulus; subthreshold stimulus.*

subminimal s. Subliminal stimulus.

subthreshold s. Subliminal stimulus.

supraliminal s. A stimulus of greater magnitude than necessary to evoke an overt response; one of greater magnitude than a liminal stimulus.

Syn., *supraminimal stimulus; suprathreshold stimulus.*

supramaximal s. A stimulus of greater energy value than necessary to produce the greatest response for that type of stimulation.

supraminimal s. Supraliminal stimulus.

suprathreshold s. Supraliminal stimulus.

threshold s. Liminal stimulus.

stint. Conformer.

stippled epiphyses (stip'ld e-pif'ih-sēs). A rare congenital condition characterized by enlargement of the epiphyses due to punctate calcium deposits with resulting deficient skeletal growth. The affected are short-limbed dwarfs with immobile joints, most of whom die by the age of three. Bilateral total cataract is frequently present. Syn., *chondrodystrophia calcificans congenita punctata; chondrodystrophia fetalis hypoplastica; congenital calcareous chondrodystrophy; dysplasia epiphysialis punctata; Conradi's syndrome.*

stippling (stip'pling). Pinpoint areas of discontinuous or devitalized corneal epithelium which, upon the application of fluorescein, will absorb the dye and be detected with the slit lamp biomicroscope as a series of discrete green dots.

Stocker's line. See under *line.*

Stokes's (stŏks'ez) **disease; law; lens; lines.** See under the nouns.

stop. The material, opaque border of an aperture, or the border of an optical element in an optical system, which limits the number of rays traversing the system. Syn., *diaphragm.*

aperture s. The stop of an optical system which, by virtue of its size and position with respect to the radiating object, is effective in limiting the bundle of light rays traversing the system.

back s. A stop in an optical system located in the image space.

field s. The stop of an optical system which limits the extent of the field of view.

front s. A stop in an optical system located in the object space.

light s. A stop, a baffle plate, or a baffling ring located between the lenses of an optical system to cut out stray light derived from the body tube or the lens mounts.

telecentric s. A stop placed at one of the focal points of an optical system.

strabilismus (stra"bih-liz'mus, strab"ih-). Strabismus. *Obs.*

strabism (stra'biz-um, strab'iz-um). Strabismus. *Obs.*

strabismal (strah-biz'mal). Pertaining to or affected with strabismus.

strabismic (strah-biz'mic). 1. Pertaining to or affected with strabismus. 2. One affected with strabismus.

strabismometer (strah"biz-mom'eh-ter). Any instrument for measuring the angle of strabismus. Syn., *ophthalmotropometer.*

Allied s. Trade name for an instrument for doing the Lancaster test.

Galezowski's s. A strabismometer consisting of a graduated horizontal bar to which are attached a nose rest, temples, and two adjustable, vertical needles, one on each side of the nose rest, which are aligned with the centers of the pupils, or some other reference point.

Laurence's s. A strabismometer consisting of a flat piece of ivory or metal with a concave graduated edge to fit against the lower eyelid to estimate the angle of strabismus.

Maddox' tangent s. Maddox cross.

strabismometry (strah"biz-mom'eh-tre). Measurement of the angle of strabismus. Syn., *ophthalmotropometry.*

angular s. Strabismometry in which the deviation is measured in degrees, as with a perimeter.

linear s. Strabismometry in which the deviation is estimated by means of a scale placed before the eyes, as with Laurence's strabismometer.

tangential s. Strabismometry in which the deviation is measured with a tangent scale.

◆

STRABISMUS

strabismus (strah-biz'mus). The condition in which binocular fixation is not present under normal seeing conditions, i.e., the foveal line of sight of one eye fails to intersect the object of fixation. Syn., *heterotropia; ophthalmotropia; squint; tropia.*

absolute s. Constant strabismus.

accommodative s. 1. Strabismus resulting from abnormal demand on accommodation, such as convergent strabismus due to uncorrected hypermetropia or divergent strabismus due to uncorrected myopia. 2. Strabismus resulting from the act of accommodating in association with a high AC/A ratio.

adventitious s. *Optometric Extension Program:* Acquired strabismus considered to be an adaptation to the stress of convergence demands.

alternating s. Strabismus in which either eye can maintain fixation. Syn., *bilateral strabismus; binocular strabismus.* **accidental a.s.** Alternating strabismus in which either eye can maintain fixation, although one eye is preferred. **convergent isoametropic a.s.** A convergent alternating strabismus associated with high hypermetropia of equal amount in the two eyes. **convergent paretic a.s.** Convergent alternating strabismus associated with paresis of the external rectus muscles. **essential a.s.** Alternating strabismus in which either eye can maintain fixation with the same facility and in which either eye is used indiscriminately.

ambiocular s. Strabismus in which both eyes are used simultaneously but in which different portions of the image of each eye are utilized to form a single composite percept, said to occur in anomalous retinal correspondence.

anatomical s. Strabismus resulting from anatomical anomalies of the orbits, the eyeballs, or the extraocular muscles and their check ligaments.

apparent s. The appearance of strabismus as induced by an abnormally small or large angle lambda, extreme variation in the shape or placement of the eyelids, the breadth of the nose, or epicanthus. Syn., *pseudostrabismus.*

s. ascendens. Strabismus sursumvergens.

basic s. Heterotropia which is of approximately the same magnitude for both far and near fixation distances.

bilateral s. Alternating strabismus.

binocular s. Alternating strabismus.

Braid's s. A simultaneous upward and inward turning of the eyes; a requested response sometimes employed as a part of the procedure to induce hypnosis.

comitant s. Concomitant strabismus.

concomitant s. Strabismus in which the angle of deviation remains constant for all directions of gaze and with either eye fixating. Syn., *comitant strabismus*. Cf. *nonconcomitant strabismus*. **primary c.s.** Concomitant strabismus not of paralytic origin. **secondary c.s.** Concomitant strabismus which follows a long standing nonconcomitant strabismus.

congenital s. Strabismus present or existing since birth.

consecutive s. Strabismus in which the deviation differs from that of a pre-existing strabismus, as may occur following surgery.

constant s. Strabismus present at all times. Syn., *absolute strabismus; continuous strabismus; fixed strabismus; permanent strabismus.*

continuous s. 1. Constant strabismus. 2. Strabismus which, when present, occurs for all distances and directions of fixation. 3. Strabismus in which the magnitude of the deviation is the same for all fixation distances.

s. convergens. Convergent strabismus. **s.c. deorso-adductorius.** Convergent strabismus in which the deviating eye turns downward on convergence. **s.c. surso-adductorius.** Convergent strabismus in which the deviating eye turns upward on convergence.

convergent s. Strabismus in which the deviating eye turns inward, so that its foveal line of sight crosses the line of sight of the fixating eye at a point nearer than the object of fixation. Syn., *esotropia; strabismus convergens; internal strabismus.*

cyclic s. Strabismus recurring at regular time intervals.

s. deorsumvergens. Strabismus in which the deviating eye turns downward, so that its foveal line of sight is below the object of fixation. Syn., *hypotropia; strabismus descendens.*

s. descendens. Strabismus deorsumvergens.

s. divergens. Divergent strabismus.

divergent s. Strabismus in which the deviating eye turns templeward, so that its foveal line of sight crosses the line of sight of the fixating eye at a point farther than the object of fixation or at a hypothetical point behind the eyes. Syn., *exotropia; strabismus divergens; external strabismus.*

external s. Divergent strabismus.

fixed s. 1. Constant strabismus. 2. Strabismus in which the magnitude of the deviation is the same for all fixation distances. 3. Strabismus in which the magnitude of the deviation is the same at all times for the same fixation distance.

s. fixus. Congenital strabismus in which both eyes are held in a fixed adducted position by fibrotic and inelastic internal rectus muscles, muscle foot plates, or check ligaments.

hysterical s. Strabismus occurring in hysteria, characterized by extreme inconstancy.

incipient s. Premonitory strabismus.

incomitant s. Nonconcomitant strabismus.

inconstant s. Intermittent strabismus.

infantile s. Spurious strabismus.

innervational s. Strabismus attributed to anomalous innervation to the extraocular muscles.

intermittent s. Strabismus which is not present at all times. Syn., *inconstant strabismus; occasional strabismus; periodic strabismus; recurrent strabismus; relative strabismus.*

internal s. Convergent strabismus.

kinetic s. Strabismus resulting from a spasm of an extraocular muscle due to an irritative lesion in the central nervous system. The onset is usually sudden and the duration temporary.

latent s. Heterophoria.

lateral s. Strabismus in which the deviating eye is turned either in or out.

manifest s. Strabismus, as distinguished from *latent strabismus.* Syn., *patent strabismus.*

mechanical s. Strabismus resulting from pressure or traction on the eyeball, as may occur from an orbital tumor.

monocular s. Unilateral strabismus.

monolateral s. Unilateral strabismus.

muscular s. Strabismus due to overdevelopment or underdevelopment of any of the extraocular muscles or to anomalies of their insertions or check ligaments.

nonaccommodative s. Strabismus not attributable to abnormal demands on accommodation.

noncomitant s. Nonconcomitant strabismus.

nonconcomitant s. Strabismus in which the angle of deviation varies with the direction of gaze and/or with the eye that fixates, due to paralysis or paresis of one or more extraocular muscles. Syn., *incomitant strabismus; noncomitant strabismus.* Cf. *concomitant strabismus.*

nonparalytic s. Strabismus not attributable to paresis or paralysis of extraocular muscles, characterized by concomitant eye movements and equal primary and secondary deviations.

occasional s. 1. Intermittent strabismus. 2. Spurious strabismus.

occlusion s. Strabismus manifested after prolonged occlusion of one eye.

optical s. Strabismus in which refractive error is considered a primary etiological factor, such as high hypermetropia or anisometropia.

paralytic s. Strabismus resulting from paralysis of extraocular muscles, often characterized by nonconcomitant eye movements, unequal primary and secondary deviations, limitation of eye movement, head tilt or turn, and diplopia.

paretic s. Strabismus resulting from paresis of extraocular muscles, characterized by an overshooting of the nonaffected eye when the affected eye fixates in the field of action of the paretic muscle.

patent s. Manifest strabismus.

periodic s. 1. Strabismus present only at certain distances or directions of fixation. 2. Intermittent strabismus. 3. Strabismus in which the magnitude of the deviation varies with the fixation distance. **direct p.s.** Strabismus in which the deviation is greater at near fixation distances than at far fixation distances, as would obtain in esotropia with a high AC/A ratio. Cf. *inverse periodic strabismus.* **inverse p.s.** Strabismus in which the deviation is greater at far fixation distances than at near fixation distances. Cf. *direct periodic strabismus.*

permanent s. Constant strabismus.

physiological s. A class of strabismus identified with faulty extraocular muscle innervation, as distinct from anatomical and optical classes of strabismus.

premonitory s. Dissociations of the eyes of infants prior to the full development of binocular fixation, occurring relatively frequently and lasting a few minutes or more. Syn., *incipient strabismus.*

psychopathic s. Strabismus attributed to psychological or emotional causes.

purposive s. Strabismus in which the magnitude of the deviation is increased so that the stimulation of the deviating eye is more peripheral, thus to facilitate suppression.

recurrent s. Intermittent strabismus.

relative s. 1. Periodic strabismus. 2. Intermittent strabismus.

spasmodic s. Spastic strabismus.

spastic s. Strabismus resulting from spasm of extraocular muscles which may be primary, of neurogenic or myogenic origin, or secondary to a paretic contralateral or ipsilateral synergist or an ipsilateral antagonist. Syn., *spasmodic strabismus.*

spurious s. The momentary, incoordinated dissociations of the eyes of normal infants prior to the full development of binocular fixation. Syn., *infantile strabismus; occasional strabismus.*

s. sursumvergens. Strabismus in which the deviating eye turns upward, so that its foveal line of sight is above the object of fixation. Syn., *hypertropia; strabismus ascendens.*

tonic s. Strabismus attributed to abnormal tonicity of the extraocular muscles.

unilateral s. Strabismus in which the same eye is always the deviating eye and the other eye is always the fixating eye. Syn., *monocular strabismus; monolateral strabismus; uniocular strabismus.*

uniocular s. Unilateral strabismus.

variable s. Strabismus in which the magnitude of the deviation is not constant.

vertical s. Strabismus in which the deviating eye is turned either up or down.

◆

strabometer (strah-bom'eh-ter). Strabismometer.

strabometry (strah-bom'eh-tre). Strabismometry.

strabotic (strah-bot'ik). Strabismic.

strabotomy (strah-bot'o-me). An operation for the correction of strabismus.

strain. A deformation of, or an internal tension in, a solid elastic body resulting from stress. In ophthalmic glass it may be induced by annealing, from a non-uniform coefficient of expansion, or from external pressure at eyewire or mounting contact points, and results in birefringence detectable with a polariscope.

Strampelli (stram-pel'e) **implant; lens.** See under *lens.*

strap. That part of a rimless bridge or endpiece that extends from the shoe over the surface of the lens. It is usually one of a pair, the other strap being on the other surface of the lens, and the two are connected by a screw which passes through holes in the two straps and a hole in the lens.

Stratton's experiment (strat'onz). See under *experiment.*

stratum (stra'tum, strā'tum). A layer.

   s. bacillorum. Layer of rods and cones of the retina.

   s. cinereum. The thin layer of gray matter in the superior colliculus, between the stratum zonale and the stratum opticum, containing small multipolar cells which synapse with the optic and corticotectal fibers. Syn., *stratum griseum.*

   s. ganglionare. Ganglion cell layer of the retina.

   s. griseum. Stratum cinereum.

   s. lemnisci. The deepest of four layers of the superior colliculus, composed of cell bodies and fibers from the stratum opticum, the spinotectal tract, and the medial lemniscus, and the fibers which either enter the fountain decussation of Meynert and connect with the nucleus of the oculomotor nerve, or enter into the tectobulbar and tectospinal tracts, or connect with the reticular formation.

   s. nerveum of Henle. Fiber layer of Henle.

   s. opticum. 1. Nerve fiber layer of the retina. 2. The third layer of the superior colliculus, between the stratum cinereum and the stratum lemnisci, composed of multipolar cells and

fibers from the optic nerve and the lateral geniculate body which enter via the superior brachium and, for the most part, terminate in the stratum cinereum.

   s. pigmenti bulbi oculi. The layer of pigmented epithelium, derived from the outer layer of the optic cup, which extends from the optic disk to the pupillary margin of the iris. It is collectively: the *stratum pigmenti retinae,* the *stratum pigmenti corporis ciliaris,* and the *stratum pigmenti iridis.*

   s. pigmenti corporis ciliaris. Pigmented layer of the epithelium of the ciliary body.

   s. pigmenti iridis. Posterior pigment epithelium of the iris.

   s. pigmenti retinae. Pigment epithelium layer of the retina.

   sagittal s., external. A layer of visual fibers of the optic radiations passing from the posterolateral extremity of the thalamus to the outer side of the posterior horn of the lateral ventricle.

   sagittal s., extreme. A layer of nerve fibers just lateral to the optic radiation fibers in the external sagittal stratum, of uncertain function.

   sagittal s., internal. A layer of nerve fibers probably from the visual association areas of an occipital cortex that terminates in the superior colliculus and elsewhere; located just external to the posterior horn of the lateral ventricle.

   sagittal s., medial. A layer of nerve fibers between the posterior horn of the lateral ventricle and the internal sagittal stratum near the optic radiations. It contains commissural fibers from the two occipital cortices via the splenium of the corpus callosum.

   s. zonale. The thin, white, superficial layer of the superior colliculus, consisting of nerve fibers, chiefly from the occipital cortex, which enter via the superior brachium.

Straub's theory (strawbz). See under *theory.*

streak. A stripe, a line, or a furrow.

   angioid s's. A bilateral degenerative affection characterized by pigmented lines or streaks in the fundi of the eyes in a pattern similar to that of blood vessels, due to degeneration of the lamina vitrea of the choroid. The streaks anastomose around the optic disk and radiate toward the equator, rarely passing it. It may occur in association with *pseudoxanthoma elasticum* (Grönblad-Strandberg syndrome).

Knapp's s's. Pigmented lines resembling blood vessels which may appear following retinal hemorrhage. Syn., *Knapp's striae*.

Moore's lightning s's. Flashes of light upon eye movement, comparable to lightning, usually vertical, almost invariably referred to the temporal side of the field and either accompanied or followed by dark spots before the eyes. It is not considered to be a precursor of any serious fundus disease.

reflex s. A shining or glistening streak seen along the retinal vessels, in ophthalmoscopy, attributed to reflection of light from the surface of the blood column.

Siegrist's s's. Chains of pigmented spots coursing along the paths of white sclerosed choroidal vessels in advanced hypertensive retinopathy. Syn., *Siegrist's spots*.

Strehl criterion; definition; ratio. See under *definition*.

Streidinger chart (stri'din-jer). See under *chart*.

Streiff syndrome. Embryotoxon.

strephosymbolia (stref"o-sim-bo'le-ah). Partial alexia in which letters, such as *b* and *d*, and words, such as *no* and *on*, which form mirror images of each other, are confused.

stress. Tension, compression, or shear within a solid elastic body such as optical glass, which results in strain detectable with a polariscope.

stretcher, cone. A hollow, tapered, rigid metal tube having a cross section shape of a given spectacle lens and mounted over a heating element for stretching and shaping the rims of plastic spectacle frames.

stria (stri'ah). 1. A streak. 2. A streak in glass caused by a variation in the refractive index, due to an imperfect mixture of the ingredients or to contamination during manufacture.

striae ciliares. Shallow dark grooves on the inner surface of the pars plana of the ciliary body extending from the ora serrata to the valleys between the ciliary processes. They are formed by the invagination of the pigment epithelium.

s. of Gennari. Line of Gennari.

Haab's striae. Branched ruptures in Descemet's membrane, due to

distension of the cornea in hydrophthalmos.

Knapp's striae. Knapp's streaks.

striae retinae. White concentric lines in the retina that form following either spontaneous or surgical retinal reattachment.

striate area (stri'āt). See under *area*.

stripes, Vogt keratoconus. Keratoconus lines.

Stroblite (strōb'līt). An argon lamp used in conjunction with fluorescein in the fitting of contact lenses and for the detection of corneal abrasions or ulcers.

stroboscope (stro'bo-skōp, strob'-). An instrument which presents, by means of intermittent illumination or shutters, a series of motionless pictures, each representing successive phases of a movement or successive instantaneous views of a moving object. See also *stroboscopic disk; stroboscopic movement*. Syn., *phenakistoscope*.

strobostereoscope (stro"bo-ster'e-o-skōp). Stereostroboscope.

stroma (stro'mah). The supporting framework of an organ or a structure, consisting primarily of connective tissue and blood vessels.

s. of the cornea. The lamellated connective tissue consituting the thickest layer of the cornea, located between Bowman's and Descemet's membranes.

s. iridis. The iridal loose connective tissue in which the sphincter pupillae muscle, nerves, and pigment cells are contained, located between the anterior border layer and the region of the dilator pupillae muscle.

s. vitreum. The gossamerlike fibrillar structure within the vitreous body, especially as seen with the slit lamp.

stromectomy, lamellar corneal (stro-mek'to-me). A surgical procedure for the treatment of myopia in which a thin layer of corneal stroma is removed to reduce the convexity of the curvature of the cornea.

Strümpell-Lorrain disease (strim'-pel-lo-rān). Familial spasmodic paraplegia.

Strümpell-Marie disease (strim'pel-mar-e'). Ankylosing spondylitis.

Studie Centrum der Toegepaste Optische Wetenschappen. See *Centre d'Étude des Sciences Optiques Appliquées*.

Studt-Abel chart. See under *chart*.

Sturge-Weber (ster'je-web'er) **disease; syndrome.** See under the nouns.

Sturm's (sturmz) **conoid; interval; lines.** See under the nouns.

Sturman monocular. See under *monocular*.

sty. 1. External hordeolum. 2. A purulent infection of a gland of the eyelid.

    Meibomian s. Internal hordeolum.

    Zeisian s. Inflammation of a gland of Zeis.

stye. Sty.

subcapsular (sub-kap'su-lar). Occurring or situated beneath the capsule of the crystalline lens.

subconjunctival (sub″kon-junk-ti′-val). Occurring or situated beneath the conjunctiva.

subconjunctivitis, epibulbar gonorrheal (sub″kon-junk″tih-vi′tis). Endogenous gonococcal conjunctivitis.

subduction (sub-duk'shun). Infraduction.

subfusional (sub-fu'zhun-al). Pertaining to intermittent stimulation at a frequency too low to produce continuous uniform sensation.

subhyaloid (sub-hi'ah-loid). Occurring or situated beneath the hyaloid membrane.

subjective. Subjective refraction.

sublatio retinae (sub-la'she-o ret'ih-ne). Detachment of the retina.

subliminal (sub-lim'in-al). Below the threshold of sensation, as a subliminal stimulus.

subluxation of the lens (sub″luk-sa′-shun). Incomplete dislocation of the crystalline lens, so that it remains in part within the pupillary aperture. Cf. *luxation of the lens.*

subocular (sub-ok'u-lar). Occurring or situated beneath the eyeball.

suborbital (sub-ōr'bih-tal). Occurring or situated beneath the orbit.

subretinal (sub-ret'ih-nal). Occurring or situated between the retina and the choroid.

subscleral (sub-skle'ral). Occurring or situated beneath the sclera.

substance, cement. An amorphous substance in the crystalline lens which binds the individual lens fibers with each other and which is also found beneath the anterior and the posterior capsule, in back of the anterior epithelium, and in a central strand occupying the anteroposterior axis of the lens, extending out to form the Y lens sutures.

substantia lentis (sub-stan'she-ah len'tis). The substance of the crystalline lens contained within its capsule.

substantia propria (sub-stan'she-ah pro'prih-ah). The main connective tissue portion or stroma of a structure, as in the cornea, the sclera, the choroid, and the iris.

subtarsal (sub-tahr'sal). Occurring or situated beneath (posterior to) the tarsus of the eyelid.

subversion (sub-vur'zhun). Infraversion.

subvitrinal (sub-vit'rih-nal). Occurring or situated beneath the vitreous body.

subvolution (sub″vo-lu'shun). An operation for pterygium in which a flap is turned over and placed so that its outer surface is in contact with the raw dissected surface.

successive contrast; induction. See under the nouns.

Suda ocular compression test. See under *test*.

Sugar's method (shoog'arz). See under *method*.

suggilation of the eyelid (sug″jih-la'shun). Ecchymosis of the eyelid.

Suker's sign (soo'kerz). See under *sign*.

sulcus (sul'kus). A furrow or groove as occurs on the surface of the brain or in bone. See also *fissure; groove.*

    calcarine s. Calcarine fissure.

    s. circularis corneae. The shallow circular groove at the margin of the posterior surface of the cornea at its junction with the sclera.

    circum-marginal s. of Vogt. A circular furrow in the iris, near the pupillary margin, due to localized senile atrophic changes.

    infraorbital s. Infraorbital groove.

    infrapalpebral s. The furrow or crease in the skin below the lower eyelid.

    lacrimal s. An infrequent extension of the tract of the nasolacrimal duct downward toward the floor of the nasal cavity, consisting of a groove sometimes bridged by a mucous membrane to form a blind tube.

    s. lacrimalis maxillae. A vertical groove on the orbital surface of the frontal process of the maxillary bone which contributes to the formation of the fossa for the lacrimal sac.

s. lacrimalis ossis lacrimalis. A vertical groove in the lacrimal bone which contributes to the formation of the fossa for the lacrimal sac.

lateral calcarine s. A lateral prolongation of the posterior calcarine fissure at the posterior pole of the occipital lobe in the area striata.

lunate s. A groove often present on the outer surface of the occipital lobe, near the occipital pole, representing the anterior edge of the area striata.

oculomotor s. A longitudinal furrow on the medial side of the cerebral peduncle from which a series of rootlets of the oculomotor nerve emerge.

orbitopalpebral s., inferior. A sulcus in the skin of the lower eyelid extending along the inferior margin of the tarsus.

orbitopalpebral s., superior. A sulcus in the skin of the upper eyelid extending along the superior margin of the tarsus.

paracalcarine s., inferior. A groove in the lingual gyrus, inferior to the area striata, which separates that area from the surrounding cortex.

paracalcarine s., superior. A groove in the cuneus, superior to the area striata, which separates that area from the surrounding cortex.

scleral s., external. The shallow circular groove at the margin of the anterior surface of the sclera at its junction with the cornea.

scleral s., internal. The shallow circular groove on the margin of the posterior surface of the sclera at its junction with the cornea.

subtarsal s. A groove on the inner surface of the eyelid, near the eyelid margin and parallel to it, which marks the junction of the marginal and the palpebral conjunctivae.

summation. The accumulative effect of stimuli presented simultaneously or successively.

binocular s. The accumulative effect of stimulating the two eyes simultaneously or alternately.

spatial s. The combining of the effect of two or more stimuli which impinge simultaneously on different retinal regions.

temporal s. The combining of the effect of two or more stimuli which impinge consecutively on the same retinal region.

sunglasses. Spectacles, or attachments to spectacles, which have absorptive lenses or otherwise reduce transmission of light to the eye.

sunlight. Light received directly from the sun. Cf. *daylight; skylight.*

Sunsensor. A trade name for a photochromic glass available in readymade sunglasses.

superciliaris (su″per-sil″e-a′ris). Corrugator supercilli muscle.

superciliary (su″per-sil′e-ar-e). Pertaining to the region of the eyebrow.

supercilium (su″per-sil′e-um). An eyebrow.

superduction (su″per-duk′shun). Supraduction.

superimposition (su″per-im″po-zish′-un). The laying or imposing of one object, pattern, or form over another. In haploscopic viewing, the common localization of the images seen by the two eyes, as a bird seen by one eye in a cage seen by the other.

superposition (su″per-po-zish′un). Superimposition.

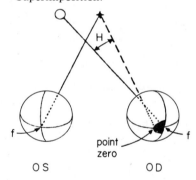

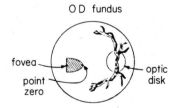

Fig. 35 Illustration of suppression. *Top,* theoretical posterior view of the eyes showing the suppression zone that might result from an esotropia of the right eye; *bottom,* ophthalmoscopic view of the right fundus illustrating the shape and location of the suppression zone in this example. (From J. R. Griffin, *Binocular Anomalies.* Chicago: Professional Press, 1976)

supertraction of the retina (su″per-trak′shun). An ophthalmoscopically apparent encroachment of retinal tissues over the blurred appearing, usually nasal, border of the optic disk. Syn., *supervolution of the retina.*

superversion (su″per-vur′zhun). Supraversion.

suppression. The lack or inability of perception of normally visible objects in all or part of the field of vision of one eye, occurring only on simultaneous stimulation of both eyes and attributed to cortical inhibition. (See Fig. 35.)

active s. Suppression occurring in the absence of binocular fixation, to avoid diplopia and confusion.

border s. 1. The reduction in perceptibility of a stimulus pattern in the perceptual region of a contrast border. 2. The suppression of perception of a pattern presented to one eye when a contrast border is viewed in the corresponding retinal area of the other eye.

central s. Suppression of images in the foveal or the macular area.

gross s. Suppression involving a large area of the visual field.

passive s. Suppression attributed to gross inequality of vision in the two eyes, as in uncorrected anisometropia.

peripheral s. Suppression of images in the peripheral retina.

saccadic s. A brief depression of vision accompanying and preceding a saccade. (Lawrence Stark)

suprachoroid (su″prah-ko′roid). 1. The outer layer of the choroid between Haller's layer and the perichoroidal space or the lamina fusca of the sclera, consisting of relatively nonvascular, loose, connective tissue containing fibroblasts, chromatophores, and reticulo-endothelial cells. Syn., *epichoroid; lamina fusca of the choroid; lamina suprachoroidea; suprachoroid layer; suprachoroidea.* 2. The outer layer of the ciliary body.

suprachoroidea (su″prah-ko-roi′de-ah). Suprachoroid.

supraciliary (su″prah-sil′e-er″e). Superciliary.

supradextroversion (su″prah-deks″tro-vur′zhun). Conjugate rotation of the eyes, upward and to the right.

supraduction (su″prah-duk′shun). 1. Upward rotation of an eye. 2. In vertical divergence testing, the upward rotation of one eye with respect to the other in response to increases in base-down prism, or the equivalent. Syn., *sursumduction.*

alternating s. Double hyperphoria.

supralevoversion (su″prah-lev″o-vur′zhun). Conjugate rotation of the eyes, upward and to the left.

supraliminal (su″prah-lim′ih-nal). Above the threshold of sensation or response, as a supraliminal stimulus.

supraobliquus (su″prah-ob-li′kwus). Superior oblique muscle.

supraorbital (su″prah-ôr′bih-tal). Occurring or situated above the orbit.

suprascleral (su″prah-skle′ral). Occurring or situated on the outer surface of the sclera.

supratrochlear (su″prah-trok′le-ar). Occurring or situated above the trochlea.

supravergence (su″prah-vur′jens). Upward rotation of an eye, the other eye remaining stationary. Syn., *sursumvergence.*

supraversion (su″prah-vur′zhun). Conjugate rotation of the eyes upward. Syn., *sursumversion.*

◆

SURFACE

surface. 1. The outside or exterior of a body. 2. A two dimensional face of a body.

abathic s. The surface of the objective frontoparallel plane horopter determined for a fixation distance at which it coincides with the apparent frontoparallel plane horopter.

aplanatic s. A refracting or reflecting surface of such shape that it brings all the rays emanating from a point source to a point image.

aspherical s. A surface which deviates from a spherical form, usually to conform to a parabola or similar curve, or to a systematically changing series of curves, often employed on a lens to correct for or to reduce certain types of aberration.

base s. In ophthalmic lenses, the standard or reference surface in a given series of lenses. Syn., *base curve.*

Cartesian s's. Cartesian ovals.

caustic s. The surface or form generated by the revolution of the caustic curve about the optical axis of the reflecting or refracting system converging the light rays; hence, the surface containing all the caustic curves.

color s. A plane section of a color solid representing all possible hue, saturation, and brightness variations at that level.

combining s. The surface of a lens on the side opposite to the base surface.

concave s. A curved surface depressed toward the center, as that of the inside of a sphere.

convex s. A curved surface elevated toward the center, as that of the outside of a sphere.

cylindrical s. 1. A surface forming either the inside or the outside of a cylinder. 2. In ophthalmic lenses, synonymous with *toric surface*.

diffusing s. A surface which scatters reflected light in all directions away from the surface. Syn., *mat surface*.

diffusing s., perfect. A surface which reflects light in accordance with Lambert's cosine law, regardless of the angle of incidence.

emergent s. The last surface in an optical system; the surface from which the light leaves the optical system.

index s. A theoretical surface relating the indices of refraction for different directions in doubly refracting crystals, so called in analogy to the ray velocity surface from which it is derived.

s. induction. Spatial induction. See under *induction*.

isochromatic s. With respect to the point of origin of a group of inphase waves in an anisotropic medium, the locus of all points for which the phase difference is a given constant.

isogonal s. The surface generated by the rotation of the Vieth-Mueller horopter about the two points of reference representing the eyes.

isoindicial s's. Surfaces corresponding to regions of the media having the same index of refraction, such as those delineating zones of the crystalline lens of the same index.

lambert s. A surface that emits or reflects light in accordance with Lambert's cosine law and hence has the same luminance at all viewing angles.

mat s. Diffusing surface.

normal velocity s. With respect to the point of origin of a group of in-phase waves in an anisotropic medium, the locus of points whose distances from the origin equal the phase velocities in the corresponding directions.

ocular s. The surface of a spectacle or contact lens worn toward the eye.

optical s. A surface at which specular reflection or uniform refraction occurs, especially one having the desired quality and designed for this purpose in an optical system.

Petzval s. A parabolic surface formed by point images of point objects, both on and off the axis, in an optical system corrected for spherical aberration, coma, and astigmatism.

plane s. A flat surface; a surface of zero curvature; one having an infinite radius of curvature.

principal s. A spherical surface, in an optical system corrected for coma, at which refraction of the emergent light may be considered to occur, its center of curvature being the secondary focal point of the system.

ray velocity s. Wave surface.

redirecting s. A surface which changes the direction of incident light, such as that of a mirror or a prism.

refracting s. A surface separating two isotropic media of different indices of refraction.

scattering s. A surface which redirects light into a multiplicity of separate, variously directed pencils.

spherical s. A surface that conforms to either the inside or the outside of a sphere; one having a single radius of curvature.

toric s. 1. A surface described by a circle rotating about a straight line in its own plane, especially about an off-center line. 2. An ophthalmic lens surface with meridians of least and greatest curvature located at right angles to each other.

wave s. 1. A wavefront. 2. The envelope of wavefronts in doubly refracting crystals representing the positions of the ordinary and the extraordinary waves at a given time, hence a surface of constant phase for waves spreading from a point source. Syn., *ray velocity surface*. **extraordinary w.s.** The wave surface in a doubly refracting substance corresponding to the loci of points of equal phase belonging to the extraordinary ray. **ordinary w.s.** The wave surface in a doubly refracting substance corresponding to the loci of points of equal phase belonging to the ordinary ray.

◆

surfacing. Grinding and polishing of the surface of a lens to a specified curvature.

surround, visual. All visible features in the immediate field of view which are not an integral part of the *visual task*, q.v., though they may influence its perceptibility.

sursumduction (sur"sum-duk'shun). Supraduction.

sursumvergence (sur"sum-vur'jens). Supravergence.

sursumversion (sur"sum-vur'zhun). Supraversion.

suspenopsia (sus"pen-op'se-ah). 1. Voluntary ignoring of the objects in the field of vision of one eye when visual attention is directed to objects in the field of vision of the other eye, as occurs when using a monocular microscope with both eyes open. 2. Suppression.

suspension (sus-pen'shun). 1. Suppression. 2. Suspenopsia.

Sutcliffe's rule (sut'klifs). See under *rule*.

◆

SUTURE

suture (su'tūr). 1. The line of junction between immovable bones, as those of the skull, or the junction itself. 2. The line of junction formed by the meeting of fibers of the crystalline lens. 3. The act, the process, or the method of stitching tissue, or the type of stitch so used. 4. The material used in stitching tissue.

ethmofrontal s. The suture between the frontal and the ethmoid bones in the orbit. Syn., *frontoethmoidal suture*.

ethmolacrimal s. The suture between the ethmoid and the lacrimal bones in the medial wall of the orbit.

ethmomaxillary s. The suture between the ethmoid bone and the orbital plate of the maxillary bone.

ethmopalatine s. The suture between the ethmoid and the palatine bones in the orbit.

ethmosphenoidal s. The suture between the ethmoid and the sphenoid bones in the orbit. Syn., *sphenoethmoidal suture*.

frontoethmoidal s. Ethmofrontal suture.

frontolacrimal s. The suture between the frontal and lacrimal bones.

frontomalar s. Frontozygomatic suture.

frontomaxillary s. The suture between the frontal process of the maxillary bone and the frontal bone. Syn., *maxillofrontal suture*.

frontonasal s. Nasofrontal suture.

frontosphenoidal s. The suture between the wings of the sphenoid bone and the frontal bone. Syn., *sphenofrontal suture*.

frontozygomatic s. The suture between the frontal and the zygomatic bones. Syn., *frontomalar suture; zygomaticofrontal suture*.

infraorbital s. The suture in the maxillary bone over the infraorbital canal.

lens s. One of the many radiating lines in the crystalline lens, formed by the meeting of systems of lens fibers. **anterior Y l.s.** The lens suture in the shape of an upright Y, formed anterior in the fetal nucleus. **posterior Y l.s.** The lens suture in the shape of an inverted Y, formed posterior in the fetal nucleus.

maxilloethmoidal s. Ethmomaxillary suture.

maxillofrontal s. Frontomaxillary suture.

maxillolacrimal s. The suture between the maxillary and the lacrimal bones, in the medial wall of the orbit.

maxillonasal s. Nasomaxillary suture.

maxillopalatine s. The suture between the orbital plate of the maxillary bone and the palatine bone, in the floor of the orbit.

maxillozygomatic s. The suture between the maxillary and the zygomatic bones. Syn., *zygomaticomaxillary suture*.

nasofrontal s. The suture between the frontal and the nasal bones. Syn., *frontonasal suture*.

nasomaxillary s. The suture between the nasal and the superior maxillary bones. Syn., *maxillo nasal suture*.

sphenoethmoidal s. Ethmosphenoidal suture.

sphenofrontal s. Frontosphenoidal suture.

sphenomalar s. Sphenozygomatic suture.

sphenopalatine s. The suture between the sphenoid and the palatine bones in the orbit.

sphenozygomatic s. The suture between the great wing of the sphenoid bone and the zygomatic bone, in the lateral wall of the orbit. Syn., *sphenomalar suture.*

zygomaticofrontal s. Frontozygomatic suture.

zygomaticomaxillary s. Maxillozygomatic suture.

◆

Swann's syndrome (swahnz). Blind spot syndrome.

Swann-Cole charts (swahn-kōl). See under *chart.*

Sweet's method. See under *method.*

Swenson's method. See under *method.*

Swindle's ghost (swin'd'lz). See under *ghost.*

Sx. Symptoms.

sycosis palpebrae marginalis (si-ko'sis pal-pe'bre mar-jih-nal'is). Sycotic blepharitis.

sycosis vulgaris (si-ko'sis vul-ga'ris). Acne mentagra.

Sylvian syndrome (sil've-an). See under *syndrome.*

symblepharon (sim-blef'ah-ron). A cicatricial attachment of the conjunctiva of the eyelid to the conjunctiva of the eyeball. Syn., *symblepharosis.*

anterior s. Symblepharon in which the tarsal or the marginal conjunctiva is attached to the conjunctiva of the eyeball but which does not involve the fornix.

posterior s. Symblepharon extending to and involving the fornix.

total s. Symblepharon forming a complete adhesion of the conjunctiva of the eyelid to the conjunctiva of the eyeball.

symblepharopterygium (sim-blef"-ah-ro-ter-ij'e-um). A symblepharon in which the cicatricial band resembles a pterygium.

symblepharosis (sim-blef"ah-ro-sis). Symblepharon.

symparalysis (sim"pah-ral'ih-sis). Simultaneous paralysis of synergistic extraocular muscles of an eye or of the yoke muscles of the eyes.

sympathetic ophthalmia (sim"pah-thet'ik of-thal'me-ah). See under *ophthalmia.*

sympathizer. A sympathizing eye.

symptom. An incidental or concomitant subjective indication of disease, disorder, or anomaly. See also *phenomenon; reflex; sign; syndrome.*

Anton's s. Subjective unawareness of one's own visual disability in cortical blindness.

Behçet, triple s. complex of. Behçet's syndrome.

Bumke's s. Absence of normal pupillary dilatation to psychic stimuli, as fear or pain, in catatonia.

Epstein's s. Failure of the upper eyelid to move downward on downward movement of the eye, occurring in premature and nervous infants.

Franceschetti's digital-ocular s. Frequent pressing of the eyeballs with the fingers, occurring in association with such congenital deformities as coloboma of the eyelids or gargoylism.

Gower's s. Abrupt intermittent oscillation of the pupil on light stimulation of the eye, occurring in tabes dorsalis.

halo s. Colored circles seen around lights in glaucoma. Syn., *rainbow symptom.*

Liebreich's s. A symptom of red-green color blindness in which light areas are reported red while dark areas are reported green.

rainbow s. Halo symptom.

Redlich's s. Redlich's phenomenon.

Stellwag's s. Stellwag's sign.

Weber's s. Weber's sign.

Wernicke's s. Hemianopic pupillary reflex.

synaphymenitis (sin-af"ih-men-i'tis). Conjunctivitis.

syncanthus (sin-kan'thus). Adhesion of the eyeball to the orbital tissues or structures.

Synchro-haploscope (sin"kro-hap'lo-skōp). A motor-activated visual training haploscope, designed by Mason, with independent control of the vergence, version, and accommodative demands.

synchysis (sin'kih-sis). Liquefaction of the vitreous body, commonly occurring in senile or myopic degeneration and often in other inflammatory or degenerative states of the eye or after trauma. It is usually associated with the development of vitreous opacities, which may be ophthalmoscopically visible, and which, when seen entoptically, move more freely than similar opacities seen when the elastic structure of the gel is maintained.

s. scintillans. The presence of numerous, bright, shiny particles in a fluid vitreous body, occurring secondarily to degenerative conditions of the eye. They appear as flat, angular, golden crystals and are considered to be composed of cholesterol. They may be hidden at the bottom of the vitreous when the eye is immobile and then suddenly float into sight when the eye is moved.

syndectomy (sin-dek'to-me). Peridectomy.

syndesmitis (sin"des-mi'tis). Conjunctivitis.

◆

SYNDROME

syndrome (sin'drōm). The aggregate signs and symptoms characteristic of a disease, a lesion, an anomaly, a type, or a classification. For syndromes not listed, see under *disease*.

A s. 1. A pattern. 2. Case type A.

ACL s. Large hands and feet and protruding jaws as in acromegaly, a type of cutis verticis gyrata, and corneal leukoma.

Acosta s. Defective light adaptation, visual scintillation, and defective color vision associated with dysacousia, defective muscle tonus, and defective breathing coordination, due to cerebral hypoxia and hyperventilation in mountain climbers. Syn., *mountain climbers' syndrome.*

Adair-Dighton s. Van der Hoeve's syndrome.

adenopharyngealconjunctival s. Acute contagious conjunctivitis and upper respiratory infection of viral origin. Syn., *APC syndrome.*

adherence s. A developmental abnormality of the extraocular muscles in which one becomes joined or adherent to another, resulting in a condition simulating paralysis or paresis. Syn., *Johnson syndrome.*

Adie s. Dilation of the pupil, usually unilateral, with sluggish response to light, darkness, accommodation and convergence, together with absence of tendon reflexes, such as the knee jerk. It is usually found in women and is of unknown etiology. Syn., *Holmes-Adie syndrome; Markus syndrome.*

adiposogenital s. Froehlich's syndrome.

Albright's s. Pigmented nevi of the skin, precocious puberty, and polyostotic fibrous dysplasia which may lead to unilateral cranial thickening and optic atrophy. Syn., *Albright-McCune-Sternberg syndrome.*

Albright-McCune-Sternberg s. Albright's syndrome.

Alport's s. Hereditary progressive nephropathy with albuminuria and hematuria and progressive bilateral nerve deafness, mostly affecting males. Cataract, spherophakia, and lenticonus are sometimes present.

Alström-Hallgren s. Pigmentary degeneration of the retina, deafness, diabetes mellitus, and frequently psychosis, considered due to inherited endocrine dysfunction. Night blindness and reduced visual acuity are primary symptoms.

Amalric's s. Deaf-mutism associated with macular dystrophy without functional loss.

Amidei's s. Strabismus, stuttering, and left-handedness, of undetermined etiology.

Andogsky's s. Cataract associated with the late stage of an allergic dermatitis, occurring as a recessive heredofamilial trait.

Angelucci's s. Vasomotor instability, tachycardia, lymphoid hyperplasia, and sometimes vernal conjunctivitis, attributed to endocrine disturbance.

angio-encephalo-cutaneous s. Sturge-Weber syndrome.

angiospastic ophthalmo-auricular s. Otosclerosis, concentric contraction of the visual fields, and increased tortuosity of the retinal vessels; a rare condition attributed to angiospasm. Syn., *Bazzana syndrome.*

anterior choroidal artery s. Monakow's syndrome.

Anton's s. Statements of visual experience although totally blind, with intellectual deterioration, especially of memory, a tendency to confabulate, and amnesic aphasia, due to bilateral destruction of cortical visual sensory area 17 or to a lesion affecting fibers from this area leading to the thalamus.

aortic arch s. Pulseless disease.

APC s. Adenopharyngeal-conjunctival syndrome.

Apert's s. Acrocephalosyndactyly.

apex s. Paresis of the third, fourth, fifth, and sixth cranial nerves and lesions of the optic nerve resulting in central scotomata, peripheral visual field defects, and sometimes papilledema, due to a large diffuse lesion at the base of the skull.

aqueduct of Sylvius s. Sylvian syndrome.

Arnold-Chiari s. Herniation of a portion of the cerebellum and medulla into the cervical portion of the spinal canal, often associated with spina bifida. Nystagmus is a usual accompaniment, typically horizontal on lateral gaze and vertical on upward gaze.

Arnold-Pick s. Apperceptive blindness and inability to fixate, associated with motor aphasia, apraxia, agnosia, and apathy, with normal eyegrounds, occurring in females aged 40 to 70, and caused by widespread cortical atrophy.

Ascher's s. Blepharochalasis, edema of the lips, and goiter without hyperthyroidism. Syn., *Laffer-Ascher syndrome.*

atresia of the foramen of Magendie s. Hydrocephalus, ptosis, papilledema and external rectus paralysis in infants due to malformation and stenosis of the foramina of Luschka and Magendie with dilation of the fourth ventricle and anomalies of the rostral vermis. Syn., *Dandy-Walker syndrome.*

Aubineau-Lenoble s. Recessive familial congenital nystagmus associated with tremors of the head and limbs, hyperreflexia, vasomotor disturbances, and fasciculations of muscles upon mechanical or cold stimulation. Syn., *nystagmus myoclonia syndrome.*

Avellis s. Horner syndrome associated with ipsilateral paralysis of the soft palate and vocal cords with occasional loss of pain and temperature sense on the contralateral side of the body.

Axenfeld's s. Embryotoxon associated with adhesions of strands of iridic tissue to a prominent Schwalbe's line; an inherited anomaly usually associated with glaucoma occurring in adolescence or early adulthood. Syn., *iridocorneal mesodermal dysplasia.*

Axenfeld-Schurenberg s. Familial congenital cyclic oculomotor paralysis alternating with spasm.

B s. Case type B.

Babinski-Froehlich s. Froehlich's syndrome.

Babinski-Nageotte s. Cerebellar hemiataxia, nystagmus, miosis, ptosis, and enophthalmos on the side of the lesion, with hemiparesis and sensibility disturbance on the contralateral side, due to involvement of the pyramidal tract, the median fillet, the inferior cerebellar peduncle, and the descending sympathetic fibers in the brain stem.

Balint's s. Ocular motor apraxia in which there is an inability to perform voluntarily fixational movements in the presence of normal reflex ocular movements, with specific inattention for visual stimuli, especially for objects in the peripheral field of vision.

Bardet-Biedl s. Laurence-Moon-Biedl syndrome.

Barré-Liéou s. Cervical spine abnormalities, cervical pain, tinnitus, vertigo, headache, and retrobulbar pain. Syn., *posterior cervical sympathetic syndrome.*

Bartenwerfer s. A congenital condition of retarded growth and spinal curvature, frequently associated with congenital dislocation of the hip, and including epicanthus, mongoloid eyelid fissures, blepharophimosis, and ocular hypertelorism.

Bartholin-Patau s. Trisomy 13 syndrome.

Bassen-Kornzweig s. Crenated erythrocytes, celiac disease, ataxia of the Friedreich type, and atypical pigmentary degeneration of the retina; a rare recessive hereditary disease.

Bazzana s. Angiospastic ophthalmo-auricular syndrome.

Beal's s. Acute follicular conjunctivitis of Beal. See under *conjunctivitis, follicular.*

Behçet's s. Recurrent ulceration of the genitalia, aphthous ulcers of the mouth, and uveitis which may affect either the anterior or the posterior segment of the eye and usually results in hypopyon. It is of unknown etiology and is attributed by some to a virus or focal infection. Syn., *triple symptom complex of Behçet.*

Behr s. Infantile optic atrophy, predominantly temporal and usually stabilizing after a few years, increased tendon reflexes usually with a positive Babinski sign, mild ataxia, mental deficiency, nystagmus, and weakness of the sphincter of the bladder with incontinence; occurring as a heredofamilial disease. Syn., *optic atrophy-ataxia syndrome.*

Benedikt's s. Ipsilateral oculomotor paralysis and contralateral tremor, spasm or choreic movements of the face and the limbs, due to involvement of the red nucleus, oculomotor nerve, and the superior cerebellar peduncle. Syn., *tegmental mesencephalic paralysis; tegmental syndrome.*

Bernard's s. 1. Ipsilateral pupillary dilation, widening of the palpebral fissure, and slight exophthalmos, with possible associated vaso-constriction, lowered temperature, and excessive sweating of the face, due to irritation of the sympathetic pathway. 2. Horner's syndrome.

Bernard-Horner s. Horner's syndrome.

Besnier-Boeck-Schaumann s. Sarcoidosis.

Bickel-Bing-Harboe s. Optic neuritis with defects of central vision associated with hyperglobulinemia, neuroses, and psychic disturbances; of unknown etiology.

Biedl's s. Laurence-Moon-Biedl syndrome.

Bielschowsky-Jansky s. Bielschowsky-Jansky disease.

Bielschowsky-Lutz-Cogan s. Anterior internuclear ophthalmoplegia.

Biemond's s. Laurence-Moon-Biedl syndrome.

Blegvad-Haxthausen s. Zonular cataract associated with osteogenesis imperfecta and anetodermia; of familial etiology. Syn., *Robstein syndrome.*

blind spot of Swann s. Esotropia in which the magnitude of the deviation is such that the image of the object of fixation falls on the optic disk of the deviating eye.

Bloch-Sulzberger s. A form of incontinentia pigmenti usually occurring either congenitally or in the first year of life, primarily affecting females, and characterized by patches of wavy streaks of slate-gray cutaneous pigmentation and other defects such as of teeth, hair, nails, and eyes. Ocular anomalies accompany about one-fourth of the cases and include pseudoglioma, cataract, strabismus, optic atrophy, nystagmus, uveitis, and chorioretinitis. Syn., *Naegli syndrome.*

blue sclera s. Eddowes' syndrome.

Boder-Sedgwick s. Progressive cerebellar ataxia commencing in infancy, sinus and pulmonary infection, slow spasmodic eye movements, fixation nystagmus, slow labored indistinct speech, and telangiectasia of the bulbar conjunctiva, of the skin in the area of the bridge of the nose, and of the external ears, occurring as a disease of strong familial incidence.

Bogorad s. Crocodile tears syndrome.

Bonnet's s. Congenital tortuosity of the retinal vessels and vascular malformations in the mid-brain.

Bonnevie-Ullrich s. Status Bonnevie-Ullrich.

van den Bosch s. Horizontal nystagmus, high myopia, choroideremia, mental deficiency, abnormal electroretinogram, and skeletal and skin anomalies; occurring as a heredofamilial disease.

Brailsford s. Morquio's disease.

Brain's s. Exophthalmos and external ophthalmoplegia in exophthalmic goiter.

Brown's tendon sheath s. An apparent paralysis of the inferior oblique muscle with an inability to elevate the eye above the horizontal plane in full adduction, limitation of movement of the affected eye in the forced duction test (q.v.) into the field of action of the inferior oblique muscle on adduction, elevation of the eye in a straight line from the inner canthus, widening of the palpebral fissure on adduction, and essentially normal motility in the temporal fields of gaze, due to a congenitally short anterior tendon sheath of the superior oblique muscle.

Burnett s. Nausea, headache, dizziness, depression, and mental confusion, with a characteristic band keratopathy and deposition of amorphous particles in the cornea, a condition due to hypercalcemia which may develop during milk-alkali therapy for peptic ulcer.

Burns s. Bilateral partial ophthalmoplegia with associated gaze paresis, rarely ptosis, and preceded by ataxia, caused by a lesion in the cerebellum. Cf. *Nothnagel's syndrome.*

C s. Case type C.

Caffey-Silverman s. Infantile cortical hyperostosis.

Capgras s. Phantom double syndrome.

carotid occlusion s. Transient monocular blindness, which may become permanent, and hemiplegia and hemianesthesia of the opposite side of the body, due to unilateral carotid artery occlusion. The most characteristic diagnostic sign is a significant difference in the retinal arterial pressure, the affected side being lower.

cat-cry s. Hypertelorism, epicanthus, and oblique palpebral fissures, associated with stunted growth and mental retardation. A congenital condition ascribed to deletion of a portion of chromosome 5. Syn., *LeJeune syndrome; cri du chat syndrome.*

cat's eye s. Vertical coloboma of the iris and choroid, an imperforate anus, microphthalmos, strabismus, and cataracts, caused by an extra chromosomal fragment. Syn., *Schmidt-Fracaro syndrome.*

cavernous sinus s. Paralysis or paresis of the third, fourth, and sixth nerves and the first division of the fifth nerve, proptosis, and possibly edema of the eyelids and the conjunctiva, due to involvement of the cavernous sinus as from thrombosis, a tumor, or inflammatory conditions. Syn., *Jefferson syndrome.*

cerebellopontine angle s. Mixed nystagmus, falling and past pointing toward the affected side, marked vertigo, tinnitus and deafness, due to a lesion in the region of the cerebellopontine angle. Extension of the lesion may involve the fifth and seventh nerves.

cervico-oculo-acoustic s. Retractio bulbi, vertebral synostosis, cervical spina bifida, labyrinthine deafness, and occasionally pterygium colli and/or torticollis; occurring congenitally as a dominant hereditary disease. Syn., *cervico-oculo-facial dysmorphia; cervico-oculo-muscular syndrome.*

cervico-oculo-muscular s. Cervico-oculo-acoustic syndrome.

Cestan's s. 1. Cestan-Chenais syndrome. 2. Raymond-Cestan syndrome.

Cestan-Chenais s. Cerebellar hemiataxia, nystagmus, miosis, ptosis, and enophthalmos on the side of the lesion, hemiparesis and sensibility disturbance on the contralateral side, ipsilateral paralysis of the soft palate and the vocal cords, due to involvement of the pyramidal tract, the median fillet, the inferior cerebellar peduncle, the nucleus ambiguus, and the descending sympathetic fibers in the brain stem.

Chandler's s. Dystrophy of the corneal endothelium, corneal edema, mild atrophy of the stroma of the iris, peripheral anterior synechiae, and glaucoma.

Charlin's s. Orbital and periorbital neuralgia, keratitis, iritis, rhinorrhea, and inflammation in the area of the nose, due to affection of the nasal, the nasociliary, and the anterior ethmoidal nerves.

Chédiak-Higashi s. Hematologic abnormalities including anomalous granulations in the polymorphonuclear leukocytes and lymphocytes, anemia, neutropenia, thrombopenia, lymphadenopathy, hepatosplenomegaly, low resistance to infection, and partial albinism with localized hyperpigmentation. Eye signs include pale fundi, photophobia, increased lacrimation, papilledema, and infiltration of ocular tissues with immature leukocytes. It is familial and results in death in childhood.

chiasmal s. Bitemporal, visual field defects and primary optic atrophy with apparently normal roentgenological findings in the sella turcica, due to involvement of the optic chiasm as by tumors or expanding aneurysms. Syn., *Cushing's syndrome.*

Christian's s. Schüller-Christian-Hand syndrome.

Claude's s. Ipsilateral, third nerve paralysis and contralateral, cerebellar ataxia or hemichorea, due to involvement of the red nucleus and the oculomotor nerve.

Claude Bernard's s. Bernard's syndrome.

clivus ridge s. Ipsilateral fixed mydriasis of the pupil, ipsilateral exotropia, and occasionally a slight ipsilateral ptosis, due to increased intracranial pressure on the oculomotor nerve in the region of the clivus ridge, caused by a space-taking lesion such as a tumor, abscess, or hemorrhage.

Cockayne s. A rare autosomal recessive progressive disease commencing in the second year of life and characterized by dermatitis, mental retardation, dwarfism, maxillary prognathism, large hands and feet, prominent ears, carious teeth, microcephaly, loss of hearing, loss of fatty tissue in the face, optic atrophy, pigmentary degeneration of the retina of the salt and pepper type primarily in the macular area, and cataracts. Syn., *Cockayne's disease.*

Cogan's s. A patchy granular type of posterior interstitial keratitis, usually bilateral, with daily variation in severity, accompanied by the vestibuloauditory symptoms of severe vertigo, nausea, vomiting, nystagmus and finally deafness.

Collins-Franceschetti-Zwahlen s. Mandibulofacial dysostosis.

s. of compression of the anterior angle of the chiasm. Unilateral blindness with temporal hemianopsia of the other eye, usually indicative of a meningioma of the tuberculum sellae.

cone dysfunction s. Subnormal visual acuity, defective color vision, and absence of the photopic flicker electroretinogram, frequently accompanied by nystagmus and photophobia, due to a generalized disturbance of the cone system.

conjunctivoglandular s. of Parinaud. Granulomatous conjunctivitis characterized by red or yellowish growths (Parinaud's conjunctivitis), swollen hardened eyelids, and swelling of the lymph glands of the neck, especially the preauricular, due to a leptothrix infection.

Conradi's s. Stippled epiphyses.

Creix-Lévy s. Retrobulbar pain, headaches, excessive lacrimation, cervical pain and excessive rhinorrhea and salivation.

cri du chat s. Cat-cry syndrome.

crocodile tears s. Lacrimation reflexly induced by gustatory stimuli to the tongue, occurring in the stage of recovery of a facial nerve injury in or proximal to the geniculate ganglion, thought to be due to misdirected regeneration of fibers which proceed to the lacrimal gland instead of to the salivary glands. Syn., *Bogorad syndrome.*

cryptophthalmos-syndactyly s. Cryptophthalmos, syndactyly, dyscephaly including meningocele, harelip and cleft palate, ear and nasal anomalies, and genital malformations such as small penis, nondescended testes in the male, and hypertrophy of the clitoris with vaginal atresia and incomplete labial development in the female; of autosomal recessive inheritance.

Cushing s. 1. Chiasmal syndrome. 2. Cerebellopontine angle syndrome.

dancing eyes and dancing feet s. Syndrome of opsoclonus and polymyoclonia.

Dandy-Walker s. Atresia of the foramen of Magendie syndrome.

Déjerine-Klumpke s. Lower radicular syndrome.

Dighton-Adair s. Van der Hoeve's syndrome.

Dimitri's s. Sturge-Weber syndrome.

Down's s. A syndrome of congenital defects including mental retardation (IQ 20 to 60), typical mongoloid facial features, protrusion of tongue, short stubby fingers and limbs, and frequently strabismus and high refractive errors; due to cytogenetic abnormality consisting of trisomy 21 or the displacement of part or all of one chromosome to another. Syn., *mongolian idiocy; mongolism.*

Dresbach s. Sickle-cell disease. See under *disease.*

Duane retraction s. Retraction of the eyeball into the orbit, associated with drooping of the upper eyelid on attempted adduction of the affected eye. Adduction is limited and, when attempted, the eye also moves upward or downward. Abduction is limited or abolished and, when attempted, the palpebral fissure may widen. It is usually unilateral, rarely affecting both eyes, and is considered to be due to congenital aberrant innervation to the lateral and medial rectus muscles which produces an anomalous co-contraction. Syn., *Türk's disease; Duane's phenomenon; retractio bulbi; retraction syndrome; Stilling-Türk-Duane syndrome.*

Duane-White s's. 1. *Convergence insufficiency:* slight exophoria at far, marked exophoria at near, and near point of convergence three inches or more. 2. *Convergence excess:* orthophoria or moderate esophoria at far and esophoria at near. 3. *Divergence insufficiency, primary:* esophoria up to 8^Δ at far and esophoria at near. 4. *Divergence insufficiency, secondary:* esophoria over 8^Δ at far and high esophoria at near. 5. *Divergence excess:* marked exophoria at far and equal or less exophoria at near. *Primary* if with normal near point of convergence and *secondary* if deficient.

dyscephalic mandibulo-oculo-facial s. Mandibulo-oculo-facial dyscephaly.

Eddowes' s. Blue sclerae associated with osteogenesis imperfecta. Syn., *blue sclera syndrome; Lobstein's syndrome; Spurway's syndrome.*

Edwards s. Trisomy 18 syndrome.

Ehlers-Danlos s. Meekrin-Ehlers-Danlos syndrome.

Elschnig s. Congenital cleft palate, hare lip, ectropion of the lower eyelids, long palpebral fissures, and downward displacement of the lateral canthi.

embryonic fixation s. Waardenburg's syndrome.

empty sella s. Gradually increasing hemianoptic or quadrantanoptic, usually bitemporal, loss of the visual fields and atrophy of the optic disks, resulting from non-tumorous enlargement of the sella turcica.

Espildora-Luque s. Sylvian syndrome.

Falls-Kurtesz s. Distichiasis, chronic lymphatic edema of the lower extremities, pterygium colli, and ectropion of the lower eyelids; a dominant hereditary disease.

Fanconi-Türler s. Familial cerebellar ataxia, seen in early infancy with uncoordinated eye movements and nystagmus.

Felty s. Chronic rheumatoid arthritis, splenomegaly, leukopenia, mild anemia, scleritis, and keratitis; occurring in the middle-aged and of unknown etiology.

Fiessinger-Leroy-Reiter s. Oculo-urethro-synovial syndrome.

Fiessinger-Rendu s. Stevens-Johnson syndrome.

Fisher's s. Symmetrical ophthalmoplegia, ataxia, and absence of reflexes, due to cranial nerve neuropathy without an accompanying fever.

Foix's s. Paresis of third, fourth, fifth, and sixth cranial nerves, due to involvement of the external wall of the cavernous sinus by a neoplasm.

Forsius-Eriksson s. Primary foveal hypoplasia, varying degrees of tapeto-retinal degeneration, myopia, and nystagmus, occurring in natives of Ahvenanmaa on Åland Islands as an inherited sex-linked condition in which the female carrier is symptom free. Syn., *Åland disease.*

Foster Kennedy s. Kennedy's syndrome.

Foville's s. Ipsilateral palsy of the abducens nerve, loss of conjugate deviation of the eyes toward the affected side, ipsilateral facial paralysis, and contralateral paralysis of the limbs, due to a pontine lesion at or above the level of the sixth nerve nucleus.

Franceschetti s. Mandibulofacial dysostosis.

Franceschetti-Gernet s. Microphthalmia without microcornea, associated with macrophakia, high hypermetropia, tapetoretinal degeneration, disposition to glaucoma, and dental anomalies; occurring as a familial disease.

Franceschetti-Zwahlen s. Mandibulofacial dysostosis.

François' s. Dyscephalia with bird face, dental anomalies, dwarfism, hypotrichosis, cutaneous atrophy, bilateral microphthalmia, and congenital cataracts; a hereditary ectodermal dysplasia.

Fränkel s. Ocular contusion syndrome.

Fränkl-Hochwart s. Pineal-neurologic-ophthalmic syndrome.

Freeman-Sheldon s. Craniocarpo-tarsal dystrophy.

Friedreich s. Friedreich's disease.

Froboese s. Myelin neuromatosis.

Froehlich's s. Adolescent obesity, especially around the shoulders and hips, soft hairless skin, genital hypoplasia, disturbed carbohydrate and fat metabolism, absence of secondary sex characteristics, and ocular signs of optic atrophy, bitemporal field defects, and delayed pupillary reaction to light, depending on the extent of the lesion. Diabetes insipidus and polyuria may also be present. The condition is due to involvement of the medial nuclei of the hypothalamus, the tuber cinereum, and neighboring structures. Syn., *dystrophia adiposogenitalis; adiposogenital dystrophy; adiposogenital syndrome; Babinski-Froehlich syndrome.*

Fuchs' s. Unilateral heterochromia of the iris, iridocyclitis with keratic precipitates, and cataract, occurring as a congenital, slowly progressive condition of unknown etiology.

Fuller-Albright s. A disease entity representing a generalized bone lesion (disseminated osteitis fibrosa) affecting the long bones, the pelvis, and the skull, and associated with patches of pigmentation on the skin. Ocular symptoms may involve a depression of the globe, pupillary dilation, occasional exophthalmos, and diplopia.

Garcin s. Unilateral defect of smell, unilateral trigeminal paresis, possible paresis of cranial nerves IX, X,

XI, and XII, and possible deafness, due to nasopharyngeal or brain stem neoplasm or meningitis.

Gasperini s. Deafness, contralateral hemiplegia, unilateral paresis of fifth, sixth, and seventh cranial nerves, nystagmus, and conjugate gaze paresis, due to a pontine lesion.

Gelineau s. A usually familial disorder of obscure etiology characterized by short diurnal attacks of uncontrollable sleep, diplopia, and transient blurring of vision.

general fibrosis s. Bilateral ptosis and paralysis of all the extraocular muscles, due to a general congenital fibrosis.

Gerstmann's s. Visual agnosia, visual apraxia, dyslexia, loss of revisualization, acalculia, agraphia, finger agnosia, confusion of laterality, occasionally astereognosis, and possibly right-sided homonymous hemianopsia and loss of optokinetic nystagmus, due to a lesion at the occipitoparietal border involving the peristriate and the parastriate areas, the angular gyrus, and the interparietal sulcus area.

Gillespie's s. Aniridia, cerebellar ataxia, and oligophrenia, occurring as an autosomal recessive condition.

Godtfredsen's s. Ophthalmoplegia, trigeminal neuralgia, and twelfth nerve paralysis, resulting from involvement of the cavernous sinus and the neck lymphatics by a neoplasm.

Goldenhar's s. Subconjunctival dermoids near the limbus, accessory auricular appendages, and auricular fistula, occurring unilaterally and considered to be due to maldevelopment of the first branchial arch. Syn., *oculoauricular dysplasia; oculo-auricular syndrome.*

Gopalan s. Nutritional amblyopia, central scotomas, sweating of the feet and aching foot paresthesia resulting from B avitaminosis; recorded primarily among prisoners of war but also may be due to diabetes.

Goppert s. Bilateral cataracts and galactosemia in infants; a congenital metabolic disorder.

Gorlin-Chaudhry-Moss s. A hereditary condition characterized by craniofacial dysostosis, hypertrichosis, dental anomalies, microphthalmia, limited upward gaze, oblique palpebral fissures, and inability to close the eyelids fully with a resultant exposure keratitis.

Gougerot-Sjögren s. Sjögren's syndrome.

Gower-Paton-Kennedy s. Kennedy's syndrome.

Gradenigo's s. Ipsilateral pain in or about the eye, in the temple, or the side of the face, facial paralysis, photophobia, lacrimation, reduced corneal sensitivity, and paralysis of the sixth nerve, due to mastoiditis extending to the tip of the petrous bone and affecting the meninges in the epidural space and the adjacent sixth nerve, Gasserian ganglion, and seventh nerve.

Gregg s. Rubella syndrome.

Greig s. Ocular hypertelorism.

Grignolo s. Erythema exudativum multiforme.

Grönblad-Strandberg s. Pseudoxanthoma elasticum occurring in association with angioid streaks, due to degeneration of elastic tissue of the skin and the lamina vitrea of the choroid.

Gruber s. Splanchnocystic dysencephaly.

Gruner-Bertolotti s. Parinaud's syndrome combined with Monakow syndrome.

Gunn's jaw-winking s. Jaw-winking.

Hallerman-Streit s. Mandibulo-oculo-facial dysmorphia.

Hallgren s. Vestibulo-cerebellar ataxia, mental deficiency, deafness, psychosis, pigmentary retinal degeneration, cataract, occasional nystagmus; a hereditary, autosomal recessive condition.

Hand's s. Schüller-Christian-Hand syndrome.

Hanhart s. Dyskeratosis palmo-plantaris, skin anomalies, and superficial corneal dendritic ulcers without loss of normal corneal sensitivity; a condition of unknown etiology.

Harada's s. Bilateral, acute, diffuse, exudative choroiditis, retinal detachment, headache, loss of appetite, nausea and vomiting, and sometimes temporary vitiligo, poliosis, and deafness; of undetermined origin, thought due to a virus infection.

Harris s. Periodic migraine.

Heerfordt's s. Bilateral parotitis, uveitis, and fever, often associated with paresis of the cranial nerves, especially the seventh, and considered to be a form of sarcoidosis. Syn., *Heerfordt's disease; uveoparotid fever; uveoparotitis.*

Heidenhain s. Presenile dementia, cortical blindness of rapid onset, and possible hemianopsia; associated with ataxia, dysarthria, athetoid movements, and generalized rigidity; due to cortical degeneration.

Hennebert's s. Attacks of spontaneous nystagmus and dizziness with exaggeration of the nystagmus when the column of air in the auditory meatus is compressed, due to a fistula in the labyrinth.

von Herrenschwand s. Sympathetic heterochromia.

Herrick s. Sickle-cell disease.

Hertwig-Magendie s. Magendie-Hertwig sign.

Hilding s. Uveo-arthro-chondral syndrome.

histoplasmosis s. See *histoplasmosis.*

van der Hoeve's s. Blue sclerae, otosclerosis, and osteogenesis imperfecta. Syn., *Adair-Dighton syndrome.*

van der Hoeve-Halbertsma-Waardenburg s. Waardenburg's syndrome.

Holmes-Adie s. Adie's syndrome.

Hooft s. Diffuse pericentral tapeto-retinal degeneration, mental retardation, and abnormalities of hair, teeth, and nails, considered to result from a primary disorder of tryptophan metabolism.

Horner's s. Unilateral miosis, slight ptosis, anhidrosis, slight enophthalmos, and flushing of the face, due to involvement of sympathetic fibers on that side. Syn., *Bernard-Horner syndrome.*

Horton s. Migraine.

Horton-Magath-Brown s. Ischemic optic neuritis, paresis of extraocular muscles, and, frequently, occlusion of the central retinal vein, associated with temporal arteritis, headaches, and hyperchromic anemia, and usually seen only in older males.

Hunter s. Dwarfism, gargoyle-like facies and other symptoms of Hurler's disease but with less severity, a life span that may extend through the fourth decade, and absence of corneal cloudiness until adulthood. It is due to an x-linked recessive mode of inheritance and characterized chemically by excessive chondroitin sulfate B and heparitin sulfate in urine and tissues. Syn., *mucopolysaccharidosis II.*

Hurler's s. Hurler's disease.

Hutchison's s. Neuroblastoma of the adrenal gland with metastases to the bones of the orbit and the skull, usually occurring in the first five years of life.

hydrostatic pressure s. Temporary loss of vision, conjunctival and retinal hemorrhages, mental confusion, and shock, as a result of blood being forced into the brain, face, and orbits by raised intravascular pressure during a supersonic bail-out by an aviator. Syn., *negative acceleration syndrome.*

hypophyseo-sphenoidal s. Ophthalmoplegia, paresis of the sympathetic, and neuroparalytic keratitis, due to involvement of the trunks of the ocular cranial nerves in the region of the cavernous sinus by an infiltrating tumor.

inferior s. of the red nucleus. Rubro-ocular syndrome.

interoculo-irido-dermato-auditive s. Waardenburg's syndrome.

inverted Y (λ) s. Inverted Y (λ) pattern.

Irvine's s. Vitreous syndrome.

Jacob s. Oculo-oro-genital syndrome.

Jacod s. Jacod's triad.

Jadassohn-Lewandowsky s. Corneal dystrophy, cataracts, thickened horny skin, mental retardation, and fingernail changes; a congenital condition mainly affecting males.

Jahnke's s. The Sturge-Weber syndrome but without glaucoma.

Jayle-Ourgaud s. Ataxic nystagmus.

Jefferson s. Cavernous sinus syndrome.

Johnson s. Adherence syndrome.

Kalischer s. Sturge-Weber syndrome.

Kearns s. Myopathic external ophthalmoplegia, cardiomyopathy, and pigmentary retinal dystrophy similar to but not characteristic of a typical pigmentary retinal dystrophy, occurring in either sex, apparently not hereditary, and with onset at ages from 3 to 25.

Kennedy's s. Ipsilateral optic atrophy with contralateral papilledema, due to direct pressure on one optic nerve with the resultant forcing of cerebrospinal fluid into the sheath of the opposite optic nerve, most commonly caused by a tumor at the base of the frontal lobe. Syn., *Foster Kennedy syndrome; Gower-Paton-Kennedy syndrome; Paton's syndrome.*

Kiloh-Nevin s. Progressive pareses of the extraocular muscles, bilateral ptosis and progressive weakness of the muscles of the face, neck, and shoulder.

Kimmelstiel-Wilson s. Renal edema, pronounced albuminuria, and frequently hypertension and diabetic retinopathy.

Klauder s. Vesicular eruption and inflammation of the mucous membranes and of the skin of trunk, face, and extremities, hemorrhagic conjunctivitis, subconjunctival ecchymoses, and sometimes pneumonia, symblepharon, or visual loss.

Klein's s. Hypertelorism, blepharophimosis, hypertrophy of the eyebrows, retrognathism, partial albinism and bilateral blue irides, high arched palate and dental anomalies, bilateral deafness, rigidities of the joints, amyoplasias, skeletal dysplasias, and syndactyly.

Klein-Waardenburg s. Waardenburg syndrome.

Kloepfer s. Optic atrophy, blindness, mental deficiency, and infantilism, occurring as a hereditary, autosomal recessive condition with onset in infancy and mortality usually by early adulthood.

Klumpke s. Lower radicular syndrome.

Konigsmark s. An autosomal, recessive, inherited condition characterized by optic atrophy, hearing loss, and juvenile diabetus mellitus.

Kornzweig-Bassen s. Bassen-Kornzweig syndrome.

Krause's s. Encephalo-ophthalmic dysplasia.

Kuf s. Early infantile amaurotic family idiocy. See under *amaurotic.*

Kurz's s. Partial or total blindness, enophthalmos, moderately dilated and fixed pupils, high hypermetropia, and progressive mental retardation.

labyrinthine s. Ménière's syndrome.

Laffer-Ascher s. Blepharochalasis, edema of the lips, and goiter without hyperthyroidism. Syn., *Ascher's syndrome.*

Laurence-Moon-Biedl s. Pigmentary degeneration of the retina, girdle-type obesity, polydactylism, hypogenitalism, and mental retardation; a heredodegenerative disease probably due to recessive mutations of two genes in the same chromosome. It is more common in males, is usually progressive, and night blindness and reduced visual acuity are primary symptoms. Syn., *Bardet-Biedl syndrome; Biedl's syndrome; Biemond's syndrome; Moon-Bardet-Biedl syndrome.*

Lawford's s. Vascular nevi of the face and scalp and glaucoma, occurring without neurologic signs or enlargement of the eyeballs.

Leber s. Leber's congenital amaurosis.

Leigh s. Muscle weakness, hypotonia or hypertonia, coordination difficulties, ataxia, and absence of pupillary reactions to light. A familial disorder mainly affecting young children and thought to be a congenital error of metabolism. Syn., *infantile subacute necrotizing encephalopathy.*

LeJeune s. Cat-cry syndrome.

Lenoble-Aubineau s. Aubineau-Lenoble syndrome.

Lhermitte's s. Paralysis of the internal rectus muscle for lateral conjugate gaze with normal function in convergence, due to a lesion in the posterior longitudinal bundle in the pons. Syn., *anterior internuclear ophthalmoplegia.*

Lignac-Fanconi s. Systemic cystinosis, dwarfism, and renal glycosuria, an autosomal recessive familial condition usually seen in early childhood and in which prognosis is poor. Needle-like cystine crystals are seen clinically in the cornea, conjunctiva, and sclera.

Lilliputian s. Micropsia and related illusory distortions of perceived object distances associated with some varieties of mental disturbance. Syn., *micropsia syndrome.*

Lindau-von Hippel s. Von Hippel-Lindau disease.

Lobstein's s. Eddowes' syndrome.

Louis-Bar s. Cerebellar ataxia and telangiectases of the conjunctiva, face, and external ears. Bronchiectases was later added to the syndrome. It is a hereditary and developmental disease classified as one of the phacomatoses group. Syn., *ataxia telangiectatica.*

Lowe s. Aminoaciduria, glycosuria, albuminuria, faulty ammonia metabolism, nephritis, renal dwarfism, mental deficiency, muscular hypotony, vitamin resistant renal rickets, congenital cataracts, and congenital glaucoma; considered to be a recessive, sex-linked, hereditary disease. Syn., *Lowe-Terry-MacLachlan syndrome; Miller syndrome; oculocerebrorenal syndrome.*

lower radicular s. Paralysis and atrophy of small muscles of the hand and forearm, ptosis, and miosis resulting from a lesion involving the inferior roots of the brachial plexus derived from roots of the eighth cervical and first thoracic nerves. Syn., *Déjerine-Klumpke syndrome; Klumpke syndrome.*

Lowe-Terry MacLachlan s. Lowe's syndrome.

maculo-labyrinthine s. Recurrent central angiospastic retinopathy and Ménière's syndrome. Syn., *Montes-Lasala syndrome.*

Magendie-Hertwig s. Magendie-Hertwig sign.

Marchesani's s. Spherophakia, myopia, and glaucoma associated with brachydactyly and short stature. Syn., *dystrophia mesodermalis congenita hyperplastica; Weil-Marchesani syndrome.*

Marfan's s. Congenital, familial, bilateral, partial dislocation of the crystalline lens associated with arachnodactyly. It occurs more frequently in males, congenital miosis is usually present, and the pupils do not respond readily to atropine.

Marie-Guillan s. Rubrothalamic syndrome.

Marin Amat s. Reverse jaw-winking.

Marinesco-Sjögren s. Bilateral congenital cataracts, oligophrenia, and spinocerebellar ataxia; a hereditary disease.

Markus s. Adie syndrome.

Maroteaux-Lamy s. An appearance similar to that in Hurler's disease, including marked skeletal changes and corneal opacities, but with normal intelligence; characterized chemically by excessive secretion of chondroitin sulfate B in the urine and transmitted as an autosomal recessive. Syn., *mucopolysaccharidosis VI.*

Martin-Albright s. Polyvisceral dystrophy.

Martorell's s. Pulseless disease.

Mauriac s. Juvenile diabetes mellitus characterized by osteoporosis, defective growth, hepatomegaly, moon face, defective fat metabolism, diabetic retinopathy, and posterior subcapsular cataracts.

medial longitudinal fasciculus s. Anterior or posterior internuclear ophthalmoplegia.

Meekren-Ehlers-Danlos s. Hyperelastic and fragile skin, hyperflexible joints, and fragile blood vessels, with resulting hematomata which sometimes develop into pseudotumors. The condition has a hereditary tendency and often affects the skin of the eyelids. Syn., *fibrodysplasia hyperelastica.*

Melkersson-Rosenthal s. Recurrent facial paralysis, recurrent edema of the face and lips, and furrows in the tongue. Associated eye signs may include swelling of the eyelids, epiphora, conjunctivitis, marginal corneal opacities, retrobulbar neuritis, or exophthalmos.

Mende s. Waardenburg syndrome.

Ménière's s. Severe vertigo, nausea, nystagmus, falling toward the affected side, tinnitus, and deafness on the affected side, due to labyrinthine involvement, cerebellopontine angle tumors, otitis media, etc. Syn., *Ménière's disease; labyrinthine syndrome.*

Meyer-Schwiekerath-Weyers s. Oculodentodigital dysplasia.

micropsia s. Lilliputian syndrome.

Mikulicz' s. Chronic, bilateral, noninflammatory, symmetrical enlargement of the lacrimal glands, enlargement of the salivary glands, especially the parotid, and swelling and drooping of the eyelids with marked narrowing of the palpebral fissures, occurring in association with another disease, such as reticulosis, sarcoidosis, tuberculosis, or syphilis.

Millard-Gubler s. Ipsilateral abducens palsy and facial paralysis and contralateral hemiplegia of the limbs, due to a nuclear or infranuclear lesion in the pons. Syn., *hemiplegia alternans facialis; Gubler's paralysis; Weber-Gubler syndrome.*

Miller s. Lowe syndrome.

Milles's s. Vascular nevi of the face and scalp and angioma of the choroid, without glaucoma.

Moebius' s. Congenital, bilateral, abducens, and facial paresis due to a lesion in the brain stem. There also may be restricted adduction, deafness, webbed fingers or toes, or absence of induced vestibular nystagmus. Syn., *congenital facial diplegia; congenital oculofacial paralysis.*

Moeller-Barlow s. Hemorrhages and hematomas of the skin and mucous membranes, bone weakness, exophthalmos, and conjunctival hemorrhages, due to vitamin C deficiency and usually occurring in the first year of life.

Monakow's s. Contralateral hemiplegia, hemianesthesia, and homonymous hemianopsia, due to occlusion of the anterior choroidal artery. Syn., *anterior choroidal artery syndrome.*

Monrad-Krohn s. Raeder syndrome.

Montes-Lasala s. Maculo-labyrinthine syndrome.

Moon-Bardet-Biedl s. Laurence-Moon-Biedl syndrome.

morning glory s. A congenital anomaly in which the optic disk appears large and pink with a funnel-shaped cupping that has a central dot of fluffy white tissue and a surrounding wide, gray, elevated annulus of chorioretinal pigment over which retinal vessels course from the edge of the disk; poor visual acuity and frequently strabismus occur.

Morquio-Ullrich s. A later stage of Morquio's disease having an added symptom of corneal clouding due to gray punctate opacities, more marked in the periphery.

mountain climbers' s. Acosta syndrome.

mucocutaneous s. Stevens-Johnson syndrome.

Naffziger s. Scalenus anticus syndrome.

negative acceleration s. Hydrostatic pressure syndrome.

Negri-Jacod s. Jacod's triad.

Nieden s. Multiple generalized telangiectases and cataract associated with aortic sclerosis and organic heart disease; of unknown etiology and affecting youths or young adults.

nondominant parietal lobe s. Spatial disorientation, confusion of laterality, dressing apraxia, hemianopsia, inability to maintain motor responses, and abnormal optokinetic responses, with intact language and mental functions; due to lesions involving the nondominant parietal lobe.

Nonne-Marie s. Marie's disease.

Nothnagel s. Third nerve paralysis with contralateral cerebellar ataxia, due to a lesion of the superior peduncle, red nucleus, and emerging oculomotor fibers. Syn., *ophthalmoplegia cerebellar ataxia syndrome.*

nystagmus blockage s. A condition in which convergence reduces nystagmus, thought to be an etiological explanation for strabismus. Nystagmus is increased upon abduction of an eye and reduced upon adduction. A marked head turning is frequent in many individuals with this condition to allow the adducted fixating eye to view with minimal nystagmus. Syn., *nystagmus compensation syndrome.*

nystagmus compensation s. Nystagmus blockage syndrome.

nystagmus myoclonia s. Aubineau-Lenoble syndrome.

ocular contusion s. Mydriasis, iridoplegia, hyphema, iridodialysis and subluxation of the crystalline lens due to blunt trauma to the anterior eyeball. Syn., *Fränkel syndrome.*

oculo-auricular s. Goldenhar's syndrome.

oculocerebrorenal s. Lowe's syndrome.

oculodentodigital s. Oculodentodigital dysplasia.

oculoglandular s. of Parinaud. Conjunctivoglandular syndrome of Parinaud.

oculo-oro-genital s. Bulbar conjunctivitis, keratitis, optic atrophy, stomatitis, glossitis, exfoliative dermatitis of the scrotum, aphthous ulceration of buccal mucous membranes, and pharyngitis, resulting from deficiency of vitamins A and B. Syn., *Jacob syndrome.*

oculopharyngeal s. Progressive ptosis and dysphagia occurring in the elderly.

oculo-urethro-synovial s. Initial diarrhea followed by urethritis, polyarthritis, and conjunctivitis, iridocyclitis, or keratitis; a rare condition of unknown etiology primarily affecting young adult males. Syn., *Fiessinger-Leroy-Reiter syndrome; Reiter's syndrome.*

oculovertebral s. Oculovertebral dysplasia.

ophthalmoplegia cerebellar ataxia s. Nothnagel syndrome.

opsoclonus and polymyoclonia s. Opsoclonus associated with skeletal myoclonus, a disease of infancy attributed to a neuroblastoma. Syn., *dancing eyes and dancing feet syndrome.*

optic atrophy-ataxia s. Behr syndrome.

orbital apex-sphenoidal fissure s. S-O syndrome.

paratrigeminal s. Raeder's syndrome.

Parinaud's s. 1. Paralysis of vertical conjugate movements of the eyes either for elevation or depression, or both, due to a lesion in the subthalmic or the upper peduncular region. Pupillary abnormalities, especially dilated pupils which fail to react to light, may be present, as may be ptosis, retraction of the upper eyelid, or paralysis of convergence. Bell's phenomenon is present. 2. Conjunctivoglandular syndrome.

Parks monofixational s. See *monofixation.*

Parry-Romberg s. Romberg's disease.

Passow s. Fifth, sixth and seventh nerve pareses, heterochromia iridis, cyclitis, Horner syndrome, kyphosis, funnel chest, spina bifida, finger anomalies, and trophic and vasomotor defects of the legs, thought to be a form of status dysraphicus.

Patau s. Trisomy 13 syndrome.

Paton's s. Kennedy's syndrome.

Pel s. Pel's crisis.

Penfield s. Lacrimation, dilation or contraction of the pupils, exophthalmus, vasodilation of the skin, rise of blood pressure, increased pulse rate, and excitability, occurring suddenly in cycles lasting minutes to hours and characteristic of hypothalamic dysfunction.

petro-sphenoidal s. Ophthalmoplegia, ipsilateral deafness, temporo-facial neuralgia, and paresis of the palate, resulting from a naso-pharyngeal carcinoma arising in the fossa of Rosenmüller and extending into the eustachian tube.

Peutz-Touraine s. Freckles or café-au-lait spots on the eyelids, nostrils, and lips, associated with intestinal polyposis, transmitted as an autosomal dominant trait and appearing in early infancy.

phantom double s. A form of schizophrenia in which the subject cannot recognize an individual in his presence and insists the person is double and even describes differences between the individual and the phantom double. Syn., *Capgras syndrome.*

pineal s. Sylvian syndrome.

pineal-neurologic-ophthalmic s. Papilledema, limitation of upward gaze, concentric visual field constriction, bilateral deafness, ataxia, and hypopituitarism, due to a tumor in the region of the pineal gland. Syn., *Fränkel syndrome.*

Piper s. Congenitally incipient growth retardation, short stature, flattened, scoop-shaped fingernails, occasional bronchiectasis, high astigmatism, and corneal dysplasia.

Posner-Schlossman s. Glaucomatocyclitic crisis.

posterior cervical sympathetic s. Barré-Liéou syndrome.

pulseless s. Pulseless disease.

Raeder's s. Involvement of the trigeminal nerve and one or more other cranial nerves, together with oculopupillary fibers, which varies with the site of the lesion. It may include ptosis, miosis, enophthalmos, and facial hyperesthesia. Severe unilateral head pain is typical and characteristically sweating is intact on the ipsilateral side. Syn., *Monrad-Krohn syndrome; paratrigeminal syndrome.*

Ramsay-Hunt s. Paralysis of the facial nerve, Bell's palsy, and herpes zoster involving the inner ear.

Raymond's s. Ipsilateral abducens palsy and contralateral hemiplegia of the limbs, due to a lesion involving the pyramidal tract and sixth nerve nucleus.

Raymond Cestan s. Paralysis of the lateral rectus muscle for conjugate gaze, sometimes associated with contralateral hemiplegia, due to a lesion of the posterior longitudinal bundle in the pons and the lower midbrain.

Refsum's s. Cerebellar ataxia, chronic polyneuritis, atypical pigmentary degeneration of the retina, night blindness, and contraction of the visual fields; a recessive hereditary disease.

Reiter s. Oculo-urethro-synovial syndrome.

retraction s. Duane's syndrome.

retraction s., vertical. Congenital paralysis of the superior and the inferior rectus muscles of the same eye, slight enophthalmos, and slight narrowing of the palpebral fissure, usually due to limiting fibrous bands in the vertical recti.

Riddoch's s. Loss of interest and attention in the homonymous half fields, due to interference in the corticothalamic connections with visual sensory area 17.

Rieger's s. Rieger's disease.

Riley-Day s. Crying without tears, corneal hypesthesia or anesthesia, sleeping with the eyelids partially open, and such dehydration symptoms as attacks of high fever, vomiting, diarrhea, broncho-pneumonia, profuse salivation, and sweating, occurring in young children. Corneal pathology may be present, especially in the lower portion, ranging from superficial involvement to severe deep keratitis. Syn., *dysautonomia; familial autonomic dysfunction.*

Robin's s. A congenital triad of temporary abnormal smallness of the chin (microgenia), abnormal smallness of the tongue with backward dislodgement, and cleft palate. Accompanying ocular anomalies may include glaucoma, retinal detachment, or high myopia.

Robstein s. Blegvad-Haxthausen syndrome.

Rochon-Duvigneaud s. Superior orbital fissure syndrome.

Rollet s. S-O syndrome.

Romberg's s. Romberg's disease.

Roth-Bielschowsky s. A type of vestibular nystagmus with absence of the fast phase and retention of the slow phase, paralysis of voluntary conjugate gaze in one direction, reflex turning of the eyes opposite that of the paralysis upon labyrinth stimulation by ear irrigation or head rotation, and full deviation of the eyes toward the side of the paralysis upon stimulation of the opposite labyrinth, resulting from a supernuclear (cerebral) lesion, particularly of the temporal lobe.

Rothmund s. Atrophy of the skin with patches of pigmentation and telangiectasis, hypogonadism, and rapidly developing cataracts, occurring in early childhood as a recessive heredofamilial trait. Syn., *Zinsser-Thomson disease.*

rubella s. Congenital nuclear cataracts, heart disease, deafness, microcephaly, and mental retardation, found in infants whose mothers contracted rubella in the early months of pregnancy. Syn., *Gregg syndrome.*

Rubenstein-Taybi s. Slight antimongoloid slant of eyes, exotropia, slightly beaked straight nose, small skull, and asymmetric arch of the eyebrows; occurring as a familial abnormality.

Rubino-Corrazza s. Uveomeningitic syndrome.

rubro-ocular s. Ipsilateral third nerve paralysis and contralateral cerebellar ataxia, due to involvement of the superior cerebellar peduncle and the inferior portion of the red nucleus. Syn., *Claude's syndrome; Nothnagel's syndrome; inferior syndrome of the red nucleus.*

rubrothalamic s. Contralateral cerebellar ataxia, nystagmus, and contralateral hemianesthesia due to involvement of the superior cerebellar peduncle and superior portion of the red nucleus. Syn., *Marie-Guillan syndrome; superior syndrome of the red nucleus.*

Rud s. Pigmentary retinopathy associated with congenital ichthyosis, infantilism, epilepsy, polyneuritis, and, possibly, hyperchromic macrocytic anemia, which may be related to congenital neuroectodermal dysplasias such as tuberous sclerosis or neurofibromatosis.

Sabourad s. Dryness, thickening, and fragility of the eyelashes and eyebrows, juvenile cataracts, spindle-shaped body hair characterized by nodules on the hair shaft, and, possibly, nail and teeth abnormalities; a familial condition primarily affecting children.

Saenger's s. Pupillary rigidity to light and delayed pupillary contraction in convergence which persists for a short period after the convergence movement has ceased.

Sanders' s. Epidemic keratoconjunctivitis.

Sanders-Hogan s. Epidemic keratoconjunctivitis.

Sanfilippo s. Moderately cloudy corneal opacities, possible albinoid fundi, mental deterioration that is severe by age five or six, and dwarfism, hepatosplenomegaly, etc.; similar to Hurler's disease but milder; occurring as a recessive hereditary abnormality of mucopolysaccharide metabolism. Syn., *mucopolysaccharidosis III.*

scalenus anticus s. Ptosis, ipsilateral miosis, loss of ciliospinal reflex, weakness of ipsilateral hand grip, and reduced muscle tonus of ipsilateral upper extremity as a result of compression of the brachial plexus and subclavian artery by the scalenus anticus muscle. Syn., *Naffziger syndrome.*

Schäfer's s. Dyskeratosis of the palms of the hands and soles of the feet, hyperhidrosis, disseminated follicular hyperkeratosis, leukoplakia of the buccal mucosa, and congenital cataract; a dominant hereditary disease.

Schaumann's s. Sarcoidosis.

Scheie s. Progressive marked corneal clouding, which may be congenital, anomalies of retinal pigment, stiff joints, coarse facial features, hirsutism, and normal or above normal intelligence; occurs as an autosomal recessive congenital abnormality of mucopolysaccharide metabolism. Syn., *mucopolysaccharidosis V.*

Schirmer's s. Vascular nevi of the face and scalp and hydrophthalmos.

Schmidt-Fracaro s. Cat's eye syndrome.

Schönenberg s. Proportional dwarfism, congenital heart defect, blepharophimosis, pseudoptosis, and occasional epicanthus.

Schüller's s. Schüller-Christian-Hand syndrome.

Schüller-Christian-Hand s. Exophthalmos, polyuria associated with diabetes insipidus, and lipoid deposits in the bones, occurring in Schüller-Christian-Hand disease. Syn., *Christian's syndrome; Hand's syndrome; Schüller's syndrome.*

Sézary s. Erythroderma and edema of the skin of the eyelids and extremities, leading in the eyelids to ectropion; a malignant reticulosis affecting elderly females.

Sforzini s. Exophthalmos, malformation of the bony orbit, stuttering, hyperplasia of the long bones with a resultant tall stature, and intestinal prolapses.

Shy-Drager s. Progressive degeneration of the nervous system of unknown etiology characterized by iris atrophy, external ophthalmoplegia, hyperactive muscle stretch reflexes, loss of sphincter control, and occasionally dysphagia. Sensory and mental states remain normal.

Siemens' s. Congenital atrophy or hypoplasia of the skin, and congenital cataract; a simple recessive hereditary disease.

Sjögren's s. 1. Failure of lacrimal secretion, keratoconjunctivitis sicca, failure of secretion of the salivary glands and mucous glands of the upper respiratory tract, and polyarthritis, usually occurring in women after menopause, due to degeneration of the glandular parenchyma followed by fibrosis, of undetermined etiology. Syn., *Gougerot-Sjögren syndrome.* 2. Bilateral congenital cataracts and oligophrenia; a recessive hereditary disease.

Sjögren-Larsson s. Congenital ichthyosis, oligophrenia, spastic paraplegia, and occasionally bilateral macular degeneration.

Sluder's s. Orbital and periorbital neuralgia, accommodative asthenopia, and sensation of the eyeball being too large for the orbit, due to irritation of the ciliary ganglion.

S-O s. External and internal ophthalmoplegia of varying degree, ptosis, hyperesthesia or anesthesia of the upper eyelid, half of the forehead and the cornea, vasomotor disturbances, impairment of vision which may result in blindness, and constant radiating pain behind the eyeball, due to a traumatic, inflammatory, or neoplastic process involving the sphenoidal fissure and the optic canal which results in pressure on the structures passing through them. Syn., *Collier's sphenoidal palsy; orbital apex-sphenoidal fissure syndrome; Rollet syndrome; sphenoidal fissure-optic canal syndrome.*

Sorsby's s. Absence or rudimentary presence of the terminal phalanges of the hands and feet and bilateral pigmented macular colobomata; a dominant familial disease.

Spannlang-Tappeiner s. A recessive hereditary condition involving zonular corneal opacities and possibly cataracts, associated with keratosis palmaris et plantaris, hyperhidrosis, and partial alopecia.

sphenoidal fissure-optic canal s. S-O syndrome.

Spurway's s. Eddowes' syndrome.

Steele-Richardson-Olszewski s. A progressive neurological disorder occurring in late middle life characterized by paralysis of voluntary downward gaze, retraction of eyelids, impairment of convergence, dysarthria, and dementia. Syn., *progressive supranuclear palsy.*

Stevens-Johnson s. An acute purulent form of erythema multiforme exudativum in which vesicles appear on the mucous membranes of the conjunctiva, mouth, nose, genitourinary orifices, and anal canal, followed by similar eruptions on the skin. It may be of toxic origin or of unknown etiology. Syn., *Stevens-Johnson disease; ectodermosis erosiva pluriorificialis; mucocutaneous syndrome.*

Stilling-Türk-Duane s. Duane's syndrome.

Streiff s. Embryotoxon.

Sturge-Weber s. Vascular nevi of the face and the scalp, epileptic convulsions, glaucoma, angioma of the brain and the meninges, calcification of the cortex of the brain, and sometimes hemiplegia, of undetermined etiology. Syn., *angio-encephalo-cutaneous syndrome; Sturge-Weber-Kalischer-Dimitri syndrome; vascular encephalotrigeminal syndrome; vascular neuro-oculocutaneous syndrome.*

subclavian steal s. Transient blindness, diplopia, vertigo, dysarthria, and unilateral numbness of the body, aggravated by exercise and caused by a reversal of blood flow through a vertebral artery as a result of stenosis of one subclavian artery just proximal to the origin of the vertebral artery, whereupon its direction of blood flow yields to the greater pressure from the opposite vertebral artery with which it is united to form the basilar artery.

superior oblique tendon sheath s. Brown's tendon sheath syndrome.

superior orbital fissure s. Ipsilateral motility disturbances of the extraocular muscles, hypesthesia of the ipsilateral cornea, ipsilateral exophthalmos, ipsilateral palpable swelling in the temporal region, partial or complete loss of the field of vision, ipsilateral disturbances of the pupillary reflexes, and frequently papilledema and edema of the eyelids and conjunctiva, usually caused by a meningioma of the sphenoid bone affecting nerves passing through the superior orbital fissure. Syn., *Rochon-Duvigneaud syndrome.*

superior s. of the red nucleus. Rubrothalamic syndrome.

Swann's s. Blind spot syndrome.

Sylvian s. Nystagmus retractorius, palsy of ocular movement, especially of elevation, tonic spasms of convergence on the attempt to look upward, and attacks of clonic convergence movements, due to a neoplasm or inflammation in the region of the aqueduct of Sylvius. Syn., *aqueduct of Sylvius syndrome; Espildora-Luque syndrome; pineal syndrome.*

tegmental s. Benedikt's syndrome.

temporal arteritis s. Temporal arteritis.

tendon sheath s. Brown's tendon sheath syndrome.

Terson's s. Subarachnoid hemorrhage and profuse bleeding into the vitreous.

Tolosa-Hunt s. Recurrent unilateral retro-orbital pain and extraocular muscle palsies, attributed to indolent inflammation of the cavernous sinus or superior orbital fissure.

Touraine s. Elastosis dystrophica.

Touraine-Solente-Golé s. Thickening of the skin, especially of the forehead, face, and eyelids, and enlargement of the extremities, particularly the hands; a hereditary mesenchymal disease commencing in the second decade of life.

Treacher Collins s. Mandibulofacial dysostosis.

trisomy D s. Trisomy 13 syndrome.

trisomy 13 s. A congenital condition in which an extra 13th autosomal chromosome is present, resulting in 47 chromosomes instead of the normal 46, and producing a variety of deformities, the most common of which are mental retardation, malformed ears, heart defects, cleft palate, deafness, polydactyly, umbilical hernia, microphthalmia, coloboma, and cataract. Syn., *Patau syndrome; trisomy D syndrome.*

trisomy 18 s. A congenital condition in which an extra autosomal chromosome is present, resulting in 47 chromosomes instead of the normal 46, and producing a variety of deformities, the most common of which are prominent occiput, short palpebral fissures, epicanthal folds, corneal opacities, microphthalmos, short neck, flexed overlapped fingers, and congenital heart anomalies. Syn., *Edwards syndrome.*

trisomy 21 s. See *Down's syndrome.*

Ullrich's s. Cranial deformities with a broad nose and small jaw, skeletal deformities of the vertebrae and extremities, visceral degeneration, and bilateral anophthalmus or microphthalmus.

Usher's s. Pigmentary degeneration of the retina associated with deafness.

uveo-arthro-chondral s. Chronic uveitis associated with dystrophy of the cartilage of ears and long bones, especially of the ribs, and joint subluxation. Syn., *Hilding syndrome.*

uveo-meningitic s. Acute bilateral uveitis associated with meningitis, of undetermined etiology. Syn., *Rubino-Corrazza syndrome.*

Uyemura s. Epithelial xerosis associated with night blindness and multiple small white round spots scattered over the retina, resulting from vitamin A deficiency.

V s. V pattern.

vascular encephalotrigeminal s. Sturge-Weber syndrome.

vascular neuro-oculocutaneous s. Sturge-Weber syndrome.

vertical retraction s. A congenital condition involving only the vertical muscles of the eye, the affected eye showing hypotropia upon looking upward and outward and hypertropia upon looking downward and outward with possible orthophoria in the primary position.

vitreoretinal retraction s. Separation of the posterior vitreous caused by traction on the internal limiting membrane of the retina by adherent vitreous fibrils accompanied by reduced vision, photopsia, scotomata, and metamorphopsia.

vitreous s. Prolapse of the vitreous into the anterior chamber following rupture of the hyaloid face, occurring weeks or months after apparently uncomplicated intracapsular cataract extraction. Subsequent changes include the formation of strandlike adhesions to the operative wound and to the retina, iris, and ciliary body, and macular degeneration, pain, and photophobia. Syn., *Irvine's syndrome.*

vitreous tug s. A complication which may manifest itself two or three weeks following cataract extraction in which one or more strands extending from the deeper parts of the vitreous are caught in the postsurgical corneal wound and give rise to an irregular pupil, vitreous detachment, retinal edema, and related visual impairment.

Vogt-Koyanagi s. Bilateral uveitis, alopecia, poliosis, vitiligo, and deafness; of undetermined etiology, probably synonymous with *Harada's disease.*

Vrolik s. A form of osteogenesis imperfecta characterized by small limbs, brittle bones, compressible skull, and blue sclerae, usually fatal in youth.

Waardenburg s. Blepharophimosis, lateral displacement of the medial canthi and the lacrimal puncta, hyperplasia of the root of the nose and the medial eyebrows, pigment anomalies, such as heterochromia iridis and a white forelock, and congenital deafness or deaf-mutism, occurring as a dominant hereditary trait. Syn., *van der Hoeve-Halbertsma-Waardenburg syndrome; interoculo-irido-dermato-auditive syndrome; Klein-Waardenburg syndrome; Mende syndrome.*

Waldenström's s. A pronounced increase of gamma globulin in the blood associated with normocytic anemia, recurrent purpura, and, usually, accompanying ocular signs of sharply reduced central vision with normal peripheral vision, due to retinal edema, hemorrhages, retinal detachment, and occasionally papilledema. Syn., *macroglobulinemia; hyperglobulinemic purpura.*

Wallenberg's s. Vertigo, nausea, vomiting, difficulty in swallowing and speaking, nystagmus, ipsilateral ataxia of the limbs, loss of pain and temperature sensibility ipsilaterally of the face and contralaterally of the body, and ipsilateral miosis, ptosis, and enophthalmos, due to occlusion of the posterior inferior cerebellar artery.

Weber's s. Homolateral ptosis, dilated and fixed pupil, divergent strabismus, and contralateral hemiplegia of the face and the limbs, due to a lesion in the region of the cerebral peduncles affecting the third cranial nerve. Syn., *Weber's paralysis.*

Weber-Gubler s. Millard-Gubler syndrome.

Weil-Marchesani s. Marchesani's syndrome.

Werner's s. Premature graying and thinning of the hair, scleroderma, especially of the face and the extremities, ulceration of the feet and the legs, bilateral cataracts, hypogonadism, osteoporosis, calcification of peripheral arteries, endocrine dysfunction, and sometimes blue sclerae and keratitis, occurring as a heredofamilial disorder.

Wernicke's s. Wernicke's disease.

Weyers-Thier s. Oculovertebral dysplasia.

Wilson's s. Wilson's disease.

Wyburn-Mason s. Dilated tortuous and intercommunicating arteries and veins of the retina and midbrain accompanied by facial nevi and mental disorders. Symptoms include hemiplegia, homonymous hemianopsia, ocular paresis, strabismus, ptosis, nystagmus, and facial palsy.

X s. X pattern.

Y s. Y pattern.

Zieve s. Jaundice which frequently has its initial appearance in the sclera, with epigastric pain, hepatomegaly, telangiectasia, and malaise; due to hypercholesterolemia and hemolytic anemia found in the later stages of alcoholism.

◆

synechia (sih-nek′e-ah). Adhesion of the iris to the cornea or to the capsule of the crystalline lens.

annular s. Posterior synechia of the entire pupillary margin of the iris. Syn., *circular synechia; ring synechia.*

anterior s. Adhesion of the iris to the cornea.

circular s. Annular synechia.

peripheral s. Anterior synechia of the root of the iris.

posterior s. Adhesion of the iris to the capsule of the crystalline lens.

ring s. Annular synechia.

total s. Posterior synechia of the entire iris.

synechotomy (sin″eh-kot′o-me). Surgical division of a synechia, as in cutting the iris free from adhesion to the capsule of the crystalline lens.

syneresis of the vitreous (sih-ner′eh-sis). Contraction of the vitreous gel with separation of some of its fluid, sometimes erroneously regarded as liquefaction. Cf. *synchysis.*

synergist (sin′er-jist). See *muscles, synergistic.*

synesthesia (sin″es-the′ze-ah). 1. Concomitant sensation of a sense other than the one being stimulated, such as

seeing a color on hearing a sound. 2. Sensation in one part of the body or of an organ, due to stimulation of another part.

synizesis pupillae (sin″ih-ze′sis pu-pil′e). Occlusion or closure of the pupil.

synkinesis, pterygoid-levator (sin-kih-ne′sis). Jaw- winking.

synkinesis, trigeminal-oculomotor (sin-kih-ne′sis). Associated movements between muscles innervated by the trigeminal and oculomotor nerves, as, for example, jaw-winking.

synophrys (sin-of′ris). Joining of the eyebrows.

synophthalmia (sin″of-thal′me-ah). Cyclopia.

synopsia (sin-op′se-ah). 1. Cyclopia. 2. Synopsy.

synopsy (sin′op-se). A type of synesthesia in which visual sensations are produced by auditory stimulation. See also *color hearing.*

Synoptiscope (sin-op′tih-skōp). A type of major amblyoscope.

Synoptophore (sin-op′to-fōr). A type of major amblyoscope.

Synoropticon (sin-or-op′tih-kon). An orthoptic instrument devised by McLaughlin for the treatment of strabismus, consisting essentially of a rectangular box, one square end containing a black field on which is a green disk centered in a complementary colored, square, red frame. Each target can be independently transilluminated by enclosed light sources and is viewed through complementary red and green filters. See also *synoroptics.*

synoroptics (sin-or-op′tiks). A technique devised by McLaughlin for the orthoptic treatment of strabismus in which the patient views the targets on the Synoropticon through complementary color filters such that the normally deviating eye sees the red square and the fixating eye the central green disk. The targets are illuminated in a prescribed sequence of flash exposures until simultaneous perception and then superimposition are elicited.

synoscope, Terrien's (sin′o-skōp). A hand-held instrument for determining the presence of simultaneous binocular vision, consisting essentially of a bar, one end of which is placed in contact with the bridge of the nose, supporting a vertical median-plane septum at the proximal end, a variable distance, vertical, transverse plate with a square aperture, and a distal pair of vertical, transverse, laterally separable plates in each of which is one half of the letter *V*.

synthesis, additive (sin'theh-sis). The formation of a color by a mixture of light stimuli of two or more other colors incident on the same area of the retina simultaneously or in rapid succession.

syntonics (sin-ton'iks). A system of corrective procedures in which selected frequencies of the visible spectrum are utilized, usually by means of color filters, with the implication of therapeutic value in the colors themselves.

syntonist (sin'ton-ist). One who practices syntonics.

syphilis, pseudogranular conjunctival (sif'ih-lis). Conjunctivitis granulosa syphilitica.

◆

SYSTEM

system. 1. A methodical arrangement of interacting or interdepending parts to subserve a common function. 2. A group of organs serving an over-all biological function, such as the nervous sytem. 3. Organized ideas, essential principles, or facts arranged in a rational dependence. 4. The body as a functional unit.

Becker s. A classification of the size of the angle of the anterior chamber between the iris and the cornea as estimated by gonioscopy, ranging from 0 for a narrow or closed angle to 4 for a wide open angle. Cf. *Scheie system* and *Shaffer system*.

boxing s. Boxing method.

CIE coordinate s. A graphic system of representing the colors in relation to each other by plotting on a plane coordinate scale the proportional values of two of the three primary colors of light (red, green, and blue) required by a standard observer to match all other colors. The value of the third primary is derived from the fact that the sum of the three is constant.

datum s. Datum method.

GOMAC s. GOMAC method.

Grolman Fitting s. The trade name for a device with adjustable scales which may be attached to an empty eyeglass frame to determine in situ the proper lateral and vertical placement of the optical centers and segments.

lens s. A combination of lenses, or lens elements, ordinarily mounted on a common axis, which may be in contact with each other or separated by transparent isotropic media, and which act together to produce an image. **Celor l.s.** Gauss objective lens. **compound l.s.** A lens system having more than two refracting surfaces, i.e., consisting of more than one lens. **simple l.s.** A lens system having only two refracting surfaces, i.e., consisting of only one lens.

M s. A system for specifying the size of a test type letter in terms of the distance in meters at which the letter subtends a visual angle of five minutes. Hence a 2 M letter subtends a five minute visual angle at a distance of 2 meters and an 0.5 M letter subtends a five minute visual angle at a distance of 0.5 meters. With a letter threshold size at 40 cm of 2 M the visual acuity is recorded as 0.4/2.0. Multiplying the M system notation by 50 converts it to a Snellen notation, e.g., $50 \times 0.4/2.0 = 20/100$.

Munsell s. A three dimensional, polar, co-ordinate system for cataloging opaque, surface, pigment colors in accordance with three psychophysical attributes called *hue* (wavelength), *chroma* (saturation), and *value* (lightness, brightness, or luminance), in which the chroma is represented in equal sensation intervals on a radial scale, hue on a circumferential scale, and value on an axial scale.

optical s. A combination of mirrors, lenses, lens elements, or prisms, ordinarily mounted in a common axis, which may be in contact with each other or separated by transparent isotropic media, and which act together to produce an image. **achromatic o.s.** An optical system designed to minimize chromatic aberration, as represented by its ability to bring the light of two fiducial wavelengths to a common focus. **afocal o.s.** An optical system of zero focal power, such that rays entering parallel emerge parallel. **aplanatic o.s.** An optical system free of both spherical aberration and coma. **Bouwers' o.s.** A catadioptric system consisting of a concave spherical mirror and a diverging meniscus lens having spherical surfaces. The lens, whose convex surface is turned toward the mirror, is located at the center of curvature of the mirror and serves to correct the spherical abberation of the concave mirror. **Cassegrain o.s.** A system designed to shorten the length of an optical unit utilizing a large, parabolic, concave mirror which receives the incident light and reflects it to a small, hyperbolic, convex mirror, located on the optical axis, which transmits it through a central hole in the large mirror to the eyepiece. **Cassegrain-Schmidt o.s.** A Cassegrain optical system with a Schmidt plate. **catoptric o.s.** An optical system in which the image forming elements are mirrors. Also spelled *katoptric*. **centered o.s.** Homocentric optical system. **coaxial o.s.** Homocentric optical system. **concurrent o.s.** An optical system in which a displacement of the object along the optical axis results in a displacement of the image in the same direction, characteristic of lens systems. **contracurrent o.s.** An optical system in which a displacement of the object along the optical axis results in a displacement of the image in the opposite direction, characteristic of mirror systems. **convergent o.s.** An optical system which bends incident light rays toward its axis, increasing the curvature of incident wavefronts. Hence, an optical system in which the first principal point is to the right of the primary focal point. **convergent (dioptric) o.s.** A convergent optical system employing refracting surfaces. **convergent (katoptric) o.s.** A convergent optical system employing reflecting surfaces. **dioptric o.s.** An optical system employing refracting surfaces. **divergent o.s.** An optical system which bends incident light rays away from its axis, decreasing the curvature of incident wavefronts, hence an optical system in which the first principal point is to the left of the primary focal point. **divergent (dioptric) o.s.** A divergent optical system employing refracting surfaces. **divergent (katoptric) o.s.** A divergent optical system employing reflecting surfaces. **Gaussian o.s.** A method of representing the paraxial properties of compound optical systems in terms of principal points and planes and focal points and planes. The concept of nodal planes and points, sometimes considered in optical systems, was introduced by Moser, but is sometimes alluded to in Gaussian optics. **hemisymmetric o.s.** An optical system consisting of two parts, the second being a magnified mirror image of the first. **holosymmetric o.s.** An optical system consisting of two parts, the second being a mirror image of the first. **homocentric o.s.** An optical system in which the elements are centered on a common axis. Syn., *centered optical system; coaxial optical system*. **orthoscopic o.s.** An optical system corrected for distortion and spherical aberration. Syn., *rectilinear optical system*. **rectilinear o.s.** Orthoscopic optical system. **reduced o.s.** An optical system in which axial distances are represented by the ratios of the actual distances to the index of refraction of the medium in which they lie. **schlieren o.s.** A combination of light source, lenses, and knife edges arranged so that the interposing of refractive index gradients in the media in the optical path, as by heat, pressure, stress, or tension, produces a change in gradient distribution pattern in the image, used especially to observe air flow as affected by such factors as heat, projectile speed, or turbulence. **telecentric o.s.** An optical system in which either the entrance pupil or the exit pupil is at infinity. **telescopic o.s.** Any optical system which transforms a cylindrical bundle of parallel rays into another cylindrical bundle of parallel rays; an afocal system. **thick lens o.s.** An optical system consisting of one or more thick lenses, e.g., a camera lens. **thin lens o.s.** An optical system consisting of two or more thin lenses, e.g., an astronomical telescope. **unreduced o.s.** An optical system in which actual distances are designated regardless of the index of refraction of the medium in which they lie. **zoom o.s.** Zoom lens.

Ostwald s. A system of specifying surface colors, based on a color match with a hypothetical ideal surface which has either (a) a constant value of spectral reflectance for the wavelength band between two spectral complementaries, and another constant value for all wavelengths outside this band, or (b) in the case of a wavelength having no spectral complementary, a constant value of spectral reflectance for all wavelengths shorter than this particular wavelength, and another constant value for all longer wavelengths. Underlying this concept of an ideal surface is the basic idea that all surface colors of the same dominant wavelength differ only in the proportions of black, white, and color which they contain, and so can be specified according to these proportions in the equation: $W + B + C = 1$. Hence the variables employed in the system and their correlates in terms of the ideal surface described are: (1) *Ostwald hue*, representative of that portion of the spectrum for which the surface has the higher reflectance value; (2) *full color content*, represented by C in the above equation and specified as the higher reflectance value minus the lower; (3) *white content*, represented by W in the equation, and specified as the lower of the two reflectance values; and (4) *black content*, represented in the equation by B, and specified as the difference between unity and the higher of the two reflectance values. By use of the *Ostwald notation*, these variables are designated for the various *Ostwald tints* and *tones* which comprise the entire array of *Ostwald colors*, consisting of several hundred chromatic and achromatic samples of various mixtures of *semichromes* with black and white.

Ridgway s. A systematic arrangement and notation for naming and specifying colors by reference to the *Ridgway Color Dictionary* (1912 edition) containing 1,113 painted samples. It is widely used for describing colors of flowers, birds, and insects and the arrangement of colors and terminology are similar to the Ostwald system.

Scheie s. A classification of the size of the angle of the anterior chamber between the iris and the cornea as estimated by gonioscopy, ranging from "wide" for a wide open angle through I, II, III, and IV for successively narrower angles in which IV is an invisible angle. Cf. *Becker system* and *Shaffer system*.

Shaffer s. A classification of the size of the angle of the anterior chamber between the iris and the cornea as estimated by gonioscopy, ranging from 0 for a "closed" angle to 4 for a "wide open" angle. Cf. *Scheie system* and *Becker system*.

Telecon s. A Galilean telescopic system in which the eyepiece is a contact lens of high concave dioptric power and the objective is a wafer of appropriate convex power cemented to the ocular side of a spectacle lens carrier.

visual approach slope indicator s. A color signaling system located at each side of the runway to guide incoming pilots. Acronym *VASIS*.

◆

SYVW. See *Save Your Vision Week*.
von Szily (fon-sil'e) **phenomenon; ring sinus; test.** See under the nouns.

T

T. Abbreviation for (1) *intraocular tension;* (2) *tropia.*

tabes dorsalis (tāb'bēz dor-sa'lis). A degenerative disease of the dorsal columns of the spinal cord, the posterior nerve trunks, and frequently certain cranial nerves, especially the optic nerve, due to neurosyphilis. Ocular symptoms include the Argyll Robertson pupil, absent or diminished pupillary dilation in response to pain, optic atrophy, visual field defects, ptosis, and paralysis of one or more of the extraocular muscles.

table. A collection or an arrangement of related data.
   color t. 1. A chromaticity diagram. 2. A systematic arrangement of colors for classification or cataloging purposes. 3. A pattern or an arrangement of colors for testing color vision. **Daae's c.t.** Seventy colored wool samples in 10 horizontal rows of 7 each, one row of which includes variations of green, another variations of red, and the others, wools of various colors which a color-deficient person may identify as shades of the same color. **Helmholtz' c.t.** 1. Helmholtz' color circle. 2. Helmholtz' color triangle. **Maxwell's c.t.** Maxwell's color triangle. **Newton's c.t.** Newton's color circle.
   Donders' t. A table of expected amplitudes of accommodation at different ages, based on Donders' data.
   Duane's t. A table, compiled by Duane, indicating maximum, minimum, and average amplitudes of accommodation at different ages.
   Neumueller's t's. Tables compiled by Julius Neumueller which indicate the expected lens correction for astigmatism, on the basis of the ophthalmometer finding, after allowing for physiological astigmatism and the effectivity of the spherical component of a lens placed 15 mm in front of the cornea.
   Whitwell's t. A table for indicating the optimal curvatures of the ocular surfaces of the correcting spectacle lenses in anisometropia to minimize aniseikonia.

TABO notation. See under *notation.*

tachistoscope (tah-kis'to-skōp). An instrument which exposes visual stimuli for a brief period of time, usually $^1/_{10}$ second or less.

Tachistoscreener, Roberts (tah-kis'-to-skrēn-er). A visual field screening instrument having a translucent screen from behind which are flashed various patterns of dots of light. A chin rest, occluder, rheostat, rotary switch for target selection, and a flash control device are provided.

tachycardia strumosa exophthalmica (tak"e-kahr'de-ah stroo-mo'sah ek"sof-thal'mih-kah). Excessively rapid heart action in exophthalmic goiter.

TAF. Transient adaptation factor.

Taillefer's valve (tā-yeh-ferz). See under *valve.*

Tait's method (tātz). See under *method.*

Tajiri method (tah-jēr'e). See under *method.*

Takayasu's disease (tah"kah-yah'-suz). Pulseless disease.

Takayasu-Ohnishi disease (tah"-kah-yah'soo-o-nish'e). Pulseless disease.

talantropia (tal″an-tro′pe-ah). Nystagmus.

talbot (tahl′but). A unit of luminous energy. One talbot per sec. = one lumen.

Talbot's (tahl′butz) **bands; effect; law; level.** See under the nouns.

Talbot-Plateau law (tahl′but-plă-to′). See under *law.*

Tamascope (tah′mah-skōp). The trade name for a projector which produces a high contrast magnified image of a contact lens on any smooth vertical surface for the purpose of inspection.

tangent centune (tan′jent sen-tūn). Prism diopter.

tangent screen. See under *screen.*

tape. A narrow strip or band of paper, cloth, metal, etc., usually calibrated.

   Holtzert t. An auxiliary tape, 1 m long, attached to Priestley Smith's tape, extending from beneath the fixating eye to the fixation target, and serving to maintain a constant fixation distance.

   Priestley Smith's t. An apparatus for determining the objective angle of strabismus, consisting of two tapes attached to a ring, one being 1 m in length and the other graduated in centimeters. One end of the meter tape is placed beneath the fixating eye and a light source is placed through the ring on the other end of the tape and positioned in the midplane 1 m from the subject. A fixation target is moved along the calibrated tape, held perpendicular to the midplane, until the corneal reflex of the light source occupies the same relative position in the deviating eye as originally in the fixating eye, the examiner's eye remaining directly above the light source.

tapeto-retinal (tah-pe′to-ret′ih-nal). Pertaining to both the tapetum and the retina.

tapetum (tah-pe′tum). Any of certain membranous layers, especially of the choroid and the retina.

   t. cellulosum. A type of tapetum lucidum consisting of several layers of highly reflecting endothelial cells in tilelike formation in the choroid of most carnivorous animals, seals, and nocturnal prosimians which gives the pupils a lustrous appearance when illuminated in the dark.

   choroidal t. A tapetum lucidum located within the deeper layers of the choroid.

   t. fibrosum. A type of tapetum lucidum consisting of wavy, tendinouslike, fibrous tissue in the choroid of most hoofed animals, elephants, whales, some monkeys, and certain fishes, which gives the pupils a lustrous appearance when illuminated in the dark.

   guanine t. A type of tapetum lucidum in which guanine crystals are the reflecting medium, found in the choroid of chondrosteans and some teleosts, and in the retina of crocodilians and some teleosts.

   t. lucidum. A reflecting structure lying behind the visual receptors, either in the pigmented epithelium of the retina or in the deep layers of the choroid, in the eyes of certain mammals, birds, and fishes which gives a shining appearance to the eyes, as is seen in cats' eyes when illuminated in the dark. It aids vision in dim illumination by reflecting light back through the visual receptors which it has already traversed, thus augmenting the effectiveness of the light stimulating the retina.

   t. nigrum. The pigment epithelium layer of the retina.

   nonocclusible t. A tapetum lucidum that is not variably obscured by pigment migration, remaining exposed to the same extent in all degrees of illumination.

   occlusible t. A tapetum lucidum that is primarily operative in dim light, being obscured in bright light by migrating pigment.

   retinal t. A tapetum lucidum in the pigment epithelium of the retina, formed by reflecting crystals such as guanine.

taraxis (tah-rak′sis). 1. Reduced vision resulting from trauma to the eye. *Obs.* 2. Mild conjunctivitis. *Obs.*

target. A pattern or an object of fixation, attention, or observation in vision testing or training.

   bird-and-cage t's. A classic pair of colligation targets, one consisting of a bird and the other of a cage, which when viewed haploscopically may appear as a bird in a cage, hence a test for simultaneous binocular vision.

   colligation t's. A pair of targets each of which is viewed monocularly and contains different components of a total picture to be perceived haploscopically, as in a stereogram.

   Helmholtz ring t. A white card on which are drawn numerous evenly spaced black, fine-line, concentric circles, to detect or demonstrate subjectively radial asymmetries of ocular image sharpness.

Lapicque's t. A small dark rectangle of height twice its width located directly above a square of the same height and twice the luminance of the rectangle, which, when moved away from the observer, are seen to become indistinguishable.

tarsadenitis (tahrs-ad″e-ni′tis). Inflammation of both the tarsus and the Meibomian glands.

tarsal (tahr′sal). Pertaining to, or situated in, the tarsus.

tarsal arches; cartilage; cyst; glands; plate. See under the nouns.

tarsectomy (tahr-sek′to-me). Surgical removal of a portion of the tarsus.

tarsitis (tahr-si′tis). Inflammation of the tarsus secondary to inflammatory processes originating in the skin and subcutaneous tissues or in the conjunctiva.

t. necroticans. Necrosis of the tarsus with perforations through the conjunctiva and subsequent scarring, due to multiple internal hordeolums occurring simultaneously in crops.

tarso- (tahr′so-). A combining form denoting or pertaining to the tarsus or to the edge of the eyelid.

tarsocheiloplasty (tahr″so-ki′lo-plas″-te). Plastic surgery of the eyelid margin.

tarsomalacia (tahr″so-mah-la′she-ah). Softening of the tarsus.

tarso-orbital (tahr″so-ōr′bih-tal). Pertaining to the tarsus and the orbital walls.

tarsophyma (tahr″so-fi′mah). Any tarsal growth or tumor.

tarsoplasia (tahr″so-pla′se-ah). Tarsoplasty.

tarsoplasty (tahr′so-plas″te). Plastic surgery of the eyelid; blepharoplasty.

tarsorrhaphy (tahr-sōr′ah-fe). A surgical operation for shortening or closing the palpebral fissure in which the upper and the lower eyelids are sutured together.

tarsotomy (tahr-sot′o-me). Surgical incision of the tarsus or of the eyelid.

tarsus (tahr′sus). A thin plate of dense fibrous and some elastic tissue in the upper and the lower eyelids, giving them their shape and firmness, located anterior to the palpebral conjunctiva and extending from the orbital septum to the eyelid margin. The tarsus is attached to the lateral and medial walls of the orbit by the lateral and the medial palpebral ligaments and to the superior and the inferior margins of the orbit by the orbital septum. The tarsus in the upper eyelid is larger than in the lower and contains approximately 25 Meibomian glands, while the lower contains approximately 20. Syn., *tarsal cartilage; tarsal plate; tarsus palpebrarum.*

t. palpebrarum. The tarsus.

task, visual. That which is to be seen in sufficient detail to enable the viewer to respond appropriately.

tattooing, corneal. Surgical embedding of fine particles of metallic salts, such as gold or platinum chlorides, into the subepithelial areas of the cornea, by means of special needles, to color the cornea for therapeutic or cosmetic reasons.

Tay's (tāz) **choroiditis; disease; dots; sign; spot.** See under the nouns.

Taylor reflectometer. See under *reflectometer.*

Tay-Sachs disease (ta-saks′). See under *disease.*

TBI. Translid Binocular Interactor.

TBUT. See *BUT.*

tears. The salty, slightly alkaline, clear, watery fluid secreted by the lacrimal gland which, together with the secretions of the conjunctival goblet cells, the Meibomian glands, the glands of Zeis, and the accessory lacrimal glands of Krause and Wolfring, serves to keep the conjunctiva and the cornea moist and to facilitate eyelid movement. The fluid contains proteins, urea, sugar, salts, lysozyme, and mucin, and is drained from the eye through the nasolacrimal duct via the lacrimal puncta.

crocodile t's. 1. A spasmodic, copious flow of tears, occurring in facial paralysis, on the tasting or chewing of food. See also *gustolacrimal reflex.* 2. False or affected tears.

technician, optometric. One trained and qualified to administer technical and clinical tests and measurements, adapt, repair, and maintain optometric materials, and/or perform related clerical duties as delegated and supervised by an optometrist for the purpose of making the optometrist's professional services more effective and/or more comprehensive. Variously called para-optometric, optometric assistant, optometric technologist, and optometric aide, especially to convey differences of qualifications and emphasis.

technique. See *method* or *test*.

Teichmann's (tĭk'mahnz) **lymphatic circle; radial vessels.** See under the nouns.

teichopsia (ti-kop'se-ah). A transient visual sensation of bright shimmering colors, such as the fortification spectrum associated with a scintillating scotoma.

telangiectasia, hereditary hemorrhagic (tel-an"je-ek-ta'ze-ah). Rendu-Osler disease.

telangiectasis of the retina (tel-an"je-ek'tah-sis). Numerous, small, sharply defined, red globules in a slightly elevated area of the fundus which may become whitish in color due to circulatory disturbance. It consists of groups of dilated capillaries, may be stationary, or progressive (Coats's disease), and is usually unilateral.

Telebinocular (tel"e-bi-nok'u-lar). A trade name for a Brewster-type stereoscope containing 5 D convex spheroprisms (base-out) for eyepieces.

telecanthus (tel-eh-kan'thus). Excessive separation of the medial canthi of the eyelids.

telecentric (tel"e-sen'trik). Pertaining to an optical system in which either the entrance pupil or the exit pupil is at infinity.

teleceptor (tel"e-sep'tor). Telereceptor.

Telecon system (tel'eh-kon). See under *system*.

teleopsia (tel"e-op'se-ah). A perceptual disturbance characterized by an apparent increase in distances; hence close objects appear to be far away.

telereceptor (tel"e-re-sep'tor). A sensory receptor of stimuli perceptually localized at a distance from the point of reception of the stimulus effect, such as visual or auditory receptors, distinguished from touch or pain receptors. Syn., *teleceptor*.

Telerotor (tel'e-ro-tor). A motor attachment which controls the flash sequence in visual training instruments (especially the Tel-eye-trainer) by means of rotating notched disks whose edges control the light switch.

telescope. An optical instrument for magnifying the apparent size of a distant object, consisting essentially of an objective (a converging lens or mirror) which collects light and forms a real image of the distant object, and an eyepiece which magnifies the image formed by the objective.

    astronomical t. A refracting telescope in which both the objective and the eyepiece are converging systems and so placed in relation to each other that the posterior focal point of the objective and the anterior focal point of the eyepiece are coincident, so that the viewed object is seen inverted. Syn., *Kepler telescope*.

    Bioptic t. Bioptic telescopic lens. See under *lens*.

    Cassegrainian t. A reflecting telescope which has a large, parabolic, concave mirror to collect light from a distant body and a small, hyperbolic, convex mirror, located on the optical axis, to transmit the light back through a central hole in the large mirror to the eyepiece or to a photographic plate.

    Dutch t. Galilean telescope.

    Galilean t. A refracting telescope in which the objective is a large converging lens and the eyepiece is a smaller diverging lens which intercepts the converging rays before they come to a focus. It forms an erect virtual image and is commonly used in opera glasses,

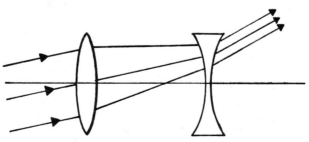

Fig. 36 Galilean telescope.

low power field glasses, and telescopic spectacles. (See Fig. 36.) Syn., *Dutch telescope.*

Gregorian t. A reflecting telescope having a large concave mirror to collect light from a distant body and a small concave mirror located on the optical axis so that its focus is coincident with the large mirror, which transmits the light back through a hole in the large mirror to the eyepiece.

Hale t. A reflecting telescope which has a large, parabolic, concave mirror to collect light from a distant body and focus it on a point on the axis where the image is directly observed.

Herschelian t. A reflecting telescope in which the parabolic concave mirror is so inclined that the image is formed near one side of the open end of the tube, to be viewed through the eyepiece.

Kepler t. Astronomical telescope.

mercurial t. A reflecting telescope in which light rays are reflected by a basin of mercury either in revolution or at rest.

mirror t., Dixon's. A magnifying telescopic spectacle lens, designed by H. Dixon in 1786, consisting of a concave mirror with a small central aperture, mounted like a spectacle lens, and a small convex mirror anterior to the aperture. The path of light is from the object to the large mirror, to the small mirror, and through the aperture to the eye.

Newtonian t. A reflecting telescope which has a large, parabolic, concave mirror to collect light from a distant body and a small diagonal plane mirror (or a prism) near the open end of the tube to reflect the light at right angles toward the eyepiece.

panoramic t. A telescope which may be oriented in various directions while its eyepiece remains stationary.

reflecting t. A telescope which employs a concave mirror as the objective.

refracting t. A telescope which employs a converging lens as the objective.

Schmidt's t. A reflecting telescope which has a large, spherical, concave mirror to collect light from a distant body, a small, spherical, convex mirror located on the optical axis to transmit the light back through a central hole in the large mirror to the eyepiece, and an optically weak, aspherical lens in the plane of the center of curvature of the large mirror to correct for spherical aberration and coma.

terrestrial t. A telescope having the optical system of an astronomical telescope except that an erecting lens (or lens system) is placed between the objective and the eyepiece to erect the image.

Trioptic t. Trioptic telescopic lens. See under *lens.*

Telesight unit (tel′eh-sīt). See under *unit.*

telestereoscope, Helmholtz′ (tel″e-ster′e-o-skōp″). An instrument, invented by Helmholtz, to produce exagerated perception of depth for distant objects. It consists essentially of a long narrow box or tube containing, on one side, two widely separated apertures for collecting light from distant objects, and, on the opposite side, two apertures, separated by an average interpupillary distance, through which the objects are viewed. Light entering through the instrument is reflected in the interior by a system of mirrors or right angle prisms to emerge through the rear apertures into the eyes.

telestereoscopy (tel″e-ster″e-os′ko-pe). Exaggeration of apparent depth relationships by the increased lateral separation of the objectives of a binocular viewing instrument.

teletraumatism, retinal (tel″e-traw′-mah-tizm). Purtscher's disease.

television trainer. See under *trainer.*

Tel-eye-trainer (tel″i-trān′er). A trade name for a Brewster-type stereoscope containing 5.00 D convex spheroprisms (base-out) for eyepieces, a housing to exclude extraneous light, and a motor attachment to provide variably intermittent illumination of the targets.

Tellais′ sign (tel′āz). See under *sign.*

telo-menotaxis (tel-o-men″o-tak′sis). A type of light-compass reaction in which the orientation of movement is governed by directional sensitivities of receptors to light and the ability to select a guiding stimulus with the inhibition of others.

teloramic (tel-or-am′ik). Weston's classification of a visual task located at a distance greater than two meters. Cf. *ancoramic; mesoramic.*

telotaxis (tel″o-tak′sis). A movement of a motile organism directly toward or away from a light source which may be mediated by a single receptor organ having a number of elements spatially distributed, enabling localization of the light source and orientation of the head and body with the light. See also *klinotaxis; menotaxis; mnemotaxis; tropotaxis.*

temperature. The degree or scalar representation of coldness or hotness.

    blackbody t. Radiation temperature.

    brightness t. Luminance temperature.

    color t. The temperature of a complete radiator (blackbody) which yields a chromaticity matching that of a given color sample or source.

    correlated color t. The colorimetric equivalence of a light source on the full-radiator (blackbody) locus, expressed in degrees of absolute temperature. Loci of equal (correlated) color temperature can be represented graphically on a chromaticity diagram.

    luminance t. The temperature of a complete radiator (blackbody) which has the same luminance for some narrow spectral region (usually at 665 mμ) as that of the source in question. Syn., *brightness temperature.*

    radiation t. The temperature, in degrees Kelvin, of a complete radiator (blackbody) which has the same total radiant emittance as that of the source in question. Syn., *blackbody temperature.*

template (tem′plit). A metal plate cut on one edge to a specific curvature for use as a gauge for the curvature of a lens grinding or polishing tool. Syn., *templet.*

temple. 1. One of a pair of shafts extending backward from the endpieces of a spectacle frame or mounting to rest against the head or the ears for the purpose of holding the frame or mounting in position. 2. The lateral portion of the head above the zygomatic arch, anterior to the ear.

    bent library t. Hollywood temple.

    t. butt. The portion or end of a temple that fastens to the endpiece.

    comfort cable t. A type of riding bow temple whose curl is made of flexible coiled cable.

    gun butt t. Spatula temple.

    Hollywood t. A library temple with a slight downward bend near its posterior end to follow the arc of the sulcus at the top of the base of the pinna, resembling a polo stick. Syn., *bent library temple; polo temple.*

    library t. A temple typically with a continuously tapering size from the small butt end to the vertically wide posterior end, and nearly straight to facilitate easy slipping of the frame on or off the face. It extends to just slightly posterior to the top of the base of the pinna and is commonly used on heavy plastic spectacle frames. Syn., *stub temple.*

    paddle t. Spatula temple.

    polo t. Hollywood temple.

    riding bow t. A temple which has a curved posterior portion designed to follow the posterior contour of the external sulcus at the base of the pinna from the top down to the lobe, originally made of relatively stiff wire.

    skull t. Any temple that holds the spectacle frame or mounting primarily by following and resting against the contour of the side of the skull behind the ear, and secondarily by following in part the contour of the sulcus at the base of the pinna. **full s.t.** A temple having a relatively rigid, posterior portion designed to follow the contour of the external sulcus at the base of the pinna from the top down along an arc of about 75° and thence extending about 2 cm tangentially downward and curved medially to follow the contour of the mastoid protuberance. **semi s.t.** A temple having a relatively rigid, posterior portion designed to follow the contour of the external sulcus at the base of the pinna from the top down along an arc of about 40° and thence extending about 2 cm tangentially downward and curved medially to follow the contour of the skull, barely reaching the top of the mastoid bone.

    spatula t. A temple having a posterior portion shaped much like a spatula, a paddle, or a gun butt, designed to rest against the side of the head at the top of the external sulcus at the base of the pinna and extending slightly back and around the contour of the head. Syn., *gun butt temple; paddle temple.*

    stub t. Library temple.

templet (tem′plet). A template.

temporal induction. See under *induction.*

tendo (ten′do). A tendon.

t. oculi. Medial palpebral ligament.

t. palpebrarum. Medial palpebral ligament.

tendon (ten'don). A dense band of fibrous connective tissue constituting the termination of a muscle, usually attaching it to a bone.

ciliary t. An annular tendon adjacent to, and blending with, the scleral spur and the meshwork of the angle of the anterior chamber, serving as a common origin for the fibers of the ciliary muscle.

lower t. of Lockwood. Lower tendon of Zinn.

lower t. of Zinn. An inferior thickening of the inner surface of the annulus of Zinn, attached to the inferior root of the small wing of the sphenoid bone, which gives origin to the inferior rectus muscle and to portions of the medial and the lateral rectus muscles. Syn., *lower tendon of Lockwood; inferior orbital tendon.*

orbital t., inferior. Lower tendon of Zinn.

orbital t., superior. Upper tendon of Lockwood.

upper t. of Lockwood. A superior thickening of the inner surface of the annulus of Zinn, attached to the body of the sphenoid bone, which gives origin to the superior rectus muscle and to portions of the medial and the lateral rectus muscles. Syn., *superior orbital tendon.*

t. of Zinn. Annulus of Zinn.

tenebrescence (ten-eh-bres'ens). A decrease in transmittance or increase in absorption of light induced by exposure to it, as in photochromic glass.

tenomyotomy (ten"o-mi-ot'o-me). Incision of a portion of the tendon of an extraocular muscle to weaken its action, in the surgical treatment of strabismus,

Tenon's (te'nonz) **capsule; fascia; membrane; space.** See under the nouns.

tenonitis (ten"on-i'tis). Inflammation of Tenon's capsule or the connective tissue within Tenon's space, occurring in either a purulent or a serous form.

tenonometer (ten"o-nom'eh-ter). Tonometer.

tenontotomy (ten"on-tot'o-me). Tenotomy.

tenoplication (ten"o-pli-ka'shun). A surgical procedure for strabismus to enhance the activity of an extraocular muscle in which the tendon is laid bare, folded forward, and sutured to a denuded sclera at a point nearer the cornea.

tenotomy (ten-ot'o-me). Incision of a tendon, as of an extraocular muscle, in the surgical treatment of strabismus.

central t. Tenotomy in which the central portion of the tendinous insertion is cut, leaving the margins intact.

controlled t. Tenotomy in which sutures are placed through the tendinous insertion before its division and then loosely attached to the sclera and externalized to permit later adjustment of the position of the muscle by loosening or tightening the sutures. Syn., *guarded tenotomy.*

fenestrated t. Tenotomy in which one or more small incisions are made in the tendon, creating openings in it.

free t. Tenotomy in which the entire tendon of the muscle is cut and not surgically reattached.

graduated t. Partial tenotomy.

guarded t. Controlled tenotomy.

marginal t. Tenotomy in which the margins of the tendinous insertion are cut, leaving the central portion intact.

partial t. Incomplete division of a tendon. Syn., *graduated tenotomy.*

Tensilon. A trade name for *edrophonium.*

tension, intraocular. Ocular tension.

tension, ocular. The resistance of the tunics of the eye to indentation, which depends on the intraocular pressure, the thickness and rigidity of the tunics, the surface area, etc., and which may be estimated digitally or with a tonometer. Abbreviated T. Cf. *intraocular pressure.*

tensor choroideae (ten'sor ko-roi'-de-e). Brücke's muscle.

tensor tarsi (ten'sor tar'si). Horner's muscle.

tenthmeter. The ten millionth part of a millimeter, hence equal to 1 Å.

teratoma (ter"ah-to'mah). A neoplasm or a tumor in which all three germinal layers are represented and which thus may be composed of skin, hair, teeth, bone, cartilage, muscle, internal organs, etc. It may affect the orbit, the lacrimal gland, etc.

Terrien's (ter'e-enz) **marginal corneal dystrophy; sign; synoscope.** See under the nouns.

Terson's syndrome. See under *syndrome.*

◆

TEST

test. 1. A trial or an examination. 2. A task or a series of tasks performed to evaluate ability, quality, strength, etc. 3. Subjection to conditions that show the character of a person or a thing in a certain particular. 4. The equipment or apparatus with which a test is made. For tests not listed here, see under *method.*

accommodation t., for glaucoma. Reading test for glaucoma.

Adler's t. A test to distinguish between color blindness and aphasia in which an individual who cannot verbally identify colors is given pairs of colors to match. Aphasia is indicated if he succeeds.

afterimage t. Hering's afterimage test.

afterimage transfer t. Brock's afterimage transfer test.

Albini's E t. A test for determining the visual acuity of children or illiterates in which the subject is given an E to hold and orient in the same direction as an indicated E on an illiterate E chart. Syn., *illiterate* E *test; rotatable* E *test; tumbling* E *test.*

alignment t. Rosenbach test.

Ammann's t. Dark filter test.

Amsler-Huber t. A test used to evaluate aqueous humor formation in which fluorescein is injected intravenously and the density of the fluorescein as it arrives in the anterior chamber is determined and plotted as a function of time.

amyl nitrite t., for glaucoma. The inhalation of amyl nitrite, preceded and followed by tonometry, said to cause little or no change in eyes with normal intraocular pressure but a considerable reduction with simple glaucoma.

anterior chamber puncture t. Kronfeld's test.

AO H-R-R t. A test for color vision consisting of pseudoisochromatic plates, each containing one or two variously located, geometric figures (circle, cross, or triangle). Four plates are for demonstration, 6 are for screening into red-green-deficient, blue-yellow-deficient, and normal, 10 are for further testing of the red-green-defici-

ent, and 4 are for further testing of the blue-yellow-deficient.

applanation outflow t. Applanation tonometry taken before, during, and after compression of the eye, an experimental procedure to determine the effect of ocular rigidity on applanation tonometry.

Asher's t. A test for ocular dominance in which the subject holds two large cards, one in each hand with arms extended, and slowly brings them closer together while he fixates the examiner's open eye until the space between the cards is so narrow that only one of the subject's eyes can be seen by the examiner, this eye being considered dominant.

attention span t. A test for determining the amount or complexity of material that can be perceived in a single brief presentation, as with a tachistoscope.

Autocross t. A test for astigmatism by means of the *Matsuura Autocross,* q.v.

Bach's t. A test for malingering in which the allegedly blind eye fixates the revolving drum of an optokinetoscope, producing nystagmus when vision is present.

Bagolini's striated glass t. A test for visual sensory and motor functioning in which a Bagolini glass is mounted in front of each eye, with the striations oriented 90° apart, while a test target and a light source are viewed. Vision of the test target is relatively unimpaired while the light source appears as two streaks at right angles to each other. The number of streaks perceived (one or two) or the positioning of the two streaks, relative to each other, indicates the state of binocularity.

Bailey's t. A test for determining visual acuity of young children consisting of a series of individual pictures in cutout form, placed near the child, which he attempts to match with identical silhouettes on a chart held at various distances and calibrated to rate the acuity in Snellen fraction values.

Bailliart's dazzling t. A test for treatment amenability of reduced central vision in which the macular area is bleached for about 15 seconds by means of a bright ophthalmoscope light beam and the time noted for subsequent recovery of the pre-test acuity. About 30 seconds is normal; longer delay indicates chorioretinal impairment. Syn., *Magder's test; photostress test.*

bar reading t. A test for the presence of binocular vision in which one or more vertical bars are interposed between the eyes and reading material, such that some portions of the print are excluded to one eye and other portions to the other eye. Perception of all the print without head movement indicates binocular vision. Syn., *Welland's test.*

bead t. A test of color vision in which a set of colored beads are sorted into four groups: red, yellow, green, and blue.

Becker's t. A test for astigmatism in which sets of three parallel lines, each set oriented in a different meridian, are viewed.

Bender-Gestalt visual-motor t. A clinical test to evaluate intelligence, emotional stability, school readiness, and visual-motor skill, consisting of nine figures which are presented singly for freely copying on blank paper.

Benton right-left discrimination t. A 32 item performance test (example, touch your right eye with your left hand) designed to assess one's ability to differentiate left from right in terms of lateral parts of his own body and in terms of those of another person facing him.

Benton visual retention t. A test to measure short term visual memory in which designs on a set of cards are to be reproduced.

Berens' Three Character t. A test for binocular vision in which the transilluminated outline of three characters, a red girl, a green elephant, and a white ball on a black background mounted at the head of a flashlight, are viewed through complementary-colored red and green filters. The simultaneous perception of all three figures indicates normal binocular vision and the absence of the girl or elephant indicates suppression of one eye.

bichrome t. Duochrome method.

Bielschowsky's afterimage t. Hering's afterimage test.

Bielschowsky's head tilting t. A test for differentiating paralysis of a superior oblique muscle from that of a superior rectus muscle, consisting of forcibly reversing the natural head tilting, i.e., tilting the head toward the side of the palsied muscle. Sharp upward movement of the affected eye indicates paralysis of the superior oblique muscle and no movement, or a downward movement, indicates paralysis of the superior rectus muscle.

bifoveal t. Cüppers' bifoveal test.

Bishop Harman diaphragm t. A test for detecting heterophoria or suppression in which a horizontal row of letters or numbers is viewed through an adjustable aperture which is narrowed until the common binocular field is eliminated and each eye sees an opposite side of the target. Overlapping of the figures indicates esophoria, separation exophoria, one group higher, hyperphoria, and perception of only one side, suppression.

black and red t. A test for malingering in which red and black letters on a white background are viewed while a red filter is before the sound eye, rendering the red letters invisible to this eye. Reading of all the letters indicates vision in the allegedly poor eye.

Blaxter's t. Bulbar pressure test.

Boberg-Ans t. Determination of corneal sensitivity with the Boberg-Ans corneal sensibilitometer, q.v.

Bodal's t. A test for color perception consisting of the sorting of colored blocks.

Boder t., for dyslexia. A test for classifying dyslexia into one of three types in terms of patterns of reading and spelling, namely, *dysphonetic, dyseidetic,* or *dysphoneidetic,* q.v.

Boström's t. A test for color vision consisting of 16 pseudoisochromatic plates, 12 containing digits, and 4 blank to detect malingering.

Boström-Kugelberg t. A test for color vision consisting of 20 pseudoisochromatic plates, 15 containing digits, 2 containing winding trails for illiterates, and 3 blank to detect malingering.

box t. A test for determining sighting ocular dominance utilizing a small box, open at both ends, having two vertical rods, one at each end, placed in the center of the open ends. The subject aligns the two rods, one behind the other, while holding the box before himself, and the examiner notes which of the subject's eyes is in line with the vertical rods.

broad H t. A test for motility of the extraocular muscles in which a fixated target is moved horizontally, and then vertically, to describe the shape of the letter H having an exaggerated horizontal dimension.

Brock's afterimage transfer t. A test to detect and measure eccentric or anomalous fixation in an amblyopic eye, in cases of normal retinal correspondence, in which only the normal eye is exposed to and fixates a vertical light and is then occluded, while the amblyopic eye fixates a central point on a horizontal scale at a specified distance. The position of the vertical afterimage in relation to the fixated point indicates the angle of eccentric fixation.

Brock's scotoma box t. A test for detecting a central scotoma utilizing two small boxes, one containing a transilluminated red disk with a central black dot and the other containing a spot of light 1 to 5 mm in diameter. The box with the transilluminated red disk is strapped to the head over the nonamblyopic eye and the head is moved to superimpose the black dot on the spot of light in the other box, which is located variously from 6 in. to 6 ft in front of the amblyopic eye. Disappearance of the spot of light on superimposition indicates a central scotoma.

Brock's string t. A test to determine binocular fixation in which one end of a string is placed against the bridge of the nose and the other fastened to a light source fixated through red and green filters, one before each eye. The perception of two strings, each the color of the filter of the opposite side, intersecting at the point of fixation, indicates normal binocular fixation. The procedure is also used in training the range of binocular fixation in strabismus.

Brock-Givner t. A test for eccentric fixation in amblyopia in the absence of anomalous correspondence, in which, immediately after a bright vertical light band is monocularly fixated at its center by only the normal eye to produce an afterimage, the normal eye is occluded and the subject notes the location of the afterimage while the amblyopic eye fixates a black spot on a white background monocularly. The apparent displacement of the afterimage from the spot is a measure of the degree of eccentric fixation. Syn., *transferimage test.*

bulbar compression t. for glaucoma. A provocative test for

glaucoma in which a weight of 25 gm is placed on an anesthetized eye for 2 minutes and tonometry is performed after 5, 15, and 35 minutes.

bulbar pressure t., for glaucoma. A provocative test for glaucoma in which a pressure of 50 gm is applied to the eye by an ophthalmodynamometer placed at the site of the insertion of the lateral rectus muscle. Tonometry is performed before the application of pressure (A), and, without removal of the tonometer, 15 seconds (B) and 4 minutes (C) after the application of pressure, and after removal of pressure (D). The percentage that the change in pressure (B − C) is of the initial pressure B, is then calculated by the formula $\frac{100(B-C)}{B}$. Values below 30% indicate glaucoma. Syn., *Blaxter's test.*

Burnham-Clark-Munsell color memory t. A test for memory color discrimination for persons with normal color vision, in which 20 colored chips are individually exposed for five seconds and, following a five second waiting period, a selection is made of the one which appears of the same color from among 43 chips mounted in a circle. The chips consist of odd numbered chips from the Farnsworth-Munsell test.

caffeine t. for glaucoma. A provocative test for glaucoma in which ocular tension is measured after 150 cc of water containing 45 gm of coffee is drunk. A rise of over 8 mm Hg in 15 to 60 minutes is considered positive. Syn., *coffee test for glaucoma.*

Cantonnet's t. Determination and measurement of phorias or tropias by means of Cantonnet's diploscope.

t. card. See under *chart.*

Carter's t. A test to determine the thresholds of color perception, in which attempts are made to identify various colored targets viewed in an instrument with a rheostat control for illumination.

catoptric t. A test for the diagnosis of cataract by observing the Purkinje images on the cornea and the lens capsule.

t. chart. See under *chart.*

chi-square t. A test to determine the statistical significance of a discrepancy between an actual and a theoretical distribution.

chromatic t. A test for perceptual ocular dominance in which a red filter is alternately placed before each of the eyes while a white light is fixated binocularly. The eye with which the light appears reddest is considered the dominant eye.

Cibis t. A test for irradiation stereoscopy in which a horizontal row of 12-cm-square white cards mounted on a dull black background is viewed from a distance of 2 m with a neutral filter before one eye. Normally the cards appear rotated about vertical axes so that the edge of each card on the filter side appears nearer.

City University color vision t. A series of ten charts each consisting of a Munsell color disk symmetrically surrounded by four Munsell color disks each of which is a color match for the central disk by subjects with either the normal, protan, deutan, or tritan type of color vision.

cobalt blue glass t. A test to determine the refractive state of the eye, in which a spot of white light is viewed through a cobalt lens. A central red spot with a blue halo indicates myopia, a blue spot with a red halo absolute hypermetropia, and a purple spot either emmetropia or faculative hypermetropia. Syn., *Landolt's cobalt blue test.*

Cochet's t. 1. A screening test for the fragility of the corneal epithelium in prospective contact lens wearers, in which a spherical surface having engraved concentric circles and radiating lines is brought to bear on the cornea by means of an adapted Goldmann applanation tonometer. The degree of fluorescein staining as observed with the slit lamp indicates the prognosis. 2. Determination of corneal sensitivity with the Cochet-Bonnet esthesiometer, q.v.

coffee t. for glaucoma. Caffeine test for glaucoma.

Cohn's t. A test for color perception in which attempts are made to identify various colored, embroidered patterns intended to confuse the red-green color blind.

cold pressor t., for glaucoma. Immersion of a patient's hand in ice water in tonometry, said to cause a rise of ocular tension in glaucomatous eyes.

color threshold t. Any color perception test which determines the minimum luminous intensity at which colored lights are correctly identified.

complementary color t. for malingering. A test for malingering in which complementary-colored red and green letters are viewed through complementary-colored red and green filters; the reading of all the letters indicates vision in both eyes.

confrontation t. A test to determine the approximate extent of the visual field in which the subject, with one eye occluded, faces the examiner at a distance of about 60 cm and fixates the opposite eye of the examiner, while the examiner extends an object beyond the peripheral limit of the visual field of the subject and slowly brings it inward until it is seen.

confrontation field t. for malingering. A test for malingering in which a test object is introduced into the temporal field of the admittedly good eye and moved toward and into the nasal field of that eye. A malingerer, being unaware that the nasal fields overlap, might not admit seeing the object as it passes the median plane.

contrast t. for color blindness. A test for color vision utilizing the principle of simultaneous contrast, e.g., the viewing of gray numbers or letters on a colored background of the same brightness through tissue paper, the letters being invisible to the color blind and appearing tinged with a color complementary to the background to the normal.

convergence t. for ocular dominance. A test to determine motor ocular dominance, in which a fixation object is brought toward the eyes, past the near point of convergence, the eye maintaining fixation being considered the dominant eye.

convex lens t. for malingering. A test for malingering in which a convex lens of about 2.50 D is placed before the admittedly good eye while a test card is moved from a position within the focal point of the lens to a position beyond it. The continued reading of the test letters beyond the focal point indicates vision in the supposedly blind eye.

Cords's stereoscopic t. A test for stereoscopic vision in which the attempt is made to align vertically two pointers enclosed in a box and viewed through an aperture, the upper pointer being stationary and the lower manually controlled.

corneal dryness t. Following fluorescein instillation into the cul-de-sac and a blink, the eyes are kept in the straightforward position with the eyelids open. Normally the first dry spot appears in about 30 seconds and is best seen with the slit lamp as a dark spot of about ½ mm diameter.

cover t., alternate. The successively alternate placement of the occluder in front of each eye without allowing interim binocular viewing, to observe the magnitude of the heterophoria or heterotropia and to measure the deviation by repeating with varying amounts of corrective prism until the heterophoric or heterotropic angle is neutralized as indicated objectively by no fixational movement or subjectively by no apparent target movement. See *objective cover test; subjective cover test.*

cover t., kinetic. An objective alternating cover test advocated by Griffin in which a fixation target is moved toward and away from the examinee between the distances of approximately 10 and 50 cm at the rate of approximately 5 cm/sec during alternate occlusion to disclose vergence related trends not so readily detected in single distance tests.

cover t., objective. A test to determine the presence and the type of phoria or strabismus, in which a point is fixated at a given test distance while an opaque cover is placed first before one eye and then the other, and then placed and removed before each eye. Diagnostic data include: the movement of the eye as it is covered, the movement of the eye to assume fixation as the cover is moved to the other eye, and the movement of the two eyes when the cover is removed. Prisms may be used with this test to neutralize eye movement and thus measure the magnitude of the deviation. Syn., *objective screen test.*

cover t., subjective. A test to determine the type of phoria, in which a point is fixated at a given test distance while the eyes are alternately occluded. An apparent lateral movement opposite to the movement of the occluder indicates esophoria, in the same direction of the occluder exophoria, and no apparent movement orthophoria. An apparent downward movement indicates hyperphoria of the eye from which the occluder is moved. Prisms may be placed in front of the eyes until the movement is eliminated to measure the magnitude of the phoria. Syn., *Duane's parallax test.*

cover t., unilateral. An objective test for determining the presence of a deviation of the visual axes and differentially diagnosing a heterophoria from a heterotropia, in which one eye is covered and uncovered with an opaque occluder while a point is fixated at a given test distance. Syn., *cover-uncover test.*

cover-uncover t. Unilateral cover test.

Crisp-Stine t. A procedure for precise determination of the astigmatic axis of the eye in which the correcting cylinder lens is placed at the presumed or approximated astigmatic axis while the axes of a crossed cylinder lens and the orientation of a pair of perpendicularly crossed lines on a test chart are meridionally inclined at 45° on either side of the axis of the correcting cylinder. When the axes of the crossed cylinder lens are reversed the subject reports for which of the two positions the crossed lines appear more nearly equally clear. The axes of the crossed lines and of the crossed cylinder lens are then rotated a few degrees toward the equalizing crossed cylinder lens axis of the same sign as the correcting cylinder and the test is repeated until equality or reversal is obtained.

crossed cylinder t. for astigmatism. A clinical test for determining the axis and the amount of astigmatism, in which a crossed cylinder lens is placed before the eye with its axes each 45° away from the axis of a presumed cylinder correction (such as the static retinoscopic finding) which is also before the eye. While letters on a distant test chart are viewed, the crossed cylinder lens is flipped over so that its axes are reversed in position. The position which provides the clearer vision indicates the direction to which the axis of the correcting cylinder should be turned. The setting of the crossed cylinder lens and the axis of the correcting cylinder are varied until vision is equally distorted in both positions, indicating the proper axis of the correcting cylinder. The crossed cylinder lens is then placed with one of its axes coincident with the axis of the correcting cylinder and the flipping of the crossed cylinder is repeated. The position which provides the clearer vision indicates the adjustment of the dioptric power of the correcting cylinder, and the point of equality of vision indicates the proper amount.

crossed cylinder t., near point. Any of several monocular or binocular clinical tests, usually performed at a 40 cm fixation distance, in which a test chart containing intersecting, parallel, horizontal, and vertical lines is viewed through the subjective finding and crossed cylinder lenses with axes horizontal and vertical. Spherical lenses are added until the lines on the test chart appear equally black or dark. The finding is compared with findings of other tests to determine the desired near point lens prescription.

cube E t. A cube having a different sized E on each of its six sides, used as test targets in the evaluation of visual acuity.

Cuignet's t. 1. The bar reading test as used to detect malingering. 2. Retinoscopy.

Cüppers' bifoveal t. A test for anomalous retinal correspondence in which a light source in the center of a Maddox cross is fixated by one eye while a small ophthalmoscopically projected target is positioned on the fovea of the other. Failure to superimpose the ophthalmoscopic target on the fixated light source indicates anomalous retinal correspondence and the magnitude of the separation is a measure of the angle of anomaly.

Cüppers' neosynoptophore t. A test for either eccentric fixation or anomalous retinal correspondence utilizing the neosynoptophore. Eccentric fixation is indicated if Haidinger's brushes are perceived to be displaced with respect to the fixation dot when both are observed by the amblyopic eye, and anomalous retinal correspondence is indicated if the Haidinger's brushes are displaced with respect to the fixation dot when one eye fixates while the other observes the Haidinger's brushes.

cycloplegic t. Cycloplegic refraction.

dark filter t. A test to differentiate functional amblyopia from organic amblyopia in which visual acuity is measured with and without a neutral density filter. A marked reduction is said to indicate organic amblyopia and a slight reduction or improvement is said to indicate functional amblyopia. Syn., *Ammann's test; neutral density filter test.*

dark room t. for glaucoma. A provocative test for glaucoma in which the patient is placed in complete darkness for one hour. An increase in ocular tension of 10 mm Hg or more is considered pathological. Syn., *Seidel's test.*

dazzling t. The determination of time required for the recovery of normal acuity following bright ophthalmoscopic illumination of the macula preceded by a period of dark adaptation.

decubitus t., for glaucoma. Measurement of the intraocular tension before and after reclining with the head lower·than feet for up to an hour, a rise of more than 6 mm Hg indicating glaucoma. Cf. *prone provocative test for glaucoma.*

diplopia t. 1. A test for the state of motility of the extraocular muscles in strabismus, in which a light source is fixated in various directions of gaze, in a darkened room, with a red filter before one eye, and sometimes with a green filter before the other, to produce diplopia. The relative separation of the diplopic images is noted, first with one eye fixating and then with the other. 2. A test for suppression, consisting of the determination of the presence or the absence of physiological diplopia.

dissociating t. Any test for measuring a phoria in which fusion is disrupted or made impossible, as by means of a prism.

distortion t. Any test for measuring a phoria in which the stimulus to fusion is eliminated by distorting the retinal image of one eye, as may be done with a Maddox rod.

Dobson's t. A binocular test for constant unilateral suppression, consisting of reading from a book printed with some letters in orange and some in black while one eye views through a filter that renders the orange letters invisible. Reading all the letters indicates no suppression in the uncovered eye.

Dolman's t. 1. A test for sighting ocular dominance, in which the subject sights an object through a pinhole in an opaque card, the eye used to sight being considered dominant. 2. Howard-Dolman test.

Donders' t. A test for color perception consisting of the identification of the colored glass sides of a lantern.

double prism t. 1. A test for malingering in which a double prism is placed before one eye with the seeing of three images indicating vision in the allegedly blind eye. 2. A test for determining the type of phoria, in which a double prism is placed before one eye and a red lens before the other while a small spot of light is fixated, the position of the red image in relation to the double white images indicating the type of phoria. 3. A test for determining the presence of cyclophoria, in which a double prism is placed before one eye while a single horizontal line is fixated, no cyclophoria existing if the resultant three line images are parallel.

drinking t. for glaucoma. Water drinking test for glaucoma.

Driver's t. A test for malingering in which a bar is interposed vertically between the patient's eyes and test letters of various sizes so that it screens the right letters from the left eye and the left letters from the right eye. The reading of all the letters indicates vision in the allegedly blind eye and the size of the letters read indicates the visual acuity.

drop ball t. A test to determine the resistance of a case-hardened lens to breakage by impact, in which a 1.56 oz steel ball, ⅞ in. in diameter, is dropped perpendicularly onto the front surface of the lens from a distance of 50 in., the lens being supported in a hollow tube by a ⅛ in. rubber washer. A variation of the test calls for a 16 mm (⅝ in.) steel ball at a height of 1 m (39 in.).

dropping t. Hering's drop test.

dry t. for contact lenses. A test for the fit of the corneal section of a fluid scleral contact lens in which the lens is inserted dry, the presence and the size of an air bubble indicating the clearance between the cornea and the lens.

Duane's diplopia t. A test for the state of motility of the extraocular muscles in strabismus, in which a light source on a black screen is fixated in various directions of gaze, in a darkened room, with a red lens before one eye to create diplopia. The patient locates, with a pointer, the position of the diplopic image of the light source for each direction of gaze, first with one eye fixating and then with the other eye fixating.

Duane's parallax t. Subjective cover test.

duction t. 1. Any test in which prism or prism effect is introduced before the eyes to create a vergence demand to a point of blur or diplopia. 2. A test to determine the limits of ocular motility of an eye by moving a fixation target in various directions of gaze with the head held stationary.

duction t., forced. A procedure performed either under local or general anesthesia to test for restriction of eye movement in which the eyeball is rotated by means of forceps pulling on the conjunctiva.

Dunnington-Berke t. A test to differentiate between a disturbance in ocular motility due to fibrous adhesions and one due to paralysis, in which forceps are attached to the muscle tendon and traction is exerted in the direction of restricted ocular motility. Easy movement of the eye in this direction indicates paralysis, and considerable resistance indicates fibrous adhesions of the antagonist.

duochrome t. Duochrome method.

duochrome star t. A test to determine the astigmatic and the spherical components of the refractive correction, consisting of an astigmatic dial composed of double stripes, at angles of 60° with each other, superimposed on a half red and half green transilluminated field. The dial is rotated until the border between red and green coincides with one of the principal meridians of the eye.

Dvorine's pseudoisochromatic t. A test for color vision which utilizes pseudoisochromatic plates.

dye t., primary. A test for the ability of tears to flow through the lacrimal duct in which a cotton-tipped applicator is placed in the nose under the inferior meatus at the opening of the nasolacrimal duct. The presence of dye on the cotton two minutes after instilling fluorescein into the cul-de-sac indicates no obstruction to tear flow.

dye retention t. A test to evaluate function of the lacrimal excretory system in which the cul-de-sac is inspected for retention of fluorescein two minutes after the dye is instilled. Normal function is indicated by absence, or a minimal amount of, fluorescein.

dye t., secondary. A test for obstruction of the nasolacrimal duct, performed immediately after a negative *primary dye test* and a negative *dye retention test*, in which a saline solution is syringed into the lacrimal sac through a needle in the lower canaliculus. Saline stained with fluorescein emitting from the nostril indicates partial obstruction of the nasolacrimal duct. Saline not stained indicates partial obstruction of the puncta or canaliculus, and no saline coming out of the nostril indicates complete obstruction of the duct.

Eames t. A battery of stereograms for the screening of visual acuity, heterophoria, and binocular vision.

Edridge-Green t. A lantern test for color perception in which seven colored filters are mounted on three disks which are rotated in succession or in combination before the aperture. A fourth disk contains a ground glass to represent mist, a ribbed glass to represent rain, and neutral glasses to represent varying intensities of fog. The diaphragm has apertures of different sizes to represent railway signals or ship lights.

edrophonium chloride tonogram t. A diagnostic procedure for myasthenia gravis consisting of continued tonometry, subsequent to the intravenous administration of edrophonium chloride (Tensilon), in which increased intraocular tension is considered positive.

electroretinographic glare t. A test for retinal responses to glare in which an electroretinogram is obtained in relation to the application of a high intensity light stimulus (photoflash) in addition to the standard photostimulation.

Ellis visual designs t. A series of patterned line drawings to be copied freehand with pencil and paper and scored by an examiner for distortions and errors to assess the level of visual perception development.

euthyscope t. The Giessen test in which euthyoscopy is used to create a foveal afterimage in the deviating eye.

Evans' t. A test to approximate the visual acuity of infants, in which metal balls of various sizes are moved on a tray by means of a magnet held underneath. The smallest ball which the eyes follow indicates the acuity.

excursion t. A test for ocular motility in which a moving target is fixated in various directions while the head remains motionless. Limitation of ocular movement or overshooting of one eye indicates paralysis or paresis of an extraocular muscle.

extension t. A test for hand dominance devised by Schilder in which, with the eyes closed, the arms are extended horizontally, with the fingers spread, the higher hand being considered dominant. Syn., *Schilder's test.*

Farnsworth D-15 t. Farnsworth dichotomous test.

Farnsworth dichotomous t. A color vision test designed primarily for industrial use to permit detection of workers unable to distinguish colors of industrial color codes. A series of 15 small disks of Munsell 5/2 papers, whose hues appear to comprise a closed circuit of colors (cf. *color circle*) for normal observers, mounted in black plastic caps, must be arranged by the subject into a smooth color series. Score sheets with dots numbered 1 to 15, arranged in a circle, are marked by drawing lines to connect the numbered dots in the order in which the caps were arranged. Normal observers and those with mild color defects make few or no errors and yield generally circular score profiles. Subjects whose score sheets show a crisscrossing of the circle are more severely defective and would be unable to use color codes effectively. The principal direction of the crisscrossing score lines identifies the type of color blindness, e.g., protanopia, deuteranopia, or tritanopia.

Farnsworth-Munsell t. A color vision test consisting of 85 small disks of colored papers selected from the Munsell 100-hue series so that they appear approximately equal in chroma and value but perceptibly different in hue for normal observers. The disks are mounted in black caps and consecutively numbered from 1 to 85. The series is divided into four parts, each in a black tray, with the caps containing the terminal colors for that part mounted at the ends of the tray. The caps are shuffled, and the subject must then arrange them into a smooth color series. Errors are scored as the sum of differences between the number of a cap and the numbers of the two caps adjacent to it and are marked on special polar coordinate scoring sheets. The profile of scores on the graph then permits diagnosis of the type and the degree of severity of the color vision defect.

Fink Near-Vision t. A visual acuity test chart calibrated for use at 14 inches and containing continuous sentences with letter sizes designating vision from 20/20 to 20/140.

Firth t. A test for visual acuity consisting of counting the lines on a series of grids, the lines being separated by a different distance in each grid.

Fischer-Schweitzer t. A test to determine the integrity of the corneal surface in which the cornea is massaged by a finger on the upper eyelid with the eyes in the straightforward position and after the instillation of fluorescein in the cul-de-sac. This is followed by the appearance on the cornea of a delicate mosaic pattern which lasts only a few seconds and appears as a honeycomb design with each polygon being about 100 to 200 microns in diameter. The pattern is difficult to demonstrate in eyes with epithelial corneal edema and is altered by trauma, band keratopathy, keratoconus, or defects of Bowman's membrane.

Fitton t. A test for strabismus in which a spot of light is fixated at 6 meters with a red filter in front of the deviating eye. Superimposition of the images indicates harmonious anomalous correspondence, normal correspondence when correcting prisms are equal to the angle of strabismus, and unharmonious anomalous correspondence when correcting prisms are not equal to the angle of strabismus. Vertical prisms are placed in front of the deviating eye when necessary to produce diplopia and their strength indicates the extent of the suppression area.

flicker fusion t. The determination of the rate of presentation of intermittent, alternate, or discontinuous photic stimuli that just gives rise to a fully uniform and continuous sensation, obliterating the flicker.

Flom-Kerr t. An afterimage test to determine the angle of anomaly in strabismus in which the center of a horizontal filament is fixated for 30 seconds at one meter by the usually fixating eye, and then after the patient is rotated 180° on a movable stool, the center of a vertical filament is fixated with the deviating eye for 20 seconds. The afterimages are then viewed on a silver screen after the patient is rotated another 90°. The screen includes a small fixation light and an inconspicuous prism diopter scale.

fluorescein t. 1. A test for the fit of contact lenses in which fluorescein is instilled between the eye and the contact lens. Under blue or ultraviolet light illumination the pattern of coloration of the fluorescein indicates the physical fit of the contact lens. 2. The instillation of fluorescein onto the surface of the eye to detect abraded, degenerated, or dying tissue by means of ocular staining.

fly t. A test for gross stereopsis consisting of a vectograph of an enlarged housefly which is viewed through Polaroid filters and appears in marked relief when stereopsis is present.

fogging t. Fogging.

forced duction t. A test for anatomical restriction of motility of an extraocular muscle, in which, under general anesthesia, an attempt is made to passively rotate the eye, by means of a muscle hook or forceps, in the field of action of its antagonist.

Foucault knife-edge t. A test to determine the optical uniformity or equivalency of different portions of a reflecting surface or of different cross-section regions of a refracting system, consisting of a pinhole light source as the object, a movable, across-the-beam, knife edge in the image plane and the pupil of the observer's eye effectively in or near the image plane. The optical variations of the mirror or system thus seen in Maxwellian view appear as variations in brightness patterns.

four color t. Pickford test.

four diopter base-out prism t. Irvine's prism displacement test, definition 1., utilizing a four diopter lens placed base-out.

four dot t. Worth's four dot test.

foveal lock t. A test of questionable validity similar in design to the Turville test but with a narrow, 21 mm wide, opaque strip instead of a wide septum, located half way between the subject and the test chart of Landolt rings at 6 m, claimed by Banks to dissociate the two eyes while they fuse the foveal images.

Fridenberg's stigmometric t. A test for visual acuity with the use of Fridenberg's chart.

FRIEND t. A test for binocular vision in which the word FRIEND, printed with letters in alternate complementary red and green colors, is viewed through complementary-colored red and green filters, one before each eye. Simultaneous seeing of all the letters indicates binocular vision. Syn., *Snellen's test*.

Frostig t. A battery of tests of visual perception for evaluating normal and neurologically handicapped children, consisting of five subgroups of tests for eye-motor coordination, figure-ground, form constancy, position in space, and spatial relations.

fundus reflex t. Retinoscopy.

Gaviola's caustic t. An adaptation of the Foucault knife-edge test to survey a parabolic mirror using a number of off-axis points to determine the radius of curvature at these points.

Giessen t. A test for anomalous retinal correspondence and the subjective angle in strabismus, in which one eye fixates a light source in the center of a Maddox cross through a red filter after a foveal afterimage has been created by stimulation of the other eye. Failure to superimpose the afterimage on the fixated light source indicates anomalous retinal correspondence, the magnitude of the separation serving as a measure of the angle of anomaly, while the separation of doubled images of the fixation target (one red and one white) serves as a measure of the subjective angle.

Goodenough-Harris Draw t. A test in which a child is asked to draw a picture of a person. At age 3 a circular form would be considered a normal response and for each extra detail 3 months is added to the intelligence score.

Goodlaw t. A test designed to indicate the limits of clear single binocular vision at 40 cm through added prism or lens power, consisting of a pair of contiguous, vertically aligned, transilluminated and oppositely polarized 3 × 3 mm squares, one containing the numeral 2 and the other the numeral 3, mounted in the center of a square 10 × 10 mm translucently illuminated field surrounded by a large, opaque black card, to be used in conjunction with oppositely polarized filters in front of the two eyes.

gradient t. A test to determine the amount of accommodative convergence associated with a 1.00 D change in accommodation at a given test distance. It is usually performed clinically by noting the change in phoria induced by adding 1.00 D convex lenses to the subjective finding, at a 40 cm test distance.

Gradle t. A test for malingering in which two Polaroid disks are placed

in front of the admittedly good eye and one in front of the other, all with polarizing axes, horizontal. If the subject continues to read when one of the pair of disks in front of the good eye is rotated 90°, malingering is indicated.

von Graefe's t. 1. A test for the determination of the type of phoria, in which fusion is made impossible by the placing of a dissociating prism in front of one eye to create diplopia. A rotary prism may be placed in front of the other eye to align the diplopic images and determine the magnitude of the phoria. 2. The past pointing test.

Gray oral reading t. A test for oral reading ability, performed binocularly and with each eye separately, utilizing five sets of cards containing reading material ranging in difficulty from primary to adult levels.

Guibor t. A test for near visual acuity performed with the Guibor chart at a fixation distance of 14 in. and in an illumination of not less than 3 footcandles.

Guy's color vision t. A screening test for color vision designed for use with children and illiterates, consisting of eight pseudoisochromatic plates each containing one or two of six letters to be identified by pointing to corresponding plastic cut-out letters.

Haidinger's brushes t. A test for eccentric fixation and/or the integrity of the macular area in which an entoptic image of a rotating brush or propeller-like pattern is generated through the polarizing properties of the retinal layers acting as an analyzer for the continuously rotating plane of polarization of incident light.

Hall's t. A test to differentiate congenital amblyopia from amblyopia ex anopsia, in which two circular red targets, 5 mm in diameter and 1½ in. apart, are viewed at a distance of about 25 in. from the eye, with the nonamblyopic eye occluded. Equal brightness of the fixated and the peripheral targets is said to indicate congenital amblyopia, and greater brightness of the peripheral target, amblyopia ex anopsia.

Halldén's t. Halldén's method.

Handy Confirmation t. An assembly of four spherical lenses, +0.50, −0.50, +0.75, and −0.75, mounted on a handle so that each lens can be held individually and conveniently in front of a tentative refractive correction lens for comparison with another of opposite power in the series, the lack of preference indicating the tentative correction to be correct.

Hardy-Rand-Rittler t. AO H-R-R test.

Harlan's t. A test for malingering in which a 6 D convex lens is placed before the admittedly good eye and a plano lens before the allegedly blind eye, in addition to the correction for ametropia. A reading card is held 6½ in. from the eyes; as the letters are read, it is slowly moved farther away, continued reading of the letters indicating vision in the allegedly blind eye.

Harman's t. Bishop Harman diaphragm test.

Harrington-Flocks t. A screening test to detect defects of the visual field, in which simple, abstract patterns of lines, dots, or crosses are presented tachistoscopically to the fixating eye, the other being occluded. The patterns are printed in fluorescent ink and are visible only when illuminated by a flash of ultraviolet radiation. A black, central, fixation spot is visible in the center of each pattern at all times.

Harris t. of lateral dominance. A group of performance and preference tests for hand, eye, and foot dominance and dexterity, designed for age six or over.

Hartmann t. A test for aberrations in a lens or an optical system, in which a diaphragm containing a series of small holes is placed in contact with the lens or the system, and photographs of a distant light source are taken from a number of positions on both sides of the paraxial focus.

head tilting t. 1. Bielschowsky's head tilting test. 2. Helmholtz' head tilting test.

Helmholtz' head tilting t. Detection and differentiation of palsies of the cyclomotor muscles utilizing Helmholtz' indicator.

Hering's afterimage t. A test to determine the state of retinal correspondence, in which first a vertical light filament is monocularly fixated at its center by one eye, and then a horizontal light filament is monocularly fixated at its center by the other eye, or vice versa. Perception of the afterimages in the form of a cross, regardless of the positions of the eyes, indicates normal retinal correspondence. Syn., *afterimage test; Bielschowsky's afterimage test.*

Hering's drop t. A test of stereoscopic vision consisting of looking through a tube or a box at a horizontal thread and determining whether little balls are dropped in front of or behind the thread.

Hertel's t. A test for color vision utilizing Hertel's plates, q.v.

Hess's t. See *Hess screen.*

Hess-Lancaster t. An ocular motility test utilizing the *Hess screen* and the projected red and green lights of the *Lancaster test.*

Hesse's t. A test for malingering, in which strong convex lenses are placed before the eyes, in addition to the correction for ametropia, while distant test letters are viewed. The convex power before the allegedly poorer eye is gradually reduced until the maximum visual acuity is determined.

Hirschberg's t. A test for approximating the objective angle of strabismus, in which the position of the reflex of a fixated light source, in line with the observer's eye, is noted on the cornea of the deviating eye. Syn., *Hirschberg's method.*

hole-in-the-card t. A test for sighting ocular dominance, in which a target is sighted through a hole in a card held in the hands, the eye used for sighting being considered dominant.

hole-in-the-hand t. A test for binocular vision, in which an object is viewed through a tube placed before one eye while a hand is held a few inches before the other eye. Seeing the object through an apparent hole in the hand indicates binocular vision, and seeing only the object or only the hand indicates its absence.

Holmgren t. A test for color vision consisting of selecting skeins of woolen yarns of various colors, shades, tints, and grays to match three standard test skeins.

homatropine t. for glaucoma. A provocative test for glaucoma in which one drop of a dilute solution of homatropine is instilled into each eye, and tonometry performed each 30 minutes for 2 hours. A rise in ocular tension of 8–11 mm Hg is considered probably pathological and a greater rise definitely pathological.

Horner's syndrome t. If a very weak, usually sub-threshold, direct acting mydriatic, such as 0.10% solution of epinephrine, produces mydriasis, whereas an indirect acting sympathomimetic, such as 1.0% hydroxyamphetamine, does not have a comparable effect, an absence of sympathetic function is indicated, as in Horner's syndrome.

Houstoun's t. A test for color vision consisting of the identification of minute spots of color on a microscope slide, or on a gray paper, which are desaturated by transmitted or reflected white light from the surrounding area by setting the microscope out of focus to various degrees.

Howard-Dolman t. A test for depth perception or stereopsis, in which the attempt is made to position a movable vertical rod, by means of a double cord pulley arrangement, to the same distance as a fixed vertical rod. The rods are housed in a rectangular box, are viewed through an aperture in the box from a 20 ft distance, are black against a white background, and the test score is usually the average error in millimeters for ten trials.

H-R-R t. AO H-R-R test.

Hughes t. Three disk test.

Humphriss immediate contrast t. Humphriss method.

Hunt-Giles t. A test to determine the distance lens correction considered best for daylight vision, consisting of the adding of convex or concave spherical lenses to the correction determined routinely, to obtain maximum acuity for black letters on a transilluminated yellow-green background.

illiterate E t. Albini's E test.

Inter-Society Color Council color aptitude t. A test of color discrimination in which individually dispensed colored chips having small saturation differences for four hues (red, yellow, green, blue) must be quickly and individually matched with one of a series of 50 fixed colored samples mounted on a panel.

Irvine's prism displacement t. 1. A test for the detection of a small angle strabismus, or for plotting the extent of a retinal inhibition or suppression area or of an absolute scotoma, in which prisms are placed momentarily before an eye. Small angle strabismus is indicated if a conjugate movement of the eyes, toward the apex of the prism, is observed when a low power prism is placed before the fixating eye, or if no eye movement is observed when the prism is placed before the deviating

eye. The extent of a suppression area in strabismus or of an absolute central scotoma with binocular alignment is measured by momentarily placing prisms of progressively increasing power, in various meridians of orientation, before the deviating or affected eye until diplopia for the fixation target is observed. 2. The area of inhibition in amblyopia ex anopsia is measured by momentarily placing prisms of progressively increasing power, in various meridians of orientation, before the fixating amblyopic eye, the other eye being occluded, until a shift in direction of the fixation target is observed. The degree to which a scotoma approaches the macular area in glaucoma is determined by momentarily placing prisms of progressively increasing power before the glaucomatous eye, the other eye being occluded, such that the image of the fixated target is momentarily shifted toward the scotomatous area, its boundary being indicated when the fixation target disappears.

Ishihara t. A test for color vision which utilizes pseudoisochromatic plates.

Ives's t. The determination of visual acuity by means of the Ives's visual acuity grating.

Jackson's t. A test for malingering, in which two cylindrical lenses, neutralizing each other, are placed before the admittedly good eye and one is rotated to blur vision while test letters are read. Continued reading of the letters indicates vision in the allegedly poor eye.

Jenning's t. A test for color perception, in which standard test skeins of green and rose are matched with green and green confusion colors and rose and rose confusion colors printed on a board. In the center of each color sample is a hole through which a stylus is thrust to register the selection of a matched color by perforating a record sheet placed beneath the board.

Jones's t. 1. Determination of the nature of hyposecretion when found to exist by Schirmer's test by repeating Schirmer's test in the dark or in dim light after anesthetizing the conjunctiva with a topical anesthetic and additionally placing a cotton-tipped applicator soaked in 5% cocaine hydrochloride for 30 seconds to the area of the conjunctiva to be in contact with the filter paper. Reflex lacrimation produced by light and irritation stimuli are thus eliminated, and basic lacrimation alone occurs which should produce 10 mm of wetting on the filter paper. 2. A test of lacrimal apparatus patency in which one drop of one per cent fluorescein is instilled into the cul-de-sac. The appearance of dye in the nose indicates normal drainage.

jugular compression t. for glaucoma. The lability test for glaucoma, with the exception of the cooling of the hand.

Kestenbaum's limbus t. A test to determine the limits of excursion of the eye in which the positions of the limbus are noted on a transparent millimeter rule as the eye is moved maximally from the straightforward position inward, outward, upward, and downward.

Kestenbaum's outline t. A modification of the confrontation test in which the test object is kept in a plane not more than 2 or 3 cm from the patient's face so that the outline of a normal visual field will be limited by the facial features.

knife-edge t. Foucault test.

Koster's cocaine t. A test used in congenital ptosis to aid in determining the presence or absence of the levator palpebrae superioris muscle. Complete or almost complete failure of the upper eyelid to elevate upon the administration of cocaine indicates absence of the muscle. Normally cocaine increases contraction of the superior palpebral muscle of Mueller which assists the levator, when present, causing elevation of the upper eyelid.

Krimsky's t. Krimsky's method.

Kronfeld's t. A diagnostic test for glaucoma consisting of paracentesis of the anterior chamber, a rise in ocular tension to 40 mm Hg, or more, being positive. Syn., *anterior chamber puncture test.*

lability t. for glaucoma. A provocative test for glaucoma, in which a pressure of 40 to 60 mm Hg is applied to the neck with a blood pressure cuff for one minute while one hand is placed in ice water. A rise in ocular tension of more than 8 mm Hg, or an increase to over 30 mm Hg, indicates glaucoma. Syn., *pressor-congestion test for glaucoma.*

Lancaster t. A test for the state of motility of the extraocular muscles in strabismus, in which the patient per-ceptually superimposes two complementary-colored slits of light, one red and one green, projected onto a screen in a darkened room while wearing red and green filters. One projected slit, the fixation target, is controlled by the examiner and is moved to various directions of gaze and the other slit is controlled by the patient. The test is conducted with first one eye fixating and then the other, for each position, and the physical separation of the slits is noted in each instance.

Landolt's broken ring t. A test for visual acuity consisting of locating the gaps in a graduated series of incomplete rings with radial thickness and gaps equal to one-fifth of their outer diameters. Syn., *Landolt C test.*

Landolt's cobalt blue t. Cobalt blue glass test.

Landolt's projection t. A test for the detection and measurement of false projection with Landolt's projectionometer.

lantern t. Any of several tests for color perception, in which transilluminated, colored glass filters are identified or matched with standard samples, e.g., the Edridge-Green test.

Lazich's t. A test for measuring eccentric fixation, employing two exposed ophthalmoscope bulbs at a distance of one meter, one of which is fixated by the amblyopic eye while the position of the other bulb is adjusted until its corneal reflection in the same eye is so located with respect to the center of the pupil as to correspond symmetrically with the relative position the reflection would have when fixated by the occluded, nonamblyopic eye.

leaf room t. A test utilizing the leaf room, q.v., for demonstrating, detecting, and measuring spatial distortions resulting from aniseikonia.

Leavell t's. A series of tests designed to determine motor-visual directional preferences and their relation to the functioning of the dominant eye, hand, and foot.

li t. A measure of the ratio of the cumulative duration of periods of visibility to that of invisibility of the printed lower-case letters li viewed at a maximum distance of resolvability during a several minute test period and under a given set of test conditions to investigate the effect of such variables as illumination, prior visual tasks, general fatigue, eccentric fixation, etc.

light patch t. A test to estimate the magnification required to aid subnormal vision, in which a circular patch of light is projected onto a graduated scale placed one meter from the patient and gradually reduced in size until it no longer appears circular. The size of the spot at this point indicates the size of the lesion, and reference to a special chart indicates the magnification needed.

Lighthouse Flash-Card Vision for Children t. A set of 24 test charts each having a black acuity test character consisting of the profile of a house, an apple, or an umbrella in equivalent Snellen fraction sizes ranging from 6/3 to 6/60.

Lighthouse near acuity t. A test for near visual acuity consisting of nine rows containing three familiar, quickly learned symbols at each acuity level. The figures are an apple, a tree, and a house calibrated for 40 cm and noted in Snellen equivalent (20/400 to 20/50) and meter size (8m to 0.5m).

Linnér's t. A diagnostic test for glaucoma in which the ratio of the coefficient of the facility of aqueous outflow as influenced by pilocarpine, which decreases outflow resistance, to that as influenced by acetazolamide, which increases outflow resistance, is tonographically determined and then compared to the ratio found for a healthy eye.

Livingston binocular gauge t. A test to determine the near point of either convergence or accommodation with the use of Livingston's binocular gauge.

Livingston's phoria t. A test to determine the type and the magnitude of phoria, in which two pairs of complementary-colored red and green slits in an internally illuminated box, one pair oriented vertically and the other horizontally, are viewed through complementary-colored red and green filters. A scale is provided for each pair of slits by which the perceptual displacement is determined.

Lüscher color t. A test said to reveal personality traits of a subject according to his serial ranking of eight colored cards in terms of "liking" or "feeling most sympathy for" their colors.

luster t. 1. A test for sensory fusion, in which a bright light source is placed against the closed eyelid of one eye while the other fixates a black dot on a uniform gray ground. Perception of a red glow over, or mixed with, the gray field indicates binocular vision; perception of either the red glow or the gray field alone indicates suppression. 2. A test for sensory fusion, in which two different surface colors, usually one chromatic and the other achromatic, are viewed in a stereoscope, one color to each eye. Perception of one color as though seen through, or mixed with, the other color indicates binocular vision.

Maddox groove t. 1. A test for measuring a phoria or a heterotropia, in which a Maddox groove is placed in front of one eye while a small light source is fixated. The groove distorts the image of the light source into a streak perpendicular to the axis of the groove, preventing fusion, and its position relative to the fixated source is determined on a tangent scale or estimated with prisms correcting the displacement. 2. A test for cyclophoria, in which a Maddox groove is placed before each eye, each axis oriented in the same meridian, while viewing a spot light source through displacing prisms. Parallelism of the resultant streaks indicates absence of cyclophoria.

Maddox prism t. A test for measuring a phoria or a heterotropia, in which the diplopic images of one eye, created with a Maddox prism, are compared with the position of the single image of the other eye.

Maddox projection t. A test for false projection, in which a black vertical line, about 1 in. long, on a large white card, is monocularly fixated at a 6 in. distance and is located by pointing on the back of the card to its apparent position. An identically located line is on the back of the card, and failure to point to it indicates false projection.

Maddox rod t. The Maddox groove test, except that a Maddox rod is used instead of a groove.

Maddox tangent scale t. 1. A test for the measurement of a phoria or a heterotropia, in which the central light source of a Maddox cross is fixated through a red filter or a Maddox rod before one eye to produce diplopia. 2. A test for determining the objective angle of strabismus, in which the fixating eye moves along the arm of a Maddox cross until the reflex of the central light source appears centered on the cornea of the deviating eye.

Maddox V t. A test, utilizing the Maddox V chart, for determining the axis of astigmatism.

Maddox wing t. A test, utilizing the Maddox wing, to measure a phoria at near.

Magder's t. Bailliart's test.

Mallett Fixation Disparity t. See under *unit*.

manoptoscope t. A test for sighting ocular dominance, in which the subject holds the base of a manoptoscope (a hollow truncated cone) against his face, covering both eyes, and views a distant object through the small end of the cone. Only one eye can fixate under this condition, and that eye is considered to be the dominant. Syn., *Parson's test*.

Mark diplopia t. A test for ocular motility consisting of a series of nine stereograms, each having an arrow with a dot above it in one half and an arrow with a dot below it in the other half. Each pair of arrows is positioned so as to provide a stimulus for fixation in a different direction of gaze, with fusion of the arrows, with a dot above and below, indicating normal motility.

Marlow's t. The occlusion of one eye for several days or more to reveal latent heterophoria (especially hyperphoria) or to determine if symptoms are related to binocular vision. Syn., *prolonged occlusion test*.

Massachusetts Vision t. A portable battery of screening tests for visual performance of school children which includes determination of visual acuity, visual acuity through a convex lens, vertical phoria at far, and lateral phorias at both near and far.

massage t. for glaucoma. A provocative test for glaucoma, in which the eyeball is deeply massaged for 1 minute, the normal eye losing one third to one half its tension and regaining it in 60 to 70 minutes, the glaucomatous eye manifesting only a slight reduction in tension, returning to the original tension rapidly, in about 30 minutes, and then rising above this level with a return to normal in about 90 minutes.

Mauthner's t. A test for color perception consisting of the identification of colored powders in vials.

Max Pfister color pyramid t. A psychological diagnostic test for personality traits in which the subject selects and arranges 24 differently colored, 2.5-cm-square paper patches into a triangular array of 15 squares, 5 at the base, and 4, 3, 2, and 1 in each succeeding layer until the pattern has been structured to the subject's greatest satisfaction.

Maxwell disk t. A test for color vision, in which a Maxwell disk containing a colored sector on a white ground is rotated at slowly increasing speeds until the color flicker disappears. The slower the speed at which the color disappears, the greater the sensitivity for color.

Meissner's t. A test for torsion of the eyes when fixating a near object, in which a taut vertical thread is placed slightly closer to, or farther from, the eyes than the point of fixation, so as to effect physiological diplopia. The thread is tilted toward or away from the eyes until the diplopic images appear parallel, indicating the type and the amount of torsion.

Meyrowitz' t. A test for color vision employing pseudoisochromatic plates.

Miles t. A test for anisodominance, q.v.

Miles A-B-C t. A test for determining the sighting dominant eye, utilizing the V-Scope and a set of cards, each of which has printed on it two round spots which differ from each other in size and shade. The subject is instructed to look through the V-Scope as each target is presented and to report which of the two spots is larger and which is darker, the examiner noting which eye is sighting. A-B-C stands for *area, brightness, comparison*.

Mills's t. A test for motor ocular dominance, in which a target is moved along the median line toward the eyes until the near point of binocular fixation is passed, the eye maintaining fixation being considered dominant.

mirror t. 1. A test for sighting ocular dominance, in which the subject sights his nose within a small circle on a mirror, the eye seeing the nose being the dominant. 2. Hirschberg's test when performed with a retinoscope mirror as the effective light source.

mirror-screen t. Travers' test.

Mitchell's stability t. A test for the ability to maintain binocular fixation on a near point target while the lateral overlapping binocular visual fields are being gradually reduced by a septum moved slowly away from the eyes along a rod in the midplane toward the target.

Mizukawa-Kamada t. A test to measure lacrimal secretion. One end of a scaled strip of filter paper is placed at the inferior lacrimal punctum and the point of absorption is noted at one minute and at five minutes.

Money Road Map t. Named after the originator, John Money, and used to evaluate the visual perceptual ability of directionality, consisting of a simulated map of a city's streets in which the examinee must visually follow a dotted line and respond to whether the line turns to the right or to the left at various street corners on the map.

Monroe Visual Three t. A visual memory test consisting of a series of 16 elementary form figures which the subject is asked to reproduce on paper following 10 seconds exposure of 4 at a time.

Morgan's infinity balance t. A modification of Turville's infinity balance test utilizing a directly viewed acuity chart and an opaque vertical strip placed midway between the chart and the viewer.

mydriasis t. for glaucoma. A provocative test for glaucoma, in which a mydriatic is instilled into the eye and ocular tension is measured at regular intervals. See also *homatropine test for glaucoma*.

Nagel's t. 1. A test for color vision, in which one half of the bipartite field in an anomaloscope is illuminated with a standard yellow, and the other half is matched with the yellow by mixing red and green. Anomalous color vision is indicated by an atypical combination of red and green. 2. A test for color vision utilizing pseudoisochromatic plates.

Nela wools t. A color perception test employing a series of finely graded colored wool skeins to be arranged in triplets with a test skein between each comparison pair, the test score being given in terms of the number of correct distinctions made.

neutral density filter t. Dark filter test.

Newton ring t. A test for the accuracy of curvature of a lens surface in which the pattern of Newton's rings, formed by placing the surface in contact with another surface of known opposite curvature, is observed.

nicotine t. for glaucoma. A test for determining the effectiveness of medical treatment for glaucoma, in which 0.5 ml of one percent nicotinic acid solution is injected intravenously and tonometry readings are taken at 15, 30, 60, 120, and 180 minute intervals. Readings within normal range and not exceeding preinjection measurement indicate success of medical treatment. Readings above preinjection measurement indicate the need for surgical treatment.

Nucholls' t. A screening test for the measurement of the limits of perception of movement in the lateral peripheral field of vision.

O'Brien t. A series of seven stereograms to be viewed in a stereoscope to detect a central scotoma, and hemianopic and quadrantanopic field defects.

Oliver's t. Any of several early techniques, described by Oliver, for testing the color sense, including a wool skein color matching test, a colored pellet matching test, and a color wheel technique for mixing the colors in various proportions.

Oppenheim's t. A test for relative hemianopsia, in which test objects are presented simultaneously on either side of a fixated point and then alternately. Perceiving the objects when presented alternately but not when presented simultaneously indicates relative hemianopsia.

optokinetic nystagmus t. 1. A test for simulated or hysterical blindness, in which the patient is asked whether the stripes on the revolving drum of an optokinetoscope are motionless or moving, the manifestation of optokinetic nystagmus being evidence of vision. 2. An objective test for visual acuity, in which the threshold for optokinetic nystagmus is determined, as with an optokinetoscope.

Osterberg bichromatic balance t. A test for determining the spherical and binocularly balanced components of the refractive correction, designed for use with the Rodenstock Rodavist projector, in which polarized targets of figures on red and green backgrounds are viewed through Polaroid filters such that each eye is independently exposed to targets having both red and green backgrounds. Spherical lens power is adjusted before each eye until all of the figures appear equally clear or distinct on both colored backgrounds.

Osterberg coincidence t. A test for measuring heterophoria, designed for use with the Rodenstock

Rodavist projector, in which polarized targets of a divided square are viewed through Polaroid filters such that each eye sees one-half of the square. The phoria is determined by the prism power required to align the two halves into a perfect square.

outlying screen deviation t. A test for determining the limits of the field of binocular fixation, in which the subject, with his head held in the straightforward position, fixates a target moved in various directions of gaze until binocular fixation is lost, as revealed by the cover test.

parallax t. 1. A subjective cover test. 2. Determination of the location of an opacity in the eye by the parallactic movement of the opacity in relation to the pupil and the lateral motion of the observer.

Parson's t. Manoptoscope test.

Pascal-Raubitschek t. A test identical to the Raubitschek test except that, in determining the power of the cylinder, the target is usually rotated 35° away from the position at which the lines in the tip of the arrowhead are equal and clearest, and concave cylinder power is then placed before the eye with its axis 20° away from the axis of the ocular astigmatism, toward the meridian of the arrow tip, and increased or decreased until the target lines again appear equally clear at the tip of the arrowhead, the cylinder thus required being the amount necessary to correct the astigmatism. Pascal preferred to rotate the target 40° and the lens 10° for high cylinders, and the target 30° and the lens 30° for low cylinders, the two values of each pair being such that twice the first plus the second equals 90°.

past pointing t. A test for anomalous fixation or for paresis or paralysis of an extraocular muscle, in which an object is fixated by the suspected eye, the other eye being occluded, in various directions of gaze and then localized by pointing to it. Failure to point accurately to the object indicates anomalous fixation, paresis, or paralysis. Syn., *von Graefe's touch test.*

Peckham's blindspot t. A test for eccentric fixation in which the blind spot of Mariotte is plotted for both the normal and amblyopic eyes, an unequal displacement of the blind spots from the fixation target being an indi-

cation of eccentric fixation. Syn., *Peckham's method.*

peephole t. for ocular dominance. A test for sighting ocular dominance, in which the patient, without using his hands, sights through a small peephole, such as that of a monocular optical instrument, the eye used being considered dominant.

perilimbal suction cup t. for glaucoma. A test used for evaluating aqueous flow and outflow resistance in the diagnosis of glaucoma, in which the aqueous outflow channels are closed for 15 minutes by a perilimbal suction cup applied under a pressure of 50 mm Hg. Tonometry is performed before suction, at its termination, and 15 minutes after termination. The rise of pressure during suction is an indication of the rate of aqueous secretion, and the fall of pressure during the 15 minutes after suction is removed is an indication of outflow resistance. Normally, pressure returns to its original level 15 minutes after termination of suction.

Perlia's t. A test for binocular depth perception in which an attempt is made to touch with a small, round, white object a similar object held by the examiner in various positions of binocular gaze. The test is performed without head movement, with white-headed pins at near, or with white balls on three foot sticks at intermediate distances.

Pettit's macula function t. A test used prior to cataract extraction to assist in the determination of macular function. It is performed with an instrument similar to a flashlight, having a central red fixation point of light and 4 surrounding white points of light so separated from the fixation point as to subtend either a one degree or a two degree angle when held 13 inches from the eye. If the 5 points of light cannot be individually resolved, the 4 white targets are shuttered and an accessory light source is used in conjunction with the red fixation target to determine the minimum separation for which the two lights may be distinguished.

phoria t., habitual. Clinical measurement of a phoria through the prescription worn prior to the examination. Cf. *induced phoria test.*

phoria t., induced. Clinical measurement of a phoria through the subjective finding. Cf. *habitual phoria test.*

photostress t. Bailliart's dazzling test.

physiological diplopia t. for ocular dominance. A test for ocular dominance in which a target is placed between the patient and a distant fixated target to produce crossed physiological diplopia for the nonfixated target, the diplopic image seen more distinctly indicating the dominant eye.

Pickford t. A test to detect red-green and yellow-blue color vision deficiencies, utilizing a specially designed anomaloscope employing colored filters to produce a variable colored stimulus which is to be compared or matched to a standard stimulus. Syn., *four color test.*

Pierce's t. A test for color perception, in which a series of colored disks of finely graded saturation difference are to be placed in the order of their saturation, the result being recorded as the number of misplacements.

pinhole t. The determination of the visual acuity through a pinhole aperture, by means of which the effect of dioptric errors is minimized.

plano-prism t. for malingering. A test for malingering, in which a lens, 6Δ base-down in its upper half and plano in its lower half, is placed before the admittedly good eye, the other eye being occluded, while a small spot of light is fixated, such that monocular diplopia results. The allegedly blind eye is then uncovered and, if vision is present, its image will fuse with the lower image of the good eye. The plano-prism lens is lowered, eliminating the lower image of the good eye, and the continuation of diplopia indicates malingering.

pointing t. for ocular dominance. A test for sighting ocular dominance, in which the patient points with the finger, or sights along an object such as a gun, at a designated target, the eye used for pointing or sighting being considered the dominant.

Pola t. An instrument used in refraction and for investigating binocular functions which presents a series of vectograms to be viewed through Polaroid filters for testing heterophoria, fixation disparity, aniseikonia, stereopsis, and visual acuity.

Pola-Mirror t. A test devised by Griffin in which a person with suppression of an eye will see that eye as blacked-out while looking at himself in a mirror through a pair of crossed polarizing viewers. Cf. *vis-à-vis test.*

Polaroid t. for malingering. A test for malingering, in which a rotatable polarized disk is viewed through Polaroid filters, such that vision may be blocked from either eye by rotating the disk.

Posner t. A test for the axis of the cylinder for correcting astigmatism based on the premise that a tilt of the eyes lags behind head tilt in which, with the correcting lens mounted in front of the eye, the head, and with it the lens, is tilted 30° toward each side while viewing a test chart; the correct axis is indicated when the chart is equally clear upon tilting toward either right or left side.

Pray's t. A test, utilizing Pray's astigmatic chart, for estimating the axis of astigmatism.

pressor-congestion t. for glaucoma. Lability test for glaucoma.

Priestley Smith tape t. A test, utilizing Priestley Smith's tape, for determining the objective angle of strabismus.

Prince's rule t. A test for determining the near point and the amplitude of accommodation, in which a Prince's rule is held against the lower orbital margin and a test chart is moved along the tape, toward the eye, until a blur is noticed.

Priscol t. for glaucoma. A provocative test for glaucoma, in which 1 ml of Priscol is injected under the conjunctiva and tonometry is performed each 15 minutes for 1½ hrs. A rise in ocular tension of 11–13 mm Hg is probably pathological, and a greater rise is considered definitely pathological.

prism adaptation t. The wearing of base-out prism slightly greater than the strabismic angle prior to extraocular muscle surgery for esotropia for an hour or more; a significant increase in angle of strabismus is considered indicative of unfavorable prognosis of surgical correction and no increase or a decrease is considered favorable.

prism t. for malingering. A test for malingering, in which a vertical prism is placed before the admittedly good eye, with its base bisecting the pupil, to produce monocular diplopia. If vision is present in the allegedly blind eye, its image will fuse with one of the images of the other eye. While the target is being viewed, the prism is moved until it is completely over the good eye, and the continuation of diplopia indicates malingering.

prism reflex t. Krimsky's method.

prolonged occlusion t. Marlow's test.

prone provocative t., for glaucoma. Measurement of the ocular tension before and after a half hour or more in the prone position, a rise of 8 to 10 mm Hg with angle closure indicating glaucoma. Cf. *decubitus test for glaucoma.*

provocative t. for glaucoma. Any diagnostic test for glaucoma which attempts to cause an abnormal elevation of ocular tension, hence, to detect a disturbance in the regulatory mechanism of intraocular pressure.

pseudoisochromatic t. Any test for color vision utilizing pseudoisochromatic plates.

pupillary reaction t. for color blindness. An objective test in which color blindness is indicated, for a portion of the visible spectrum, by an insufficient pupillary constriction on stimulation of the retina with that wavelength.

push-up t. 1. A test for determining the near point of convergence, in which a test target is moved toward the eyes in the midsagittal plane until binocular fixation is lost. 2. A test for determining the near point of accommodation, in which a test target is moved toward the eyes until a beginning blur is noted.

Rabkin t. A test for color vision utilizing Rabkin polychromatic plates, q.v.

railway signal t. A test for color vision, in which standard red and green signal colors are displayed through various sized diaphragms, to simulate various viewing distances, and through five neutral filters of different densities, to simulate varying conditions of visibility from clear atmosphere to heavy fog.

random-dot stereogram t. of Julesz. See *stereogram, random-dot, Julesz.*

Randot t. A test based on the principle of the Julesz stereograms, using a series of vectographs in a folder similar to the Titmus Stereo Tests, having on the right side, 6 random dot stereograms of various shapes which indicate 600 seconds of arc at 40 cm and, on the upper left side, 8 diamond-shaped targets similar to those in the Wirt test and indicating 400 to 20 seconds of arc of stereoacuity. The lower left side has 3 lines of similar stimuli ranging from 400 to 100 seconds of arc levels.

Raubitschek t. A test for determining the axis and the amount of astigmatism with a rotatable target of two parabolic lines in an arrowhead pattern, parallel at one end and each diverging from the other through 90°, used as follows: While the target is viewed through fogging lenses, it is rotated until the lines are equal and clearest at the tip of the arrowhead, 90° from this position being the axis of the concave correcting cylinder; an arbitrarily selected cylinder power, e.g., −1.00 D, is placed before the eye at a specific off-axis amount, e.g., 30°, which will make the target appear to be off axis; the target is rotated until the lines again appear equal and clearest at the arrowhead tip, the amount of this rotation being referred to a prepared table to obtain the cylinder power.

Rayleigh's t. A test for color vision, in which a spectral red and green are mixed to match a spectral yellow. Anomalous color vision is indicated by an atypical combination of red and green.

RDE (Random-Dot E) t. A test utilizing Julesz random-dot stereograms which contain a tumbling E pattern observable only through the stereoscopic sense.

reading t. for glaucoma. A provocative test for glaucoma, in which fine print is read for 45 min., a rise of ocular tension of 10–15 mm Hg being considered positive. Syn., *accommodation test for glaucoma.*

reclining t., for glaucoma. A provocative test in which the subject reclines with head lower than feet for one hour with a rise of intraocular tension of 6 mm Hg being considered positive.

red disk t. 1. A test for determining suppression or diplopia by which a bright light at near is fixated while a red lens is before one eye. Perception of one white light indicates suppression and of one white and one red indicates diplopia. 2. The identification of a paretic muscle by measuring the distances between the diplopic images produced by a red disk, in various positions of gaze, the distance increasing in the field of the paretic muscle.

red-green t. 1. A test for determining the spherical component of the refractive correction for an eye, in which spherical lenses are placed before the eye until black test targets, one-half on a green background and one-half on a red background, appear equally black or clear. 2. Lancaster test.

Reed-Van Osdal t. A test for sighting ocular dominance, in which an opaque card, with a round hole in its center, is held with both hands and raised to sight a specified distant object through the hole, the eye used for sighting being considered the dominant.

retinal rivalry t. for ocular dominance. A test for ocular dominance, in which retinal rivalry-inducing patterns are viewed, the dominant eye being that whose image predominates in the fluctuations.

Ring Fusion t. A test for binocular vision, in which a projected target of three dots, two red and one green, surrounded by a vertically broken white ring, is viewed through complementary-colored red and green filters, such that one eye sees the two red dots and the white ring and the other eye sees the green dot and the white ring. The perception of the pattern of the original formation indicates normal binocular vision; the three dots and the circle sections, but not in a circular pattern, binocular vision without fusion; and two red dots and a circle section only, or one green dot and a circle section only, suppression of one eye.

ring t. for ocular dominance. A test for sighting ocular dominance, in which a target is sighted through a ring held in the hands, the eye used for sighting being considered the dominant.

Robinson Cohen t. A test for determining the axis and the amount of astigmatism, in which, with a fogging lens before the eye, the crossed lines on a Robinson Cohen slide are rotated to the position at which the blacker line appears blackest, this position being a principal meridian. An alternate method is to rotate the crossed lines until they appear equally black, the principal meridians being located midway between them (45° away). The amount of astigmatism is determined by equalizing the blackness of the crossed lines, when they are located in the principal meridians, with cylindrical lenses.

Ronchi t. A test similar to the Foucault knife-edge test but using, instead of the knife-edge, a transmission grating of a few lines per mm near the focus of the mirror or refractive system, which is illuminated by a point source at infinity so that the eye, observing the mirror or system in Maxwellian view, sees a series of overlapping images of the source with interference fringes, which are deformed according to the spherical aberration present.

Rosenbach t. A test for sighting ocular dominance, in which the patient, with both eyes open, lines up a pencil or a small stick, held at arm's length, with a mark on a distant wall. The eye with which the pencil is aligned is considered to be the dominant. Syn., *alignment test.*

Rosner Visual Analysis Skills T. Trade name for a visual-motor test designed to evaluate perceptual, form-copying ability consisting of a series of line drawings to be replicated on a dotted grid printed on an otherwise blank page. Abbreviation *Rosner TVAS.*

rotatable E t. Albini's E test.

scalar t., of light. The approximate optical description of a field of light in terms of a single complex scalar wave function rather than by specification of the magnitude of the electromagnetic field vectors and polarization as functions of position and time.

Scheerer's entoptoscope t. The entoptoscopic examination of the blood corpuscles in the perifoveal capillaries to assess the integrity of retinal circulation.

Scheiner's t. A test for determining the monocular near point of accommodation, in which a small target, observed through two laterally separated pinholes placed before the eye, is moved toward the eye until it appears double, the nearest point at which the target can be seen single being the near point.

Schilder's t. Extension test.

Schirmer's t. 1. A test to measure lacrimal secretion, in which one end of a 5 × 25 mm strip of filter paper is placed in the inner angle of the lower cul-de-sac, over the inferior lacrimal punctum, the moistening of 2 to 3 mm of the paper per minute being considered normal. 2. A test to determine the cause of reflex hypolacrimation. Either an onion or ammonia is smelled (or a cotton-tipped applicator containing one of these substances is moved about in the middle turbinate) while a strip of filter paper is inserted into the lower fornix, as in Schirmer's test. Moistening of the paper within two minutes indicates a "fatigue block" for conjunctival stimuli but not from nasal sensory nerves. No moistening indicates complete failure of the secretory mechanism.

Schmidt-Rimpler t. A test for malingering, in which the patient is instructed to look at his hand; the blind will look directly at it, the simulator will usually look in a different direction.

Schneller t. The balancing of the perceived sharpness of the two perpendicular arms of a T chart or clock dial with spherical lenses while viewing the chart through one's astigmatic correction and a crossed cylinder lens.

Schwarting three-point t. A three-step test to determine the paretic muscle in strabismus. The first step is to determine which eye shows hypertropia; second, whether the deviation is greater on elevation or depression; third, whether looking to the right or to the left produces a greater deviation. Findings are referred to a table, as follows:

1. Hypertropia

Right Eye	or	*Left Eye*
RIR		LIR
RSO		LSO
LSR		RSR
LIO		RIO

2. Greater deviation

Eyes Up	or	*Eyes Down*
RSR		LIR
RIO		LSO
LSR		RIR
LIO		RSO

3. Greater deviation

Eyes Right	or	*Eyes Left*
RSR		LSR
RIR		LIR
LIO		RIO
LSO		RSO

Cf. *Parks-Hardesty three-step method.*

screen t. A subjective or an objective cover test.

screen comitance t. A diagnostic test for paralysis of the extraocular muscles, in which the primary and the secondary deviations are objectively measured in each of the six cardinal directions of gaze by means of prisms and a cover test. An occluder is placed before one eye, with a prism behind it, while the other eye fixates, and then is moved to occlude the previously fixating eye. Prism power is varied until the uncovered eye makes no fixation movement. The test is then repeated with the other eye fixating.

screen and parallax t. The subjective cover test.

Seidel's t. Dark room test for glaucoma.

shadow t. Retinoscopy.

Shtremel's t. A test for malingering, in which the patient slowly moves his head from one side to the other. In the blind, the eyes move with the head; hence their remaining relatively stationary indicates the presence of vision.

Simultan t. See *Simultantest.*

simultaneous prism cover t. A test to determine the angular extent by which the deviating eye in strabismus misses fixation, in which a prism equal in power to the estimated deviation is placed in front of the deviating eye with simultaneous occlusion of the fixating eye. The prism power which neutralizes the movement of the deviating eye upon occlusion of the fixating eye is a measure of the deviation.

Sjögren's hand t. A visual acuity test comprised of seven square cards, each showing a different size black handprint with extended fingers on a white background, representing visual acuities ranging from 20/15 to 20/200 at 20 feet. They may be held with the fingers pointing in any direction, the subject being required to identify their orientation.

Sloan's achromatopsia t. A test to investigate differences in color vision deficiencies in achromatopsia, in which six Munsell colors of high chroma are to be matched to one of a series of 15 grays. Cone and rod monochromats can be distinguished in that their matches agree, respectively, with those computed from photopic and scotopic luminosity functions.

Sloan's color threshold t. A

color-naming test in which eight lights simulating aviation signal colors are to be identified when shown at eight intensities ranging from a low value near the chromatic threshold to a maximum 128 times as bright.

Snellen's t. 1. A test for visual acuity utilizing Snellen's test chart. 2. FRIEND test.

Southern California Figure-Ground t. A perceptual test for evaluating visual figure-ground discrimination, consisting of a series of plates each having six line drawings paired with matching plates having a composite of three figures, the criterion being to pick which three, out of the six figures, are included in the composite drawing.

Spache binocular reading t. A test to determine the relative participation of each eye in binocular reading, utilizing stereograms containing reading material printed such that some words are seen by both eyes and some by only one eye when viewed in a stereoscope.

Spraing's t. A multiple choice matching test to determine the effect of the motor component in a perceptual-motor task consisting of a series of cards, each having 12 choices, one of which matches the Bender-Gestalt test card being evaluated.

Star t. A visual acuity test consisting of a series of Landolt rings arranged in vertical, horizontal, and oblique rows, in a star formation, to detect differences in acuity thresholds as related to the meridional location of the test targets, as may occur in amblyopia ex anopsia.

Stevens' t. A test for measuring a phoria, in which fusion, for a fixated spot source of light, is disrupted by distorting one image with a pinhole disk and a + 20.00 D sphere placed before one eye.

Stilling t. A test for color perception utilizing pseudoisochromatic plates.

STYCAR t's. A series of visual acuity "Screening Tests for Young Children and Retardates," employing selected script letters, capital letters, or small toys which are presented either at 10 feet or at 20 feet and identified by naming, tracing in the air, or matching with key cards or toys close at hand.

Suda ocular compression t. A provocative test for glaucoma, in which 50 gm pressure is applied to the eye for 10 minutes. A postcompression tension of over 8 mm Hg indicates glaucoma.

swinging flashlight t. Repetitive alternate illumination of the two pupils with a flashlight while the patient fixates a distant object, at a frequency which elicits pupillary contraction when a healthy eye is illuminated and dilation while an afflicted eye is illuminated, a diagnostic response of dynamic anisocoria.

von Szily t. A test for malingering in alleged uniocular blindness in which the visual field is plotted with both eyes open; seeing of the target on the blind spot of one eye indicates that vision is present in the other.

Thibaudet's t. A test for malingering, in which the patient fixates a test chart so constructed that the separations between the component parts of the larger figures subtend smaller visual angles than the separations of the component parts of the smaller figures. Recognition of the details of the larger figures, and not of the smaller, indicates malingering.

Thiel's t. for glaucoma. A provocative test for glaucoma, in which 2.0 gm of potassium fluorescein is administered orally, the appearance of the dye in the anterior chamber shortly thereafter indicating glaucoma.

Thorington t. A test for the measurement of a near point phoria, in which a calibrated chart, with a light source placed behind an opening corresponding to the zero on the scale, is fixated with a Maddox rod placed in front of one eye. The number through which the streak appears to pass indicates the type and the amount of phoria.

three disk t. A test to differentiate between true and false macular sparing in visual field loss, in which three white disks, each about 10° in diameter and arranged one above the other, are moved from the blind to the seeing portion of the visual field. False macular sparing is indicated by seeing the disks simultaneously and by a shift of the blind spot of Mariotte toward the blind side. True macular sparing is indicated by seeing the central disk before the other two and with no shift of the blind spot of Mariotte. Syn., *Hughes test.*

three needle t. A near point test for stereopsis, in which two fixed vertical rods in the same plane, with a movable one in between, are viewed through slits or small apertures, the observer judging whether the center rod is placed nearer or farther than the others.

tilting plane t. A test for the measurement of aniseikonia, in which a universally rotatable plane surface target is viewed, usually through an aperture, and manually adjusted until it appears to lie in a plane perpendicular to the direction of gaze. A scale attached to the apparatus indicates the error in degrees.

Titmus stereo t. A set of vectographic stereograms which includes a fly test and modifications of the Wirt test for measuring stereopsis.

TNO t. for stereoscopic vision. Random dot stereograms prepared as anaglyphs that evoke a depth perception of otherwise hidden figures when stereoscopic vision is present. The test consists of 3 screening plates with a disparity of 33 minutes of arc and a series of quantitative plates allowing six different depth levels ranging in disparity from 15 to 480 seconds of arc.

Tokyo Medical College t. A test for color vision consisting of 13 pseudoisochromatic plates divided into four groups. Group I consists of five plates designed to detect deficient redgreen color perception of either deutan or protan types, group II of two plates to detect tritan deficiency, group III of three plates to distinguish between deutans and protans, and group IV of three plates to distinguish between three different degrees of red-green color perception deficiency in those who fail group I.

TOPPER t. A test for stereopsis and fusion by means of a vectogram of which the two photographic images of a shield-and-spear-carrying character named TOPPER are printed on separate sheets of oppositely polarized gelatin film to permit variation of the vergence stimulus independent of the stereopsis-inducing disparity.

touch t. of von Graefe. Past pointing test.

transferimage t. Brock-Givner test.

Travers' t. A test for the determination and the measurement of suppression areas, in which one eye directly fixates a target on a tangent screen, the other eye fixates a light source on another screen placed to the side and perpendicular to the first, perceptually superimposed on the directly fixated screen by means of reflection from a mirror. The field of the directly fixated screen is explored by a test target for any disappearance of the target or the light source. Syn., *mirrorscreen test.*

Tschermak's afterimage t. Hering's afterimage test.

Tschermak's congruence t. A test for measuring the subjective angle of strabismus, consisting of the binocular viewing of a small, illuminated, white cross with a vertical red line above the vertical limb, monocularly shielded so as to be seen by one eye, and a vertical green line below the vertical limb, monocularly shielded so as to be seen by the other eye. The localization of the red and green lines in relation to the cross indicates the subjective angle.

tumbling E t. Albini's E test.

Turville's infinity balance t. A test for equalizing the visual acuity of the two eyes in which an opaque vertical strip or septum is placed in the center of a mirror so as to allow each eye to

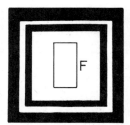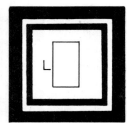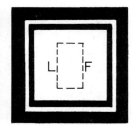

Fig. 37 Turville's infinity balance test. *Left*, view of right eye; *center*, view of left eye; *right*, view with binocular vision. (From H. W. Gibson, *Textbook of Orthoptics.* Kent, England: Hatton Press, 1955)

see only one lateral half of the image of a reflected test chart. The test may also be used for measuring vertical fixation disparity if the two halves do not appear on the same level. (See Fig. 37.) Abbreviated *TIB*. Cf. *Morgan's infinity balance test*.

t. type. See under *type*.

V t. Maddox V test.

Vasculat t. for glaucoma. A provocative test for glaucoma, in which 1 ml of Vasculat is injected under the conjunctiva and tonometry is performed after 60, 90, and 120 min. A rise in ocular tension of 11–14 mm Hg is probably pathological, and a greater rise is considered definitely pathological.

Velhagen's t. A test for color vision utilizing Velhagen's plates, q.v.

Verhoeff's t. A test for stereopsis utilizing Verhoeff's stereopter.

vis-à-vis t. A test devised by Griffin in which two cross-polarizing filters are used for detection of suppression. For example, with suppression of the right eye of the examinee the left eye of the examiner will appear blacked out. (See Fig. 38.) Cf. *Pola-mirror test*.

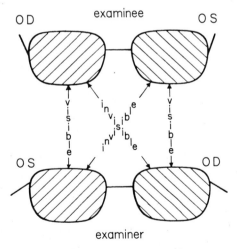

Fig. 38 Illustration of the effect of polarization of light in the vis-à-vis test for suppression.

walking t. A test for anomalous spatial localization in strabismus, in which, with the normal eye occluded, the subject is asked to walk straight toward a distant object and the path taken is observed.

water drinking t. for glaucoma. A provocative test for glaucoma, in which the patient, after fasting, drinks 1 liter of water, and tonometry is performed every 15 min for 1 hr. A rise in ocular tension of 9.00 mm Hg or more, or to 33 mm Hg or more, indicates glaucoma.

Welland's t. Bar reading test.

Whittington's t. A test for visual acuity, in which a letter E is held by the patient and is oriented in the same directions as various-sized letter Es on a test chart, the letters on the chart being rotatable so that they may be placed in any position.

Wight's t. A variation of the Newton ring test in which the number of rings per unit of diameter is taken to indicate the variance of curvature between the test and standard surfaces.

Wilbrand's t. A diagnostic test used in hemianopsia, in which prisms are suddenly placed before the eyes, while a small spot on a uniform background is fixated, to displace its images onto the blind sides of the retinae. According to Wilbrand, an abrupt refixation movement is diagnostic of a cerebral lesion, while the absence of this movement indicates a lesion in the optic tract.

Williams' lantern t. A test for color perception consisting of the identification of transilluminated colored filters exposed in sequence by means of movable shutters.

Wiltberger's t. A screening test for color perception utilizing six charts, each containing one horizontal and three vertical glossy color strips on a medium gray ground. The color of the afterimage of the horizontal strip, obtained by fixating it for about 20 sec, is compared to the vertical strips, and the one it matches best is said to indicate the type of color vision.

Wirt t. A near point test for the threshold of stereopsis, in which a vectogram consisting essentially of a series of groups of four dots is viewed through Polaroid filters. One dot in each group appears displaced toward the observer, the displacement decreasing with each successive group, and the last group in which it is detected indicates the threshold. Syn., *Wirt stereotest*.

Wold sentence copying t. A test for perceptual motor speed in which a sentence consisting of 29 words having 110 symbols is copied, the number of letters copied per minute being the subjective score.

Wood's color aptitude t. A test for color memory, in which a series of colored test patterns are individually viewed and then replaced by a set of four response plates from which one or none is selected as duplicating the same colors as the initial test pattern, regardless of differences in the pattern itself.

Worth's eccentric fixation t. A gross test to detect eccentric fixation, in which angle kappa (lambda) is measured for each eye, a difference between them indicating eccentric fixation.

Worth's four dot t. A test for binocular vision, in which four dots, one white, one red, and two green on a black background, are viewed through complementary red and green colored filters, such that one eye sees the red and the white dot and the other eye sees the two green dots and the white dot. Four dots seen in the pattern of the original formation indicate normal binocular vision, five dots binocular vision without fusion, and two red dots only, or three green dots only, suppression of one eye.

Worth's ivory ball t. A test to measure visual acuity in very young children, in which 5 balls, ranging in size from ½ to 1½ in., are thrown on the floor, one by one, about 6 yd in front of the child. He is encouraged to retrieve the balls, the smallest which excites his interest providing an estimate of visual acuity.

Worth-Ramstein t. A near point test for binocular vision and fusion consisting of four polarized symbols, a dot, two crosses, and a diamond, colored white, green, and red, which are viewed either through Polaroid filters or through complementary-colored red and green filters. Simultaneous perception of the four symbols in their original formation indicates normal binocular vision. It is one of the tests incorporated in the Freeman Near Vision Unit.

Young's t. A test to determine the state of macular function in an eye affected with cataract, consisting of the viewing of illuminated holes in a disk. The diagnosis is based on the number of holes perceived.

Young's threshold t. A clinical test for the determination of the threshold for light or color, used especially for the early detection of glaucoma. The subject observes gray or colored spots of varying intensities, on white cards bound into five albums, one each for gray, yellow, blue, red, and green. The threshold is indicated by the card on which the spot is first perceived.

Zagora rod t. A test for depth perception, similar to the Howard-Dolman, in which the top movable half of a vertical rod is aligned with the bottom stationary half, such that one continuous rod is perceived, thus involving height as well as depth judgment.

◆

Tester, Retinal Visual Acuity. Trade name for an instrument utilizing laser light to place a variable interference fringe on the retina to test the potential capability of seeing independent of refractive anomalies or moderate opacities.

tetartanopia (tĕ-tahr″tah-no′pe-ah). Tetartanopsia.

tetartanopsia (tĕ-tahr″tah-nop′se-ah). 1. Homonymous quadrantanopsia. 2. G. E. Mueller's term for a type of blue-yellow blindness, in which there are two neutral points, one in the yellow and one in the blue of the normal spectrum, which appear as white. Both red and green are seen normally and can be differentiated while blue and yellow are confused.

tetracaine hydrochloride (tet′rah-kān hi″dro-klo′rīd). A chemical compound closely related to procaine useful in 0.5% solution as a local anesthetic on the cornea.

tetrachromatism (tet″rah-kro′mah-tizm). 1. Normal color vision according to the Hering theory of four primary colors. 2. Hering's theory of color vision.

tetrafilcon A. The nonproprietary name of a hydrophilic material of which contact lenses are made.

tetrahydrozoline hydrochloride (tet″rah-hi-droz′o-lēn hi″dro-klo′rīd). A sympathomimetic drug available in 0.12% to 0.05% concentration in over-the-counter products as an ophthalmic decongestant.

tetranopsia (tet″rah-nop′se-ah). Quadrantanopsia.

tetrastichiasis (tet″rah-stih-ki′ah-sis). An anomalous condition in which there are four rows of eyelashes on a single eyelid.

thalamus (thal'ah-mus). One of a pair of ovoid masses of gray matter, about 1½ in. long, whose medial surface forms a portion of the lateral walls of the third ventricle in the diencephalon of the forebrain. The anterior extremity forms the posterior boundary of the foramen of Monro and the posterior end, the pulvinar, overhangs the midbrain and continues laterally into the external geniculate body. The internal capsule separates it above and laterally from the lenticular nucleus. It is a relay station for sensory pathways ending in the cerebral cortex, receives fibers from the cortex, and is connected with the tegmentum and with fibers of the optic tract.

   optic t. The thalamus.
thaumatrope (thaw'mah-trōp). A disk having on each face a picture representing a different portion of an object or a scene or a different stage in the movement of an object. When rotated so that both sides are alternately and rapidly viewed, the effect of a whole object or scene, or of a moving object, is obtained.
thelaziasis (the"la-zi'ah-sis). Infestation of the conjunctival sac with the nematode *Thelazia callipaeda.*
theliocapsularis (the"le-o-kap"su-lār'-is). Senile exfoliation of the capsule of the crystalline lens.

◆

THEORY

theory. 1. The general or abstract principles of a science or an art, as distinguished from the application of that science or art. 2. A general principle or formula, derived from an analysis of related facts to explain a phenomenon, which is generally more plausible than a hypothesis.
   Abbe's t. The theory of resolution with coherent illumination, in which the diffracting properties of both the illuminated object and the aperture of the lens are considered to contribute to the form of the image.
   active excretory t. Metabolic pump theory.
   across-neuron t. The theory that the activity of a single neuron cannot be considered as the neural representation of a stimulus, but that the encoding of relative amounts of neural activity in many parallel neurons at several stages of the visual pathway is involved.

   Adams' t. A theory of color vision, derived from that of Hering, which postulates a receptor system of rods and three types of cones, red, white, and blue. The receptors contain photosensitive pigment of different spectral properties and are associated with ganglion cells whose fibers relay impulses for three opponent color systems, white-black, red-green, and blue-yellow. The rods and white cones synapse directly with white optic nerve fibers and give rise to a sensation of white, the blue and red cones first modulate the response of the white cones by means of assumed lateral connections and then synapse with blue and red optic nerve fibers, respectively. Only an excess of a red or a blue response over a white response can reach the red or blue optic nerve fiber and so produce a red or blue sensation, while a white response in excess of a red or blue response results in a red optic nerve response, the negative of red (green), and a blue optic nerve response, the negative of blue (yellow).
   additive t. Young-Helmholtz theory.
   aim intent t. Voluntary eye movements do not cause a perception of apparent movement of objects whose images are moving across the retina, as such movement signals are cancelled by central signals from the brain which command the eyes to move. Cf. *inflow theory.* Syn., *outflow theory.*
   air t. of space perception. Point theory of space perception.
   Allen's t. A theory that every color stimulates all three primary color sensations, thereby causing a sensation of whiteness underlying and inseparable from color, thus explaining achromatic vision at high and low intensities, nonsaturation of colors, contrast, and complementary colors.
   alteration of response t. A postulation that uniform continuous response to continuous visual stimulation is effected by groups of parallel circuits activated in a sequential coordinated manner, each group going through a cycle of activity and recovery before again responding.
   antichromatic t. Hartridge's antichromatic theory.
   Arlt's t. The theory that myopia is caused by pressure of the extraocular muscles in convergence impeding the outflow of blood from the eye through

the vortex veins, resulting in congestion and increased intraocular pressure.

Aubert's t. A theory which postulates two pairs of "pure" colors, viz., red and green, yellow and blue, each member of the pair being capable of evoking its appropriate sensation when combined with either or both members of the other pair, but failing to do so if combined with the other member of its own pair.

Bach's t. Lenticular theory for colobomata.

Barnet's t. The theory that color vision is analogous to hearing, in that wavelengths of light may be differentiated similarly to the wavelengths of sound.

Behr's t. The theory that tissue fluid in the optic nerve normally flows from the eye toward the skull because the pressure is normally higher in the eye, and that choked disk results from a reversal of this flow when the pressure in the eye becomes lower than in the skull.

Brücke's t. The theory that the binocular perception of depth is due to continuous motion of the eyes, alternately increasing and decreasing convergence, which integrates successively the different aspects of the two scenes as seen by the two eyes.

Buffon's t. The theory that strabismus is due to reduced vision in one eye and that this eye deviates to avoid the disturbance arising from blurred vision.

capillary attraction t. of lacrimal flow. The theory that tears are drained by capillary attraction of the canaliculi.

Carmona y Valle's t. The theory that accommodation is accomplished by the compression of the periphery of the crystalline lens by the action of the circular fibers of the ciliary muscle on the fibers of the zonule of Zinn. This compression is said to act on soft peripheral portions of the lens, forcing the central portion of the lens to become more convex.

central dip t. of resolution. The theory that at threshold visual resolution the peaks of the light distributions of two adjacent point targets are separated by an intervening central dip in light distribution of fixed proportion. In the Rayleigh criterion for resolution, q.v., this is about 10% of the peak height.

Chavasse's t. The theory that strabismus is due to interference preventing normal development of the reflex acts involved in binocular vision, or if normally developed, hindering or abolishing them. The interference may be sensory, motor, or central, and congenital or acquired.

Cogan-Kinsey t. Osmotic pump theory.

Cohn's t. The theory that myopia is caused by the effects of excessive accommodation during near work in school.

Collins' t. Vascular theory for colobomata.

color constancy t. The constancy of perceived color of a reflecting surface under different illuminants depends upon a perceptual evaluation of the quality and quantity of the illumination (Helmholtz, Bartlett, Koffka, Woodworth, Judd, Beck) or upon the sensitivities and adaptations of the color response mechanisms (Hering, Helson, Cornsweet).

compression t. (of lacrimal flow). The theory that tears are drained by the action of the orbicularis oculi muscle on the lacrimal sac in the opening and closing of the eyelids. When the eyelids are closed, the lacrimal sac is compressed, forcing the tears into the lacrimal duct; when the eyelids are opened, the tears are sucked into the lacrimal sac through the canaliculi.

corpuscular t. Newton's theory.

Cramer's t. The theory that the increased convexity of the crystalline lens in accommodation is due to contraction of the iris exerting pressure on the periphery of the lens and to contraction of the ciliary muscle, which pulls the choroid forward to compress the vitreous against the posterior surface of the lens.

Cüppers' t. The theory that eccentric fixation is due to a pre-existing anomalous retinal correspondence in that the shift of the straight-ahead principal visual direction from the central fovea of the deviating amblyopic eye to an extrafoveal area, exhibited under binocular conditions, continues to operate monocularly when the amblyopic eye attempts to fixate; hence monocular fixation is with the retinal site which corresponds directionally to the foveal center of the fixating eye.

Dartnall's t. The theory that the absorption curve of visual purple for low intensities and the absorption curve for bleached visual purple at higher intensities are the physiological correlates of the scotopic and photopic luminosity curves, respectively, and that the displaced luminosity curve in the protan may be accounted for by some abnormality in the environment of the receptor, such as an unusual *pH* value.

decreased tension t. of accommodation. Any theory that accommodation is due to decreased tension of the suspensory ligament on action of the ciliary muscle, as in Helmholtz' theory of accommodation.

dialysation t. The theory that the aqueous humor is a dialysate from the blood of the capillaries of the ciliary body in thermodynamic equilibrium with the blood.

dichromatic t. Any theory which postulates a two component system for the explanation of color vision dichromatism.

Dieffenbach's t. The theory that strabismus is due to a peripheral disturbance of the extraocular muscles.

distention t. The theory that retinal detachment in high myopia is due to elongation of the anteroposterior axis of the eyeball, assisted by an accompanying hyperemia.

Doman-Delacato t. The theory that ontogenetic development consists of an invariant sequence of stages, and that proficient motor functioning at higher levels is dependent upon successful completion of lower levels.

dominator-modulator t. A theory of color vision in which a particular sense cell called the *dominator* is responsible for the brightness aspect of vision, chromatic effects being introduced by other receptors modulating the dominator response.

Donders' t. of accommodation. A maximal contraction of the ciliary muscle is required to produce maximal accommodation at any age, and each fraction of the actual range of accommodation corresponds to an equal fraction of the entire contractibility of the ciliary muscle. Hence, a greater amount of ciliary muscle contraction is required to produce a unit change in accommodation than was required at a younger age or the ability of the ciliary muscle to contract is diminished in some manner. Cf. *Hess's theory.*

Donders' t. of strabismus. The theory, attributed to Donders, that strabismus is due to uncorrected refractive errors, that hypermetropia is the cause of esotropia, and that myopia the cause of exotropia.

Druault's t. The theory that the vitreous humor is originally mesodermal, derived from ingrowing vessels, and that, as the eye grows, a secondary, ectodermal vitreous is formed from the retinal surface. The secondary vitreous displaces the primary toward the center of the eye and thus forms Cloquet's canal.

Duane's t. The theory that strabismus is caused by excessive or insufficient nerve impulses from a convergence or divergence center in the brain.

duplicity t. The theory that visual sensation stems from two independent receptor systems in the retina, one said to be composed of rods and the other of cones, the former mediating achromatic sensations at very low levels of intensity, the latter mediating vision at higher levels of intensity and capable of distinguishing colors. Syn., *von Kries duplicity theory.*

Ebbecke's t. The theory that the successive reappearances of afterimages with abrupt changes in illuminance levels of the total retina are dependent on the continued effectiveness of the initial stimulus, even for several hours, and the otherwise balanced inhibitory and counterinhibitory mechanisms of local adaptation and simultaneous contrast, respectively.

Edridge-Green t. of color vision. A speculative theory that the cones alone are the visual receptors and that rods merely secrete visual purple which flows via small channels into the fovea, where stimulation by light sets up vibrations which are transmitted via the optic nerve to two independent centers in the brain, a light center and a color center, where perceptual analysis takes place. The light center is supposed to be more primitive, the color center evolving later, with subsequent evolution of subcenters for differentiation of seven specific colors. Color blindness is atavistic, resulting from central failure of development.

Edridge-Green t. of myopia. The theory that myopia is caused by increased intraocular pressure from obstruction of the flow of lymph out of the eye during bending, straining, or lifting.

Einstein's t. The theory that (*a*) the uniform motion of translation cannot be detected by an observer stationed on the moving system from observations confined to the system, and (*b*) the velocity of light in space is a constant, independent of the relative velocity of the source and the observer.

electromagnetic t. Maxwell's theory.

electrostatic t. The theory that differential permeability of the cornea is due to static electrical charges on its surface which propel appropriately charged ions through its cell membranes.

emission t. Newton's theory.

empiristic t. See *empiricism.*

Enoch's t. The theory that anomalous anatomical composition or disturbed orientation of the central retinal receptors may be an etiological factor in amblyopia.

evolutionary t. Ladd-Franklin theory.

Exner's t. The theory that the illusion of movement of a stationary object, occurring after prolonged viewing of an object moving in one direction, is due to streams of afterimages.

Fick's t. The theory that protanopia and deuteranopia are due to the absence of either the red- or the green-sensitive photopigments, that in protanopia both the red and the green receptors contain green-photosensitive pigment, and in deuteranopia both the red and the green receptors contain red-photosensitive pigment.

field t. The theory that the neural functions and processes with which the perceptual facts are associated in each case are located in a continuous medium, and that the events in one part of this medium influence the events in other regions in a way that depends directly on the properties of both in their relation to each other.

filtration t. The theory that the formation of aqueous humor is by filtration from the capillaries of the ciliary body which are permeable to crystalloids but not to colloids of the blood plasma; hence, the filtered fluid would be devoid of proteins, whereas crystalloids and other substances would be in the same proportion as in the blood.

Fincham's t. The theory that in accommodation the anterior surface of the crystalline lens assumes a conoidal shape, with increased convexity primarily in the pupillary area, due to the elasticity of the anterior capsule and to the relative thinness of the anterior capsule in the pupillary area, an elaboration of Helmholtz' theory. The reduction of the amplitude of accommodation with age is due to sclerosing of the lens substance, such that it changes less in form for a given pressure of the capsule.

first order t. Theory of Gauss.

Förster's t. The theory that myopia is caused by stretching of the eyeball in excessive convergence, and that its increase can be prevented by the use of full correcting lenses or abducting prisms.

Fourier's t. A theory, developed by the French physicist, Fourier, showing that it is possible to describe any complex periodic wave form as the sum of a specific series of sine and cosine waves. The amplitudes, phases, and frequencies of these waves are a characteristic of the original wave form and constitute a full description of it.

Frieberg's t. The theory that tears are drained by the action on the canaliculi of the opening and closing of the eyelids. When the eyelids are closed, the canaliculi are compressed, forcing the tears into the lacrimal sac; when the eyelids are opened, the tears are sucked into the canaliculi from the conjunctival sac.

fusion faculty t. Worth's theory.

t. of Gauss. The theory that, for tracing paraxial rays through a lens system, the system may be analyzed in terms of six cardinal planes, two principal planes, two nodal planes, and two focal planes. Syn., *first order theory.*

genetic color t. Ladd-Franklin theory.

Gibson's texture gradient t. of space perception. The theory that all three dimensions are represented on the retina, since distant features of a scene are projected on the retina as smaller than nearby ones, this gradation forming a texture gradient by means of which all features within it are given size and location. Cf. *point theory of space perception.*

Goethe's t. A very subjectively derived explanation of color phenomena tending to relegate colors as phenomenal attributes inherent in the light stimulus or in the substance reflecting or transmitting the light, and hypothesizing the admixture of dark with light as the essential determining factor, with blue and yellow as the extremes on the dark to light scale, whence other colors could also be described as mixtures of these two colors.

Göthlin's t. A theory postulating that the impulse for a given color sensation releases to some extent an inhibition for the complementary color within the same area, to account for the fact that a mixture of two spectral primaries is less saturated than the matching monochromatic hue until spectral primary is added to the latter.

von Graefe's t. The theory that strabismus is due to a congenital or acquired anomaly of the ligament and muscle system of the eye, and that a disturbance in this relationship causes a predominance in one group of muscles or an insufficiency in the antagonistic group.

Granit's t. The theory that the seven relatively narrow, electroretinographic, response curves obtained by Granit, which he called *modulator curves*, might be related to the fibers of the optic nerve in such a way as to constitute three systems of receptors, by virtue of their clustering in three groups corresponding to the three main parts of the spectrum associated with three-receptor theories of color vision.

Harris' t. Metabolic pump theory.

Hartridge's antichromatic t. A postulation to account for the apparent compensation for chromatic aberration of the eye, in which the depressed sensitivity for the blue and yellow fringes of the retinal image is attributed to a neurological mechanism.

Hartridge's t. of color vision. A theory of color vision postulating seven types of receptors, six (orange, yellow, green, blue-green, blue, and blue-violet) having single response curves on the spectral scale and one, crimson, having two, one at each end of the spectral scale. Syn., *polychromatic theory.*

Hartridge's t. of visual acuity. The theory that the resolving power of the retina is facilitated by the ability of each cone to detect gradations of light intensity, not as an all-or-none receptor.

Hasner's t. The theory that myopia is caused by a stretching of the eyeball due to pulling on the posterior pole by the optic nerve.

Hecht's photochemical t. The theory that the action of light on the retinal receptors decomposes a photosensitive substance into two photochemical products which act as catalysts in a secondary reaction which results in nerve impulses.

Hecht's t. of visual acuity. The theory that the increase in visual acuity with increased illumination is due to an increase in the number of retinal receptors activated; that the retinal receptors have varied light thresholds and react individually according to the all-or-none law.

Helmholtz' t. of accommodation. The theory that in accommodation the ciliary muscle contracts, relaxing the tension of the suspensory ligament and allowing the crystalline lens to become more convex, especially its anterior surface, due to its own elasticity. The choroid aids in maintaining the tension of the suspensory ligament on the crystalline lens in its unaccommodated state and the contraction of the ciliary body pulls the choroid forward, releasing the tension. Syn., *decreased tension theory; relaxation theory.*

Helmholtz' t. of color vision. Young-Helmholtz theory.

Helmholtz' empiristic t. See *empiricism.*

Henderson's t. The theory that tension of the suspensory ligament on the crystalline lens is maintained chiefly by the longitudinal and the radial fibers of the ciliary muscle, that the contraction of the circular fibers overcomes this tension and slackens the suspensory ligament in accommodation, that both sympathetic and parasympathetic innervation are involved in accommodation, and that presbyopia is due to sclerosis of the connective tissue of the ciliary body.

Henschen's t. The theory that sensory fusion occurs in the middle stratum of three strata which compose the superficial layer of the area striata, that the fibers from the temporal retina of the eye on the same side terminate in the outer stratum and the fibers from the nasal retina on the opposite side terminate in the inner stratum, and that fibers from the corresponding points of these two strata stimulate the same cell in the middle stratum.

Hering's t. of color vision.
The theory that postulates three primary retinal substances, each responsible for one mutually antagonistic pair of color sensations, red-green, yellow-blue, or white-black, and that light falling on the retina, depending on its wavelength composition, causes a breakdown (catabolism) or synthesis (anabolism) of one or more of these substances, causing transmission of one or neither of each pair of sensations to the brain. Syn., *opponent colors theory.*

Hering's nativistic t. See *nativism.*

Hering's t. of retinal projection. The theory that the estimation of distance between points in the field of vision depends on the chord connecting the retinal images of the points and not on the angular distance between them, an explanation of the optical illusion of empty spaces appearing smaller than subdivided spaces.

Hering's t. of stereoscopic vision. The theory that stereoscopic vision is based on retinal disparity and that the appreciation of this disparity is an innate physiological process.

Hess's t. The same amount of ciliary muscle contraction will produce a unit change in accommodation at any age. Cf. *Donders' theory of accommodation.*

van der Hoeve's t. The theory that strabismus is caused by the failure of the summation of all the reflexes affecting the extraocular muscles to produce a nearly orthophoric position, the resultant diplopia acting as a stimulus to move the nonfixating eye to a position of greater deviation to facilitate suppression.

Holm's t. The theory that myopia is caused by overgrowth of the eyeball, that the tonus of the ciliary body regulates the growth of the eye, and that the increased innervation from prolonged reading acts as a growth-promoting factor.

Houstoun's t. A theory which postulates two types of cones, a red-green type and a yellow-blue type, each capable of responding to stimulation with two alternative frequencies or modes of electric discharge, each discharge frequency corresponding to its appropriate color sensation, with a third, less clearly postulated system to account for white, gray, and black.

Hubbard-Kropf t. A theory of the nature of *meta*-rhodopsin and its relation to rhodopsin, according to which *meta*-rhodopsin consists of a mixture of thermally stable rhodopsin, thermally stable *9-cis* rhodopsin, and thermally unstable compounds of opsin with *all-trans* retinene and additional retinene isomers other than *11-cis* and *9-cis*; that the absorption of one quantum of light isomerizes the chromophore of either rhodopsin or *9-cis* rhodopsin to the *all-trans* configuration, but while the *all-trans* retinene is still attached to the opsin, a second quantum of light may cause isomerization to still another configuration. If the new stereoisomer thus formed is either *11-cis* or *9-cis*, then rhodopsin or *9-cis* rhodopsin will be reformed.

Hurvich-Jameson t. A quantified version of the Hering theory of color vision. It postulates a system of three independent photosensitive materials in the retina which mediate between the incident light and the three opponent color neural response systems; it relates the total mechanism to the physical variables of stimulus wavelength and energy levels and to their dependence on adapting and surrounding stimulation.

Huygens' t. The theory that light is propagated through space in waves and that space is filled with a luminiferous ether which penetrates and permeates all matter. The ether is composed of tiny elastic particles whose mutual impacts are transmitted from one to another and act as the vehicle for the light waves. Syn., *undulation theory; wave theory.*

hydraulic t. of accommodation. The theory that the increased convexity of the crystalline lens in accommodation is due to compression of the aqueous humor against its periphery, causing the anterior pole to bulge forward, as a result of contraction of the ciliary muscle compressing the aqueous humor in the posterior chamber, where it is confined by the constricted pupil.

increased tension t. of accommodation. Any theory that accommodation is due to increased tension of the suspensory ligament on action of the ciliary muscle, as in Tscherning's theory of accommodation.

inflow t. Eye movements do not cause a perception of apparent movement of objects whose images are moving across the retina, because such movement signals are cancelled by feedback signals from the extraocular muscles to the brain. Cf. *aim intent theory.*

Ivanoff's t. The theory that night myopia is due to chromatic aberration, the Purkinje phenomenon, and a voluntary effort to accommodate to eliminate spherical aberration.

Ives's t. The theory that flicker or intermittent vision is a perceptual process involving three steps; a reversible photochemical reaction; diffusion of substances formed by the photochemical reaction; and a constant critical value of the rate of change of a transmitted reaction which must be exceeded before the perception of flicker can occur.

Javal's t. The theory that strabismus is caused by a functional anomaly of binocular vision and not by primary involvement of the extraocular muscles.

Kant's nativistic t. See *nativism.*

Keiner's t. The theory that convergent strabismus is due to an inherited retardation of the development of the myelin sheaths of nerve fibers in the visual pathways, thus delaying the acquisition of binocular reflexes.

Keith's t. The theory that myopia is caused by a growth disorder occasioned by the conditions civilization has imposed on man.

Kinsey-Cogan t. Osmotic pump theory.

Koenig's t. The theory of color vision that visual purple is the excitant of the rods at low intensity levels and hence the basis of achromatic vision, that visual yellow, the first product of bleaching of visual purple with higher intensities, is the basis of the blue sensation also carried out by the rods and absent from the fovea, that red and green sensations are accomplished by differential absorption of the pigment cells of the pigment epithelium, dichromatism being due to coincidence of the elementary sensation curves, and that the cones serve only as a dioptric mechanism to concentrate light on the pigment epithelium.

Kölliker's t. The theory that the cornea is derived entirely from mesodermal tissue which in the embryo migrates between the surface epithelium and the lens vesicle.

von Kries duplicity t. Duplicity theory.

von Kries t. of color vision. The supposition that the sensations of vision may be aroused by two different mechanisms, perhaps operating both in series and in parallel, more or less independent of each other, only one of which has the tripartite structure of the trichromatic system, whereas the other reacts to its stimulus in a simple monotone, wherefore the "colorless sensation has some outstanding physiological significance." Syn., *theory of zones; zonal theory.*

Ladd-Franklin t. A theory of color vision which postulates an evolutionary development of receptor substances from an initial "whiteness" detector, presumed to persist in the rods and the peripheral cones, from which are derived, by molecular change, two paired substances that serve as detectors of blue and yellow, the latter of which is further changed into paired substances that serve to detect red and green, whence mixtures of red and green are perceived as yellow, and mixtures of yellow and blue are perceived as white. Types of color blindness are thus regarded atavistically as incomplete recapitulations of evolutionary development. Syn., *evolutionary theory; genetic color theory; tetrachromatic theory.*

Land's t. A theory for color vision which postulates a series of retinal-cerebral systems (retinexes), each having retinal receptors with the same peak sensitivity to a given band of the spectrum. The retinal receptors for each retinex operate as a cooperative unit, independent of other retinexes, and form, through cerebral liaison, an image corresponding to the optical image on the retina but differing in terms of lightness from the images of the other retinexes. The image of the same object in each retinex has its own rank order in relation to lightness, its rank order being different in each retinex and dependent on the interaction of the spectral absorption curve of the receptors with the spectral absorption curves of all objects in the field of vision. The image from each retinex becomes superimposed, and the comparison of the rank order of lightness for the image of the same object from each retinex results in a designation of color for that object, color being the correlation number for several rank orders of lightness.

Landolt's t. The theory that strabismus is due to the topographical anatomy of the eyes, i.e., to mechanical factors.

Langworthy's t. The theory that the sphincter pupillae muscle acts against a tonal background maintained by the blood volume of the iris and the natural elasticity of its blood vessels, and that, when the sympathetic nervous system is stimulated, the arterioles and the capillaries constrict, forcing out the blood, which reduces the mass of the iris and causes the pupil to dilate.

lattice t. Maurice's theory.

Leber's t. Migration theory.

lenticular t. for colobomata. The theory that a typical coloboma is due to an abnormally large crystalline lens which mechanically prevents closure of the embryonic fissure. Syn., *Bach's theory.*

Levinsohn's t. The theory that myopia is caused by stretching of the eyeball, resulting in increased axial length, from tilting the head forward.

lid closure t. The theory that tears are drained by being forced into the lacrimal puncta by the eyelids on closure.

Lindner t. The theory that myopia is caused by weakening of the choroid and the sclera, due to a transudation of blood elements from the choroidal vessels into the surrounding tissues during near work.

linked-receptor t. of color vision. The theory that there may be a greater number of types of receptors in the retina than there are types of response mechanisms, and that pairs or groups of two or more receptors may be "linked" together to elicit a single type of response, resulting in a polychromatism of the retina with trichromatism of vision.

Lomonosov's t. The theory for color vision postulating three primary types of particles of light consisting of mercury, salt, and sulphur which are responsible for sensations of red, yellow, and blue when stimulating preferentially sensitive particles in the optic nerve which are also composed of mercury, salt, and sulphur, all other colors being a mixture of these three. One of the earliest attempts to explain color

vision, advanced by Lomonosov in 1756 and subsequently modified by Young.

Lorentz t. The theory that the oscillation of charged particles inside the atom is the source of light.

Lotze's t. of local signs. The theory that each point on the retina, when stimulated, will give rise to a specific sense of direction, that this is an innate phenomenon not dependent on previous experience.

Luneburg's t. A theory of binocular spatial localization formulated on non-Euclidean, hyperbolic geometry, whence visual space is said to be non-Euclidean in character.

Lythgoe's t. The theory that the increase in visual acuity with increased illumination is due to a decrease in the dimensions of the retinal receptor fields.

Mackenzie's t. The theory that strabismus is due to a functional anomaly of the areas in the brain and the nerves which associate the actions of the extraocular muscles.

Manz's t. Mesoblastic theory for colobomata.

Maurice's t. The theory that corneal transparency is based on the orderly and symmetrical arrangement of the collagen fibrils in the corneal stroma, which are of uniform diameter, arranged in a two-dimensional lattice pattern, of equal spacing and with the interspaces being less than one wavelength of visible light. Under these conditions, each line of fibrils will correspond to a diffraction grating and interference will suppress the scattering of light in any direction except that of the incident beam. Syn., *lattice theory.*

Maxwell's t. The theory that light consists of electromagnetic waves. Syn., *electromagnetic theory.*

McDougall's t. A color vision theory postulating four mediating systems, corresponding to red, green, blue, and white, each including an appropriate light-sensitive substance at the receptor level and each terminating in one of four appropriate, bilaterally represented, cortical centers, with presumed inhibitory interaction mechanisms between the cortical centers for the three color primaries and with inductive and integrative mechanisms between all four systems at the retinal level.

mesoblastic t. for colobomata. The theory that a typical coloboma is due to blockage of the fetal fissure by the normally migrating vascular formative mesodermal tissue. Syn., *Manz's theory.*

metabolic pump t. The theory that the normal relative deturgescence or normal water content of the cornea is maintained by the active excretion or "pumping" of tissue fluid and electrolytes from the corneal stroma through the endothelial and epithelial cells, and that this excretion requires cellular energy and is therefore a metabolic process. Syn., *active excretory theory; Harris' theory; Potts-Maurice theory.*

migration t. The theory that sympathetic ophthalmia is caused by migration of the pathogenic agent through the lymph canals of the optic nerve. Syn., *Leber's theory.*

modulation t. for color vision. The theory that color sensation is mediated by variations in the temporal pattern of afferent optic nerve impulses, rather than by types of receptors or by the subdivision of neural pathways.

Morgan's t. of accommodation. The theory that accommodation is due in part to the blood volume of the ciliary body, which affects the pull on the suspensory ligament, and that a decrease in the blood volume of the ciliary body with age produces a decreased response of the ciliary muscle.

Morgan's t. of anomalous correspondence. The theory that anomalous retinal correspondence represents an adaptive adjustment derived from an innervational pattern or position sense of the deviating eye with respect to the other eye, rather than an adaptation of the local direction signs of the retina.

Mueller's t. of color vision. A theory employing the concept that an equality, a similarity, or a difference in the condition of sensations corresponds to an equality, a similarity, or a difference in the condition of psychophysical processes, and postulating four chromatic retinal substances correlated with red, yellow, green, and blue that are chemically altered by the action of light so as to transmit impulses corresponding to their modifications to cerebral substrata of actual sensations for which there are six basic values (red, yellow, green, blue, white, and black), the resulting sensation being derived from a complex linkage system between the four types of peripheral retinal substances and the six central value processes.

Mueller's t. of strabismus. The theory that strabismus is due to a false or displaced macula in the one eye.

Nagel's empiristic t. See *empiricism.*

nasal aspiration t. The theory that tears are drained by a sucking action created by changes in pressure in the nasal cavity due to breathing.

nativistic t. See *nativism.*

neurogeometric sensory feedback t. The theory that all major characteristics of visual behavior are ascribable not to the receptor, the motor system, or learning, but to the spatial or geometric properties of neural feedback control systems linking the sensory and motor systems of the body.

Newman's t. The theory that myopia is caused by the effects of excessive accommodation on the choroid, decreasing its nutrition by pulling and tensing, so that it becomes weakened.

Newton's t. The theory that light consists of a flight of invisible, rapidly moving particles projected from a light source, the size of the particles varying with the apparent color and moving in a substance called *ether*, which varies in density for different media. Syn., *corpuscular theory; emission theory.*

noise t. The theory for the basis of the brightness difference threshold in which the fluctuations in absorption of quanta per unit area of the retina, corresponding to the background, constitute the noise against which the signal (stimulus) must be detected; hence the number of quanta from the signal, to be detected, must sufficiently exceed that of the background noise.

Norris' t. The theory that myopia is caused by "abuse" of the eyes leading to congestion and softening of the coats of the eyeball so that they stretch under normal intraocular pressure.

opponent colors t. Hering's theory of color vision.

opponent process t. Any theory postulating retinal substances which respond with opposing reactions, such as anabolic and catabolic reactions. See *Hering's theory of color vision* and *Hurvich-Jameson theory.*

osmotic pump t. The theory that the normal relative deturgescence or normal water content of the cornea is maintained by a difference in osmotic pressure between the corneal stroma and the hypertonic tear fluid and aqueous humor which bathe the intact epithelium and endothelium; hence, tissue fluid entering the corneal stroma through the limbal capillaries is continually passed through the endothelium and epithelium. Syn., *Cogan-Kinsey theory.*

Otero's t. The theory that night myopia is due to a combination of the aberrations of the eye (spherical and chromatic) and the posture of the accommodative mechanism at low levels of illumination.

outflow t. Aim intent theory.

Palmer's t. The theory for color vision, advanced by G. Palmer in 1777, that there are three color components in white light, red, yellow, and blue, and three corresponding retinal receptor systems preferentially sensitive to these three colors, that a sensation of white results from uniform agitation of the three systems, and that color sensations result from nonuniform agitation. Total color blindness results from failure of the three systems to respond differentially, and partial color blindness is due to impairment of one or two of the three systems.

Parinaud's t. 1. Two retinae theory. 2. The theory that strabismus is caused by a defect in the brain centers controlling the eyes. 3. The theory that choked disk results from edema of the brain, due to tumor, which spreads through the optic nerve to the papilla.

Petzval t. The theory that for eliminating the curvature of a stigmatic image produced by a system of two thin lenses, in contact or separated, the sum of the product of the refractive indices and the focal lengths of the two lenses must equal zero.

photon t. Einstein's theory of photoemission that a light beam acts as a stream of particles (photons).

physical t. of color vision. Young-Helmholtz theory of color vision.

Piéron's t. A theory for color vision postulating three types of cone, each containing a single pigment, and a fourth supplementary cone receptor concerned with the reception of luminosity and containing a mixture of the three pigments.

Planck's t. The theory that radiation is intermittent and spasmodic and operates by definite quanta or units of energy in the case of both emission and absorption. Syn., *quantum theory.*

point t. of space perception. The theory that objects are aggregations of points and that all positions in the frontal plane are localized in relation to that of the point of fixation. Cf. *Gibson's texture gradient theory.* Syn., *air theory of space perception.*

Polyak's t. The theory that the receptor mechanism responsible for color perception does not lie in the retinal cones, as they are identical in their chemical properties, morphological structure, and synaptic relationships, and that the synthesis and compounding of colors may involve the bipolar and the ganglion cell layers.

polychromatic t. Hartridge's theory of color vision.

pore t. The theory that the differential permeability of the cornea is due to sievelike pores in the structure of the cornea which permit passage of molecules and ions of limited size.

Posey's t. The theory that myopia is caused by the shape of the skull, which determines the conformation of the orbit and, in turn, the eyeball.

Potts-Maurice t. Active excretory theory.

projection t. The theory that an object is localized in space along a line representing the pathway of light traveled from the object to the retina and that in binocular fixation an object is localized at the point of intersection of two lines, one to each retina.

psychological t. of color vision. Hering's theory of color vision.

quantum t. Planck's theory.

quantum t. of color vision. Any theory of color vision postulating the quantal energy difference of different wavelengths as the initial or fundamental factor in color differentiation.

Rayleigh's t. The theory that an optical system will be free of spherical aberration when the difference between the optical paths of a paraxial ray and a marginal ray leading to a selected focus is less than one-quarter of a wavelength.

relaxation t. of accommodation. Helmholtz' theory of accommodation.

replacement t. Verhoeff's theory.

rivalry t. The theory that single, binocular vision is obtained through rapid, alternate perception of the two monocular images, that each monocular image is periodically suppressed and replaced by the other.

Roaf's t. The theory that color vision is mediated by three types of receptors, one being stimulated by the entire visible spectrum, one by the red end to 490 mμ (blue-green) and one by the red end to 580 mμ (yellow-green). Thus long wavelengths stimulate all three receptor types, medium, two receptor types, and short, one receptor type, the differentiation presumed to be due to color filters in the receptors.

Ronchi's t. The theory that night myopia is due to the chromatic aberration of the eye, the Purkinje phenomenon, and to the action of the pupil when it dilates in low levels of illumination. The dilatation allows the crystalline lens to move forward so that its periphery presses on the iris, forcing the central portion of the lens to bulge and become more convex.

Rydberg's t. The theory of color vision that the outer segment of the cones consists of uniform double layers of protein and lipoid lamellae which act as an interference color filter, and that each cone will react only to the one, two, or three spectral wavelengths which are able to form standing waves in its protein lamellae. Hence, the thickness of the lamellae must be an integer multiple of the half-wavelengths of these colors.

sac dilation t. The theory that tears are drained by the action of the orbicularis oculi muscle on the lacrimal sac in the opening and closing of the eyelids. When the eyelids are closed, the lacrimal sac expands, sucking in tears, and when the eyelids are opened, the lacrimal sac is compressed, forcing the tears into the lacrimal duct.

Schenck's t. A theory employing the evolutionary concept of development of color vision, largely identical to Ladd-Franklin's, and postulating an original cone substance resembling the rod substance, which underwent a "pan-chromatization," making it relatively sensitive to long waves, subsequently but independently differentiating into blue and yellow components, with the final stage of differentiation being that of the yellow component into red and green subcomponents, whence types of color blindness were identified categorically with absence of the cone mechanism, failure of pan-chromati-

zation, and/or failure of the yellow cleavage process.

Schmidt-Rimpler t. The theory that choked disk results from congested cerebrospinal fluid in the skull being forced into the intervaginal spaces of the optic nerve, causing edema of the nerve and the papilla.

Schober's t. The theory that the largest portion of night myopia is due to an increase in accommodation caused by the effort to see under low levels of illumination, that under these conditions the dioptric stimulus to accommodation is not adequate to fix its amount.

Schoen's t. The theory that accommodation is due to contraction of the ciliary muscle exerting pressure on the equator of the crystalline lens which causes the surfaces to bulge, increasing the total refractive power of the eye.

Schöler's t. The theory that the vitreous humor is entirely mesodermal in origin and can be considered to be a specialized form of connective tissue.

secretion-diffusion t. The theory that the aqueous humor is formed by secretion from the epithelium of the ciliary body and by diffusion from the blood vessels of the iris.

secretory t. The theory that the aqueous humor is formed by secretion from the epithelium of the ciliary body.

Shaxby's t. A theory postulating that the different quanta of energy contained in the different wavelengths striking the cones are the basis for color differentiation, and not the cone structures or connections themselves (single neural connections of each cone with the brain being assumed).

Sherrington's t. The theory that sensory fusion is the result of a psychic process at some higher brain level, and that the two monocular images are complete and independent sensations until they are united at this level. When the two monocular sensations are alike, the resulting binocular perception does not differ from either; when they are slightly dissimilar, the result is intermediate between the two; and when they differ widely, rivalry results.

siphon t. The theory that tears are drained by a passive flow from the eye into the nose by a siphoning action.

solvent t. The theory that the differential permeability of solutes through the cornea is effected by the cell membranes having the property of dissolving the solutes.

Speciale-Circincione t. The theory that the vitreous humor is derived from the ectoderm of the crystalline lens and the retina.

Steiger's t. The theory that myopia is caused by a chance association of inherited variables, such as the curvature of the anterior surface of the cornea and the axial length of the eye; that all refractive errors are due to normal biologic variations.

Stiles t. A color vision theory based on the assumption of five fundamental receptor mechanisms with specific spectral sensitivities and with the activity of each mechanism related to both test and background wavelength.

Stilling's t. of myopia. The theory that myopia is caused by pressure of the superior oblique muscle on the eyeball in convergence, the pressure varying with the position of the trochlea, resulting in congestion and increased intraocular tension.

Stilling's t. of strabismus. The theory that strabismus is due to the topographical anatomy of the eyes, i.e., to mechanical factors.

Straub's t. The theory that the state of refraction of the eye is caused by the psyche, that those who wish to see well at a distance are emmetropic and those overly attracted to near objects become myopic.

tetrachromatic t. Ladd-Franklin theory.

third-order t. The theory that the deviation of the path of a ray from that prescribed by the theory of Gauss may be expressed mathematically by the Seidel formulae, and that, for a lens to be free of all aberration, all of the formulae would have to be simultaneously and individually equal to zero.

three component t. Young-Helmholtz theory.

Tornatola's t. The theory that the vitreous humor is derived from ectoderm, probably from the retinal layer of the optic cup.

transudation t. The theory that the aqueous humor is formed by a pressure filtration from the blood of the ciliary body and the iris.

trichromatic t. Young-Helmholtz theory.

trireceptor t. Any theory which postulates that color vision is accomplished by means of three kinds of retinal receptors, each mediating one of the three primary hue sensations.

Troland's t. A theory postulating five "molecular resonators" which may be selectively ionized by appropriate wavelengths to give rise to respective sensations of red, green, blue, yellow, and white, for which the positive ions represent the psychophysical correlates, with the further postulation that antagonistic relations between blue and yellow, and between red and green, represent ionization phenomena occurring in a "complementation substance" in the ganglionic retinal cells, while other ion combinations result in fused or additive sensations.

Tscherning's t. The theory that accommodation is due to contraction of the ciliary muscle, which tightens the suspensory ligament and pulls the choroid forward, causing the vitreous humor to exert pressure on the posterior surface of the crystalline lens. Since the periphery of the lens is held taut by the suspensory ligament, the pressure of the vitreous causes the anterior pole of the lens to bulge forward, increasing its convexity. Syn., *increased tension theory.*

Turner's t. The theory that myopia is caused by toxins from a diseased condition of the nose or the throat, producing waterlogging of the choroid and the sclera and an increase in the bulk of the vitreous humor, with a resultant stretching of the eyeball without change in intraocular tension.

two retinae t. The theory that the retina is composed of two distinct neural mechanisms, the rods of the peripheral retina primarily responsible for distinguishing light and dark, concerned with scotopic vision, and the cones of the central retina responsible for distinguishing color and form, concerned with photopic vision. In the evolutionary development of the eye the retinal receptors were capable only of distinguishing light from dark. Later some receptor cells became more complex, and color and form vision became possible, although these cells lost sensitivity to low levels of illumination. Syn., *Parinaud's theory.*

ultrafiltration t. The theory that the formation of aqueous humor is by filtration through the capillary walls, primarily from the capillary bed of the ciliary body.

undulation t. Huygen's theory.

vascular t. for colobomata. The theory that all colobomata are due to failure of formation of blood vessels in the mesoderm surrounding the optic cup which prevents fusion of the embryonic fissure. Syn., *Collins' theory.*

Verhoeff's t. The theory that the single percept arising from binocular vision consists of a constantly changing mosaic containing parts of each monocular image. Syn., *replacement theory.*

Vogt's t. The theory that myopia is caused by overgrowth of the eyeball, that the size of the retina controls the size of the eye, and that in myopia the retina has an excessive inherent growth potential.

Walls's t. A theory postulating that each of three types of color receptors, if isolated, would be capable of invoking a pure hue sensation appropriate to itself, but that each receptor responds to all wavelengths, whence the dominant hue sensation is invoked by the maximally stimulated receptor, while the common response of all three receptors produces a certain degree of desaturation.

wave t. Huygen's theory.

Wiener's t. The theory that myopia is caused by an endocrine disturbance.

Wolfrum's t. The theory that the primary vitreous is the result of the original adhesions between the neural and surface ectoderm in the region of the lens plate, that as these two surfaces separate, protoplasmic processes are pulled out between them and an intermediate substance is formed by interlacing fibrils from this source.

Worth's t. The theory that a fusion faculty or fusion sense controls the position of the eyes for binocular fixation and that the absence or imperfect development of this fusion faculty is the essential cause of strabismus. Syn., *fusion faculty theory.*

Wright's t. A theory that the receptor subdivision responsible for color perception resides in the presumed triplicate neural connection of each cone to three separate nerve pathways by means of three different bipolar cells.

Wundt's t. A theory postulating two relatively independent processes, one, a uniform photochemical process mediating achromatic perception, related to wavelength only as an intensity function, and the other, a polyform photochemical process mediating the gradations of color perception by changes associated with wavelength variance.

Young's t. of accommodation. The theory that accommodation results from a change in form of the crystalline lens.

Young's t. of color vision. Young-Helmholtz theory.

Young-Helmholtz t. The theory that three different, independent types of receptors or receptor components mediate all color sensations by their individual and combined activities, and that these types correspond to three color primaries. Syn., *additive theory; Helmholtz' theory of color vision; three component theory; trichromatic theory; Young's theory of color vision.*

Zeeman's t. The theory that strabismus is caused by the failure or retardation of normal sequential development of the conditioned reflexes involved in coordinated eye movements.

t. of zones. Von Kries theory of color vision.

◆

thermokeratoplasty (ther″mo-ker′ah-to-plas″te). Reshaping of the corneal surface by means of a heated, approximately 115°C, concave or flat probe about 3 to 7 mm in diameter applied gently at the desired site.

thermoluminescence (ther″mo-lu″-mih-nes′ens). The emission of light by a substance when heated, but not incandescent.

theta (θ). The Greek letter used as a symbol for *angle of latitude* in the field of regard. (Fry)

thiamine (thi′ah-min). Vitamin B_1.

Thibaudet's test (te-bo-dāz′). See under *test.*

thickness. The degree or extent to which something is thick; measurement in the third dimension; the dimension from one surface to its opposite.

apparent t. Reduced thickness.

axial t. Thickness of a lens as measured along the optical axis. Syn., *polar thickness.*

center t. Thickness of a lens either at its optical center or at its geometrical center.

optical t. The product of the thickness of an optical material and its index of refraction.

point t. Thickness of a lens expressed in points, 1 point being equal to $^1/_5$ mm.

polar t. Axial thickness.

reduced t. Axial thickness of a lens divided by its index of refraction. Syn., *apparent thickness.*

strap t. The thickness of an ophthalmic lens at the hole or point over which the strap of a rimless mounting fits.

Thiel's test (thēlz). See under *test.*

Thiéry's (tyĕ"rēz') **figure; visual illusion.** See under the nouns.

Thies's sign (thĕs'ez). See under *sign.*

third dimension. The dimension of depth as contrasted to the dimensions of width and length, or the percept of distance away from an observer.

Thollon prism. See under *prism.*

Thomas' chart (tom'as). See under *chart.*

Thompson's (tom'sonz) **circles; disease; formula.** See under the nouns.

Thomsen's disease (tom'senz). See under *disease.*

Thomson (tom'sen) **effect; scattering.** See under the nouns.

Thorington (thōr'ing-ton) **chart; prism; test.** See under the nouns.

Thorpe contact lens. See under *lens, contact.*

Thouless effect; ratio. See under the nouns.

threshold. 1. The least stimulus value that will excite a response or a just noticeable difference in response. 2. Statistically, the central tendency in a range of stimulus values at which occurs a transition in a series of sensory judgments. Syn., *limen.*

absolute t. The least stimulus value that will produce a response or cause a transition from no sensation to sensation. Syn., *stimulus threshold.*

achromatic t. Light threshold.

brightness difference t. The smallest difference in luminous intensity that can be perceived as a difference in brightness. Syn., *light difference.*

chromatic t. The minimum intensity of a specified wavelength of light that gives rise to a sensation of color. Syn., *specific threshold.*

color t. Chromatic threshold.

differential t. The smallest difference between two stimuli that for a given individual gives rise to a perceived difference in sensation. Syn., *just noticeable difference.*

discrimination t. The smallest detectable change in a sensory stimulus.

double point t. Two point threshold.

flicker fusion t. Critical fusion frequency.

general t. Light threshold.

light t. The absolute threshold for the perception of light. It varies with the state of dark adaptation, location of the retinal area stimulated, size of the stimulus, spectral composition of the stimulus, etc. Syn., *light minimum; achromatic threshold; general threshold.*

linear t. of distance discrimination. Threshold of stereopsis expressed in terms of the linear difference in distance of the test objects.

movement t. 1. The minimum movement of an object that can be perceived. 2. The maximum speed at which an object moving between two points can be perceived as moving. 3. The minimal conditions necessary for inducing phi movement.

pause t. The shortest time interval between two pulses of light that will provide for the perception of two flashes, or the shortest interruption in otherwise continuous light that can be perceived as such.

photochromatic t. The lowest luminance at which hue is perceived.

relational t. The ratio between two stimulus values when their difference is just noticeable.

resolution t. The threshold of ability to resolve or perceive separately two small, nearly adjacent objects observed simultaneously; the minimum separable.

size t. The minimum perceptible size of an object, usually defined in minutes of arc. See *visual acuity.*

specific t. Chromatic threshold.

t. of stereopsis. The smallest difference between the two binocular parallactic angles subtended at two objects which just gives rise to a perceptible difference in distance of the two objects from the observer; the smallest difference in retinal disparity created by two objects, in space, which gives rise to a just perceptible difference in distance. Syn., *lower threshold of stere-*

opsis; stereoacuity. **lower t. of s.** Threshold of stereopsis. **upper t. of s.** The largest difference between the two binocular parallactic angles subtended at two objects which gives rise to a perceptible difference in distance of the two objects without producing physiological diplopia; the greatest difference in retinal disparity created by two objects in space which gives rise to a perceptible difference in distance without producing physiological diplopia, i.e., the retinal disparity is within Panum's area.

> **stimulus t.** Absolute threshold.

> **two point t.** The minimum separation at which two points are perceived as two. Syn., *double point threshold.*

thromboangiitis obliterans (throm"-bo-an"je-i'tis ob-lit'er-ans). Buerger's disease.

thrombosis (throm-bo'sis). The formation or presence of a thrombus.

thrombus (throm'bus). A plug or clot in a blood vessel or in the heart, formed by coagulation of the constituents of the blood and remaining at the site of its formation.

Thygeson's superficial punctate keratitis. See under *keratitis, punctate.*

thyrotoxicosis (thi"ro-tok"sih-ko'sis). Graves' disease.

TIB. Turville's infinity balance test.

Tibbs binocular trainer. See under *trainer.*

tic douloureux (tik"doo"loo-roo'). Sudden, spasmodic, painful muscular twitching in the face. Syn., *trigeminal neuralgia.*

Tiedemann's nerve (te'de-manz). See under *nerve.*

Tillaux, spiral of (te-yo'). See under *spiral.*

Tillyer lens (til'yer). See under *lens.*

tilt, face. Head tilt.

tilt, head. 1. A deviation of the head from its upright position, especially as a clinical symptom. 2. A forward or backward tilt of the head, as distinguished from *shoulder tipping.* Syn., *face tilt.*

time. The period during which a condition, a process, or an action continues or occurs.

> **accommodation t.** The time interval required to change the accommodation from one dioptric level to another. Positive or negative accommodation time relates to increase or decrease of accommodation, respectively.

> **action t.** 1. The time interval required, following the latent period, for a sensation or response to reach its maximum intensity. 2. The minimum duration required of a stimulus to give a maximum effect.

> **blanking t.** The interval of time between a flashed stimulus and a subsequent flash of light which totally prevents perception of the former.

> **breakup t.** The time interval between a complete blink and the appearance of the first dry spot on the cornea following topical application of fluorescein and viewed under magnification in cobalt-blue filtered light. Abbreviation *BUT.*

> **cortical t.** The period of time (about 33–35 msec) between a flash of light and the appearance of the positive electroencephalogram potential.

> **fixation t.** 1. The time required for the eye to change fixation from one point to another. 2. The time during which the eye steadily fixates an object.

> **fixation response t.** The time interval between the onset of an extrafoveal stimulus and the beginning of eye movement to fixate the stimulating target. Syn., *eye reaction time.*

> **nystagmic t.** The time interval between the observed onset of induced nystagmus and the observed termination.

> **perception t.** The maximum period of time between a flashed stimulus and a subsequent flash of light which interferes with perception of the former.

> **persistence t.** 1. The time during which a response continues after termination of the stimulus. 2. The duration of the darkness interval at the critical flicker frequency.

> **reaction t.** The time between the onset of a stimulus and the response. **eye r.t.** Fixation response time.

> **recognition t.** The time between the onset of a stimulus and its identification.

> **regression t.** The time, in reading, in which a readjustment fixation is made at the beginning of a new line or in which words previously fixated in the same line are refixated.

> **retinal t.** The period of time (about 25 msec) between a light flash and the beginning of the *b*-wave of the electroretinogram.

retino-cortical t. The period of time required for an impulse to travel the entire afferent visual pathway, beginning in the retina and terminating in the visual cortex; the cortical time minus the retinal time.

wearing t. The length of time a contact lens can be worn continuously without discomfort, blurredness, haze, abrasion, edema, injection, or other subjective or objective signs of damage or unfavorable tissue reaction.

tinea favosa (tin'e-ah fa-vo'sah). Favus.

tinea tarsi (tin'e-ah tar'si). Mycotic blepharitis.

tint. 1. A mixture of white with a color, thus the antonym of *shade*. 2. Any color lighter than median gray. 3. A slight coloring; a pale or faint tinge of any hue. 4. A term descriptive of a difference in hue only, as, "A yellower tint of green." 5. To color slightly; to tinge.

Ostwald t's. In the Ostwald color system, mixtures of semichromes with white.

tintometer, Lovibond (tin-tom'eh-ter). An empirical colorimeter in which light from the sample is matched with light passed through a combination of red, yellow, and blue filters that are numbered approximately in proportion to their densities. The color of the sample is then specified (in the Lovibond system) by three numbers representing the sums of all glasses of each of the three colors inserted into the instrument to obtain a match.

tipping, shoulder. A tilting of the head toward one shoulder, especially as a clinical symptom.

tissue. A group of cells of similar structure and their intercellular substance.

border t. of Elschnig. A ring of white fibrous tissue and neuroglia around the optic nerve, separating it from adjacent sclera and the choroid.

intercalary t. of Elschnig. Connective tissue and neuroglial elements surrounding the central retinal vessels in the lamina cribrosa.

intermediate t. of Kuhnt. A ring or partial ring of glial tissue around the optic nerve and separating it from the adjacent retina.

pore t. of Flocks. Endothelial meshwork of Speakman.

Tolosa-Hunt syndrome. See under *syndrome.*

tone, color. 1. A perceptual attribute of color variously corresponding to hue, color, or lightness. 2. A variation of a color other than a change of hue. 3. In the Ostwald system, the black content of a color.

affective c.t. The emotional affective tone associated with the perception of different colors, thought to be a learned response, whence green, e.g., may be a soothing color.

Ostwald c.t's. In the Ostwald color system, mixtures of semi-chromes with black.

tongs, tourmaline. Two plates of tourmaline crystal, mounted parallel to each other on a tonglike handle, providing for variable separation and rotation about a common axis perpendicular to their surfaces, serving as a polarizer and analyzer.

tonicity (to-nis'ih-te). The condition of normal tone or tension of muscles.

tonofibrils (ton'o-fi"brilz). Delicate fibers found in the cytoplasm of epithelial cells, such as those of the cornea.

tonogram (to'no-gram). The recorded changes in tonometer readings obtained during tonography.

Tonographer, Mueller (to-nog'rah-fer). A Mueller Electronic Tonometer coupled to a strip-chart recorder, used in tonography.

tonography (to-nog'rah-fe). The determination of the rate of outflow of aqueous humor under the continuous pressure exerted by the weight of a tonometer over a 4 to 5 min period, as represented in a series of changes or a continuously recorded change in tonometer readings.

constant pressure t. Tonography in which the intraocular pressure is maintained approximately constant by incremental increases in plunger load corresponding to changes in tonometer readings. Syn., *isotonography.*

edrophonium chloride t. See *test, edrophonium chloride tonogram.*

◆

TONOMETER

tonometer (to-nom'eh-ter). An instrument for determining ocular tension, usually by measuring the impressibility of the tunics of the eye, so as to evaluate intraocular pressure.

applanation t. A tonometer in which the ocular tension is determined either by the force required to flatten a constant area of the cornea, as with the Goldmann tonometer, or by the area flattened by a constant force, as with the Maklakov tonometer.

Bailliart t. An impression tonometer using a calibrated spring instead of weights, with corneal and scleral direct reading pressure scales and interchangeable footplates for corneal or scleral use.

corneal t. A tonometer applied to the anterior surface of the cornea.

Crescent Electronic t. The trade name for an indentation tonometer of the Schiötz type equipped with a transistorized circuit and an electronic readout, used in tonometry or tonography.

Draeger t. A hand-held applanation tonometer which indicates ocular tension by the force required to applanate a corneal area of constant size and having a counterweight mechanism permitting measurements independent of patient position. It contains a microscope with a built-in scale, a light source to illuminate both the applanated area and the scale, an adjustable support for steadying the instrument against the forehead, and a motor-controlled, spring-loaded lever arm for adjusting the force on the plunger.

Durham t. An applanation tonometer which indicates ocular tension by the air pressure required to flatten a fixed small area of the cornea or sclera in the center of an area flattened by the footplate. It consists essentially of a diaphragm-covered flat footplate having a pneumatic sensing nozzle in its center, an air pump, bottled gas, a pneumatic-to-electric transducer, and a combined amplifier and strip recorder.

electronic t. Any tonometer with an electronic readout, usually a meter or strip recorder.

Fick's t. An applanation tonometer in which the area of application is held constant while the pressure is varied.

Gambs t. The trade name for an applanation tonometer of the Goldmann type.

Goldmann t. An applanation tonometer consisting essentially of a transparent plastic footplate, a pair of juxtaposed prisms with bases in opposite directions, a coil spring and lever system to apply force to the prisms and footplate, and a dial calibrated in centimeters of mercury. The edge of the contact area is rendered visible by the instillation of fluorescein into the tears and is seen through the prisms and a blue filter, with a slit lamp microscope, as two light green semicircles on a blue ground. Force is varied until the semicircles interlock, so that the inner edge of the upper coincides with the inner edge of the lower.

Gradle t. A type of impression tonometer.

Halberg t. A hand-held applanation tonometer consisting of a transparent plunger weight combined with a lens system and a millimeter scale which permit direct viewing and measuring of the diameter of the applanated area.

Harrington t. A modified Schiötz tonometer with a transparent plastic footplate and a circular dial which magnifies the readings four times that of the Schiötz instrument.

Husted t. An impression tonometer which evaluates ocular tension through the closed eyelid by determining the compression required on a spring-loaded plunger to produce an indentation of 3.5 mm, a direct reading being obtained from a scale on the spring-enclosing barrel.

impression t. A tonometer which measures the depth of the impression produced by a plunger of small bearing area carrying a known weight. The excursion of the plunger is read from a calibrated scale. Syn., *indentation tonometer.*

indentation t. Impression tonometer.

MacKay-Marg Electronic t. A tonometer having a flat plunger, in the center of the flat footplate of the probe, sensitive to displacements of less than one micron and which measures the ocular tension in the center of a small area of the cornea flattened by the footplate. It electrically records on a scaled strip the counter force required to resist displacement of the plunger, to keep it flush with the footplate, and thus to flatten the corneal area in contact with the plunger.

Maklakov's t. One of a set of five applanation tonometers ranging in weight from 5–15 gm and consisting of a dumbbell-shaped metal cylinder balanced on the cornea with the aid of a loop on a handle. One end is for the right eye and one for the left, and each end has a flat disk of polished glass which is coated with a dye prior to placement on the cornea. The area of the cornea flattened is indicated by the smallest diameter of the area of dye removed, measured by holding a transparent plastic scale against the end plate and by referring this finding to a table.

McLean t. An indentation tonometer, similar in construction to the Schiötz tonometer, in which a weighted plunger is placed on the cornea and the ocular tension is read directly from an attached scale calibrated in millimeters of mercury.

micro-transfiguration t. An electrical recording tonometer consisting of a synthetic resin footplate and plunger both of which are slightly concave and through which the resistant force of the cornea is measured by an electric strain gauge and recorded on a moving time scale.

Mueller Electronic t. The trade name for an indentation tonometer of the Schiötz type equipped with an electronic readout, used principally in tonography.

Perkins t. A portable, hand-held tonometer utilizing essentially the features of the Goldmann applanation tonometer.

Schiötz t. An impression corneal tonometer which consists essentially of a footplate, a weighted plunger, and a measuring scale to record the vertical movement of the plunger.

scleral t. An impression tonometer applied to the surface of the sclera.

Souter's t. A tonometer in which the area of application is constant while the pressure is increased until the plunger produces the slightest recognizable indentation of the cornea.

Tonair t. A pneumatic tonometer in which a probe of fixed mass applanates an area of the surface of the cornea or sclera in excess of that of the central plunger of the instrument, and air pressure supplied by a chamber behind the central plunger is increased until the force against the posterior plunger surface just exceeds the force of the eye against its front surface. At this point air escapes from the chamber, resulting in a constant pressure serving as a measure of the ocular tension read from a dial calibrated in millimeters of mercury.

Tonomat t. Trade name for a Maklakov type tonometer.

vibration t. See *Vibra-Tonometer.*

Wolfe t. A modified Bailliart tonometer, especially intended for use on the sclera.

◆

tonometry (to-nom'eh-tre). Measurement of ocular tension with a tonometer.

applanation t. See under *tonometer.*

ballistic t. Tonometry in which photographs are made of the oscillations in the recoil of a minute hammer striking the cornea under standard conditions.

differential t. The use of different weights on the plunger in successive measurements with an impression tonometer.

digital t. Estimation of the ocular tension by applying light pressure to the eyeball through the upper eyelid with the fingers.

impression t. See under *tonometer.*

tonotics (to-not'iks). A method of visual training which stresses rotations of the eyes, performed for short periods of time with frequent rest periods.

tonus (to'nus). The slight continuous contraction present in muscles not undergoing active movement.

ophthalmokinetic t. Tonus imparted to the extraocular muscles by stimuli originating in the semicircular canals of the inner ear.

ophthalmostatic t. Tonus imparted to the extraocular muscles by stimuli originating from the otoliths in the inner ear.

top, Benham's. A disk, half black and half white, with a number of concentric black arcs on the white sector, which, when rotated, elicits a variety of chromatic color sensations. Syn., *Benham's disk.*

top, Maxwell's color. A device for studying the effects of additive color mixing, consisting of a spinning top with a flat surface on which various colors are placed in sectors.

top, Munsell. A three dimensional representation of colors in the Munsell system in which the series of neutrals, from white through gray to black, form the central core, and the various hues are arranged in circles of increasing saturation around the central gray of the same lightness.

Topalanski's sign. See under *sign*.

Topogometer (to-pog'om-eh-ter). A device attached to the front of a keratometer which provides a movable fixation target for measuring corneal curvature at points other than at the line of sight, the displacement of the fixation target from the optical axis of the instrument being indicated by a horizontal and vertical scale.

topometer (to-pom'eh-ter). An instrument for photographing, from both front and side views, the position of a pair of lenses mounted in front of the eyes.

Toposcope (top'o-skōp). An instrument used to measure the curvature characteristics of a contact lens by the use of moiré fringes. The fringes are created by nearly superimposing the reflected or refracted image of a grating upon a second grating attached to a microscope.

Toposcope, Corneal (top'o-skōp). An instrument used to measure corneal curvatures from limbus to limbus by the use of moiré fringes.

topotaxis (top'uh-tak-sis). Directional movements of a motile organism in response to light stimulation. See also *klinotaxis; tropotaxis; telotaxis; menotaxis; mnemotaxis; phototaxis; scototaxis*.

toric (tor'ik). 1. Pertaining to, resembling, or shaped like a surface, or a segment of a surface, described by a circle rotating about a straight line in its own plane, especially about an off-center line. 2. Pertaining to a lens which has one surface with meridians of least and greatest curvature located at right angles to each other. 3. A toric lens.

Tornatola's theory (tōrn"ah-to'-lahz). See under *theory*.

toroidal (to-roi'dal). 1. Pertaining to, resembling, or shaped like a surface, or a segment of a surface, described by a circle rotating about a straight line in its own plane, especially about an off-center line. 2. Pertaining to a lens which has one surface with meridians of least and greatest curvature located at right angles to each other.

torpor retinae (tōr'por ret'ih-ne). Lack of response of the retina to stimuli of normal threshold value.

Torres-Ruiz implant; lens. See under *lens*.

torsiometer (tōr"se-om'eh-ter). An instrument for measuring torsion, cycloductions, or cyclophorias.

torsion (tōr'shun). Rotation, or more specifically cyclorotation, of the eye around an anteroposterior axis such as the fixation axis. See also *extorsion; intorsion; dextrotorsion; levotorsion; angle of torsion*.

false t. The apparent cyclorotation associated with a change in direction of regard from the primary position to a tertiary position, which occurs when movement of the eye is analyzed in terms of azimuth and elevation (Helmholtz system) or in terms of longitude and latitude (Fick system). When the movement is analyzed in terms of the rotation of the eye around Listing's axis, no cyclorotation or torsion is found; hence, the cyclorotation found by other means of analysis is called false torsion.

fusional t. Torsion induced by cyclofusional stimuli.

minus t. Torsion in which the upward extension of the vertical retinal meridian rotates temporally from the true vertical.

negative t. Torsion in which the eye rotates in the direction opposite to that of the hands of a watch which it fixates.

plus t. Torsion in which the upward extension of the vertical retinal meridian rotates nasally from the true vertical.

positive t. Torsion in which the eye rotates in the same direction as the hands of a watch which it fixates.

secondary t. False torsion.

true t. Torsion representing an actual rotation of the eye around its line of sight with respect to a given system of axes for specifying eye movements; distinguished from *false torsion*.

tort. In reference to the eye, to rotate about an anteroposterior axis, i.e., to a position of torsion.

torticollis (tōr"tih-kol'is). Head tilting; twisting of the neck, producing an unnatural position of the head.

congenital t. Torticollis present from birth, due to primary contracture of the sternocleidomastoid muscle of one side. It is differentiated from *ocular torticollis* in that it is more pronounced, the head cannot be passively straightened, and conjugate ocular movements are normal.

neurogenic t. Torticollis due to irritation of the spinal accessory nerve.

ocular t. Torticollis which serves to compensate for hyperphoria or for paresis or paralysis of one or more of the vertically acting extraocular muscles. It is differentiated from congenital torticollis in that it is less pronounced, no true contracture of the sternocleidomastoid muscle is present, the head can be passively straightened, and conjugate ocular movements may be abnormal.

tortoise shell. Shell plates from the hawksbill turtle used in the making of spectacle frames.

Touraine's syndrome; systemic elastorrhexia. Elastosis dystrophica.

Touraine-Solente-Golé syndrome. See under *syndrome.*

tourmaline (tŏŏr'mah-lin, -lēn). A mineral crystal, a silicate of boron and aluminum, which polarizes light by absorbing the ordinary ray and transmitting the extraordinary ray.

Tournay's pupillary reflex (tŏŏr-nāz'). See under *reflex.*

toxoplasmosis (toks"o-plaz-mo'sis). A disease caused by infection with the protozoan parasite *Toxoplasma* and occurring in a number of forms. The congenital or infantile type, which produces encephalitis, is especially associated with chorioretinitis, appearing bilaterally as deep, heavily pigmented, necrotic lesions affecting both macular and peripheral areas, and with secondary optic nerve atrophy. There is extensive connective tissue proliferation from the lesions, the retina surrounding the lesions remains normal, and the ocular media remain clear.

Toynbee's corpuscle (toin'bēz). Corneal corpuscle.

trabecula (trah-bek'u-lah). A small column, fiber, or bundle of fibers in the framework of an organ.

bridge trabeculae. A fine net of fibrillar tissue spanning the opening of some of the crypts of the iris.

corneoscleral trabeculae. Corneoscleral meshwork.

uveal trabeculae. Uveal meshwork.

trabeculectomy (trah-bek"u-lek'to-me). Surgical removal of a portion of the trabecular meshwork to facilitate aqueous humor outflow in glaucoma.

trabeculodialysis, anterior (trah-bek"u-lo-di-al'ih-sis). A surgical procedure for glaucoma in which the corneoscleral trabeculae are detached from the overlying sclera, allowing free communication of the canal of Schlemm with the anterior chamber.

trabeculotomy (trah-bek"u-lot'o-me). Surgical incision of the trabecular meshwork to create a communication between the anterior chamber and outflow channels, for the treatment of glaucoma.

trachoma (trah-ko'mah). A chronic, contagious, viral infection of the conjunctiva and the cornea characterized by the formation of conjunctival follicles, papillary hypertrophy, pannus, and subsequent cicatrization. The course of the disease may be classified into four stages: (1) Infection of the epithelium of the conjunctiva and the cornea followed by subepithelial infiltration, formation of minute follicles, mild conjunctivitis, and inclusion bodies in epithelial scrapings. (2) Inflammatory reaction in the subepithelial tissues and the tarsal plate with the formation of larger follicles, papillae, and pannus. This stage lasts from several months to several years and mainly affects the upper eyelids, giving them a granular appearance resembling that of a raspberry. (3) Necrosis of subepithelial tissue leading to extensive and deforming cicatrization. (4) Subsidence of the disease with the persistence of scar tissue and the sequellae of ptosis, trichiasis, entropion, symblepharon, corneal opacities, and xerosis of the conjunctiva and the cornea. It responds favorably to sulfanilamide treatment. Syn., *Egyptian conjunctivitis; granular conjunctivitis; Egyptian ophthalmia; granular ophthalmia; military ophthalmia; war ophthalmia.*

Arlt's t. The granular form of trachoma.

trachomatous (trah-ko'mah-tus). Pertaining to, of the nature of, or affected with trachoma.

tracing, ray. Tracing of the paths of selected light rays through a schematic representation of a longitudinal section of an optical system.

◆

TRACT

tract. 1. A bundle or collection of nerve fibers in the brain or the spinal cord. 2. A system of organs serving a special purpose, such as the digestive tract.

anterior accessory optic t. of Bochenek. A bundle of decussated optic nerve fibers from the retina, found in some subprimates, which originates at the posterior chiasma and courses through the cerebral peduncle to terminate at the subthalamic nucleus. Syn., *anterior accessory optic bundle of Bochenek; anterior accessory fasciculus of Bochenek.*

corticobulbar t. A group of fibers, arising in the motor cortex, which synapse in motor nuclei of the cranial nerves throughout the brain stem and subserve voluntary control of skeletal muscles. The cells of origin are the large pyramidal cells (including the giant cells of Betz) located in the fifth layer of the cerebral cortex. All fibers of the tract pass through the corona radiata, twist their way in such a fashion as to occupy a particular locus in the internal capsule, and then pass downward into the base of the cerebral peduncle, with the individual fibers splitting off at the appropriate level to go to the nuclei of the III, IV, V, VI, VII, IX, X, XI, and XII cranial nerves. Syn., *corticonuclear tract.*

corticomesencephalic t. Voluntary fibers of the corticobulbar tract that arise in the frontal eye field, descend as a portion of the pyramidal system, decussate within the pons, and terminate with the motor nuclei of cranial nerves III, IV, and VI.

corticonuclear t. Corticobulbar tract.

corticotectal t. A group of fibers originating from cell bodies located in the striate, the parastriate, and the peristriate areas of the visual cortex in the occipital lobe. The fibers pass between the pulvinar and the geniculate bodies of the thalamus, course through the brachium of the superior colliculus and synapse in the tectal region of the midbrain with fibers of either the tectobulbar or colliculonuclear tracts to bring impulses ultimately to the nuclei of the extraocular muscles. It also contains fibers from the peristriate area which are involved in the accommodation near pupillary reflex. Syn., *occipitomesencephalic tract.*

Darkschewitsch's t. A bundle of nerve fibers that leave the optic tract, proceed to the habenular ganglion, pass through the posterior commissure, and end in the contralateral oculomotor nucleus. Their use in the indirect or consensual pupillary reflex is not established.

geniculocalcarine t. A group of axons, conveying visual impulses, which arise in the lateral geniculate body and pass out in a fan-shaped manner to terminate in the area striata of the occipital lobe. Syn., *optic radiations of Gratiolet.*

geniculocortical t. Geniculocalcarine tract.

occipitomesencephalic t. Corticotectal tract.

optic t's. The centralward continuation of the optic nerves beyond the optic chiasm, by which the visual impulses travel from the optic chiasm to the brain. From the posterolateral angle of the chiasm, the optic tracts run lateral and backward, each taking the form of a rounded band, running at first between the tuber cinereum and the anterior perforated substance behind which it is continued posteriorly as a flattened band sweeping around the cerebral peduncles in close association with the posterior cerebral artery. Reaching the posterolateral aspect of the optic thalamus, each breaks into two roots: (1) a lateral and larger root which ends in the lateral geniculate body; (2) a medial and smaller root which runs to the lateral geniculate body.

opticotectal t. Nerve fibers from the optic tract which run to the superior colliculus via the superior brachium.

posterior accessory optic t. of von Gudden. Transverse peduncular tract.

pyramidal t. The corticospinal and corticobulbar tracts.

spinal t. of the trigeminal nerve. A nerve tract located in the medulla and the cervical cord, composed of sensory fibers of the trigeminal nerve which terminate in the nucleus of the spinal tract of the trigeminal nerve, transmitting pain and temperature impulses from the head area.

tectobulbar t. A group of fibers arising from cell bodies located in the superior colliculus of the tectum which cross in the dorsal tegmental decussation and descend to their termination in three locations: (1) the motor nuclei of the lower part of the medulla oblongata; (2) the pontine nuclei; and (3) the reticular formation of the brain stem.

tectopontine t. A group of nerve fibers originating in the superior colliculus, and some in the inferior colliculus, of the tectum which, together with the tectospinal and tectobulbar tracts, crosses in the fountain decussation of Meynert and descends to synapse with pontine nuclei.

tectospinal t. A group of nerve fibers originating in the superior colliculus, and some in the inferior colliculus, of the tectum which, together with the tectobulbar and tectopontine tracts, crosses in the fountain decussation of Meynert and descends to synapse with motor neurons in the spinal cord that supply skeletal muscles. It conveys impulses mediating reflex postural movements in response to auditory and visual stimuli.

transverse peduncular t. A tract, present in about 30% of humans, which originates from the optic tract, travels transversely over the ventral surface of the cerebral peduncle and enters the midbrain near the exit of the oculomotor nerve. Syn., *posterior accessory optic tract of von Gudden.*

uveal t. The iris, the ciliary body, and the choroid considered collectively.

vestibulo-ocular t. A tract of homolateral and contralateral nerve fibers arising from the vestibular nuclei, which ascends in the medial longitudinal fasciculus to the nuclei of the oculomotor, the trochlear, and the abducens nerves. The tract mediates reflex movements of the head and eyes.

visual t. Visual pathway.

◆

tractus hyaloideus (trak'tus hi"ah-loid'e-us). Membrana plicata of Vogt.

tractus opticus (trak'tus op'tih-kus). Optic tract.

Trainer, Alpha Brightness Enhancement. Trade name for an instrument which is essentially a modification of the *Translid Binocular Interaction Trainer* to provide colored lights and adjustability of light intensity.

Trainer, Aperture-Rule. Trade name of an instrument for orthoptic fusional training consisting of a calibrated, pedestal-mounted rod at the distal end of which is a holder for a card with two laterally separated patterns or figures. These are to be fused or seen superimposed by visual alignment through a single rectangular aperture in an opaque card placed intermediately between the pattern card and the eyes for convergence training, or through a pair of similarly placed rectangular and laterally separated apertures for divergence training.

trainer, television. An antisuppression visual training device consisting either of two perpendicularly oriented Polaroid filters or of complementary-colored red and green filters mounted side by side and attached in front of a television screen, such that, when viewed through appropriate filters, a portion of the television picture is visible only to one eye and another portion is visible only to the other eye.

trainer, Tibbs binocular. A visual training instrument consisting of three wood leaves, hinged together at one end as in a book, with a plane mirror on each face of the middle leaf. With the middle leaf held to the nose as a septum, a target placed on the inner face of one outer leaf is seen by one eye by reflection from the mirror and is perceived as though originating on the inner face of the other outer leaf, on which the projected image may be traced, or superimposed or fused with a second target seen directly by the other eye.

Trainer, Translid Binocular Interaction. Trade name for an orthoptic training instrument consisting essentially of two very small light bulbs to be held in gentle contact with the two closed eyelids and flashed alternately at about 7 to 10 cycles per second. Abbreviation *TBI trainer.* Cf. *Alpha Brightness Enhancement Trainer.* Syn., *Translid Binocular Interactor.*

Trainer, Van Orden. A visual training device consisting essentially of a target holder mounted at one end of a rod, with transilluminated targets, and two pairs of lens cells at the other end, one fixed and one vertically adjustable so that it may be flipped down in front of the fixed cells to vary accommodative demand.

training, visual. The teaching and training process for the improvement of visual perception and/or the coordination of the two eyes for efficient and comfortable binocular vision. Cf. *orthoptics.* Syn., *visual therapy; vision therapy; vision training.*

chiastopic v.t. See *chiastopic fusion.*

diplopia v.t. Visual training to eliminate peripheral suppression by inducing awareness of physiological or pathological diplopia. Syn., *peripheral visual training*.

distance motivation v.t. Visual training to improve distance visual acuity in which test type is brought toward the eyes until it is distinguished, the attempt then being made to continue reading as it is moved back.

orthopic v.t. See *orthopic fusion*.

peripheral v.t. Diplopia visual training.

plus-acceptance v.t. Visual training to increase negative relative accommodation, positive fusional reserve convergence, or manifest hypermetropia in which the attempt is made to see clearly through increasing amounts of convex lens power introduced binocularly.

pointer v.t. Visual training to improve hand and eye coordination and spatial localization, or to eliminate suppression, in which the patient locates objects in a stereogram, a vectogram, or an anaglyph, with pointers.

primary v.t. Visual training of monocular functions.

secondary v.t. Visual training to establish or improve sensory fusion.

specific v.t. 1. Visual training to establish or improve motor fusion. 2. Visual training to establish or improve any specific visual function.

transcurve. The curve on the posterior surface of the transitional zone of a scleral contact lens.

transformation. A shift from one mode of appearance to another, e.g., from film to surface color, brought about by a change in the physical conditions of viewing or by a change in the mental set of the observer.

transillumination (trans"ih-lu"mih-na'shun). Illumination transmitted through a wall, usually translucent, especially to illuminate the interior of a body cavity or organ.

transition. Transitional zone.

Translid Binocular Interactor. Trade name for a photostimulator with two small alternately flashing bulbs separated by approximately the patient's interocular distance and held in contact with the closed eyelids to transilluminate the retinas at a frequence of 9 Hz. Abbreviation *TBI*. Syn., *Translid Binocular Interaction Trainer*.

translucence (trans-lu'sens). The con-dition of being translucent; partial transparency.

translucent (trans-lu'sent). Pertaining to a medium which transmits light diffusely so that objects viewed through it are not clearly distinguished; partially transparent.

translucid (trans-lu'sid). Translucent.

transmission. 1. The passing of radiant energy through a medium or space. 2. The ratio of the amount of radiant energy leaving the last surface of an optical system to the amount of radiant energy incident on the first surface.

diffuse t. Transmission in which the emitted light is scattered in all directions.

regular t. Transmission in which the direction of the emitted light bears a definite relationship to the direction of the incident light.

transmissivity (trans"mih-siv'ih-te). The internal transmittance for a unit thickness of a nondiffusing substance.

atmospheric t. The ratio of directly transmitted light per unit distance in the atmosphere from a projected or signal source to that identically transmitted in vacuum.

transmissometer (trans"mih-som'eh-ter). An instrument for measuring transmittance of radiant energy.

transmittance (trans-mit'ans). The ratio of radiant flux transmitted through a body to that incident on it. Syn., *transmission factor*.

diffuse t. The ratio of diffusely transmitted flux leaving a surface or medium to incident flux.

directional t. Transmittance determined in a given direction.

hemispherical t. The total luminous flux emerging from the surface of a transilluminated layer of translucent or transparent material divided by the total incident flux.

internal t. The ratio of the flux incident on the second surface of a medium to that transmitted by the first.

luminous t. The ratio of luminous flux transmitted by the object to the incident luminous flux.

radiant t. Transmittance.

regular t. The fraction of incident flux transmitted through a medium without being scattered.

spectral t. Transmittance for a specific wavelength of incident flux.

specular t. The proportion of the flux of a collimated beam transmitted through a turbid medium without deviation.

transmittancy (trans-mit'an-se). The ratio of the transmittance of a solution to that of the solvent in equivalent thickness.

transocular (trans-ok'u-lar). Extending across the eyeball.

transparency. 1. The state or quality of being transparent. 2. A picture to be viewed by the aid of light transmitted through it.

transparent. Pertaining to a medium having the property of transmitting light so that objects can be seen through it.

transplantation, cornea (trans-plan-ta'shun). The operation of transplanting healthy corneal tissue to replace opaque or diseased corneal tissue removed from another eye or rotated in the same eye. See *keratoplasty.*

transplantation, vitreous. A surgical procedure for retinal detachment in which donor vitreous is injected into the vitreous chamber.

transpose. To alter or change the mathematical form of representation of the focal properties of an ophthalmic lens, specifically from the sphere-combined-with-minus-cylinder form to the sphere-combined-with-plus-cylinder form, or vice versa.

transposition. The act of transposing. See also *transpose.*

trans-retinene. See *retinaldehyde.*

Trantas' dots (tran'tas). See under *dot.*

Traquair's concept (trah-kwārz). See under *concept.*

traumatic (traw-mat'ik). Pertaining to, of, or caused by, an injury.

Travers' test (trav'erz). See under *test.*

Treacher Collins syndrome (trĕch'er kol'inz). Mandibulofacial dysostosis.

tree, color. A three dimensional representation of all colors, chromatic and achromatic, in an orderly arrangement according to their hue, value, and chroma (or saturation). The achromatic series of black, grays, and white constitutes the "trunk" or axis of the tree, the various hues are arranged circumferentially around this axis, and chroma or saturation is represented as the radial distance from the axis. See also *color sphere.*

Treleaven's method (tre-lev'ens). See under *method.*

trepanation (trep"ah-na'shun). Trephining.

trephining (tre-fi'ning, -fe'ning). Removal of a circular button or disk of tissue.

   corneoscleral t. Trephining at the superior corneolimbal junction into the anterior chamber under a conjunctival flap, followed by an iridectomy at the trephine hole, for glaucoma.

   limboscleral t. Trephining at the superior scleral limbal junction into the anterior chamber under a conjunctival flap, followed by an iridectomy at the trephine hole, for glaucoma. Syn., *limbosclerectomy.*

triad (tri'ad). A group of three related symptoms or signs.

   Basedow's t. The three cardinal symptoms of exophthalmic goiter: exophthalmos, goiter, and tachycardia. Syn., *Merseburg triad.*

   Charcot's t. The three cardinal symptoms of multiple sclerosis: nystagmus, intention tremor, and staccato speech.

   Hutchinson's t. A syndrome found in congenital syphilis consisting of notched teeth (Hutchinson's teeth), interstitial keratitis, and deafness.

   Jacod's t. Total ophthalmoplegia, amaurosis, and trigeminal neuralgia from involvement of cranial nerves two through six by a tumor in the region of the cavernous sinus and the chiasm. Syn., *Negri-Jacod syndrome.*

   Merseburg t. Basedow's triad.

trial case; frame; lens. See under the nouns.

triangle, Arlt's. Arlt's sign.

triangle, Birren's constant hue. A systematic arrangement of tints and shades of a single hue based on the Ostwald color system; it specifies for each hue sample the percentages of white and of black mixed with the pure color. Thus, the designation 7–57 indicates that this sample is a mixture of 7% white, 57% black, and 36% color.

triangle, color. A chromaticity diagram whose coordinates are represented on a triangle with three primary colors assigned to apices, and mixtures of these primaries represented by nonapical points whose positions designate the proportion of each primary in the mixtures.

   Helmholtz'c.t. A chromaticity diagram similar to Maxwell's color triangle, but having two real spectral primaries at two of its apices and an imaginary third primary at the other apex, whereby the locus of all spectral colors is represented by a curved line inside the triangle. Syn., *Helmholtz' color table.*

Koenig's c.t. A chromaticity diagram similar in principle to Helmholtz' color triangle, based on measurements of spectral mixtures and employing three imaginary primaries of greater saturation than spectral red, green, and blue.

Maxwell's c.t. A chromaticity diagram whose coordinates are represented on an equilateral triangle with three real color primaries assigned to the apices and each mixture of a pair of colors designated by a "center of gravity" point on the line connecting the colors mixed. Since real primaries are employed, many of the spectral and near-spectral colors are represented by extrapolated points outside the triangle. Syn., *Maxwell's color table.*

Ostwald c.t. An arrangement of colors of a single constant Ostwald hue in a triangle with black, white, and an Ostwald semichrome at the corners, and orderly variations of black content, white content, and full color content within the triangle.

Young's c.t. The color triangle as originally conceived by Young, with three primaries represented at the apices and mixtures represented by points within the triangle.

triboluminescence (tri"bo-lu"mih-nes'ens). The emission of light by friction.

TRIC. Acronym for *trachoma* and *inclusion conjunctivitis.*

trichiasis (trih-ki'ah-sis). Inversion of the eyelashes resulting in impingement on the eyeball and subsequent irritation.

trichiniasis (trik"ih-ni'ah-sis). Trichinosis.

trichinosis (trik"ih-no'sis). A disease due to infestation with *Trichinella spiralis* produced by eating undercooked pork containing this nematode parasite, characterized by muscular and abdominal pain, nausea, diarrhea, fever, and stiffness and swelling of the muscles. Eye signs include edema of the eyelids, subconjunctival petechiae, chemosis, and encystment of the larvae in the extraocular muscles causing ocular immobility because of pain on movement. Syn., *trichiniasis.*

trichomegaly (trik"o-meg'ah-le). A condition in which the eyelashes are abnormally long.

trichosis carunculae (trih-ko'sis kah-rung'ku-le). Abnormal growth of hair on the caruncle.

trichroic (tri-kro'ik). Pertaining to trichroism.

trichroism (tri'kro-iz"em). The property of a substance, especially crystal, which exhibits a different color from each of three different directions of view.

trichromacy (tri-kro'mah-se). Trichromatism.

trichromasy (tri-kro'mah-se). Trichromatism.

trichromat (tri'kro-mat). One having trichromatism.

trichromate (tri'kro-māt). Trichromat.

trichromatic (tri"kro-mat'ik). Requiring the use of three color mixture primaries to match all perceived hues. Syn., *trichromic.*

trichromatism (tri-kro'mah-tizm). Color vision in which mixtures of three independently adjustable primaries (e.g., red, green, and blue) are required to match all perceived hues. Syn., *trichromacy; trichromasy; trichromatopia; trichromatopsia; trichromatic vision.*

anomalous t. A form of defective color vision in which three primary colors are required for color matching, but the proportions of primaries in the mixture-matches are significantly different from those required in normal trichromatism. It occurs in three forms: *protanomaly, deuteranomaly,* and *tritanomaly.* Syn., *partial dichromatism; anomalous trichromasy; anomalous trichromatic vision; color weakness.*

deuteranomalous t. Deuteranomaly.

protanomalous t. Protanomaly.

tritanomalous t. Tritanomaly.

trichromatopia (tri"kro-mah-to'pe-ah). Trichromatism.

trichromatopsia (tri"kro-mah-top'se-ah). Trichromatism.

trichromator (tri-kro'ma-tor). A colorimeter which isolates three selected spectral bands and combines them for color-matching investigation.

trichorrhexis nodosa (trik"o-rek'sis no-do'sah). A rare condition, of unknown etiology, in which the hairs show regularly spaced swellings and tend to break at them. It is congenital and may involve the eyelashes as well as the hair of the scalp.

trichromic (tri-kro'mik). Trichromatic.

trident, visual. The collective visual field of birds of prey of approximately

180°, consisting of a central binocular field derived from the common straight-ahead projection of the temporal foveae and two lateral uniocular fields, each associated with a laterally projecting central fovea.

trifocal (tri-fo'kal). See under *lens.*

trigeminus (tri-jem'ih-nus). The trigeminal nerve.

Trioptic lens. See under *lens.*

triplet (trip'let). A combination of three lenses.

    aplanatic t. A microscopic lens consisting of a double convex crown glass lens, cemented between two concave flint glass meniscus lenses, which provides magnification relatively free from chromatic aberration and distortion.

    Hastings' t. A series of aplanatic triplets of different magnifying powers, designed by C. S. Hastings.

triplokoria (trip"lo-ko're-ah). The abnormal condition of three pupils in one eye.

triplopia (trip-lo'pe-ah). The condition in which a single object is perceived as three rather than as one.

triptokoria (trip"to-ko're-ah). Triplokoria.

tristichia (tris-tik'e-ah). Tristichiasis.

tristichiasis (tris"tih-ki'ah-sis). The anomalous condition of three rows of eyelashes. Syn., *tristichia.*

tritan (tri'tan). One having tritanopia or tritanomaly. Syn., *tritanoid.*

tritanoid (trit"ah-noid', tri"tah-). 1. One having color vision of the tritanopic or tritanomalous type; a tritanomal or a tritanope. Syn., *tritan.* 2. Of, pertaining to, or having the characteristics of tritanopia or tritanomaly. Syn., *tritanous.*

tritanomal (trit-an'o-mal, tri-tan'-). One having tritanomaly.

tritanomaly (trit"ah-nom'ah-le, tri"tah-). A rare type of defective color vision in which an abnormally large proportion of blue must be mixed with green in order to match a standard blue-green stimulus. Very few cases of tritanomaly have been described, so details of its characteristics are not well known. Syn., *tritanomalous trichromatism.*

tritanope (trit'an-ōp, tri'tan-). One having tritanopia or defective color vision of the tritanopic type.

tritanopia (trit"ah-no'pe-ah, tri"-tah-). A form of dichromatism in which all col-

ors can be matched by suitable mixtures of only a red primary and a green (or blue) primary. Brightness (luminosity) of all colors is within normal limits. Sensitivity to differences in hue of blues, blue-greens, and greens is greatly reduced, but discrimination of short wavelength violets appears to be superior to that of normal observers. A neutral point occurs at about 570mμ in the spectrum. Acquired tritanopia occurs as the result of retinal disease or detachment. Congenital tritanopia is rare; its incidence is estimated as between 1 in 13,000 and 1 in 65,000, the higher frequency being more probable. The mode of inheritance is not yet known, but is unlike that of the protanoid and deuteranoid defects, although a slight sex difference has been shown. Syn., *blue blindness; blue-yellow blindness; tritanopic vision.*

    small-area t. A normal reduction in color discrimination for the blue wavelengths found for color fields of small angular subtense (approximately twenty minutes of arc or less) stimulating the central fovea. Under these stimulus conditions, all colors can be matched by a mixture of two primaries, and purplish blues and greenish yellows are confused with neutral and with each other.

tritanopic (trit"ah-nop'ik, tri'tah-). Pertaining to or having tritanopia.

tritanous (trit'ah-nus, tri'tah-). Tritanoid.

trochlea (trok'le-ah). A ringlike structure of fibrocartilage attached to the trochlear fossa of the frontal bone through which passes the tendon of the superior oblique muscle. It is lined by endothelium and to it is attached the fascial sheath of the muscle.

trochlear (trok'le-ar). Pertaining to the trochlea or the trochlear nerve.

trochlearis (trok"le-a'ris). The superior oblique muscle.

troland (tro'land). A unit of retinal illumination equal to that produced by viewing a surface having a luminance (photometric brightness) of 1 candela per square meter through a pupil having an area of 1 square mm, originally called *photon* by Troland and later renamed in his honor to differentiate it from a photon of light energy.

Troland's theory (tro'landz). See under *theory.*

Troncoso (tron-ko'so) **goniolens; contact lens.** See *goniolens, Troncoso.*

tropia (tro'pe-ah). Strabismus.

tropicamide (troh-pik'ah-mīd). A parasympatholytic drug used as a mydriatic and cycloplegic.

tropo-menotaxis (tro"po-men-o-tak'-sis). A type of light-compass reaction in which the orientation of movement is governed primarily by the intensity of the light or by the summated intensities of more than one light. See also *telomenotaxis*.

tropometer, Steven's (tro-pom'-eh-ter). An instrument for measuring the extent of rotation of an eye, consisting essentially of a head rest, a metal box with a circular aperture containing a transparent glass disk with a central fixation dot, a mirror in the box at a 45° angle behind the glass disk, and a telescope viewing system attached to the box. An aerial image of the fixating eye is focused on a graduated disk in the telescope, and the excursions of the eye are measured with the graduations on the disk.

tropophorometer (tro"po-fo'rom-eh-ter). An instrument with two universally adjustable arms effectively pivoted at the respective centers of rotation of the two eyes and each equipped with a fixation light visible only to the corresponding eye at a distance of 38 cm. The positions of the two lights provide a measure of the vertical and lateral angles of the phoria or tropia when adjusted to eliminate fixational movement with alternate occlusion.

Troposcope (tro'po-skōp). A type of major amblyoscope.

tropotaxis (tro"po-tak'sis). Movement of a motile organism toward or away from light as mediated by two symmetrical light receptors which simultaneously detect differences of light intensities from a single source, thus serving to orient the organism in the proper direction. See also *klinotaxis; telotaxis; menotaxis; mnemotaxis*.

Troutman's air space doublet. See under *doublet*.

Troxler's (troks'lerz) **effect; phenomenon.** See under *phenomenon*.

trueing. The restoring of a desired curvature to a worn lens-grinding tool.

Tru-Scope. The trade name for an instrument that projects either a 12× or a 20× magnified image of a contact lens onto a calibrated viewing screen for the purpose of inspection.

Tschermak's (cher'makz) **diagram;**

rectangle; test. See under the nouns.

Tschermak-Seysenegg visual illusion. See under *illusion, visual*.

Tscherning (chern'ing) **ellipse; filters; theory.** See under the nouns.

tube. A hollow cylindrical structure; something resembling a cylindrical structure; something with a tube or tubelike part as its chief feature.

Bowman's t's. Artifacts in stained corneal sections, originally thought to be spaces between the lamellae of the corneal stroma.

Gershun t. A long straight tube blackened on the inside so that as diffused light enters at one end, the amount of light emerging at the other end, where a photocell may be placed, is a function of the length of the tube and its diameter.

Gratama's t's. A pseudoscope used in the detection of malingering.

photoelectric t. A vacuum or gas-filled tube which produces electrical current when radiant energy is received on its sensitive surface (cathode). It may be used with either a galvanometer or an electrometer for photometric measurements.

photomultiplier t. Photomultiplier.

Wessely's t's. A device used to detect malingering, consisting essentially of two viewing tubes slightly converged toward each other, through which a distant object is fixated. Physiological diplopia produced by placing an object in front of the tubes indicates vision in both eyes.

tubercle (tu'ber-kl). 1. A small nodule or protuberance. 2. The nodular lesion produced by the tubercle bacillus.

infraoptic t. A roughness on the small wing of the sphenoid bone between the optic foramen and the sphenoidal fissure, to which is attached lower tendon of Zinn.

lacrimal t. A tubercle on the anterior lacrimal crest where the frontal process of the superior maxillary bone becomes continuous with the lower orbital margin.

lateral orbital t. A small elevation on the orbital surface of the zygomatic bone, just within the outer orbital margin and about 11 mm below the frontozygomatic suture. It gives attachment to the check ligament of the lateral rectus muscle, the ligament of

Lockwood, the lateral palpebral ligament, and the aponeurosis of the levator palpebrae superioris muscle. These combined attachments form the *lateral retinaculum of Hesser.* Syn., *Whitnall's tubercle.*

muscular t. A small bony tubercle, on the small wing of the sphenoid bone below the optic foramen, which frequently marks a point of origin of the extraocular muscles.

Whitnall's t. Lateral orbital tubercle.

zygomatic t. A tubercle on the frontosphenoidal process of the zygomatic bone, beneath the frontozygomatic suture.

tuberous sclerosis (tu'ber-us skle-ro'-sis). Bourneville's disease.

tucking. A surgical procedure for shortening an extraocular muscle for the correction of strabismus, in which a portion of the tendon of the muscle is folded on itself and sutured in position.

tularemia, oculoglandular (too"lah-re'me-ah). Infection with the bacterium *Pasteurella tularensis*, transmitted to humans from rabbits or other rodents, characterized by acute inflammation and chemosis of the conjunctiva, small, yellow, necrotic ulcers primarily on the tarsal conjunctiva, high fever, headaches, vomiting, and involvement of the parotid, preauricular, submaxillary, and cervical glands. Syn., *Ohara's disease.*

tunic (tu'nik). A membrane, or a layer of tissue, covering an organ or a part of the body.

fibrous t. of the eye. The outer layer of the eyeball, consisting of the cornea and sclera.

Haller's t. Haller's layer.

nervous t. of the eye. The retina.

vascular t. of the eye. The uvea.

tunica (tu'nih-kah). A tunic.

t. adnata oculi. 1. The bulbar conjunctiva. 2. The conjunctiva.

t. albuginea oculi. The sclera.

t. chorioidea. The choroid.

t. conjunctiva bulbi. The bulbar conjunctiva.

t. conjunctiva palpebrarum. The palpebral conjunctiva.

t. cornea pellucida. The cornea.

t. dura. The sclera.

t. fibrosa lentis. Fibrous tissue surrounding the embryonic crystalline lens.

t. fibrosa oculi. The outer layer of the eyeball, consisting of the cornea and the sclera.

t. interna oculi. The retina.

t. nervosa oculi. The retina.

t. ruyschiana. The choriocapillary layer of the choroid.

t. uvea. The uvea.

t. vasculosa choroideae. The uvea.

t. vasculosa lentis. The vascular network surrounding the embryonic crystalline lens, derived anteriorly from branches of the annular vessel and posteriorly from branches of the hyaloid artery. It normally degenerates and disappears prior to birth. **persistent t.v.l.** Persistent hyperplastic primary vitreous.

t. vasculosa oculi. The uvea.

t. vitrea. The hyaloid membrane.

tuning. See *adisparopia.*

Tuohy contact lens (too'e). See under *lens, contact.*

Turay (tu'ra). A trade name for a one-piece bifocal lens.

Türk's (tĕrks) **disease; line.** See under the nouns.

turn, face. Head rotation.

turn, head. Head rotation.

Turner's theory. See under *theory.*

Turville's test (tur'vilz). See under *test.*

tutamina oculi (tu-tam'ih-nah ok'-u-li). The protective appendages of the eye, as the eyelids, the eyelashes, and the eyebrows.

Twinsite (twin'sīt). A trade name for a one-piece bifocal lens.

twirl, sphere. A − .25 D spherical lens and a + .25 D spherical lens so mounted on a handle that spinning or twirling the handle alternates first one and then the other before the eye, providing a sudden change of spherical power while a distant test object is observed.

Twyman and Green interferometer (twi'man). See under *interferometer.*

tyloma conjunctivae (ti-lo'mah kon"-junk-ti've). A localized cornification of the conjunctival epithelium, occurring in xerosis of the conjunctivae. Syn., *keratosis conjunctivae.*

tylosis (ti-lo'sis). Hypertrophic blepharitis.

Tyndall's (tin'dalz) **cone; effect; light; phenomenon.** See under the nouns.

type, case. See under *case*.

type, test. Letters, figures, or characters used in vision testing.

Bjerrum t.t. Black test letters on a gray background used for testing retinal sensitivity in persons suspected of having retinal or optic nerve pathology.

Jaeger t.t. A numbered arrangement of words and phrases in various sizes of ordinary printer's type on a chart, for testing visual acuity at given reading distances.

Landolt t.t. Incomplete rings of various sizes, similar to the letter C in appearance, used as test targets for visual acuity, especially in children and illiterates. The width of each ring and the break in its continuity are each one fifth of its over-all diameter. The breaks are placed in different positions with their locations to be identified by the observer, and the identification of breaks subtending 1 minute of arc corresponds to 20/20 vision.

Pray's t.t. Assorted, relatively large letters, each hatched with lines in a given, different meridian, whence the most distinctly seen letter indicates, by the orientation of its hatching lines, the principal meridian of the astigmatism of the viewing eye.

Sheridan-Gardiner t.t. A modification of the STYCAR test employing only seven symmetrical letters, AHOTUV and X, to permit use of a mirror to double the test distance.

Snellen t.t. A series of letters for testing visual acuity, each so constructed that it can be enclosed in a square five times the thickness of the limbs composing the letter. Each limb, and the separation between, subtends a visual angle of one minute at a specified distance, hence each entire letter subtends a visual angle of 5 minutes at this distance. See also *Snellen fraction*.

Weiss's t.t. Test type arranged so that each type size represents an equal decimal interval of visual acuity from the preceeding and following ones, whence the acuity is expressed as .9, .8, etc.

typhloid (tif'loid). Pertaining to or having defective vision.

typhlolexia (tif'lo-lek'se-ah). Word blindness.

typhlology (tif-lol'o-je). The science that deals with blindness; the scientific study of blindness, its causes, effects, etc.

typhlosis (tif-lo'sis). Blindness.

typoscope (ti'po-skōp). A rectangle of dull black material having a central rectangular aperture of a size allowing two or three lines of type to be seen through it when laid against a printed page. It is used by persons having subnormal vision to aid vision by excluding extraneous light reflected from the surface of the paper.

U

U. Symbol for *reduced object vergence*.
U′. Symbol for *reduced image vergence*.
u. Symbol for *object distance*.
u′. Symbol for *image distance*.
Uhthoff's sign (oot′ofs). See under *sign*.
Ulbricht sphere. Integrating sphere. See under *sphere*.

◆

ULCER, CORNEAL

ulcer, corneal (ul′ser). Pathological loss of substance of the surface of the cornea, due to progressive erosion and necrosis of the tissue.

c.u. of acne rosacea. A corneal ulcer, either marginal or central, resulting from the rupturing of a vesicle, in rosacea keratitis. It has a tendency to recur, is resistant to treatment, and after repeated attacks the entire cornea may become scarred and vascularized.

ameboid c.u. Geographic corneal ulcer.

atheromatous c.u. A rapidly progressing corneal ulcer occurring in an old leucomatous scar which has undergone degeneration. Perforation followed by panophthalmitis often takes place.

catarrhal c.u. A crescent-shaped ulcer near the limbus associated with catarrhal conjunctivitis. The conjunctiva opposite the ulcer is usually swollen and chemotic, and capillary vascularization often extends from the pericorneal arcades.

chronic serpiginous c.u. A rodent corneal ulcer.

creeping c.u. A serpiginous corneal ulcer.

dendritic c.u. A branching linear-shaped, corneal ulcer occurring in herpes simplex of the cornea. The ends of the branches are typically club-shaped, it is slow in healing, and is accompanied by pain, lacrimation, and photophobia.

eczematous c.u. Phlyctenular corneal ulcer.

fascicular c.u. A corneal ulcer which commences at a phlycten, in phlyctenular keratoconjunctivitis, and creeps toward the central area of the cornea. As the circular edge advances centrally, the peripheral portion is healing, and a straight sheath of blood vessels from the conjunctiva follows in the furrow created by the ulcer. It never perforates, usually remains superficial, and the blood vessels gradually disappear after the ulcer heals.

geographic c.u. A sharply demarcated, irregularly shaped, superficial corneal ulcer formed in the late stage of herpetic keratitis by loss of the epithelium between the branches of a dendritic ulcer; so named because its outline resembles the map of a continent. Syn., *ameboid corneal ulcer*.

hypopyon c.u. 1. A serpiginous corneal ulcer. 2. A severe suppurative corneal ulcer accompanied by hypopyon. Syn., *panmural fibrosis*.

indolent c.u. A shallow, superficial ulcer, usually located centrally in the cornea, occurring in debilitated children. It is unaccompanied by vascularization and infiltration, causes little reaction or few symptoms, and shows little tendency to spread or to heal.

internal c.u. An ulcer involving the posterior surface of the cornea, usually with loss of the endothelium and Descemet's membrane in the affected area, and typically occurring in association with inflammatory involvement of the cornea or uvea.

marantic c.u. A superficial corneal ulcer typically of long duration and with a delay in scar formation, occurring with little or no infiltration and in association with metabolic disturbances of the cornea or with chronic debilitating disease.

metaherpetic c.u. A small, round or oval, superficial, corneal ulcer which follows the healing of a dendritic ulcer.

Mooren's c.u. Rodent corneal ulcer.

phlyctenular c.u. A corneal ulcer, resulting from the breakdown of a corneal phlycten, which may heal without leaving an opacity or may progress to a fascicular corneal ulcer. Syn., *eczematous corneal ulcer; scrofulous corneal ulcer.*

pneumococcal c.u. Serpiginous corneal ulcer.

rodent c.u. A painful, chronic, superficial ulcer of unknown etiology, occurring in elderly people, which commences near the limbus and may partially or completely surround the cornea and slowly progress centrally until the entire cornea is involved. Its advancing border characteristically has a grayish, crescentic, thickened, overhanging ledge. Syn., *chronic serpiginous corneal ulcer; Mooren's ulcer; ulcus corneae rodens.*

Saemisch's c.u. Serpiginous corneal ulcer.

scrofulous c.u. Phlyctenular corneal ulcer.

serpent c.u. Serpiginous corneal ulcer.

serpiginous c.u. A severe, disk-shaped, corneal ulcer, caused by the pneumococcus, characterized by a marked tendency to spread in one direction and usually associated with diffuse keratitis, iridocyclitis, and hypopyon. It has a gray sloughing base and a yellow crescentic advancing border, increases rapidly in depth as well as in extent, usually starts with an abrasion, more commonly affects the elderly or the debilitated, and may result in perforation of the cornea. Syn., *creeping corneal ulcer; hypopyon corneal ulcer; pneumococcal corneal ulcer; Saemisch's corneal ulcer; serpent corneal ulcer; ulcus corneae serpens.*

trachomatous c.u. A superficial indolent ulcer appearing at the advancing margin of a trachomatous pannus.

◆

ulcer, Jacob's (ul'ser). A basal-celled carcinoma or rodent ulcer of the eyelid, typically commencing with a raised nodular border and indurated base, which extends superficially and deeply and erodes the surrounding tissue of the face and the nose.

ulcus (ul'kus). An ulcer.

u. corneae rodens. Rodent corneal ulcer.

u. corneae serpens. Serpiginous corneal ulcer.

u. eczematosum. Phyctenular corneal ulcer.

ulerythema ophryogenes (u-ler''ih-the'mah of''re-o'jens). A chronic disease of the skin of the eyebrows marked by redness, hard conical elevations at the base of the hair, and loss of hair.

Ullrich's syndrome. See under *syndrome.*

Ultex (ul'teks). A trade name for a one-piece bifocal or trifocal lens.

ultramicroscope. A microscope utilizing the diffraction of a pencil of high intensity illumination by otherwise invisibly small particles in colloidal suspension so that they appear as bright spots against a dark background. Syn., *dark-field microscope.*

ultrasonogram, orbital (ul''trah-son'o-gram). A composite photograph of the serial recordings of the echoes of ultrasound waves reflected from structures of the eye or orbit occupying successive horizontal planes, primarily to detect and localize tumors.

ultrasonography, orbital (ul''trah-son-og'rah-fe). The production and study of the orbital ultrasonogram. Syn., *orbital echography.*

ultrasonography, time amplitude (ul''trah-son-og'rah-fe). A technique for determining anteroposterior ocular dimensions by oscilloscopic display of the ultrasound echo from each ocular media interface as a vertical sweep on a horizontal time scale.

ultraviolet (ul''trah-vi'o-let). Radiant energy of wavelengths shorter than the violet end of the visible spectrum and longer than the roentgen radiations, usually considered to be wavelengths of from 400 to 200 mμ.

umbilication of the lens (um-bil"-ih-ka'shun). A developmental abnormality of the crystalline lens consisting of a shallow gutter or depression in its posterior surface.

umbo. 1. A rounded protuberance, or the corresponding depression, as, e.g., the central portion of a lenticular lens. 2. The apex or pole of a spherical lens surface. 3. The small central concavity of the foveola.

umbra (um'brah). The part of the shadow of an opaque body receiving no illumination from the source of reference. Cf. *penumbra.*

umbraculum (um-brak'u-lum). A flap-like contractible structure protruding from the iris margin of the hyrax and some cetaceans. It may be extended almost to occlude the pupillary aperture or be retracted to be free of it.

umbrascopy (um-brahs'ko-pe). Retinoscopy.

Umstimmung. See *adisparopia.*

uncut. Pertaining to an ophthalmic lens with both surfaces finished but not edged to its desired size and shape.

undercorrection. 1. Ophthalmic lens power less than that required to correct or neutralize a refractive error. 2. An aberration of a lens or an optical system in which the marginal rays intersect the optical axis at a point nearer the lens than the paraxial rays; the spherical aberration normally present in a lens.

unifocal (u"nih-fo'kal). Pertaining to or having a single focus.

uniform density. See *lens, uniform density.*

Uni-Form lenses. See under *lens.*

unilateral. Affecting, pertaining to, or located in one side or half of the body with reference to the midsagittal plane.

uniocular (u"nih-ok'u-lar). Pertaining to, identified with, having, or performed with one eye. Syn., *monocular.*

Union Nationale des Optometristes et Opticiens de Belgique. An association of Belgian opticians and optometrists founded in 1954. In Flemish, National Verbond des Optometristen en Opticiens van Belgie.

l'Union Nationale des Syndicats d'Opticiens de France. The major ophthalmic optical organization in France, its membership consisting essentially of retail optical establishments which are primarily engaged in

dispensing, with occasional sight-testing.

unit. 1. A specific amount or quantity used as a standard measurement. 2. A distinct part of an aggregate whole. 3. A single thing or person, or a group regarded as an individual member of an aggregate of groups.

Aloe distance u. A Galilean telescopic system with an adjustable focus, which is hooked over a spectacle lens for distance viewing in subnormal vision, providing 3× magnification.

Aloe reading u. A Galilean telescopic system, providing 2.2× magnification, which is hooked over a spectacle lens for near viewing in subnormal vision.

angstrom u. A unit of wavelength of radiant energy, one unit being equal to one ten-millionth of a millimeter. Symbol: A or Å.

C u. Retinal elements in fish which give rise to graded changes in the resting potential as a function of the wavelength stimulating the retina, being opposite in polarity for red and green and for yellow and blue. Syn., *chromatic unit.*

chromatic u. C unit.

Freeman Near Vision U. A triangular-shaped instrument presenting transilluminated, near point test targets on each of its three faces which may be either hand held or attached to a phoropter near point rod. The targets are polarized to permit monocular testing under binocular conditions and include a red-green test for determining and balancing the near point addition, the Worth-Ramstein test for checking binocular vision and fusion, a graduated Landolt ring chart, a reading chart, and a heterophoria test used in conjunction with a Maddox rod.

Giles-Archer color perception u. A device for testing color vision deficiencies and central scotomata, consisting of a lantern with various size apertures and a series of color filters.

L u. Retinal elements in fish which give rise to the same type of polarity change in the normal resting potential for all wavelengths, a graded change of potential occurring as a function of light intensity. Syn., *luminosity unit.*

luminosity u. L unit.

Mallett Near Fixation Disparity Test U. A hand-held, transilluminated test target consisting of a small, central fixation spot with two short, adjacent, vertical, cross-polarized, line segments, one directly above and the other directly below, to be observed for lateral vernier misalignment through a pair of cross-polarized filters in front of the eyes.

Osterberg Bino near vision test u. A hand-held, self-illuminated device for testing visual acuity and binocular functioning at various reading distances, with targets mounted in a rotatable disk so as to be individually exposed, and an attached tape for measuring the test distance.

Telesight u. Trade name for prism binoculars mounted and hinged to be worn over conventional glasses or raised when not in use.

UNOOB. See *Union Nationale des Optometristes et Opticiens de Belgique.*

UNSOF. See *l'Union Nationale des Syndicats d'Opticiens de France.*

Updegrave's method (up'de-grāvz). See under *method.*

uranin (u'rah-nin). Sodium fluorescein used in dilute solution as a dye which fluoresces under black light, for determining the fit of contact lenses, and for the detection of external pathology, such as corneal or conjunctival abrasions or ulcers, the affected areas staining a yellow-green.

Ur-O-Vue. A trade name for an instrument used in the inspection of contact lenses consisting essentially of a self-contained light source, an optical system providing 14× magnification, and a viewing screen on which either the shadow image of the edge profile or the image of the transilluminated lens itself may be observed.

Usher's syndrome. See under *syndrome.*

utrocular (u-trok'u-lar). Pertaining to the ability to judge which eye is perceiving. See also *utrocular discrimination.*

uvea (u've-ah). The pigmented vascular coat of the eyeball, consisting of the choroid, the ciliary body, and the iris, which are continuous with each other.

uveitis (u"ve-i'tis). Inflammation of the uvea.

anaphylactic u. Uveitis resulting from reaction to a foreign protein such as a bacterial protein.

anterior u. Iridocyclitis.

atopic u. Uveitis caused by hypersensitivity of the tissues to an allergen, not by a local organismal infection.

atrophic u. A recurring uveitis in blind degenerated eyes that is presumed to be due to toxins liberated by tissue necrosis.

u. of Boeck's sarcoid. Sarcoidosis affecting the uveal tract, especially the iris, although it may also invade the choroid.

Förster's u. Diffuse syphilitic inflammation of the entire uveal tract.

granulomatous u. Nonpurulent, endogenous uveitis characterized by nodular or tuberclelike lesions on the iris, mutton-fat deposits on the anterior lens capsule, marked tendency to the formation of posterior synechia, and frequently Koeppe's nodules. The onset is insidious rather than acute, and it may be due to infection with any of a variety of nonpyogenic agents, as in toxoplasmosis, actinomycosis, sarcoidosis, syphilis, or tuberculosis.

heterochromic u. Heterochromic cyclitis of Fuchs.

nongranulomatous u. Nonpurulent, endogenous uveitis in which the onset is usually acute and marked by ciliary congestion, photophobia, and lacrimation. There are no nodules and little tendency to the formation of posterior synechia. Aqueous flare is usually pronounced, small pinpoint deposits are on the posterior surface of the cornea, but neither mutton-fat deposits nor Koeppe's nodules are present. It mainly affects the anterior uvea only, is usually of short course with prompt recovery, and is considered due to physical, toxic, or allergic causes.

peripheral u. A form of granulomatous uveitis which commences in the region of the pars plana or ora serrata. It may emanate from inflammation of the ciliary body or of the peripheral choroid, or may result from perivasculitis of the peripheral retinal blood vessels.

phacoanaphylactic u. Inflammation of the uveal tract occurring after extracapsular cataract extraction or a needling operation, presumed to be an allergic reaction to one's own liberated lenticular proteins.

phacolytic u. Uveitis secondary to hypermature cataract and due to permeation of liquefied cortical material through the lens capsule.

phacotoxic u. Inflammation of the uveal tract attributed to toxic reaction to liberated lens proteins following cataract surgery or, in hypermature cataract, to liquefied cortical material which has permeated the lens capsule.

sympathetic u. Sympathetic ophthalmitis.

uveoparotitis (u″ve-o-par″o-ti′tis). Chronic bilateral parotitis, uveitis, fever, and often paralysis of the cranial nerves, especially the seventh, occurring characteristically in young people and considered to be a form of sarcoidosis. The uveitis is generalized and usually includes a nodular iridocyclitis. Other ocular manifestations may include keratitis, optic neuritis, cata-

ract, and glaucoma. The disease is self-limiting, and the only permanent disability is visual impairment. Syn., *Heerfordt's disease; uveoparotid fever; Heerfordt's syndrome.*

uveoscleritis (u″ve-o-skle-ri′tis). Inflammation of both the uvea and the sclera.

uveoscopy (u″ve-os′ko-pe). Biomicroscopic examination of the iridocorneal angle, the iris, and the anterior ciliary body with a Goldmann gonioscope and illumination localized by means of fiber optics.

Uyemura syndrome. See under *syndrome.*

V

V. Abbreviation for *vision*.

VA. Abbreviation for *visual acuity*.

vaccinia, ocular (vak-sin′e-ah). A virus infection with smallpox vaccine which may accidentally occur on the eyelids, the conjunctiva, or the cornea as a result of careless inoculation from a vaccine pustule located elsewhere. On the eyelid, it appears as a pustular eruption which may ulcerate, on the cornea as a marginal infiltration, an interstitial pustule, or a disciform keratitis, and on the conjunctiva as a membranous conjunctivitis with extensive ulceration. The condition is usually accompanied by fever and swelling of the preauricular and the postauricular glands.

vagina (vah-ji′nah). A sheath or sheath-like structure.

v. bulbi. Tenon's capsule.

v. oculi. Tenon's capsule.

vaginae nervi optici. The sheaths of the optic nerve.

valence (va′lens). The capacity of a visual stimulus to evoke a color sensation, as contrasted with its capacity to evoke brightness.

validity. The extent to which a test measures what it is intended to measure; the relevancy to the task for which a test is proposed as a criterion. Cf. *reliability*.

value. 1. The relative worth, importance, or degree of usefulness. 2. Brightness or lightness of a color.

C v. The coefficient of facility of aqueous outflow.

corneal eccentricity v. A mathematical specification of the deviation of the corneal surface from circular toward another conic section shape, e.g., ellipsoid.

F v. The rate of aqueous outflow.

mired-shift v. The amount a filter alters the color temperature of a source, expressed in mireds.

Munsell v. In the Munsell system, the portion of the notation corresponding to lightness and specified on a scale ranging from 1 (black) to 10 (white). It is approximately equal to the square root of the reflectance expressed in per cent.

nu (ν) v. The reciprocal of the dispersive power of optical glass. Syn., *Abbe's number*. See *optical constringence*.

P_o v. The magnitude of the intraocular pressure just prior to tonometric measurement.

P_t v. The magnitude of the intraocular pressure during tonometry.

P_v v. The average pressure in the small episcleral veins or in the aqueous veins near the limbus.

retinomotor v. A value assigned to a retinal receptor which indicates its angular distance and radial direction from the foveal center, or other point of reference. It provides information as to the angular extent and direction an eye must rotate to assume fixation of an image stimulating the receptor.

target v. The attention-drawing attribute of an object in the field of vision, especially as applied to traffic signs, signals, and markers.

tristimulus v's. The amounts of each of three primaries required to match a color. Symbols: X; Y; Z. **spectral t.v's.** Tristimulus values, symbols: $\bar{x}(\lambda)$, $\bar{y}(\lambda)$, $\bar{z}(\lambda)$, per unit wavelength interval per unit radiant flux of the colors of the spectrum, adopted by the CIE. They are tabulated as functions of wavelength throughout the spectrum and are employed for the evaluation of radiant energy as light. The $\bar{y}$ values are identical with values of spectral luminous efficiency for photopic vision.

V v. See *nu value*.

valve. A structure for closing an orifice or a passage or for preventing the backward flow of fluid.

    v. of Béraud. Valve of Krause.

    v. of Bianchi. Plica lacrimalis.

    v. of Bochdalek. A fold of mucous membrane at the punctum of the lacrimal canaliculus.

    v. of Cruveilhier. Plica lacrimalis.

    v. of Foltz. A fold of mucous membrane in the vertical protion of the lacrimal canaliculus, near the lacrimal punctum.

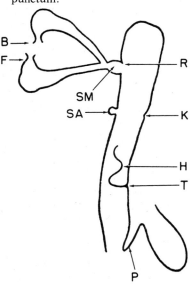

Fig. 39 Valves of nasolacrimal duct: (B) Valve of Bochdalek, (F) Valve of Foltz, (SM) Sinus of Maier, (R) Valve of Rosenmueller, (SA) Sinus of Arlt, (K) Valve of Krause, (H) Valve of Hyrtl, (T) Valve of Taillefer, (P) Plica lacrimalis. (From S. Duke-Elder, *Textbook of Ophthalmology*, vol. V. London: Henry Kimpton, 1952)

    Hasner's v. Plica lacrimalis. (See Fig. 39.)

    Huschke's v. Rosenmueller's valve.

    v. of Hyrtl. A pseudovalve consisting of a fold of mucous membrane between the valves of Krause and Taillefer in the nasolacrimal duct.

    v. of Krause. A pseudovalve consisting of a fold of mucous membrane at the junction of the lacrimal sac and the nasolacrimal duct. Syn., *valve of Béraud*.

    Rosenmueller's v. A crescentic fold in the lacrimal duct near its junction with the lacrimal sac. Syn., *Huschke's valve*.

    Taillefer's v. A pseudovalve consisting of a fold of mucous membrane above the plica lacrimalis in the nasolacrimal duct.

van Bogaert. See under *Bogaert*.

van der Heijde. See under *Heijde*.

van der Hoeve. See under *Hoeve*.

Van den Bosch syndrome. See under *syndrome*.

Van Orden star method; star; trainer. See under the nouns.

Vaquez' disease (vak'āz). See under *disease*.

varicoblepharon (var"ih-ko-blef'ah-ron). A dilated or varicose vein of the eyelid.

varicula (vah-rik'u-lah). An enlarged and tortuous vein of the conjunctiva.

vasa (vah'sah). Vessels.

    v. hyaloidea propria. Branches of the hyaloid artery of the fetal intraocular blood system which fill the vitreous cavity and anastomose with each other and with the posterior tunica vasculosa lentis.

    v. sanguinea retinae. The retinal blood vessels.

    v. vorticosa. The vortex veins.

vasculosa lentis (vas-ku-lo'sah len'tis). Tunica vasculosa lentis.

vase, Rubin's. A line drawing which may be perceived either as a vase or as two oppositely oriented human profiles.

VASIS. Acronym for *visual approach slope indicator system*.

vault. The dome-shaped inner surface of the corneal section of a scleral contact lens.

VCP. Visual comfort probability.

vectogram (vek'to-gram). A polarized stereogram consisting of two photographic images printed on opposite sides of a gelatin film with their axes of polarization at right angles to each other, to be viewed through Polaroid filters so that one image is seen only by one eye while the other is seen only by the other eye. Syn., *vectograph*.

vectograph (vek'to-graf). Vectogram.

Vectoluminator (vek"to-lu'mih-na"-tor). An instrument for transilluminating vectographs to be viewed through Polaroid filters at a near fixation distance.

vector-electronystagmography (vek"-tor-e-lek"tro-nis-tag-mog'-rah-fe). See under *electronystagmography*.

vector-electro-oculography (vek"-tor-e-lek"tro-ok"'u-log'rah-fe). See under *electro-oculography*.

Vego Graph. The trade name for an instrument that projects a magnified image of a contact lens onto a calibrated viewing screen for the purpose of inspection.

veils, congenital vascular, in the vitreous. Retinoschisis.

veil, prepapillary. Prepapillary membrane.

veil, Sattler's. Mistiness of vision usually accompanied by seeing colored halos around lights, resulting from wearing contact lenses and attributed to corneal edema. Syn., *Fick's phenomenon*.

veiling, dimple. Fogging of vision due to dimpling of the cornea in the pupillary area.

◆

VEIN

vein. A tubular vessel which conveys blood toward, or to, the heart. Like arteries, the walls of veins are composed of three coats, the tunica adventitia, the tunica media, and the tunica intima, though typically thinner. Many veins also have valves.

angular v. A vein, formed by the junction of the frontal and the supraorbital veins, which courses obliquely downward on the side of the root of the nose, about 8 mm medial to the inner canthus, to the level of the lower margin of the orbit, where it becomes the anterior facial vein. Its tributaries are an orbital branch, the superior and inferior palpebral veins, the supraorbital vein, and the frontal vein.

annular v. An annular vessel.

aqueous v's. Small vessels which transmit aqueous humor from the canal of Schlemm to episcleral, conjunctival, and subconjunctival veins.

central retinal v. A vein formed by the confluence of the superior and inferior retinal veins at about the level of the lamina cribrosa, lying temporal to the central retinal artery. After running a short course within the optic nerve, it leaves slightly posterior to the entrance of the central retinal artery and empties into the superior ophthalmic vein, the cavernous sinus, or rarely, the inferior ophthalmic vein.

chiasmal v., superior. One of two venous trunks which drain blood from the superior portion of the optic chiasm and empty into the anterior cerebral vein.

chorio-vaginal v's. Veins, lying in a stratum behind the retinal vessels, which drain a large portion of the posterior choroid and leave the eyeball in the region of the optic disk to course into the pia mater of the optic nerve.

ciliary v's., anterior. Veins which drain the anterior portion of the ciliary body, deep and superficial scleral plexuses, anterior conjunctival veins, and episcleral veins to empty into the muscular veins.

ciliary v's., posterior. 1. The vortex veins. 2. A few small veins which occasionally accompany the posterior ciliary arteries and drain the posterior region of the sclera.

cilioretinal v. A rare retinal vein which disappears at the optic disk margin instead of in the central retinal vein and drains into the ciliary system. Syn., *marginal vein*.

conjunctival v's., anterior. Veins which drain capillaries of the bulbar conjunctiva near the limbus and the superficial scleral plexus to empty into the anterior ciliary veins.

conjunctival v's., posterior. Veins which drain capillaries of the nonlimbal bulbar conjunctiva and the fornix to empty into the palpebral veins.

emissary v's. 1. Veins connecting the intracranial venous sinuses and the extracranial veins which function as added drainage channels for the venous blood of the brain, especially if the inner cranial pressure is temporarily increased. As they pass through the cranial wall, they receive tributaries from the diploë. 2. Veins joining the ciliary plexus with the episcleral veins. There are usually four to six in number, arranged circularly and symmetrically between the limbus and the equator.

episcleral v's. Veins which receive blood from the outer layer of the sclera, aqueous humor from the aqueous veins, and empty into the anterior ciliary and vortex veins.

ethmoidal v., anterior. A vein which drains the anterior ethmoidal air cells, the frontal sinus, the nose, and the dura mater, and passes through the anterior ethmoidal canal to empty into the superior ophthalmic vein.

ethmoidal v., posterior. A vein which drains the posterior ethmoidal air cells, the nose, and the dura mater, and passes through the posterior ethmoidal canal to empty into the superior ophthalmic vein.

facial v., anterior. A vein, commencing as a direct continuation of the angular vein at the root of the nose, which runs obliquely downward and backward until it meets the posterior facial vein, near the angle of the mandible, to form the common facial vein.

facial v., common. A vein formed by the confluence of the anterior and posterior facial veins, draining into the internal jugular vein at about the level of the hyoid bone.

facial v., deep. A vein connecting the pterygoid venous plexus and the anterior facial vein, of which it is considered a tributary.

facial v., posterior. A vein formed by the union of the superficial temporal and internal maxillary veins which descends in the substance of the parotid gland and divides into an anterior branch, which joins with the anterior facial vein to form the common facial vein, and a posterior branch, which unites with the posterior auricular vein to form the external jugular vein.

frontal v. A vein originating on the forehead as a venous plexus and communicating with the anterior division of the superficial temporal vein. It descends near the midline of the lower forehead as a single trunk; at the root of the nose it joins the supraorbital vein to form the angular vein.

lacrimal v. A vein which arises from the lacrimal gland, corresponding in its course to the lacrimal artery, and drains into the superior ophthalmic vein.

laminated v. A vein, consisting of a joined episcleral vein and an aqueous vein, in which blood and aqueous humor flow side by side.

marginal v. Cilioretinal vein.

muscular v's. Veins which drain extraocular muscles. Those of the rectus muscles receive the anterior ciliary veins. The upper muscular veins empty into the superior ophthalmic vein and the lower empty into the inferior ophthalmic vein.

nasofrontal v. A vein anastomosing with the angular vein at the orbital margin and emptying into the superior ophthalmic vein.

ophthalmic v., inferior. A vein extending from the anterior facial vein, over the inferior orbital margin, and continuing as a venous network on the floor of the orbit. It runs backward on the inferior rectus, dividing into two branches, one passing through the inferior orbital fissure to join the pterygoid plexus, the other passing through the superior orbital fissure to terminate in the cavernous sinus, usually in common with the superior ophthalmic vein. It receives branches from the inferior rectus and the inferior oblique muscles, the lacrimal sac, the eyelids, and the two inferior vortex veins.

ophthalmic v., superior. The largest orbital vein, formed in the upper part of the medial angle of the orbital margin by a communication with the frontal, the supraorbital, and the angular veins. It runs backward and somewhat laterally to the superior orbital fissure, where it meets the inferior ophthalmic vein and drains into the cavernous sinus. Its tributaries are the anterior ethmoidal, the posterior ethmoidal, the muscular, the lacrimal, the central retinal, the superior vortex, and usually the inferior ophthalmic veins.

optico-ciliary v. An uncommon retinal vein which drains a part of the choroid. It may appear abruptly at or near the disk margin, passing over the disk and draining into the central retinal vein, or it may drain into the central retinal vein behind the lamina cribrosa. Syn., *retinociliary vein.*

palpebral v's. Veins in the upper and lower eyelids, arranged in pretarsal and retrotarsal plexi or in venous arcades, which empty into the angular, the anterior facial, the supraorbital, the superior ophthalmic, the inferior ophthalmic, the lacrimal, and the superficial temporal veins.

papillary v., inferior. A vein formed in the region of the optic disk by the junction of the main retinal veins from the inferior temporal and inferior nasal quadrants and which, by confluence with the superior papillary vein within the optic disk, forms the central retinal vein.

papillary v., superior. A vein formed in the region of the optic disk by the junction of the main retinal veins from the superior temporal and superior nasal quadrants, and which, by confluence with the inferior papillary vein within the optic disk, forms the central retinal vein.

postcentral v. of Kuhnt. A branch of the central retinal vein which extends posteriorly in the center of the optic nerve to the optic foramen.

posterior central v. Postcentral vein of Kuhnt.

preinfundibular v. A semicircular venous arch on the inferior surface of the optic chiasm which courses anteriorly around the infundibulum, interconnects with the superior plexus of the optic chiasm, and empties into the basal veins.

recipient v. An episcleral vein which joins with an aqueous vein to form a laminary vein.

retino-ciliary v. Optico-ciliary vein.

supraorbital v. A vein which communicates with the superficial temporal vein and courses along the superior orbital margin to join the frontal vein at the medial angle of the orbit to form the angular vein. It sends a branch through the supraorbital notch to the superior ophthalmic vein.

v. of Vesalius. An emissary vein which passes through the foramen of Vesalius, medial to the foramen ovale in the great wing of the sphenoid bone, and forms a communication between the pterygoid plexus and the cavernous sinus.

vortex v's. Four, or more, veins formed by the confluence of four large whorls of veins in the choroid which drain blood from the iris, the ciliary body, and all of the choroid and leave the eyeball via canals in the sclera. They emerge slightly posterior to the equator of the eyeball and the superior and inferior veins drain into the superior and inferior ophthalmic veins, respectively. Syn., *vasa vorticosa; posterior ciliary veins; venae vorticosae.*

Velhagen's charts; plates; test. See under the nouns.

velocity of light. See *speed of light.*

velonoskiascopy (ve"lo-no-ski-as'ko-pe). A subjective method of determining ametropia, in which a very thin rod, held near to the eye, is moved across the pupil while a distant, small, light source is fixated. In myopia the perceived shadow of the rod will appear to move with the rod, in hypermetropia opposite to the movement of the rod, and in emmetropia no shadow is seen. Syn., *autoretinoscopy; rhabdoscopy.*

vena. A vein.

venography, orbital (ve-nog'rah-fe). Radiography of the veins of the orbit performed subsequent to injecting a contrast material into the angular vein, the frontal vein, or the supraorbital vein.

venting. Providing for or effecting the circulation of tear fluid under a contact lens by virtue of its design in relation to its riding position and movements.

aperture v. Venting facilitated by one or more fenestrations in a contact lens.

chamfer v. Venting facilitated by one or more grooves or channels on the posterior surface of the contact lens.

primary v. Venting facilitated by the design and selection of the conventional variables of the contact lens, such as base curve radius, peripheral curve radii, optical zone diameter, and size and shape of the lens.

secondary v. Venting facilitated by techniques employed in addition to those of primary venting, as, for example, apertures, grooves, ballasts, or truncations.

ventricle, optic (ven'trih-kl). The cavity of the optic vesicle.

VEOG. Visually evoked occipitogram.

Verdet constant. See under *constant.*

vergence (ver'jens). 1. A disjunctive rotational movement of the eyes such that the points of reference on the globes move in opposite directions, as in convergence, cyclovergence, or sursumvergence. 2. The dioptric or wavefront characteristic of a bundle of light rays, as when emanating from a point source (divergence) or directed toward a real image point (convergence).

accommodative v. See *accommodative convergence.*

fusional v. A vergence movement of the eye occurring as a response to disparate or unfused binocular stimuli, or the range or extent of such movement with respect to given conditions of reference. **reserve f.v.** Fusional vergence in excess of that required for the fixation distance, clinically measured by vergence-inducing prisms from the fusional demand point to the limit of clear, single, binocular vision.

image v. The vergence of the light leaving an optical surface, expressed in terms of the curvature of the wavefront, usually in diopters. **reduced i.v.** The reciprocal of the reduced image distance, hence the index of refraction of the image medium divided by the image distance. It is conventionally designated by the symbol U'.

jump v. See *jump duction.*

object v. The vergence of the light entering an optical surface, expressed in terms of the curvature of the wavefront, usually in diopters. **reduced o.v.** The reciprocal of the reduced object distance, hence the index of refraction of the object medium divided by the object distance. It is conventionally designated by the symbol U.

relative v. Fusional vergence measured and/or specified with reference to the position of the eyes corresponding to the normal fusional demand for a given testing distance. Its extent is clinically determined by the amount of vergence-inducing prism effect through which single, binocular vision can be maintained.

tonic v. The continuous vergence response maintained by the extraocular muscle tonus, hence absent in paralysis and in death and diminished during sleep or narcosis; the amount of vergence in effect when fixating a distant object with accommodational and fusional impulses absent.

vergens (ver'jenz). Vergence.

v. deorsum. Deorsumvergence.

v. sursum. Sursumvergence.

verger, Maddox prism (ver'jer). A pair of prisms of equal power, mounted in a frame so that one prism is before each eye, to rotate in opposite directions by equal amounts to give variable prismatic effect over a range from zero to the sum of the prism powers.

Verhoeff's (ver'hefz) **chart; circle; membrane; rings; test; theory; stereopter.** See under the nouns.

version (ver'zhun). A conjugate movement of the eyes such that their meri-

dians or lines of reference move in the same direction.

vertex (ver'teks). 1. The point of intersection of the principal axis with a reflecting or refracting surface. 2. A point of reference on the surface of a lens used in specifying the distance of the surface from another optical element in the system, ordinarily a point centered in the lens aperture.

vertex depth; distance; focal length; power; refraction. See under the nouns.

vertexometer, projection (ver"teks-om'eh-ter). An instrument for determining the vertex refractive power, cylinder axis, optical centers, and the prismatic effect of ophthalmic lenses with the test pattern, reference marks, and scales in view on a ground glass screen instead of in an eyepiece.

vertigo (ver'tih-go, ver-ti'go). The sensation that one is revolving in space or that fixed objects in space are revolving about one.

epidemic paralyzing v. Gerlier's disease.

ocular v. Vertigo attributed to an ocular or oculomotor disorder.

Vertometer (ver-tom'eh-ter). A trade name for an instrument which determines the vertex refractive power, the cylinder axis, the optical center, and the prismatic effect of ophthalmic lenses.

vesicle (ves'ih-kl). 1. A small bladder or sac containing fluid. 2. A small blister. 3. A small cavity.

Greeff's v's. Collections of protein-rich fluid beneath the ciliary epithelium, associated with the production of plasmoid intraocular fluid.

lens v. A hollow spherical body of a single row of cells, formed by invagination of the lens plate into the optic cup, after formation of the lens pit, at about the fourth week of embryonic life; the forerunner of the adult crystalline lens.

optic v. One of a pair of ventrolateral, hollow, evaginations of the neural ectoderm of the forebrain, derived from the optic pits after closure of the embryonic neural groove, which subsequently invaginate to form the optic cups. Syn., *primary optic vesicle.* **secondary o.v.** Optic cup.

vessel. A canal or tube containing and conveying blood or lymph.

annular v. An embryonic vessel appearing at about the fourth week which circles the edge of the optic cup and branches to form the anterior portion of the tunica vasculosa lentis, variously considered to be an artery and a vein.

lymphatic v's., posttarsal. A plexus of lymphatic vessels, located in the palpebral conjunctiva of the eyelid posterior to the tarsus, which communicate with pretarsal lymphatic vessels through the tarsus. They drain the conjunctival and the Meibomian glands and empty into the submaxillary lymph nodes.

lymphatic v's., pretarsal. A plexus of lymphatic vessels, located in the eyelid anterior to the tarsus, which communicate with the posttarsal lymphatic vessels through the tarsus. They drain the skin and adjacent structures and empty into the preauricular and parotid lymph nodes.

radial v's. of Teichmann. Radial lymphatic vessels in the region of the limbus which receive from the lymphatic circle of Teichmann and drain into larger subconjunctival lymphatic vessels.

sentinel v's. Dilated and tortuous episcleral vessels representing a neovascularization in response to an underlying choroidal tumor.

vf. Abbreviation for visual field.

VI. Visibility index.

VIA. Vision Institute of America. See *Vision Service Plan.*

Vibrating Localizer. A visual training instrument designed by Bangerter to teach spatial localization with the assistance of auditory clues, in the preliminary treatment of amblyopia ex anopsia. It is hand held against a screen and creates a buzzing sound and vibration which is localized and touched from the opposite side of the screen. A light source in the instrument is added to the stimulus when the site of sound and vibration has been successfully localized, and finally only the light source is presented.

Vibra-Tonometer. A tonometer which electronically modifies the force of a driven plunger until it is in equilibrium with the counter force of the elastic recoil of the tissue of the cornea, this equalizing force being recorded on a milliammeter.

Vicq d'Azyr's band (vik daz-arz'). Line of Gennari.

VICTORS. See *Vision Improvement Centers to Optimize Remaining Sight.*

Vieth-Mueller (vēth-mūl'er) **circle; horopter.** See under the nouns.

view. 1. That which may be seen, usually implying an extent of delineation; the sight presented to the eye. 2. The act of seeing. 3. A sketch, a picture, or other artificial reproduction of a scene. 4. To see.

dissolving v. The effected dimming or fading out of a projected image as it is replaced by another view, by means of a stereopticon or in a motion picture.

Maxwellian v. The appearance of a lens or a lens aperture filled with light of uniform intensity, obtained when the light is focused at the entrance pupil of the observing eye. Under these conditions the amount of light entering the eye is not affected by the size of the pupil.

viewfinder. An optical or sighting device attached to, or part of, a camera or other optical recording system to show the area of the field that will be included in the picture.

viewing, eccentric. Fixation with an off-center retinal site and with the subjective awareness that the eye is not aimed directly at the target, as may occur with an absolute central scotoma.

vifilcon A. The nonproprietary name of a hydrophilic material of which contact lenses are made.

vignetting (vin-yet'ing). 1. A graduated reduction in illumination at the edges of an image due to a series of stops in the lens system selectively blocking obliquely incident light 2. The photographic process of gradually blending the picture with the surrounding ground.

Vincent's sign (vin'sents). Argyll Robertson pupil.

violet. 1. The hue attribute of visual sensations typically evoked by stimulation of the normal human eye with radiation of wavelengths of the visible spectrum shorter than 450 mμ. 2. Any hue predominantly similar to that of the typical violet.

visual v. Porphyropsin.

violle (vi'ōl). A photometric unit equal to the luminous intensity of one square centimeter of platinum at its temperature of solidification, found experimentally to be 20.17 candelas.

VIP. See *Vision Information Program.*

Virchow's corpuscle (fēr'kōz). A corneal corpuscle.

visibility. 1. The degree, state, or quality of being visible. 2. The range of vision for objects under existing conditions of atmosphere, light, etc. 3. Luminosity. 4. The degree of clearness of the atmosphere as represented on a meteorological scale.

visibility coefficient; curve; factor; meter. See under the nouns.

visible. Capable of being perceived or distinguished through the sense of vision.

visie (vis'ih, ve'zih). 1. A careful look, as when aiming or aligning. 2. The front sight of a gun or of a similar aiming system.

visile (viz'il). 1. Of or pertaining to vision; readily recalling visual impressions. 2. A visile person; one who visualizes readily.

◆

VISION

vision. 1. The special sense by which objects, their form, color, position, etc., in the external environment are perceived, the exciting stimulus being light from the objects striking the retina of the eye; the act, function, process, or power of seeing; sight. 2. That which is seen. 3. To look at; to see. 4. A visual hallucination. 5. The quality of seeing; visual acuity.

achromatic v. Total color blindness.

after v. See *aftervision*.

alternating v. Vision considered as a process in which the impulses from each eye are alternately inhibited or suppressed while the impulses from the other eye are utilized.

ambient v. Vision mediated primarily by the peripheral retina and subserving directional localization and the recognition of motion. Cf. *focal vision.*

ambiocular v. Vision as obtained in ambiocular strabismus.

arhythmic v. Vision equally suited for both high and low levels of illumination, as in most teleost fishes, frogs, crocodiles, ungulates, or wolves. See also *crepuscular, diurnal,* and *nocturnal vision.*

averted v. Observation of a target with peripheral vision.

bifoveal v. Binocular vision involving the foveas of both eyes.

binocular v. 1. Vision in which both eyes contribute toward producing a single fused percept. 2. Vision occur-

ring as a coordinated, integrated, or simultaneous function of both eyes. **grades of b.v.** Degrees of fusion. See under *fusion.* **single b.v.** Vision in which both eyes contribute toward producing a single fused percept.

black v. A perversion of vision in which objects appear blackish, or darker than normal, as may occur in bromide intoxication.

blue v. Cyanopsia.

central v. Foveal or macular vision. Syn., *direct vision.*

chromatic v. 1. Vision in which the color sense is present, as distinguished from *achromatic vision.* 2. Chromatopsia.

color v. Chromatic vision.

cone v. Vision or vision attributes identified with cone function. Cf. *duplicity theory; photopic vision.*

crepuscular v. Vision suited only for twilight levels of illumination, as is said to occur in some snakes. See also *arhythmic, diurnal,* and *nocturnal vision.*

cyclopean v. Binocular vision regarded or schematically represented in terms of the hypothetical cyclopean eye.

daylight v. Photopic vision.

deuteranomalous v. Deuteranomaly.

deuteranopic v. Deuteranopia.

dichromatic v. Dichromatism.

direct v. Central vision.

distance v. Vision or visual acuity for objects at distances representing reasonably approximate dioptric equivalents of infinity, the distance of 20 ft or 6 m being commonly accepted for clinical purposes.

distance of distinct v. See under *distance.*

diurnal v. 1. Vision especially suited for daylight, occurring in animals whose retinae predominately or entirely contain cone cells, as in lizards, birds, and squirrels. See also *arhythmic, crepuscular,* and *nocturnal vision.* 2. Photopic vision.

double v. Diplopia.

eccentric v. Peripheral vision.

entoptic v. Illusory perception of images or patterns in the external visual field, derived from sensory stimulation by shadows or other optical effects of structures or objects inside the eye, or induced by nonphotic disturbances of the receptor system.

environmental v. Environmental optics.

extrafoveal v. 1. Vision resulting from stimulation of the retina, exclusive of the fovea; peripheral vision. 2. Macular vision, other than foveal.

field of v. See under *field*.

focal v. Vision mediated primarily by the central retina and subserving form perception. Cf. *ambient vision*.

fogged v. 1. Vision artificially blurred, generally by the use of convex lenses in excess of the power required for best vision. 2. Vision hazed by an affection of the ocular media.

form v. Perception of shape.

foveal v. Vision resulting from stimulation of the fovea.

green v. Chloropsia.

gun barrel v. Tunnel vision.

halo v. Vision in which colored or luminous rings are perceived around lights.

haploscopic v. Vision as obtained by presenting separate fields of view to the two eyes so that they may be seen as a single, superimposed, integrated, or fused field.

indirect v. Peripheral vision.

industrial v. The branch of visual care identified or concerned with visual problems of industrially classified occupational groups, involving evaluation of visual ability, prescribing corrective lenses and protective ocular devices, and determining the optimum environment for visual efficiency.

intermittent v. 1. Vision resulting from intermittent stimulation, as from a series of light pulses. 2. Vision in which objects alternately appear and disappear, as may occur in intermittent suppression or when an absolute threshold is approached.

iridescent v. Vision in which colors are perceived around the borders of an image. Syn., *rainbow vision*.

low v. Subnormal vision.

macular v. Vision resulting from stimulation of receptors in the region of the macula lutea.

mesopic v. Vision said to be intermediate or transitional between photopic and scotopic vision, identified with levels of illumination approximately between 0.001 and 10 cd/m². Syn., *mesopia; twilight vision*.

mobile v. Lawson's term for vision occurring just before, and just after, the blackout period of a blink, i.e.,

as the upper eyelid moves across the pupil. Cf. *static vision*.

monochromatic v. Monochromatism.

monocular v. Vision or visual acuity as a function of one eye only or of each eye separately.

motorist v. The branch of visual care identified or concerned with visual problems of automobile drivers, driver licensing, and vehicle and highway design.

multiple v. Vision in which more than one image of a single object is perceived. Syn., *polyopia*.

naked v. Visual acuity as measured without an ophthalmic lens or any other corrective device before the eye; unaided visual acuity.

near v. Vision or visual acuity for objects at distances corresponding to the normal reading distance, clinical standards varying from about 33 to 40 cm, usually specified from the spectacle plane.

night v. 1. Scotopic vision. 2. Vision which improves in dim light; day blindness.

nocturnal v. 1. Vision especially suited for low levels of illumination, as at night, occurring in animals whose retinae predominately or entirely contain rod cells, such as in cats, alligators, and rats. Cf. *arhythmic, crepuscular,* and *diurnal vision*. 2. Scotopic vision.

v. null. Vision characterized by unawareness of abnormal scotomata in the visual field. Cf. *vision obscure*.

v. obscure. Vision characterized by awareness of abnormal scotomata present in the visual field. Cf. *vision null*.

oscillating v. Vision in which objects appear to swing back and forth. Syn., *oscillopsia*.

panoramic v. Vision as obtained in animals whose eyes are so laterally located or divergently oriented as to make their monocular fields complementary and continuous, with a minimum of overlapping.

paracentral v. Vision resulting from stimulation of the retina immediately surrounding or near the fovea or the macula.

parafoveal v. Vision resulting from stimulation of the retina immediately surrounding or near the fovea.

peripheral v. 1. Vision resulting from stimulation of the retina exclusive of the fovea or the macula. Syn., *eccentric vision; indirect vision*. 2. Vision resulting from stimulation of receptors at or near the periphery of the retina.

persistent v. Aftervision.

photopic v. Vision attributed to cone function, normally identified with higher levels of illumination, approximately 10 cd/m² or more, and characterized by the ability to discriminate colors and small detail. Syn., *photopia; daylight vision*.

Pick's v's. Visual hallucinations or visual space distortions resulting from a lesion involving the medial longitudinal fasciculus.

protanomalous v. Protanomaly.

pseudoscopic v. Vision in reverse stereoscopic relief or as obtained with a pseudoscope.

rainbow v. Iridescent vision.

range of v. 1. The linear distance from far to near through which objects can be seen. 2. The angular extent of the visual field. 3. The range of illumination through which vision is possible.

recurrent v. Perception of the series of negative and positive afterimages after the exciting stimulus has terminated.

red v. Erythropsia.

rod v. Vision or vision attributes identified with rod function. Cf. *scotopic vision; duplicity theory*.

scotopic v. Vision attributed to rod function, normally identified with levels of illumination below approximately 0.001 cd/m², characterized by the lack of ability to discriminate colors and small detail, and effective primarily in the detection of movement and low luminous intensities. Syn., *scotopia; night vision*.

shaft v. Tunnel vision.

simultaneous v. Binocular vision.

solid v. Vision characterized by the perception of relief or depth.

speed of v. See under *speed*.

static v. Lawson's term for vision occurring during the interblink period. Cf. *mobile vision*.

stereoscopic v. Stereopsis.

subnormal v. Vision considered to be inferior to normal vision, as represented by accepted standards of acuity, field of vision, or motility, and uncorrectable by conventional lenses, or the branch of visual care identified with its

correction or rehabilitation by special aids or techniques. Cf. *blindness*. Syn., *low vision*.

telescopic v. Tunnel vision.

tetartanopic v. Tetartanopsia.

tetrachromatic v. Tetrachromatism.

v. training. See under *training*.

travel v. A classification of low vision deemed adequate to enable one to go from place to place with a minimum of special mobility aids, presumably a central resolution threshold of at least 1° and a visual field diameter of 50°.

trichromatic v. Trichromatism. **anomalous t.v.** Anomalous trichromatism.

tritanomalous v. Anomalous trichromatism.

tritanopic v. Tritanopia.

tubular v. Tunnel vision.

tunnel v. 1. Vision in which the visual field is concentrically contracted and constant in diameter irrespective of the testing distance, as if looking through a tube, usually attributed to hysteria or malingering. Syn., *gun barrel vision; shaft vision; telescopic vision; tubular vision*. 2. Vision in which the visual field is severely contracted.

twilight v. Mesopic vision.

violet v. A perversion of vision in which objects appear violet, sometimes occurring as a consequence of toxic amblyopia.

white v. A perversion of vision in which objects appear whitish, as covered with snow, as may occur in digitalis intoxication.

yellow v. Xanthopsia.

◆

Vision Improvement Centers to Optimize Remaining Sight. A low-vision program of the Veterans Administration designed to provide care on a regional basis to visually impaired veterans to enable them to function as efficiently as possible. Acronym: VICTORS.

Vision Information Program. A corporation founded in 1959 to process vision certificate forms for optometrists to fill out and give to their patients to inform them of their visual capabilities, with duplicate copies filed in a central bureau to be mailed to individual patients upon expiration of individually anticipated effective time periods.

Vision Institute of America. See *Vision Service Plan.*

Vision Service Plan. An association of vision service corporations founded in 1964 to facilitate exchanges of information relative to problems, actuarial experience, and policies involving prepaid vision care contracts and services. Formerly the Vision Institute of America.

Vision Tester, Titmus. A visual screening instrument containing targets for measuring visual acuity, phorias, fusion, stereopsis, and color perception. It consists essentially of a Brewster-type stereoscope, an internally illuminated rotating drum for holding up to 12 targets, and an adjustment to simulate either a near or a far testing distance.

visionics (vizh"e-on'iks). The study of aiding vision with electronic devices.

visual. Pertaining to vision.

visual achievement; acuity; agnosia; agraphia; amnesia; analysis; angle; aphasia; apparatus; apraxia; autokinesis; reflex arc; axis; cells; centers; concession; cone; cortex; direction; discrimination; dominance; efficiency; fibers; field; green; laterality; line; memory; pathway; plane; point; projection; purple; red; skill; space; tract; training; violet; white; yellow. See under the nouns.

Visual Stimulator. A trade name for a visual testing apparatus which provides binocular or monocular light stimuli with variations in light intensity, spectral distribution, flicker frequency, and duration of single light pulses.

visualization. The act or the faculty of forming a mental visual image of an object not present to the eyes, or the image itself.

visualize. To form a mental visual image of an object not present to the eyes.

visualness. The visual aspect or attribute of a percept not initiated by the visual mechanism, as, e.g., the visually identified attribute of a tactually sensed object, brought about by experience and association.

visuo- (vizh'u-o-). A combining form denoting *vision.*

visuoauditory (vizh"u-o-aw'dih-tōr"e). Both visual and auditory; pertaining to seeing and hearing.

visuognosis (vizh"u-og-no'sis). Recognition and interpretation of visual stimuli.

visuometer (vizh"u-om'eh-ter). An instrument designed by Smee to measure the separation of the lines of sight by the separation of a pair of parallel cylindrical apertures through each of which a distant object appears centered by each of the two eyes, respectively.

visuopsychic (vizh"u-o-si'kik). Pertaining to the visual association areas of the occipital cortex, Brodmann's areas 18 and 19.

visuosensory (vizh"u-o-sen'sor-e). Pertaining to the visual sensory area of the occipital cortex, Brodmann's area 17.

visus (vi'sus). Vision.

    v. brevior. Myopic vision.

    v. coloratus. Chromatopsia.

    v. debilitas. Asthenopia.

    v. decoloratus. Achromatopsia.

    v. defiguratus. Distorted vision.

    v. dimidiatus. Hemianopsia.

    v. duplicatus. Diplopia.

    v. muscarum. Vision in which spots are seen before the eyes.

    v. reticulatus. Vision in which the field appears sievelike, due to scotomata.

    v. senilis. Presbyopia.

    v. triplex. Triplopia.

Visuscope (vizh'u-skōp). An instrument designed to determine the type of monocular fixation in amblyopia, consisting essentially of an ophthalmoscope adapted with a small, central, opaque, fixation target which projects a shadow onto the retina, the position of the shadow in relation to the fovea indicating the type of fixation.

visuum (vizh'u-um). The two eyes, their extrinsic muscles and other contents of the orbits, the nerves, the pathways, and the visual cortex, considered collectively. Syn., *visual apparatus.*

vitamin A. A fat-soluble vitamin found in fish liver oils, liver, eggs, milk, and milk products, and in some vegetables and fruits. Deficiency in the diet causes inadequate production and regeneration of rhodopsin, resulting in night blindness, and disturbed metabolism of epithelial tissue, resulting in keratomalacia, xerophthalmia, and lessened resistance to infection through epithelial surfaces.

vitamin B₁. A water-soluble vitamin present in small quantities in most edible plant and animal tissues and more abundantly in milk, yeast, unrefined cereal grains, liver, heart, kidney, and pork. It is necessary in carbohydrate metabolism, and a deficiency in the diet results in peripheral neuropathy, such as beriberi with the accompanying eye signs of nystagmus, ptosis, extraocular muscle paresis, corneal dystrophy, and optic atrophy. Its deficiency is considered a primary cause of nutritional amblyopia. Syn., *aneurine; thiamine.*

vitamin B₆. Pyridoxine.

vitamin B₁₂. Cyanocobalamin.

vitamin C. Ascorbic acid.

vitamin D. A group of fat-soluble vitamins involved in the absorption of phosphates and calcium salts from the alimentary canal to increase the supply of calcium and phosphorus in the blood for producing and maintaining bone and teeth structure. It is found in fish liver oils, to a lesser extent in milk, eggs, and butter, and is produced by the action of ultraviolet radiation on foods containing sterols, or of sunlight on the body. Deficiency in the diet in children results in rickets and, in adults, osteomalacia, either of which may have associated cataract. Excessive therapeutic doses may impair renal function and produce metastatic calcifications with involvement of the conjunctiva, cornea, and sclera.

vitamin G. Riboflavin.

vitiligo (vit″ih-li′go). A disease of the skin characterized by patches of depigmentation of various sizes and shapes.

    v. of the choroid. Absence of pigment in the choroid with the choroidal circulation and underlying sclera being easily visible.

    v. iridis. The condition of small, white, depigmented areas on the iris.

vitrectomy (vih-trek′to-me). Surgical removal of a portion of the vitreous body.

vitrein (vit′re-in). A residual protein of the collagen-gelatin type in the vitreous humor, which partially accounts for the gel state of the vitreous body. Syn., *vitrosin.*

vitrella (vih-trel′ah). A specialized cell in the compound eyes of arthropods which secretes the crystalline cone of the ommatidium. Syn., *retinophore.*

vitreocapsulitis (vit″re-o-kap″su-li′-tis). Hyalitis.

vitreous (vit′re-us). The vitreous humor or body.

    anterior v. Fibrillar protoplasmic adhesions between the lens vesicle and the surface ectoderm of the 12 mm human embryo. It loses its connection with the lens vesicle in the 13–14 mm stage and soon disappears.

    v. body. See under *body.*

    v. chamber. See under *chamber.*

    detached v. Vitreous separated from its normal attachments, due to shrinkage from degenerative or inflammatory conditions, trauma, myopia, or senility.

    fluid v. Vitreous which is liquefied due to inflammatory or degenerative conditions of the eye. Ophthalmoscopically visible opacities are usually an accompaniment. See also *synchysis.*

    v. humor. See under *humor.*

    hyaloidean v. Primary vitreous.

    v. membrane. See under *membrane.*

    persistent hyperplastic primary v. A congenital condition occurring in full term infants characterized by a fibroplastic retrolental mass formed by a persistent primary vitreous and remnants of the hyaloid vascular system and tunica vasculosa lentis. It is usually unilateral, occurs in a microphthalmic eye, and distinguishing features include a white pupil, shallow anterior chamber, elongated ciliary processes, visible blood vessels in the iris, a partially or totally absorbed crystalline lens, and retinal detachment due to adhesions.

    plasmoid v. A vitreous humor containing protein forming a diffuse, dust-like cloud or aggregating into clumps, a condition which may occur when the capillaries of the ciliary body are dilated with cyclitis, choroidal tumors, or chorioretinitis.

    primary v. The first vitreous formed in the embryo, consisting of a mass of fibrils between the inner wall of the optic cup and the lens vesicle, derived from neuroectoderm (optic cup), surface ectoderm (lens vesicle), and mesoderm. It becomes vascularized by the hyaloid artery and its branches (vasa hyaloidea propria), and its development ends with the appearance of the hyaline capsule of the crystalline lens at about the 13 mm stage. As the secondary vitreous develops, a line of condensation between it and the primary vitreous forms the walls of the hyaloid canal to which the primary vitreous is restricted. Syn., *hyaloidean vitreous.*

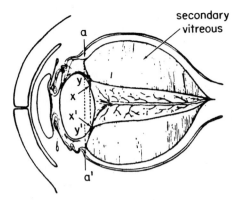

secondary
vitreous

Fig. 40 Diagram of the secondary vitreous around the primary vitreous. *xx'* marks the site of the arcuate line; *yy'* marks the site of Egger's line, and *aa'* indicates the peripheral boundary of the secondary vitreous. (From A. N. Barber, *Embryology of the Human Eye.* St. Louis: C. V. Mosby, 1955)

secondary v. Avascular vitreous formed around the primary vitreous in the embryo from the 13 mm stage to the 65–70 mm stage. It consists of a mass of densely packed, fine fibrils derived from the inner layer of the optic cup (neuroectoderm), although there may be a few fibrils derived from the lens vesicle in its central portion. (See Fig. 40.)

tertiary v. Vitreous fibrils derived from the neuroepithelium at the margin of the optic cup in the region of the ciliary body, commencing at the 65–70 mm stage of the embryo and giving rise to the zonule of Zinn.

vitreum (vit're-um). The vitreous humor.

vitric (vit'rik). Pertaining to or appearing like glass.

vitrics (vit'riks). The study of glass and glass manufacture.

vitrina (vih-tri'nah). The vitreous humor.

v. oculi. The vitreous humor.

vitritis (vit-ri'tis). Hyalitis.

vitrosin (vit'ro-sin). Vitrein.

Vogt's (fōgts) **cataract; floury cornea; mosaic degeneration; limbus girdle; lucid interval; subluxated lens; line; membrana**

plicata; sign; keratoconus stripes; theory. See under the nouns.

Vogt-Koyanagi syndrome (fōgt-ko-yah-nah'ge). See under *syndrome*.

Vogt-Spielmeyer disease (fōgt-spēl'-ma-er). Batten-Mayou disease.

Voigt effect (voit). Magnetic double refraction.

Volk conoid lens. See under *lens*.

Volkmann's (fōlk'mahnz) **center of rotation; disks.** See under the nouns.

Volunteers for Vision. A program organized in 1965 to enable volunteers to assist in determining the visual needs of underprivileged children by visual screening techniques and referring those needing professional attention through the appropriate channels.

von Frey. See under *Frey*.

von Graefe. See under *Graefe*.

von Gudden. See under *Gudden*.

von Herrenschwand. See under *Herrenschwand*.

von Hippel. See under *Hippel*.

von Kries. See under *Kries*.

von Mises. See under *Mises*.

von Noorden-Burian. See under *Noorden-Burian*.

von Reuss. See under *Reuss*.

von Szily. See under *Szily*.

vortex, lens. The configuration formed by the elongated extensions of the cells of the subcapsular epithelium of the crystalline lens which arc anteriorly from the region of the equator.

Vossius (vos'e-us) **ring cataract; ring opacity; ring.** See *cataract, Vossius ring*.

Vrolik syndrome. See under *syndrome*.

V-Scope. A truncated paper cone, so folded that it must be pressed between the two hands to keep it open, used for determining sighting dominance by sighting through it at a target. See also *Miles's A-B-C test*.

VSP. See *Vision Service Plan*.

Vu-Tach. A trade name for a near point tachistoscope with six exposure speeds from $1/100$ to 1.0 per second, used to improve speed and span of comprehension in reading.

W

Waardenburg's syndrome (vahr'-den-burgz). See under *syndrome.*

Waardenburg-Jonkers corneal dystrophy. See under *dystrophy, corneal.*

Wachendorf's membrane (vahk'en-dorfs). The pupillary membrane.

Wadsworth (wahds'wurth) **mirror; prism.** See under the nouns.

wafer. A very thin meniscus lens designed to be cemented to a larger lens to form a bifocal lens.

Wagner's disease. Vitreoretinal degeneration.

Waidner-Burgess standard. See under *standard.*

Wald cycle (wahld). See under *cycle.*

Waldenström's syndrome (vahl'den-stremz). See under *syndrome.*

Waldeyer's gland (vahl'di-erz). See under *gland.*

Walker's (wok'erz) **chart; color disk.** See under the nouns.

Wallace chart (wol'is). See under *chart.*

Wallach's rings. See under *ring.*

Wallenberg's syndrome (vahl'en-bergz). See under *syndrome.*

walleye. Leukoma of the cornea.

walleyed. Having divergent strabismus.

Walls's theory (wawlz'ez). See under *theory.*

Walser shell. See under *shell.*

wand, Branchaud. A hand-held device for testing and training pursuit fixation movements consisting essentially of a miniature neon lamp, flickering at a rate of 120 times per second, mounted at one end of a 14 in. black plastic rod which houses an electrical connection to the lamp. Deviations from accurate fixational pursuit are indicated when the subject detects flicker.

Wartenberg's sign (wor'ten-bergz). See under *sign.*

warts, Hassall-Henle. Hassall-Henle bodies.

warts, Henle's. Hassall-Henle bodies.

waterfall, James's. A device for creating a waterfall visual illusion, consisting of a pattern of alternate black and white, horizontal, parallel stripes which may be moved continuously in one direction against a stationary background of the same pattern.

wave. A periodic or systematic fluctuation, modulation, pulsation, or undulation, or one of a series of such variations.

    A w. Alpha rhythm.

    a w. A small negative dip in the electroretinogram following the latent period, after the onset of the stimulus.

    alpha w. Alpha rhythm.

    w. amplitude. See under *amplitude.*

    b w. A tall positive wave of brief duration in the electroretinogram immediately following the *a* wave.

    c w. A relatively long, slowly rising wave in the electroretinogram immediately following the *b* wave.

    d w. A small positive hump in the electroretinogram, higher than the *c* wave, which follows the latent period at the cessation of the stimulus.

    electromagnetic w. A wave produced by the oscillation of an electric charge, characterized by a varying electric field at right angles to the direction of propagation and a varying magnetic field at right angles to both.

w. frequency. See under *frequency*.

light w. 1. In the wave theory of light propagation, a single pulse or disturbance in a space of one wavelength of the advance of the disturbance in a medium. 2. A wave of radiant energy, between approximately 380 and 760 mμ, that gives rise to visual sensation on stimulating the retina. **coherent l.w.** Light waves having a constant phase difference, as when derived from the same source. **intensity of l.w.** The amount of energy, as represented in a light wave, that flows per second across a unit area perpendicular to the direction of propagation, directly proportional to the product of the velocity and the square of the amplitude. **noncoherent l.w.** Concurrent light waves not having a constant phase difference, as when derived from different sources. **phase of l.w.** See under *phase*. **plane l.w.** A light wave having a plane wavefront. **secondary l.w.** A light wave generated by the oscillations of the bound charges of an atom or a molecule induced by incident light waves. **spherical l.w.** A light wave having a spherical wavefront.

longitudinal w. A wave in which the direction of vibration is parallel to its direction of propagation, e.g., a sound wave.

w. number. See under *number*.

w. surface. A wavefront.

transverse w. A wave in which the direction of vibration is perpendicular to its direction of propagation, e.g., a light wave.

waveform. The graphical or mathematical representation of the form of a wave.

wavefront. An imaginary surface representing the locus of points in wave motion for which, at a given instant, the phase is the same.

strip division of w. The subdivision of a wavefront into strips of infinitesimal width, parallel to the slit source, for the theoretical analysis of the diffractional contribution of each portion.

wavelength. The distance in the line of advance of a wave from any one point to the next point at which, at the same instant, the phase is the same.

blaze w. For a given angle of incidence, the wavelength for which the direction of reflectance from the groove face of a diffraction grating is identical to the angle of diffraction.

complementary w. A complementary color designated in terms of its dominant wavelength.

dominant w. The spectral wavelength which, on proper mixing with white, will match a given sample of color.

wavelet. In the wave theory of light propagation, one of the infinitesimal component wave elements considered to originate at any point on a wavefront, integrating with its fellow wavelets from all other points on the same wavefront to constitute a further advanced wavefront.

weakness, color. Defectivity of color vision characterized by a diminished sensitivity to color or lowered ability to discriminate small differences in hue; usually considered synonymous with *anomalous trichromatism*.

web, terminal. A thin cytoplasmic structure, just anterior to and lining the posterior cellular membrane (the posterior limit) of the corneal mesothelium.

Weber's (va'berz) **law; phenomenon.** See under the nouns.

Weber's (web'erz) **paralysis; sign; symptom; syndrome.** See under the nouns.

Weber-Fechner law (va'ber-fek'ner). See under *law*.

Weber-Gubler syndrome (web'er-goob'ler). See under *syndrome*.

Wendesky inhibition. See under *inhibition*.

wedge, optical. A gradient filter.

weeping. 1. Excessive lacrimation. 2. Exuding fluid, as from a raw surface.

primary w. Lacrimation due to direct stimulation or irritation of the lacrimal gland.

psychic w. Lacrimation associated with emotional states or physical pain.

reflex w. Weeping in response to neurogenic stimulation, as irritation of the cornea or the conjunctiva, glare, vomiting, etc.

Weil's disease (vīlz). See under *disease*.

Weil-Marchesani syndrome. See under *syndrome*.

Weiss's (vīsz'ez) **reflex; ring; sign; test type.** See under the nouns.

Welland's test (wel'andz). Bar reading test.

Welsh Four-Drop Aspheric lens; Welsh zero error method (of refraction). See under the nouns.

Werner's (ver'nerz) **figures; syndrome.** See under the nouns.

Wernicke's (ver'nih-kēz) **aphasia; disease; triangular field; prism; pupillary reaction; pupillary reflex; sign; symptom; syndrome.** See under the nouns.

Wertheimer-Benary visual illusion. See under *illusion, visual.*

Wessely's phenomenon. See *anaphylactic keratitis.*

Wessely's tubes (ves'lēz). See under *tube.*

Westheimer function; method. See under the nouns.

Westphal, pseudosclerosis of (vest'fahl). Wilson's disease.

Westphal's sign (vest'fahlz). See under *sign.*

Westphal-Piltz (vest'fahl-piltz) **phenomenon; reaction; reflex.** Orbicularis pupillary reflex.

wet-cell. A chamber with optically flat transparent walls containing a saline solution through which an immersed soft contact lens can be inspected or measured.

Weyers-Thier syndrome. Oculovertebral dysplasia.

Weymouth-Anderson hypothesis (wa'muth-an'der-sen). See under *hypothesis.*

Wheatstone stereoscope (whēt'stōn). See under *stereoscope.*

wheel, color. Color circle.

white. 1. An achromatic color of maximum lightness or minimum darkness representing one limit of the series of grays; the complement or opposite of *black.* 2. The attribute of visual sensations typically evoked by stimulation of the normal human eye by a mixture of radiant energy of different wavelengths approximating in physiological action that which is characteristic of daylight. The ideal white is obtained when a normally illuminated surface reflects all the light incident on it.

    visual w. Leukopsin.

White's absorption cell. See under *cell, absorption.*

whiteness. 1. A positive perceptual attribute of any surface or part thereof which has higher reflectance than its surroundings, whiteness being induced by the dimmer surround. 2. The degree of approach to that extreme or limit of the series of grays known as *white.* 3. Suggesting *white,* e.g., the tint of a color.

Whitnall's (hwit'nalz) **ciliary mass; tubercle.** See under the nouns.

Whittington's (hwit'ing-tons) **stereoscope, test.** See under the nouns.

Whittle's hypothesis. See under *hypothesis.*

Whitwell's table. See under *table.*

Whytt's reflex (hwits). See under *reflex.*

Widesite (wīd'sīt). 1. A trade name for a series of corrected curve lenses. 2. A trade name for a series of fused bifocal lenses.

Widmark's conjunctivitis (wid'-mahrks). See under *conjunctivitis.*

Wieger's ligament (ve'gerz). Hyaloideo-capsular ligament.

Wien's law (vēnz). See under *law.*

Wiener's theory (wēn'erz). See under *theory.*

Wight's test. See under *test.*

Wilbrand's (vil'brahntz) **exhaustion visual field; phenomenon; test.** See under the nouns.

Wilder's sign (wil'derz). See under *sign.*

Williams' refractometer; test. See under the nouns.

Willis' circle (wil'is). See under *circle.*

Wils-Edge. See *mounting, Wils-Edge.*

Wilson's (wil'sunz) **disease; phenomenon; phorometer.** See under the nouns.

Wilson-Brocq disease. See under *disease.*

Wiltberger's test (wilt'ber-gerz). See under *test.*

window. An opening for the admission of light or air.

    entrance w. Entrance port.

    exit w. Exit port.

    Hering w. A device to demonstrate color contrast, consisting essentially of a black shutter with two openings, one containing a white ground glass, the other a colored glass. Shadows formed on a white surface by a black rod in the beams from the two openings are compared. See also *colored shadow experiment.*

wing, Maddox. A hand-held instrument for measuring a phoria at near, consisting of a target containing an intersecting vertical and horizontal tangent scale, a horizontal arrow pointing to the left and a finger pointing upward, a septum, and two slit apertures, one for each eye. In viewing the target one eye sees the arrow and the finger, the other sees the tangent scale, and the numbers to which the finger and the arrow appear to point indicate the magnitude of the vertical and horizontal components of the phoria.

wink. To momentarily close the eyelids, especially of only one eye; the act itself.

winking. The brief closing of the eyelids, especially of one eye. Cf. *blinking.*

    jaw w. See under *jaw-winking.*

    pterygoid w. Paradoxical movements of the upper eyelids occurring in association with movements of the muscles of mastication; a rare congenital anomaly.

    rectus muscle w. Paradoxical movements of the upper eyelids occurring in association with movement of a rectus muscle; a rare congenital anomaly.

Winslow's stars (wins'lōz). See under *stars.*

WinterHaven Perceptual Copy Forms. A series of seven line drawings, circle, cross, square, triangle, divided rectangle, horizontal diamond, and vertical diamond (Gesell forms), presented singly to be freely copied and interpreted as an indication of a child's developmental readiness for classroom achievement.

wires, cross. Cross-hairs.

Wirt stereotest; test. See under *test.*

Wissenschaftliche Vereinigung für Augenoptik und Optometrie e.V. A German association of professionally qualified Augenoptiker (ophthalmic opticians/optometrists) formed in 1968 by the merger of the Deutsche Gesellschaft für Optometrie and the Wissenschaftliche Vereinigung für Augenoptik primarily for educational, scientific, and social purposes.

wl. Abbreviation for *wavelength.*

WNL. Within normal limits.

Wold test. See under *test.*

Wolfe tonometer (woolf). See under *tonometer.*

Wolfring's gland (vōlf'ringz). See under *glands.*

Wolfrum's theory (volf'rumz). See under *theory.*

Wollaston's (wool'as-tonz) **doublet; lens; loupe; polarizer; prism.** See under the nouns.

Wood's filter; glass; light; sign; test. See under the nouns.

word blindness. Alexia.

worm, blinding. *Onchocerca volvulus.* See *onchocerciasis.*

Worshipful Company of Spectacle Makers. A guild or company chartered in England in 1629 and continuing presently as an examining body for the qualifying of candidates for fellowships, diplomas, certificates, awards, and practice privileges in ophthalmic optics, optical dispensing, and optical technicianry. Abbreviation: *SMC.*

Worst's goniotomy lens. See under *lens.*

Worth's (worths) **amblyoscope; deviometer; test; theory.** See under the nouns.

Worth-Ramstein test. See under *test.*

wrapped. Pertaining to the state of a hydrophilic contact lens when it conforms to the shape of the eye. Cf. *wrap factor.*

Wratten filters (rat'en). See under *filter.*

Wright's (rīts) **colorimeter; theory.** See under the nouns.

Wrisberg, intermediate nerve of (ris'berg). See under *nerve.*

writing, mirror. Writing which appears normal when viewed in a mirror, or the act of writing in this manner. Syn., *retrography.*

Wundt's (voondts) **experiment; figure; visual illusion; theory.** See under the nouns.

Wundt-Lamanski law (voondt-lahman'ske). See under *law.*

WVAO. See *Wissenschaftliche Vereinigung für Augenoptik und Optometrie e.V.*

Wyburn-Mason syndrome. See under *syndrome.*

X

x. Abbreviation for *axis* in an astigmatic lens formula.

xanthelasma (zan"thel-az'mah). A condition characterized by the presence of rounded or oval, dull yellow, slightly elevated, flat plaques containing foam cells, in the skin of the eyelids. The lesions are usually located near the inner canthi and usually commence on the upper eyelid. It is benign and chronic, occurs primarily in the elderly, and most frequently affects females. Syn., *xanthelasma palpebrarum; xanthoma palpebrarum.*

xanthocyanopia (zan"tho-si"ah-no'-pe-ah). Xanthocyanopsia.

xanthocyanopsia (zan"tho-si"ah-nop'-se-ah). Anomalous color vision in which yellow and blue are distinguished, but not red or green.

xanthocyanopsy (zan"tho-si"ah-nop'se). Xanthocyanopsia.

xanthogranuloma, ocular juvenile (zan"tho-gran"u-lo'mah). Intraocular nevoxanthoendothelioma.

xanthokyanopy (zan"tho-ki-an'o-pe). Xanthocyanopsia.

xanthoma palpebrarum (zan-tho'-mah). Xanthelasma.

xanthomatosis (zan"tho-mah-to'sis). A systemic disorder of fat metabolism characterized by the formation of lipoid tumors in bone, skin, internal organs, etc.

    x. corneae. Dystrophia adiposa corneae.

    cranio-hypophysial x. Schüller-Christian-Hand disease.

    essential hyperlipemic x. Essential familial hyperlipemia.

    x. lentis. A rare, late, degenerative change in cataract due to fatty impregnation of the crystalline lens.

xanthophane (zan'tho-fān). A yellow pigment in the retinal receptor cells of some animals.

xanthophose (zan'tho-fōz). A subjective sensation of yellow light or color.

xanthophyll (zan'tho-fil). A yellow photopigment found in plants, a carotenoid of the formula $C_{40}H_{54}(OH)_2$, its chemical derivatives being active in photosynthesis of plant metabolism.

xanthopsia (zan-thop'se-ah). A condition in which all objects appear tinged with yellow, as may occur in picric acid or santonin poisoning and jaundice. Syn., *yellow vision.*

xanthopsin (zan-thop'sin). An intermediate product of the decomposition of rhodopsin on exposure to light, following the breakdown of transient orange and prior to the formation of retinene. Syn., *indicator yellow; visual yellow.*

xanthosis of the retina. A generalized yellowish discoloration of the posterior pole of the fundus sometimes appearing with diabetic retinopathy.

xenophthalmia (zen"of-thal'me-ah). Conjunctivitis due to trauma or to a foreign body.

xeroderma pigmentosum (ze"ro-der'mah pig-men-to'sum). A progressive pigmentary degeneration of the skin, frequently familial, marked in the first years of life by the appearance of small telangiectases and freckles, particularly in areas exposed to sunlight. Later atrophic patches appear, followed by warty growths, ulcerations, and carcinoma. It frequently affects the eye, and, when involving the conjunctiva, characteristically is manifested as nodules similar to phlyctenules or pingueculae, at the limbus, which ulcerate. Exposure keratitis is common as a result of shrinkage and contracture of the skin of the eyelid margins. Syn., *angioma pigmentosum atrophicum; atrophoderma pigmentosum; Kaposi's disease; melanosis lenticularis progressiva.*

xeroma (ze-ro'mah). Xerosis of the conjunctiva.

xerophthalmia (ze"rof-thal'me-ah). Xerosis of the conjunctiva.

xerosis of the conjunctiva (ze-ro'sis). A dry, thickened, degenerative condition of the conjunctiva due to failure of its own secretory activity. It commences with localized lusterless, dry patches which may increase in size and number and coalesce with accompanying opacification, keratinization, and wrinkles. It may be due to local disease, trauma, systemic nutritional disturbance, or exposure. Syn., *conjunctivitis arida; ophthalmoxerosis; scheroma; xeroma; xerophthalmia.*

epithelial x. of the conjunctiva. Xerosis of the conjunctiva initially confined to the epithelial layers, due to a systemic nutritional disturbance such as vitamin A deficiency. Accompanying symptoms may be keratomalacia or night blindness.

parenchymatous x. of the conjunctiva. Xerosis of the conjunctiva affecting all its layers, occurring as a sequel to trauma or local disease, such as pemphigus, trachoma, membranous conjunctivitis, etc.

superficial x. of the conjunctiva. Epithelial xerosis of the conjunctiva.

XT. Constant exotropia at far.

XT'. Constant exotropia at near.

Y

YAG. Yttrium aluminum garnet, a crystal used in some solid state lasers.

yellow. 1. The normal visual sensory hue correlate of wavelengths of approximately 578 mμ, or any hue predominantly similar, located between red and green on the spectral scale, classified as one of the psychologically unique colors, and occurring as a complement of blue. 2. Any substance or pigment of yellow color.

   indicator y. Lythgoe's term for an intermediate product in the breakdown of rhodopsin, thought to be *xanthopsin*.

   y. sighted. Said to display an abnormally high color sensitivity to yellow or a tendency to see all objects tinged with yellow.

   y. spot. Macula lutea.

   visual y. Xanthopsin.

Young's experiment; optometer; test; theory; color triangle. See under the nouns.

Young-Helmholtz theory (yung-helm'hōltz). See under *theory*.

Z

Zagora rod test (zah-gōr′ah). See under *test*.

Zahn, Johann, polyspherical lens. See under *lens*.

Zeeman's (za′mahnz) **effect; theory.** See under the nouns.

Zeis's gland (zīs′ez). See under *gland*.

Zeiss loupe (zīs). See under *loupe*.

Zelex. A trade name for a molding compound used in taking eye impressions in the fitting of impression contact lenses.

Zenger prism. See under *prism*.

Zentralverband der Augenoptiker. A long-established association of virtually all licensed German ophthalmic opticians who are owners of retail optical establishments, serving the interests of its members in economic, legal, legislative, administrative, and educational affairs, and public relations.

Zeune's law (zu′nēz). See under *law*.

Ziegler prism scale (zēg′ler). See under *scale*.

Zieve syndrome. See under *syndrome*.

Zinn's (zinz) **annulus; artery; circle; corona; ligament; membrane; tendon; zone; zonule.** See under the nouns.

Zinsser-Thomson disease. Rothmund syndrome. See under *syndrome*.

zoetrope (zo′eh-trōp). A hollow cylinder containing on its inside surface a series of pictures representing the successive stages in the movement of objects or persons. The pictures are viewed through slits in the cylinder while it is rapidly revolving, so that each picture is seen individually and instantaneously and the effect of animation is obtained.

Zöllner's (zel′nerz) **figure; visual illusion; lines.** See under the nouns.

zona (zo′nah). A zone.

   z. ciliaris. The ciliary zone.

   z. ophthalmica. Herpes zoster ophthalmicus.

zone. An arbitrarily or differentially delimited area or region.

   capillary z. of the choroid. Choriocapillaris.

   chromatic z's. Color zones.

   ciliary z. The peripheral region of the anterior surface of the iris located between the root of the iris and the collarette. It has been divided by Fuchs into an inner smooth area, a middle furrowed area, and a marginal cribriform area next to the ciliary body. Syn., *greater ring of the iris; greater ring of Merkel.*

   color z's. Regions of the visual field differentiated according to chromatic response, usually determined by means of the perimeter with various color targets.

   z. of comfort. Area of comfort.

   z's. of the crystalline lens. The embryonic nucleus, the fetal nucleus, the infantile nucleus, the adult nucleus, and the cortex of the crystalline lens.

   z's. of discontinuity. Zones of varying optical density in the crystalline lens or cornea, as seen in slit lamp biomicroscopy.

   equidistant z. The zone in space between the anterior and posterior limits of the apparent frontoparallel plane horopter. Anteroposterior displacement of a nonfixated target within this space will still be judged as lying in the same plane as the fixation target, hence the displacement is less than the threshold of stereopsis.

Fresnel's z. Half-period zone.

half-period z. Any one of a series of concentric zones on a wavefront of monochromatic light whose successive contingent borders are each one-half wavelength farther or nearer from a given point of reference exterior to the wavefront surface and in its advancing path. Syn., *Fresnel's zone.*

interpalpebral z. The portion of the cornea and the sclera not covered when the eyelids are opened.

iso-indicial z's. Zones of an optical medium, especially of the crystalline lens, having the same index of refraction.

lacrimal prism z. That part of the tear layer along the eyelid margin which resembles a prism in cross-section.

marginal z. of the optic cup. Marginal layer of the optic cup.

nuclear z. The region of the crystalline lens containing an aggregation of nuclei of cells of the anterior epithelium located beneath the anterior capsule.

optical z. of contact lens. The central, optically useful, portion of a contact lens which corresponds to the area occupied by the base curve.

optical z. of cornea. The central third of the cornea.

z. of plateaus and furrows. The zone of the conjunctiva containing Stieda's plateaus and Stieda's grooves.

pupillary z. The central region of the anterior surface of the iris located between the collarette and the pupillary margin. Syn., *lesser ring of the iris; lesser ring of Merkel.*

retinal z's. Regions of the retina corresponding to those of the visual field, which are differentiated according to chromatic response or other function.

z. of single clear binocular vision. In the graphic representation of the functional relationships between accommodation and convergence on a coordinate system, the region enclosed by the extremes of accommodation and convergence that can be elicited while maintaining binocular fusion and clear retinal imagery. Clinically, these extremes or limits may be determined haploscopically, or by varying combinations of binocular fixation distance, binocularly added concave or convex lenses, and base-in or base-out prism until blurredness or diplopia is reported. (See Fig. 41.)

z. of specular reflection. In slit lamp biomicroscopy, a surface area at which specular reflection occurs, appearing as a dazzling light reflex with irregularities or defects in the surface appearing as dark areas in the bright region.

trabecular z. Trabecular band.

transitional z. The annular portion of a scleral contact lens which

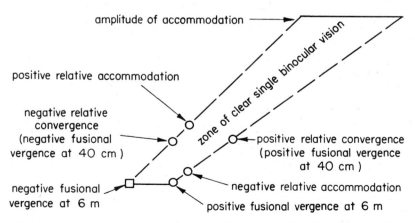

Fig. 41 Zone of clear, single, binocular vision. (From J. R. Griffin, *Binocular Anomalies.* Chicago: Professional Press, 1976)

joins the corneal section with the scleral section. Syn., *transition*.

z. of Zinn. Zonule of Zinn.

zonule (zōn'ūl). A little zone.

z. of Zinn. The suspensory apparatus of the crystalline lens consisting of a series of noncellular extensions which originate in the orbicularis ciliaris and the corona ciliaris of the ciliary body and insert into the capsule of the lens at and near its equator. The tension of these fibers varies with the state of contraction of the ciliary muscle and thus determines the degree of convexity of the lens. Syn., *suspensory ligament*.

zonulolysis (zōn″-u-lo-li'sis). Dissolving of the fibers of the zonule of Zinn by an enzyme instilled into the aqueous humor to facilitate surgical removal of the crystalline lens.

zonulotomy (zon″u-lot'o-me). Surgical division of the zonule of Zinn.

zoom lens. See under *lens*.

zoster ophthalmicus (zos'ter of-thal'-mih-kus). Herpes zoster ophthalmicus.

Zuber effect. See under *effect*.

ZVA. See *Zentralverband der Augenoptiker*.

zylonite (zi'lo-nīt). A cellulose nitrate thermoplastic material used in spectacle frames.